MW00358367

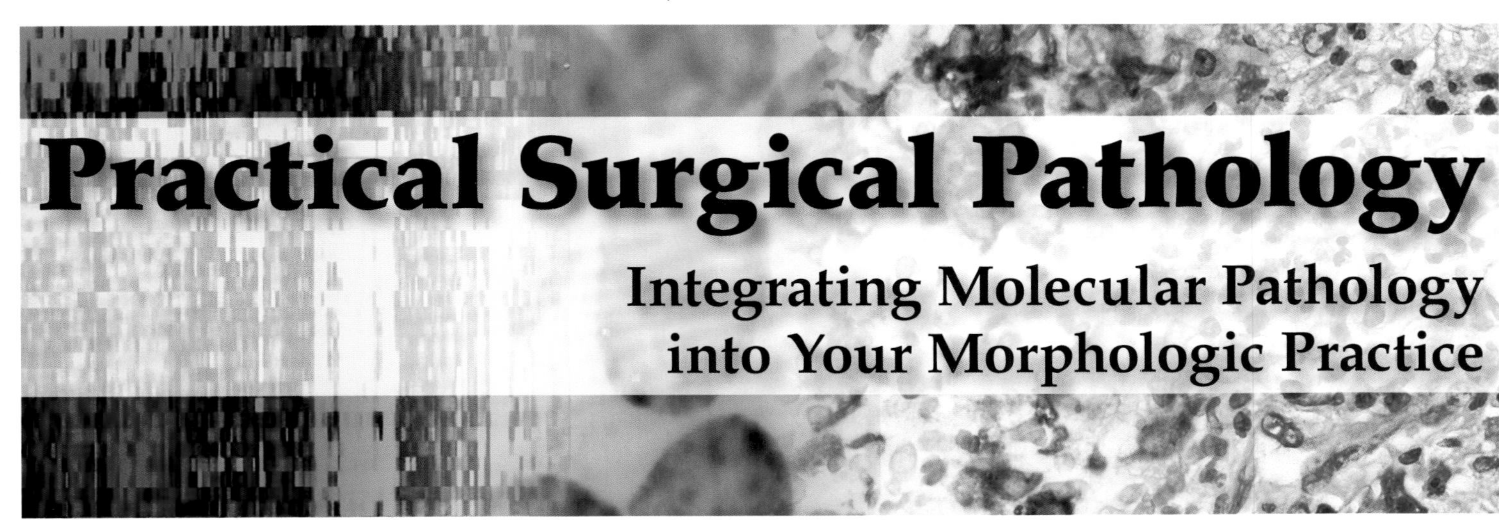

Kirk Heriot, MD, PhD

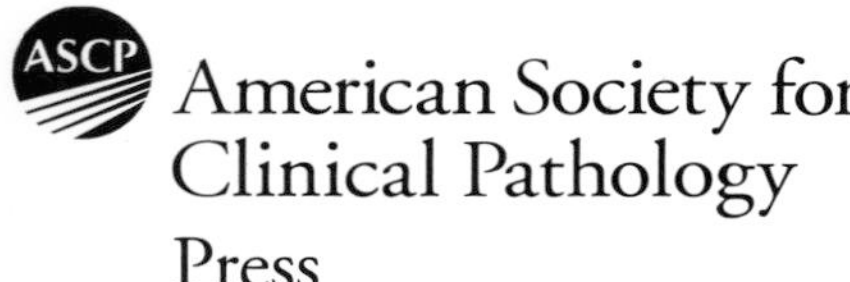

Publishing Team
Aimee Algas (editorial)
Adam Fanucci (illustration)
Erik Tanck (production)
Joshua Weikersheimer (publishing direction)

Notice
Trade names for equipment and supplies described herein are included as suggestions only. In no way does their inclusion constitute an endorsement or preference by the American Society for Clinical Pathology. The ASCP did not test the equipment, supplies, or procedures and therefore urges all readers to read and follow all manufacturers' instructions and package insert warnings concerning the proper and safe use of products.

17 16 15 14 13   5 4 3 2 1

Printed in Hong Kong

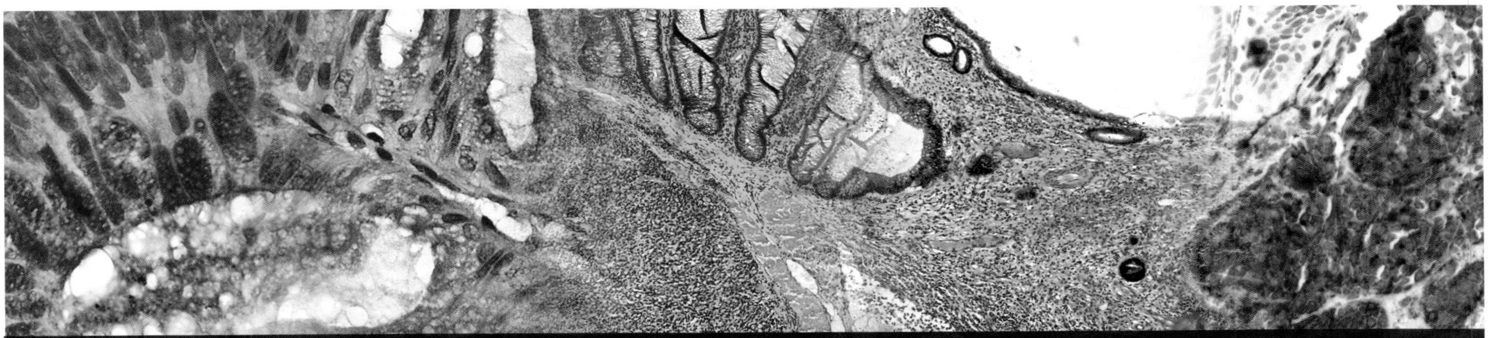

Practical Surgical Pathology

Integrating Molecular Pathology into Your Morphologic Practice

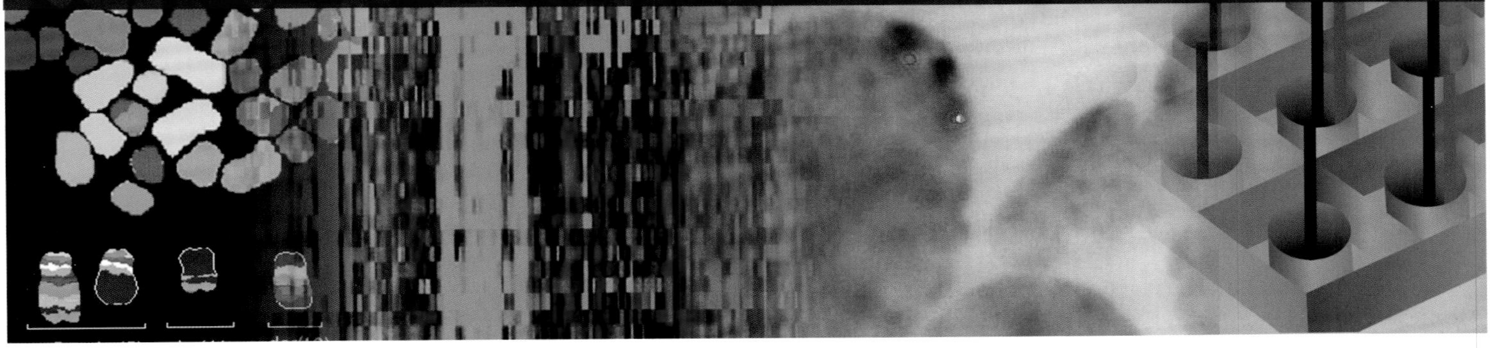

***Kirk Heriot*, MD, PhD**
Pathologist & Laboratory Medical Director
Thompson Health
Canandaigua, NY

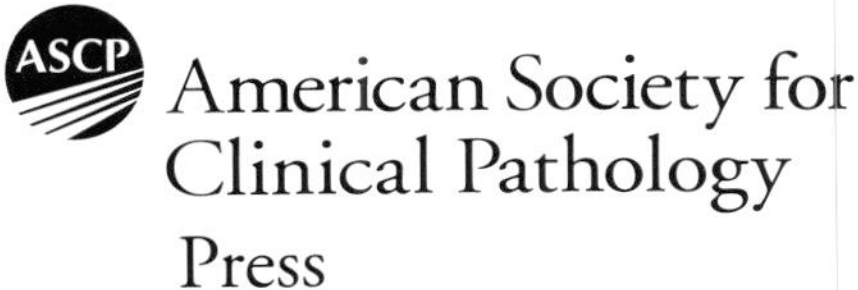

Dedication

This work is dedicated with gratitude to my parents, Henry and Mary Heriot, who instilled a love of learning in me, with love to my sons Adam and Neil, who have inspired me, and with humility to my wonderful teacher, David Jones, MD, the epitome of a scholar and a gentleman.

Acknowledgments

No one can ever thank all of the myriad people who contribute to one's personal and professional development, but a few people have been vital mentors and role models for me. The attending physicians in the pathology department at the State University of New York Upstate Medical Center in Syracuse gave me a wonderful experience as a resident, and opened my eyes to the vast world of pathology. I especially thank these four mentors and role models, all of whom were not only superb pathologists, whose standard I continue to strive for, but also first class gentlemen:

David Jones, MD
Frederick Davey, MD
Douglas Nelson, MD
Rolla Hill, MD

I am indebted to Drs Katherine Warpeha, Charlotte Brown, Amanda Toland, and Judith Connett for fact-checking portions of the manuscript and making many helpful corrections and comments. I am additionally indebted to John Gerlach, PhD, of Michigan State University for granting me access to the excellent material in his courses. 3 wonderful librarians—Lana Rudy, Cathy Carey, and Jane Seelman—obtained many articles for me and never tired of my repeated requests. I thank my partner, Dr William Dean, for his excellent patient care and enormous personal support throughout our long and productive association.

Very special thanks to Joshua Weikersheimer of the ASCP, a scholar of integrity whose knowledge of content creation and bookmaking is endless and whose knowledge of life is inspiring. This book is immeasurably better because of Joshua's constant support, guidance, and suggestions.

The credit for any praise this work is fortunate enough to receive belongs entirely to these most excellent people. I am merely the instrument through which they have come together to speak.

Kirk Heriot

Image Contributors

David Czuchlewski, MD
University of New Mexico
Albuquerque, NM
f1.8, i8.46, i8.58, i8.76, i8.77, i10.17, i10.18, i10.24, i10.25-i10.28, i10.38, i10.39, i10.52, f45.14

John D'Souza, MD
ACM Laboratory
Rochester, NY
f1.6, i16.25, i16.26, f45.12, f45.15

Richard Mac DeMay, MD
University of Chicago
Chicago, IL
i5.1, i30.16-i30.18

Celeste Lamberson, MS, MT(ASCP)
SUNY Upstate Medical University
Syracuse, NY
f4.2, i25.10, f45.17, f46.13, f46.14

Robin LeGallo, MD
University of Virginia Health Science Center
Charlottesville, VA
i2.21-i2.24, i2.27, i2.28, i2.49, i2.58, i2.64, i2.72, i2.74, i2.75

Paul Rothberg, PhD
University of Rochester Medical Center
Rochester, NY
i10.41, i10.42, f23.1, f41.1, f45.9, f46.1, f46.2, f46.12

Larry Lemon, CT(ASCP)^{CM}
ASCP Asset Warehouse
Indianapolis, IN
i19.15, f45.19, f45.21, f45.26, f47.6, f47.7

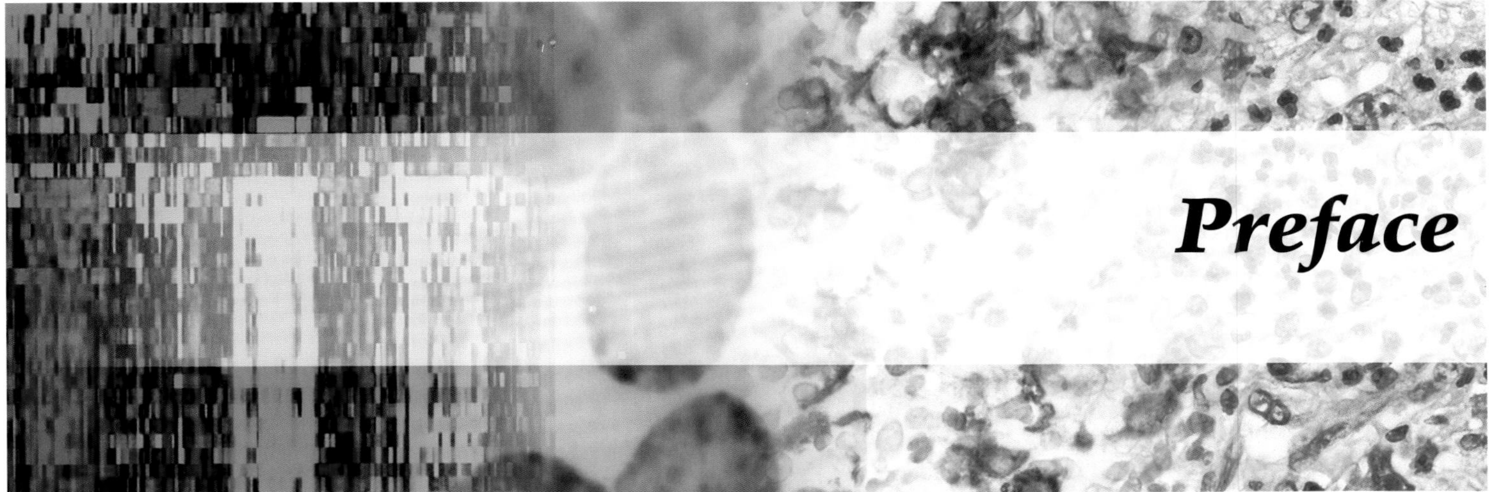

Preface

The primary audience for this work is the practicing pathologist and those studying to be pathologists, and it has 4 objectives. The first objective is to function as a convenient reference for problematic situations that are commonly encountered in the daily practice of surgical pathology. I believe there is a need for an accessible single volume that quickly addresses 95% of the difficult situations a pathologist is likely to encounter. The second objective is to present recent developments in surgical pathology, especially those that relate to molecular techniques, and to provide a thorough integration of morphologic and molecular diagnosis. The third objective is to render a reasonably comprehensive treatment of molecular pathology and the new tools that are revolutionizing our profession, in a stepwise manner, beginning with basic molecular biology. The fourth objective is to provide a clear and succinct general reference that can be read cover-to-cover, in the very limited time available to practicing pathologists, for general education.

The intent is to blend a survey of the literature with my own experience to offer a useful guide to daily practice in a rapidly evolving discipline. My hope is that by omitting the common and simple entities that are very unlikely to be challenging, and the very rare entities that are unlikely to be encountered, a more practical, readable, and accessible work has resulted. This view of pathology is intended to allow busy readers to feel anchored and secure in the rapidly shifting ground beneath their feet.

In keeping with the desire for a shorter and more accessible work that focuses on recent developments, references have been generally restricted to review articles, foundational papers, and recent publications that propose and support fundamental changes in practice. I have generally omitted citations for assertions that most would consider uniformly accepted, and which are likely to be found in other books. I apologize to those whose work could not be cited because of the spatial limitations.

The integration of traditional morphologic pathology with newer molecular concepts has been especially challenging. I have chosen to discuss specific findings in molecular pathology for each organ system with the corresponding discussion of morphologic pathology, so as to provide a complete and integrated discussion of all aspects of pathology for each organ system in one location, while placing the detailed treatment of cell and molecular biology, and its applications, at the end of the work. No approach or organization is perfect, and I have no doubt that others might have done it differently, but my hope is that this approach permits the most complete discussion of individual entities, while the final chapters provide a standalone guide to molecular pathology.

No book is ever perfectly accurate or complete, and readers are invited to share any thoughts regarding the accuracy, comprehensiveness, or "user-friendliness" of the discussion. This work was born of the personal experience of its author, and can be augmented and improved by the personal experience of its readers.

Kirk Heriot

Special User Notes

Geneticists express gene names as italicized capital letters, while proteins are expressed in nonitalicized capital letters. This work uses capitalized italics for gene names, and nonitalicized small letters for protein names with a few exceptions due to convention (eg, MLH1, MSH2, ATP7B, etc).

We have implemented in this text a new reference citation system that takes advantage of the accessibility of universal online identification numbers for publications. PubMed identification numbers (PMID) are used for journal articles, and international standard book numbers (ISBN) are used for books throughout the body of this text. We also make available a complete list of traditional reference citations. Download either HeriotSurgicalPathologyRef.xlsx or HeriotSurgicalPathologyRef.pdf at www.ascp.org/PressUpdates.

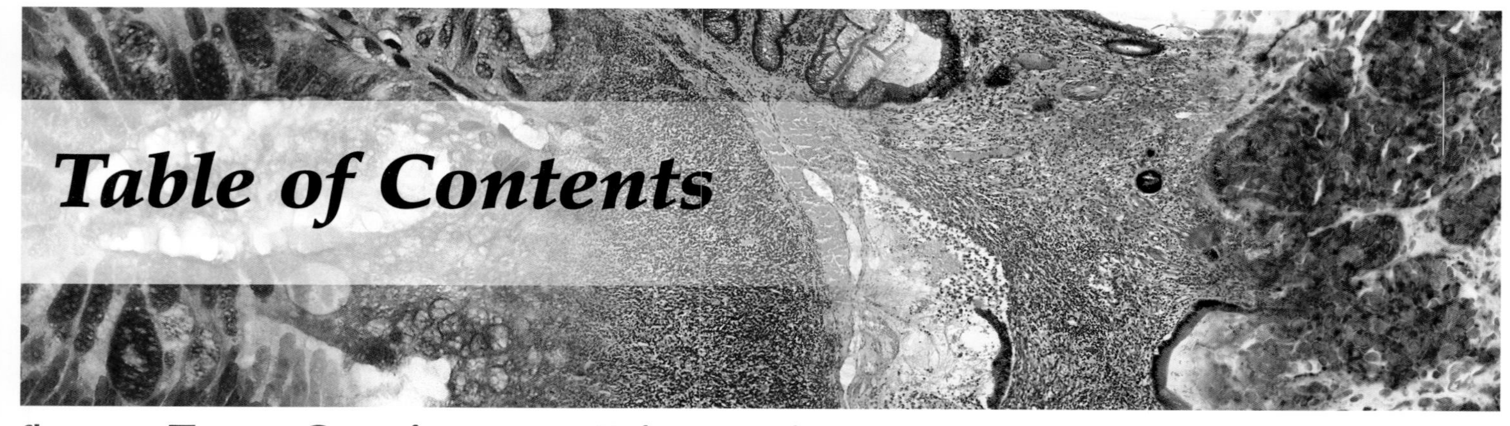

Table of Contents

Chapter 1: *From Specimen to Diagnosis: Techniques & Methods in Pathology* . . . 1

Light Microscopy Remains the Foundation . . . 1
Formalin Reacts with Water, and the Resulting Methylene Glycol Is the Actual Fixative . . . 1
Hematoxylin & Eosin Are Used Throughout the World, Making Slides Interchangeable among Laboratories . . . 1
A Variety of Lenses Are Available to Correct Spherical & Chromatic Aberration . . . 2
The Microscopic Appearance of Tissues Is Largely an Artifact . . . 3
Malignant Cells Tend to Share Certain Morphologic Characteristics . . . 4
A Suggested Algorithm for the Microscopic Examination of a Specimen . . . 4
Immunohistochemistry . . . 4
Most Antigens That React with Monoclonal Antibodies Have CD Designations . . . 5
There Are a Number of Detection Methods in Immunohistochemistry . . . 5
Immunohistochemical Stains Must Be Interpreted with Caution . . . 6
Molecular Studies . . . 7
In Situ Hybridization . . . 7
Polymerase Chain Reaction . . . 8
Core Points for Techniques & Methods . . . 9

Chapter 2: *Soft Tissue* . . . 10

Soft Tissue Masses May Be Composed of Many Types of Tissues, and Each Type Has Benign Mimics . . . 10
Many Soft Tissue Neoplasms Are Associated with Specific Cytogenetic Abnormalities . . . 10
Benign Sarcoma-Like Proliferations . . . 10
Tumors of Fat . . . 12
Tumors of Muscle . . . 14
Vascular Tumors . . . 14
Reactive Vascular Lesions . . . 15
Developmental Vascular Lesions . . . 15
Benign Vascular Neoplasms . . . 15
Low-Grade Malignant Vascular Neoplasms . . . 15
Angiosarcomas . . . 16
Nerve Sheath Tumors . . . 16
Cartilaginous Tumors . . . 17
Benign & Low-Grade Malignant Fibrous Histiocytomas . . . 18
Undifferentiated Pleomorphic Sarcoma (High-Grade Malignant Fibrous Histiocytoma) & Related Neoplasms . . . 18
Unusual Soft Tissue Neoplasms . . . 19
Core Points for Soft Tissue . . . 20
Synoptic Atlas . . . 21

Chapter 3: *Bone & Joint* . . . 30

Traumatic & Degenerative Conditions . . . 30
Arthritis . . . 30
Osteonecrosis . . . 31
Metabolic Bone & Joint Disease . . . 31
Masses & Neoplasms of Bones & Joints . . . 31
Location & Radiographic Appearance Are Indispensable in the Diagnosis of Bone & Joint Masses . . . 31
Core Points for Bone & Joint . . . 33
Synoptic Atlas . . . 34

Chapter 4: *The Breast* . . . 38
Benign Processes That Mimic Invasive Carcinoma . . . 38
Nonpapillary Intraductal Proliferations . . . 39
Macropapillary Intraductal Proliferations. . . . 41
The Breast Biopsy: Potentials & Limitations . . . 42
Assessment of Invasive Ductal Adenocarcinomas. . . . 43
Unusual Forms of Invasive Ductal Adenocarcinoma . . . 47
Intralobular Proliferations . . . 49
Invasive Lobular Adenocarcinomas . . . 49
Stromal Proliferations . . . 50
Stromal Changes Secondary to Therapy . . . 51
Core Points for Breast . . . 51
Synoptic Atlas . . . 52

Chapter 5: *The Neuroendocrine System & Paragangliomas* . . . 60
Core Points for the Neuroendocrine System & Paragangliomas . . . 61
Synoptic Atlas . . . 62

Chapter 6: *The Endocrine System* . . . 63
The Thyroid Gland . . . 63
Inflammatory & Autoimmune Conditions of the Thyroid . . . 63
Mass Lesions of the Thyroid, Neoplastic & Nonneoplastic . . . 63
Nodular & Multinodular Hyperplasia . . . 63
Papillary Carcinoma . . . 64
Follicular Neoplasms . . . 65
Medullary Carcinoma . . . 66
Unusual Forms of Thyroid Carcinoma. . . . 66
Nonepithelial Neoplasms of the Thyroid . . . 66
Fine Needle Aspiration of the Thyroid. . . . 66
Frozen Sections of the Thyroid . . . 67
The Parathyroid Gland. . . . 67
The Adrenal Glands . . . 68
The Normal Adrenal Cortex. . . . 68
Adrenal Cortical Masses . . . 68
Neoplasms of the Adrenal Medulla . . . 68
Core Points for the Endocrine System. . . . 69
Synoptic Atlas . . . 70

Chapter 7: *Normal Immune Function & the Inflammatory Response* 76
Innate Immunity Is Rapid but Nonspecific . . . 76
Acute Inflammation. . . . 76
Cytokines . . . 81
Cell Adhesion Molecules. . . . 84
Healing & Repair . . . 86
Collagen . . . 86
Elastin . . . 86
Glycosaminoglycans (GAGs) . . . 87
Fibronectins . . . 87
Sequence of Events in Wound Healing . . . 87
Adaptive Immunity & Normal Lymph Node Function . . . 88
The Human Leukocyte Antigen (HLA) System. . . . 89
T-Cell Receptor Gene Rearrangement . . . 94
Activation of B Cells . . . 99
Assessment of Clonality . . . 104
Peripheral Tolerance . . . 105
Mechanisms of Cell-Mediated Immunity . . . 105
Mechanisms of Humoral Immunity . . . 105
The Immune Response to Viruses . . . 106
The Immune Response to Parasites . . . 106
Hypersensitivity Reactions. . . . 106
Vaccines & DNA Vaccines . . . 106
Core Points for Normal Immune Function & the Inflammatory Response . . . 107

ISBN 978-089189-5886

Chapter 8: *Lymph Node Pathology* 108

Benign Causes of Lymphadenopathy 108
Metastatic Neoplasms in Lymph Nodes 109
Immunohistochemistry in Lymphomas 109
Hodgkin Disease 109
Classical Hodgkin Disease 110
Nodular Lymphocyte Predominant Hodgkin Disease (NLPHD) 111
Non-Hodgkin Lymphomas (NHLs) 111
World Health Organization Classification of B-Cell Neoplasms 112
The "Small Cell" Lymphomas. 112
Diffuse Large Cell B-Cell Lymphomas. 116
Burkitt & Burkitt-Like Lymphomas 117
Lymphoproliferative Disorders in Immunocompromised Patients 118
T-Cell & Natural Killer Cell Neoplasms 119
WHO Classification of T-Cell Neoplasms 119
Very Rare Neoplasms of Lymph Nodes 121
Core Points for Lymph Node Pathology 122
Synoptic Atlas 123

Chapter 9: *The Spleen* 134

Benign Lesions of the Spleen 134
Malignant Lesions of the Spleen 135
Core Points for the Spleen. 135
Synoptic Atlas 136

Chapter 10: *Bone Marrow* 138

Nonneoplastic Processes in the Marrow 138
Metastatic Carcinoma, Hodgkin Disease, & Lymphomas 138
The Myelodysplastic Syndromes (MDSs) 138
Acute Myelogenous Leukemia (AML) 140
Chronic Myeloproliferative Neoplasms 142
Myelodysplastic/Myeloproliferative Neoplasms. 146
Acute Lymphoid (Lymphoblastic) Leukemia (ALL) 146
The Bone Marrow in Chronic Lymphoid Leukemia. 147
Multiple Myeloma & Other Immunosecretory Disorders 148
Unusual Conditions Found in the Marrow or Blood 149
Core Points for Bone Marrow 150
Synoptic Atlas 151

Chapter 11: *The Ear & the Eye* 159

The Ear 159
The External Ear. 159
The Ear Canal 159
The Middle Ear 159
The Inner Ear 160
The Eye 160
Lesions of the Conjunctiva, Cornea, & Eyelids 160
Neoplasms of the Eye. 160
Other Pathologic Processes of the Eye 161
Core Points for the Ear & the Eye 161
Synoptic Atlas 162

Chapter 12: *The Oral Cavity* 165

Inflammatory Lesions 165
Odontogenic Cysts 165
Other Nonneoplastic Mass Lesions of the Oral Cavity 166
Benign Odontogenic Neoplasms 166
Proliferations of Squamous Epithelium 167
Core Points for The Oral Cavity 168
Synoptic Atlas 169

Chapter 13: *The Salivary Gland* . . . 173
Nonneoplastic Processes . . . 173
Benign Salivary Neoplasms . . . 173
Malignant Salivary Neoplasms . . . 174
Core Points for the Salivary Glands . . . 175
Synoptic Atlas . . . 176

Chapter 14: *The Nose, Sinuses, Oropharynx, & Nasopharynx* . . . 179
Inflammatory & Infectious Reactions . . . 179
Benign Neoplasms & Neoplasm-Like Conditions . . . 179
Malignant Sinonasal Neoplasms . . . 180
Malignant Neoplasms of the Nasopharynx . . . 181
Malignant Neoplasms of the Oropharynx . . . 181
Wegener & Its Differential Diagnosis . . . 181
Core Points for the Nose, Sinus, & Pharynx . . . 182
Synoptic Atlas . . . 183

Chapter 15: *The Larynx & Trachea* . . . 186
Nonneoplastic Processes . . . 186
Laryngeal Neoplasia & Intraepithelial Neoplasia . . . 186
Core Points for the Larynx & Trachea . . . 187
Synoptic Atlas . . . 188

Chapter 16: *The Lung* . . . 191
Nonneoplastic Lung Masses . . . 191
Benign Lung Masses . . . 191
Malignant Lung Neoplasms . . . 192
Non-Small Cell Lung Carcinomas (NSCLCs) . . . 192
Metastatic Carcinomas to the Lung . . . 193
Mutations in Non-Small Carcinomas of the Lung . . . 194
Neuroendocrine Carcinomas of the Lung, Including Small Cell Carcinoma . . . 195
Rare Malignant Lung Neoplasms . . . 197
Unusual Inflammatory Lung Conditions . . . 197
Interstitial Lung Disease . . . 198
Core Points for the Lung . . . 200
Synoptic Atlas . . . 202

Chapter 17: *The Pleura* . . . 209
Mesothelial Cells vs Metastatic Carcinoma . . . 209
Malignant Mesotheliomas & Their Mimics . . . 209
Solitary Fibrous Tumors . . . 210
Core Points for the Pleura . . . 210
Synoptic Atlas . . . 211

Chapter 18: *The Mediastinum* . . . 213
Nonneoplastic Anterior Mediastinal Lesions . . . 213
Epithelial Neoplasms of the Anterior Mediastinum . . . 213
Nonepithelial Neoplasms of the Anterior Mediastinum . . . 214
Middle & Posterior Mediastinal Lesions . . . 215
Core Points for the Mediastinum . . . 215
Synoptic Atlas . . . 216

Chapter 19: *Blood Vessels* . . . 219
Core Points for Blood Vessels . . . 221
Synoptic Atlas . . . 222

ISBN 978-089189-5886

Chapter 20: *The Esophagus* 224
Gastroesophageal Reflux Disease (GERD) & Barrett Esophagus 224
Dysplasia in Barrett Esophagus 226
Inflammatory Conditions in the Esophagus Unrelated to Barrett 227
Carcinomas of the Esophagus 227
Core Points for the Esophagus 228
Synoptic Atlas 229

Chapter 21: *The Stomach* 232
Normal Histology of the Stomach 232
Gastritis 232
Helicobacter Gastritis 233
Nonneoplastic & Polypoid Conditions of the Stomach 233
Gastric Lymphoid Proliferations 234
Gastric Dysplasia 234
Gastric Adenocarcinoma 234
Gastric Stromal Tumors 235
Core Points for the Stomach 236
Synoptic Atlas 237

Chapter 22: *Nonneoplastic Intestinal Disorders* 241
Gluten-Sensitive Enteropathy (Celiac Disease) 241
Unusual Small Bowel Conditions 242
Inflammatory Bowel Disease 242
Dysplasia in Ulcerative Colitis 244
Diversion Colitis & Pouchitis 245
Collagenous Colitis & Lymphocytic Colitis 245
Ischemic Colitis 246
Mucosal Prolapse Syndromes & Conditions Resulting from Mucosal Injury 246
Displaced Epithelium vs Invasive Adenocarcinoma 247
Infectious Colitis 247
The Appendix 248
Unusual Conditions in the Bowel 249
Core Points for Nonneoplastic Intestinal Disorders 249
Synoptic Atlas 251

Chapter 23: *Intestinal Neoplasms* 257
Intestinal Stromal Neoplasms 257
Intestinal Lymphoid Proliferations 257
Colonic Polyps & Adenocarcinoma 258
Dysplasia in Adenomatous Polyps 259
Colorectal Cancer Screening 259
The Colectomy Specimen 260
Intestinal Carcinomas with Neuroendocrine Differentiation 260
Unusual Intestinal Neoplasms 261
Molecular Pathology in Colorectal Cancer 261
The Anal Canal 262
Core Points for Intestinal Neoplasms 262
Synoptic Atlas 263

Chapter 24: *The Pancreas* 269
Developmental Anomalies 269
Nonneoplastic Conditions of the Pancreas 269
Pancreatic Neoplasia 270
Core Points for the Pancreas 271
Synoptic Atlas 272

Chapter 25: *The Gallbladder & the Nonneoplastic Liver* 274
The Gallbladder 274
Normal Hepatic Histology 274
Approach to the Liver Biopsy 275
Duct Obstruction & Atresia 275
Iron Overload Syndrome & Hereditary Hemochromatosis 275
Wilson Disease 276
α-1-Antitrypsin (α1AT) Deficiency 277
Acute Hepatitis 277
Viral Hepatitis 277
Autoimmune Liver Disease 279
Primary Sclerosing Cholangitis 279
Primary Biliary Cirrhosis 279
Autoimmune Hepatitis 280
Alcoholic & Nonalcoholic Fatty Liver Disease (NAFLD) 281
Cirrhosis 282
Drug-Induced Hepatitis 282
Unusual Forms of Hepatitis 282
Graft vs Host Disease & Transplantation Pathology of the Liver 283
Core Points for the Gallbladder & the Nonneoplastic Liver 284
Synoptic Atlas 285

Chapter 26: *Liver Masses & Neoplasms* 291
Benign Hepatic Masses 291
Hepatocyte Dysplasia 292
Hepatocellular Carcinoma (HCC) on Core Biopsy 292
The Clearly Malignant Biopsy of a Liver Mass: Hepatocellular Carcinoma or Another Tumor Type? 293
Nonepithelial Primary Liver Neoplasms 294
Core Points for Liver Masses & Neoplasms 295
Synoptic Atlas 296

Chapter 27: *The Placenta* 301
Development of the Placenta 301
Gross Examination of the Placenta 302
Microscopic Examination of the Placenta 303
What Constitutes Products of Conception? 305
Testing in Pregnancy 305
Core Points for the Placenta 306
Synoptic Atlas 307

Chapter 28: *Gestational Trophoblastic Disease* 309
Abnormalities of Intermediate Trophoblasts 310
Choriocarcinoma 311
Core Points for Gestational Trophoblastic Disease 311
Synoptic Atlas 312

Chapter 29: *The Vulva & Vagina* 315
Benign Cysts of the Vulva & Vagina 315
Inflammatory/Infectious Processes of the Vulva & Vagina 315
Benign Neoplasms of the Vulva 316
Vulvar & Vaginal Intraepithelial Neoplasia (VIN & VAIN) 316
Vulvar Carcinoma 317
Glandular Cells in the Vagina 317
Core Points for the Vulva & the Vagina 317
Synoptic Atlas 318

Chapter 30: *The Cervix* 321
Cervical Intraepithelial Neoplasia 321
The Pap Smear 323
Invasive Squamous Cell Carcinoma of the Cervix 324
Endocervical Lesions 325
Core Points for the Cervix 326
Synoptic Atlas 328

ISBN 978-089189-5886

Chapter 31: *The Endometrium* . . . 333

Normal Histology & Dating . . . 333
The Effect of Exogenous Hormones on the Endometrium . . . 334
Endometritis . . . 334
The Endometrium in Dysfunctional Uterine Bleeding . . . 335
Endometrial Metaplasia . . . 335
Endometrial Hyperplasia . . . 335
Endometrial Adenocarcinoma . . . 336
Unusual Types of Endometrial Adenocarcinoma . . . 337
Endometrial Stromal Proliferations . . . 338
Core Points for Endometrium . . . 339
Synoptic Atlas . . . 340

Chapter 32: *The Myometrium* . . . 346

Adenomyosis . . . 346
Uterine Smooth Muscle Neoplasms . . . 346
Core Points for Myometrium . . . 347
Synoptic Atlas . . . 348

Chapter 33: *The Ovary & Fallopian Tube* . . . 350

Normal Function & Histology . . . 350
Nonneoplastic Stromal Processes . . . 350
Epithelial Ovarian Neoplasms . . . 351
Serous & Mucinous Epithelial Neoplasms . . . 351
Epithelial Tumors of Low Malignant Potential . . . 351
Serous LMP Neoplasms . . . 352
Mucinous LMP Neoplasms . . . 352
Endometrioid Adenocarcinoma of the Ovary . . . 353
Primary Ovarian Adenocarcinoma vs Metastatic Adenocarcinoma . . . 353
Other Ovarian Epithelial Neoplasms . . . 354
Sex Cord-Stromal Neoplasms . . . 354
Ovarian Germ Cell Tumors . . . 356
Unusual Ovarian Neoplasms . . . 357
The Fallopian Tube . . . 357
Nonneoplastic Conditions of the Fallopian Tube . . . 357
Neoplasms of the Fallopian Tube . . . 357
Core Points for the Ovary & Fallopian Tube . . . 358
Synoptic Atlas . . . 359

Chapter 34: *The Peritoneum* . . . 363

The Normal Serosa, Reactive Fibrosis, & Inclusion Cysts . . . 363
Mesothelioma & Mesothelial Hyperplasia . . . 363
Pseudomyxoma Peritonei . . . 364
The Secondary Müllerian System . . . 364
Unusual Peritoneal Neoplasms . . . 365
Core Points for the Peritoneum . . . 365
Synoptic Atlas . . . 366

Chapter 35: *The Kidney* . . . 367

Nonneoplastic Conditions . . . 367
Congenital Disorders . . . 367
Vascular Changes in the Kidney . . . 367
Chronic Pyelonephritis . . . 367
Other Commonly Encountered Nonneoplastic Renal Conditions . . . 368
The Thrombotic Microangiopathy Conditions . . . 368
The Kidney in Transplantation . . . 368
Benign Renal Neoplasms . . . 369
Malignant Renal Neoplasms . . . 370
Core Points for the Kidney . . . 373
Synoptic Atlas . . . 374

Chapter 36: *The Bladder & Urethra* 377

Inflammatory Conditions of the Bladder 377
Benign Neoplasms & Neoplasm-Like Conditions of the Bladder & Urethra 377
Urothelial Dysplasia & Carcinoma in Situ 378
Papillary Urothelial Lesions 378
Invasive Urothelial (Transitional Cell) Carcinoma 379
Unusual types of Urothelial Carcinoma 379
Subtle Forms of Urothelial Carcinoma 380
Screening for Urothelial Carcinoma 380
Core Points for the Bladder & the Urethra 381
Synoptic Atlas 382

Chapter 37: *The Prostate Gland* 384

Prostate Cancer Screening 384
The Prostate Biopsy 385
Mimics of Prostatic Adenocarcinoma 387
Immunohistochemistry of Prostatic Tissue 387
Prostatic Intraductal Neoplasia (PIN) 388
The Prostate Biopsy after Treatment for Carcinoma 389
The Radical Prostatectomy 389
The Transurethral Resection 390
Prostatic Carcinoma in Metastatic Sites 391
Prevention of Prostate Carcinoma 391
Core Points for the Prostate 391
Synoptic Atlas 392

Chapter 38: *The Testes* 395

Normal Development & Structure of the Testis 395
Disorders of Testicular Development & Location 395
The Testis in Infertility 396
Nonneoplastic Conditions 396
Testicular Neoplasms 396
Germ Cell Neoplasms 396
Sex Cord-Stromal Neoplasms 399
Other Testicular Neoplasms 399
Core Points for the Testes 400
Synoptic Atlas 401

Chapter 39: *The Penis & Scrotum* 403

Normal Anatomy 403
Nonneoplastic Conditions 403
Neoplasms of the Penis 403
Core Points for the Penis & the Scrotum 404
Synoptic Atlas 404

Chapter 40: *The Skin* 405

Normal Structure of the Skin 405
Cutaneous Neoplasms & Masses 405
Benign Epidermal Hyperplasia 405
Epithelial Neoplasms 406
Nonepithelial Neoplasms 406
Cutaneous Lymphoproliferative Disorders 407
Joint WHO/EORTC System for Primary Cutaneous Lymphomas 408
Cutaneous T-Cell Lymphoid Proliferations 408
Cutaneous B-Cell Lymphoid Proliferations 409
Melanocytic Proliferations 409
Inflammatory Skin Lesions (Dermatoses) 412
Acute & Chronic Dermatitis 413
Bullous/Vesicular Disorders 414
Other Autoimmune Disorders of the Skin 415
Infectious & Granulomatous Conditions of the Skin 415
The Panniculitis Conditions 415
Core Points for the Skin 416
Synoptic Atlas 417

ISBN 978-089189-5886

Chapter 41: *The Central Nervous System* 423
Nonneoplastic Disorders of the CNS 423
Neoplasms of the Sella & Suprasellar Region 423
Neoplasms of the CNS 424
Inflammatory & Degenerative Conditions of Muscles 425
Core Points for the Central Nervous System 426
Synoptic Atlas 427

Chapter 42: *Anatomic Pathology Quality Assurance* 429
Mistakes of Identification 429
Mistakes of Omission 430
Mistakes of Interpretation 430
Mistakes of Documentation 432
The Anatomic Pathology Quality Assurance Program 432
Surgical Pathology "Critical" Values—What To Do? 433
Core Points for Quality Assurance 434

Chapter 43: *Clinical Genetics* 437
Mendelian Inheritance 437
Y-linked Inheritance 439
Bayesian Analysis in Mendelian Inheritance 439
Mitochondrial Inheritance 442
Non-Mendelian Inheritance Secondary to Multifactorial Inheritance 443
Chromosome Banding & Cytogenetics 444
Linkage & Association: Tracing a Gene 447
Association Studies 447
The Evolution of the X & Y Chromosomes 450
Core Points for Clinical Genetics 451

Chapter 44: *Molecular Pathology I: Foundations* 452
Historical Background 452
The Structure of DNA 453
Distinction between Prokaryotes & Eukaryotes 453
Life Is Based On 2 Sugars, 5 Bases, and a Phosphate Group 453
Each Cell Contains As Much As a Meter of DNA, Packed in an Intricate Series of Structures 456
The Cell Cycle Consists of Phases and Has Specific Regulatory Checkpoints 457
DNA Replication 457
There Are Many Forms of DNA Polymerase, in Both Prokaryotes & Eukaryotes 458
There Are Many Enzymes That Repair Damaged or Mismatched DNA 458
Mitosis Is the Separation of the Duplicated Chromosomes to Opposite Poles of the Cell 458
DNA Transcription & Translation 459
Transcription Requires 1 of Several Forms of RNA Polymerase, a Promoter Site on the DNA, and a Number of Transcription Factors 459
Eukaryotic RNA Undergoes Modifications after Transcription, the Most Important of Which Is the Splicing of Introns 461
Only a Minority of mRNA Is Ever Translated into Protein 462
Translation Involves Relative Motion between the Nascent Polypeptide Chain and 3 Critical Sites on the Ribosome 463
Many Properties of Proteins Come from Posttranslational Modification 464
Like RNA, the Fully Developed Proteins Must Be Transported to the Correct Intracellular Location 464
So What Is a Gene? 466
Mobile Genetic Elements 466
A Large Amount of DNA is Repetitive, and There Are Different Types of Repetitions 468
Core Points for Molecular Pathology I: Foundations 468

Chapter 45: *Molecular Pathology II: Techniques* . . . 469

Early Nucleic Acid Studies . . . 469
Nucleic Acid Extraction & Measurement . . . 469
Blotting . . . 470
Types of Electrophoresis . . . 470
Nucleases . . . 471
Cloning . . . 472
Vectors . . . 472
Gene Modification . . . 475
Amplification Techniques . . . 476
Polymerase Chain Reaction . . . 476
Other Methods of DNA Amplification . . . 482
Isothermal Nucleic Acid Amplification Techniques . . . 484
Signal Amplification Techniques . . . 485
Melting Curve Analysis . . . 486
In Situ Hybridization & FISH . . . 486
Limitations of FISH . . . 487
FISH Preparation . . . 487
FISH Limited to Characterized Abnormalities . . . 489
Multiple Probe FISH . . . 493
Comparative Genomic Hybridization . . . 493
Multicolor FISH & Spectral Karyotyping . . . 495
DNA Sequencing . . . 497
Newer Methods of DNA Sequencing Based on Synthesis, Not Termination . . . 498
Bioinformatics & Public DNA Databases . . . 500
Need for Faster, Cheaper DNA Sequencing and Annotation of the Genome . . . 500
Repetitive DNA . . . 501
Microarrays . . . 503
Molecular Techniques: Closing Comments . . . 508
Core Points for Molecular Pathology II: Techniques . . . 508

Chapter 46: *Molecular Pathology III: Applications & Diagnoses* . 509

Regulatory, Ethical, and Legal Issues in Molecular Pathology . . . 509
Oncogenes & Tumor Suppressor Genes . . . 510
Oncogenes Are Normal and Necessary Genes That Have Undergone a Gain of Function Mutation That Facilitates Cancer . . . 511
Tumor Suppressor Genes Undergo a Loss of Function Mutation to Facilitate Cancer . . . 512
Hereditary Cancer Syndromes . . . 513
HNPCC Is One of the Best Understood Hereditary Cancer Syndromes . . . 514
Familial Adenomatous Polyposis Is Another Major Hereditary Colon Cancer Syndrome . . . 516
Hereditary Diffuse Gastric Cancer Syndrome Predisposes to Both Diffuse Gastric Cancer and Lobular Breast Cancer through Loss of E-Cadherin . . . 517
BRCA1 & *BRCA2* Are Involved in DNA Repair . . . 517
Multiple Endocrine Neoplasia Type 2 is a Rare Form of Hereditary Cancer Syndrome That Is Associated with an Oncogene, Not a Tumor Suppressor Gene . . . 517
Molecular Testing in Infectious Disease . . . 518
Chlamydia . . . *518*
Neisseria gonorrhoea . . . *519*
Enterococcus . . . *519*
Staphylococcus aureus . . . *520*
Enterobacteriaceae, Extended Spectrum β-Lactamases, and Carbapenem-Resistant Enterobacteriaceae . . . 521
Macrolide Resistance . . . 521
Clostridium difficile . . . *521*
Tuberculosis . . . 522
Strain Typing & Molecular Epidemiology . . . 522

ISBN 978-089189-5886

Viruses 523
The Human Immunodeficiency Virus 524
The Hepatitis Viruses. 525
The Human Papillomavirus Family 526
The Human Herpesvirus Family 528
The Polyomavirus Family 529
The Influenza Viruses 529
The *Enterovirus* Genus 530
Molecular Testing for Other Pathogenic Organisms 530
Molecular Testing of Infectious Diseases—Closing Comments 531
Pharmacogenetics. 531
Most Enzymes of Phase 1 Metabolism Are Members of the Cytochrome P450 System 532
Pharmacogenetics of Drugs Not Metabolized by CYP. 533
The Central Nervous System in Dementia 534
Other Causes of Dementia Share Clinical and Histologic Characteristics with AD 535
Prion Disease—Infectious Proteins? 536
Applications of Microsatellite Analysis 536
Identity Testing 536
The Principles of DNA Profiling Are Very Similar to Those of Paternity Testing. 537
There Are Many Other Applications of Microsatellites 538
Single Nucleotide Polymorphisms 538
The Tendency for SNPs to Remain Together during Evolution Is the Basis of the HapMap 540
Molecular Pathology of Inherited Disorders 540
Cystic Fibrosis 541
Spinal Muscular Atrophy 543
Inherited Hypercoagulability 543
Achondroplasia, Hypochondroplasia, and Craniosynostosis Syndromes 543
Muscular Dystrophy 544
Neurofibromatosis 545
Osteogenesis Imperfecta 545
Hearing Loss 545
Genetic Screening in Ashkenazi Jews 546
Trinucleotide Repeat Disorders. 547
Trinucleotide Repeat Disorders Have Anticipation and Grey Zones 547
Core Points for Molecular Pathology III: Applications & Diagnoses 548

Chapter 47: *Molecular Pathology IV: Frontiers & Personalized Medicine* 549

Epigenetic Regulation of the Genome 549
Transcription: Key to Complexity 551
Study of Gene Expression Begins Functional Genomics 552
Proteomics 553
Mass Spectrometry (MS). 554
Proteomics 555
Molecular Phenotyping of Cancers 556
Breast Cancer Is the Best Developed Example of Molecular Phenotyping 556
Molecular Pathology: Closing Comments. 558
Core Points for Molecular Pathology IV: Frontiers & Personalized Medicine 559

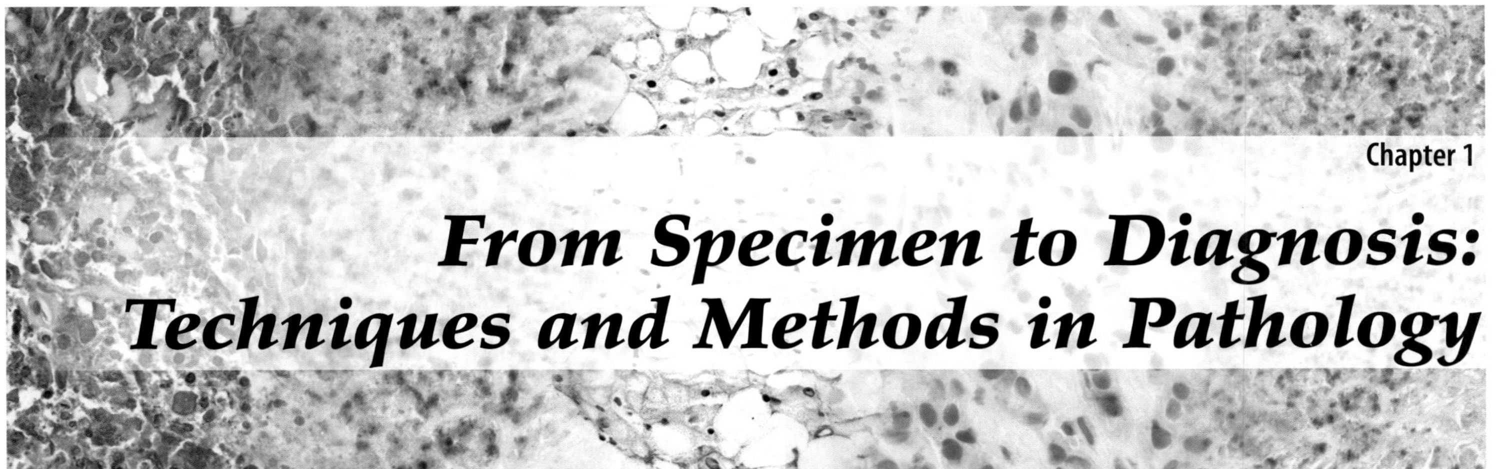

Chapter 1

From Specimen to Diagnosis: Techniques and Methods in Pathology

Light Microscopy Remains the Foundation

There are 4 principal forms of examination that are employed sequentially on a specimen, in the order in which they were discovered: gross examination, examination by light microscopy, immunohistochemistry, and molecular/cytogenetic studies.

A gross examination is the first level of study of a specimen and is the only study performed in a few simple situations. A good gross examination is certainly a critical part of the overall evaluation because the gross specimen can never be perfectly reconstructed in the state in which it was received. Slides and paraffin blocks can be retrieved and reexamined, but no one other than the person performing the gross examination will ever see the specimen exactly as it was received. That said, however, no comments are made on this topic in this work because the skills involved are basic and rarely challenging. Several excellent grossing manuals are available, and compendiums are included in many large textbooks.

Light microscopy is the second level of study on a specimen and still constitutes the bulk of the pathologist's contribution to patient care and the bulk of the text in pathology books that are not specifically dedicated to 1 of the other 3 levels of study. Light microscopic study begins with tissue fixation, which is necessary to preserve the structure of cells. Because cells are water-based, the fixative must be water soluble. The most popular fixative in pathology is formalin, an aqueous solution of formaldehyde gas, which is buffered to physiologic pH by sodium phosphate (this is called neutral buffered formalin). Neutral buffered formalin, though marketed as 10%, is actually only about 4% formaldehyde, because it is 10% of a solution containing 37% formaldehyde gas.

Formalin Reacts with Water, and the Resulting Methylene Glycol Is the Actual Fixative

In water, the formaldehyde (CH_2O) reacts with water to produce methylene glycol (CH_4O_2) [PMID19886758]. Glycols are a type of alcohol (ie, compounds containing a hydroxyl, or –OH group) in which there are 2 hydroxyl groups. The reaction of formaldehyde and water is as follows:

$$CH_2O + H_2O \rightarrow CH_4O_2$$

The structure of methylene glycol is ($HO{-}CH_2{-}OH$). Thus, the reactive moieties in formalin fixation are 2 hydroxyl (–OH) groups, not 1 aldehyde (–CHO) group. The conversion to methylene glycol is important because it allows 1 molecule of formaldehyde to react with more than 1 protein, thereby cross-linking proteins, which would be impossible with a single reactive aldehyde group.

After fixation, the specimen is processed through a variety of fluids, the object of which is to remove all of the water and replace it with paraffin, a type of wax that is hard at room temperature, so that it can be sectioned. The process begins with alcohol (usually a mixture of methyl, ethyl, and isopropyl), as alcohol is miscible in both water and organic solvents. After increasing concentrations of alcohols, the sample is exposed to xylene or another purely organic compound. After saturation with the organic compound, the tissue can then be impregnated by paraffin, after which it is firm enough to section.

Hematoxylin and Eosin Are Used Throughout the World, Making Slides Interchangeable among Laboratories

After sectioning, the tissue must be deparaffinized before it can absorb dye. Paraffin removal is achieved by heating, followed by sequential immersions in organic solvent, alcohol, and water. The standard stain of histopathology is a combination of hematoxylin and eosin (known all over the world as H&E). In an H&E stain, the hematoxylin stains the nucleus while eosin stains the proteins of the cytoplasm.

Hematoxylin has been used in histopathology since the early 20th century and is now entering its second century as the most important stain in medicine. Hematoxylin is obtained from the heartwood of the tree *Haematoxylum campechianum*, a logwood tree that is native to southern Mexico, Central America, and the West Indies. It was used as a textile dye by the Mayans and Aztecs, then by Europeans before its medical use was discovered. The actual dyeing agent is hematein, an oxidized form of hematoxylin. Several varieties of hematoxylin are available, varying in the compounds that are used as mordants (metallic agents that permit adherence of the dye to the target molecules). In most uses, either aluminum or iron is used as a mordant [PMID16195172]. A shortage of hematoxylin in the 1970s engendered a search for synthetic analogs, but these have been only partially successful.

Because it is a basic dye, and because nucleic acids make the nucleus acidic, hematoxylin stains the nucleus. The precise target of hematoxylin depends on the pH, the nature of the fixative and solution, and the mordant used, but it appears to complex with proteins that are associated with nucleic acids rather than with the nucleic acids themselves [PMID11473818].

There are 2 approaches to nuclear staining with hematoxylin. The first approach, called progressive, attempts to stain the tissue just long enough for adequate staining of the target molecules. The second approach, called regressive, deliberately overstains the tissue and then uses acid alcohol to leach out excess hematoxylin, a process oddly called differentiation. Differentiation is terminated by removal from the acid alcohol and restoring the tissue to a neutral or basic pH. The restoration of a basic pH also imparts a bluish color to the hematein. If done properly, regressive staining avoids the problem of different portions of the nucleus requiring different lengths of time in hematoxylin and results in a more uniform degree of staining [Carson ISBN978-0891895817].

Eosin is an aniline dye (ie, based on aniline, an aromatic compound similar to benzene) and, therefore, is not soluble in water. In typical use, it is dissolved in alcohol, requiring an alcohol rinse between the water-soluble hematoxylin and eosin. Interestingly, eosin is a bromine derivative of the important fluorescent dye fluorescein and is itself strongly fluorescent, though this property is not used in histopathology. If fluorescence is desired, the parent compound fluorescein is used. In the staining of proteins, the amino acids arginine, histidine, and lysine electrostatically bind to the carboxylic and phenolic groups of eosin (at acidic pH, tryptophan also binds the dye) [PMID11078585].

H&E is often supplemented with a variety of special stains, collectively called cytochemical stains, that are also based on color, but which highlight particular types of tissue instead of just the nucleus or the cytoplasm in general. Examples include the trichrome stain, which stains collagen blue; Gomori methenamine silver (GMS), which causes some pathogenic organisms such as fungi and *Pneumocystis* to appear black; and periodic acid-Schiff (PAS), which conveys a pink-red color to glycogen and complex carbohydrate macromolecules that are found in basement membranes and in some pathogenic organisms.

A Variety of Lenses Are Available to Correct Spherical and Chromatic Aberration

Single-lens microscopes are not made now because compound microscopes, which use 2 sets of lenses, offer much greater magnification. The 2 difficulties to be overcome with compound microscopes are spherical aberration and chromatic aberration. Spherical aberration occurs because light rays that strike the lens at its periphery are refracted more than those that strike the lens at its center. Therefore, there is no single point of focus. Spherical aberration does not depend on the wavelength of the incident light, only on the location on the lens where the light strikes it.

Spherical aberration is corrected by a combination of lenses such that variations in refraction cancel each other out. Simple combinations are called achromatic lenses, or achromats. The simplest achromat is a doublet. Most achromats correct spherical aberration for 1 wavelength, usually green. Apochromatic lenses, or apochromats, are more complex combinations that offer better correction and correct for 2 wavelengths, green and blue. Planapochromatic lenses (planapochromats) are the most sophisticated and effective of lens combinations. They produce a flat field (the term "plan" refers to a flat field) and correct spherical aberration in 4 colors [PMID14719324]. High-power apochromats and planapochromats often have correction collars to compensate for variations in coverslip thickness (such variations are not a problem at lower power).

Chromatic aberration is also a failure of the lens to focus all of the incident light to the same point, but here, the lens fails to focus light of different wavelengths to the same point. The different components of white light will be refracted to a different degree, with light of shorter wavelengths being refracted to a greater extent, focusing onto a plane that is closer to the lens.

Chromatic aberration is often corrected by a combination of 2 techniques. The first is to use lenses that contain fluorite, which reduces the amount of aberration of the lens. The second method is to use lens in combination, as is done in the correction of spherical aberration. Better correction for chromatic aberration is successively provided by achromatic, apochromatic, and planapochromatic lenses, as was the case for spherical aberration. Achromatic lenses correct color aberration in 2 wavelengths (usually red and blue), apochromats correct in 3 wavelengths (usually red, blue, and green), and planapochromats in 4 [James ISBN978-9024719006]. Fluorite objectives are intermediate in quality between achromats and apochromats, and correct both spherical and chromatic aberration in 3 wavelengths [PMID14719324].

The lenses are only 1 component of the optical system of a microscope. They work in conjunction with condensers and diaphragms, which ensure a uniform intensity of light throughout the field. Before there is any magnification, a special lens called the substage condenser collects the light from the source and focuses it onto the slide, ensuring even distribution and parallel alignment of light rays [PMID14719326]. Because the condenser is a lens, it produces spherical and chromatic aberration, and achromatic lenses, correcting for spherical and chromatic aberration, are used in high-quality condensers.

The iris diaphragm works with the substage condenser to illuminate the specimen in a uniform manner. August Köhler (1866-1948; also spelled "Koehler") developed the procedure for the precise alignment of all of the components that ensures an evenly-lit field in which the light source cannot be seen, and "Köhler illumination" refers to an optical system that is optimized in this manner. The details and procedure for attaining Köhler illumination are available for the intrepid [PMID14719326].

The 3 parameters that are important in a light microscope are magnification, resolution, and numerical aperture. Magnification is the simplest of these, and in understanding its implications, it is only necessary to realize that magnification is limited by resolution, the smallest distance between 2 objects for which they can still be discerned as separate, and that higher magnification means a smaller field of view.

Numerical aperture (NA) is a more difficult concept. After the light moves through the specimen, it diverges into an inverted cone, with the apex of the cone being the specimen and the base being the objective. 1/2 of the angle at the apex of this cone is usually called μ, although other Greek letters such as θ or α are also used. NA = n(sin[μ]) [PMID14719326], where n is the index of refraction (ie, a measure of how much light is refracted) of the *medium* (not of the lens). For air, n=1.0, and the NA is simply the sine of 1/2 the angle at the apex of the cone.

Without the use of oil, the NA increases with increasing magnification because higher-power objectives are closer to the specimen, and the angle μ and its sine are greater. A higher percentage of the light that passes through the specimen enters the lens. The NA is a measure of the light-gathering capacity of the lens. A higher NA implies greater light-gathering capacity [PMID14719326]. The theoretical maximum of μ is 90°, and the theoretical maximum for sin[μ] is 1.0, since the sine of 90° is 1.0. Without the use of oil, a high-power objective contacting the slide has a theoretical maximum NA of 1.0.

Oil immersion lenses have a higher NA not only because they are closer to the slide, but also because oil has a higher index of refraction than air. For most immersion oils, n=1.51. Because oil immersion lenses are not much closer to the slide than a 40× objective, they have a higher NA primarily because of the higher index of refraction of oil.

The resolution depends on NA and wavelength, and is usually given by the formula

$$R=0.61\lambda/NA$$

where λ is the wavelength of the light. A higher NA of the objective will lead to better resolution (ie, a lower number) as well as better light-gathering capacity. For practical purposes, the resolution of a light microscope is about 0.5 μm, roughly the size of most bacteria.

Light that enters the specimen, like any electromagnetic radiation, is composed of alternating electric and magnetic fields vibrating in all planes. In rare cases, it is desired to have the light that enters the specimen vibrate in only 1 plane by first passing it through a polarizer, creating polarized light. Polarized light appears essentially identical to ordinary light, but if the polarized light emerging from the specimen is passed through a second polarizer that is perpendicular to the first, the light is completely quenched and the field is dark. Some structures, especially if of foreign origin, are birefringent, meaning that they will rotate a beam of polarized light. Birefringent material is identified by placing 1 polarizer below the specimen and a second above it, at a right angle, so that no light reaches the eyepieces. If a birefringent structure is in the specimen, the polarized light that emerges from it will be rotated and will no longer be completely perpendicular to the second polarizer, so the light will not be completely quenched. Birefringent material is bright against a dark background.

The Microscopic Appearance of Tissues Is Largely an Artifact

In histopathology, we labor against a number of compelling handicaps. First, fixation kills the cells, so we never examine living tissue. Considerable effort has been expended searching for a way to image living cells in medical practice, but success has been elusive. Dark-field microscopy, phase contrast microscopy, and Nomarski optics are all techniques, taking advantage of light scattering or differences in the indices of refraction among different portions of the cytoplasm, that attempt to visualize living cells. These methods are important in many research applications, but their use in routine medical practice is very limited and, even in the best case, is restricted to cells that have not been fixed (eg, blood smears), because formalin fixation kills cells.

The simplest method employed to visualize living cells is dark field microscopy. In traditional bright-field microscopy, the light source, the specimen, and the optics are all in a line. In the most common version of dark field microscopy, this linear arrangement is maintained, but an opaque disk is inserted above the condenser. This disk blocks the light from directly entering the specimen, but light, like all electromagnetic radiation, spreads out as it travels, so some light enters the specimen from the sides. Some of this light is then scattered vertically and enters the eyepieces. This "roundabout" illumination of the specimen makes it appear bright against a dark background. Dark-field microscopy permits the examination of cells that have not been stained and therefore may be living, since staining kills cells. However, dark field microscopy can only be used for cells that have not been fixed (eg, blood smears). Nothing is accomplished by examining paraffin-processed tissue in dark field microscopy.

Phase contrast microscopy makes use of the fact that different parts of the cell, including the cytoplasm or different organelles, have different indices of refraction. The higher the index of refraction in a medium, the more the light will be retarded as it passes through it. This causes interference, wherein the peaks and troughs of adjacent light rays tend to cancel each other out, resulting in a dark field. Less refractive structures will retard light less, resulting in less interference and a relatively brighter field. Because of its granularity, the cytoplasm typically has a high refractive index and will appear dark relative to most organelles. A more advanced version of phase contrast microscopy is differential interference (Nomarski) microscopy. However, these techniques are used only in special situations, primarily in research. In medical practice, we are forced to make educated guesses about disease processes from the study of dead cells.

The second handicap is that fixation and paraffin processing cause artifacts in the appearance of cells and tissues. Life is based on water, but the pathologist studies dehydrated, wax-impregnated structures that are in fact casts of cells. Many of the primary, foundational histologic findings are actually artifacts that would not be seen if the abnormal cells could be seen in their pristine state in vivo.

The third handicap is that light microscopy has severe limitations in the degrees of magnification and resolution that can be attained. Electron microscopy, based on the shorter wavelengths of electrons, offers much greater magnification and resolution, but cannot be used in routine medical practice.

The fourth handicap is that pathology is based on the visualization of a single plane, with essentially no depth (a typical section is about 6 μm in thickness). The experienced pathologist has learned that this difficulty can be mitigated by obtaining deeper sections into the paraffin block, but true 3-dimensional structure cannot be studied.

The fifth handicap against which the pathologist labors is that any staining, be it H&E or a special stain, stains only a small part of the cell. Most of the structures of a cell are invisible to us at any magnification and with any staining technique.

ISBN 978-089189-5886

Histopathology is a limited and artificial snapshot of a small portion of the dynamic, changing disease process.

Malignant Cells Tend to Share Certain Morphologic Characteristics

Although the microscopic appearance of specimens is largely an artifact, standardized fixation, staining, and examination techniques have made these artifacts reproducible among laboratories, so that the morphologic characteristics of most malignant cells have been well characterized and can be readily detected. The precise criteria for malignancy depend on the specific tissue and the clinical situation, as we will encounter throughout this work, but in general, on routine H&E stains, malignant neoplasms have at least 1 of the following characteristics:

- Increased cellularity
- Enlarged nuclei that are hyperchromatic (indicating increased chromatin), pleomorphic (ie, variable), or that have prominent nucleoli (indicating increased protein synthesis)
- Increased mitotic activity or abnormal mitotic figures
- Necrosis
- Failure of the cells to form normal structures (eg, failure of glandular cells to form glands, or the formation of incompletely-formed glands in an adenocarcinoma or failure of endothelial cells to form well defined blood vessels in an angiosarcoma)
- Destruction of adjacent normal tissue
- In a lymphoid lesion, evidence of monoclonality

For any tumor, clinical evidence of destructiveness or of a metastasis is an indication of malignancy, but these may not be known to the examining pathologist.

A Suggested Algorithm for the Microscopic Examination of a Specimen

The clinical situation figures heavily into the overall interpretation, but the pathologist is well advised to construct a preliminary opinion without knowing the clinical circumstances, to ensure that his or her opinion is not prejudiced by this information. Before this preliminary opinion is finalized, however, the clinical findings must be taken into account, and the final pathologic diagnosis must be contextually correct. Errors are minimized when the clinician and the pathologist first think independently, then confer and think together.

It is useful to construct an algorithm in the study of a specimen. A useful series of questions to be asked sequentially is the following:

- What was the gross appearance?
- What is the tissue type?
- Is there a pathologic process at all?
- If so, is it inflammatory or neoplastic?
- If it is neoplastic, is it benign or malignant?
- If it is malignant, what is the type of malignancy, and what other useful information about the cancer can be gleaned?

Every site has 1 or more nonneoplastic processes that simulate neoplasia. The false impression of neoplasia can result from the presence of a clinical mass, a mass identified at gross examination, or microscopic findings of increased cellularity or cellular atypia. Nonneoplastic simulators of malignancy can be reactive, developmental, infectious, iatrogenic, or idiopathic [PMID9739546].

Numerous recommendations for the surgical pathology report ("checklists") have been published for virtually every type of specimen that the pathologist is likely to receive. The College of American Pathologists and the Association of Directors of Anatomic and Surgical Pathology have been leaders in this important area. In addition to their published recommendations, a comprehensive series of guidelines is also included in Dr Rosai's excellent text [Rosai ISBN0-32301342-2]. The most recent and comprehensive guidelines for most tumor types are those from the College of American Pathologists, available to members on their website at www.cap.org/cancerprotocols.

These recommendations are commendable because they make it less likely to omit an important finding and they can be quicker for the clinician to digest, but they have 2 potential difficulties. The first is that they can potentially circumvent a thorough thought process, such as the above series of questions. For example, one may be tempted to "get going" on a checklist for a neoplastic process without properly excluding an inflammatory process. Second, the pathologist may be able to make important points that are not included in a checklist. Indeed, the role of a pathologist is 2-fold: to observe and describe the findings in a particular specimen, and to synthesize all available information that might be relevant to the case. Examples of this second role include any information that is not morphologic, such as information from molecular pathology, discussing possible syndromes, possible characteristics of a tumor that might affect therapy or prognosis, characteristics of a particular case that are unique to that patient, and the integration of information from the patient's medical record or from the clinical laboratory. This important second function as a synthesizer of relevant information cannot be fulfilled through a checklist.

One approach is to use checklists to ensure that all critical observations are included, but to supplement the report with a comment or description that discusses unique aspects of the case or provides additional information. **The important points are that, first, the report must include certain observations, and checklists can help ensure this, but second, some degree of narration and synthesis is often beneficial.**

Immunohistochemistry

The third level of study, used in only a minority of cases, is immunohistochemistry. Numerous immunohistochemical stains will be described throughout this text, and there are a number of books on the field [Buchwalow ISBN978-3642046087, Dabbs ISBN978-0443066528, Taylor ISBN978-0721601823], but here we will review the basic principles. Immunohistochemistry is based on the identification of specific proteins by labeled antibodies and was understood before the development of monoclonal antibodies. Indeed pneumococcal antigens were identified in cells by using an antibody attached to a fluorescent molecule as early as 1942 [Coons 1942]. However, the modern era of routine immunohistochemistry emerged from the development of monoclonal antibodies [PMID1172191]. Rarely, traditional polyclonal antibodies will be used in diagnosis, but monoclonal antibodies are by far the rule. Immunohistochemistry is now used in all types of tissues from all body sites.

Most Antigens That React with Monoclonal Antibodies Have CD Designations

In immunohistochemical nomenclature, the term "CD," for "cluster of differentiation" or "cluster designation," is often used. Soon after monoclonal antibodies were employed, it was recognized that there were groups of antibodies that were made in different laboratories and that reacted with the same antigen. It was difficult to know precisely which antibodies reacted to which antigens, and to which epitopes (the actual portion of the antigen that is recognized by a single antibody) on which antigens. To analyze large amounts of data emerging from the then-recent technology, the CD nomenclature was developed at the First International Workshop and Conference on Human Leukocyte Differentiation Antigens (HLDA) in Paris in 1982. It was decided that antigens that were well characterized and that reacted to a group of antibodies were to be considered members of the same CD. Typically, antigens of the same CD had slightly different epitopes that slightly different monoclonal antibodies reacted to.

For an antigen to receive a CD number, it must be well characterized and there must be at least 2 monoclonal antibodies that will bind to it. If an antigen is reasonably well characterized but falls short of the criteria for a CD designation (eg, only 1 monoclonal antibody is known to bind to it), it may be denoted with a "w," as in "CDw198." Tables of CD numbers are updated constantly on a variety of web sites.

The term "CD" more properly refers to an antigen that binds to 1 or more related antibodies (as in, "The cells of this tumor express CD X"), but in common usage, it may also refer to the antibody (as in, "The cells of this tumor bind CD X"). If CD terminology is not employed, the entity cited may refer to either the antigen or to the antibody, but in most cases, it refers to the antigen. For example, p53 is an antigen, not an antibody. When we say a tumor is positive for p53, we mean that it will bind to a monoclonal antibody specific for that antigen. The antibody 1801 is an antibody that stains the p53 protein. Some tumors stain *for* p53 *with* 1801. No one says a tumor is "positive for 1801." On the other hand, many melanocytic lesions are said to express HMB-45, but there is no antigen of that name. If we say that a tumor is positive for HMB-45, we are actually saying that it has a protein called gp100 that binds to a monoclonal antibody called HMB-45. While many will say that a neoplasm stains *for* HMB-45, it is more properly said to stain *with* HMB-45. Fortunately, terminology is rarely a problem in practice.

While the nature of most antigens used in immunohistochemistry is reasonably well understood, there are a few antigens whose nature has not been well elucidated. For example, Ki-67 is a protein that is associated with and apparently essential for mitosis. Although its precise function is unclear, it is a reliable marker for cells that are committed to mitosis, even if a mitotic apparatus is not morphologically apparent [PMID10653597].

Formalin fixation, and the protein crosslinking that results from it, may render some antigens unrecognizable to antibodies, compromising immunohistochemical evaluation [PMID19886755]. The first step in immunohistochemistry of formalin fixed, paraffin-embedded tissue is often a pretreatment that renders the antigens more accessible. Pretreatment antigen retrieval techniques (usually heat, sometimes enzymatic) can break crosslinks and expose sites that were previously inaccessible to antibodies.

There Are a Number of Detection Methods in Immunohistochemistry

Unlike hematoxylin and eosin, and the cytochemical stains, immunohistochemical stains are not based on making certain parts of a cell or certain types of tissue appear as a particular color. Rather, they are antigen-antibody reactions that are based on the presence of a *specific amino acid sequence*. The method of detection in immunohistochemistry is either fluorescent or chromogenic. In fluorescent detection, the antibody is attached to a fluorescent compound (ie, one that absorbs light and then emits it at a longer wavelength), and its binding is detected by fluorescence microscopy. In chromogenic detection, developed independently by 2 groups in 1966 [PMID4958634, PMID17121392], the antibody is attached to an enzyme, usually peroxidase or alkaline phosphatase. If the target antigen is present, after the antigen-antibody reaction, the antibody and enzyme will be bound, and the reaction catalyzed by the enzyme leads to a brown or red color, depending on the details of the enzyme system, in the tissue.

Either fluorescent or chromogenic detection can be primary or indirect (secondary). In the primary detection method, the primary antibody is be directly labeled with the fluorochrome or enzyme. In indirect detection, a second antibody that is reactive to the first antibody is employed, and the detection fluorochrome or enzyme is attached to this second antibody. Because multiple secondary antibody molecules can bind to 1 primary antibody molecule, amplification of the signal can be achieved in an indirect system.

Another indirect detection system, introduced in 1981 [PMID6167159, PMID6166661], is based on secondary antibodies that are attached to biotin. Avidin, a compound that binds biotin tightly, is conjugated to peroxidase and allowed to react to the biotin on the second antibody. If the target antigen is present, the first antibody will bind, then the secondary antibodies, attached to biotin, will bind to the first antibody, and finally, the avidin-enzyme complex will bind to the biotin. This is called the avidin-biotin complex (ABC) method and permits appreciable amplification. Streptavidin has largely replaced avidin, because the latter molecule occasionally binds nonspecifically, and the use of streptavidin results in a lower background.

There are newer methods showing great promise for increasing both sensitivity and specificity of detection. For example, in chain polymer-conjugated technology, the secondary antibody is attached to a dextran chain to which are affixed many peroxidase molecules, allowing significant amplification.

In all of these systems, depending on what chromogen the peroxidase or alkaline phosphatase enzyme is allowed to react with after all antibody reactions are completed, the color is usually brown or red. If diaminobenzidine (DAB) is used as the chromogen, a brown color results. If aminoethylcarbazole (AEC) is used, a red color results. Because the color depends on the detection method and not on the target antigen, all immunohistochemical stains that employ the same technique and chromogen will be the same color, and it is therefore essential to properly label the slides for the antigen under study. If a histotechnologist mislabels an H&E or a trichrome as a PAS stain, it is easy for the pathologist to recognize the error because the colors seen will not be expected for the indicated stain. But if a keratin immunohistochemical stain is mislabeled as an S100 protein, the error may not be detected because the pathologist will see tumor cells with brown cytoplasm in either case.

With 2-color immunohistochemical staining, it is possible to stain the same section for 2 antigens, with a different color for each antigen. 2-color immunohistochemical staining can be performed sequentially or simultaneously. In sequential staining, the primary antibody for 1 of the 2 target antigens is applied and the process is carried to completion, after which the process is repeated with the application of the second primary antibody and a chromogen of a different color. In 1 form of simultaneous 2-color immunohistochemistry, both primary antibodies are added at the same time, but the secondary antibodies are conjugated to enzymes whose chromogens produce different colors. 2-color methods are excellent when one wishes to identify 1 antigen associated with 1 type of tissue and a second antigen associated with another type. For example, in prostate biopsies, the basal layer that is characteristic of benign glands can be stained 1 color and an enzyme that is characteristic of dysplasia and carcinoma can be stained with another color.

Immunohistochemical Stains Must Be Interpreted with Caution

Any use of immunohistochemistry requires an understanding of several concepts. The problematic areas in immunohistochemistry have been reviewed [PMID16998317], but in my experience, 6 potential pitfalls are commonly encountered in immunohistochemistry.

1. Both positive and negative controls must be run. The positive control is run on commercially obtained tissue, known to contain the antigen of interest, in exactly the way as the patient's sample. Its purpose is to ensure that the target antigen, if present, will stain and that a negative result is valid. The negative control is of equal importance. The negative control is run on the patient's tissue, but omits the second antibody. Its purpose is to ensure that any staining has resulted from the presence of the target antigen, and not from nonspecific staining. Immunohistochemical stains often have focal, weak nonspecific staining that can be misinterpreted as a true positive if comparison is not made to the negative control. The positive control verifies negative results and the negative control verifies positive results.

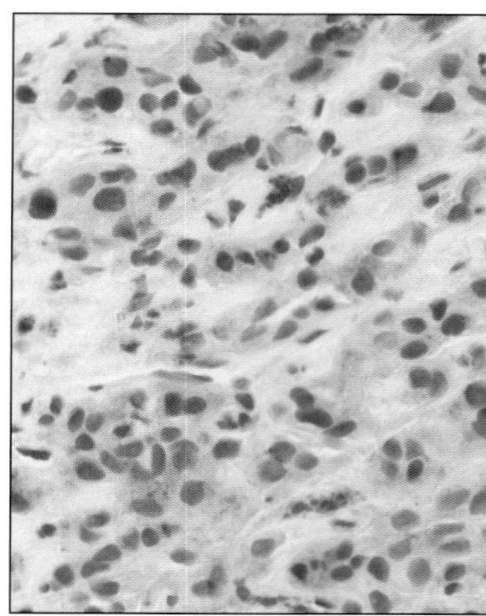

f1.1 A negative immunohistochemical stain for estrogen receptor in a breast carcinoma. Artifactual staining in the cytoplasm might cause this stain to appear positive were it not understood that ER is a nuclear stain.

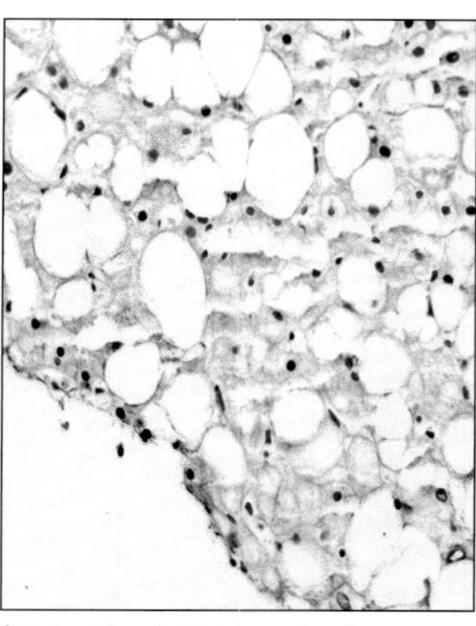

f1.2 A cytokeratin 20 stain employed on a metastatic carcinoma in the liver. The benign hepatocytes on the edge might appear positive, but hepatocytes are negative for cytokeratin 20.

2. If the target cells stain negatively for all antigens, some positive staining within the tissue must be shown to verify that there has been sufficient fixation and acceptable processing to allow immunohistochemical staining to take place in the tissue. Vimentin staining of the connective tissue or CD31 staining of the endothelial cells are often employed in this capacity. All neoplasms have some connective tissue and blood vessels, and if the tumor cells are negative for all antigens, positivity for either vimentin or CD31 ensures immunogenicity.
3. The expected location of a positive reaction in the cell should be known. The early immunohistochemical stains were almost all cytoplasmic. This has led to 2 potential errors: that the cytoplasm is the only place one need look for positivity, and that any staining of the cytoplasm is a positive stain. In addition to cytoplasmic staining, nuclear staining and cell membrane staining are common patterns. If the target antigen is normally found in either of these 2 locations, cytoplasmic staining should be considered negative f1.1. Staining in the wrong intracellular location, even if intense, should be considered negative, and the positive control must be carefully reviewed to ensure that the staining is in the correct location. In rare cases, a fourth pattern of staining, perinuclear, is encountered. In some of these unusual cases, this perinuclear staining is a well-demarcated dot immediately adjacent to the nucleus, in which case it can be reasonably well identified, but in other cases, perinuclear staining is in the form of a thin rim of staining around the nucleus, in which case its differentiation from general cytoplasmic staining can be difficult.
4. Care should be taken in interpretation of tissue near the edges of a section, as there is often artifactual positivity in this location f1.2.
5. Necrosis often causes artifactual positivity f1.3, and stains should be interpreted only in well-preserved areas.
6. Uniformity of interpretation is difficult with immunohistochemical stains. What appears clearly positive to one observer might be borderline to another. What appears

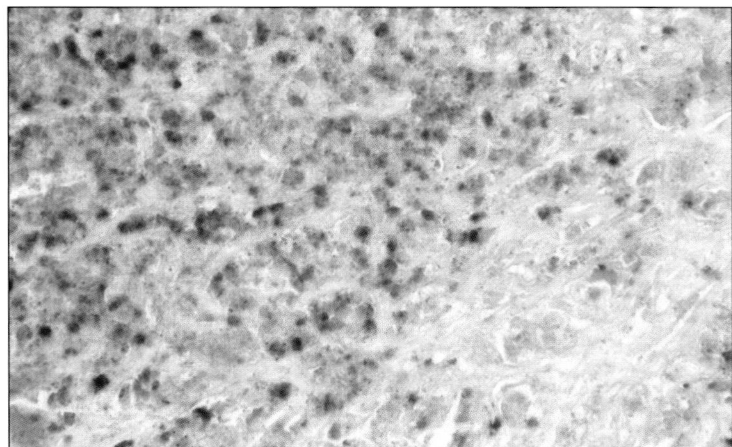

f1.3 An immunohistochemical stain for estrogen receptor that shows artifactual positivity because of necrosis. The tumor was actually ER negative.

to be of borderline significance to one observer might be of no significance to a second observer and of definite significance to a third. Immunohistochemical stains are not usually approached in a quantitative manner, except when digital imaging technology is used [PMID21370029], but there are 2 manual scoring systems that attempt to address interobserver variation: the H-score and the Allred score. The H-score is obtained by counting multiple fields and determining whether the cells stain negatively (0), weakly (1+), moderately (2+), or strongly (3+). The percentage of cells at each staining intensity is determined and the H-score is obtained by the following formula [PMID9059351]:

$$\text{H-score} = (\text{\% cells at 1+ intensity}) + 2\times(\text{\% cells at 2+ intensity}) + 3\times(\text{\% cells at 3+ intensity})$$

The Allred score is also a composite that takes into account both the percentage of cells that stain and the degree to which they stain. In the Allred system, the number of cells that stain is classified from 0 to 5. The intensity of the staining is rated from 1 to 3. These 2 numbers are then added [PMID18631198]. For example, if 10% of cells stain, the first number would be 1. If that staining is minimal, the second number would be 1, for an Allred score of 2. On the other hand, if 90% of cells stained, the first number would be 5, and if most of those cells stained strongly, the second number would be 3, for an Allred score of 8.

The sixth potential difficulty with immunohistochemical stains is that there is a tendency to jump to a conclusion based only on immunohistochemical results, without realizing that few stains are truly specific for one tissue type. For example, some muscle tumors will stain with keratin, normally an epithelial marker, and if an observer is not careful and aware, a spindle cell tumor with keratin staining may be called a carcinoma when it is in fact a myosarcoma. For this reason, immunohistochemical stains should almost always be employed in panels or groups. Reliance on a single stain is likely to be more harmful than helpful. In this example, the inclusion of vimentin, a marker for nonepithelial mesenchymal processes, and actin, a muscle marker, would have prevented a misdiagnosis of carcinoma. There is never any one stain that identifies a process as malignant (ie, there is no "cancer antigen").

While immunohistochemistry is no longer considered experimental, its findings must be considered along with the H&E morphology and the report should indicate that this

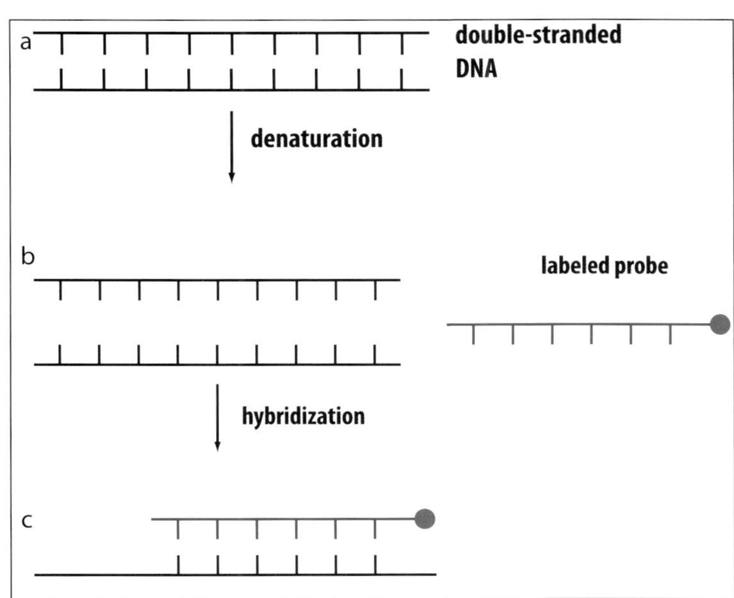

f1.4 The principle of hybridization and gene probes. In **a**, there is double-stranded DNA that contains the sequence of interest. In **b**, after denaturation, a portion of nucleic acid with a reporter molecule, called a probe, is added, after which the DNA is returned to conditions that favor hybridization. In **c**, if the target sequence is present, the probe will bind to it and this binding will be detectable by the reporter molecule, usually by fluorescence.

has been done, with a phrase to the effect of "putting the immunohistochemical results in conjunction with the H&E appearance."

Even with testing beginning to shift to the DNA level, immunohistochemistry remains a huge and growing field, with many variables, new technologies, and exciting possibilities.

Molecular Studies

Examination at the molecular level and information derived from cytogenetic studies are the fourth level of investigation of a specimen. This huge field is the future of pathology and receives its own series of chapters (44-47), but 2 molecular techniques—FISH and PCR—are referred to throughout this work and are briefly discussed here, to be followed by more detailed discussions in Chapter 45.

In Situ Hybridization

Hybridization—the binding of a probe to a target—can occur in solution, or on a number of commercially available substrates. Here, we consider ISH, in which hybridization of a sequence of nucleic acid (bound to a reporter probe to a target sequence) occurs in the cell of interest **f1.4**. The advantage of ISH is that the results can be correlated with morphology because the precise location of the target nucleic acid within a cell can be determined. In the case of some viruses, it is possible to determine if the viral nucleic acid has integrated in to the host DNA or not.

ISH often uses a fluorescent-labeled probe that binds to a target. This is FISH. FISH grew out of the use of fluorescent compounds that adhere to individual proteins to identify both the intracellular location of the protein and follow its movement in the cell. After this technology, involving only proteins, was mastered, fluorescent probes that bound to nucleic acids were developed. In FISH, the probe is a specifically designed

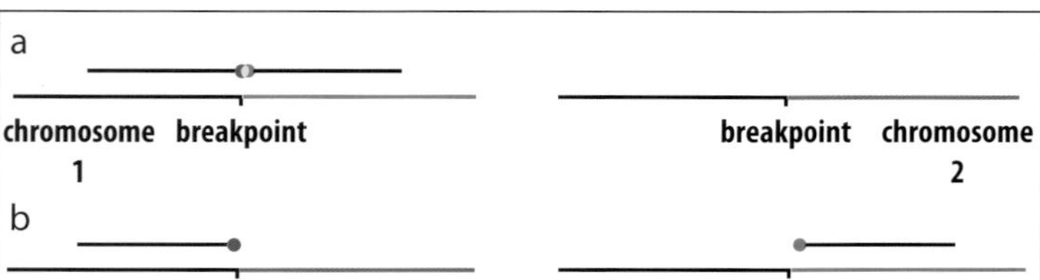

f1.5 Break apart FISH strategy. **a** depicts 2 normal chromosomes. In chromosome 1 the DNA to the left of the breakpoint is black, while the DNA to the right of the breakpoint is red. In chromosome 2, the DNA to the left of the breakpoint is black while the DNA to the right of the breakpoint is green. Sequences of DNA that are complementary to the sequences immediately on either side of the breakpoint, labeled with fluorescence probes of different colors, come to rest immediately on either side of the breakpoint. If there is no translocation, the 2 colors are too close together to resolve and appear as a single color (yellow). In **b**, there has been a reciprocal translocation. Both chromosomes have broken and the green portion of chromosome 2 and the red portion of chromosome 1 have changed places. In this case, the 2 probes bind to complementary sequences that are now on different chromosomes. Their separate colors, green and red, are readily apparent.

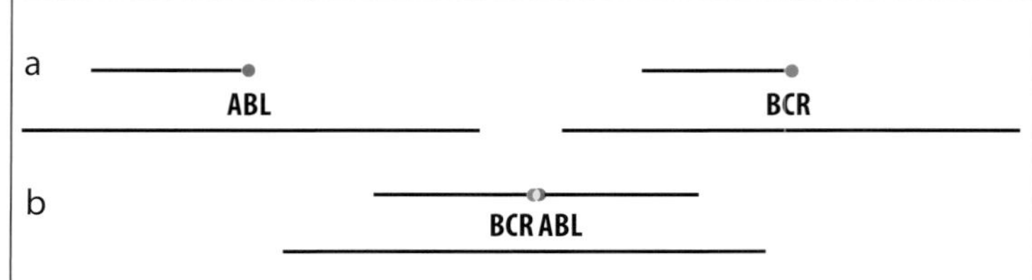

f1.7 Dual-fusion FISH strategy.
a a probe with a red fluorochrome is specific to the ABL locus on chromosome 9 and a probe with a green fluorochrome is specific to the BCR locus on chromosome 22. In the normal state, where there has not been a translocation, the colors are widely separated.
b If there has been a translocation, the 2 colors are brought together and are either seen as immediately juxtaposed or as a merged single color (yellow).

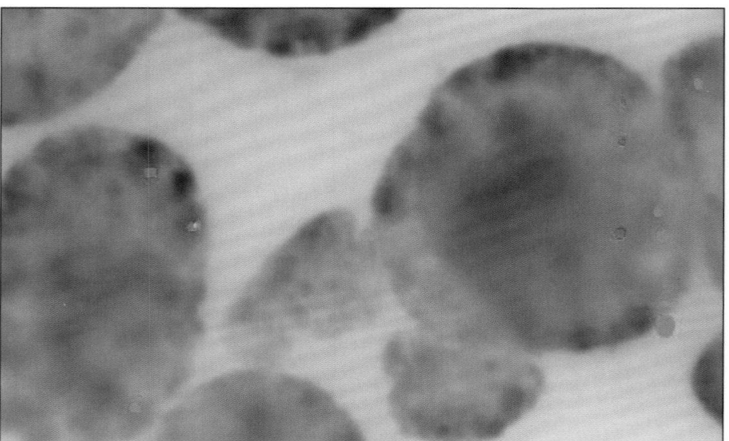

f1.6 Break apart FISH. Note the separation between the red and green signals.

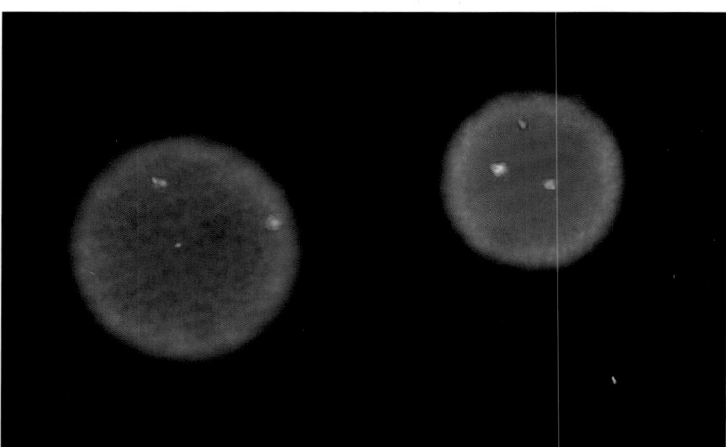

f1.8 Dual-fusion FISH study confirming the t(9;22) in a case of CML. In the normal case, the red and green signals remain separate, but in a translocation, they are fused, as is seen by the yellow signal.

sequence of nucleic acid—usually DNA—that is labeled with a fluorescent compound and the target is DNA or RNA from the patient to be tested. After exposure of the patient sample to the probe and a washing step, the presence of the fluorochrome in the sample indicates that the target sequence is present **f1.4**. Because fluorescence microscopy is required, the target may have a weak fluorescent counterstain to permit it to be seen. In using FISH to search for translocations, a common procedure is to employ DNA probes that are specific for the portions of DNA that are on either side of the possible translocation, not for the abnormal DNA itself. In one form of testing, a different color conjugate is used for each side. In normal situations, where there is no translocation, the 2 colors are so close together that they merge into a single, intermediate color. In situations where the translocation has occurred, the 2 colors are separated and will appear as 2 distinct colors (this is called break apart FISH) **f1.5**, **f1.6**. The process can also be reversed, so that in the normal situation, the probes are hybridized to areas that should be far apart, with 2 distinct colors. If there has been a translocation, it will bring the 2 colors together and merge them into a new color (this is called double fusion strategy) **f1.7**, **f1.8**. We will consider FISH much more extensively in Chapter 45.

Polymerase Chain Reaction

Few advances have fundamentally changed DNA technology as profoundly and quickly as PCR [PMID3472723]. PCR begins with the use of an elevated temperature—about 94°C—to separate the 2 strands, a process called melting. In the presence of new bases and appropriate conditions of ionic strength, primers that bind to the regions of the DNA adjacent to the area to be amplified are then added. The temperature is then lowered to permit the primers to anneal to the single-stranded DNA molecules (the exact temperature employed during this step will influence the specificity of primer binding), and DNA polymerase is added. The primers then hybridize at both ends of the target sequence. The DNA polymerase then creates a short complementary strand whose length is determined by the distance between the primers. The temperature is then elevated to denature the new DNA molecules, and the process is repeated, using both the old and the new DNA molecules as templates. At the beginning

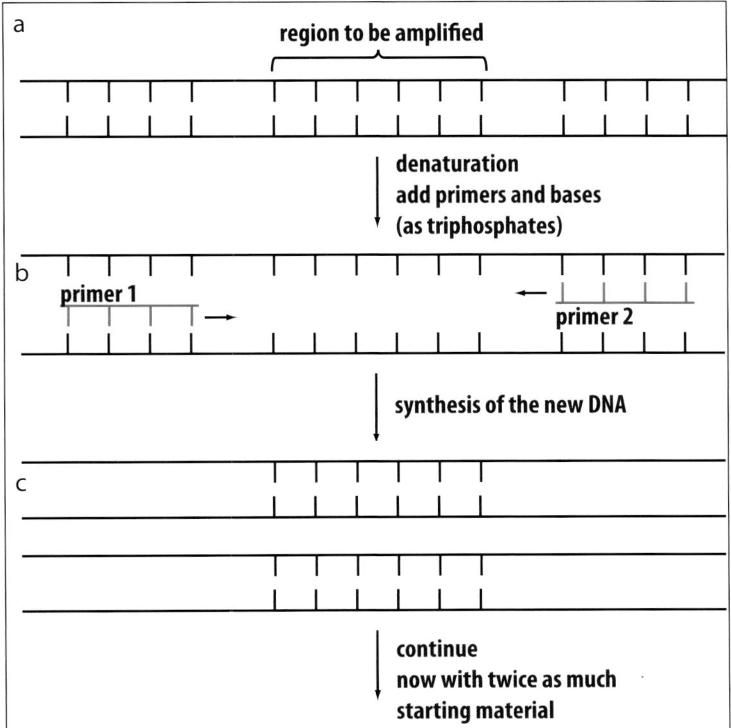

f1.9 Polymerase chain reaction. **a** depicts the native double stranded DNA with the region of interest that is to be amplified. In **b**, after denaturation and the addition of primers and bases, the primers bind to the portions of the DNA that are adjacent to the region to be amplified. In **c**, after the process goes to completion, there are 2 copies of the region of interest, 1 derived from each of the original strands. Not indicated in this figure is the need for thermocycling. The DNA must be heated to achieve denaturation, but then cooled to permit binding of the primer and the synthesis of new DNA strands.

of this second cycle, there are twice as many copies of the desired DNA sequence compared to the starting material **f1.9**. These continual cycles of raising the temperature to denature, lowering it to permit primer annealing, allowing synthesis of complementary strands between the primers, and raising it again doubles the amount of the desired DNA sequence with each cycle. There are many forms of PCR, and this technique will be much more extensively discussed in Chapter 45.

Core Points for Techniques and Methods

- Sequential approach to the examination of a specimen—gross, microscopic, immunohistochemical, molecular.
- Formalin fixation: after interaction with water, methylene glycol is the actual fixative.
- Hematoxylin & eosin stain nucleus and cytoplasm, respectively.
  - o Supplement with cytochemical stains that highlight particular types of tissue.
- Spherical aberration: light rays from the periphery of the lens are refracted more than those from the center.
- Chromatic aberration: the lens focuses light of different wavelengths to slightly different points.
- Microscopic appearance of tissues is largely an artifact, but the artifacts are reproducible and the general morphologic characteristics of malignant cells are well understood.
- Immunohistochemistry: based on the presence of specific antigens.
  - o Numerous detection systems, involving amplification of the original signal.
  - o Results are difficult to quantify, but several systems have been described.
  - o Pitfalls: staining in the wrong location, edge artifact, and staining in necrotic tissue.
- In situ hybridization: allows the identification of specific mutations, often in paraffin-fixed tissue.
  - o But is limited to those mutations that have been characterized.
  - o Reporter molecule is usually fluorescent (FISH).
  - o Many uses, variations, and elaborations on FISH.
  - o Used for translocations, deletions, and inversions.
  - o Has been expanded into comparative genomic hybridization, multicolor FISH/spectral karyotyping, and microarrays.
- PCR: First and most common nucleic acid amplification method.
  - o Many forms, most important of which are reverse transcriptase, quantitative, and allele-specific.

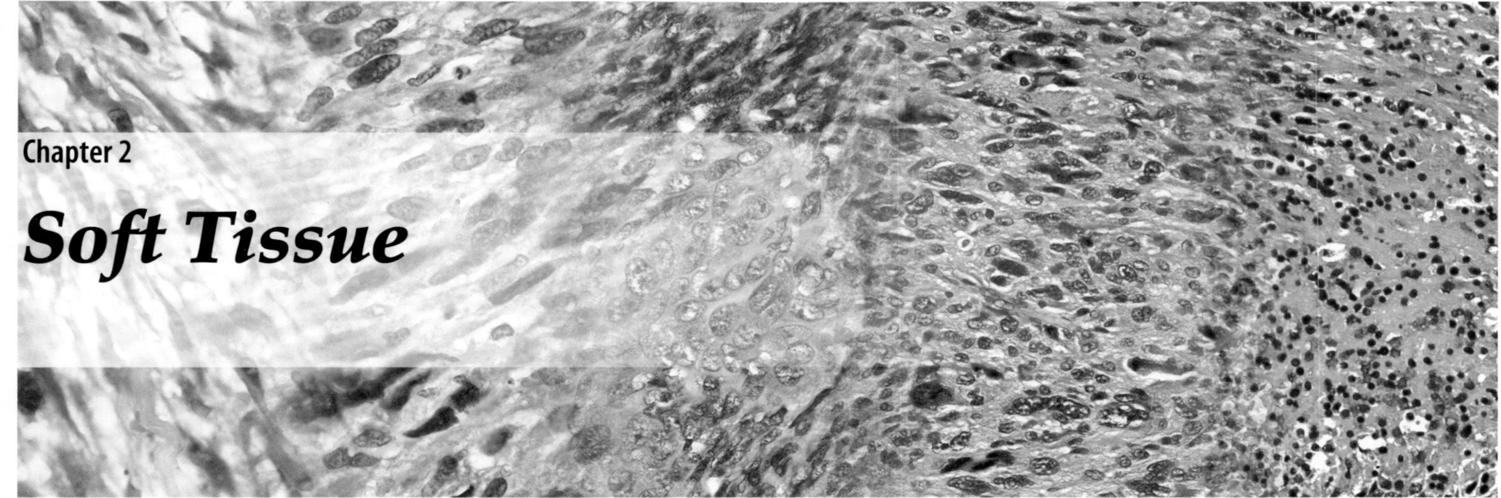

Chapter 2 Soft Tissue

The current World Health Organization classification of soft tissue neoplasms [Fletcher ISBN978-9283224136], as well as the time-honored text originally written by Dr Enzinger [Weiss ISBN978-0323046282], provides more detailed discussions of soft tissue processes. Here, we will consider the most common entities and general principles.

Soft Tissue Masses May Be Composed of Many Types of Tissues, and Each Type Has Benign Mimics

Because of the many nonneoplastic, reactive conditions in soft tissue, and the many benign neoplasms, the initial approach to soft tissue masses must be stepwise and must include from the beginning the possibility of a reactive condition or benign neoplasm. In soft tissue lesions more than in any other type, the series of questions outlined in Chapter 1 must be employed. Is the process neoplastic? Many nonneoplastic conditions may simulate a sarcoma nearly to perfection, and mistakes are made in the evaluation of soft tissue lesions by assuming that they are neoplasms when they are not.

If the process is neoplastic, is it benign or malignant? Once the diagnosis of malignancy is secure, and a sarcoma is suspected, the next question is, "Does the process take place in an organ, such as breast, uterus, lung, etc, rather than in soft tissue?" Apparent sarcomas occurring in organs rather than in soft tissue are probably spindle cell carcinomas with sarcomatous metaplasia. These may have a paucity of epithelial elements and initially appear to be a pure sarcoma, but the golden rule of sarcomas in organs is that an apparent sarcoma in an organ is much more likely to be a sarcomatoid carcinoma than a true sarcoma. An assiduous search for epithelial differentiation by immunohistochemistry will usually (but not always) reveal the fundamental epithelial nature of the process.

Once the diagnosis of sarcoma is secure, it is usually helpful to employ a location description such as "superficial," "deep," or "intramuscular." Several systems of grading sarcomas have been proposed, all more or less based on a combination of differentiation, necrosis, and mitoses. It is important to note, however, that there are limitations in the grading of sarcomas that are not encountered in the grading of carcinomas. First, grading is not suitable on core biopsy material because of the great heterogeneity of sarcomas. Second, though most sarcomas in adults are amenable to grading, some are not. Third, sarcomas in children are more difficult to grade and pediatric myosarcomas are especially difficult to grade [PMID17090186].

The efficacy of neoadjuvant (ie, prior to resection) treatment effect in sarcomas is assessed somewhat differently from carcinomas. In the latter tumor type, the central responsibility is to search for necrosis, but in sarcomas, one should compare to the pretreatment biopsy and look for increased differentiation as much as for necrosis.

Many Soft Tissue Neoplasms Are Associated with Specific Cytogenetic Abnormalities

A final preliminary comment on soft tissue neoplasms, before we consider individual entities, is that approximately 20% of them have been associated with apparently specific cytogenetic alterations [PMID19787372]. Indeed, with the exception of hematopoietic proliferations, there is no other group of tumors for which so much progress has been made at the molecular level. The Chromosomes and Morphology (CHAMP) Collaborative Study Group correlates cytogenetic abnormalities with morphological changes and with specific types of tumors, and has had more success in soft tissue neoplasm than in other types of tumors [PMID11793371, PMID8579124, PMID9591630]. Good reviews of the cytogenetic findings in soft tissue tumors that are detectable by fluorescence in situ hybridization (FISH) are available [PMID19851129, PMID21128778].

Benign Sarcoma-Like Proliferations

The fascia, a layer of connective tissue between the subcutaneous tissue and the muscle, is the site of a number of reactive conditions that can simulate a sarcoma. Foremost among these is nodular fasciitis. Nodular fasciitis occurs in the subcutaneous tissue or fascia and often demonstrates zonation, with a hypocellular center, a myxoid middle zone, and a hypercellular periphery. There may be microcysts and rare giant cells. The characteristic cell is bipolar, and there are scattered stellate cells. Nuclei are large, often with prominent nucleoli i2.1, but they are uniform. If the observer subtracts the nucleolus in the mind's eye, much of the concern for malignancy is abated. The low-power appearance is reminiscent of tissue culture i2.2. Lymphocytes and macrophages are common, but neutrophils and plasma cells are rare. Large numbers of the latter cell types raise suspicion for an inflammatory malignant fibrous histiocytoma.

Variant forms of nodular fasciitis occur in many sites. Intradermal, cranial, and intravascular variants have the same appearance as nodular fasciitis. Fibro-osseous pseudotumor (reactive periostitis) is a variant that occurs mostly in the digits and that resembles osteosarcoma. Proliferative fasciitis is a variant that has large, ganglion-like cells but is otherwise similar to nodular fasciitis. In proliferative myositis, these ganglion-like cells separate muscle fibers into a "checkerboard" pattern.

Atypical decubital fibroplasia (also called ischemic fasciitis) usually occurs over bony prominences in debilitated patients but may also be seen adjacent to areas of prosthetic implants. Atypical decubital fibroplasia typically also has large ganglion-like cells i2.3 and can resemble sarcoma, but also often has areas of fibrosis, degeneration, and fibrin deposition i2.4, in which case it may resemble a degenerative schwannoma. In addition to the characteristic location over weight-bearing areas or areas that have been traumatized by surgery, atypical decubital fibroplasia is also typically found in the subcutaneous tissue, a more superficial location than most sarcomas. Areas of fibrin deposition and the appropriate location are particularly important clues.

Before diagnosing any of these reactive conditions, a myxoid neoplasm should be excluded. Nodular fasciitis-like lesions can also occur in the viscera, in which case they are probably better diagnosed as inflammatory myofibroblastic tumor (a true neoplasm formerly called inflammatory pseudotumor or plasma cell granuloma).

Like nodular fasciitis, myositis ossificans often demonstrates a zonation in which the central area resembles the cellular areas of nodular fasciitis, and calcification, often with bone formation, as seen in the periphery. The benign ossifying fibromyxoid tumor of soft tissue is often multilobated, with bland cells in a fibromyxoid matrix and calcium or bone at the periphery. It resembles a chondromyxoid fibroma of bone.

Eosinophilic fasciitis often presents as a mass and consists of subcutaneous fibrosis with eosinophils. It is commonly believed to be a form of morphea and may be called morphea profundus [PMID21151540]. Eosinophilia-myalgia syndrome is eosinophilic fasciitis in combination with pain and has been linked to tryptophan ingestion.

There are several unusual entities that are related to the reactive fasciitis group. The postoperative spindle cell nodule is usually in the vagina, urethra, or bladder, and is discussed in Chapter 36. The pleomorphic fibroma is a proliferation of atypical, but benign fibroblasts in the dermis. A collagenous fibroma (also called desmoplastic fibroma) is characterized by a paucicellular, densely collagenous stroma, and may be an old pleomorphic fibroma that has lost its characteristic atypical cells.

Before leaving the topic of fasciitis, special mention should be made of necrotizing fasciitis, an inflammatory condition that is unlikely to present as a mass. Necrotizing fasciitis is usually caused by Group A *Streptococcus*, but other bacteria have been implicated (mostly *Clostridium* species). There is little inflammation in necrotizing fasciitis, and the diagnosis is primarily clinical.

The aggressive angiomyxoma and the angiomyofibroblastoma are similar entities that differ from the simple myxoma in their greater cellularity and extensive vascularity. Both are primarily found in the deep tissues of the vulva in young women and are considered to be benign neoplasms, without metastatic potential, though the aggressive angiomyxoma has greater potential for local recurrence. The aggressive angiomyxoma and the angiomyofibroblastoma have overlapping histologic features and are characterized by delicate vessels in a myxoid stroma. Both of these neoplasms have moderate cellularity, with spindle or stellate cells that may stain for desmin or actin, reflecting myoepithelial properties.

Angiomyxomas are not well circumscribed and have occasional thick-walled vessels, with focal hyalinization of vessel walls. The angiomyofibroblastoma has a similar appearance, but lacks thick-walled or hyalinized vessels, and may have alternating areas of hypocellularity and hypercellularity. The hypercellular areas of the angiomyofibroblastoma may have minimal myxoid change, and may resemble a smooth muscle, a nerve sheath tumor, or a hemangiopericytoma. Immunohistochemical staining for HMGA2 favors an aggressive angiomyxoma over an angiomyofibroblastoma [PMID20551826], but these histologic and immunohistochemical differences notwithstanding, the distinction between these entities is made primarily on the basis of the greater circumscription of the angiomyofibroblastoma [PMID19430941].

The principal differential diagnosis for these entities is the family of benign myxoid neoplasms, primarily the myxoid neurofibroma and the myxoid leiomyoma. The latter is a particularly troublesome differential because of its positivity for muscle markers. It is wise to exclude an aggressive angiomyxoma/angiomyofibroblastoma before diagnosing any myxoid neoplasm in the genital area.

"Inflammatory myofibroblastic tumor" is a new term for inflammatory pseudotumor, reflecting the current opinion that it is a true neoplasm that is benign or a low-grade malignancy. The stroma may be hypercellular i2.5, myxoid, hypocellular and fibrous i2.6, or a combination of these. Some cases are quite vascular, simulating a vascular lesion. The myofibroblast is usually rare and difficult to identify amid all of the inflammatory and endothelial cells, but should be apparent as an oval to spindle cell with more vesicular chromatin (ie, the chromatin is primarily on the periphery of the nucleus, making the nuclear center clear) than the usual fibroblast i2.7. Actin stain may be needed to find these cells, but about 1/3 may also stain for keratin (but not for EMA). 50% are positive for ALK [PMID17938159].

The hypercellular cases of inflammatory myofibroblastic tumor may resemble a fibrohistiocytic proliferation. Plasma cells are commonly found in cases with a fibrous stroma but are less common in the myxoid variant. Some cases of plasma cell variant of inflammatory myofibroblastic tumor appear to be part of the IgG4 syndrome (discussed in Chapter 24) [PMID16426926], and for that reason, I recommend serum IgG4 levels, an immunohistochemical stain for IgG4 on the tissue, and the clinical exclusion of sclerosing conditions at other sites, especially the pancreas, before the diagnosis of a plasma-cell-rich variant of inflammatory myofibroblastic tumor is made.

The fibrous cases of inflammatory myofibroblastic tumor may resemble a fibromatosis but form a more discrete mass. It is wise to consider the inflammatory myofibroblastic tumor in any case of an apparently circumscribed fibromatosis.

ISBN 978-089189-5886

The inflammatory myofibroblastic tumor may also resemble nodular fasciitis, and the myofibroblast is similar to the bipolar or stellate cells in the nodular fasciitis family. The immunohistochemical profiles are also similar unless the inflammatory myofibroblastic tumor expresses ALK. Masses that resemble nodular fasciitis, but are in an odd location or in the viscera, may be inflammatory myofibroblastic tumors. The inflammatory myofibroblastic tumor has local recurrence potential, but no significant metastatic potential.

Fibromatosis is a locally recurring, but nonmetastasizing proliferation of fibroblasts or myofibroblasts, and can occur in a variety of sites. Fibromatoses have greater cellularity in their early period i2.8, with diminishing cellularity and more collagen with time i2.9. By the time of resection, there is often variable cellularity, with some areas having moderate fibroblastic cellularity, while other areas are more collagenous. At all stages in its evolution, fibromatosis has little pleomorphism i2.10, in contrast to the malignant fibrous histiocytoma, and minimal mitotic activity, in contrast to a fibrosarcoma.

Fibrosarcomas are rarely diagnosed in adults now that improved immunohistochemical and cytogenetic methods have placed most such neoplasms into another category [PMID20829680], but they are a consideration in fibromatoses that have nuclear atypia or are mitotically active. Well differentiated fibrosarcomas typically have greater cellularity and slightly greater nuclear atypia than fibromatosis, and are also distinguished from benign fibroblastic proliferations by mitotic activity i2.11. The distinction between a fibromatosis and a well differentiated fibrosarcoma is one of the situations in which mitotic activity is a major consideration (others include smooth muscle tumors, nerve sheath tumors, hemangiopericytomas, and granular cell tumors).

The topic of mitotic figures will arise many times, and there is considerable interobserver variation in the counting of mitoses [PMID10804295], so we will consider several concepts now. 3 comments can be made concerning the counting of mitotic figures in any situation. The first concerns what should and should not be counted as a mitotic figure. To be counted as a definitive mitotic figure, 5 criteria must be fulfilled [Baak ISBN978-0387114316, PMID1592381]. First, there must be a projection, or "pole." Second, this projection must be "hairy," or fuzzy. Third, the projection must emanate from a dense structure that is identifiable as chromatin. Fourth, there must be no nuclear membrane. Fifth, the cell must appear viable, so as not to mistake karyorrhexis for a mitotic figure.

The second comment concerns the variation that is occasionally seen from one microscope to another in the size of a high-power field. The usual diameter encompassed by a high-power field is approximately 0.5 mm, resulting in a surface area of approximately 0.2 mm^2, and this is the surface area that is assumed in this work whenever the phrase "high-power field" is used. The third comment concerns how to count mitotic figures in tumors for which the number varies significantly from one area to another within the tumor. In general, the area of greatest activity should be counted.

In fibromatosis, there is focal staining with smooth muscle actin (SMA), indicative of a myofibroblastic origin rather than a strict proliferation of fibroblasts. Fibromatosis may resemble a solitary fibrous tumor but will be negative for CD34, while solitary fibrous tumors are generally negative for actin and positive for CD34 [PMID1592381], bcl-2 [PMID9669348], and CD99 [PMID19929175].

Fibromatoses have abnormalities in the *APC* tumor suppressor pathway (tumor suppressor genes are discussed in Chapter 46). These abnormalities lead to nuclear accumulation of the β-catenin protein, so fibromatoses often demonstrate nuclear staining for β-catenin, which is useful in separating them from gastrointestinal stromal tumor and sclerosing mesenteritis, which are negative for β-catenin [PMID12360044]. The differentiation of mesenteric fibromatosis from sclerosing mesenteritis is particularly challenging. In addition to staining for β-catenin, it is helpful to remember that sclerosing mesenteritis is an inflammatory condition, often caused by abdominal trauma, that eventuates in fibrosis through the normal reparative process. There will usually be areas of fat necrosis or inflammation in addition to areas of fibrosis. By contrast, mesenteric fibromatosis is an idiopathic process characterized by generalized fibrosis without a history of trauma, or areas of inflammation or necrosis. In addition, sclerosing mesenteritis typically spares the wall of the bowel, whereas mesenteric fibromatosis does not.

There are 2 confusing and antiquated terms associated with the fibromatoses. "Desmoid" is an old term that was used for a fibromatosis that was not on the hands or the feet. This term is best avoided now, especially since it was equated with low-grade fibrosarcoma in the past. The term "aggressive fibromatosis" is rarely used now, since all fibromatoses are locally aggressive. Postoperative radiation may be clinically helpful in fibromatosis.

Tumors of Fat

Lipomas usually are usually at least partially encapsulated, though the capsule may not be evident if the entire tumor is not removed intact. Lipomas have lipid vacuoles of uniform size. There are numerous types of lipoma. It is rarely necessary to distinguish between them, but an acquaintance with the different types helps to prevent a misinterpretation as a sarcoma.

There are 2 types of spindle cell lipomas, those with a predominantly myxoid stroma i2.12 and those with a predominantly fibrous stroma i2.13, though many cases will have areas of both types of stroma. The amount of fat in either type of spindle cell lipoma is variable and may be surprisingly minimal, causing the tumor to simulate a neoplasm of another type. Adding to this potential diagnostic challenge is that spindle cell lipomas of either type may be punctuated by occasional atypical cells.

If there is little fat and a predominance of fibrous septae, the fibrous type of spindle cell lipoma may resemble an atypical lipoma/well differentiated liposarcoma. The combination of minimal fat and cellular atypia may cause the fibrous variant of a spindle cell lipoma to resemble an undifferentiated pleomorphic sarcoma (UPS; formerly called malignant fibrous histiocytoma, or MFH). The myxoid type of spindle cell lipoma may resemble a neurofibroma, a resemblance that is heightened by the frequent presence of mast cells, or a UPS/MFH of the myxoid type (myxofibrosarcoma). In difficult cases, the spindle cells in spindle cell lipomas usually stain for CD34 [PMID20559119].

The fibrous type of spindle cell lipoma is closely related to the sclerosing lipoma, and some use these terms synonymously, while others reserve the term "sclerosing lipoma" for those cases in which the mass is primarily composed of paucicellular, sclerotic collagen, with minimal adipose tissue. Another related entity is the so-called fibrolipoma. The fibrous type of spindle cell lipoma, the sclerosing lipoma, and the fibrolipoma all have a mixture of fat and fibrous tissue, and the distinction between them is subjective and largely academic as long as a sarcoma diagnosis is avoided.

The pleomorphic lipoma is small (usually not exceeding several centimeters), encapsulated, and occurs on the chest, upper back, shoulders, and head and neck. It has minimal vascularity, few lipoblasts, and a characteristic alarmingly atypical cell called a floret cell i2.14 that makes the lesion appear initially to be an unmistakable sarcoma. The major differential diagnoses are a liposarcoma and an UPS/MFH, but in addition to its encapsulation, the atypical cells in a pleomorphic lipoma are of a particular type. Floret cells are generally multinucleated, often with the nuclei located on the periphery of the cell. Although there may be a collagenous background, the fibrous septae that are characteristic of an atypical lipoma/well differentiated liposarcoma are absent, and the atypical cells tend to occur randomly in the fat. After one sees a few cases of pleomorphic lipoma, the diagnosis generally follows easily from the location, size, encapsulation, and characteristic nature of the atypical cells and their distribution in the stroma. The pleomorphic lipoma overlaps with a spindle cell lipoma [PMID17890910] and its floret cells may be positive for CD34.

2 unusual types of lipoma are the angiolipoma and the hibernoma. All fat is vascular, and there is subjectivity as to whether or not a lipoma is truly of the angiolipoma type. To my mind, the diagnosis of angiolipoma can be made when the capillaries of the tumor, if removed from the fat, would initiate a diagnosis of hemangioma. An apparent angiolipoma that is within muscle is better regarded as an intramuscular hemangioma, which often has adipose tissue. Because hibernomas are derived from brown fat (ie, with many mitochondria), they have granular cytoplasm.

Lipomas in young children are likely to be lipoblastomas. Some lipoblastomas have an immature appearance, with a very myxoid stroma, while others are more differentiated and resemble lipomas. Many lipoblastomas have both patterns i2.15. If an apparent lipoma in a child has myxoid areas, it may be a differentiated lipoblastoma, especially if it has a micronodular architecture, though this distinction is academic. Much more important is that if a tumor in a young child resembles a myxoid liposarcoma, it is likely to be an immature lipoblastoma.

The term "atypical lipoma" has largely replaced the term "well differentiated liposarcoma" because a pure well differentiated liposarcoma has minimal metastatic potential and poses only a risk of local recurrence. The term "well differentiated liposarcoma" remains in use, especially in the retroperitoneum, the inguinal area, and the paratesticular area.

The atypical lipoma/well differentiated liposarcoma has fibrous septae within the fat. Although there may be rare atypical cells in the lobule, in practice, the diagnosis is much easier to make by focusing on the fibrous septae. These septae are of increased cellularity and will contain scattered atypical cells that may or may not be recognizable as adipocytes i2.16. Additionally helpful features are that these tumors are not encapsulated and have fat vacuoles of varying size. The distinction from a lipoma is best noted in the lack of a capsule, the hypercellular septae, the atypical cells in the septae, the rare atypical adipocyte in the lobule, and the variation in the size of the cytoplasmic fat vacuoles. Of these, the atypical cells in the fibrous septae are the most useful differentiating feature.

There are several types of atypical lipoma/well differentiated liposarcoma, of which the sclerosing and inflammatory forms are most commonly encountered. The sclerosing atypical lipoma is a variant in which the fibrous septae occupy most of the tumor and fat is rare. One must note the small amount of fat that is present and the atypical cells that are in the fibrous tissue. The inflammatory type of atypical lipoma/well differentiated liposarcoma contains many lymphocytes and plasma cells. This can resemble an inflammatory myofibroblastic tumor but will have more fat and more atypical stromal cells than the latter entity. If the observer subtracts the lymphocytes and plasma cells in the mind's eye, he or she will see a routine atypical lipoma/well differentiated liposarcoma. Clusters of chronic inflammatory cells within apparently bland fibroadipose tissue suggest this type of atypical lipoma.

The myxoid liposarcoma is relatively hypocellular with uniform nuclei, in contrast to the myxoid UPS/MFH and has an arborizing vascular pattern colloquially referred to as "chicken feet" i2.17. A pure myxoid liposarcoma has a tendency for local recurrence, but minimal metastatic potential. However, the myxoid liposarcoma is often mixed with a higher-grade component that can metastasize. Because the nuclei of this higher-grade component are often rounded, these sarcomas have traditionally been called round cell liposarcoma i2.18, but in newer terminology, these lesions are called higher-grade myxoid liposarcomas or cellular myxoid liposarcomas because the higher-grade component may not have round nuclei.

The key feature in higher-grade myxoid liposarcomas is that there are areas of greater cellularity, and the cells have nuclei that are slightly enlarged but still relatively uniform and less cytoplasm that is more eosinophilic and granular. There is less extracellular material, the classic vascular pattern is not as prominent, and the mitotic rate is higher. Grade 2 myxoid liposarcomas have <25% hypercellular areas while grade 3 tumors have >25%. Examples of newer terminology that might be used in a report include the following:

- Grade 1 myxoid liposarcoma (pure classic myxoid liposarcoma with minimal metastatic potential)
- Grade 2 myxoid liposarcoma (<25% of the tumor is composed of areas of higher cellularity; some metastatic potential)
- Grade 3 myxoid liposarcoma (>25% of the tumor is of high cellularity; formerly called round cell liposarcoma; aggressive behavior expected)

Generally speaking, a dedifferentiated malignant neoplasm is a tumor that has a mixture of well to moderately differentiated, readily identifiable areas mixed with very poorly differentiated, difficult to recognize regions, whereas a poorly differentiated tumor consists entirely of high-grade areas with poorly differentiated features. A dedifferentiated liposarcoma has some areas that are readily identifiable as a well differentiated liposarcoma/atypical lipoma i2.19a and other areas which are more atypical and not readily recognizable as lipomatous i2.19b. Often, there is an abrupt transition between the 2 areas, though this feature is not required for the diagnosis.

Some consider dedifferentiated liposarcoma to be a type of pleomorphic liposarcoma, but most reserve the term "pleomorphic liposarcoma" for tumors in which the entire tumor is high grade, with little lipomatous differentiation anywhere. In this more common usage of the term, the pleomorphic liposarcoma consists entirely of high-grade areas and resembles a pleomorphic UPS/MFH throughout its extent. This type is diagnosed by finding the rare identifiable malignant lipoblast, which will have cytoplasmic vacuoles (usually multiple and small) i2.20.

Based on cytogenetic and immunohistochemical findings, well differentiated liposarcoma and dedifferentiated liposarcoma may be opposite ends of one form of lipomatous malignancy, while myxoid/round cell lipomas are of a different type [PMID22301498]. Ring or giant chromosomes involving chromosome 12 are seen in the well differentiated liposarcoma/atypical lipoma family, leading to amplification of the *MDM2* gene i2.21, i2.22, while myxoid and round cell liposarcomas often have a translocation involving che *CHOP* (also called *DDIT3*) gene on chromosome 12 i2.23. Although the translocation may rarely fuse *CHOP* with the *EWS* gene, more often the fusion partner is a related gene called *FUS* (or *TLS*) on chromosome 16p11 [PMID18517278] i2.24. It is not known if the different breakpoints have clinical significance.

Tumors of Muscle

The choice of muscle immunohistochemical markers depends on the target tissue. Nuclear staining with myogenin and myosin are good markers for skeletal muscle [PMID16861966]. Desmin is an intermediate filament largely restricted to muscle and will stain both skeletal and smooth muscle neoplasms [PMID15558188]. Actin is an excellent muscle marker, and there are isoforms that are relatively specific for smooth muscle or skeletal muscle [PMID3307744]. Smooth muscle actin (SMA) is sensitive and relatively specific for smooth muscle, though it also stains myofibroblastic lesions such as nodular fasciitis and fibromatosis, as well as some rhabdomyosarcomas. SMA is often the preferred marker for smooth muscle lesions and for myofibroblastic lesions.

Rhabdomyosarcomas (RMS) are divided into the embryonal, alveolar, and pleomorphic types. The cells in embryonal rhabdomyosarcoma have little cytoplasm, with no discernible cross striations, but enough cytoplasm and sufficient differentiation to have eccentric nuclei, and some cells may be spindled i2.25. There may be some myxoid change in the stroma. Botryoid RMS is a type of embryonal rhabdomyosarcoma that occurs near a lumen or space and has an appreciable myxoid stroma. Cellularity in a botryoid RMS is higher just under the epithelium (the cambium layer).

Although it is true that the alveolar type of rhabdomyosarcoma tends to have fibrous septae, with loosely cohesive clusters of cells, this type of RMS is not defined by the architecture, but rather by the morphology of individual tumor cells. In the alveolar type, the cells have almost no cytoplasm and essentially no differentiation i2.26. Indeed, there is a solid type of alveolar RMS that lacks septae. Alveolar RMS has a poorer prognosis than embryonal RMS and often has either t(1;13) or t(2;13) [PMID18973919]. Both of these involve the *FOX01* (*FHKR*) gene. The former translocation results in a *PAX2-FOX01* fusion gene and the latter in a *PAX7-FOX01* fusion gene i2.27, i2.28.

The pleomorphic type of rhabdomyosarcomas is rare and occurs mostly in adults. This type generally resembles the UPS/MFH, though there are occasional cases of discernible muscle differentiation i2.29.

The Intergroup Rhabdomyosarcoma Study has recommended that the traditional classification—embryonal, alveolar, and pleomorphic—be replaced by a 2-tiered system wherein favorable rhabdomyosarcomas are those of the embryonal type or which are well differentiated based on the combination of nuclear atypia, necrosis, and mitoses. The unfavorable group consists of those of the alveolar type or those that are poorly differentiated and resemble UPS/MFH [PMID8625211].

Leiomyomas may occur in any location because of the prevalence of smooth muscle in the walls of blood vessels, the lining of the gastrointestinal and respiratory tracts, etc. Leiomyosarcomas can be deceptively bland in many locations, and one should exclude a leiomyosarcoma before making a diagnosis of leiomyoma in soft tissue. Atypia is helpful in this distinction, but assessment of mitotic activity is essential. The number of mitotic figures permitted in a benign diagnosis of a smooth muscle neoplasm varies with the anatomic location. In the skin and subcutaneous tissue, deeper lesions are more likely to metastasize [PMID19694881].

A caveat in counting mitoses in smooth muscle neoplasms is to be sure that a soft tissue muscle tumor is not a proliferation of myofibroblasts, as the number of mitotic figures is less important in myofibroblastic tumors. Myofibroblasts often have shapes other than the fusiform shape characteristic of muscle cells (eg, stellate). Myofibroblasts also often have vesicular nuclei and less eosinophilic cytoplasm. Their actin positivity is usually peripheral and not diffuse, and they may stain for ALK, which is not expected in pure muscle tumors.

Vascular Tumors

Common endothelial markers are CD31 and CD34, which have largely replaced factor 8/von Willebrand factor (vWF). Of these 2, CD31 (platelet-endothelial cell adhesion molecule-1; PECAM-1) is more specific for endothelium, as CD34 also stains a number of other entities and is the most commonly used endothelial marker. FLI-1, a marker used for the Ewing/PNET family, also stains most benign and malignant vascular neoplasms, including Kaposi [PMID11474291]. FKBP12, a cytosolic protein that binds the immunosuppressant drug tacrolimus, is also a good vascular marker [PMID12502928]. D2-40 stains endothelium and appears to preferentially stain lymphatic endothelium [PMID12218087].

Vascular lesions may be reactive, developmental, benign neoplasms, or malignant neoplasms, and the terminology can be confusing, especially since some of it has recently changed, and slight differences in nomenclature indicate very different entities. To further confuse matters, many entities have more than 1 name.

Reactive Vascular Lesions

The pyogenic granuloma is now considered to be a lobular capillary hemangioma, meaning that it is a true neoplasm, but it is included here because it there remains considerable feeling that it is reactive and the acute inflammation is often more impressive than the vascularity.

A Masson hemangioma is an organizing thrombus with sufficient recanalization to simulate a hemangioma. It has well defined papillae, which are not generally seen in true hemangiomas, and can be seen to conform to the annular contour of the thrombosed vessel.

Bacillary angiomatosis is seen primarily in immunocompromised patients, especially those with HIV. It resembles a pyogenic granuloma or granulation tissue, with abundant numbers of vessels and neutrophils. There may be scattered eosinophils, but there is a clear predominance of neutrophils. It is often polypoid. Bacteria are demonstrable in bacillary angiomatosis with special stains such as a tissue gram stain or Warthin Starr, and can sometimes be seen on H&E. Bacillary angiomatosis is caused by several members of the *Bartonella* family, including *Bartonella henselae*, the cause of cat scratch disease in immunocompetent patients. *Verruca peruana* is a closely related entity with a very similar appearance, but is caused by a different member of the *Bartonella* family.

Developmental Vascular Lesions

A flame nevus is a developmental anomaly characterized by ectatic capillaries. The clinical terms "salmon patch" and "port-wine stain" both refer to types of flame nevus. The salmon patch usually involutes, while the port-wine stain tends to have deeper involvement of the dermis, does not involute, and may rarely be associated with systemic syndromes.

An arteriovenous malformation is another developmental vascular lesion that can be difficult to distinguish from a hemangioma. If such a distinction is clinically important, most immunohistochemical stains will not help, but hemangiomas stain for GLUT-1, whereas developmental lesions and vascular malformations generally do not [PMID10665907].

Benign Vascular Neoplasms

In addition to the common hemangioma, there are a number of unusual forms, 3 of which are described. A tufted hemangioma is simply a lobular hemangioma with dilated capillaries surrounding each lobule. A glomeruloid hemangioma has dilated capillaries, into which project additional vascular proliferations that impart the appearance of a renal glomerulus. Cellular hemangioma (also called strawberry nevus and formerly called juvenile hemangioma or juvenile hemangioendothelioma) occurs before the age of 1 and is benign, despite its cellularity and frequent mitotic figures.

There are 2 enigmatic processes that are vascular and have large numbers of eosinophils: angiolymphoid hyperplasia with eosinophilia (also called epithelioid hemangioma) and Kimura disease. These 2 entities were once thought to be synonymous, but are now understood to be distinct [PMID21382284]. Angiolymphoid hyperplasia with eosinophilia presents as cutaneous papules, primarily in the head and neck, usually without adenopathy or systemic symptoms. The characteristic histologic triad of vascular prominence, lymphocytes, and eosinophils is suggested by the name, and it also has plump endothelial cells with an epithelioid appearance. While commonly included among the benign vascular neoplasms, it is of unclear nature, and some feel that it may be a lymphoproliferative disorder [PMID20507406].

Kimura disease is an entity of unknown nature, primarily found in Asia. It occurs in lymph nodes and is characterized by great numbers of eosinophils, often forming microabscesses and infiltrating germinal centers. Because there is often increased vascularity, Kimura disease may resemble and is often confused with angiolymphoid hyperplasia with eosinophilia, but the former is nodal while the latter is cutaneous. Kimura disease is associated with generalized adenopathy, nephrotic syndrome, and/or peripheral eosinophilia [PMID21423602].

Low-Grade Malignant Vascular Neoplasms

Kaposi sarcoma is associated with human herpesvirus 8 (HHV-8). The histologic appearance of Kaposi sarcoma changes with time. In the macular stage, the histologic changes are subtle, and both the clinician and the pathologist may mistake the lesion as a dermatosis. There is a modest proliferation of thin walled, angulated capillaries i2.30, especially around adnexa. There may be hemosiderin. The patch stage is more diagnostic, with more obvious blood vessels that are angulated and dissect between collagen fibers. These vessels often proliferate around venules or some small vessels may protrude into the lumen of larger vessels (promontory sign). This stage may resemble a well differentiated angiosarcoma, as dissection of stroma is also a major finding in angiosarcoma. But even a well differentiated angiosarcoma will have at least focal atypia and more crowding of nuclei. In the tumor stage of Kaposi sarcoma, there are clusters of spindle cells that appear to "stream" together in an organized manner i2.31. The cells often contain eosinophilic hyaline globules. Lymphocytes and plasma cells are commonly seen. A clue to the diagnosis of well developed Kaposi sarcoma is a proliferation of bland spindle cells, resembling a fibrous tumor, with admixed blood or hemosiderin. Kaposi sarcoma may be negative for factor 8 but is usually positive for CD34, CD31, and FLI-1. The acid test is the demonstration of HHV-8. While usually regarded as a low-grade angiosarcoma, the malignant nature of Kaposi sarcoma is not universally accepted [PMID18976452].

The spindle cell hemangioma (formerly called spindle cell hemangioendothelioma) is a benign entity that is discussed here because it may resemble Kaposi sarcoma. Unlike Kaposi sarcoma, the spindle cell hemangioma has larger vessels, resembling a cavernous hemangioma, in addition to the spindle component. Also, even the Kaposi-like areas generally have a few round endothelial cells. The spindle cell hemangioma has vacuolated endothelial cells (which can resemble fat) that are not found in Kaposi sarcoma, and it also lacks the lymphoplasmacytic response and hyaline globules that are often seen in Kaposi.

The term "hemangioendothelioma" was introduced by Mallory in 1908 and refers either to vascular tumors that behave as a low-grade malignancy or have sufficient cellularity to suggest possible low-grade malignant behavior. The *retiform* hemangioendothelioma is a dermal or subcutaneous

ISBN 978-089189-5886

neoplasm whose vascular channels dissect collagen, resulting in a low-power appearance that resembles the rete testis. It has moderately atypical nuclei that are often apical. Metastases are very rare, but some regard this tumor as a low-grade angiosarcoma. The *epithelioid* hemangioendothelioma is sclerotic and can be mistaken for a sclerosing carcinoma, especially in the liver. Septated vacuoles, characteristic of endothelial cells, and nuclei that face each other, as if trying to form a vascular channel, are clues to the vascular nature of this entity. The epithelioid hemangioendothelioma is considered a low-grade malignancy and is discussed in more detail in Chapters 16 and 26, concerning the lung and liver, as these are common locations of this entity. The *infantile* hemangioendothelioma is a vascular neoplasm found in the liver of young children, and is also discussed in the Chapter 26 .

To my mind, we would be well served to remove the term "hemangioendothelioma" and simply classify vascular tumors as benign, malignant (well differentiated, moderately differentiated, or poorly differentiated), or of indeterminate or low-grade malignancy, with a comment on cellularity and terminology. This would not only remove the plethora of confusing terms such as "epithelioid hemangioendothelioma," "retiform hemangioendothelioma," "juvenile hemangioendothelioma," and "infantile hemangioendothelioma," it would also leave the clinician with a simpler, more understandable diagnosis and comment in vascular neoplasms.

Although most hemangiopericytomas will behave in a benign manner if completely excised, many feel that they are low-grade malignancies, so they are included in this section. Hemangiopericytomas have traditionally been regarded as tumors of pericytes, the cells that are adjacent to the endothelial cells, because it is easy to see the neoplastic cells surrounding endothelial cells. However, origin from the pericyte has never been proven and most now feel that they arise more from fibroblast-like cells [PMID16359532]. Hemangiopericytomas are cellular tumors that have dilated, thin-walled vessels. An important key feature is that the vessels are not only dilated, but they also branch **i2.32**. Close study of the vessels will show that they are lined by a single layer of endothelial cells, immediately adjacent to which is the proliferation of cells that are slightly plumper **i2.33**. Both the characteristic cell type—a small spindle cell—and the vascular pattern should be present throughout the tumor for the diagnosis of hemangiopericytoma to be considered. This tumor is closely related to and perhaps synonymous with the solitary fibrous tumor, which is discussed in Chapter 17.

Unfortunately, there is no immunohistochemical marker that is specific for the actual neoplastic cells of hemangiopericytoma—whatever their nature. CD34 stains hemangiopericytomas/solitary fibrous tumor, but in many cases, the staining is more prevalent in the endothelial cells and is lackluster in the actual tumor cells. CD31 does not stain the actual tumor cells, but can be helpful in highlighting the adjacent endothelial cells and confirming that the neoplastic cells are adjacent to, but distinct from the endothelial cell.

Hemangiopericytoma is one of the tumors for which mitotic activity is the major differentiating factor in assessing malignancy, but unfortunately, no clear number has been agreed on for the diagnosis of a malignant hemangiopericytoma. Opinions have ranged from 1 to 5 mitotic figures per 10 HPF. In problematic cases, it is reasonable to indicate an uncertain malignant potential.

Angiosarcomas

Well differentiated angiosarcomas can be subtle and diagnostically challenging. They have freely anastamosing and branching vessels with slight crowding of endothelial cells and mild nuclear atypia. The low-power clue is a slightly more complex architecture, with vessels that dissect the stroma and anastomose **i2.34**. This should elicit a search for the endothelial hyperplasia (often with microtufting), atypia, and occasional mitoses that secure the diagnosis **i2.35**. Angiosarcomas are poorly demarcated, and one should be wary of the diagnosis of angiosarcoma in any encapsulated or circumscribed lesion.

The epithelioid variant of angiosarcoma can be diagnostically challenging because the endothelial nature of the neoplastic cells is not readily apparent **i2.36**. Immunohistochemical stains will clarify the nature of the cells, but the pathologist must realize that these stains are needed, and he or she must further realize that vascular markers must be included in the panel. Moreover, the epithelioid variant of angiosarcoma may have keratin or EMA positivity in addition to positivity for vascular markers and vimentin [PMID21164288], and can therefore simulate both a carcinoma and a sarcoma of another type if the immunohistochemical panel does not include vascular markers. In the sclerosing variant, the vascular histogenesis of the neoplasm may again be difficult to appreciate, and septated vacuoles and nuclei facing each other are important clues. If the stroma is sclerotic, or if the lesion is in the liver, the lower grade epithelioid hemangioendothelioma should be excluded before diagnosing an epithelioid or sclerosing angiosarcoma.

Nerve Sheath Tumors

Both a schwannoma and a neurofibroma arise from the nerve sheath. Their distinction is usually not clinically important and they can generally be lumped together under benign peripheral nerve sheath tumor. What matters is that these be distinguished from malignant peripheral nerve sheath tumors (MPNSTs). Schwannomas are encapsulated, whereas neurofibromas are not. Schwannomas often have areas of alternating greater and lesser cellularity (Antoni A and B areas), with foci of fascicle formation. Fascicle formation may result in 2 fascicles that are juxtaposed and separated by a small amount of stroma (Verocay body) **i2.37**. They tend to have serpiginous nuclei **i2.38** and thick-walled vessels **i2.39**. Neurofibromas often have a myxoid background **i2.40** or thin collagen fibers that appear to have been dropped onto the field **i2.41**. They commonly contain scattered mast cells **i2.42**. Either a schwannoma or a neurofibroma may contain fat, but there is also a fibrolipomatous hamartoma of nerves that is not a nerve sheath neoplasm (a hamartoma is a nonneoplastic overgrowth of tissues that are normally found in a site).

There are 2 forms of schwannoma that particularly simulate an MPNST: the degenerative (ancient) schwannoma and the cellular schwannoma. Degenerative changes in a schwannoma include cystic formation, hyaline fibrosis, and occasional very atypical nuclei **i2.43**, which are a source of confusion. Like all schwannomas, and in contrast to an MPNST, degenerative schwannomas are encapsulated. A degenerative schwannoma should be excluded in any tumor with nuclear pleomorphism if it is encapsulated, or if the pleomorphism is only focal.

The cellular schwannoma is usually found near the vertebral column, mediastinum, or pelvis, or in the retroperitoneum, and this diagnosis deserves consideration for any unusual cellular spindle cell neoplasm in one of these locations. Like the degenerative schwannoma, the cellular schwannoma may have focal nuclear atypia, but unlike the former neoplasm, the cellular schwannoma may also have an appreciable numbers of mitoses. It is the only benign nerve sheath neoplasm that is routinely mitotically active. The observer is thus confronted with an alarming combination of cellularity, focal atypia, and mitotic activity. However, generalized nuclear atypia is not present, and some features of an ordinary schwannoma, such as Antoni A and B areas, thick-walled vessels, or Verocay bodies, are often recognizable somewhere i2.44.

Importantly, both a degenerated and a cellular schwannoma are encapsulated neoplasms. In addition to lack of encapsulation and more generalized atypia of the MPNST, appreciable necrosis suggests the possibility of a malignancy. Generalized atypia, necrosis, and poor circumscription without encapsulation are indicative of MPNST. Mitoses are helpful unless the differential diagnosis is between a cellular schwannoma and an MPNST.

In situations where it is clear that there is a sarcoma, nerve sheath origin can be suspected by looking for alternating hypocellular and hypercellular regions, serpiginous nuclei, nuclei that are bullet-shaped (though the identification of this feature requires a perfectly longitudinally sectioned nucleus), Verocay bodies i2.45, whorls, thick-walled vasculature i2.46, greater cellularity around vessels, or heterologous elements. A negative S100 stain is not helpful, as some MPNSTs do not stain for S100 [PMID10549251], but a positive stain suggests that a sarcoma is of nerve sheath origin. Equally important is negative staining for markers that suggest a different histogenesis, such as actin or CD117. Rarely, one will encounter a purely epithelioid variant of the MPNST that simulates a carcinoma, especially if there is keratin positivity, as is sometimes seen in MPNSTs [PMID10549251]. A history of neurofibromatosis type 1 (NF1) favors a nerve sheath origin for a sarcoma, as 1/2 of such tumors arise in patients with NF1 [PMID22084762].

Coming from the other direction, if it is clear that a tumor is of nerve sheath origin, and the question concerns its benign or malignant nature, the considerations are encapsulation, mitoses, atypia, and necrosis. Encapsulation virtually disqualifies a nerve sheath neoplasm from malignancy, but lack of encapsulation does not imply malignancy since common neurofibromas are not encapsulated, and even among benign encapsulated nerve sheath tumors, the sampling may not demonstrate the capsule. But even allowing for the possibility that a sampling may not demonstrate a capsule, and further allowing for the mitotic activity of a cellular schwannoma, the apparent absence of a capsule, in conjunction with 1 mitosis per 20 high-power fields, significant generalized atypia, and necrosis secures the diagnosis of malignancy in a nerve sheath neoplasm to the satisfaction of most observers.

Malignant peripheral nerve sheath tumors can resemble spindle cell melanomas both on H&E and on initial immunohistochemical stains (vimentin positive, S100 positive, HMB-45 negative). A more complete immunohistochemical panel, encompassing additional melanoma markers, such as Melan-A, are often needed. It is also helpful to look for epidermal involvement or areas of more classic melanoma in spindle cell melanoma.

The perineurioma is a distinctive nerve sheath tumor. If intraneural, it has a characteristic appearance of bland spindle cells surrounding individual axons, resulting in an onion-skin appearance. If extraneural, it is a whorled proliferation of bland spindle cells resembling a meningioma. Perineurioma are strongly positive for epithelial membrane antigen (EMA) and negative for S100. 92% stain with claudin-1 (the claudins are a family of proteins associated with tight junctions) [PMID12459629].

Unlike most neuromas, the palisaded encapsulated neuroma is a true neoplasm, not merely a disorganized mass of axons, but it is associated with Schwann cell hyperplasia and appears to be a combination of axonal hyperplasia with a benign nerve sheath neoplasm [PMID20237984]. A Bodian stain (for axons) or an immunohistochemical stain for neurofilament proteins (intermediate filaments found in neurons) may be needed to distinguish this entity from a routine nerve sheath neoplasm. A dermal location favors a palisaded encapsulated neuroma over a nerve sheath neoplasm, as the latter is generally found in the subcutaneous or deeper tissue. Indeed, a high percentage of cases of palisaded encapsulated neuroma are seen in skin biopsies.

Cartilaginous Tumors

Before approaching the true cartilaginous tumors, it is important to note that a variety of neoplasms that are not fundamentally cartilaginous may have cartilaginous elements. For example, a metaplastic carcinoma must be excluded before making the diagnosis of chondrosarcoma in an organ, and an MPNST with heterologous elements must be excluded before the diagnosis of chondrosarcoma is made in soft tissue.

The myxoid chondrosarcoma may be intraskeletal or extraskeletal, and has relatively uniform nuclei. The myxoid chondrosarcoma often has a multinodular architecture i2.47, with thin cords of cells radiating from the periphery of the lobule to the center, in a myxoid background i2.48.

The myxoid chondrosarcoma poses particular problems because many other mesenchymal tumors have a myxoid component or areas of chondroid metaplasia. Myxoid liposarcoma, myxoid nerve sheath tumors, and the myxoid type of spindle cell lipoma are only a partial list of the potential mimics. Generous sampling will usually uncover areas that are less confusing and reveal the fundamental nature of the tumor.

The myxoid variant of spindle cell lipoma tends to be in subcutaneous tissue, superficial to the usual location of a chondrosarcoma. Myxoid liposarcomas pose a particularly challenging differential in the diagnosis of myxoid chondrosarcoma. Cytogenetic findings may help. Myxoid liposarcomas often have a translocation involving the *CHOP* gene on chromosome 12, while myxoid chondrosarcomas tend to have t(9;22)(q22;q12), which results in the fusion of the

EWS gene on chromosome 22 with *NR4A3* (also called *TEC*, *CHN*, or *NOR1*) gene on chromosome 9 [PMID10359536] **i2.49**. Until cytogenetic differences become more firmly characterized, or in those many situations in which cytogenetic information cannot be fully obtained, location and H&E finding remain essential in the distinction. Myxoid liposarcomas tend to occur in the retroperitoneum, the inguinal area, and the leg, and have a characteristic arborizing network of capillaries.

Other types of chondrosarcoma occur primarily in bone and are therefore considered in Chapter 3.

Benign and Low-Grade Malignant Fibrous Histiocytomas

The fibrous histiocytoma family of tumors is discussed last among the common types of soft tissue tumors to emphasize that they are diagnoses of exclusion, not to be made until H&E and immunohistochemical stains have failed to identify a cell or origin for a mesenchymal tumor. The term "fibrous histiocytoma" is undoubtedly a misnomer, since origin from the histiocyte (macrophage) has never been shown.

Benign forms of fibrous histiocytoma tend to be superficial and cytologically bland. Caution is warranted in making the diagnosis of a benign fibrohistiocytoma when the mass is deeper than the subcutaneous tissue, because deep fibrohistiocytoma-like masses may behave in a malignant manner despite an innocuous histologic appearance.

The dermatofibroma, the dermatofibrosarcoma protuberans, and the atypical fibroxanthoma are usually considered to be benign or low-grade malignant dermal fibrohistiocytic lesions, but are encountered as cutaneous masses and are therefore discussed in Chapter 40.

Undifferentiated Pleomorphic Sarcoma (High-Grade Malignant Fibrous Histiocytoma) and Related Neoplasms

Undifferentiated pleomorphic sarcoma (UPS) is the currently preferred name for malignant fibrous histiocytomas (MFHs) [PMID16359532]. The latter term is inappropriate since, despite occasional focal staining for the macrophage marker CD68, origin from neither the histiocyte nor the fibroblast can be shown. In deference to both tradition and new information, this work will designate these sarcomas as UPS/MFH.

These tumors may be a final common dedifferentiated pathway of many types of mesenchymal neoplasms. Gene expression analysis, discussed in Chapter 45, has shown that whereas other types of sarcomas have a distinct profile of mRNA expression, the UPS/MFH does not, further suggesting that this is a heterogeneous group of sarcomas [PMID17464315]. Until the matter is eventually clarified, malignant mesenchymal proliferations that do not fit clearly into another category on H&E examination after extensive sampling, which stain for vimentin and for which there is no immunohistochemical or cytogenetic evidence of a specific tissue type, can be placed in the category of UPS/MFH. The immunohistochemical panel employed must be extensive, addressing all other types of sarcoma and including actin, S-100, and bcl-2, CD99, and CD34 (to exclude a malignant solitary fibrous tumor/ hemangiopericytoma). It is also desirable to include epithelial markers, as poorly differentiated carcinomas with sarcomatous metaplasia may appear to be sarcomas. Finally, before the diagnosis of UPS/MFH is made, the periphery of the tumor should be examined for a more differentiated morphology.

Of the numerous types of UPS/MFH, the storiform-pleomorphic type is the most common [PMID21424079]. The neoplastic cells may be spindled or histiocytoid, and there are usually pleomorphic giant cells that are also malignant **i2.50**. The pattern is usually focally storiform (intersecting fascicles, often in a cartwheel arrangement) **i2.51**. A pleomorphic liposarcoma should be excluded by looking for vacuolated cells before making a diagnosis of pleomorphic UPS/MFH.

The inflammatory UPS/MFH is highly aggressive and has a background of neutrophils, eosinophils, macrophages, lymphocytes, or plasma cells. It is no longer considered imperative that neutrophils be present for the diagnosis, but if these cells predominate, an aggressive clinical course is the rule. This type of UPS/MFH may not have many pleomorphic cells, and those that are present may not be of the same type as those seen in the storiform-pleomorphic variety, but rather may have large nuclei with a vesicular chromatin pattern **i2.52**. Because of the inflammatory infiltrate and the absence of giant cells, this highly malignant tumor can look deceptively bland at first glance. This tumor is usually in the retroperitoneum and is easily confused with tumors from another class, such as liposarcoma, or—if lymphoid cells outnumber neutrophils—lymphoma or inflammatory myofibroblastic tumor. If neutrophils are the predominant inflammatory cell, this tumor can also be confused with a benign inflammatory lesion such as an abscess or an acute pyelonephritis that has extended into the retroperitoneal soft tissue. The inflammatory UPS/MFH must be excluded in any mesenchymal retroperitoneal mass with acute or chronic inflammation.

The myxoid UPS/MFH is a low-grade myxoid UPS/MFH that is now called the myxofibrosarcoma, again in an attempt to avoid nomenclature that implies knowledge of histogenesis that is not present. The difficulty, however, with the term "myxofibrosarcoma" is that it is easily confused with fibromyxoid sarcoma, a different entity that is not part of the UPS/MFH family. The neoplastic cells in the myxoid UPS/MFH may have a stellate shape and are less pleomorphic than the nuclei of the storiform-pleomorphic type of UPS/MFH, but still more than those of a myxoid liposarcoma **i2.53**. It is further distinguished from the latter tumor by its thicker vessels, which are more curved and less arborizing.

There are a variety of giant cell tumors of soft tissue that are benign (eg, the common giant cell tumor of tendon sheath) or of intermediate malignancy, but the fully malignant giant cell tumor of soft tissue appears equivalent to the giant cell UPS/MFH. The giant cell UPS/MFH is distinct from the giant cell tumor of bone. In the latter tumor, the mononuclear cells are malignant and the giant cells are benign. Indeed, the giant cells in the giant cell tumor of bone have been identified as benign osteoclasts [PMID17013643]. In contrast, in the giant cell type of UPS/MFH, both the giant cell and mononuclear components are malignant **i2.54**. Moreover, the giant cell UPS/MFH may also have some of the smaller neoplastic giant cells that are seen in the storiform-pleomorphic type.

Nevertheless, the giant cell tumor of bone and giant cell UPS/MFH in the bone can appear very similar. A giant cell tumor arising *in* the bone should be considered a giant cell tumor *of* bone and not an UPS/MFH unless the evidence is compelling or there is a history of a giant cell UPS/MFH of soft tissue. In questionable cases, it might help to prove that the giant cells do or do not have the characteristics of osteoclasts.

The angiomatoid UPS/MFH is subcutaneous, is of intermediate grade, and usually occurs in younger patients. This neoplasm usually does not have the nuclear pleomorphism that is generally characteristic of the UPS/MFH, but rather has nodules of histiocyte-like cells, often surrounded by lymphocytes. The name derives from the fact that it is often cystic and hemorrhagic, with many apparent vascular spaces. But these spaces are not lined by endothelial cells. Because of its more superficial location, its less aggressive behavior, and its dilated pseudovascular spaces, some believe it is not a member of the UPS/MFH family and prefer the term "angiomatoid fibrous histiocytoma." This type of UPS/MFH can look much like the aneurysmal type of dermatofibroma, but has a subcutaneous rather than dermal location, a nodular appearance, and a lymphoid cuff.

Unusual Soft Tissue Neoplasms

As mentioned in the discussion of fibromatosis, most apparent fibrosarcomas are actually sarcomas of another type. The diagnosis of fibrosarcoma is one of exclusion, based on absence of epithelial, lymphoid, or melanocytic differentiation, positive staining for vimentin, no other staining that would suggest a specific histogenesis (eg, muscle markers or S100), and the lack of characteristic features of the UPS/MFH family, such as tumor giant cells or a storiform growth pattern.

The fibromyxoid sarcoma (fibromyxosarcoma) is distinct from the myxofibrosarcoma and is not a member of the UPS/MFH family. Its stroma is more collagenous and less myxoid than that of a myxofibrosarcoma. Fibromyxoid sarcomas may be very bland, with no atypia and very rare mitoses. They are very difficult to recognize and many cases have been recognized only after recurrence or metastasis. The fibromyxoid sarcoma may appear notoriously similar to neurofibromas, perineuriomas, or fibromatosis. A fibromyxoid sarcoma should be considered if a bland myxoid lesion is recurrent, has metastasized, has considerable collagen i2.55, collagen in a circular pattern i2.56, alternating areas of fibrous and myxoid foci i2.57, areas of hyalinization, areas of rosetting around collagen, or nests of mucin [PMID3673943]. It should also be excluded if an apparent myxofibrosarcoma is collagenous, a soft tissue neoplasm away from the genital area appears to be an angiomyxoma or an angiomyofibroblastoma, or an apparent fibromatosis is in an unusual area or has uneven cellularity. The fibromyxoid sarcoma often has translocations involving the *FUS* gene [PMID21536545] i2.58.

Because many sarcomas may have a myxoid component, the differential diagnosis of myxoid mesenchymal neoplasms is extensive and often difficult. FISH is useful in many cases of a problematic myxoid tumor, as many of these tumors are associated with characteristic cytogenetic abnormalities, typically involving the *DDIT3* (12q13), *FUS* (16p11), or *EWS* (22q12) genes. For example, almost all myxoid liposarcomas have translocations involving *DDIT3* and *FUS*, but not *EWS*. 70-95% of low-grade fibromyxoid sarcomas have a balanced translocation between the *FUS* gene on 16p11 and the *CREB3L2* gene on 7q34. This is typically seen as t(7;16)(q34;p11), which can be detected by FISH in paraffin material and is extremely helpful in confirming this very difficult diagnosis. About 1/2 of extraskeletal myxoid chondrosarcomas have translocations of *EWS*, often seen as t(9;22)(q31;q12) [PMID18162764].

Granular cell tumors have a distinct eosinophilic granularity of the cytoplasm resulting from numerous lysosomes in the cytoplasm i2.59 (in contrast to Hürthle cells, in which the cytoplasm is denser, and which have large numbers of mitochondria). Granular cell tumors are positive for S100 and CD68. In granular cell tumors, the determination of benign from malignant is very difficult. Necrosis, generalized nuclear pleomorphism i2.60, and a tendency towards irregularly shaped or spindled nuclei may suggest malignancy, but this is one of the tumors (with hemangiopericytoma, smooth muscle tumors, unencapsulated nerve sheath tumors, and fibrous proliferations) whose potential is historically based substantially on mitotic rate, though the number of mitotic figures needed to make a granular cell tumor malignant is not universally agreed on. Some believe that only the presence of metastases can truly determine the malignant examples of granular cell tumor. The size of the neoplasm is not a factor.

Synovial sarcomas may be biphasic or monophasic. The biphasic, epithelioid/spindle cell tumor is rare, but has a distinctive morphology i2.61, i2.62, while the diagnosis of the monophasic variant is more difficult. A monophasic synovial sarcoma should be excluded in any tumor that resembles a hemangiopericytoma/solitary fibrous tumor, as both the cell type and the vascular pattern of these tumors are similar, with small, spindled cells with minimal nuclear pleomorphism i2.63a and dilated, branching vessels i2.63b. However, the appearance of a monophasic synovial sarcoma is variable, and some cases will not have a hemangiopericytoma-like vasculature i2.63c or may have larger, more ovoid nuclei i2.63d, in which case they may resemble a malignant peripheral nerve sheath tumor (MPNST) more than a hemangiopericytoma.

85% of synovial sarcomas have t(X;18)(p11.2;q11.2), resulting in fusion of the *SYT* gene from chromosome 18 to *SSX1* or *SSX2* from the X chromosome (usually to the *SSX1* in a biphasic synovial sarcoma and to *SSX2* in the monophasic form). This is detectable at the DNA level by FISH, using a probe for *SYT/SSX* i2.64. The protein product of this transcript can be detected by immunohistochemistry in paraffin sections in 85% of cases of synovial sarcoma, where it will be a nuclear stain. While this translocation has been reported in MPNST, its presence in a sarcoma essentially secures the diagnosis of a synovial sarcoma. In cases where testing for this translocation cannot be performed, synovial sarcomas usually stain for vimentin, keratin, epithelial membrane antigen, bcl-2, and calponin [PMID18626152]. Staining for TLE1 has more recently been reported [PMID21571956]. The most difficult part of correctly diagnosing a monophasic synovial sarcoma is to think of it, and it is important to perform studies for t(X;18) if possible, and the aforementioned immunohistochemical stains if this is not possible, for any sarcoma that cannot be clearly shown to fit into another category.

It is wise to consider both extranodal sinus histiocytosis with massive lymphadenopathy (SHML; also called Rosai-Dorfman disease) and Langerhans cell histiocytosis (LCH; formerly called histiocytosis X) whenever there are large numbers of histiocytic cells. SHML, described in 1969 [PMID5782438], is characterized by large numbers of histiocytic cells i2.65, often associated with plasma cells and fibrosis i2.66. 1/2 of patients with SHML have evidence for an autoimmune disorder [PMID2180012].

Langerhans cell histiocytosis is a rare neoplasm composed of Langerhans cells, antigen-presenting cells discussed in Chapter 7 i2.67a, i2.67b, i2.67c, i2.67d. It usually occurs in bone, but may rarely be found in soft tissue. The histiocytic cells in both SHML and Langerhans cell histiocytosis are positive for S100 i2.67e, but Langerhans cells are also positive for CD1a i2.67f, which is more specific than S100 [PMID21697965]. Fibrosis and plasma cells are seen less common in LCH than in SHML, and SHML is also positive for CD68 and CD14, markers not seen in LCH. An actin stain might be included to exclude an inflammatory myofibroblastic tumor, which may also have fibrosis and plasma cells.

2 rare neoplasms often have a multinodular architecture—the epithelioid sarcoma and the clear cell sarcoma of soft tissue. Epithelioid sarcoma often presents on the forearm of young adults as multiple subcutaneous nodules, each of which consists of a mixture of rounded to spindled cells enveloped by a cuff of fibroblasts and inflammatory cells i2.68. There is often central necrosis i2.69. The epithelioid morphology of the tumor cells and the necrosis may cause these sarcomas to resemble granulomas.

The clear cell sarcoma of soft tissue is distinct from the clear cell sarcoma of the kidney, which is a pediatric neoplasm. It occurs primarily in the distal extremities of young adults. Although the clear cell sarcoma of soft tissue demonstrates melanocytic differentiation and has been designated as a melanoma of soft tissue, it is distinct from a conventional melanoma and is less aggressive than a thick cutaneous melanoma [PMID20418233]. It has small nodules of tumor within a fibrous stroma i2.70. The tumor cells have round to oval nuclei, prominent nucleoli, and clear to eosinophilic cytoplasm i2.71. In addition to the clear cells, there is often a spindle cell component and occasionally scattered giant cells. Like a number of soft tissue neoplasms, clear cell sarcomas often have a translocation involving the *EWS* (*EWSR-1*) gene [PMID22510762] i2.72.

Peripheral neuroectodermal tumor (PNET) is closely related to Ewing sarcoma and Ewing sarcoma/PNET is envisioned as a family, with Ewing sarcoma being essentially undifferentiated, while PNET has some evidence of neuroendocrine differentiation by the presence of rosettes i2.73, electron microscopy, or immunohistochemistry, but the clinical significance of distinguishing between the two neoplasms has not been established [PMID15939194]. Both tumors express MIC 2, a glycoprotein corresponding to CD99, though CD99 is not specific for this class of tumor [PMID21267687]. The Askin tumor is a PNET of the chest wall.

Ewing sarcoma/PNET results from translocations between the *EWS* (also called *EWSR1*) gene and a member of the *ETS* family, which is a family of transcription factors [PMID19920188] i2.74. Usually, there is usually a t(11;22), which results in fusion of the *EWS* gene from chromosome 22 with the *FLI-1* (or *Fl-1*) from the long arm of chromosome 11 (11q). *FLI-1* is a member of the *ETS* family whose transcription is potentiated when it is adjacent to the *EWS* gene. Immunohistochemistry for the FLI-1 protein is more specific for PNET/Ewing than CD99, though FLI-1 also stains endothelial cells, either normal or neoplastic.

The second most common cause of PNET/Ewing is a translocation involving *EWS*, and a member of the *ETS* family is one involving *ERG* on chromosome 21 rather than *FLI-1*. 3 other members of the *ETS* family may rarely be involved. All of these less common translocations result in Ewing sarcoma/PNET and will be missed with *EWS/FLI-1* FISH probe or reverse transcriptase PCR for that transcript. Translocations involving the *EWS* gene to locations *not* involving members of the *ETS* family are implicated in extraskeletal myxoid chondrosarcoma, clear cell sarcoma, a few cases of myxoid liposarcoma, and desmoplastic small round cell tumor [PMID22510762] i2.75.

Lymphoblastic lymphoma may also be CD99+ and must be excluded before diagnosing the Ewing sarcoma/PNET family (by lymphoid markers and TdT). Neuroblastomas are also in the differential diagnosis of Ewing sarcoma/PNET. Neuroblastomas and Ewing sarcoma/PNET are both nonepithelial neuroendocrine tumors (see Chapter 5 for a discussion of this concept), and immunohistochemical stains may be needed to separate them. Neuroblastomas are negative for CD99 and FLI-1, and are positive for neurofilament triplet. They are more convincingly positive for neuroendocrine markers such as chromogranin, synaptophysin, and CD56. Urinary catecholamines may also help in the diagnosis of neuroblastoma.

Lymphomas may occur in soft tissue, usually concurrent with or after presentation in a more usual site, such as a lymph node or bone marrow. Occasionally, however, lymphomas may present in or be restricted to soft tissue. However, even in these unusual cases, they are diagnosed as in other sites and as discussed in Chapter 8.

Core Points for Soft Tissue

- Benign mimics must first be excluded.
  - Pitfall: the presumption that a cellular mesenchymal proliferation is malignant when it is reactive.
  - Pitfall: the presumption that a spindle cell neoplasm in an organ is a sarcoma when it is a metaplastic carcinoma.
- Cytogenetics or FISH are often important.
- Grading of sarcomas: based on resemblance to normal tissue, mitoses, and necrosis.
  - Grading should not be done on a biopsy.
- Tumors of the so-called fibrous histiocytoma family, the undifferentiated pleomorphic sarcoma (formerly called malignant fibrous histiocytoma), and fibrosarcoma are diagnoses of exclusion.

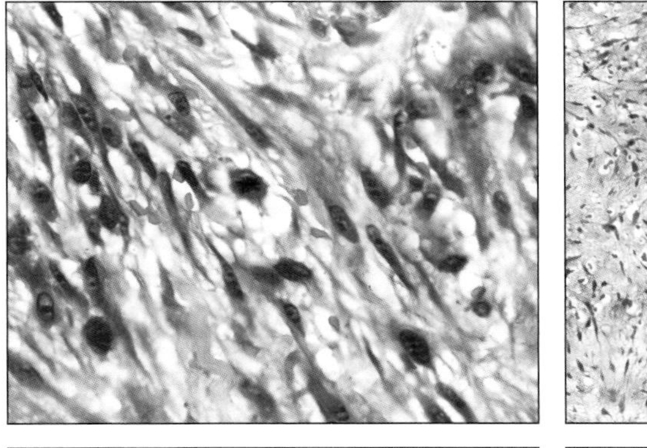

i2.1 Nodular fasciitis with prominent nucleoli and mitotic activity

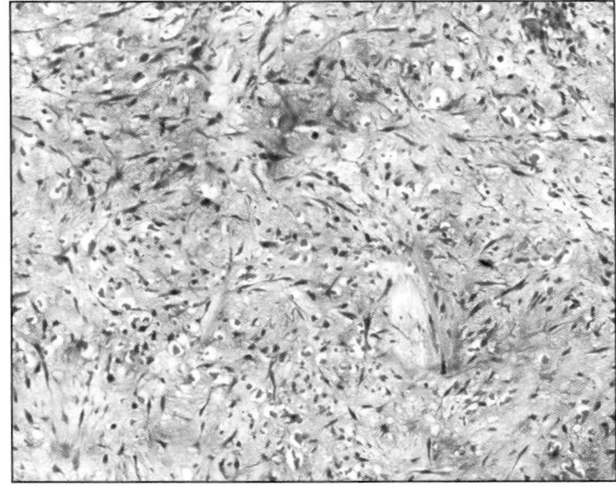

i2.2 Nodular fasciitis with a myxoid stroma a tissue culture appearance

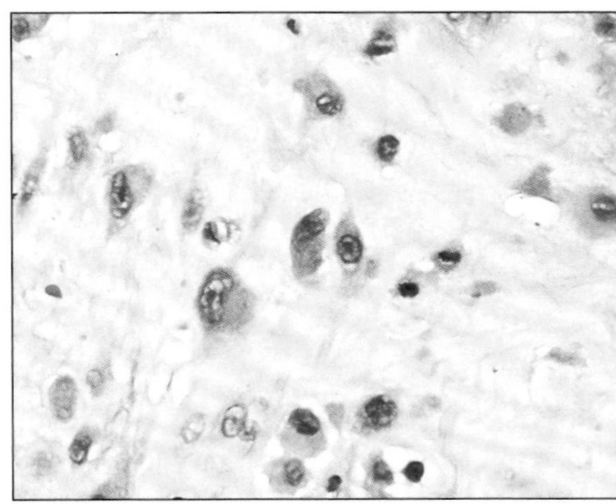

i2.3 Atypical decubital fibroplasia with large cells resembling ganglion cells

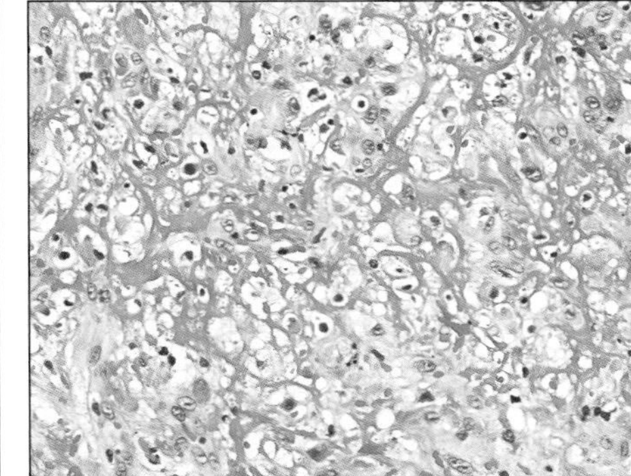

i2.4 Atypical decubital fibroplasia with fibrin deposition

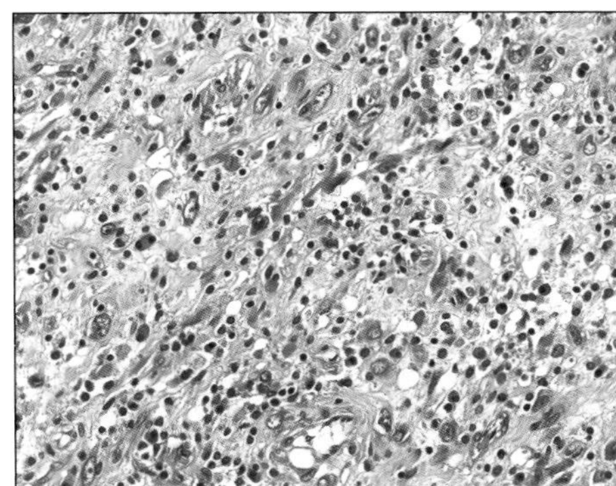

i2.5 Inflammatory myofibroblastic tumor with a hypercellular stroma

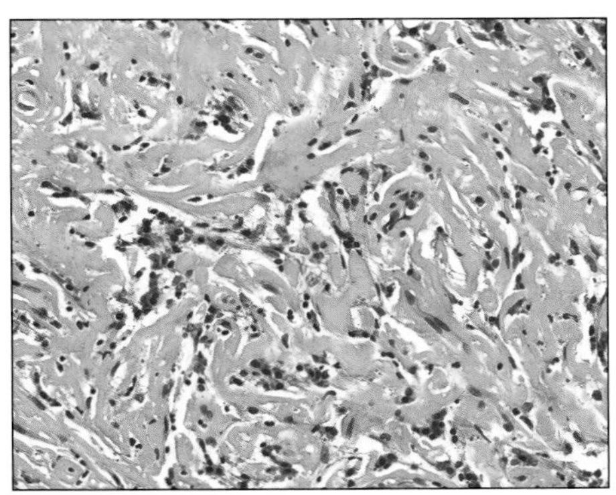

i2.6 Inflammatory myofibroblastic tumor with a hypocellular collagenous stroma

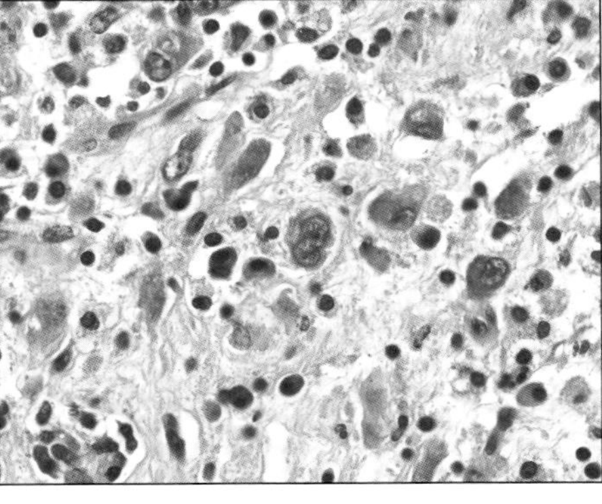

i2.7 The neoplastic cells in inflammatory myofibroblastic tumor may be difficult to appreciate because they are outnumbered by nonneoplastic background cells, but they have characteristics of both muscle cells and fibroblasts, with small nucleoli. Note the numerous plasma cells, which are typically seen in this neoplasm.

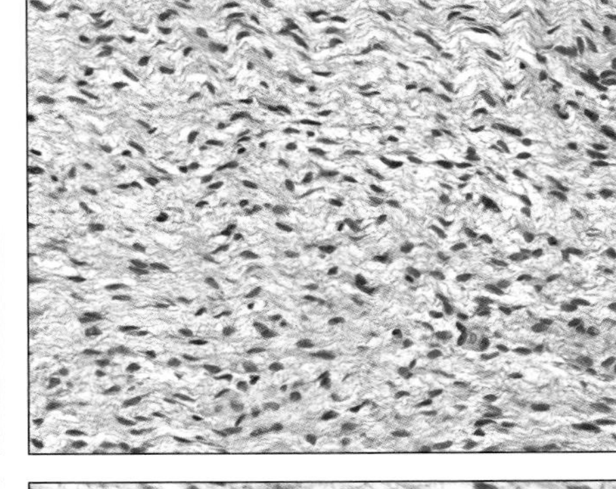

i2.8 Fibromatosis with appreciable cellularity. There is nuclear uniformity and minimal mitotic activity.

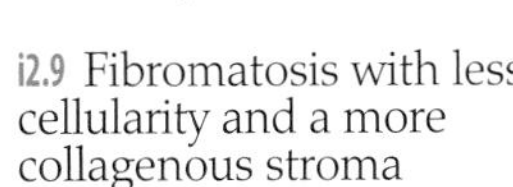

i2.9 Fibromatosis with less cellularity and a more collagenous stroma

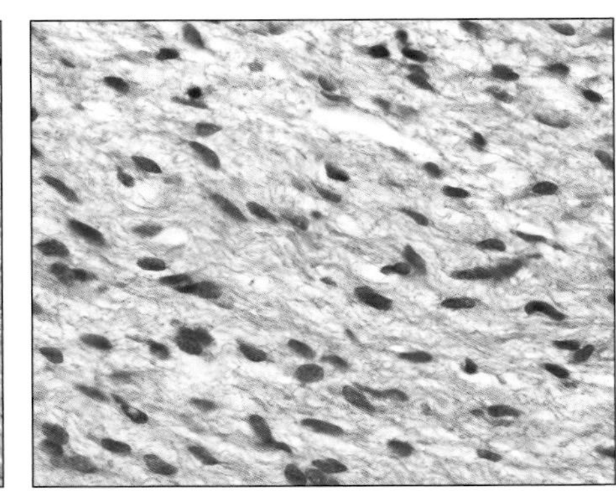

i2.10 The nuclear uniformity of fibromatosis (note also the minimal mitotic activity)

ISBN 978-089189-5886

i2.11 A well differentiated fibrosarcoma with moderate nuclear pleomorphism and occasional mitosis

i2.12 Spindle cell lipoma with myxoid stroma

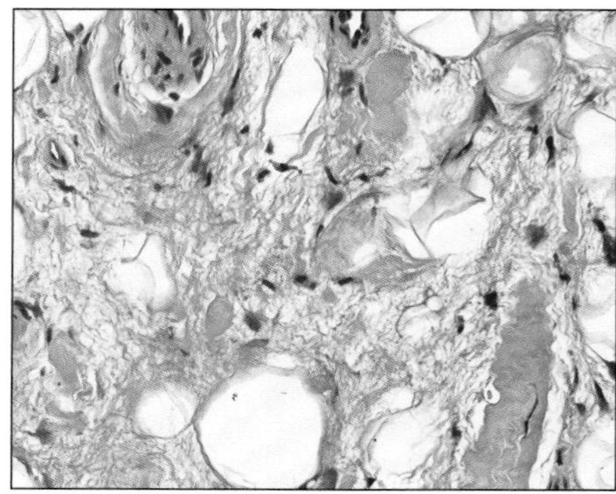

i2.13 Spindle cell lipoma with fibrous stroma

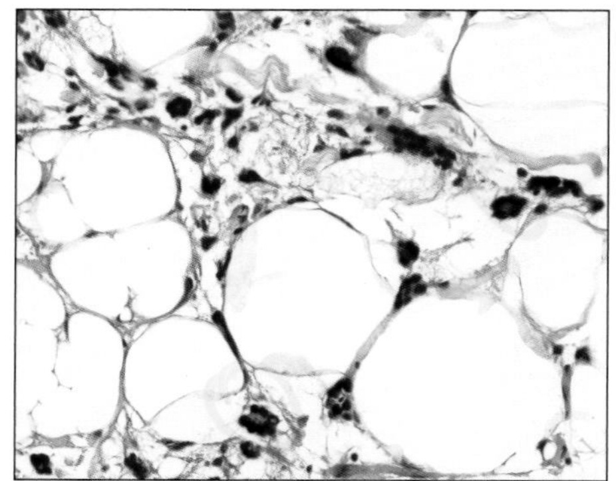

i2.14 Pleomorphic lipoma with atypical nuclei and multinucleated floret cells

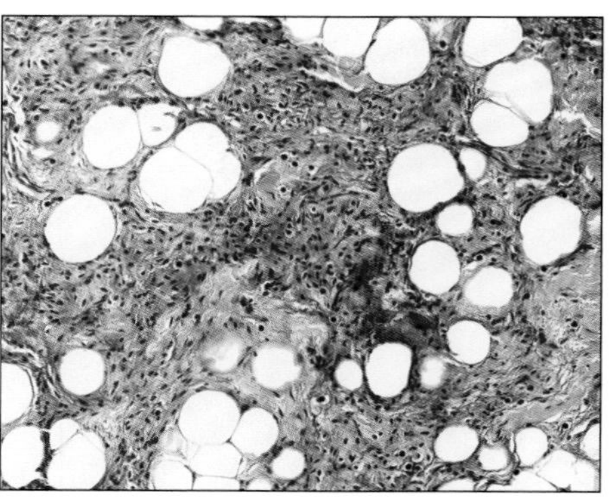

i2.15 Lipoblastoma in a child with myxoid areas resembling a myxoid liposarcoma. Note arborizing capillaries in the center, also resembling a myxoid liposarcoma. More differentiated areas of the lipoblastoma, resembling a mature lipoma, are seen on the periphery.

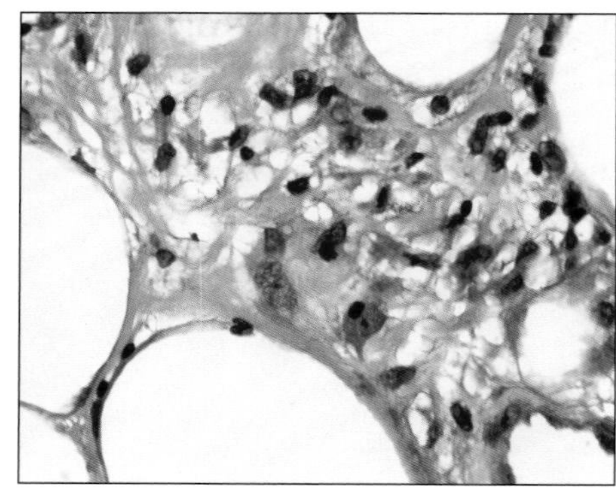

i2.16 Atypical lipoma with atypical cells in the fibrous septae

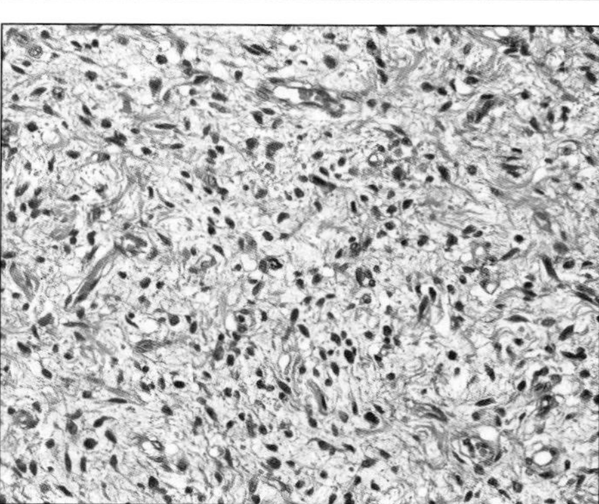

i2.17 Low-grade myxoid liposarcoma with arborizing capillary network

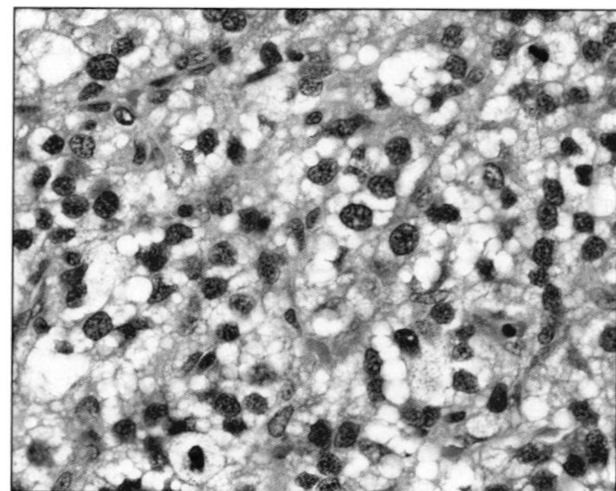

i2.18 High-grade (round cell) liposarcoma with larger neoplastic cells and indistinct vascular pattern

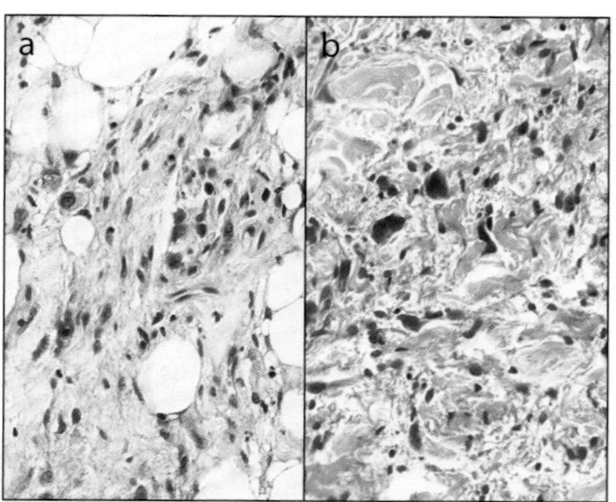

i2.19 **a** Dedifferentiated liposarcoma. There is an atypical cell in a septa, as is seen in atypical lipoma. **b** More cellular areas of a dedifferentiated liposarcoma with atypical nuclei that, out of context, are not clearly of adipocyte origin

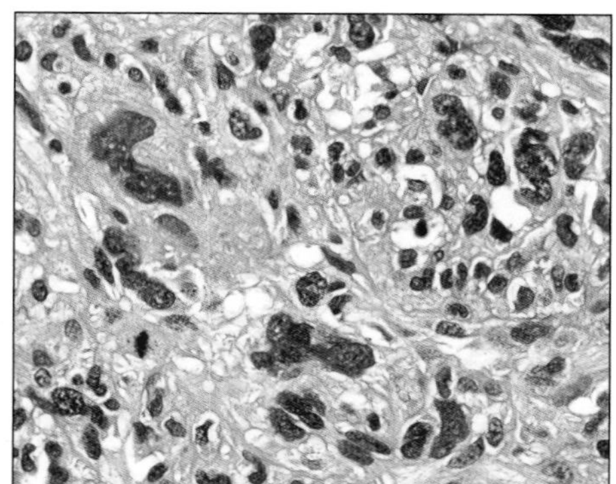

i2.20 Pleomorphic liposarcoma with very atypical nuclei throughout. The neoplasm is recognized as lipomatous because of the small residual fat vacuoles.

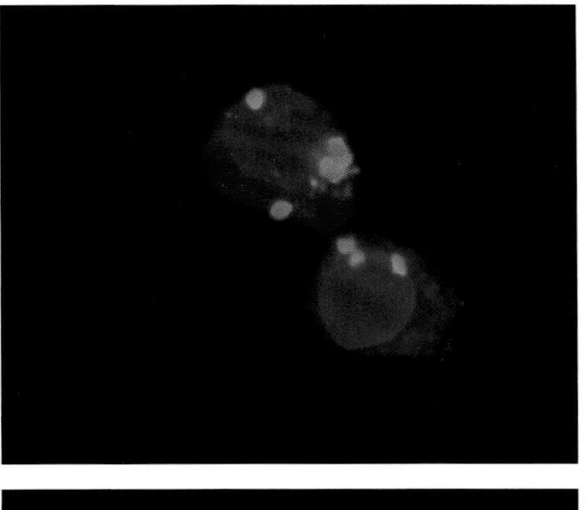

i2.21 Well differentiated liposarcoma with *MDM2* amplification. *MDM2* is amplified as a homogenously staining region as seen by coalescing red signals. Centromere 12 probe shows 2 green signals indicating that the increased expression of *MDM2* is not because of an increase in copy number of this chromosome.

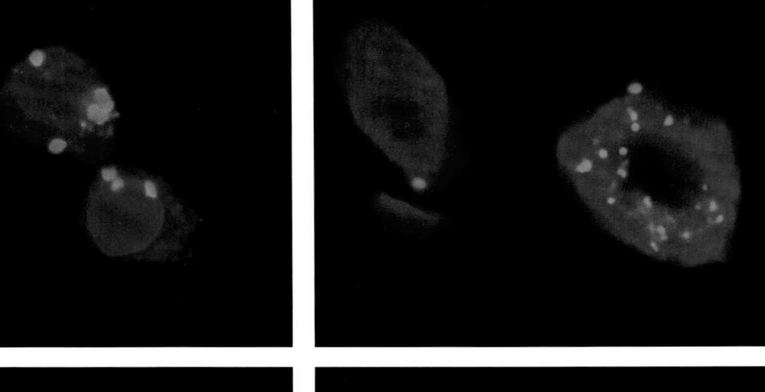

i2.22 Well differentiated liposarcoma with *MDM2* amplification. *MDM2* is amplified as small extrachromosomal fragments called double minutes, seen as multiple red signals throughout the cell. Centromere 12 probe shows 2 signals consistent with 2 copies of chromosome 12.

i2.23 Myxoid liposarcoma with a *DDIT3* rearrangement seen as one intact gene fluorescing yellow and one disrupted gene seen as split green and red signals.

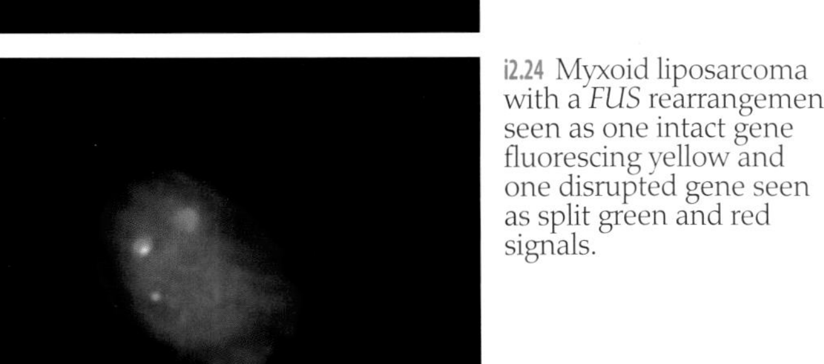

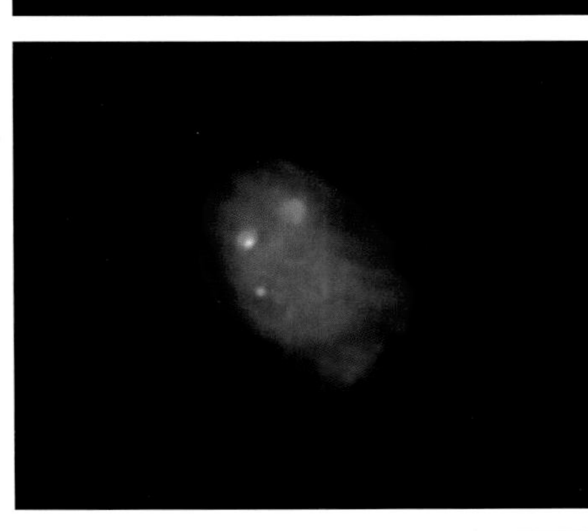

i2.24 Myxoid liposarcoma with a *FUS* rearrangement seen as one intact gene fluorescing yellow and one disrupted gene seen as split green and red signals.

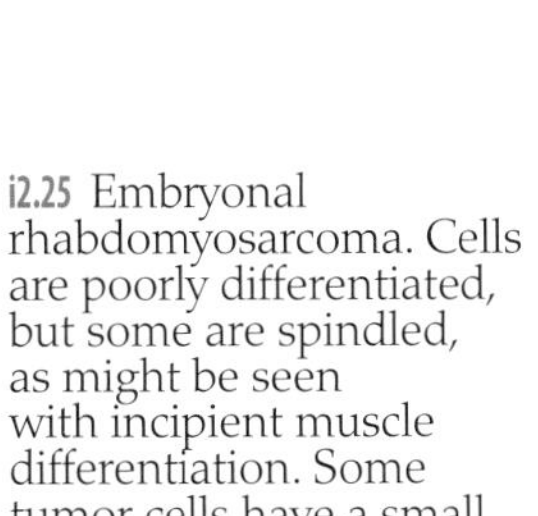

i2.25 Embryonal rhabdomyosarcoma. Cells are poorly differentiated, but some are spindled, as might be seen with incipient muscle differentiation. Some tumor cells have a small amount of eosinophilic cytoplasm.

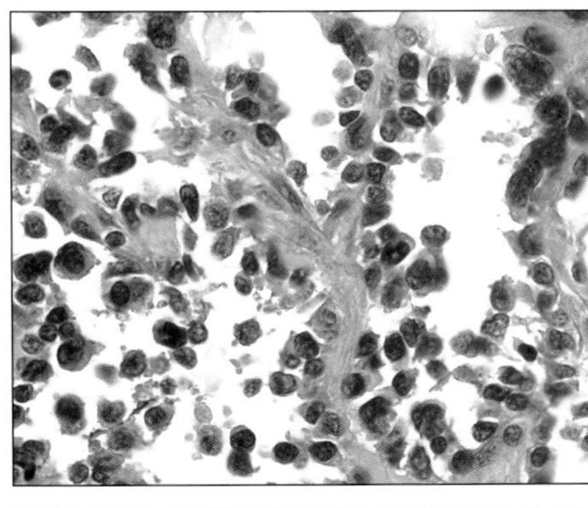

i2.26 Alveolar rhabdomyosarcoma. There are clusters of dyscohesive tumor cells between fibrous setae, but the important finding is that the individual cells are round, with very little cytoplasm and no differentiation towards muscle.

i2.27 Alveolar rhabdomyosarcoma with a *FOXO1* (*FHKR*) rearrangement seen as a central intact fused yellow signal and split red and green signals.

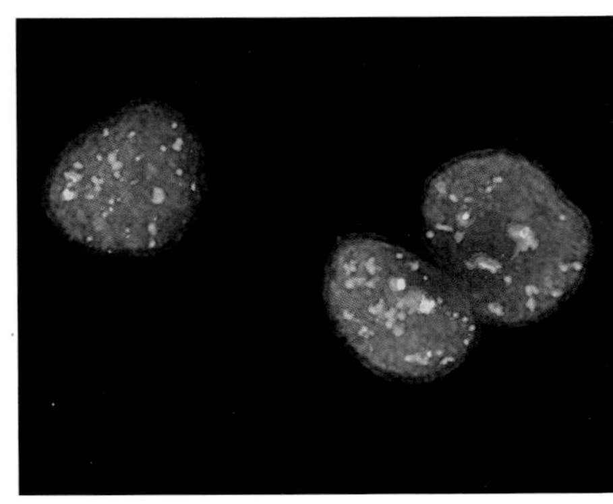

i2.28 Alveolar rhabdomyosarcoma with a t(1;13)(p36:q14). FISH shows 3 intact genes and multiple copies of the 3' green probe indicating amplification of the disrupted *FOXO1* gene. Amplification is common in this variant translocation and rarely seen with the more frequent t(2;13)(q35;q14). (touch prep)

i2.29 Pleomorphic rhabdomyosarcoma, with much larger and more atypical nuclei than are seen in embryonic or alveolar rhabdomyosarcoma

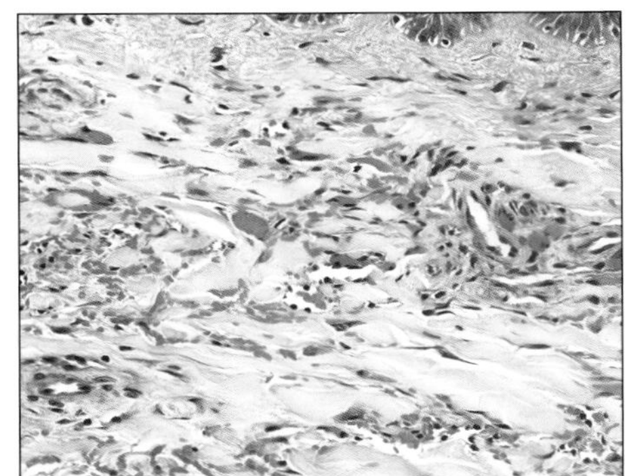

i2.30 Early Kaposi sarcoma, corresponding to a clinical macular stage, with disordered, thin-walled blood vessels. Because of poor endothelial integrity, there is extravasation of erythrocytes into the tissue.

ISBN 978-089189-5886

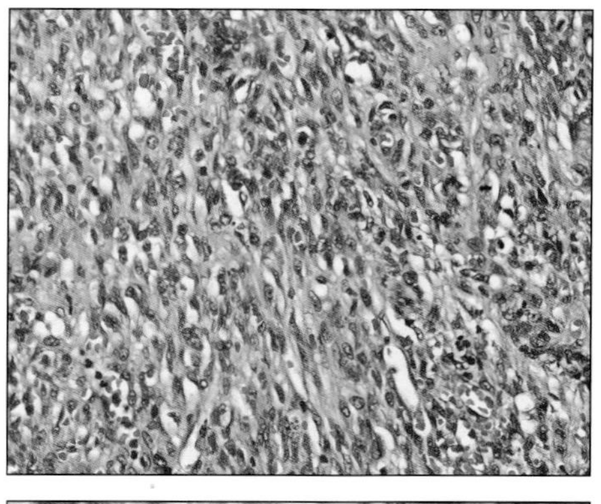

i2.31 The tumor stage of Kaposi sarcoma, with fascicles of neoplastic endothelial cells

i2.32 The thin-walled, branching blood vessels that are characteristic of a hemangiopericytoma

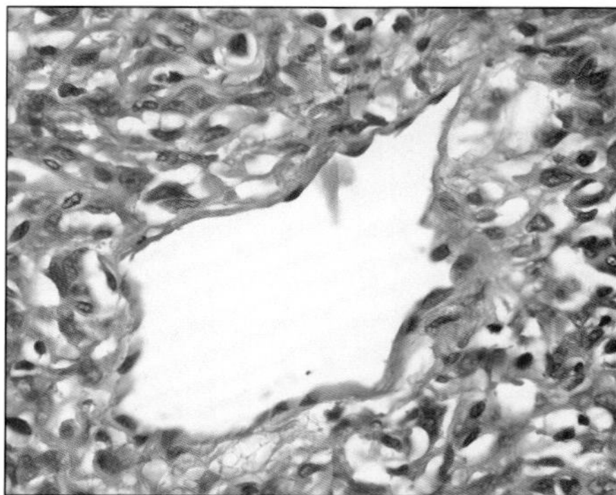

i2.33 The neoplastic cells of a hemangiopericytoma adjacent to the smaller, nonneoplastic endothelial cells binding the blood vessels. This juxtaposition has led to the supposition that the neoplastic cell is the pericyte, which is normally adjacent to the endothelial cell.

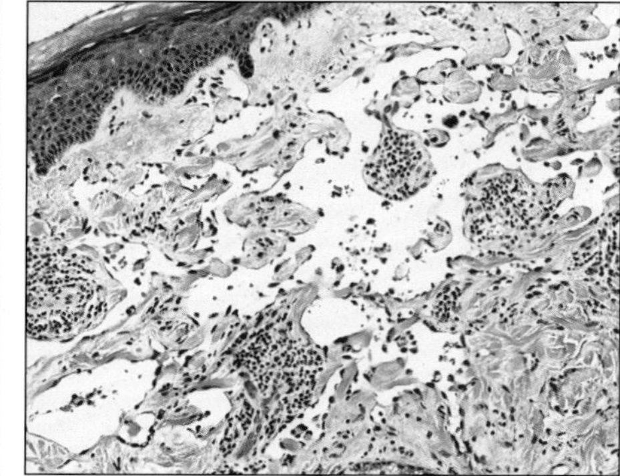

i2.34 A well differentiated angiosarcoma, with vascular channels that appear to dissect into the stroma

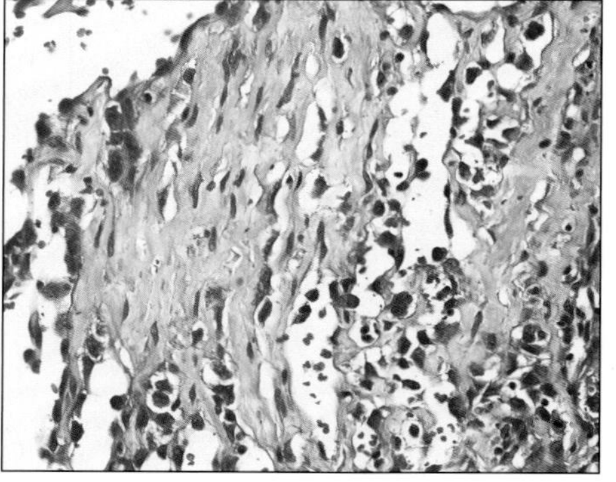

i2.35 A high-grade angiosarcoma with endothelial hyperplasia, nuclear crowding, nuclear atypia, and neoplastic cells that form microtufts

i2.36 Epithelioid angiosarcoma. The neoplastic cells form vaguely defined vascular channels, but immunohistochemical stains are necessary for proper identification.

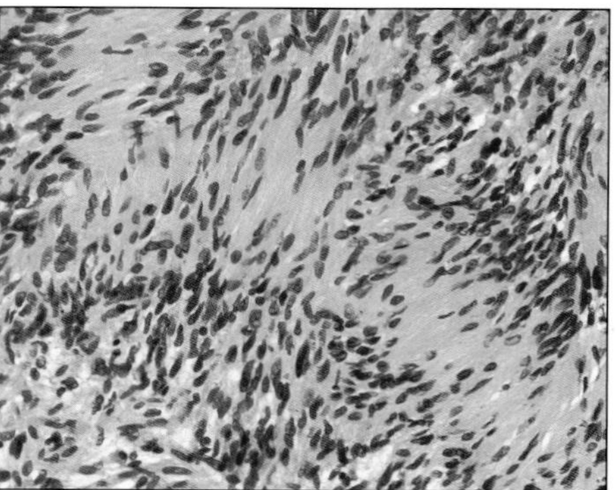

i2.37 A schwannoma with a Verocay body, where two areas of greater cellularity, often in the form of vesicles, are separated by a hypocellular area

i2.38 Serpiginous nuclei are often seen in schwannomas.

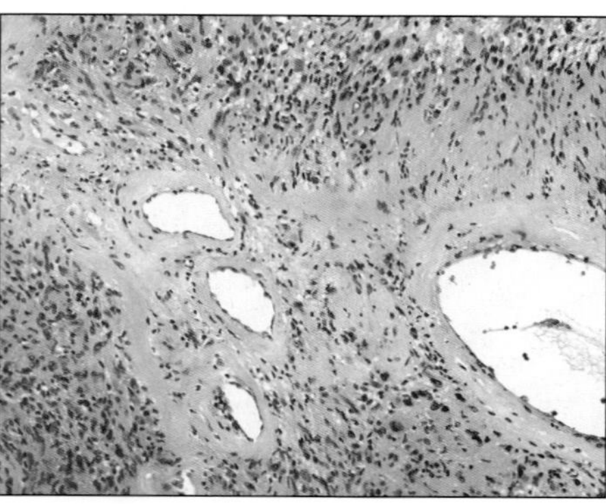

i2.39 Schwannomas often have blood vessels with thickened, hyalinized walls.

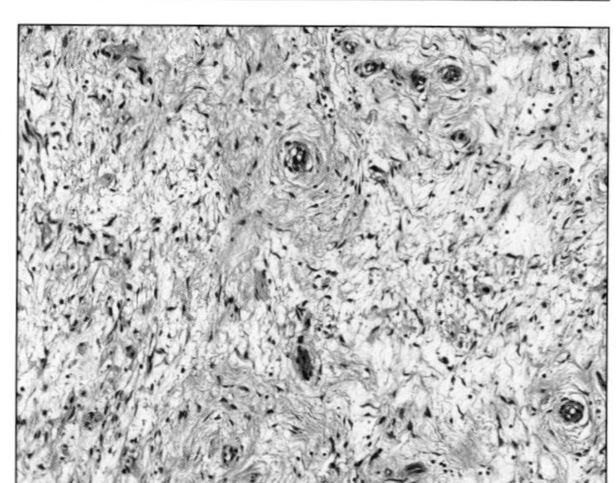

i2.40 An edematous or myxoid stroma is often seen in neurofibromas.

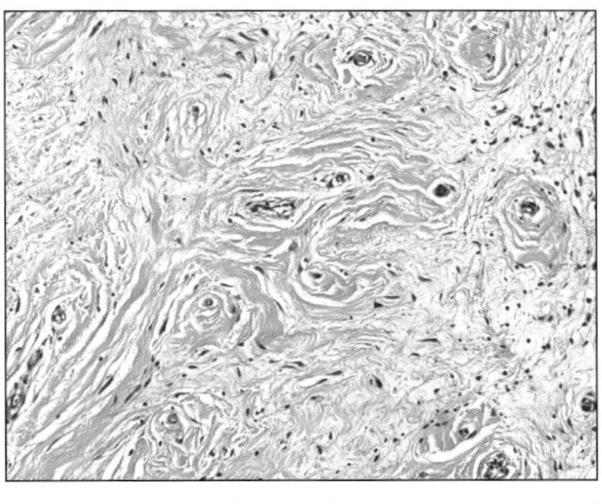

i2.41 Neurofibromas often have foci of thin collagen fibers.

i2.42 For unknown reasons, neurofibromas usually contain mast cells.

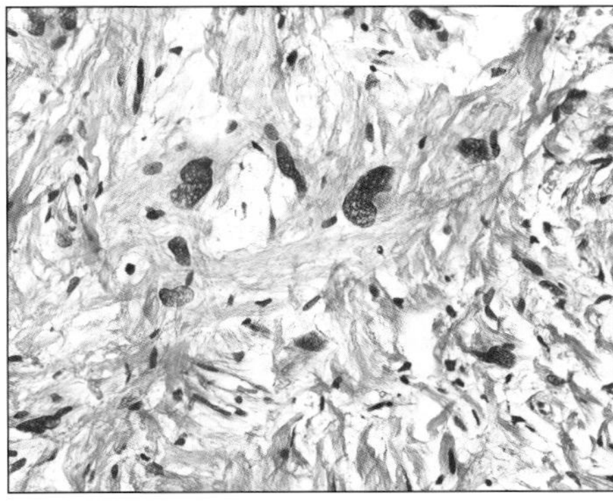

i2.43 A degenerative (ancient) schwannoma may have appreciable focal nuclear atypia, but it does not have generalized atypia.

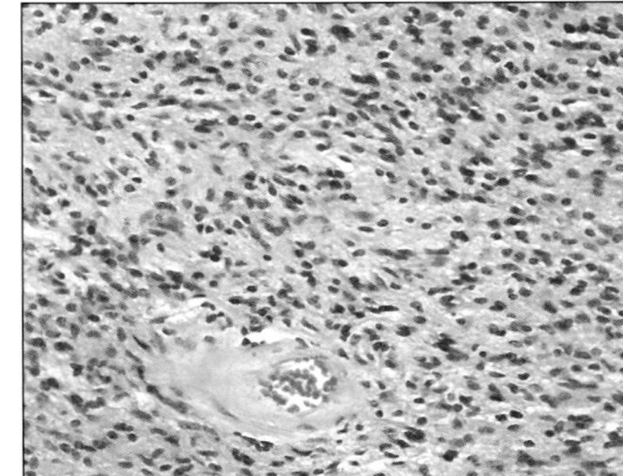

i2.44 A cellular schwannoma may have alarming cellularity and appreciable mitotic activity, but it remains encapsulated and does not have generalized atypia. In addition, it typically retains some features of a common schwannoma. In this example, the blood vessel has a slightly thickened, hyalinized wall.

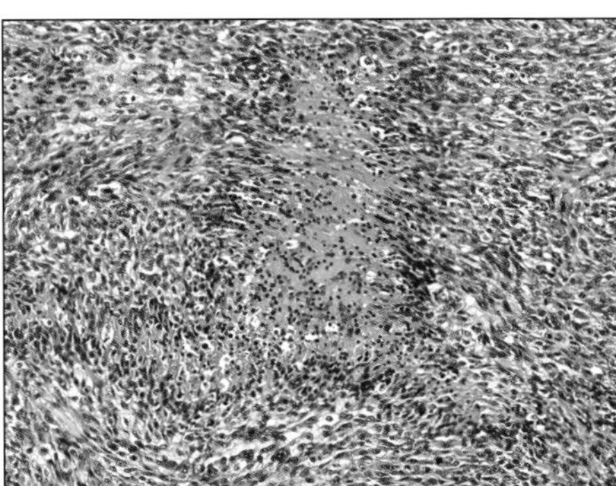

i2.45 A sarcoma in which the presence of a Verocay body suggests nerve sheath origin

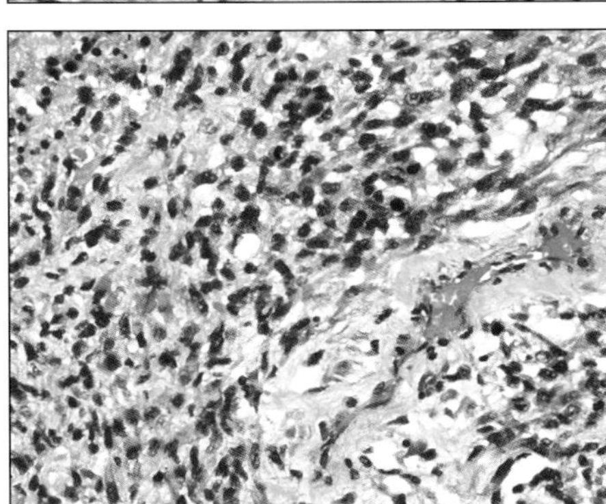

i2.46 A sarcoma in which a thickened, hyalinized vascular wall suggests nerve sheath origin

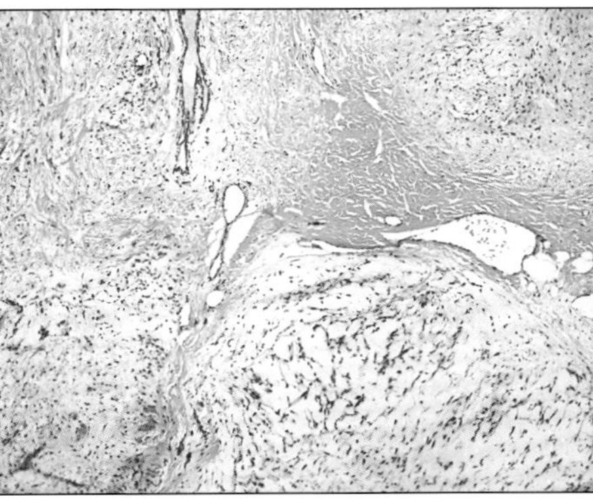

i2.47 A low-power illustration of a myxoid chondrosarcoma, illustrating the multinodular architecture

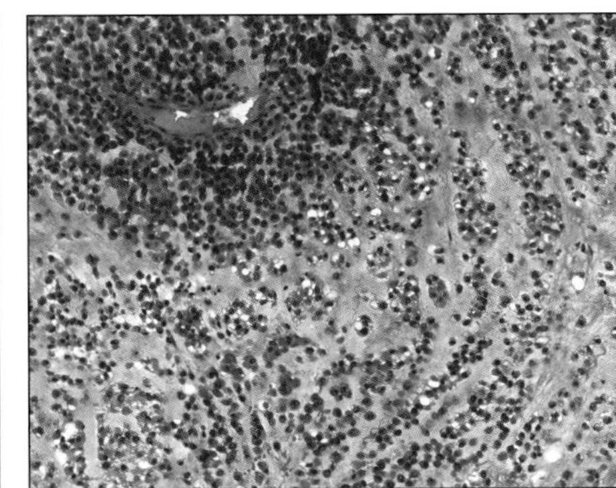

i2.48 A myxoid chondrosarcoma in which neoplastic cells appear to radiate from a hypercellular area in the center of a nodule towards the periphery

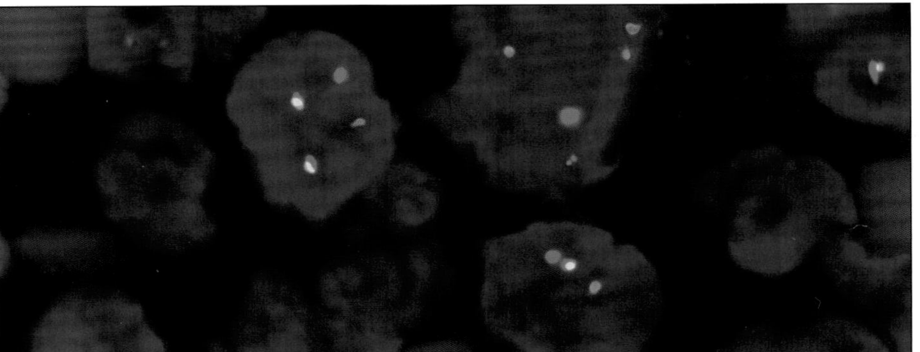

i2.49 Break apart FISH study of *EWSR1* in an extraskeletal myxoid chondrosarcoma showing 2 intact genes fluorescing as yellow signals and a single copy of the disrupted genes seen as split green and red signals.

ISBN 978-089189-5886

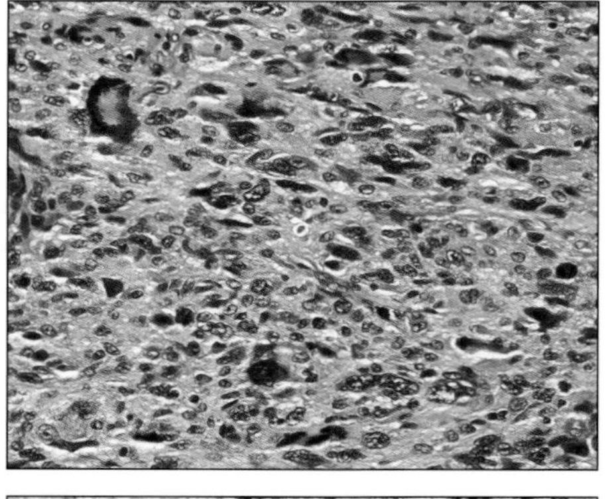

i2.50 An undifferentiated pleomorphic sarcoma, with characteristic giant cells

i2.51 The storiform-pleomorphic type of undifferentiated pleomorphic sarcoma often has fascicles that intersect each other.

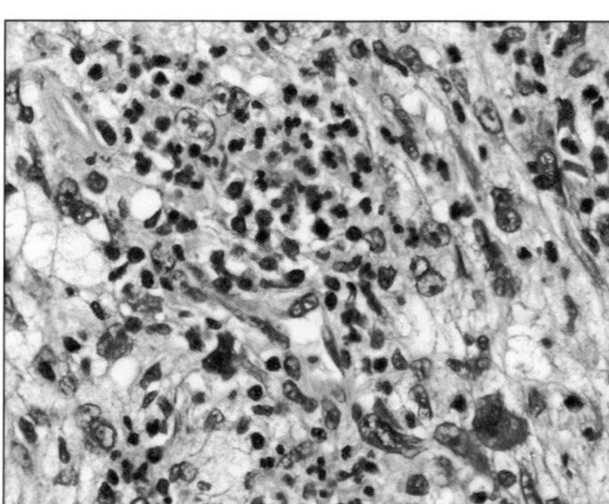

i2.52 The inflammatory form of undifferentiated pleomorphic sarcoma generally contains numerous neutrophils and is characterized by neoplastic cells with only 1 nucleus, with a vesicular chromatin pattern and occasional nucleoli.

i2.53 The neoplastic cells of a myxoid UPS are often stellate shaped. While they are less pleomorphic than in other forms of UPS, they are more pleomorphic than in a myxoid liposarcoma. Note the abnormal mitotic figure in the center.

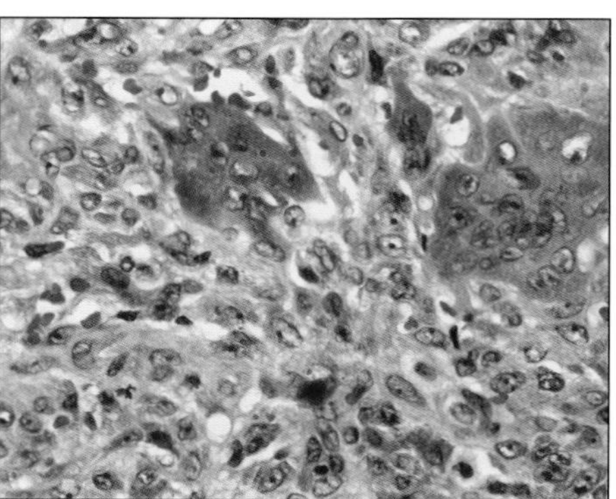

i2.54 A giant cell UPS. Note that the nuclei in the mononuclear cells and in the giant cells have an identical appearance and appear malignant.

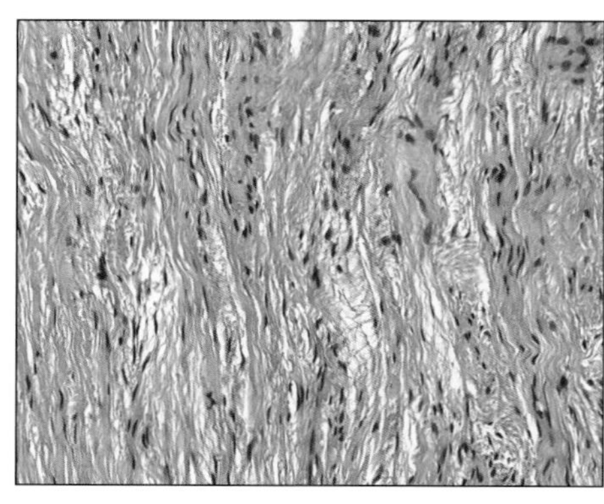

i2.55 A fibromyxoid sarcoma with a more collagenous stroma than is typically seen in the UPS family

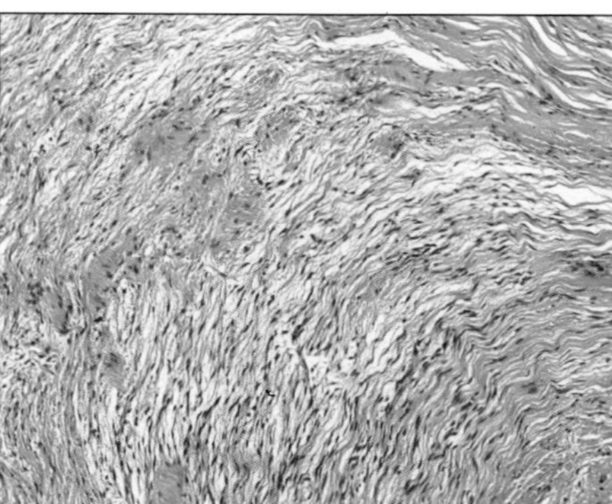

i2.56 A fibromyxoid sarcoma with collagen fibers in a circular outline

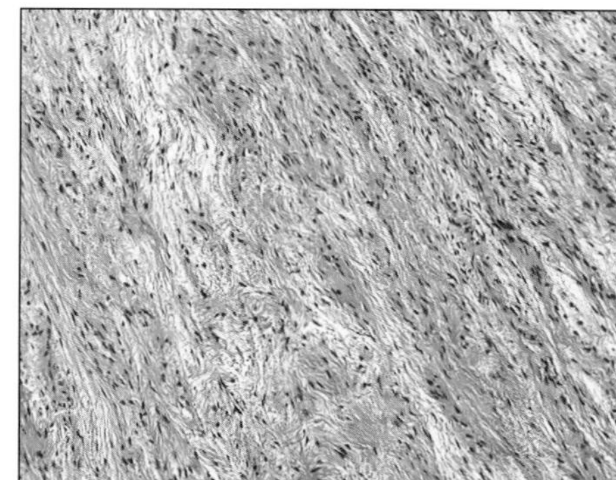

i2.57 A fibromyxoid sarcoma with alternating areas of dense collagenous stroma and looser, myxoid stroma

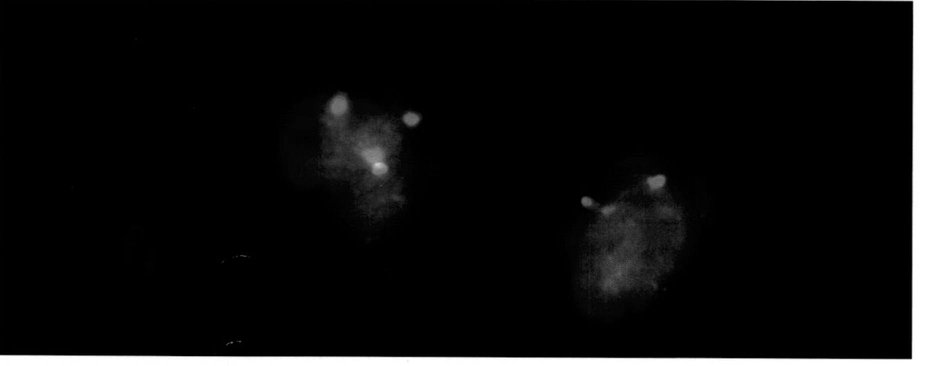

i2.58 Low-grade fibromyxoid sarcoma with a *FUS* rearrangement. The center cells shows a fused red and green signal indicating an intact gene and a split red and green signal consistent with a *FUS* disruption.

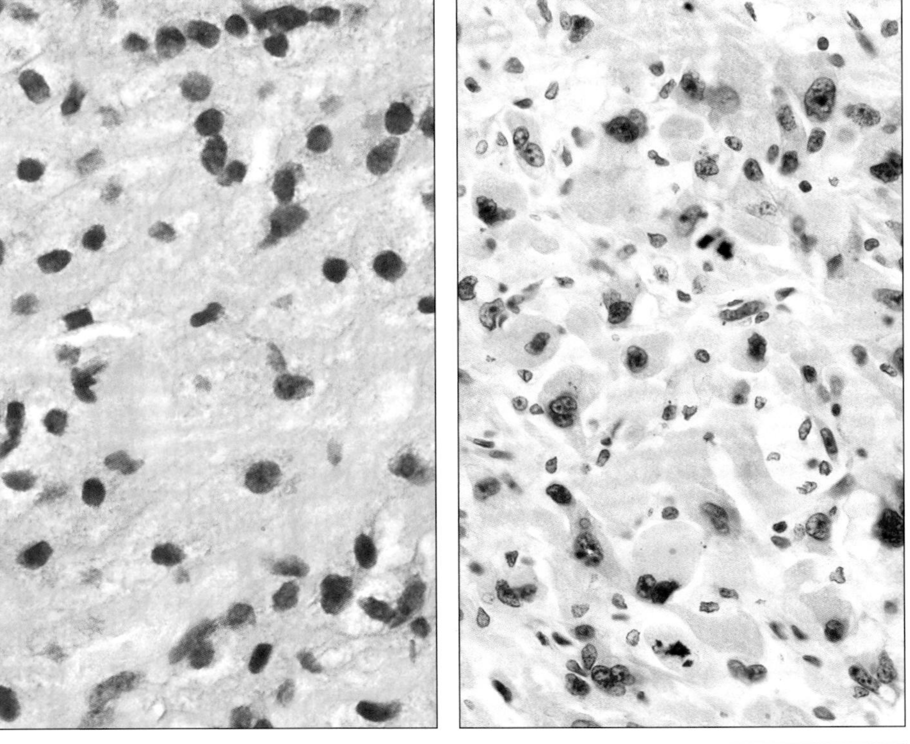

i2.59 A granular cell tumor with eosinophilia and granularity of the cytoplasm.

i2.60 A malignant granular cell tumor with generalized nuclear enlargement, pleomorphism, and spindled or irregularly shaped nuclei.

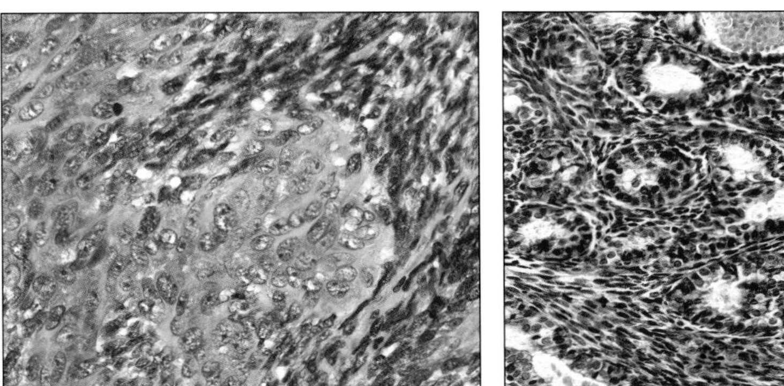

i2.61 Biphasic synovial sarcoma with clusters of round, epithelioid cells in a spindle cell background

i2.62 Biphasic synovial sarcoma with clusters of round, epithelioid cells in a spindle cell background

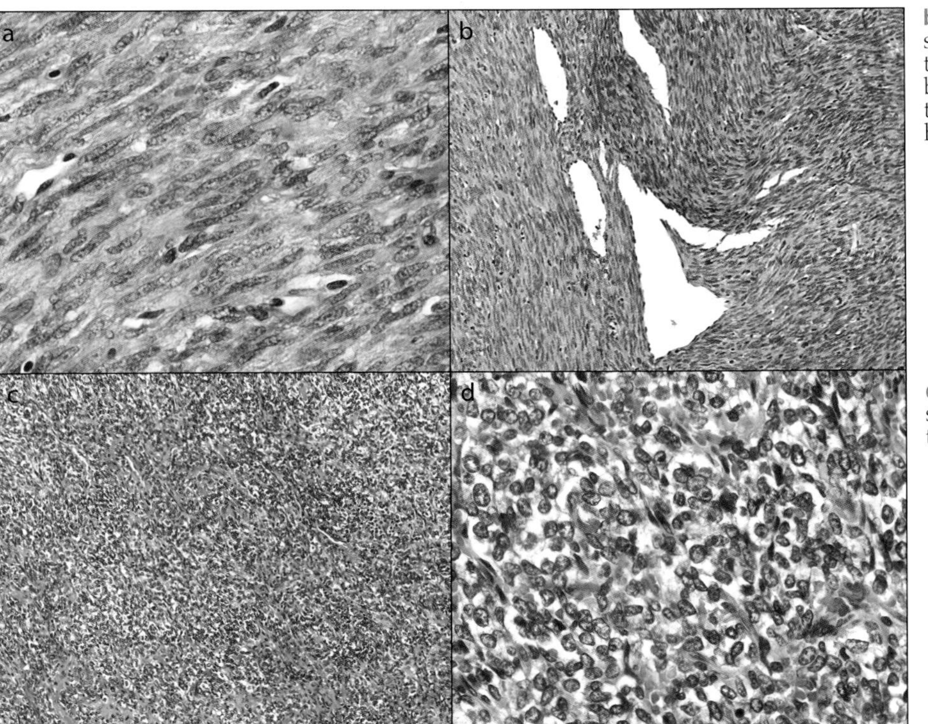

i2.63 **a** A monophasic synovial sarcoma with relatively uniform neoplastic cells with spindled nuclei

b A monophasic synovial sarcoma with dilated, thin-walled, branching blood vessels similar to those seen in a hemangiopericytoma

c A monophasic synovial sarcoma that does not have a hemangiopericytoma-like vascular pattern

d A monophasic synovial sarcoma with ovoid, rather than spindled nuclei

ISBN 978-089189-5886

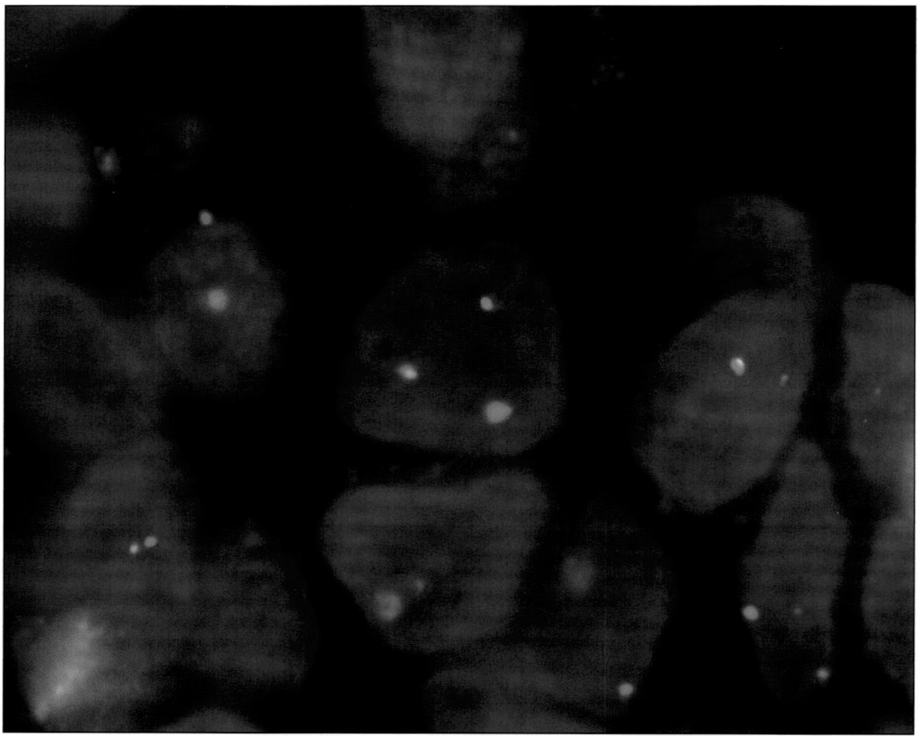

i2.64 Synovial sarcoma with a *SYT* rearrangement. The intact gene shows a fused red and green signal and the split yellow and green signals indicates a *SYT* disruption.

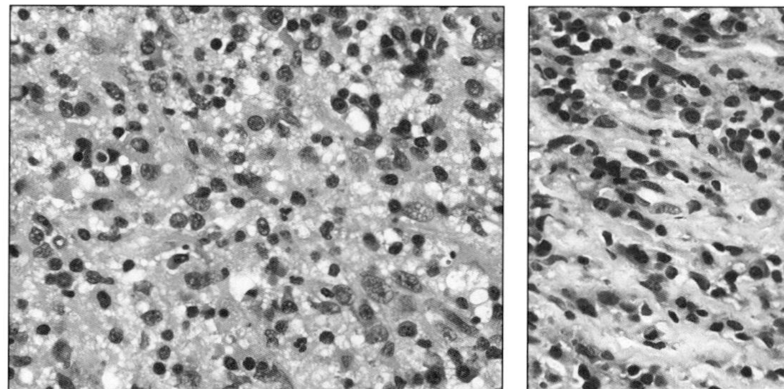

i2.65 Rosai-Dorfman disease, with clusters of histiocytic cells

i2.66 Rosai-Dorfman disease with plasma cells and fibrosis

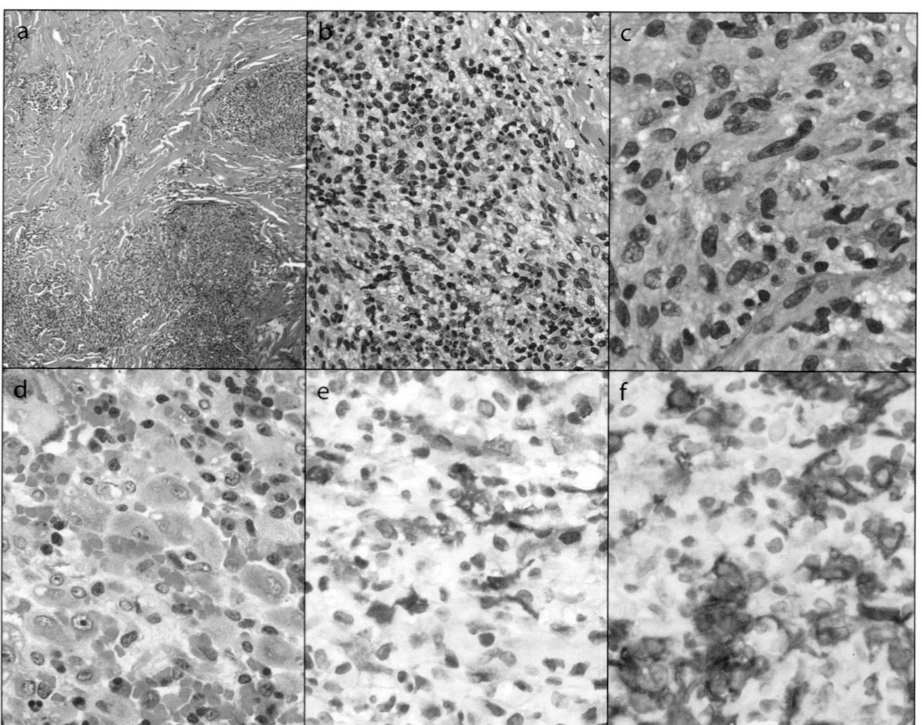

i2.67 **a** Langerhans cell histiocytosis in soft tissue. This low-power view illustrates a multinodular pattern.
b A higher-power view of the same process as in image i2.67a illustrating the eosinophils that typically accompany Langerhans cells and account for the old name of "eosinophilic granuloma"
c A high-power view of the Langerhans cells illustrating that the nucleus is often somewhat spindled relative to the nucleus of an ordinary macrophage
d Langerhans cells histiocytosis with histiocytic cells that are morphologically similar to, but immunohistochemically distinct from, common histiocytes or those seen in Rosai-Dorfman disease.

d (cont) Note the eosinophils and the melanin pigment in the upper left that is characteristic of Langerhans cells, as they are typically found in the skin and may take up some melanin pigment during their antigen presenting function (discussed in Chapter 7).
e An S100 stain of the same case as in image i2.67a. This stain highlights the Langerhans cells and demonstrates the extensive cytoplasmic processes that are important in their function as antigen presenting cells in the immune system.
f A CD1a stain of the same case as in image i2.67a, highlighting the Langerhans cells in a membranous staining pattern

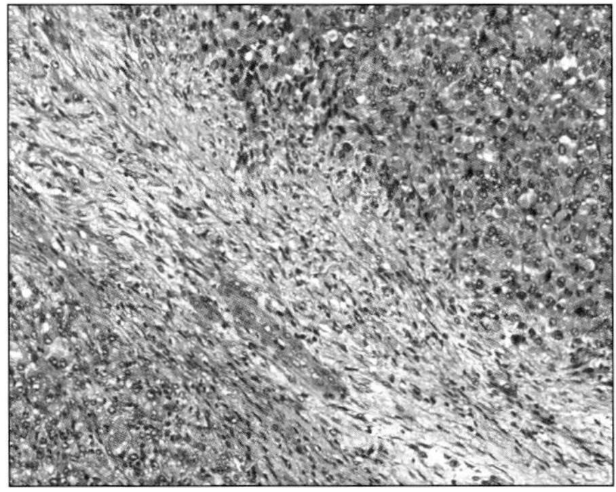

i2.68 Epithelioid sarcoma. The neoplastic cells form nodules which are separated by fibrous septae that contain inflammatory cells.

i2.69 The central necrosis that is typical of nodules of epithelioid sarcoma and which may lead to a misinterpretation of a necrotizing granulomatous process.

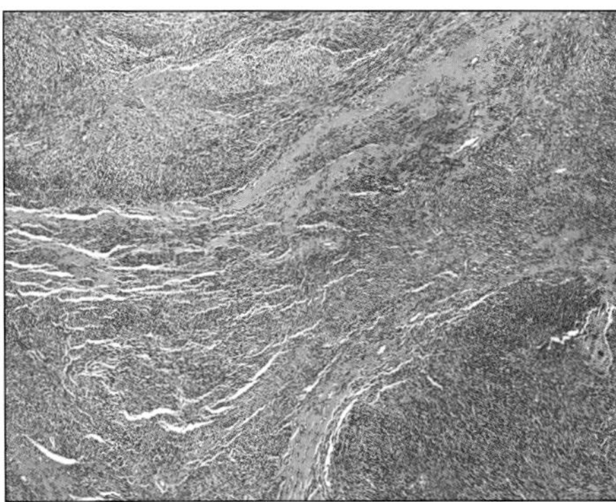

i2.70 A low-power view of a clear cell sarcoma, illustrating the multinodular architecture

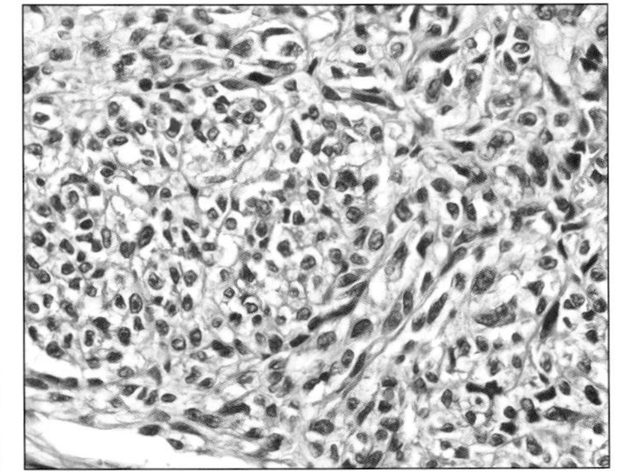

i2.71 A high-power view of a clear cell sarcoma, illustrating the relatively uniform nuclei and clear cytoplasm that are characteristic of the sarcoma

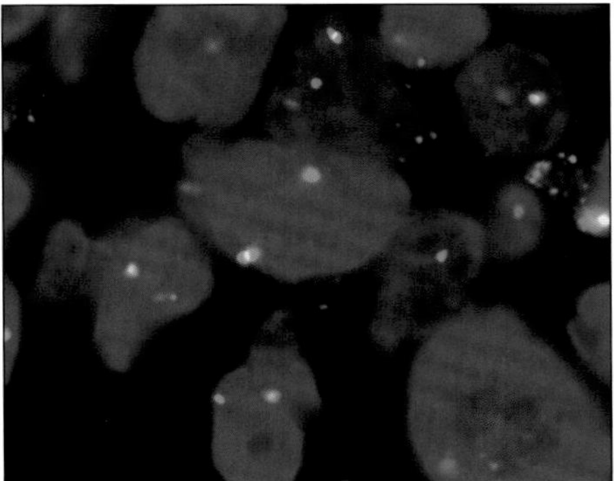

i2.72 Clear cell sarcoma with a *EWSR1* rearrangement showing one intact gene fluorescing as a yellow signal and split red and green signals.

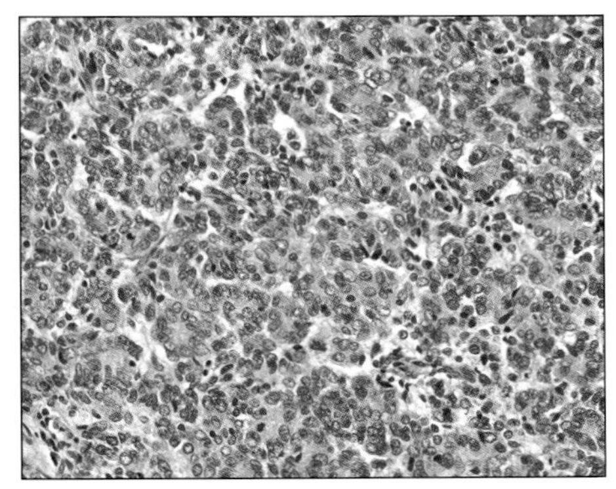

i2.73 A primitive neuroectodermal tumor with some rosette formation

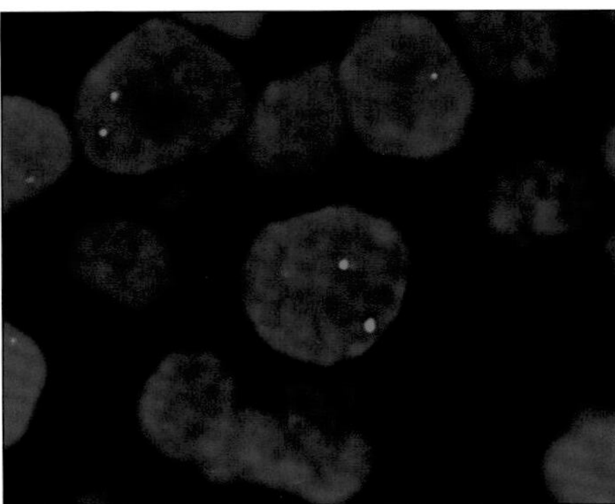

i2.74 Ewing sarcoma with a *EWSR1* rearrangement. The intact gene shows a fused red and green signal and the split red and green signals indicates a *EWSR1* disruption.

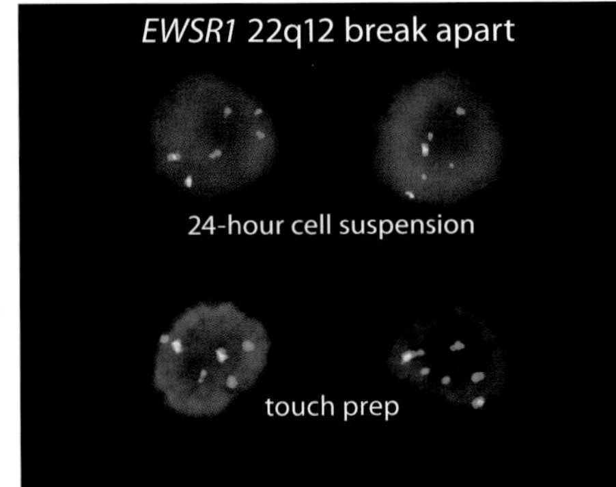

i2.75 Break apart FISH study for *EWSR1* in a desmoplastic small round cell tumor showing a variant signal pattern with 2 intact genes fluorescing as fused yellow signals and 2 disrupted genes with split red and green signals. This often corresponds to tumor tetraploidy on metaphase spreads.

ISBN 978-089189-5886

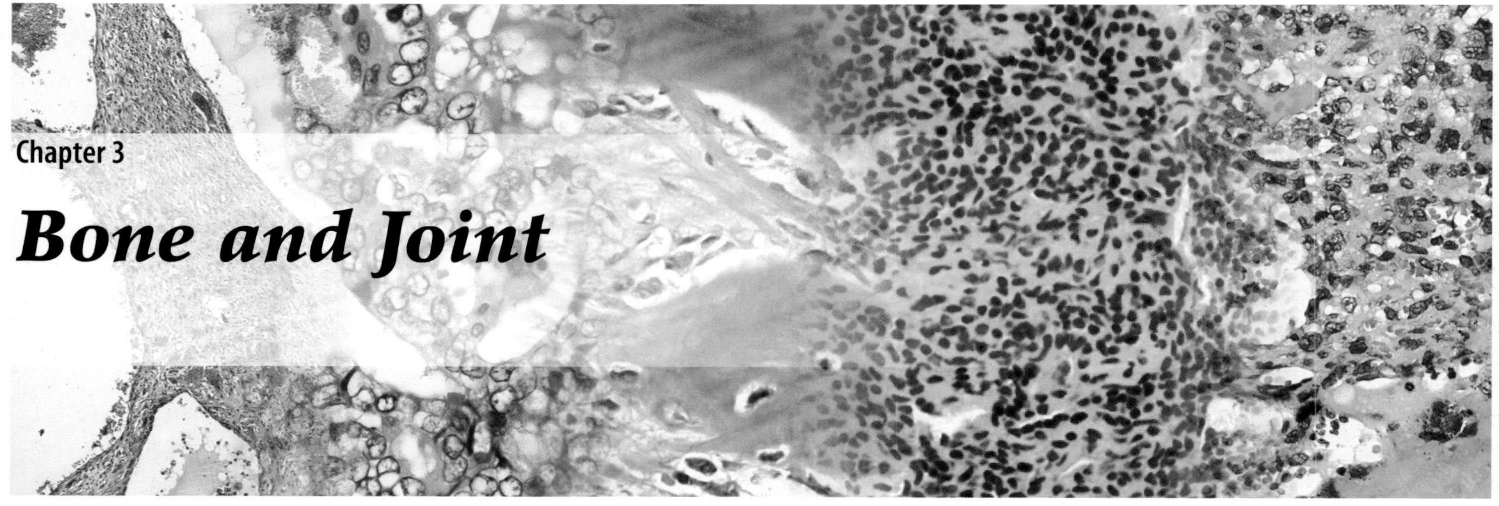

Traumatic and Degenerative Conditions

A meniscus is an intrarticular plate of fibrocartilage found in some joints, especially the knee, where 2 menisci sit on top of the tibia and are attached to the joint capsule. The meniscus is an important part of the joint and in the knee can bear up to 50% of the weight. For this reason, meniscectomy changes the weight-bearing dynamics of a joint and is not to be undertaken lightly. Repair of a torn meniscus is to be preferred, but is difficult, especially in adults.

A bursa is a flattened portion of synovium with a connective tissue core. Bursas are located wherever there is motion, and serve to diminish friction. They also function as cushions to reduce pressure affects, but unlike menisci, they do not bear weight. They are avascular, but can become inflamed or infected, like any synovial tissue, in which case they can acquire vascularity. They may also become an enclosed sac filled with viscous fluid.

A ganglion cyst is a myxoid degeneration in or herniation of the joint capsule or tendon sheath. It has no lining. "Baker cyst" is a generic term for any cyst of the popliteal fossa. Most of these are distended bursas, but some are herniations of synovial lining into the joint capsule, and a few are ganglion cysts, in which case there is no lining. The presence of a Baker cyst usually means some degree of damage to the synovium.

A neuroma is a disorganized proliferation of axons, often secondary to trauma. The most common neuroma is a Morton neuroma, on the bottom of the foot at the base of the toes. Because Morton neuroma is caused by abnormal weight distribution over a prolonged time, there may also be arterial thickening and occlusion, as well as Schwann cell or fibroblastic proliferation.

Carpel tunnel syndrome is caused by any process that compresses the median nerve during its passage through the carpel tunnel. Although some cases are secondary to amyloid deposition, most have more prosaic causes, such as arthritis or fibrosis.

Arthritis

Portions of bone removed for osteoarthritis (also called degenerative joint disease) are often not sent to the pathologist, since the diagnosis is readily made by clinical and radiologic criteria. In those cases that are sent for examination, there is thinning and disruption of the articular cartilage, with a particular form of fragmentation called fibrillation, that is characterized by vertical linear fissures i3.1. Osteophyte (bone spur) formation, secondary to abnormal weight bearing, is often seen.

The exposed bone is denser and more cortical, with fewer trabeculae (eburnation; i3.2. In addition to eburnation, there may be evidence of injury in the subchondral bone, with alterations in the shape and contour of the bone, along with loss of bone substance elsewhere because of shifts in weight bearing. There may also be subchondral bone cysts.

Additional findings in osteoarthritis may include a diminution of basophilic staining in cartilage, loss of chondrocytes, as indicated by empty lacunae, and evidence of regeneration, as seen by multiple chondrocytes within a lacuna. These are all indications of injury to the cartilage.

Although osteoarthritis is noninflammatory in its origin, there may be secondary hyperplasia and chronic inflammation of the synovium. In contrast to rheumatoid arthritis, the synovial inflammation is a secondary finding rather than the etiologic event and is milder. There is no pannus formation in osteoarthritis.

A Charcot joint is secondary to any loss of neural function and results in severe osteoarthritis and deformity from unawareness of pain over a period of years. Ischemia, often secondary to diabetes, is a common cause of Charcot joints.

In contrast to osteoarthritis, in rheumatoid arthritis, the etiology is primary inflammation of the synovial lining, resulting in a pannus which attacks the articular cartilage and may erode into the capsule. There may be secondary chronic inflammation in the subchondral bone. Rheumatoid arthritis is also a diagnosis made primarily by clinical and radiographic criteria (and also by the presence of serologic evidence of autoantibodies or rheumatoid factor), and the pathologist rarely makes a contribution. Even in those cases in which the pannus is biopsied or resected for therapeutic purposes, the pathologist will be unable to see the actual attack of the synovium on the cartilage, but rather will simply see pronounced synovial hyperplasia, usually with a papillary architecture, along with an intense lymphoplasmacytic infiltrate i3.3. Only very rarely does the pathologist see the actual attack of the pannus on the articular cartilage i3.4. About 20% of patients with rheumatoid arthritis will have rheumatoid nodules, areas of necrosis surrounded by inflammatory cells, either in the synovium or in extrasynovial sites.

Osteonecrosis

Osteonecrosis is not a specific diagnosis. It has numerous causes, including ischemia (clinically, avascular necrosis), trauma, infection (osteomyelitis), sickle cell disease, and steroid use. Osteonecrosis is a pathological diagnosis whose etiology can only be determined by clinical and radiographic correlation. Osteonecrosis of any etiology is characterized by fragments of devitalized bone, called sequestrum. Sequestrum lacks osteoblasts in lacunae and often has a fragmented, "moth-eaten" appearance i3.5. Sequestrum is surrounded by new bone called involucrum. However, osteonecrosis can often be diagnosed more readily and with greater sensitivity by fibrosis and fat necrosis of the marrow i3.6. If the diagnosis is based on finding fat necrosis in the marrow, the differential diagnosis is serous atrophy, which is characterized by a gelatinous, amorphous extracellular material in the bone marrow, seen in patients with cachexia of any cause (often in AIDS patients). Serous atrophy does not indicate osteonecrosis.

The terms "osteonecrosis" and "osteomyelitis" are often used synonymously and may overlap in the sense that osteonecrosis of any cause is likely to be accompanied by some degree of inflammation. Likewise, in chronic osteomyelitis, long-standing infection and inflammation are likely to result in at least focal osteonecrosis. More correctly, however, osteomyelitis refers to osteonecrosis that is caused by an inflammatory process, often secondary to an infectious agent. As is the case for osteonecrosis of any etiology, the findings in the marrow are often more diagnostic than those in the trabeculae. In acute osteomyelitis, mature neutrophils are seen in the marrow in far greater numbers than usual and to the exclusion of other marrow elements. In chronic osteomyelitis, the same is true for lymphocytes and plasma cells i3.7. The histologic diagnosis of osteomyelitis—an inflammatory cause of osteonecrosis—should be made with caution if there is a clinical history of fracture or radiographic evidence of avascular necrosis, as the history and radiographic findings suggest a specific alternative cause for the osteonecrosis.

Metabolic Bone and Joint Disease

Paget disease (osteitis deformans) is rarely biopsied because the diagnosis is established by clinical and radiographic criteria. In the early stages, there is a combination of osteoblastic and osteoclastic activity, with a hypervascular stroma. The bony trabeculae are disorganized, and the collagenous matrix is also disordered, resulting in woven bone. Later stages have a more fibrotic stroma, with less activity of osteoblasts and osteoclasts i3.8. There is thickened, relatively inactive bone with jagged cement lines [PMID14676639].

Most, but not all patients with gout have hyperuricemia, and the kidney is almost always affected. Deposits in the joint may erode into bone i3.9a, i3.9b. Because uric acid crystals are water soluble and will largely dissolve in processing, their distinction from calcium pyrophosphate crystals (clinically causing pseudogout) can be challenging. If present in sufficient numbers after processing, urate crystals form gouty tophi that are pale on H&E and appear as needle-shaped crystals in polarized light i3.9c, while calcium pyrophosphate is deeply basophilic on H&E i3.10 and consists of rhomboid crystals in polarized light i3.11. It is helpful to roll the fresh tissue on a slide and examine it under polarized light before placing the tissue in fixative.

Another form of crystal deposition is calcium hydroxyapatite, which is seen in metastatic calcification (secondary to metabolic abnormalities), dystrophic calcification (secondary to tissue damage), and tumoral calcinosis (a rare condition of unknown etiology, but associated with elevated phosphate levels).

One of the exciting developments in bone pathology is improved treatment for osteoporosis. Beyond a reasonable calcium intake, increased calcium does not prevent osteoporosis. Estrogens have been disappointing when used for this purpose. Exercise is beneficial, but a series of drugs shows great promise.

Bisphosphonates are analogues of pyrophosphate that bind to the hydroxyapatite matrix of bone. When taken up by osteoclasts, bisphosphonates inhibit osteoclast enzymes that require pyrophosphate, reducing the effectiveness of the bone resorptive pathway [PMID21258058]. There are 4 bisphosphonates currently approved: alendronate (Fosamax), etidronate (Didrocal), risedronate (Actonel), and zoledronic acid (Reclast). The last of these can be given once a year intravenously. Bisphosphonates are also used in some metabolic diseases of bone, such as Paget disease, and in osteolytic bone metastases. A newer treatment, promising but still under evaluation, is Denosunab, a monoclonal antibody to a protein called RANKL (receptor activator of NFκB ligand) [PMID22688622].

Another class of drugs showing promise is based on an increased understanding of the interplay between osteoblasts and osteoclasts. Osteoblasts secrete 2 proteins that lead to an increase in osteoclasts, providing negative feedback on themselves. The first of these stimulates macrophage proliferation. The second is RANKL that binds to the receptor activator of NFκB (RANK) on macrophages and stimulates a transcription factor called NFκB. Increased activity of NFκB facilitates macrophage differentiation into osteoclasts. A monoclonal antibody that binds to and inhibits RANKL shows promise in the treatment for osteoporosis [PMID20872215].

Masses and Neoplasms of Bones and Joints

Synovial chondromatosis, osteochondritis dessicans, and loose bodies are commonly encountered conditions that may clinically simulate a neoplasm. Synovial chondromatosis is the formation of cartilage, sometimes with bone, within the synovium i3.12. These bodies may occasionally be extruded into the joint space. Osteochondritis dessicans is a separation of a fragment of cartilage from subchondral bone. The fragment may or may not completely detach. "Loose bodies" is a general term for any unattached cartilaginous or bony fragment in the joint space. Many loose bodies are secondary to synovial chondromatosis or osteochondritis dessicans, but other causes include detached osteophytes and damaged menisci.

Location and Radiographic Appearance Are Indispensable in the Diagnosis of Bone and Joint Masses

There are 2 imperatives in the diagnosis of bone masses. The first is that specific entities tend to have specific locations. For example, one would almost never diagnosis an osteosarcoma

ISBN 978-089189-5886

in the hand because a reactive periostitis is far more likely. The second is that radiographic correlation is essential. While the pathologist can no longer be expected to personally and expertly review the radiographic studies, she or he should confer with the radiologist and reach a diagnosis that is reasonable to both specialists.

The localized form of giant cell tumor of tendon sheath (also called nodular tenosynovitis), is a commonly encountered benign neoplasm, usually small and encapsulated, usually occurring in the hand, and characterized by scattered giant cells in a fibrous background. The tendon sheath fibroma lacks giant cells, but is probably a variant of the localized giant cell tumor of tendon sheath [PMID7777476].

There is a more pronounced and generalized process that primarily affects the knees, hips, and ankles and appears to be related to the localized giant cell tumor of tendon sheath, but the terminology of this process can be confusing. When confined to the synovium, it is often called pigmented villonodular synovitis (PVNS), a benign, but potentially locally aggressive neoplasm. PVNS exhibits papillary synovial hyperplasia, marked chronic inflammation, hemosiderin deposition, and giant cells **i3.13a**, **i3.13b**. It often requires synoviectomy and is prone to local recurrence, but the ultimate prognosis is good. The extra-articular form, in a bursa or a tendon sheath, is generally called diffuse tenosynovial giant cell tumor and is the diffuse counterpart of the localized giant cell tumor of tendon sheath [PMID18794322, PMID10757395]. Unlike the localized form of giant cell tumor of tendon sheath, the diffuse form is not encapsulated and tends to occur in younger adults [Weiss ISBN978-0323046282]. Abnormalities of the short arm of chromosome 1 have been shown in some cases [PMID10392632].

PVNS/diffuse tenosynovial giant cell tumor often has hemosiderin macrophages but is distinguished from bleeding secondary to such entities as hemophilia by the clinical history and presentation, and by the presence of numerous giant cells. Although osteoarthritis and rheumatoid arthritis may have synovial inflammation and villous hyperplasia, these are more pronounced in PVNS/diffuse tenosynovial giant cell tumor. Synovial reactions in osteoarthritis usually do not have giant cells, and neither type of arthritis has the striking combination of inflammation, hemosiderin, synovial hyperplasia, and giant cells that is characteristic of PVNS/diffuse tenosynovial giant cell tumor.

Hematologic neoplasms of bone are discussed in Chapter 10. Some bone tumors occur more often in soft tissue and are discussed there. Here, only a few brief comments about intraosseous masses that are either likely to be encountered in general practice or are often misunderstood will be made. For a much more detailed discussion including chondrosarcomas, osteosarcomas, their variant forms and their mimics, the World Health Organization, whose numerous classifications are becoming the gold standard in many body sites and are referred to throughout this work, considers bone tumors in the same volume as soft tissue neoplasms [Fletcher ISBN978-9283224136].

The aneurysmal bone cyst (ABC) develops in young people, often in the long bones or in the vertebra. The ABC has a cellular stroma, with many giant cells and dilated vessels **i3.14a**, **i3.14b**. It may resemble a giant cell tumor of bone or a telangiectatic osteosarcoma, but there will not be generalized significant nuclear atypia [PMID140511]. The nature of the ABC is unclear. Historically, it has been regarded as a reactive lesion of unknown etiology, but many different translocations have been described, all of which activate the ubiquitin-specific protease-6 (*USP6*) gene on chromosome 17p13 by placing it next to an active promoter [PMID15026324, PMID15735689, PMID16382110]. The product of *USP6* is involved in the remodeling of actin microfilaments [PMID12612085]. While the mechanism by which *USP6* upregulation leads to ABC is unclear, the strong association of translocations involving a specific gene with the ABC suggests that at least some cases may be neoplastic.

The unicameral (also called simple or solitary) bone cyst is also primarily seen in the long bones of young people. Its lining may have a few giant cells, but is much simpler and less cellular than that of an ABC.

The giant cell tumor of bone consists of 3 cell types—mononuclear stromal cells that are the neoplastic component, mononuclear histiocytic cells that appear to be recruited to and not involved in the origin of the lesion, and multinuclear giant cells **i3.15a**, **i3.15b** [PMID17013643]. The giant cells in the giant cell tumor of bone are the most conspicuous cell type but are benign osteoclast-like cells, thought to be formed from the fusion of the mononuclear macrophages that have migrated into the lesion. The mononuclear stromal cells are the neoplastic component, and although they are of unclear nature, they are mesenchymal, not hematopoietic. Indeed, since it is well established that the giant cells are not the neoplastic component, it has been suggested that the name of the tumor be changed [PMID15612014]. The behavior of the giant cell tumor of bone is notoriously unpredictable, and no reliable histologic prognostic criteria have been developed.

The conventional chondrosarcoma of bone is usually not a diagnostic difficulty and is not discussed here other than to caution that a chondroid variant of osteosarcoma must be excluded. 2 benign tumors that can mimic chondrosarcoma are the chondromyxoid fibroma and the chondroblastoma. Radiographic findings are central, as the chondromyxoid fibroma and the chondroblastoma tend to be circumscribed, while chondrosarcomas are not. A histologic clue to a chondromyxoid fibroma is lobules of chondromyxoid material separated by fibrous stroma with occasional giant cells. They may have mild nuclear atypia, and often occur in the tibia [PMID15612014].

The term "chondroblastoma" was coined by Jaffe and Lichtenstein in 1942 [PMID19970672]. The chondroblastoma occurs mostly in the second decade, primarily in the long bones (often in the tibia) and is often painful. It has a mixture of relatively bland mononuclear and giant cells, as well as foci of cartilage. There is calcification between cells that has a "chicken wire" appearance **i3.16** [PMID7332302]. The chondromyxoid fibroma is characterized by lobules of tumor cells, in a myxochondroid matrix, separated by a fibrous stroma **i3.17**. The chondroblastoma and the chondromyxoid fibroma deserve consideration whenever a lesion in or around bone appears to be a low-grade chondrosarcoma but is histologically circumscribed or radiographically benign.

The mesenchymal chondrosarcoma and the dedifferentiated chondrosarcoma are unusual entities that occur in bone and occasionally in soft tissue, and should not be confused with a poorly differentiated chondrosarcoma. Poorly differentiated chondrosarcomas have high-grade nuclei *throughout their extent* i3.18, without a dimorphic appearance. If they have areas that do not form cartilage, they have the same high-grade nuclei in those areas as in the cartilaginous areas. Mesenchymal chondrosarcomas and dedifferentiated chondrosarcomas, on the other hand, have cartilage that appears benign or like a low-grade chondrosarcoma, along with a high-grade noncartilaginous component i3.19.

The principal distinction between the mesenchymal chondrosarcoma and a dedifferentiated chondrosarcoma is the nature of the noncartilaginous component. In the mesenchymal chondrosarcoma, the noncartilaginous component has the appearance of a hemangiopericytoma i3.20 or a small cell carcinoma i3.21 and there is usually a hemangiopericytoma vascular pattern. A dedifferentiated chondrosarcoma is characterized by a low-grade cartilaginous tumor that transitions abruptly into a high-grade sarcoma that has the appearance of an undifferentiated pleomorphic sarcoma/malignant fibrous histiocytoma i3.22. A mesenchymal chondrosarcoma and a dedifferentiated chondrosarcoma should be considered whenever a tumor has a dimorphic population, with a component of benign-appearing or low-grade malignant cartilage and a second component of much higher grade. If there are high-grade nuclei everywhere, without a lower-grade component, the tumor is more likely to be a poorly differentiated chondrosarcoma or another sarcoma with chondroid metaplasia, such as an osteosarcoma or a nerve sheath tumor, than either a mesenchymal chondrosarcoma or a dedifferentiated chondrosarcoma.

Little will be said of the conventional osteosarcoma because it is usually not a diagnostic dilemma, and only 3 points will be made. First, there are several reactive conditions that are easily confused with osteosarcoma. The diagnosis of osteosarcoma should be made with great care in the hands and feet because fibro-osseous pseudotumor (reactive periostitis) is common in these locations and may have a histologic appearance that is very alarming i3.23. Bizarre parosteal osteochondromatous proliferation of bone (BPOP; also called Nora lesion) is another benign condition with alarming histology, occurring primarily in the hands and feet i3.24, that can easily be confused with an osteosarcoma, especially of the parosteal type [PMID11779053].

The differential diagnosis for a well differentiated osteosarcoma also includes fibrous dysplasia. In addition to the absence of significant nuclear atypia in fibrous dysplasia, its disorganized trabeculae are referred to as "fishhook" or "Chinese characters" i3.25. If this differential diagnosis is particularly difficult, it may help to recall that fibrous dysplasia is associated with a specific mutation in the *GNAS* gene [PMID21354047].

A healing fracture, with pronounced osteoblastic reactive atypia, can simulate a well differentiated osteosarcoma so perfectly that only radiographic and clinical correlation can prevent a serious diagnostic error i3.26a, i3.26b.

Second, there are unusual forms of osteosarcoma that can be confused with other entities. The parosteal osteosarcoma is a type of well differentiated osteosarcoma that has long arrays of reasonably normal bony trabeculae in a fibrous stroma. In a parosteal osteosarcoma, cellularity and nuclear atypia are usually minimal i3.27a or moderate i3.27b, but may rarely be more pronounced i3.27c. The parosteal osteosarcoma is not to be confused with the periosteal type of osteosarcoma, which is a higher grade tumor that is largely cartilaginous.

The telangiectatic variant of osteosarcoma is characterized by dilated vascular spaces, containing blood, lined by malignant cells that produce osteoid i3.28 [PMID6950802]. This form of osteosarcoma may be subtle and can resemble an aneurysmal bone cyst i3.29a. Again, radiographic and clinical correlations are indispensable, but the key histologic feature in the distinction of a telangiectatic variant of osteosarcoma from benign mimics is the increased cellularity and nuclear atypia that is focally present in the cells lining the spaces i3.29b.

Third, osteosarcomas are often treated with neoadjuvant radiation or chemotherapy, in which case after resection, the pathologist is called upon to evaluate the effect of this therapy. Effective neoadjuvant therapy may cause partial i3.30 or nearly complete i3.31 necrosis of the tumor and the osteoid it produces.

Core Points for Bone and Joint

- Evaluation of masses of bones and joints requires rigorous correlation with the location and the radiographic findings.
- Osteoarthritis: diagnosed by clinical and radiographic findings.
- Rheumatoid arthritis: diagnosed by clinical and radiographic findings with a positive rheumatoid factor or antinuclear antibody.
- Metabolic diseases of bone and joint: diagnosed by clinical and laboratory findings, though the pathologist can confirm deposition of urate or calcium pyrophosphate crystals.
- Osteonecrosis: often best diagnosed in the marrow.
  - Cause usually cannot be determined by morphology alone.
  - Osteomyelitis is an infectious/inflammatory cause of osteonecrosis.
- Cytogenetics is becoming important.
  - Translocations of the ubiquitin-specific protease-6 (*USP6*) gene on chromosome 17p13 in the aneurysmal bone cyst.
  - Activating mutations in the *GNAS* gene in fibrous dysplasia.

ISBN 978-089189-5886

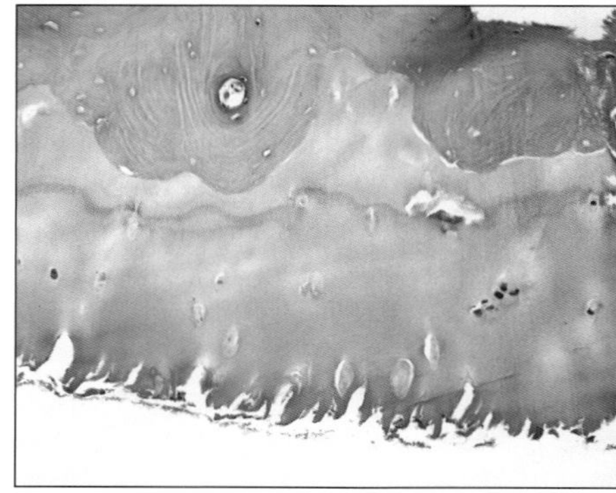

i3.1 Early osteoarthritis with fibrillation of the articular cartilage

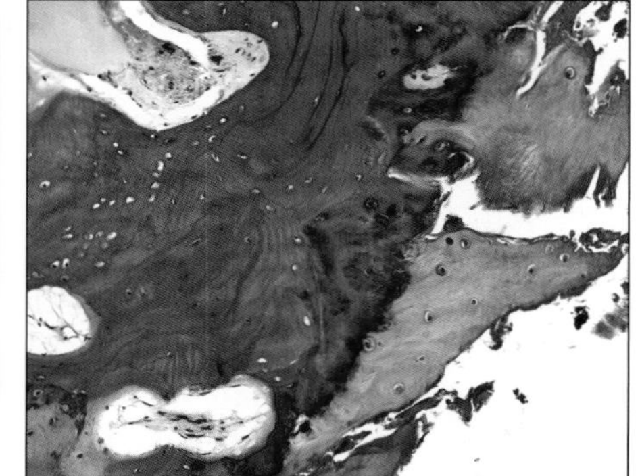

i3.2 Well developed osteoarthritis with eburnation of the subchondral bone. Note the irregular cement lines of the bone. This photograph also illustrates the tide mark, which is an area of calcification of the articular cartilage that is immediately adjacent to the bone.

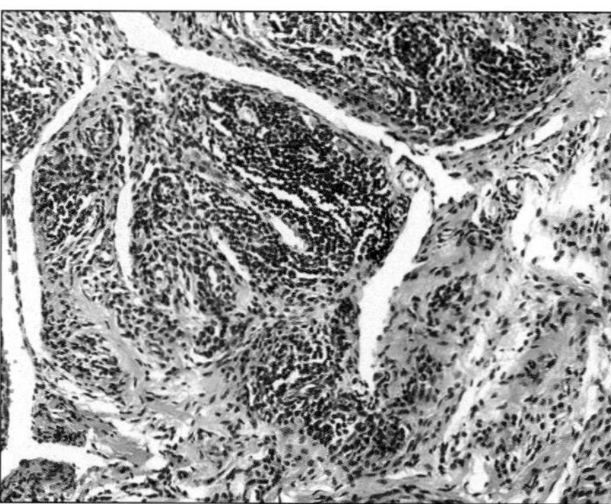

i3.3 A pannus with an intense lymphoplasmacytic inflammatory infiltrate

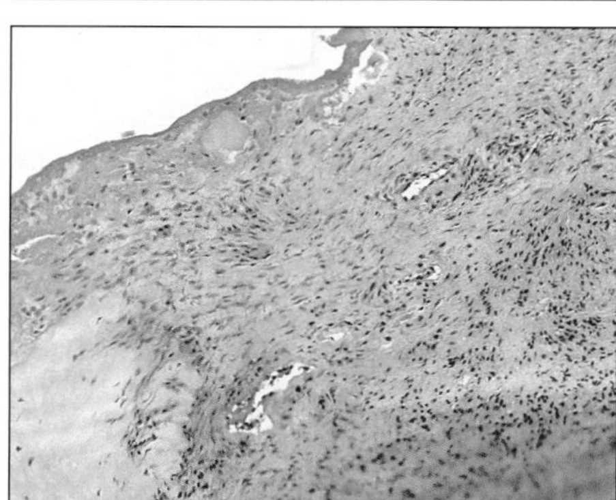

i3.4 A pannus attacking articular cartilage.

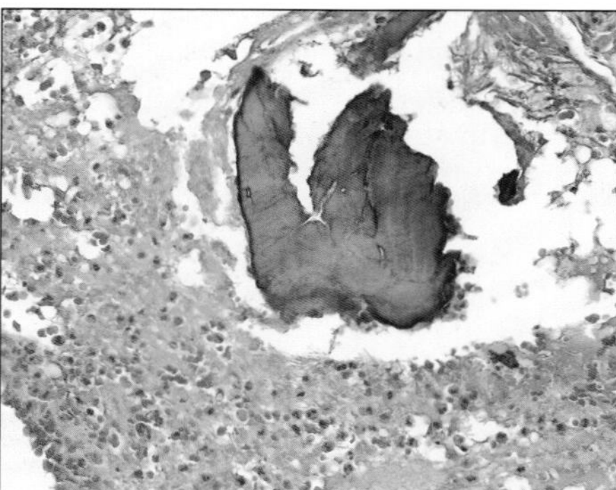

i3.5 A fragment of devitalized bone in osteonecrosis. Note the "moth-eaten" appearance and the lack of osteoblasts in lacunae.

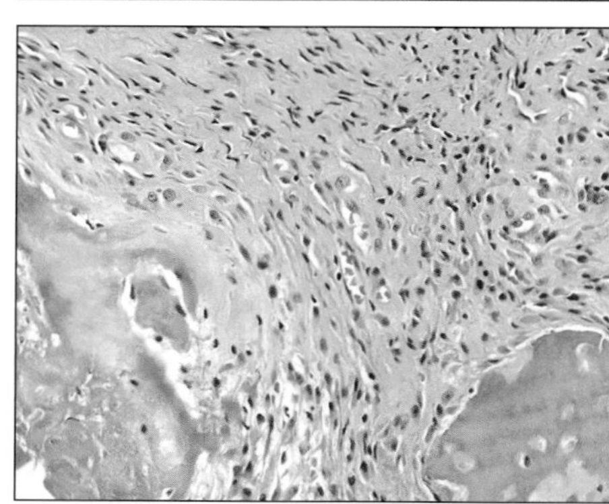

i3.6 Osteonecrosis. There are 2 devitalized trabeculae of bone in the lower portion, but note also the fibrosis of the bone marrow.

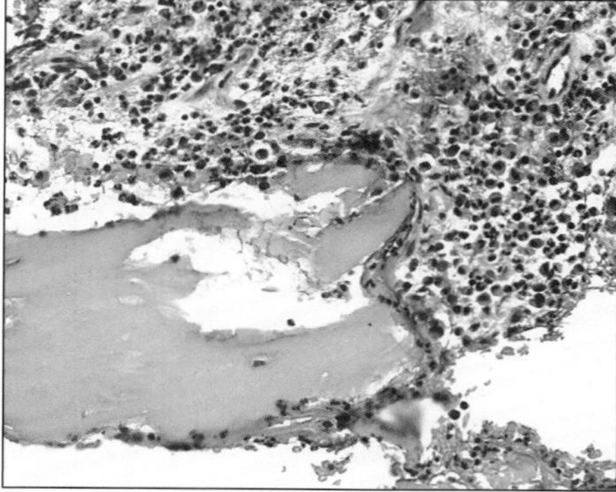

i3.7 Acute and chronic osteomyelitis with inflammatory cells surrounding a fragment of devitalized bone

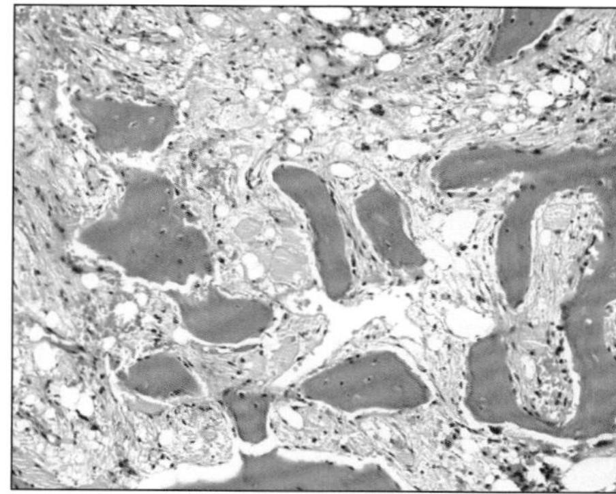

i3.8 Late-stage Paget disease with a fibrotic stroma and disorganized, woven bone

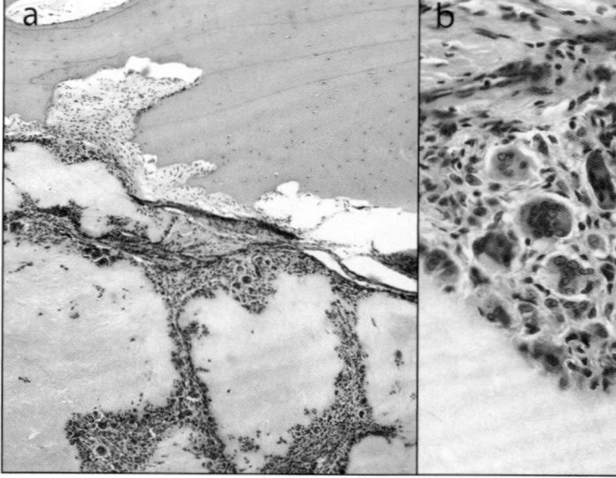

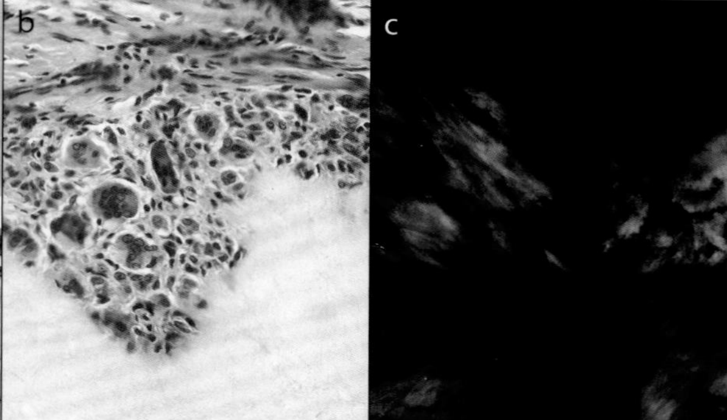

i3.9 **a** Deposition of uric acid crystals (gout) in the bone, eroding bony trabeculae
b A higher power view of the same process as in i3.9a. The uric acid crystals have largely dissolved out, but the giant cell reaction to them is readily seen. Sometimes, enough of the uric acid crystals remain after processing to be recognized as a gouty tophus.

c Uric acid crystals, with their characteristic needle configuration, seen under polarized light

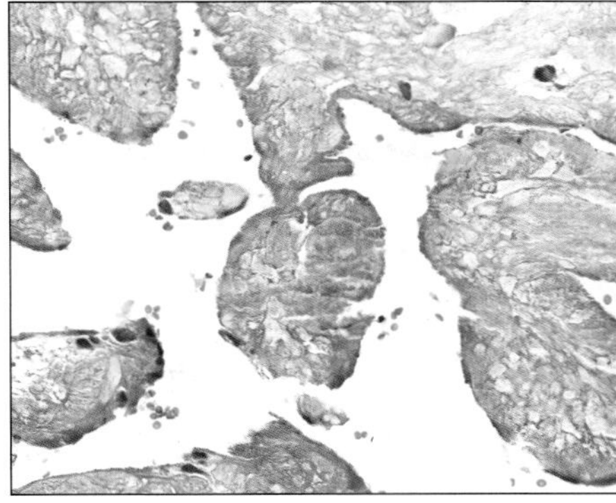

i3.10 The basophilic deposits that are characteristic of calcium pyrophosphate

i3.11 The rhomboid crystals of calcium pyrophosphate, seen under polarized light

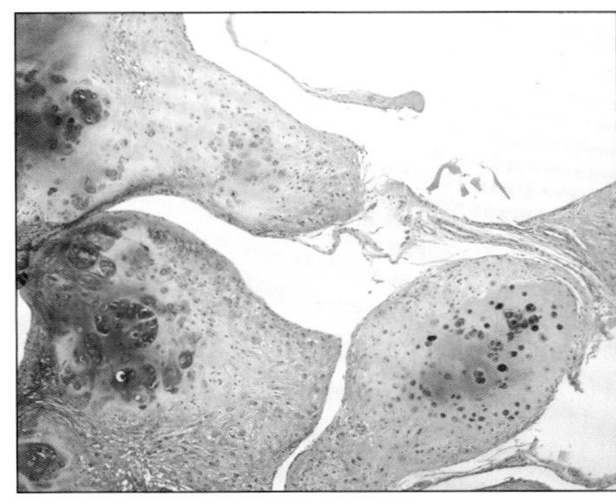

i3.12 Synovial chondromatosis, with metaplastic cartilage within synovial tissue

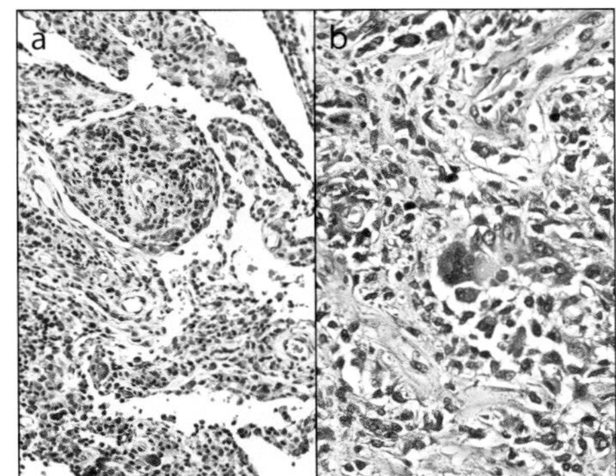

i3.13 **a** Pigmented villonodular synovitis, with synovial hyperplasia, chronic inflammation, and hemosiderin deposition **b** Pigmented villonodular synovitis with hemosiderin, chronic inflammation and giant cells

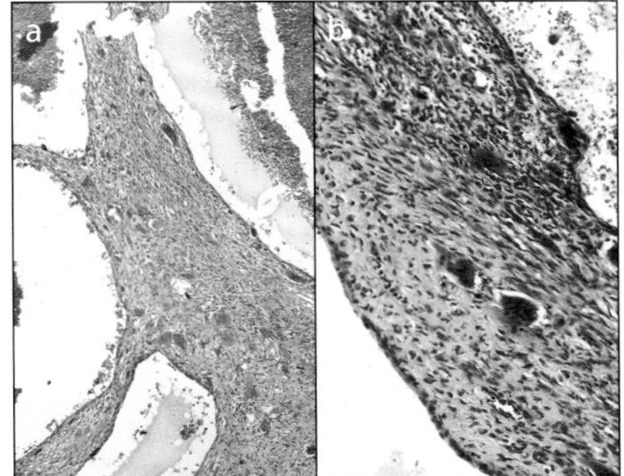

i3.14 **a** An aneurysmal bone cyst (ABC) with dilated blood-filled spaces separated by fibrous septae with giant cells **b** A higher power view of an ABC, illustrating the giant cells, fibroblasts, and chronic inflammatory cells that are characteristic of the septae in an ABC

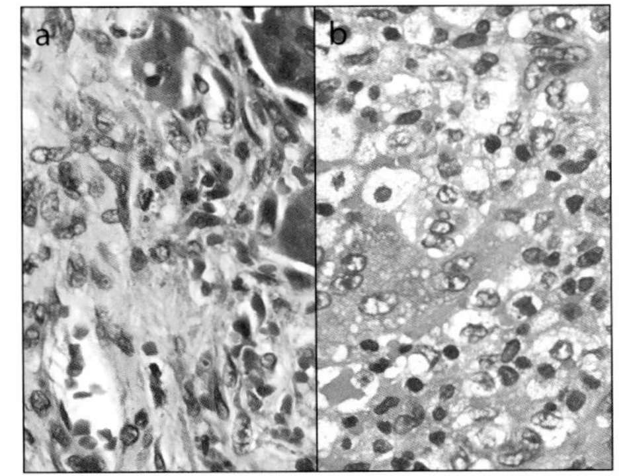

i3.15 **a** A giant cell tumor of bone, illustrating the greater pleomorphism of the nuclei in the mononuclear cells (left) relative to the more uniform and innocuous nuclei in the giant cells (right) **b** A giant cell tumor of bone illustrating the histiocytes that give rise to the nonneoplastic giant cells. Note the innocuous nuclei relative to the neoplastic mononuclear cells in i3.15a.

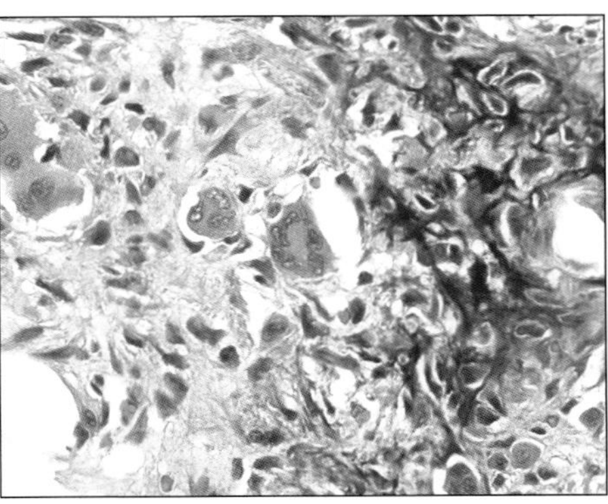

i3.16 A chondroblastoma with giant cells and a "chicken wire" pattern of calcification

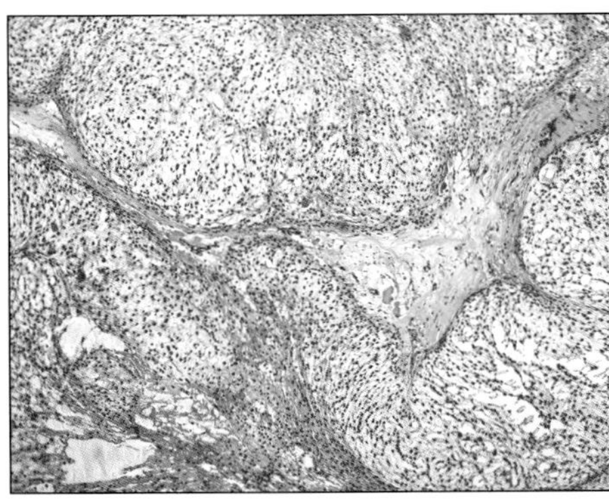

i3.17 A low-power view of a chondromyxoid fibroma illustrating the multinodular architecture

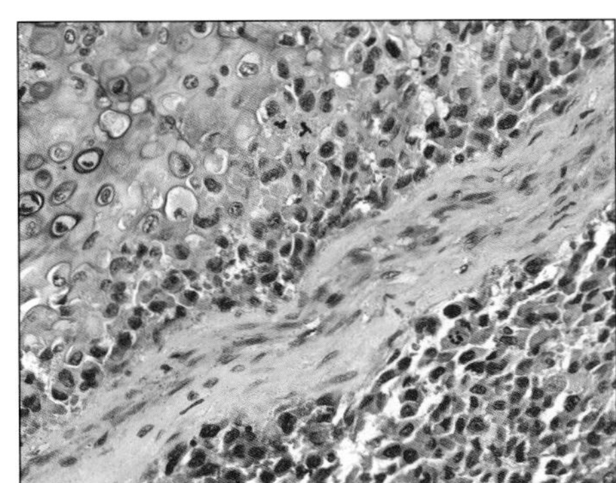

i3.18 A poorly differentiated chondrosarcoma with pleomorphic nuclei in the areas that form cartilage (upper left) as well as in the areas that do not (lower right). Note the tripolar mitotic figure in the cartilaginous area.

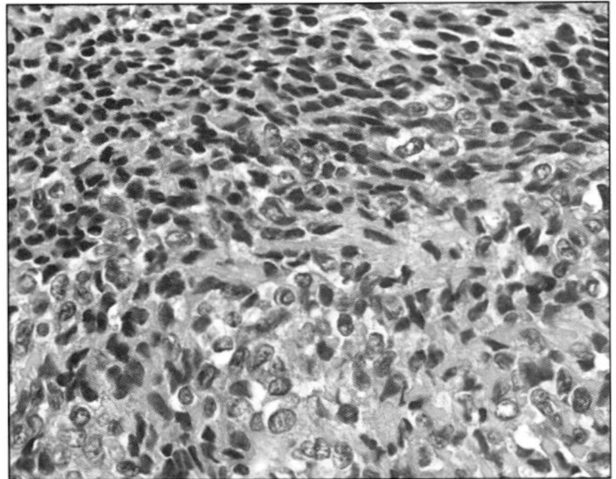

i3.19 A mesenchymal chondrosarcoma. Note the different nuclear morphologies in the cartilaginous area at the bottom and the noncartilaginous area at the top.

ISBN 978-089189-5886

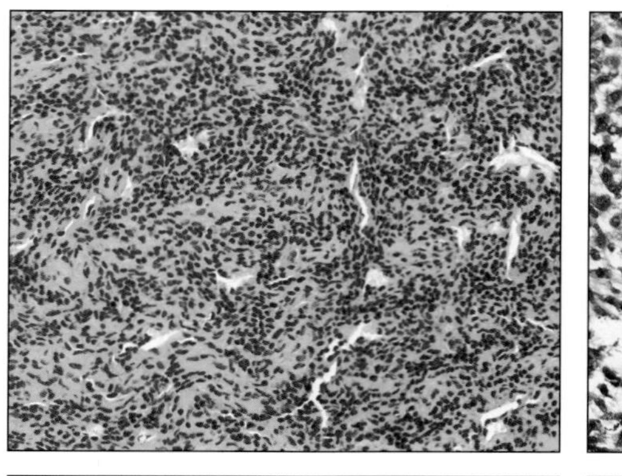

i3.20 The noncartilaginous area of a mesenchymal chondrosarcoma with a hemangiopericytoma-like appearance

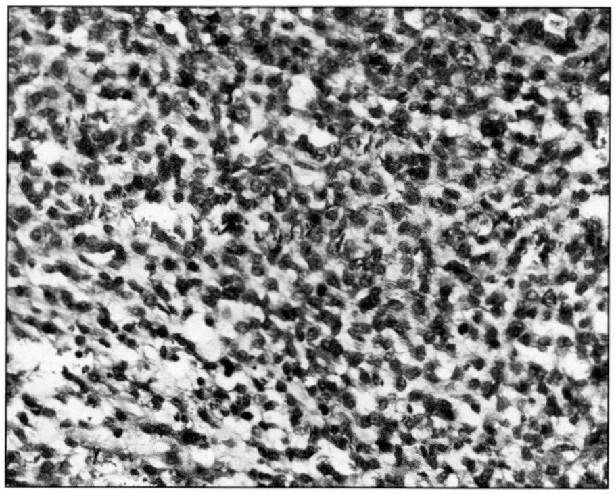

i3.21 The noncartilaginous area of a mesenchymal chondrosarcoma with a small cell carcinoma appearance

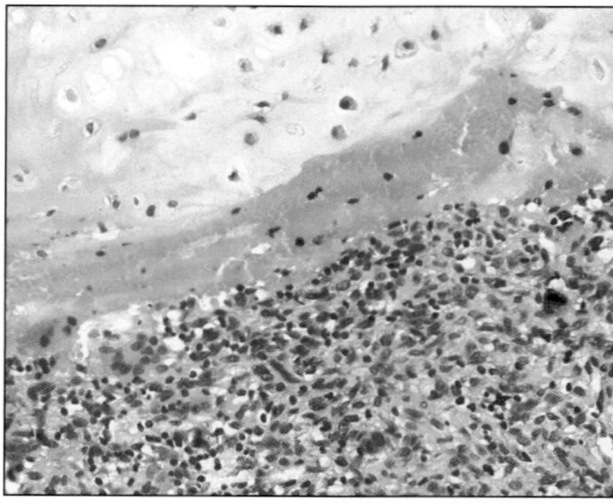

i3.22 A dedifferentiated chondrosarcoma. In the upper left, the appearance is that of a well differentiated chondrosarcoma or possibly even a benign chondroma, but in the lower right, the appearance is that of a high-grade sarcoma.

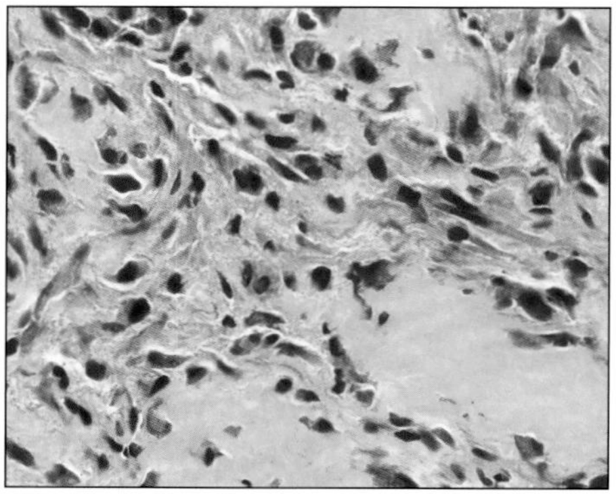

i3.23 Reactive periostitis. Note the alarming atypia and osteoid, which can easily result in an incorrect diagnosis of osteosarcoma. In addition to the location and radiographic findings, an additional reassuring feature is that many of the atypical cells have eccentric nuclei, a feature of osteoblasts.

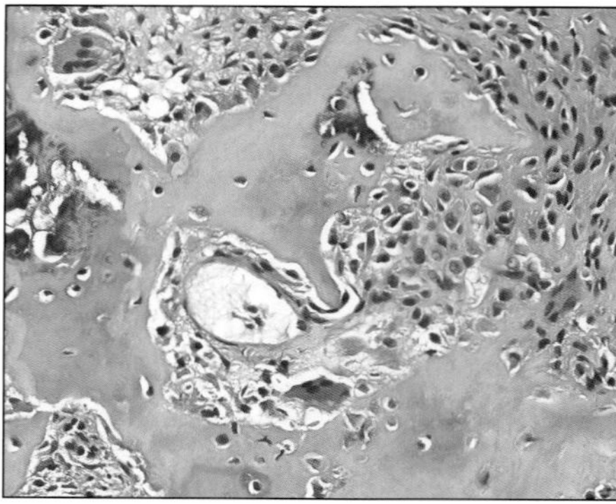

i3.24 Bizarre parosteal osteochondromatous proliferation of bone-simulating osteosarcoma

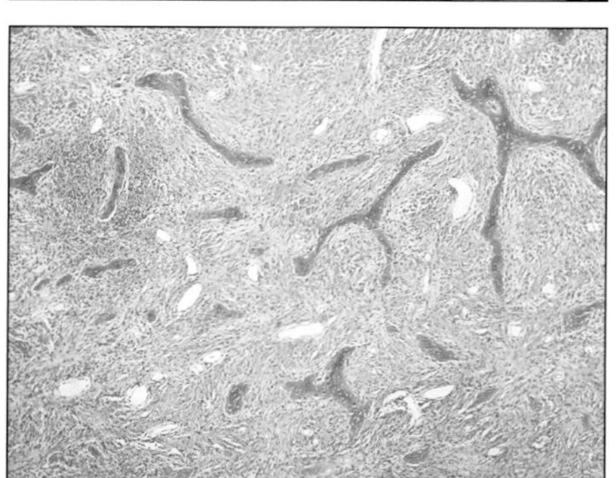

i3.25 Fibrous dysplasia, with disorganized trabeculae, consisting of woven bone with a "fish hook" or "Chinese characters" appearance

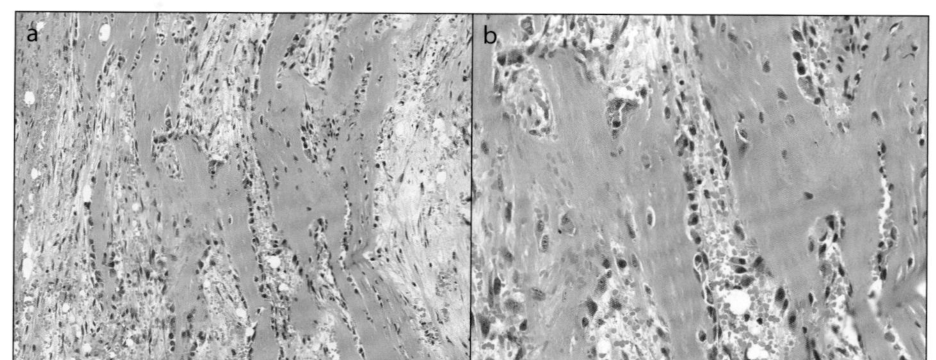

i3.26 **a** A healing fracture in a femoral head. There is extensive, confluent osteoblastic hyperplasia.

b A higher-power view of the same case as in i3.26a, highlighting the increased cellularity and reactive atypia that simulates a well differentiated osteosarcoma. A helpful feature is that some of the osteoblasts maintain an eccentric nucleus, as seen in the center.

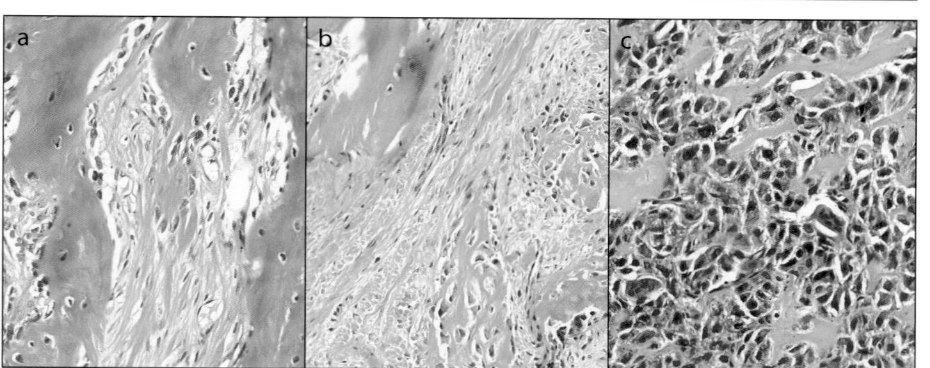

i3.27 **a** A well differentiated parosteal osteosarcoma. Note the alternating osteoid and fibrous tissue, with deceptively minimal atypia.

b A parosteal osteosarcoma that is more cellular and less differentiated than in i3.27a.

c A parosteal osteosarcoma with obviously increased cellularity and significant nuclear atypia

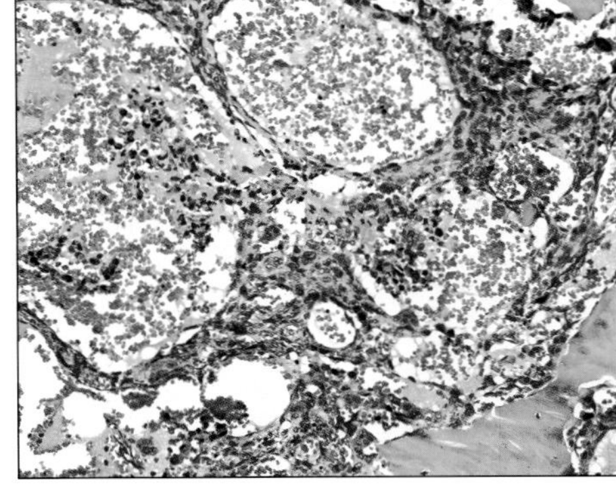

i3.28 A telangiectatic variant of osteosarcoma, with dilated, blood-filled spaces, separated by stroma containing malignant cells, simulating an aneurysmal bone cyst

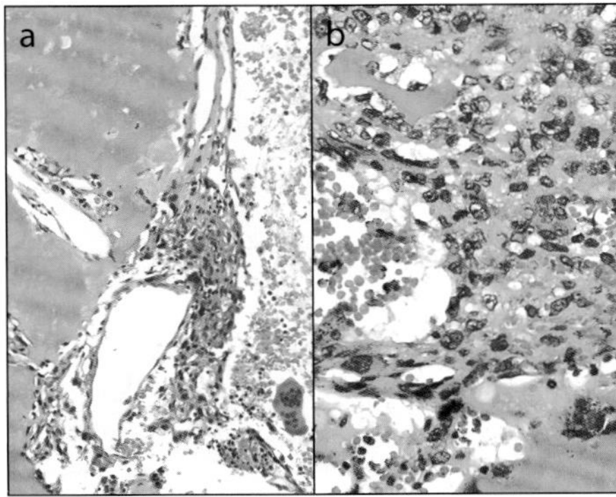

i3.29 **a** Another telangiectatic osteosarcoma closely simulating an aneurysmal bone cyst.
b A telangiectatic osteosarcoma with increased cellularity

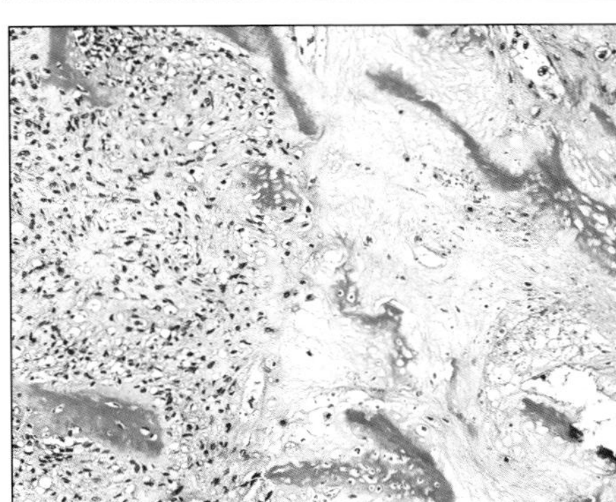

i3.30 An osteosarcoma resected after neoadjuvant radiation and chemotherapy, with partial tumor necrosis evident on the right

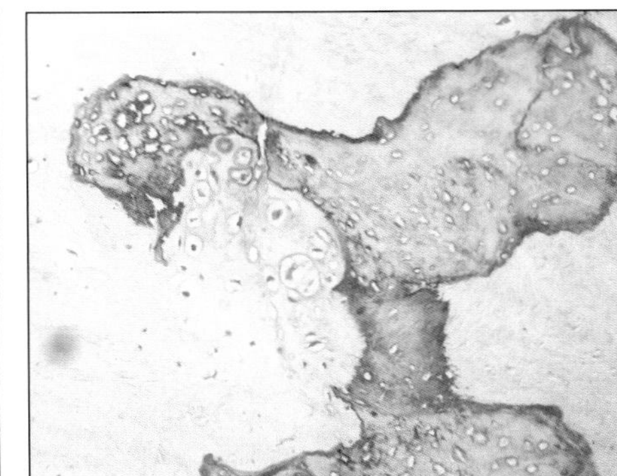

i3.31 An osteosarcoma resected after neoadjuvant radiation and chemotherapy with complete necrosis of the neoplastic cells and the osteoid they produced

ISBN 978-089189-5886

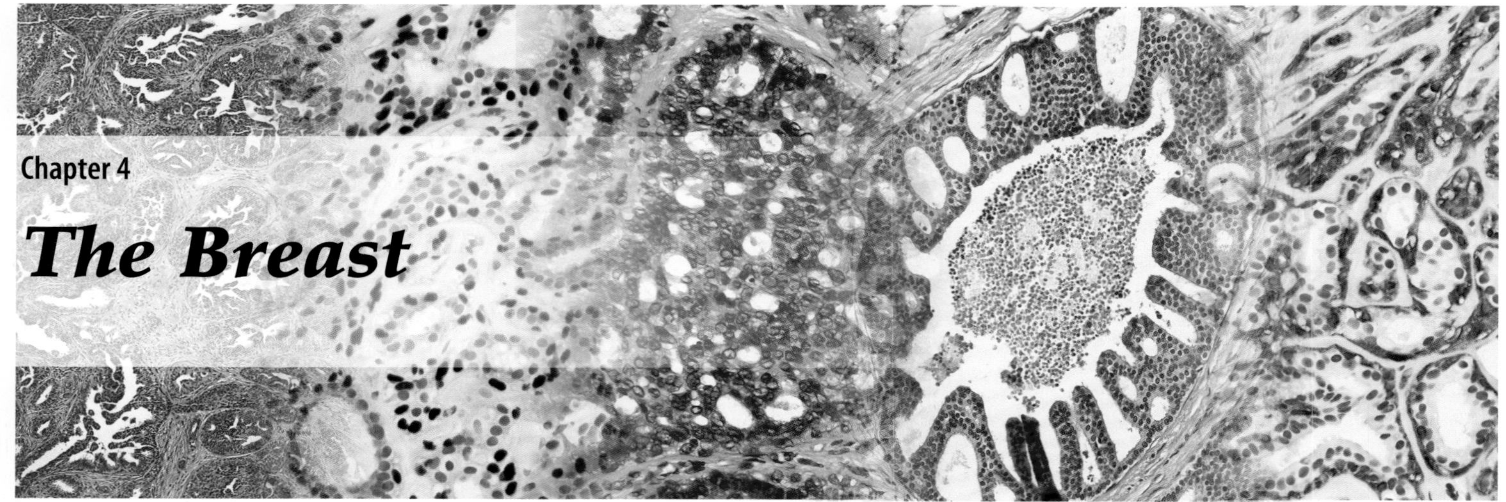

Chapter 4

The Breast

Benign Processes That Mimic Invasive Carcinoma

The most common benign simulator of breast cancer is adenosis. Adenosis exists in both a localized and generalized or florid form. The localized form has a cellular proliferation of acini, often accompanied by stromal cells, and frequently has a low-power "whorled" appearance i4.1. The florid form has multiple such nodules, often with coalescence, that may result in a clinically distinct mass i4.2. Because the proliferation and crowding of lobules in florid adenosis distorts the normal lobular architecture, it may resemble infiltrating carcinoma. The diagnosis of carcinoma—even a minute focus of carcinoma—should be made with caution when it is within or adjacent to an area of adenosis. A helpful feature is that a focus may appear to be infiltrative at high power, but at lower power, it seems more circumscribed. If a putatively invasive area is encircled in the imagination and has a fundamentally smooth contour, a diagnosis of florid adenosis may be more appropriate. Very close examination of the nuclei in this area will disclose that they are smaller than in most cases of carcinoma, even lobular carcinoma.

The distinction of florid adenosis from carcinoma is particularly challenging on a thin needle biopsy, which unlike a mammotome, affords little opportunity to appreciate the retained lobular architecture of adenosis. Indeed, on a needle biopsy, florid adenosis may so strongly resemble carcinoma that immunohistochemical stains are not even thought to be necessary to support a malignant diagnosis. Thin needle biopsies of cellular benign breast masses are a trap in waiting i4.3. In these biopsies, where the overall architecture and circumscription cannot be assessed, the presence of a myoepithelial layer underneath the epithelium strongly suggests a benign process. Myoepithelial cells have small, often spindled nuclei and generally clear cytoplasm, but they may be indistinct on H&E, and immunohistochemical stains may be needed. Nuclear staining for p63 i4.4 and cytoplasmic staining for calponin i4.5, actin, or myosin heavy chain are often used to demonstrate a myoepithelial layer [PMID16575508, PMID21263240]. Low molecular weight cytokeratins 5/6 (CK5/6) are also used as cytoplasmic stains for myoepithelial cells. While CK5/6 is well established in the identification of a basal layer in the prostate and may work well in the breast, to my mind, these low molecular weight keratins are problematic for myoepithelial cells in the breast because some breast cancers (called basal-type) are well known to express these 2 keratins. Whatever stains are used, in evaluating these stains, it should be remembered that the normal myoepithelial layer is discontinuous. A well formed myoepithelial layer is a strong point for a benign process, but the inability to demonstrate a continuous myoepithelial layer in a small problematic focus does not prove invasion.

The greatest challenge in biopsies of benign, cellular breast lesions is to appreciate the need to obtain immunohistochemical stains. The clues that an apparent carcinoma may contain myoepithelial cells and requires immunohistochemical stains to exclude a benign lesion include:

1. The apparent infiltration of clusters of cells with any indication of a dimorphic population, such as cells on the periphery that have clear cytoplasm or smaller uniform nuclei
2. The apparent infiltration of glands whose lining is multilayered
3. Infiltration largely as rounded clusters, as neoplastic glands tend to be flattened or misshapen, while those of adenosis are usually more rounded
4. Infiltration by cells with clear cytoplasm or small, spindled nuclei
5. The absence of an in situ component

The demonstration of an intact, well developed basement membrane by immunohistochemical stains for type 4 collagen and laminin—components of basement membranes—may also be helpful in the distinction of florid adenosis from carcinoma [PMID3817761], though this approach is not used as often as the identification of myoepithelial cells.

The term "apocrine adenosis" has been used in different ways [PMID19147303] and is somewhat confusing, as apocrine metaplasia and adenosis often occur together as part of the spectrum of fibrocystic changes. In apocrine adenosis, there is often myoepithelial hyperplasia in addition to adenosis and apocrine metaplasia, accounting for the alternative name of adenomyoepithelial adenosis. Apocrine adenosis is a combination of adenosis, apocrine metaplasia, and myoepithelial hyperplasia. The difficulty in distinguishing this process from carcinoma may be augmented by the prominent nucleoli of apocrine cells i4.6, but the clue to a benign diagnosis, or the need for immunohistochemical stains, is circumscription i4.7.

The tubular adenoma is rarely specifically diagnosed, but refers to a benign, circumscribed proliferation of innocuous glands whose increased cellularity may simulate an invasive carcinoma i4.8. Its circumscription and innocuous-appearing nuclei usually make immunohistochemical stains unnecessary, but if needed, the identification of myoepithelial cells as described above, is recommended.

Microglandular adenosis (MGA) is an unusual entity that is felt by some to be related to adenosis of the usual type, but by others to be a distinct process that may be an early form of tubular carcinoma because of its apparently infiltrative pattern i4.9. MGA usually (but not always) has only 1 layer of epithelial cells, without a myoepithelial layer. There are eosinophic secretions in the lumens, and the cytoplasm is often clear i4.10. In microglandular adenosis, the glands have an infiltrative pattern, but the nuclei appear benign. If the differential diagnosis is between microglandular adenosis and carcinoma, myoepithelial cells can be sought by immunohistochemistry, as MGA occasionally has a few such cells and their presence is a strong indicator of a benign process, though a negative stain has no meaning. A search for a confluent basement membrane may be informative, as this is retained in microglandular adenosis but is generally lost in invasive carcinoma. Occasionally a periodic acid-Schiff (PAS) stain may sufficiently highlight the basement membrane [PMID19824997], but more often immunohistochemical staining for either collagen type 4 or laminin will be needed [PMID11494007] (immunohistochemical stains are more sensitive and the pink color of a PAS stain blends into the pink color of the background fibrous tissue). In equivocal cases, or situations where the immunohistochemical stains and H&E are not concordant, a diagnosis of atypical MGA can be rendered.

A complex sclerosing lesion (radial scar) usually has a central sclerotic zone with triangular-shaped collections of ducts radiating outward, giving a contracted "purse string" appearance i4.11. In difficult cases, the immunohistochemical demonstration of a myoepithelial layer is a point for a benign process, as is the demonstration of a basement membrane around the problematic glands [PMID3817761].

Special caution must be used in diagnosing carcinoma in the nipple and areola, as this area is the site of several forms of benign proliferative disease, and the areola has sebaceous glands that are related to the lactiferous ducts and that may give rise to skin appendage tumors that can be confused with those arising in the breast parenchyma. The most common diagnostic dilemma in this region is the so-called nipple adenoma, which was elucidated by my teacher, David Jones, in 1955 [PMID14352171] as a florid, cellular, and complex papillomatosis of the nipple ducts, often associated with hyperplasia of the adjacent ducts and increased stromal cellularity i4.12. Although initially worrisome, the appearance is that of an increased number of ducts, each of which has hyperplasia and papillomas, rather than true infiltration, and nuclei are unremarkable.

Nonpapillary Intraductal Proliferations

In assessing intraductal proliferations, it is helpful to first look for nuclear atypia. If this is pronounced, the diagnosis of high-grade ductal carcinoma in situ (DCIS, also called intraductal carcinoma) can be made without consideration of architectural features i4.13. Necrosis is often taken as an additional diagnostic criterion of high-grade DCIS, but it is not a criterion and its significance is simply that it should heighten the search for significant nuclear atypia.

If there is no high-grade nuclear atypia, then *both* a characteristic nuclear morphology and an architectural pattern are needed for the diagnosis of low-grade DCIS. Low-grade intraductal carcinomas of all types are composed of a monomorphic population of cells with relatively uniform, evenly spaced, round nuclei, in one of several recognized growth patterns. In contrast, a benign intraductal proliferation (hyperplasia) is likely to have oval nuclei separated by irregular distances i4.14. If there are secondary lumens, they are irregularly shaped. Hyperplasias are characterized by a process colloquially called "streaming," in which the intraluminal epithelial cells to "run together" in a direction that is more parallel to the wall of the duct than the normal perpendicular arrangement i4.15.

There are several patterns to low-grade DCIS, all of which have cells with rounded, hyperchromatic nuclei, which are paradoxically *more* uniform than in intraductal hyperplasias (possibly reflecting clonal origin). In the cribriform type of low-grade DCIS, the nuclei are more evenly spaced and cytoplasmic boundaries are sharper than in hyperplasias. There is no streaming. It is often said that the spaces are rounder and more sharply defined in DCIS, as if they had been "punched out" by a rounded cookie cutter. This is true, but the real difference between the spaces of hyperplasia and those of cribriforming low-grade DCIS concern the cells around the lumen. In cribriforming low-grade DCIS, the cells are palisaded around the lumen. They have a basal nucleus and apical cytoplasm, resulting in a radial orientation around the lumen i4.16. The result is that in low-grade DCIS, there is a more orderly radial arrangement around the lumen than in hyperplasia.

In micropapillary low-grade DCIS ("micropapillary" refers to tiny papillae with very subtle fibrovascular cores), there is nuclear uniformity and hyperchromasia, as is the case for other forms of low-grade DCIS. There is often a club-like appearance, with the apical portion of the papillae being wider than the portion near the duct wall, in contract to the tapering appearance of most benign micropapillae i4.17. Whereas benign micropapillary proliferations rarely distend the duct or acinus, micropapillary carcinoma often does. The milieu is often helpful. In micropapillary carcinoma, there is often an associated proliferation, close to the problematic micropapillary focus, that is compatible with nonpapillary DCIS, whereas benign micropapillations are often associated with benign hyperplasias in the adjacent tissue.

Additional features, usually less helpful, are that benign micropapillae are relatively uniform in size and shape, whereas their malignant counterparts show more variability. Benign micropapillae are cohesive, whereas their malignant counterparts are dyscohesive, with exfoliation of cells into the lumen. In benign micropapillae, there is maturation, with the cells at the tip being smaller than those at the base, while there is uniformity throughout the micropapillae in micropapillary DCIS. The "Roman bridge" form of low-grade intraductal carcinoma is a variant of the micropapillary type in which there is connection between the micropapillae at their tips i4.18.

The least common type of low-grade DCIS is the solid type, which must be distinguished from high-grade DCIS. In the solid type of low-grade DCIS, there is nuclear monotony, as is the case for all forms of low-grade DCIS of nuclei, rather than the large and variable nuclei of high-grade DCIS.

Special mention should be made of the entity called "clinging carcinoma," first described by Azzopardi [PMID2548274] and now called "flat epithelial atypia" or "flat intraductal neoplasia." Flat epithelial atypia is characterized by a single layer of cells with high-grade nuclei lining the duct i4.19. These cells fulfill the criteria for high-grade DCIS and are considered as such by some observers, but because there is only a single layer of such cells and the architectural features of all other forms of DCIS are lacking, some prefer to regard this as a form of atypical hyperplasia. It now appears that this finding does indicate an increased incidence of invasive carcinoma, vindicating Azzopardi's thinking [PMID20306828, PMID20306829].

Considerable variation in the diagnosis of problematic intraductal lesions has been shown among so-called "expert" breast pathologists [PMID1847606]. To my mind, this study not only indicates the extremely difficult nature of difficult intraductal proliferations, but also exposes the fallacy that the so-called "expert" supersubspecialist pathologist is necessarily superior to the general pathologist. Clearly, the case for the esteemed academic specialist is heavily diluted when these individuals cannot agree among themselves. Neither the clinician nor the general pathologist should search for a "magical guru" who can provide "the" answer in diagnostically difficult situations, but should rather seek a thorough understanding of current knowledge, with a willingness to indicate and accept the uncertainty that is sometimes an inherent and inescapable part of medicine. Since this study, standardization in the interpretation of difficult lesions has improved with better immunohistochemical stains, but these stains strengthen the case for the general pathologist, as they are readily available to all pathologists and provide a far more standardized algorithm than was heretofore possible.

There is a consensus that a diagnosis of low-grade DCIS requires some degree of geographical extent. While high-grade DCIS can be diagnosed in a single duct of any size, the diagnosis of low-grade DCIS generally requires that >1 minute focus be present. Some suggest that the total extent of the process be 0.2 cm (2 mm) or more, while others suggests that 3 or more ducts be involved.

There is considerable confusion over the term "atypical hyperplasia." It is not clear if this is a true, reproducible stage in the progression of carcinoma, or if it simply represents a variety of patterns that cannot be unanimously accepted as benign or malignant. To diagnose atypical hyperplasia (ADH), some require the full diagnostic criteria of DCIS, but insufficient extent (less than 2 mm or <3 ducts i4.20, while others do not require that any part of the questionable area resemble fully developed DCIS and will diagnose ADH for a proliferation that has some characteristics of DCIS, but no part of which clearly fulfills the criteria for DCIS—for example, intraductal proliferations that lack both the nuclear atypia of a high-grade DCIS and the architectural characteristics of a low-grade DCIS i4.21a, i4.21b.

Once DCIS and atypical hyperplasia have been excluded, the process is diagnosed as an intraductal hyperplasia of the usual type. Previously, hyperplasias were graded as mild, moderate, or severe, depending on the degree of epithelial proliferation and the extent to which the duct was filled. For example, >4 layers of epithelial cells was considered to be moderate hyperplasia. Newer thinking pays less attention to the degree of proliferation and simply seeks to differentiate the process from atypical hyperplasia. If there is no atypia and no architectural features of any form of DCIS, such that the diagnosis of DCIS is not tenable even for a part of the intraductal process, the diagnosis should be hyperplasia of the usual type. Because the extent of the proliferation is not critical, no comment need be made as to whether the process is mild, moderate, or severe. The term "florid" can be used if the ducts are nearly completely filled but the criteria for atypical ductal hyperplasia and intraductal carcinoma are not fulfilled. However, the process can simply be designated as hyperplasia of the usual type without comment on the cellularity because if there is no atypia, the malignant potential is minimal for any cellularity (1.5 times normal) [PMID11914619].

While all carcinomas develop along a continuum that defy distinct "breakpoints," the risk for invasive cancer is clearly greater for ADH than for usual hyperplasia, suggesting that the clinically important breakpoint is between any hyperplasia of the usual type—of any cellularity—and atypical hyperplasia, not between atypical hyperplasia and intraductal carcinoma. There is little need to differentiate between ADH and low-grade DCIS because such a distinction is arbitrary, subject to substantial interobserver variation, and the biologic potential of the 2 processes is similar. Indeed, there is a proposal to conflate atypical ductal hyperplasia and low-grade intraductal carcinoma together under the designation of intraductal neoplasia grade 1 (ie, to essentially consider ADH as a low-grade DCIS) [PMID17058097].

In situations that are equivocal between ADH/DCIS and usual intraductal hyperplasia, obvious apocrine metaplasia is often taken as a reassuring indicator, but this is not a primary criteria. In equivocal situations, a focus of streaming favors usual hyperplasia. Processes that run along the ductal system and undermine or replace the normal epithelium of ducts or lobules suggest ADH/DCIS.

The presence or absence of a myoepithelial layer, while of immense value in identifying subtle manifestations of invasive carcinoma, may not be definitive in the assessment of intraductal lesions because many foci of intraductal carcinoma retain some degree of myoepithelial cells around the periphery. However, myoepithelial cells are often attenuated or partially lost in a population of neoplastic cells, and the clear presence of a well defined myoepithelial layer is a reassuring finding in situations where other criteria have not yielded a definitive diagnosis, especially if they can be found accompanying a problematic epithelial proliferation into the lumen and not just on the periphery. The presence of a myoepithelial layer in excluding ADH/DCIS is most helpful in macropapillary intraductal processes, where a benign process can be assumed if myoepithelial cells are found throughout the proliferation.

High molecular weight keratin (CK903; also called 34βE-12) is generally present in hyperplasia of the usual type and is absent in 90% of cases of ADH/low-grade DCIS. Likewise, cytokeratins 5 and 6 are found in nearly all cases of usual ductal hyperplasia but are rarely seen in ADH/DCIS [PMID15252316], but as we will see in our discussion of molecular phenotyping of breast cancers in Chapter 47, those invasive carcinomas that do express cytokeratins 5 and 6 (ie, have a basal phenotype) tend to be negative for estrogen and progesterone receptors and negative for *HER2* overexpression, and may be more aggressive [PMID17146782].

To my mind, the diagnosis of either ADH or DCIS on a biopsy should generally prompt a complete excision. The sole exception to this appears to be a situation where there is a biopsy of microcalcifications (not a mass) and *both* of the following 2 conditions are met: there are only 1 or 2 foci in the biopsy that most observers would classify as atypical ductal hyperplasia and not DCIS *and* postbiopsy mammogram reveals no residual calcifications at all [PMID19095574].

The pathologist often encounters a situation in which extensive intraductal carcinoma, with nearly confluent clusters of intraductal tumor, must be differentiated from early invasion. Because foci of intraductal carcinoma generally retain some myoepithelial cells (though this layer may be attenuated), the immunohistochemical demonstration of a well defined myoepithelial layer suggests absence of invasion. The same panel of antibodies employed in distinguishing florid adenosis from invasion is recommended in this situation. Likewise, basement membrane material is generally intact in intraductal carcinoma and attenuated, but not necessarily lost altogether, in invasive foci, and in my experience, a well defined and essentially continuous basement membrane layer may also suggest the absence of invasion.

While immunohistochemistry can be of great help in addressing this question, the pathologist must again remember the twin caveats: The myoepithelial layer is discontinuous and myoepithelial cells may not be readily demonstrable in noninvasive cases, and invasive cases may still have some amount of basement membrane. The experienced observer weaves together the H&E appearance, the general presence or absence of a myoepithelial layer, and perhaps the degree of basement membrane formation into a determination of the degree of invasion, if any. In cases that remain problematic after the application of immunohistochemical stains, a useful rule on H&E examination is to lean away from invasion if the putative invasive focus is very close to a focus of DCIS because of the possibility that the focus of putative invasion is actually a tangential section through DCIS simulating invasion. If invasion can be confidently established, but extends <1 mm into the stroma, the term "microinvasion" can be used.

A number of detailed classifications of DCIS have been proposed, based primarily on nuclear grade and the presence or absence of necrosis. Of these, the Van Nuys system [PMID7723550] and the Nottingham system [PMID8380275] are the most commonly used. The Van Nuys system was been expanded into a prognostic index [PMID8635094] that factors in size and margin status, and was subsequently updated to include patient age [PMID14553846]. However, at the end of the day, the exclusion of small foci of invasion and margin status seem to be the most important considerations because the incidence of lymph node metastases from high-grade DCIS is only about 1% [PMID20210234] and that of low-grade DCIS is negligible. Recently, higher numbers of lymph node metastases in high-grade DCIS have been suggested, ranging from about 4% if the DCIS is negative for p16, cyclooxygenase-2, and Ki-67 to about 20% if the DCIS is positive for all 3 markers [PMID20427430], but there is always the difficulty of an unappreciated small focus of invasion in these studies, and even if the validity of these markers and these higher numbers are verified, the principal difficulty with DCIS with negative margins is the risk of local recurrence, not metastases.

If a focus of DCIS is estrogen receptor positive, attenuation of estrogen effect, either by receptor blockade or by inhibition of the aromatase enzyme involved in estrogen production, seems to reduce local recurrence, but with this exception, no additional studies beyond H&E seem to have routine relevance in DCIS at this writing. Even allowing for discontinuous foci, a margin of 1 cm (10 mm) appears adequate for DCIS and if achieved, likely obviates the need for radiation therapy in most cases [PMID10320383].

Macropapillary Intraductal Proliferations

Benign papillomas usually have uniform nuclei, less cellularity, prominent fibrovascular cores with only a few fronds i4.22, less nuclear crowding, and a simpler architecture than intraductal papillary carcinoma, but none of these criteria are absolute. Benign papillomas maintain a 2-cell population, epithelial and myoepithelial i4.23.

Papillary intraductal carcinomas tend to have delicate fibrovascular cores with numerous, thin, or variable papillations that are much longer than they are wide i4.24. Nuclear crowding, atypia, enlargement, or hyperchromatism are suggestive of malignancy, as are numerous mitoses i4.25. Intraductal papillary carcinomas tend to have a monomorphic population of cells without myoepithelial cells i4.26.

An important clue to the possibility of an intraductal papillary carcinoma is nuclear crowding. Such crowding may impart either stratification or columnarity to the cells i4.26, and for this reason, columnar cells that are oriented perpendicularly to the core, with or without stratification, while not diagnostic of papillary DCIS, should elicit a search for other features. In problematic cases, the appearance of epithelium that is in proximity to the papillary process can be helpful. If the epithelium in the portion of the duct wall not involved by the papillary proliferation is clearly innocuous, one can lean toward a benign diagnosis for the whole duct, whereas an intraductal papillary carcinoma might be favored if the remaining epithelium resembles nonpapillary DCIS. Likewise, if the adjacent ducts are benign, the problematic duct is probably best regarded as benign, whereas it is likely malignant if surrounded by malignant intraductal proliferations of any sort.

The term "intracystic papillary DCIS" is somewhat unclear, but usually refers to papillary DCIS in a dilated duct [PMID20306827]. The only significance of this is that it is more likely to present as a mass. The term "solid papillary carcinoma" refers to a large, cellular intraductal papillary carcinoma whose intraductal location and papillary nature may not be immediately obvious, causing concern for invasive carcinoma i4.27a. On close examination, subtle fibrovascular cores can be seen i4.27b, but the primary clue to this process is that low-power examination shows a well circumscribed process, suggesting a dilated dust i4.27c [PMID20340006].

ISBN 978-089189-5886

In equivocal cases, the best test currently available is the presence or absence of myoepithelial cells, as the demonstration of these cells in reasonable numbers essentially precludes a malignant diagnosis. A number of markers have been proposed to highlight myoepithelial cells in papillary lesions, but as discussed earlier in benign mimics of invasive carcinoma, a combination of nuclear staining for p63 and cytoplasmic staining for smooth muscle actin, calponin, and myosin heavy chain offer the greatest combination of sensitivity and specificity [PMID17525625].

As is always the case, immunohistochemical stains must be interpreted in conjunction with the H&E appearance and the presence of myoepithelial cells in breast lesions does not guarantee benignity since the myoepithelial cells at any location within a duct or lobule may persist as carcinoma spreads to that location from another focus in the duct. Myoepithelial cells will also be found in the rare cases of myoepithelial carcinoma. Likewise, their absence does not ensure malignancy if the H&E appearance does not suggest carcinoma.

An intraductal papillary proliferation may be clearly benign in some areas but suspicious or clearly malignant in others i4.28. Immunohistochemical staining for myoepithelial cells may parallel this appearance, being demonstrable in the benign-appearing areas and absent in the areas of concern. After the presence of a focus of DCIS is established within a papilloma, there are differences in terminology, but good agreement on basic concepts. Tavassoli uses the term "atypical papilloma" if the criteria for DCIS are satisfied in <1/3 of the lesion, and "carcinoma within a papilloma" when the involved area is between 33% and 90% of the papillary mass [PMID13680220], but has more recently avoided the term "carcinoma" in such situations in favor of "ductal intraepithelial neoplasia" for foci occurring in a papilloma [PMID19492881]. Page feels that any area that could be regarded as DCIS elsewhere and is larger than 3 mm should be called "DCIS within a papilloma," while such areas that are smaller than 3mm should be called "ADH within a papilloma" [PMID8674001]. Either of these nomenclatures is perfectly acceptable, and there are advantages to each, but to my mind, there are 2 central points. First, the same cytologic, architectural, *and size* criteria should apply in a papillary lesion as elsewhere, and if the criteria for low-grade DCIS are met, I favor a diagnosis of low-grade DCIS within a papilloma because the use of different nomenclatures for foci within and not within papillomas is likely to confuse the clinician. Second, to my mind, a patient should not be labeled with a "cancer" diagnosis—even in situ—if the size criteria for DCIS are not met.

Papillary intraductal carcinomas may invade beyond the duct in which they arose, resulting in stromal invasion and a truly invasive carcinoma. As is the case for any form of DCIS, it can be difficult to determine if there is focal invasion immediately adjacent to the duct. The clues to focal stromal invasion in papillary intraductal carcinoma are those employed in other situations—irregularly shaped or angulated clusters of atypical cells and a desmoplastic stromal reaction, though the latter finding may be difficult to appreciate in the breast, where the stroma is often fibrotic. In questionable situations, immunohistochemical proof of loss of myoepithelial cells in a small cluster of cells suggests stromal invasion.

The Breast Biopsy: Potentials and Limitations

The breast biopsy begins with a suspicious finding on a mammogram or an MRI. Mammographically suspicious findings are reported using the BIRADS (Breast Imaging-Reporting and Data System) developed by the American College of Radiology [PMID17164080]. This system is as follows:

0: Incomplete or compromised study.

1: Negative.

2: A findings that is comfortably felt to be benign; normal surveillance indicated.

3: A finding that is probably benign, but a followup within 4-6 months is suggested.

4: A suspicious finding; biopsy should be considered.

5: A highly suspicious finding; biopsy indicated.

6: A finding that has been shown to be malignant by biopsy.

Carcinoma of the breast is rising in incidence and will now affect 1 in 9 women at some point in their lives. Mammography (and increasingly MRI) in conjunction with biopsy remains our best defense against this alarming trend. The breast biopsy has performed admirably in the early diagnosis and treatment of breast cancer, but there are several caveats in forming conclusions about a breast mass or areas of radiographic abnormality from a biopsy.

A useful way to minimize both overdiagnoses and underdiagnoses is to remember that the breast biopsy—like any biopsy—simply serves to stratify patients into 3 categories—clearly positive, clearly negative, and a third group for which a definitive diagnosis cannot be rendered at the time.

The third group of breast biopsies—those that are indeterminate—include 2 broad situations. The first group of indeterminate biopsies is those cases in which there is atypical breast tissue, such that it can safely be assumed that the area of interest has been sampled, but the interpretation of the biopsy is problematic, even after following the algorithms and special stains discussed above. While there are a variety of situations in which interpretation of a breast biopsy can be inconclusive, 2 of the most frequent areas of problematic interpretation involve papillary lesions and foci of atypical ductal hyperplasia.

Papillary lesions that are identified on aspiration or core biopsy material are challenging, and there is not yet a clear consensus on this matter. Some believe that any papillary process identified in such a sample, even if it appears clearly benign, should prompt an excision [PMID19492881, PMID15569209]. On the other hand, because stereotactic (mammotome) biopsies remove much more tissue, an argument can be made that histologically benign-appearing papillary lesions biopsied by this means might be followed without excision if the postprocedure mammogram suggests no residual lesion. If the patient and her physician cannot reach a clear decision on the next step, immunohistochemical stains that suggest benignity may permit a "wait and see" approach, provided that the lesion does not enlarge or become radiographically more worrisome, but because papillary lesions are often heterogeneous, and there may be unsampled areas of atypia or carcinoma adjacent to benign areas that were sampled, this approach is potentially problematic. In any case, in a core biopsy or fine needle aspiration (FNA) with any papillary process, it is generally wise to comment that a focal papillary carcinoma cannot be excluded with complete certainty in that material, even if myoepithelial cells are found, and to recommend either an excision or close surveillance.

Also in this first group of indeterminate biopsies, in which the target has been sampled but interpretation is problematic, are those that have atypical ductal hyperplasia. As discussed above, excision is prudent unless the biopsy was done for microcalcifications, there are only 1 or 2 foci of ADH, and there are no residual calcifications. Even in this situation, some are more comfortable with an excision. As mentioned, florid hyperplasia of the usual type is no longer considered a major risk factor, but the difficulty with this diagnosis on a biopsy is the possibility that there may be a more significant process that was not sampled, especially if the biopsy was of a distinct mass. These situations must be individualized, but clearly, there must either be an excision or surveillance.

The second group of potentially indeterminate breast biopsies consists of those situations in which the biopsy is clearly benign, but there is the possibility that the target may not have been sampled. There are a variety of situations in which the pathologist can suspect that the target area may not have been sampled, and should therefore take care to avoid imparting a false sense of security, but 3 situations are commonly encountered and deserve special mention. The first is a biopsy for a mass in which there is normal breast tissue that would not seem to form a clinical mass, in which case it is prudent to comment that the tissue is benign, but verification that the target was sampled is needed.

The second concerns biopsies that are benign, but do not have breast parenchyma (eg, contain only fat). In these cases, it is problematic as to whether the clinical mass is mesenchymal or the biopsy captured only surrounding fibroadipose tissue (eg, does the patient have a lipoma, or did the biopsy sample only adipose tissue adjacent to a neoplasm?). In these cases, a comment should be made that the mass may be a mesenchymal lesion, such as a lipoma, but that clinical correlation is needed to ensure that the target area was sampled.

The third situation in which the biopsy is benign but there is a hazard of a false negative are those biopsies done for microcalcifications and no calcifications are seen in the biopsy. In these cases, I recommend a comment on the presence or absence of calcifications in the biopsy so that the physician who performed the biopsy can ensure that the target area was sampled. However, the primary defense against a false negative from failure to sample the target area lies with the physician performing the biopsy, not with the pathologist. The physician performing a biopsy for calcifications should radiograph both the tissue removed before it is sent to pathology to ensure that it contains the target calcifications, and also the patient after the procedure to ensure that calcifications are no longer present or are reduced in number. This postprocedure double-radiographic examination is superior to radiographing the paraffin blocks because there may be tissue in the patient, adjacent to that which was removed, that may contain calcifications that are of greater concern, in which case the pathologist's affirmation of calcifications in the paraffin blocks may lead to a false sense of security regarding specimen adequacy. Only the radiologist can confirm that the most significant calcifications were sampled.

About 10% of microcalcifications are of the calcium oxalate type, and cannot be detected on H&E examination. These are birefringent, requiring examination with polarized light to be detected, and are usually associated with benign processes [PMID2589947]. While the pathologist should comment on the presence or absence of calcifications, he or she should not be expected to determine, based on either paraffin block radiography or microscopic examination, if the target was sufficiently sampled.

Assessment of Invasive Ductal Adenocarcinomas

It is generally recommended to remove each inked margin in a lumpectomy en bloc, transect it at right angles, then place each fragment in the cassette on its side. If the tissue contains tumor, it can then be determined how close it is to the margin, whereas simply laying the tissue face down in a cassette prevents the examiner from determining the distance of the tumor from the margin. Some advocate fixing lumpectomy specimens overnight prior to taking margins. While this delays the case for a day, some feel this provides better morphology. The caveat here, however, is that if this procedure is employed, it might be prudent to ink and section or incise the tumor to allow fixative to access to the tumor to permit prompt fixation.

Any breast specimen that has been radiographed prior to being sent to the laboratory is likely to have distorted dimensions, especially in the dimension that was compressed. This compression may compromise the assessment of margins and a comment regarding this distortion and its possible effect on the assessment of margins might be made in these situations. Evaluation of margins in lumpectomy specimens may also be complicated by the fact that the ink applied to the specimen by the pathologist often runs into crevices that are caused by the trauma of excision, thus coating surfaces that are not true margins. A third area of concern in margin assessment is that cautery artifact (linear streaking of cells and chromatin) clearly indicates a surgeon's margin, but does not necessarily indicate a final margin, as surgeons often "back out" and excise around an area that was previously penetrated. Thus, a surface may have both cautery artifact and India ink and still not be a final margin. A fourth difficulty is that the final assessment of margins is done in a 2-dimensional microscopic field, which does not perfectly reflect the 3-dimensional ramifications of the ductal system. No absolute numbers have emerged for minimum requirements for a margin to be considered negative, but in general, it should be negative by at least 2 mm [PMID20073613] and preferably by 5 mm [PMID17439024]. Even if these margins are achieved, postoperative radiation therapy is generally given in lumpectomy cases. It is generally prudent to report the margin status of the invasive and in situ components separately.

The submission of separate margins by the surgeon from the cavity after the lumpectomy has been advocated as a method of assessing margins that is superior to attempting to obtain margins from the lumpectomy itself [PMID16327435]. These separate margins from the cavity should overlap as much as possible, inked, cut at right angles, and submitted for

ISBN 978-089189-5886

paraffin processing. Frozen section evaluation of margins is discouraged [PMID11707625].

From time to time over the years, the entity "extensive intraductal component" has received attention as an indicator of more extensive or multifocal disease, or a process that is more likely to extend to the margins. This continues to be a matter of controversy. While some maintain that the finding of extensive DCIS may indicate a greater likelihood of multicentric disease, suggesting a possible mastectomy, to my mind, such cases should not be handled differently, except that particularly close attention should be paid to the margins.

Cryoprobe-assisted lumpectomies, in which the area of concern and a surrounding cuff are preoperatively frozen, will facilitate recognition and removal of the abnormal area by the surgeon, who faces the simpler task of removing an iceball, but will introduce frozen artifact that is likely to compromise definitive assessment of tumor grade and margin status. It may also be more difficult to perform hormone receptor or Her2 studies on tissue that has been frozen since the freezing process may compromise the antigenicity of the relevant proteins. In addition, although definitive data are not yet available, it is possible that preoperative freezing may compromise the lymphatic drainage from the area, in cases in which a sentinel lymph node biopsy is to be undertaken before the freezing.

Tumor invasion into lymphatic spaces **i4.29** increases the risk of both local recurrence and distant metastases in node-negative cases [PMID21171081]. Intuitively, one might think that such invasion is irrelevant in node-positive cases, since the neoplasm must have gained access to the lymphatic system, but even in these cases, lymphatic invasion increases the risk of both local recurrence and distant metastases [PMID20564641].

Lymphatic invasion should not be diagnosed in the immediate vicinity of the tumor mass because it is very difficult to differentiate between lymphatic invasion and retraction of tumor from the surrounding stroma secondary to formalin fixation and paraffin processing **i4.30**. In questionable situations, immunohistochemistry for vascular markers can improve detection of lymphatic invasion. In particular, the vascular marker D2-40 is reported to stain lymphatic endothelium more than that of blood vessels [PMID12218087]. Because D2-40 may occasionally stain myoepithelial cells (though less strongly than lymphatic endothelium), the addition of the myoepithelial marker p63 may prevent weak staining of myoepithelial cells by D2-40 from being misinterpreted as lymphatic invasion [PMID20042851].

Of the many attempts to prognosticate the behavior of invasive ductal carcinomas, the most successful has been the Scarff-Bloom-Richardson system, which takes into account nuclear pleomorphism, mitotic activity, and gland formation. Elston and Ellis have issued a modified Scarff-Bloom-Richardson system which is commonly used [PMID1757079]. In this system, gland formation is assessed as follows: >75% of cells forming tubules is a 1, 10-75% is a 2, and <10% is a 3. In mitotic counts, with a microscope whose 40× is about 0.25 mm^2, 0-9 mitoses per 10 high-power fields (HPF) is a 1, 10-19 is a 2, and 20 or more is a 3. In Chapter 1, we saw that there is variation among observers in the counting of mitoses [PMID10804295], and we examined the criteria for a mitotic figure [PMID1592381, Baak ISBN978-0387114316]. Because mitoses often vary considerably in different areas of a tumor, I recommend selecting areas with the highest activity and counting more than 1 set of 10 HPFs. In the Scarff-Bloom-Richardson system, nuclei are assessed as grade 1, 2, or 3 in the usual (albeit poorly reproducible) fashion. A total score of 5 or less signifies a well differentiated tumor, scores of 6 and 7 are indicative of a moderately differentiated carcinoma, and scores of 8 and 9 indicate poorly differentiated tumors. In addition to the Scarff-Bloom-Richardson system, the Nottingham index has been expanded to include invasive ductal carcinomas and is a combined grade/stage system that combines tumor size and grade with lymph node status [PMID18543079].

The term "micrometastasis" refers to a deposit <0.2 cm **i4.31**. There is disagreement about the significance of micrometastases, with some studies suggesting that they are inconsequential and others indicating that they affect prognosis [PMID20190185]. We may need to await more information concerning the molecular classification of breast cancer before settling this matter, as the molecular profile of an individual micrometastasis may be important. Exceptionally small metastatic deposits (<0.2 mm) are called nanometastases. While the significance of micrometastases is unclear, nanometastases are unlikely to change prognosis [PMID19457697].

Sentinel lymph node examination, in which the lymph node or nodes that are most likely to be positive are identified by dye and/or scintillation methods and then removed and examined, has dramatically changed the surgical treatment of breast cancer and greatly reduced the morbidity of axillary dissection. Only 16% of patients will have a negative sentinel node and a positive node elsewhere in the axilla [PMID18216523]. At this writing, a uniform consensus on the procedure for examining sentinel nodes has not emerged. Immunohistochemical stains will detect an occasional positive sentinel lymph node that was missed on H&E, but in cases of ductal carcinoma, these cases usually involve micrometastases, so the consequences to the patient, if any, of the false negative H&E examination are unclear [PMID11859211]. Moreover, a keratin positive cell in a node does not necessarily imply a metastasis, and immunohistochemical staining of a sentinel lymph node can result in a false positive.

Reverse transcriptase-PCR for mammaglobin, prolactin-inducible protein, CK19, mucin 1, and CEA had a higher sensitivity and specificity than either serial sections or immunohistochemical stains in identifying metastatic deposits in sentinel lymph nodes [PMID16213901, PMID19469912] but it is not clear that any minute deposits this methodology might uncover have clinical significance.

Frozen section or imprint study of sentinel nodes is occasionally undertaken for the purpose of immediately preceding to an axillary dissection if the intra-operative examination is positive, though there is a false negative rate of up to 15% in intra-operative sentinel lymph node evaluation [PMID19131285], much higher than in most frozen sections. There are 2 potential problems with an intraoperative examination of a sentinel node. First, not all agree that a positive sentinel node must necessarily prompt an axillary dissection in all cases. Sentinel lymph node excision *in lieu of* a complete axillary dissection has been found to be safe and effective in many cases. The incidence of involvement of nonsentinel axillary lymph nodes in situations where the sentinel node has a micrometastasis is <50% and is often zero [PMID20846864]. Moreover, new data suggest that patient care may not be improved by an axillary dissection even if a sentinel node with a *macrometastasis* is found [PMID21523451, PMID21440434]. Even if a complete axillary dissection following the identification of a positive sentinel node discloses additional positive nodes, the procedure does not appear to improve long-term patient care if systemic endocrine therapy or chemotherapy is used [PMID21304082].

It remains to be seen whether the identification of a positive sentinel node by either frozen or paraffin section study should necessarily be followed by a full axillary dissection, and in all probability, the answer to this question will be different for different patients and for tumors with different molecular profiles. Second, very rarely, there may be small deposits of benign ectopic epithelium in an axillary node, and paraffin-processed sections will be needed to differentiate these from metastatic deposits.

While in theory, there is the possibility of saving the patient a second surgery if a sentinel node is shown to be positive at the time of surgery, in practice it is not this simple, and there is much to be said for collecting all thoughts for a day or two before proceeding with a full dissection, given the potential morbidity secondary to impaired lymphatic drainage.

Yet another potential difficulty with axillary dissection decisions based on sentinel node study is that some patients whose axillary lymph nodes are all negative will have positive internal mammary nodes. The probability of this depends on the location of the tumor, being no >1% for tumors in the upper outer quadrant, but as high as 29% for medial tumors [PMID18684584]. In a significant minority of patients with medial tumors, the entire concept of axillary dissection, with or without a sentinel node and with or without frozen section, is of questionable benefit.

If a sentinel node is examined, no special handling—in the form of frozen section/imprint, extra levels, or immunohistochemistry—is indicated [PMID21247310], but it is wise to consider keratin stains when looking for metastatic lobular carcinoma in lymph nodes, as this type of carcinoma often has smaller cells and is more difficult to detect on H&E examination [PMID16497870].

Unlike many other hormones, estrogen and progesterone do not bind to receptors on the cells surface, but rather diffuse through the plasma membrane (their steroid structure permits this) to bind to receptors in the nucleus. These receptors are part of the nuclear receptor superfamily of proteins that also includes the receptors for thyroid hormone, glucocorticoids, vitamin D, and retinoic acid. The normal breast has positivity for estrogen receptor, but mostly in the terminal duct/lobular unit (TDLU), and even there, only about 35% of cells are positive [PMID16417654]. Most breast carcinomas have increased expression of the estrogen receptorm, and blockade of this receptor or, more recently, inhibition of estrogen synthesis, is beneficial in these cases.

The American Society of Clinical Oncology and the College of American Pathologists recommend testing for estrogen and progesterone receptors in any invasive carcinoma, and further recommend hormonal treatment if >10% of tumor cells have positivity for estrogen receptor. Cases in which between 1 and 10% of tumor cells are positive may or may not be hormonally treated, depending on the individual case. Hormonal therapy is rarely indicated if <1% of tumor cells are positive for estrogen receptor [PMID20524868]. About 8% of breast carcinomas will change their estrogen receptor expression in metastatic foci, usually from positive to negative [PMID20939012], suggesting that ER should also be retested in a recurrence or metastasis.

A β form of the estrogen receptor has been identified [PMID8769313]. The β form appears to be more widespread than had been believed [PMID20494112]. These 2 versions of the receptor are encoded on different chromosomes. They have similar affinity for estradiol, but the response may be different [PMID19967775]. In 2009, it was shown that expression of the β form of the estrogen receptor is a favorable prognostic indicator if the α form is also present [PMID19703124], and in 2011, it was shown that patients with the β form of the receptor benefit from receptor blockade with or without concomitant expression of the α form [PMID21204712]. At this writing, testing for the β form is available, but not generally performed in routine assays. It is to be hoped that testing for both forms of the receptor will soon become commonplace.

In premenopausal patients, the ovaries are the main source of estrogen, and receptor blockade, usually with tamoxifen, remains the mainstay of hormonal therapy for estrogen receptor positive carcinomas in these patients. Tamoxifen binds about equally well to the α and β forms of the estrogen receptor. Raloxifene (Evista), a second generation estrogen receptor modulator, also binds both forms, but binds more to the α form [PMID19817711]. Raloxifene is antiestrogen in the breast, appears beneficial in the treatment of some cases of osteoporosis, and seems to lack the weak estrogen activity in the endometrium [PMID15270657], but its use is largely restricted to nonneoplastic conditions. Rarely, oophorectomy is employed in younger patients.

Because tamoxifen is a weak estrogen agonist (ie, it has weak estrogen effect) rather than a complete antagonist [PMID16681767], it could actually cause a slight increase in estrogen activity in older women whose baseline estrogen activity is minimal. Rare tamoxifen-associated endometrial adenocarcinomas have been reported in postmenopausal patients [PMID16147692]. For this reason, reduction of estrogen synthesis is the more common approach in postmenopausal women. Aromatase inhibitors block the synthesis of estrogen from androgens in the adrenal, the principal site of estrogen synthesis in the postmenopausal patient. Anastrozole (Arimidex) is the most often used aromatase inhibitor and is generally preferable to receptor blockers in older patients, except in cases of osteoporosis [PMID19889200]. The inhibitor exemestane (aromasin) may be of prophylactic benefit in postmenopausal patients who are at high risk [PMID21639806].

Clinicians must balance the desired antiestrogen activity of these and other estrogen receptor modulators against the side effects and possible benefits in other tissues, but this is a very difficult task because the in vivo activity of any drug depends on a variety of factors, including the binding of cofactors, inhibitors, and the microenvironment. Because these factors will vary among different tissue types, drugs do not always behave the same way in all tissues, and one must be careful in extrapolating in vitro data to patients.

Human epidermal growth factor receptor type 2 (Her2 or Her2/neu) is a normal protein, encoded by the *HER2* (*HER2/neu*) gene. The Her2 protein is related to epidermal growth factor receptor and functions to transmit growth or mitogenic signals to the interior of the cell. Like most growth factors, Her2 is a transmembrane protein whose extracellular portion binds an intercellular messenger ligand and whose intracellular portion contains a tyrosine kinase (ie, an enzyme that adds a phosphate group to tyrosine residues on proteins that are part of a signaling pathway, activating them and causing them to modify the next protein in the signaling pathway). Binding of ligand to the extracellular portion of Her2 activates the intracellular tyrosine kinase, setting in motion an enzymatic cascade that activates the cell.

There are 2 major types of tyrosine kinases. The first type, of which Her2 is an example, is part of a single transmembrane protein that is usually encoded by a single gene. These are called receptor tyrosine kinases. Other members of the receptor tyrosine kinase family include epidermal growth factor receptor (EGFR) and platelet derived growth factor receptor (PDGFR).

The second group of tyrosine kinase enzymes, called cytoplasmic tyrosine kinases, is entirely intracellular. They are close to the inner surface of the plasma membrane and can receive input from an external receptor via other proteins, but unlike receptor tyrosine kinases, are not directly attached to the receptor. Important members of the cytoplasmic tyrosine kinase family include Abl (important in chronic myelogenous leukemia), ZAP-70 and a related protein called Syk (important in signaling in T and B lymphocytes, respectively), and the Janus kinase (JAK) family (important in some chronic myeloproliferative neoplasms).

There are 2 therapeutic approaches to receptor tyrosine kinases: blocking the receptor and inhibiting the enzyme that the receptor is attached to. Her2 is overexpressed in approximately 25% of breast carcinomas, usually from amplification of the DNA. Trastuzumab (Herceptin) is a monoclonal antibody (the generic name of any medication based on a monoclonal antibody ends in "mab") that binds to the exterior portion of this receptor, and is therapeutically valuable in those cases that overexpress this protein. Trastuzumab blocks the extracellular portion of Her2, preventing activation of the tyrosine kinase by blocking the initiating signal. Lapatinib (Tykerb) inhibits the kinase itself, even if the extracellular domain has been activated and holds promise because many patients whose tumors overexpress Her2 and who initially respond to trastuzumab will become refractory to that drug. Lapatinib also inhibits the tyrosine kinase activity of EGFR.

At this time, Her2 is assayed either by immunohistochemistry for the protein or by fluorescence in situ hybridization (FISH) for the *HER2* DNA. The action of the Her2 protein is discussed in Chapter 46. Historically, 3% of cases that are negative for the Her2 protein by immunohistochemistry can be shown by FISH to have amplification of *HER2* DNA, though the clinical significance of this is not established. In addition, 1+ or 2+ Her2 positivity by immunohistochemistry may be reported as equivocal and tested by FISH for overexpression of the *HER2* gene **f4.1**, **f4.2**. Some investigators believe that equivocal Her2 immunohistochemical results indicate tumor heterogeneity [PMID21934215].

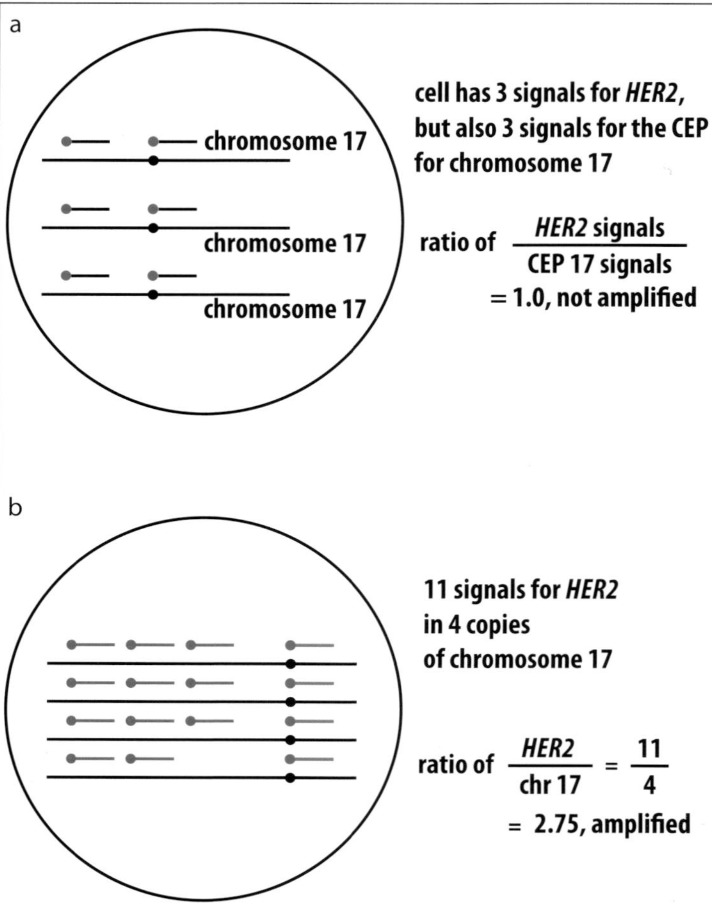

f4.1 *HER2* testing by FISH. The *HER2* gene is on chromosome 17, the centromere of which is indicated by the black dot. In **a**, the cell has 3 copies of chromosome 17 (increased copy number of this chromosome is relatively common in breast cancer). This is determined by a chromosome enumerator probe (CEP) that binds to the centromere and which is green in this illustration. A sequence complementary to the *HER2* focus carries a fluorescent probe of a different color from the CEP (red in this illustration). In **a**, there are 3 copies of the *HER2* gene in the cell instead of the expected 2 copies, but there are also 3 copies of chromosome 17, as determined by the CEP for that chromosome. The ratio of HER2 signals to chromosome 17 is unchanged, and an increase in the number of *HER2* genes resulting from a copy number increase in chromosome 17 does not count as amplification. In **b**, there are 4 copies of chromosome 17 in the cell, but the number of *HER2* genes is increased even compensating for this. There are 11 signals from the *HER2* probe and 4 from the CEP for chromosome 17, resulting in a ratio of 2.75, which is amplification.

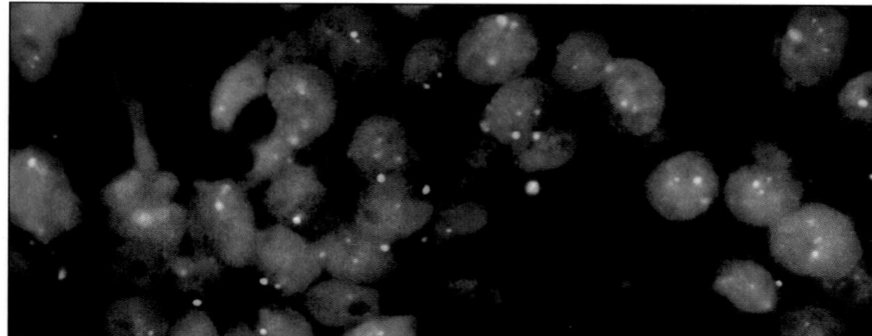

f4.2 A dual-color FISH study in breast cancer. The red signals indicate *HER2* DNA sequences and the green signals indicate a chromosome enumerator probe (CEP) for chromosome 17, the chromosome containing the *HER2* locus. The ratio of *HER2* signals to CEP signals is 2.33, indicating slight amplification. Modified from [PMID19019769] with permission.

Concordance between immunohistochemistry for the Her2 protein and FISH testing for the *HER2* gene has improved and is 95% at this writing [PMID21685042]. An automated quantitative analysis of immunohistochemical results appears promising in this regard [PMID19722747].

The FDA approved a chromogenic in situ hybridization assay (SPoT-Light) in July 2008. Chromogenic assays have excellent potential to be faster, cheaper, and also provide a permanent signal (fluorescence decays with time). An early study showed only a 94% concordance with FISH [PMID17908324], but a 2011 study demonstrated a 98% concordance rate [PMID21173138]. In addition, quantitative reverse transcription polymerase chain reaction assay for *HER2* mRNA shows promise [PMID18343783].

In general, *HER2* DNA or Her2 protein status should be determined on a resection specimen, as opposed to a biopsy, because tumors are often heterogeneous and there may be areas in a resection that are more likely to be positive for Her2 (such as high-grade areas). The exception to this, of course, is when neoadjuvant therapy (ie, chemotherapy given before surgery) is expected. However, even in these situations, if the *HER2* status on the biopsy is equivocal or negative, testing should be repeated on the resection, even if neoadjuvant therapy was given in the interim [PMID19483670].

A metastatic focus, if available at the time of presentation or initial testing, is even better for *HER2* testing, and also for estrogen and progesterone receptor testing, because the metastatic deposit is more representative of the actual tumor that the oncologist will be confronting. In about 20% of cases, the *HER2* status in a recurrence or metastatic focus will differ from that of the primary site. In most of these cases, the metastatic or recurrent site will show overexpression, whereas the original tumor did not. It is therefore important to reassess *HER2* status in a recurrence or metastasis [PMID17973263], as is the case for ER.

The occasional difference in immunohistochemical properties between a primary tumor and its metastatic sites is likely a reflection of the finding that in many cases, there are different clones within a given tumor [PMID10214356], some of which are more likely to give rise to metastases than others. Different intratumoral clones have been shown for *HER2* expression [PMID17319852] and for the expression of estrogen and progesterone receptors [PMID20368555]. While the clinical significance of tumor heterogeneity remains to be established, its immediate impact is to increase interobserver variability in interpretation of testing.

Because suboptimal fixation of the tumor may result in diminished or even artifactually negative staining [PMID19734848], resection specimens should be promptly sectioned to expose the tumor to the fixative. If there is a question concerning the preservation of a resection specimen, the tumor and the surrounding tissue can be stained for keratin, vimentin, and CD31. Strong staining for these markers in appropriate tissues indicates that fixation is adequate and that the negative results for ER, PR, or Her2 overexpression are valid and not an artifact of poor fixation. There have been suggestions that prolonged periods of formalin exposure may lessen *HER2* recovery, but a more recent study indicates that this is not true [PMID20855640].

Paget disease of the nipple, caused by the migration of tumor cells up the lactiferous ducts and into the epidermis, does not affect treatment or prognosis and therefore need not be a major concern for the pathologist. The sole value of identifying Paget disease is that it is rarely the means by which an initial diagnosis of cancer is made in a patient who has a lesion on or near the nipple, but no known mass. Paget cells can be subtle on H&E examination and immunohistochemical stains may be needed. CAM 5.2, EMA, Her2, and CEA all tend to preferentially stain Paget cells in the epidermis [PMID19130406].

In cases where neoadjuvant chemotherapy has been given, the pathologist is called upon to assess the effects of the regimen after resection. Fibrosis in the site of the tumor may indicate some responsiveness to the neoadjuvant therapy, but fibrosis is common in the breast, especially around a tumor, so tumor necrosis is a more reassuring finding.

Breast carcinoma in metastatic sites is easily confused with carcinomas from other organs. Most problematic situations regarding possible metastatic breast carcinoma involve its distinction from metastatic adenocarcinomas from the lung, endometrium, or from nonmucinous ovarian adenocarcinoma, as all of these tumors are positive for cytokeratin 7 and negative for cytokeratin 20. Estrogen or progesterone positivity in a tumor of unknown primary points away from the lung, but is not helpful in the distinction from adenocarcinomas of the endometrium and ovary, which may also be ER or PR positive. Moreover, even if a breast carcinoma is initially positive, it may be negative after metastasizing. Although GCDFP-15 stains only a minority of breast carcinomas, it is essentially specific for breast. Mammaglobin is a more sensitive but less specific marker for breast carcinoma than GCDFP-15. For example, 55% of breast carcinomas stain for mammaglobin, vs only 23% for GCDFP-15, but mammaglobin also stains 8% of nonbreast tumors, vs essentially no such staining for GCDFP-15 [PMID17145637]. GCDFP-15 and mammaglobin staining, especially the former, strongly suggest a breast primary, but negativity is not helpful. Thyroid transcription factor 1 (TTF-1) is helpful in the differentiation of lung and breast carcinomas, as it is frequently positive in lung carcinomas and only rarely positive in breast carcinomas. TTF-1, as the name implies, will also stain thyroid carcinomas, but this is usually not in the differential diagnosis. PE-10 (SP-A), a stain for lung surfactant, may also help, as it is essentially specific for non-small cell carcinomas of the lung, though it is of suboptimal sensitivity [PMID11956814]. WT1 stains 92% of ovarian serous carcinomas, but very few ovarian neoplasms of another type and few breast carcinomas [PMID16006803].

Reliable and specific serum markers to monitor treatment and progression of breast cancer have been elusive. At this writing, Ca 15-3 [PMID16410341] and CA 27.29 [PMID11239757] show promise.

Unusual Forms of Invasive Ductal Adenocarcinoma

A number of unusual forms of invasive breast carcinoma are recognized and described in detail in the WHO classification [Tavassoli ISBN978-9283224129], but unusual forms of breast carcinoma are often coexist with a more traditional form. While there is no uniform opinion as to how much of a tumor should be of a particular morphology before the entire tumor is so designated, most would hold that at least 75% of a tumor should be of a special type before that specific designation is used.

The invasive micropapillary adenocarcinoma is usually mixed with 1 or more other forms of invasive carcinoma, but is aggressive and prone to lymph node metastases in its pure state [PMID14717664].

Mucinous (colloid) carcinoma is a form of invasive ductal adenocarcinoma that is characterized by pools of mucin, within which are clusters of neoplastic cells, generally with low-grade nuclei **i4.32**. In its pure form, mucinous carcinoma is thought to be slightly less aggressive than conventional invasive ductal carcinoma [PMID20962055], but routine breast carcinomas often have mucinous areas and there is no survival advantage unless the entirety of the tumor is of mucinous.

The so-called medullary carcinoma of the breast is a form of invasive ductal carcinoma that has highly pleomorphic nuclei, intermingled with lymphocytes and with minimal gland formation **i4.33**, but a clinical course that belies the alarming nuclear morphology. Additional criteria for this diagnosis are sharp circumscription **i4.34** and an essential absence of an intraductal component [PMID18566570]. Many (but not all) studies have indicated that if a carcinoma fulfills *all* of these criteria, it can be called a pure medullary carcinoma and may have a less aggressive course. Although medullary carcinoma is an invasive ductal carcinoma, Bloom-Richardson grading is not generally used because it would result in an inappropriately high number. Some favor dispensing with this category because of the rarity of its pure state and poor agreement in diagnosis among different observers, but others continue to accept it as a distinct entity if all criteria are met. A more reproducible characterization of medullary carcinoma will hopefully be forthcoming from developments in molecular pathology, but until the matter is clarified, it seems prudent to insist that a neoplasm meet all of the criteria of medullary carcinoma before making the diagnosis, and even then to comment that a less aggressive course cannot be guaranteed and clinical stage is still the most important prognostic criterion. Carcinomas that fulfill some, but not all, of the criteria of a medullary carcinoma (the so-called atypical medullary carcinoma) have a minimal, if any, survival advantage. In these cases, it seems prudent to make a diagnosis of ductal carcinoma, with Bloom-Richardson grading, and comment that there are medullary features.

Tubular carcinoma is a subtype of the well differentiated invasive ductal carcinoma that scores a 1 on a scale of 3 for each of the criteria used in the Bloom-Richardson system—nuclear pleomorphism, mitotic activity, and gland formation—thus achieving a total score of only 3 of 9 **i4.35**. Because a score of 5 or less is well differentiated, the terms "tubular carcinoma" and "well differentiated carcinoma" are not quite synonymous. Tubular carcinoma is the most differentiated form of breast carcinoma. Indeed, it can be difficult to distinguish tubular carcinoma from adenosis or a complex sclerosing lesion. Tubular carcinomas have an infiltrative pattern and often have angulated outlines with small protrusions **i4.36**. They often coexist with either higher-grade invasive areas or a DCIS component, but in many cases, the distinction can only be made by the presence or absence of a myoepithelial cell layer.

Metaplastic breast carcinoma (formerly called carcinosarcoma or carcinoma with sarcomatous metaplasia) may have an inconspicuous epithelial component and may simulate a sarcoma. Chondrosarcoma-like areas are common. Although metaplastic carcinomas are high-grade by definition, there may be surprisingly little nuclear pleomorphism in the mesenchymal component, making the diagnosis of metaplastic carcinoma particularly challenging when it presents as a pure sarcomatoid variant, without any epithelioid cells. If the mesenchymal component predominates and consists of spindle cells without cartilage, a benign mesenchymal process, such as a myofibroblastoma or fibromatosis, may be considered. A negative CD34 points away from a myofibroblastoma, while a negative β-catenin points away from fibromatosis. In the absence of nuclear atypia, clues to the malignant nature of a mesenchymal-predominant metaplastic carcinoma include the presence of occasional atypical epithelial cells, increased mitotic activity, or infiltration. Any of these findings suggest a need for immunohistochemical characterization. While myoepithelial cells may stain for keratin, especially CK5/6, staining with multiple epithelial markers such as CK5/6, CAM5.2, AE1/AE3, CK903, CK7, and epithelial membrane antigen heavily favors a metaplastic carcinoma over a mesenchymal process **i4.37a**, **i4.37b** [PMID12047767, Rosen ISBN978-0781771375]. In addition, p63, normally a myoepithelial marker, can be very helpful, as pure adenocarcinomas and sarcomas of the breast are negative, while metaplastic carcinoma is positive in slightly >1/2 of cases **i4.38** [PMID16484002]. The diagnosis of metaplastic carcinoma is especially challenging on biopsy material **i4.39a**, **i4.39b**.

Although about 10% of these carcinomas will be completely negative for all keratins, 90% will have some staining for at least one epithelial marker. In addition to staining for p63, 90% of pure sarcomatoid carcinomas stain for CD29, another myoepithelial marker, suggesting a myoepithelial origin for some of these neoplasms, and negativity for myoepithelial markers has been recommended in the absence of any keratin staining before a diagnosis of a pure sarcoma in the breast is made [PMID15725803].

Apocrine lesions are rarely malignant. Indeed, the presence of apocrine metaplasia is often a reassuring sign. Clues to the presence of the rare apocrine carcinoma are an infiltrative pattern and atypia that goes well beyond the prominent nucleoli that are inherent in apocrine cells, including stratification, 3-fold enlargement of some nuclei relative to others, overly prominent or multiple nucleoli instead of a single central nucleolus, and coarse chromatin **i4.40**. It is acceptable—and often prudent—to recognize an intermediate category of apocrine proliferation of uncertain potential [PMID19147303].

Adenoid cystic carcinoma and infiltrating cribriform carcinoma are additional unusual forms of invasive ductal adenocarcinoma and can look very much alike. Adenoid cystic carcinoma has a myoepithelial component and thus has 2 cell types, vs the single cell type of infiltrating cribriforming carcinoma, though immunohistochemical staining may be needed to identify the myoepithelial component. The presence of intraductal cribriform carcinoma suggests that the invasive component is likely cribriform carcinoma. Another diagnostic difficulty with invasive cribriform carcinoma is its distinction from extensive intraductal carcinoma of the cribriform type. The presence of irregularly shaped clusters of tumor cells suggests invasion, but immunohistochemical staining for myoepithelial cells or basement membrane components may be needed.

Secretory carcinoma is seen mostly in children. It has a favorable prognosis and is characterized by minimal nuclear pleomorphism and abundant cytoplasm i4.41, occasionally with intraluminal secretions.

Intralobular Proliferations

In the normal breast, the acini that empty into a terminal duct form a lobule i4.42. Intralobular proliferations are conceptually more challenging than their intraductal counterparts. Ewing first noticed that some epithelial proliferations in the breast are centered in the lobule rather than in the duct [Ewing 1919]. In 1941, Foote and Stewart understood the essential characteristic of lobular carcinoma in situ—that there is a uniform population of cells that expands the lobule [PMID19970575]. Since then, lobular lesions have been divided into simple lobular hyperplasia, atypical lobular hyperplasia (ALH), and lobular carcinoma in situ (LCIS). Another terminology refers to these processes as lobular neoplasia grades 1, 2, and 3, respectively [PMID209887, PMID19642738]. Regardless of nomenclature, simple lobular hyperplasia is likely a variant of normal and clinically inconsequential. It is characterized by a mild increase in the number of epithelial cells ling the acini, without nuclear atypia or expansion i4.43. Atypical lobular hyperplasia (LN2) demonstrates the complete filling of some acini, with expansion i4.44A and i4.44b.

The essential diagnostic criteria of LCIS (LN3) are still those enumerated by Page, expanding on the observations of Ewing, Foote, and Stewart. All 3 of the following features must be present: There must be a complete replacement of the normal cells in the lobule by a single population of uniform cells with small nuclei, these cells must completely fill all acini in the lobule, and they must distend at least 1/2 of the acini **i4.45a**, **i4.45b** [Page ISBN978-0443022401]. While rare cases of LCIS with pleomorphism are seen (presumably the in situ counterpart to the pleomorphic variant of infiltrating lobular carcinoma), LCIS usually demonstrates substantial nuclear uniformity. The acini are filled and distended with a single population of small cells with relatively uniform nuclei. In cases where it is difficult to determine if the process is ALH (LN2) or LCIS, pagetoid spread to ducts favors LCIS over ALH.

It had been thought that LCIS is only a marker for increased risk of invasive carcinoma, not an actual precursor. The rationale for this was that the risk was equal bilaterally, but data from Page et al have shown that the ipsilateral risk for invasive lobular carcinoma is significantly higher than the contralateral risk in patients diagnosed with atypical lobular hyperplasia or LCIS [PMID12531579], leading to a newer opinion that atypical lobular hyperplasia and lobular carcinoma in situ are true precursor lesions, similar to DCIS. Some feel that watchful waiting for these patients may not be appropriate [PMID16604564], while others have concluded that LCIS (and therefore presumably ALH also) can be radiographically followed without excision, provided that there is no nuclear pleomorphism, there is no radiologic concern, and that the remaining breast tissue can be followed well by mammography [PMID18348299, PMID18660792].

Whereas it is generally agreed that the "breakpoint" in ductal processes is between ADH and DCIS on the one hand from usual hyperplasia on the other, there is not yet a corresponding consensus in lobular processes. Page et al [PMID12531579] suggests that the important diagnostic "breakpoint" is not between ALH and LCIS, but between simple lobular hyperplasia and ALH/LCIS, as is the case for ductal processes. Shaaban et al reached a similar conclusion when they found a very high relative risk for invasive carcinoma in patients with ALH [PMID11914619]. On the other hand, another study concluded that ALH carries a smaller risk of invasion than LCIS and can in most cases be monitored radiographically. In this study, about 1/4 of biopsies with LCIS had invasive carcinoma on resection, but no cases of ALH had invasion [PMID20431477].

In biopsy material, LCIS must be distinguished from intralobular spread from DCIS. Indeed, nuclear atypia in a lobule may be the only indication of a ductal carcinoma in an unsampled area of the breast. In lobular extension of DCIS, the cells are generally more pleomorphic **i4.46a**, **i4.46b** and there may be a second population of smaller, residual benign lobular cells, whereas LCIS is usually a single population of less pleomorphic cells. In cases in which it is unclear if there is a primary lobular process or an extension of a ductal process, E-cadherin tends to stain the cells in ductal processes, but not those of lobular origin [PMID20586632]. Cadherins are a superfamily of transmembrane proteins, the external portion of which binds to their counterparts from other cells, facilitating intercellular adhesion. Of the approximately 20 such proteins, the most important are those in epithelial (E-cadherin) and neural cells (N-cadherin). E-cadherin is generally maintained in ductal processes and lost in lobular processes.

Columnar cell lesions of the breast are a group of disorders of the TDLU that are often associated with microcalcifications. In simple columnar cell change of the TDLU, the normal 2-layered epithelium is replaced by a single layer of columnar cells, often with apical snouts i4.47. In columnar cell hyperplasia, the epithelium consists of 2 or more layers of such cells. The most important manifestation of the columnar cell spectrum in the TDLU is columnar cell change or hyperplasia with atypia, which is considered a flat epithelial atypia (ie, a form of low-grade in situ carcinoma) by the WHO, analogous to flat atypia at the ductal level [PMID16169223]. At the same time, however, the precise nature of flat epithelial atypia at the lobular level is unclear. The risk of progression to invasive cancer appears low [PMID12927037, PMID19287465], and it is not clear how aggressively these lesions should be treated [PMID19089736].

Before leaving the discussion of intralobular processes, mention should be made of the old term "blunt duct adenosis." This term is best not used now because it has different meanings to different people. To most people, it referred to dilatation of acini, sometimes with columnar metaplasia.

Invasive Lobular Adenocarcinomas

Invasive lobular carcinoma often has a slightly different histologic appearance from its ductal counterpart, with smaller cells, less cytoplasm, and more uniform nuclei i4.48. Occasionally, there is abundant, distinctly vacuolated cytoplasm, sometimes called the signet ring form of lobular carcinoma i4.49.

The growth pattern of lobular carcinoma is also slightly different, with less gland formation, single-file infiltration (so-called "Indian filing") i4.50 and occasionally a "targetoid" arrangement in which the neoplastic cells infiltrate in a vague circular pattern over a larger area than can be explained by an attempt to form glands. Invasive lobular carcinomas are traditionally held to have a slightly better prognosis than those of ductal origin, but clinical stage remains the key prognostic indicator for all breast carcinomas, followed by histologic grade. The pleomorphic and solids variants of lobular carcinoma often occur together i4.51 and are more aggressive than the routine form.

In practice, many carcinomas, called tubulolobular, arise from the terminal duct/lobular unit (TDLU) and have morphologic and immunohistochemical characteristics of both ductal and lobular carcinomas. These carcinomas often express both E-cadherin, typical of ductal origin, and cytokeratin 903 (high molecular weight), more typically seen in carcinomas of lobular origin [PMID15577677]. Despite this hybrid point of origin, occasional duct formation, and mixed immunohistochemical profile, tubulolobular carcinomas are often considered to be a type of lobular carcinoma.

Other than designating the rare pleomorphic and solid forms of invasive lobular carcinoma, which are both more aggressive than the usual variety, lobular carcinomas are not generally graded. The Nottingham system has also been adapted for use with invasive lobular carcinomas, though there is uncertainty as to its prognostic value in lobular neoplasms [PMID20828724].

It may be that loss of E-cadherin, with subsequent compromise of intercellular adhesion, is a fundamental defect in lobular carcinoma and in diffuse gastric carcinoma. In these tumors, E-cadherin is lost from the cell membrane and inappropriately expressed in the cytoplasm [PMID11345240], though interestingly, 16% of invasive lobular carcinomas maintain membranous expression of E-Cadherin and presumably have a defect in the cytoskeletal proteins it interacts with [PMID20871222]. While the lobular or ductal origin of an invasive breast cancer is rarely clinically important, cases of lobular carcinoma of the breast that are candidates for *BRCA1* and *BRCA2* testing and are negative for these mutations should be tested for mutations in *CDH1*, the gene that codes for E-cadherin.

A final comment on invasive lobular carcinoma is that a neuroendocrine carcinoma can resemble a lobular carcinoma, so immunohistochemical stains can be considered if an apparent lobular carcinoma has a slightly unusual appearance.

Stromal Proliferations

Juvenile papillomatosis is an exuberant form of fibrocystic changes found in younger patients and is characterized by epithelial hyperplasia and intraductal papillomatosis i4.52, i4.53, but also by dilated ducts (microcysts). The latter feature often predominates i4.54, resulting in the ineloquent moniker "Swiss cheese disease" for this process.

The stroma of juvenile fibroadenomas is usually more cellular than that of common fibroadenomas i4.55a, i4.55b, but the principle feature is that they tend to grow rapidly. But the stroma of a juvenile fibroadenoma is not as cellular as a phyllodes tumor and it has more epithelial hyperplasia. The term "fibroadenomatoid hyperplasia" is preferred to "fibroadenomatosis" for those situations in which a vaguely defined fibroadenoma-like process extends throughout a biopsy or resection.

Phyllodes (also spelled "phylloides") tumors are occasionally still called by their original name, "cystosarcoma phyllodes," though this term is no longer recognized by the World Health Organization. While phyllodes tumors have some overlapping histologic features with fibroadenomas, the relationship, if any, between the 2 entities has never been clarified. The distinction between them can be difficult and is usually made by the presence of epithelium-lined stromal projections resembling leaves i4.56; the name is derived from the Greek word "phullon," meaning "leaf"), by the greater stroma to epithelium ratio i4.57, possible stromal atypia, or occasional mitoses in a phyllodes tumor. A cellular stroma, or one with >2 mitoses per 10 HPF, suggests a phyllodes tumor.

It is debatable whether there are any truly benign phyllodes tumors or whether all are low-grade malignancies, since all have some tendency to recur if not completely excised and metastases may rarely occur. The prediction of either local recurrence or metastases is notoriously difficult. More than 30 years ago, Azzopardi recognized that aggressive behavior correlated with infiltrative margins, stromal overgrowth without an epithelial component i4.58, nuclear atypia i4.59, and >3 mitoses per 10 HPFs [Azzopardi ISBN978-0721614632]. More recent studies have confirmed this opinion and shown that the factors that increase the likelihood of local recurrence are infiltration, mitoses, higher cellularity, and nuclear atypia. These characteristics, plus size, necrosis, and overgrowth of the stromal component increase the risk of metastases, though these remain very rare [PMID19415945].

If a needle biopsy or FNA is equivocal as to fibroadenoma vs phyllodes tumor, it can be called fibroepithelial lesion with cellular stroma i4.60a, i4.60b, and should be excised, as only an excision can exclude a phyllodes tumor. Likewise stromal mitotic activity in a biopsy or FNA should elicit a recommendation for excision, as this finding introduces the possibility of a phyllodes tumor [PMID18417670].

If a needle biopsy discloses an obvious fibroadenoma, with no concern for a phyllodes tumor, it can be left alone and watched if it is less than about 4 cm, but if it is larger or is enlarging, many would suggest excision, even if the diagnosis seems assured on biopsy [PMID2048612]. The reasons for this are that there may be unsampled areas of greater concern and there is the theoretical possibility of transformation into a phyllodes tumor (though this has not been documented).

Diabetic mastopathy is usually a discrete mass, seen in longstanding type I diabetes mellitus, characterized by fibrosis, aggregates of lymphocytes i4.61, and possibly epithelioid stromal cells i4.62, although the latter is inconstant and not necessarily specific for diabetes [PMID1612578].

The so-called hamartoma (fibroadenolipoma) of the breast consists of fibrous tissue and glands, often with dilated ducts. It has the appearance of fibrocystic change, but is said to differ therefrom by the presence of adipose tissue i4.63 and the more common clinical presentation as a mass.

The myofibroblastoma is a rare benign spindle cell neoplasm that usually occurs in the breast. It is demarcated and often encapsulated, and has no significant nuclear atypia.

It may be cellular i4.64 or may have a densely collagenous stroma i4.65. A myofibroblastoma should be considered when there is an apparent phyllodes tumor that is small, is encapsulated, or lacks an epithelial component. A myofibroblastoma should also be excluded if the H&E appearance suggests a leiomyoma, spindle cell lipoma, neurofibroma, or solitary fibrous tumor. Myofibroblastomas are positive for CD34, actin, and desmin.

The following features are typical of benign breast hemangiomas [PMID18171415]:

1. They tend to be smaller than 2 cm.
2. Their vessels are lined by flat endothelium without atypia or cellular crowding i4.66.
3. Their vascular channels do not anastomose, as they often do in angiosarcomas.
4. They do not dissect between or push aside collagen fibers i4.66.
5. 50% of hemangiomas are near an artery.
6. Hemangiomas are sometimes surrounded by or intermingled with smooth muscle.
7. Hemangiomas do not disturb the architecture of the breast i4.67.

If a benign appearing vascular proliferation inserts itself between acini and tends to push them apart, suspect a low-grade angiosarcoma. An angiosarcoma should also be suspected if there is any palpable mass. In problematic cases, a Ki-67 immunohistochemical stain may help, as it tends to disclose the higher proliferation that is characteristic of angiosarcomas [PMID17425381].

Stromal Changes Secondary to Therapy

A final comment on stromal processes in the breast concerns those that are largely caused by therapy. Fat necrosis caused by previous surgery is a leading cause of a clinically worrisome mass after lumpectomy or mastectomy. Should masses caused by fat necrosis be excised, they are of considerable concern grossly, as they are firm and may be calcified [PMID8480933, PMID19234281]. Microscopically, fat necrosis is relatively easy to identify i4.68, but the reactive fibroblasts and endothelial cells that are present may also be of concern i4.69 [PMID3141983], and occasionally immunohistochemical stains will be needed to exclude carcinoma.

Changes caused by radiation therapy may also be difficult to distinguish from residual/recurrent carcinoma. Radiation therapy in any tissue causes fibrosis, glandular atrophy, and dilated capillaries [PMID19721835]. In the breast, a clue to radiation change is atrophic lobules i4.70 in which there is concentric fibrosis around the lobule or the acini therein i4.71. Individual epithelial cells of the lobule may be quite atypical, but there is no infiltration.

Angiosarcomas of the breast may arise after radiation therapy for carcinoma, but most postirradiation vascular lesions are benign. A range of benign vascular proliferations, ranging from cellular hemangiomas/lymphangiomas to postirradiation atypia of endothelial cells without an increase in the number of vascular channels i4.72, may occur after radiation therapy. Most of these benign vascular proliferations will not progress to angiosarcoma [PMID17357996]. Postirradiation vascular atypia may resemble a well differentiated angiosarcoma. Whereas angiosarcomas of the breast are generally positive for Myc protein by immunohistochemistry, or for amplification of the *MYC* gene by FISH, postirradiation vascular atypia will be negative [PMID22121953].

Like angiosarcomas in other sites, those in the breast often have a more benign appearance at the periphery. As is the case anywhere, vascular channels which anastomose freely or in an architecturally complex manner are a clue to a possible angiosarcoma and should elicit a search for endothelial hypercellularity or atypia. Moderately differentiated angiosarcomas have obvious nuclear atypia, but still form recognizable vessels i4.73, while poorly differentiated angiosarcomas may form masses with little or no recognizable vessel formation i4.74.

Core Points for Breast

- Florid adenosis vs invasive carcinoma:
  - Particularly difficult on biopsy.
  - Demonstration of myoepithelial (ME) cells helpful.
  - P63 stains the nuclei of ME cells.
  - Stains for ME cell cytoplasm include calponin and myosin heavy chain.
- "Breakpoint" in intraductal proliferative lesions is between ADH/DCIS from any form of usual ductal hyperplasia.
- "Breakpoint" in lobular processes is likely between atypical lobular hyperplasia/lobular carcinoma in situ from any lesser lobular proliferation.
- Low-grade DCIS:
  - Specific architectural patterns (eg, cribriform, micropapillary)
  - Regular nuclear spacing
  - Paradoxically, nuclear uniformity
  - More than one focus of such a process should be identified for the diagnosis.
- High-grade DCIS: compelling nuclear atypia.
  - Often has central necrosis, but this is not a diagnostic criterion.
  - No quantitation requirements for the diagnosis.
- Cellular intraductal papilloma vs papillary intraductal carcinoma: immunohistochemical demonstration of myoepithelial cells secures the diagnosis of a benign process.
- Invasive breast carcinoma:
  - Size of tumor
  - Specific type
  - Grade
  - Presence or absence of angiolymphatic invasion
  - Assessment of margins
    - May report margin status of invasive component separately from that of in situ component.
    - 0.5 cm of normal breast tissue is negative margin.
    - No consensus if <0.5 cm.
    - Prudent to report anything <0.2 cm as equivocal or close to the margin.
- Most common genetic syndromes involving breast carcinoma are *BRCA1/2* and the E-cadherin gene *CDH1*.

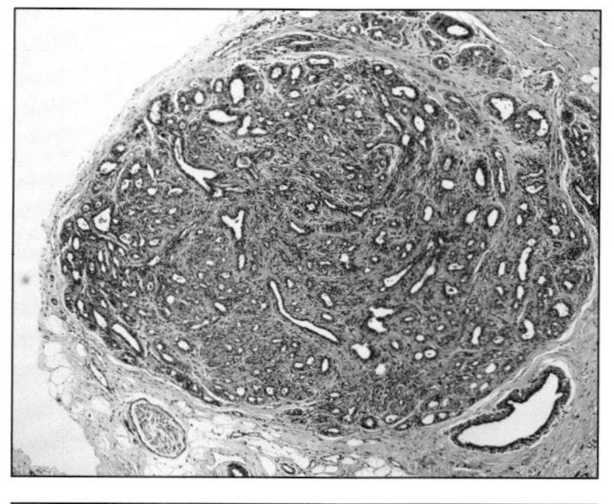

i4.1 A nodule of adenosis. Note the sharp circumscription.

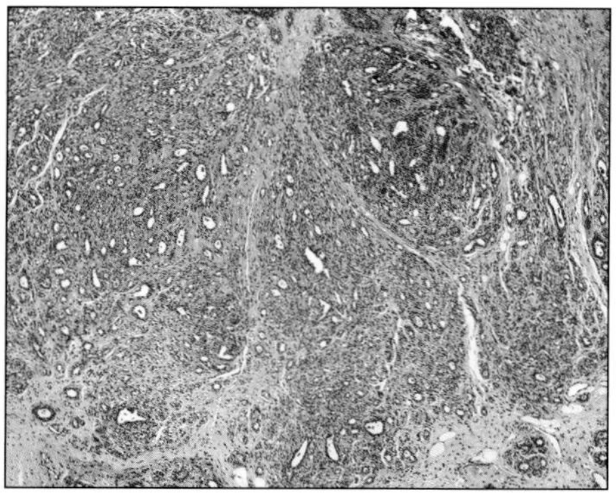

i4.2 Multiple coalescing nodules of adenosis, forming a clinically worrisome mass. Note the circumscription of the individual masses.

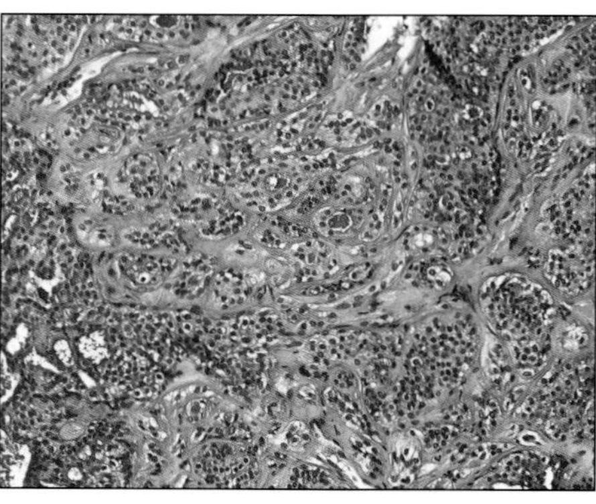

i4.3 A needle biopsy of a distinct breast mass with worrisome cellularity and what appears to be an infiltrative pattern

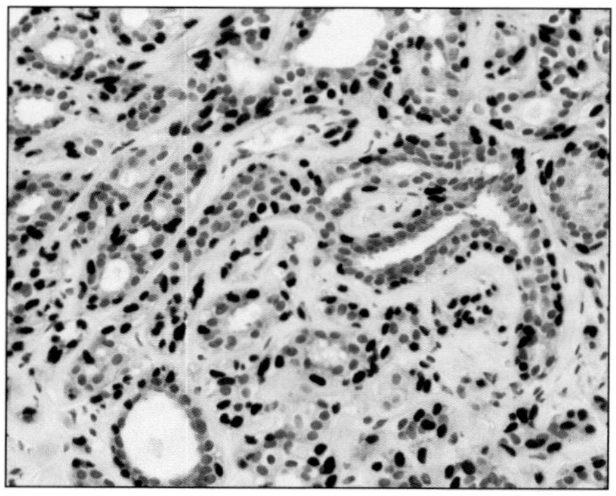

i4.4 The same biopsy as in i4.3 stained for p63, identifying the nuclei of a myoepithelial layer, suggesting a diagnosis of adenosis rather than invasive carcinoma

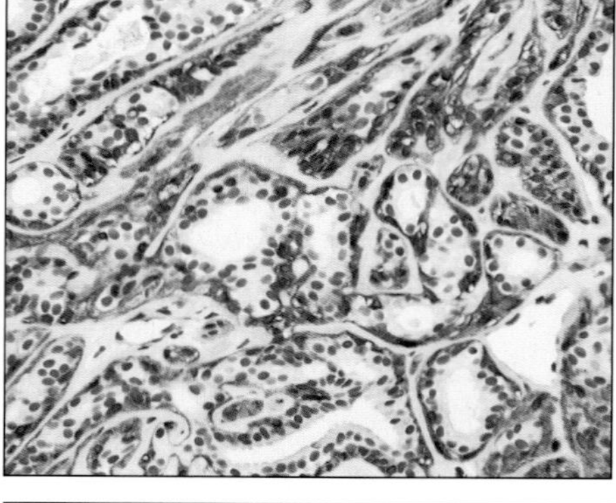

i4.5 The same biopsy as in i4.3 stained for calponin, identifying myoepithelial cytoplasm. The identification of a myoepithelial layer by both p63 and calponin secures a diagnosis of adenosis rather than invasive carcinoma.

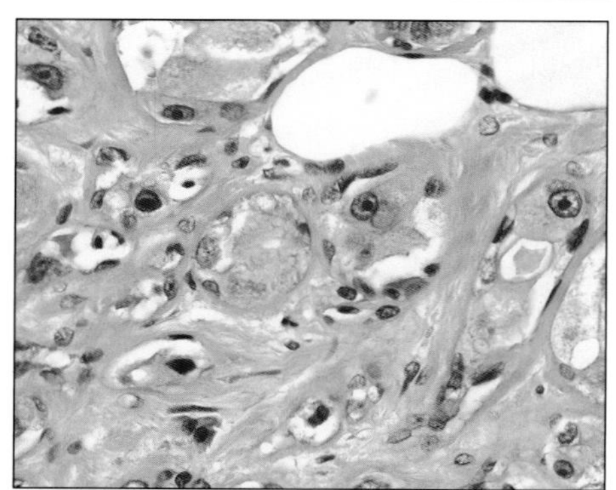

i4.6 Sclerosing adenosis with apocrine metaplasia. The nuclear enlargement, and in particular, the prominent nucleoli, can easily cause a misdiagnosis of carcinoma.

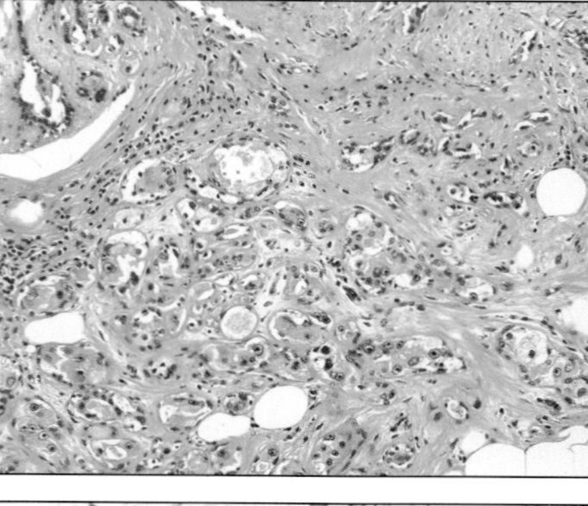

i4.7 The same specimen as in i4.6, but shown at lower power to illustrate the circumscription of the process

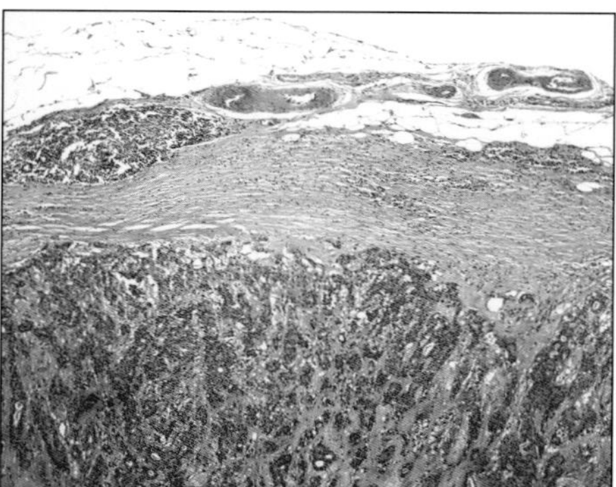

i4.8 A so-called tubular adenoma, another process of extensive cellularity that can simulate a carcinoma unless attention is given to its circumscribed overall architecture

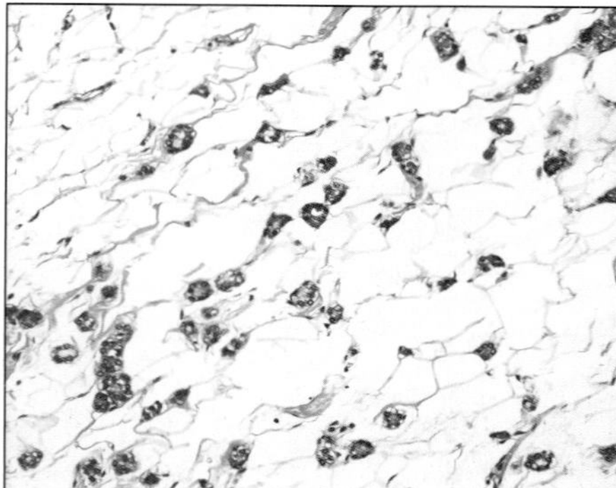

i4.9 Microglandular adenosis simulating a tubular carcinoma because of the infiltrative pattern

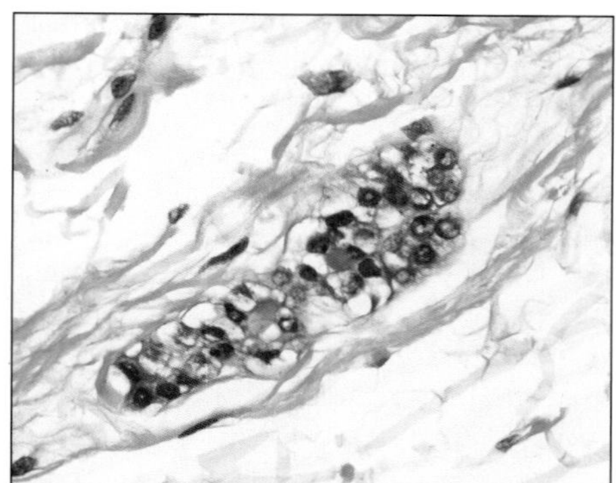

i4.10 Microglandular adenosis often have clear cytoplasm and eosinophilic secretions in the lumens.

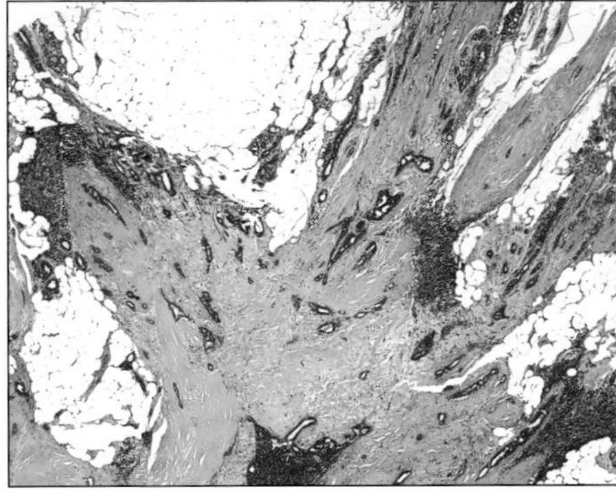
i4.11 A complex sclerosing lesion (radial scar) photographed at low power to illustrate the stellate shape, but overall circumscription of the process

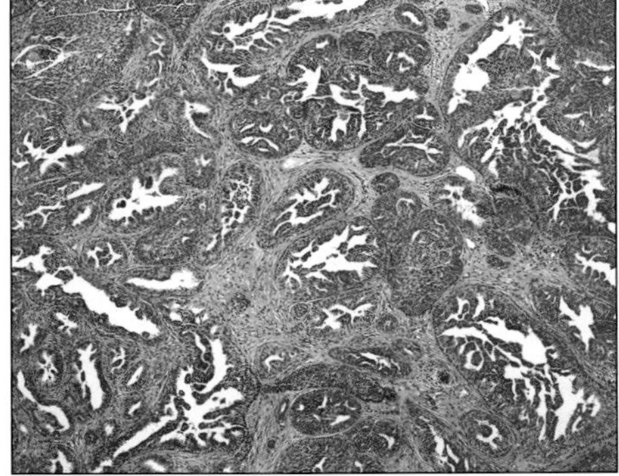
i4.12 A complex epithelial proliferation of hyperplasia and papillomatosis in the lactiferous ducts of the nipple (nipple adenoma). If each duct is studied separately, the process in it will be resolved as benign.

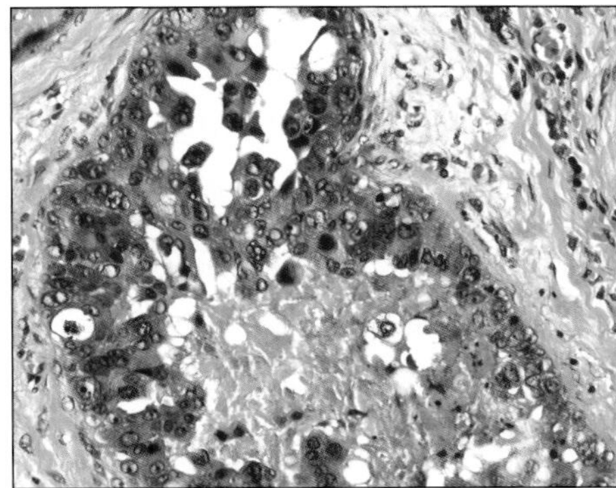
i4.13 High-grade intraductal carcinoma, with obvious nuclear pleomorphism. Neither the architecture of the intraductal proliferation nor the amount need be considered in diagnosis of high-grade intraductal carcinoma.

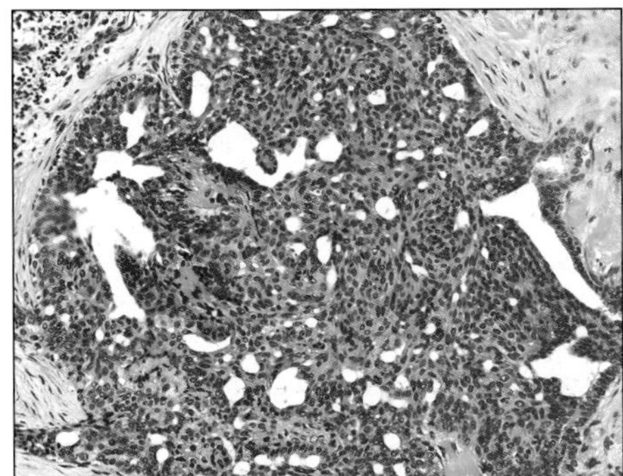
i4.14 Florid hyperplasia of the usual type. Although the duct is nearly completely filled, the epithelial cells lack pleomorphic nuclei and the secondary lumens are irregularly shaped. Even at low power, myoepithelial cells, with spindled nuclei, can be identified.

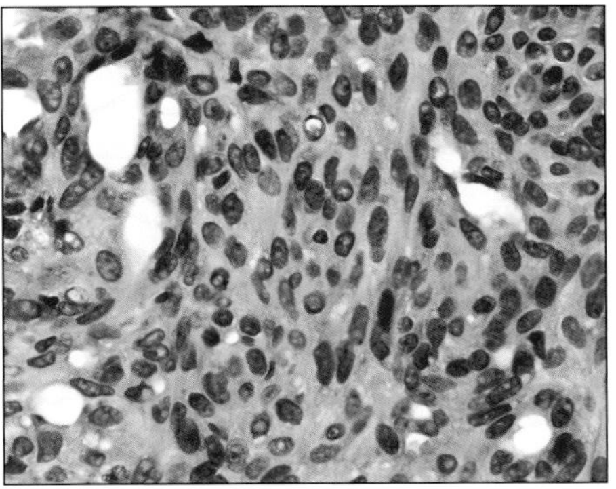
i4.15 A high-power view of the process depicted in i4.14, in which epithelial and myoepithelial cells appear to form a vague fascicle (streaming).

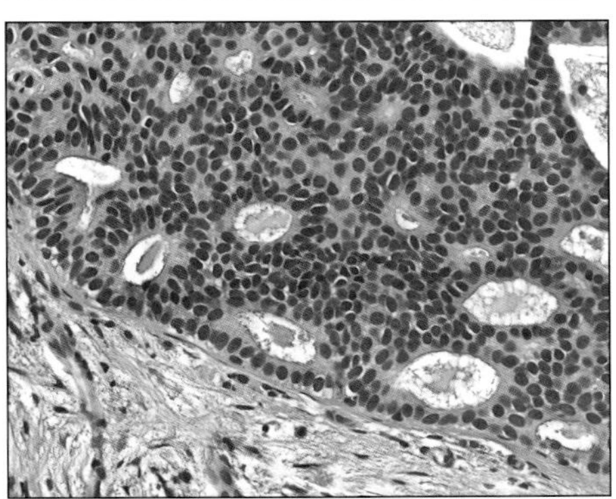
i4.16 Low-grade intraductal carcinoma of the cribriform type. In contrast to the hyperplasia depicted in i4.14, note the monomorphic population of cells, without myoepithelial cells. Note also the generally uniform and well demarcated se condary lumens formed by a sharp radial distribution of tumor cells. The nuclei are generally relatively evenly spaced, in contrast to the nuclei of hyperplasia.

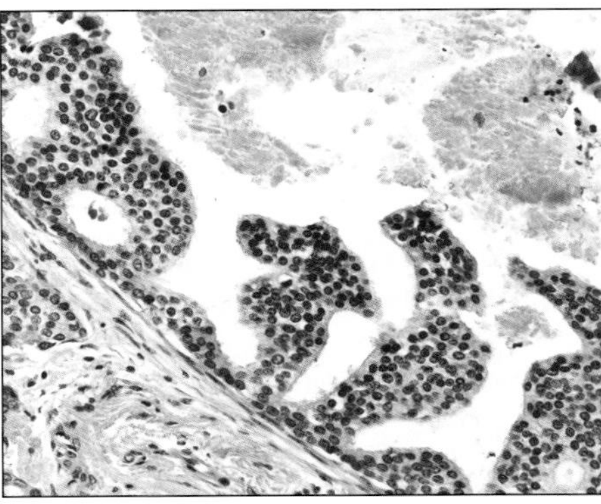
i4.17 Low-grade intraductal carcinoma of the micropapillary type. Note the relatively uniform nuclei, the monomorphic population of cells within the micropapillae, without myoepithelial cells, and the broadened tip of some of the micropapillae.

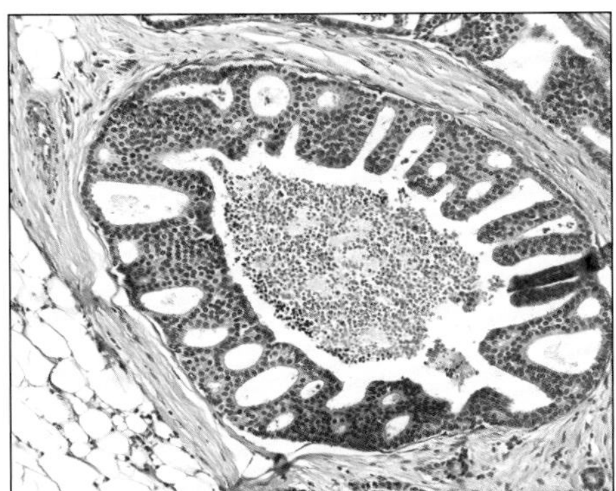
i4.18 The micropapillary type of low-grade intraductal carcinoma in which the tips of the papillae are connected, forming so called "Roman bridges"

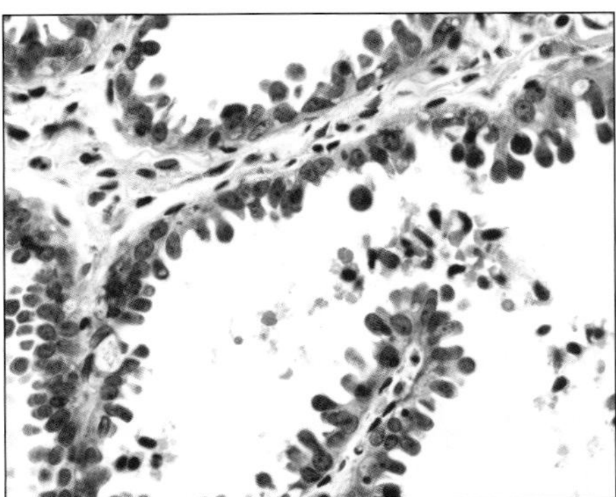
i4.19 Flat epithelial atypia (formerly called clinging carcinoma) in which the ducts are lined by a single layer of very atypical cells. While there is debate whether this is a form of atypical hyperplasia or a form of intraductal carcinoma, it is clear that this finding increases the risk of invasive carcinoma.

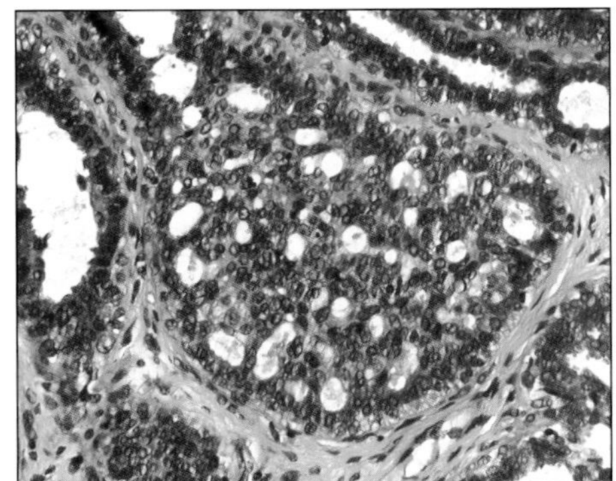
i4.20 A problematic breast proliferation that received a consensus diagnosis of atypical hyperplasia because this was the only duct involved, despite the fact that the criteria for low-grade intraductal carcinoma of the cribriform type are essentially fulfilled

ISBN 978-089189-5886

i4.21 a A cellular, complex intraductal epithelial proliferation, which at low power lacks the nuclear uniformity, even spacing, and well defined round secondary lumens of low-grade cribriform intraductal carcinoma

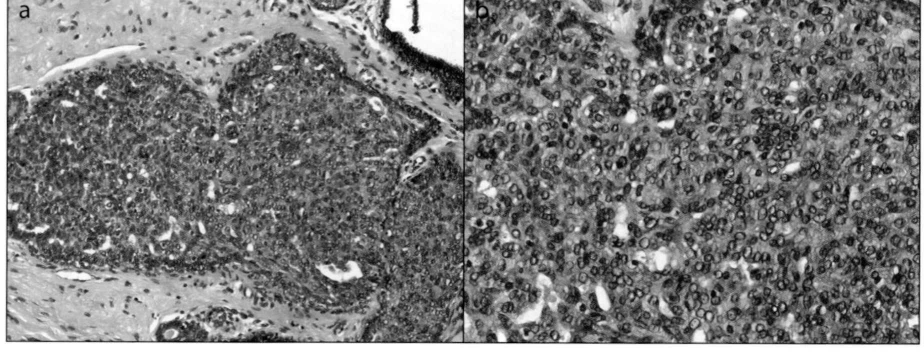

b Higher magnification confirms that although this is a cellular proliferation (reflexively more worrisome than common hyperplasia) that does not fulfill either the nuclear or architectural characteristics of any form of low-grade intraductal carcinoma. This case received a consensus diagnosis of atypical hyperplasia because there were numerous ducts with this appearance.

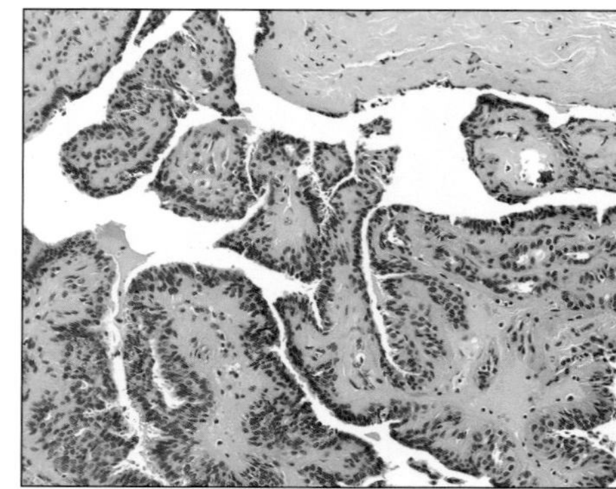

i4.22 Benign intraductal papilloma with well developed fibrovascular cores and low cellularity.

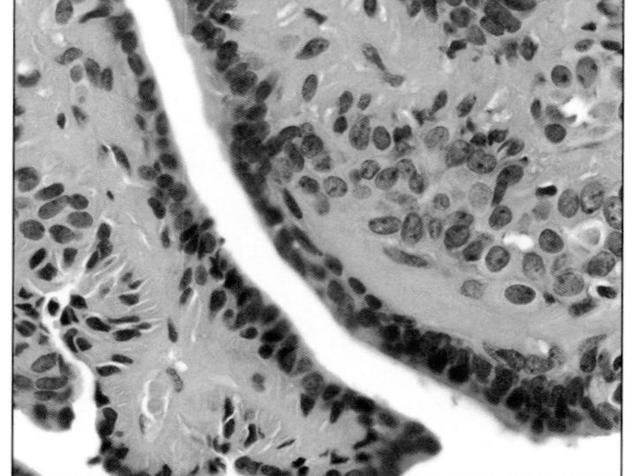

i4.23 A high-power view of the process in i4.22 illustrating the retention of the spindle-shaped myoepithelial cells

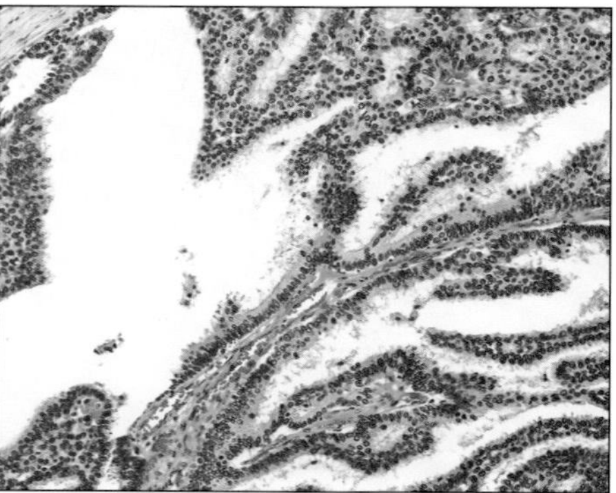

i4.24 Papillary intraductal carcinoma with a complex architecture consisting of numerous thin papillations

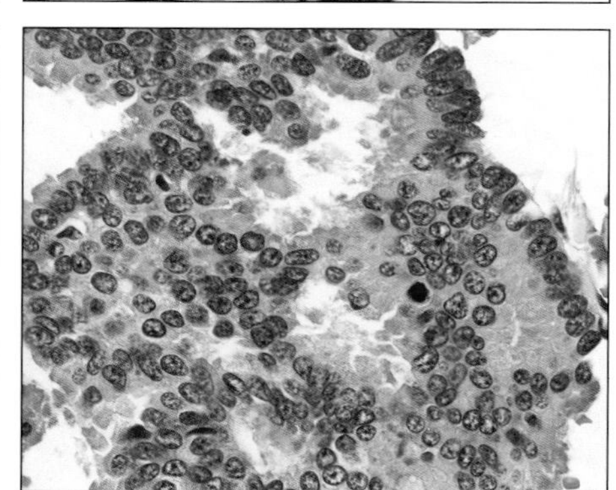

i4.25 Papillary intraductal carcinoma with areas of hypercellularity, with numerous epithelial cells that are not directly connected to a papilla. Note the mitotic figure in the right center.

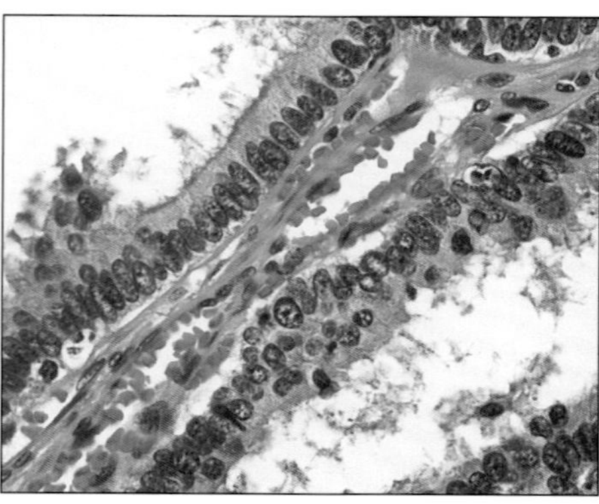

i4.26 Papillary intraductal carcinoma demonstrating the lack of myoepithelial cells compared to the benign papilloma in i4.23, which retains myoepithelial cells

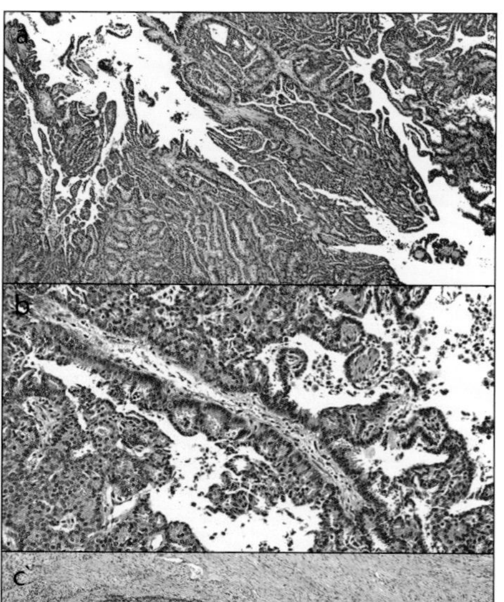

i4.27 a Papillary intraductal carcinoma of great cellularity with small, subtle fibrovascular cores, which out of context can simulate invasive carcinoma

b The same process as in i4.27a, but subtle fibrovascular cores, suggesting a papillary process, can be seen.

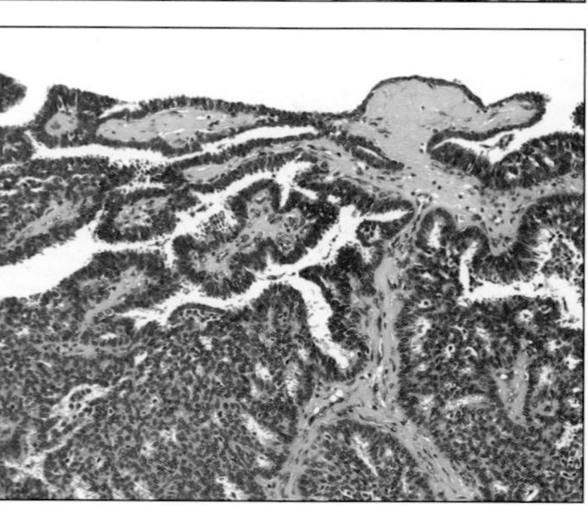

i4.28 The upper portion of this intraductal papillary proliferation appears entirely benign, with well developed fibrovascular cores and low cellularity, but in the lower portion of the process there is much greater cellularity and architectural complexity.

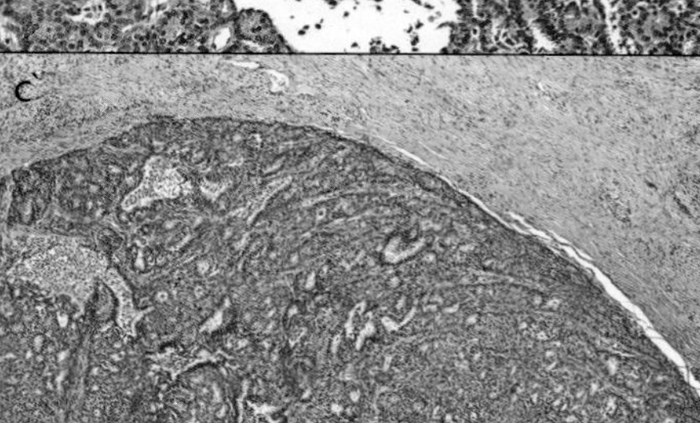

c The same process as in i4.27a, but this low-power view demonstrates circumscription and shows that the process is occurring in a dilated duct.

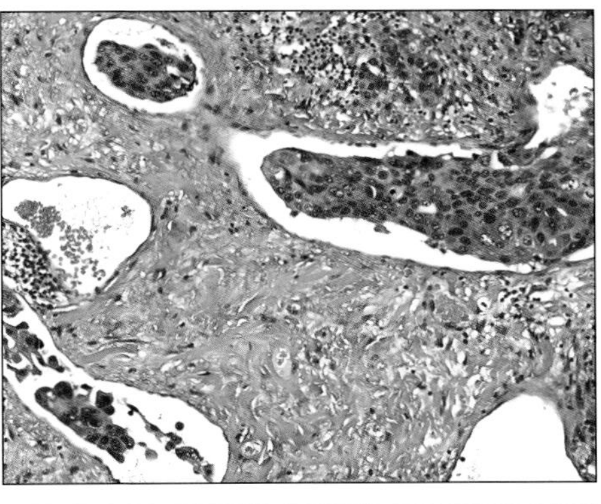

i4.29 Lymphatic invasion of an invasive carcinoma

i4.30 Small clusters of tumor cells, within the main tumor mass, that simulate lymphatic invasion because of retraction artifact

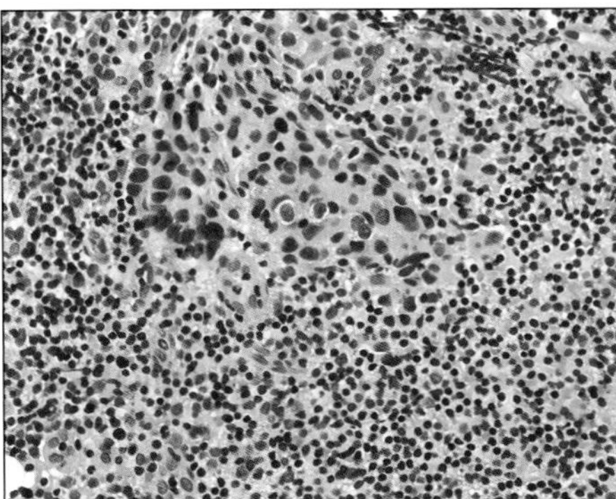

i4.31 A micrometastasis of breast carcinoma to an axillary lymph node

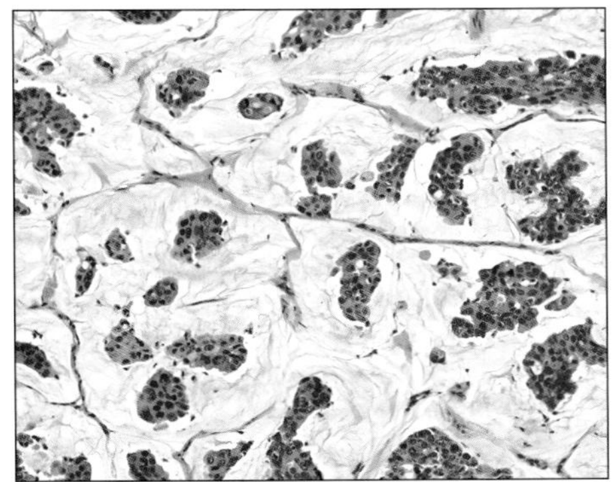

i4.32 Mucinous (colloid) carcinoma of the breast

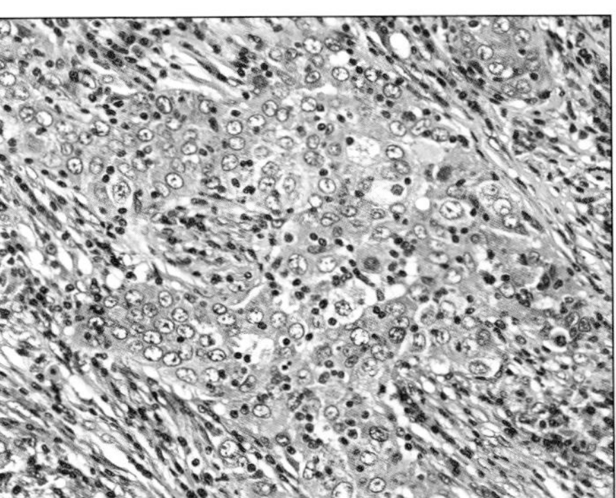

i4.33 Medullary carcinoma of the breast with pleomorphic nuclei, minimal gland formation, and lymphocytes. Note the absence of an intraductal component.

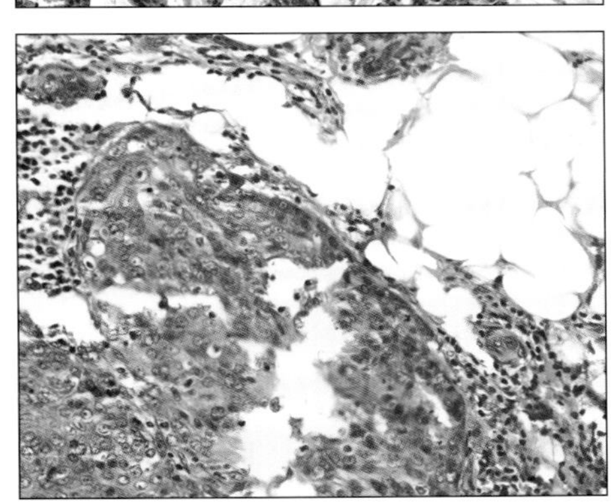

i4.34 Medullary carcinoma of the breast with sharp circumscription

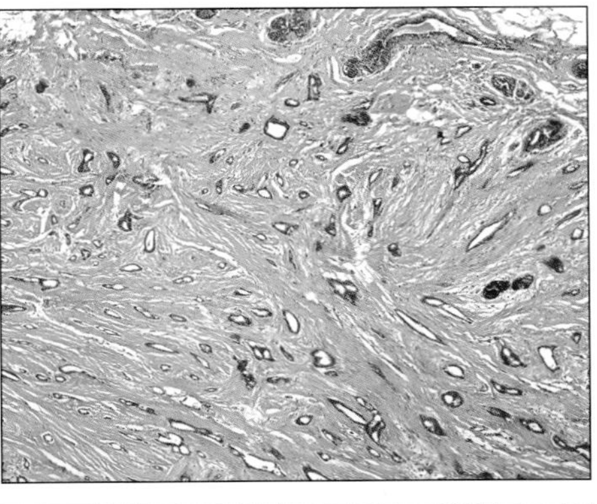

i4.35 Tubular carcinoma of the breast with small, angulated glands and minimal nuclear pleomorphism. Although the individual glands appear innocuous, note the infiltrative pattern.

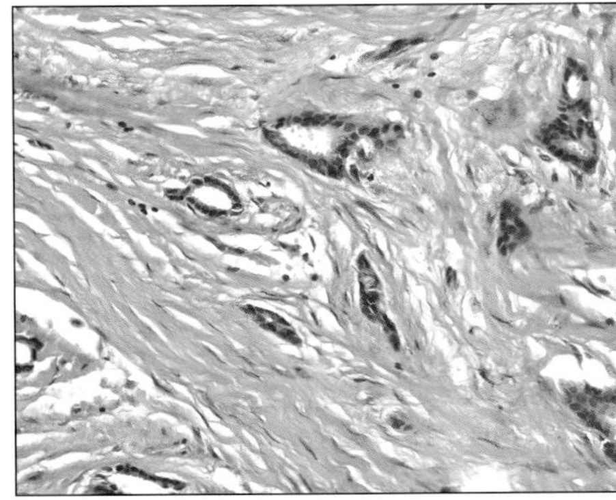

i4.36 A high-power view of tubular carcinoma of the breast, demonstrating the angulated outline with occasional protrusions

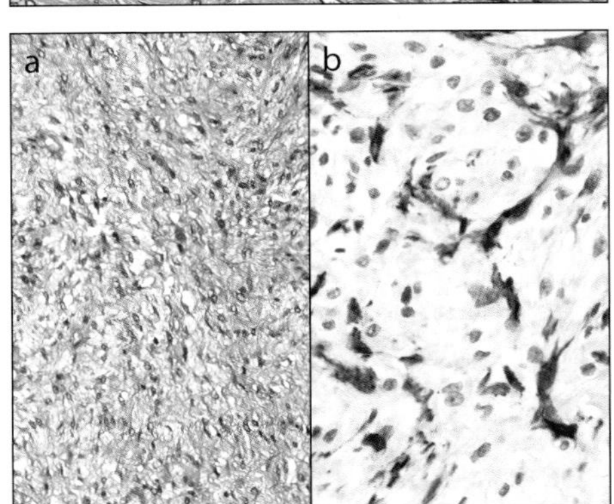

i4.37 **a** A metaplastic carcinoma of the breast with a benign-appearing stromal component. **b** Same case as in 4.37a with positive immunohistochemical staining for cytokeratin 7, identifying the stromal component as having epithelial characteristics

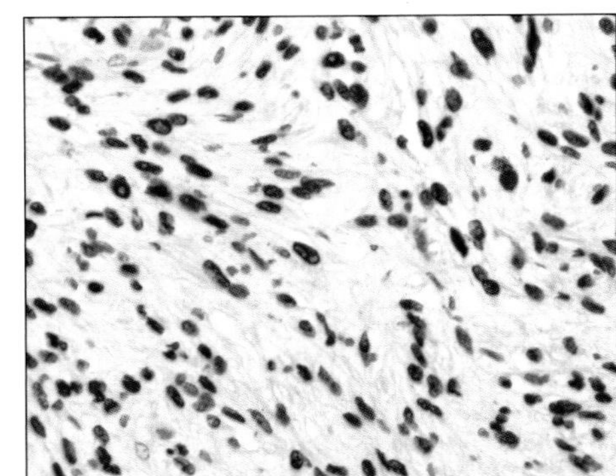

i4.38 The same case as in i4.37 with p63 staining of the nuclei, additional evidence of a metaplastic carcinoma

ISBN 978-089189-5886

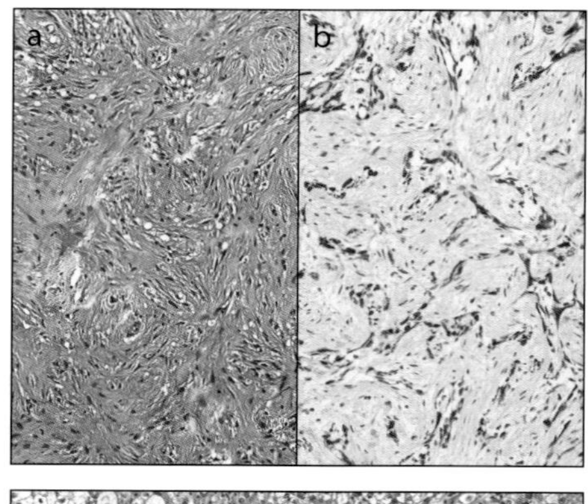

i4.39 **a** A metaplastic carcinoma on a biopsy. **b** The same biopsy as i4.39a with staining for cytokeratin 7, confirming an epithelial component

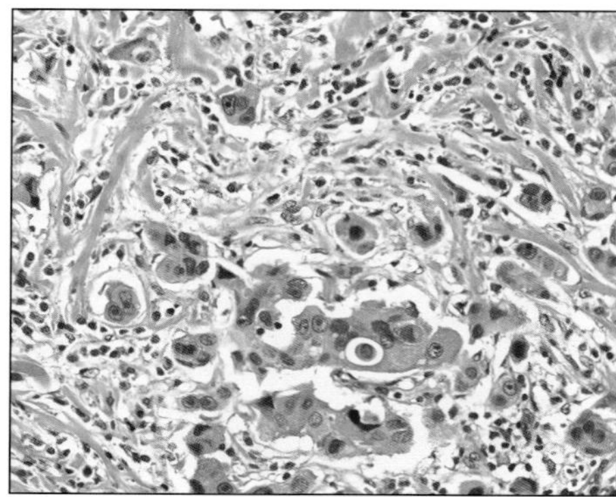

i4.40 Apocrine carcinoma of the breast. The individual cells are more pleomorphic than in apocrine metaplasia, but the important finding is the infiltrative nature of the process.

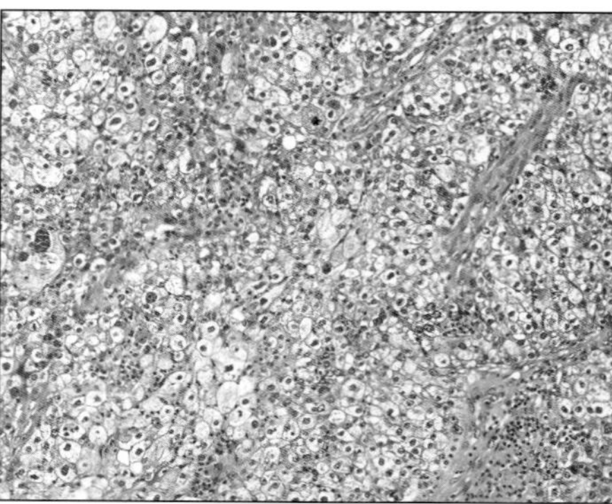

i4.41 Secretory carcinoma of the breast. Note the relatively uniform nuclei and abundant clear cytoplasm. This case occurred in a young adult.

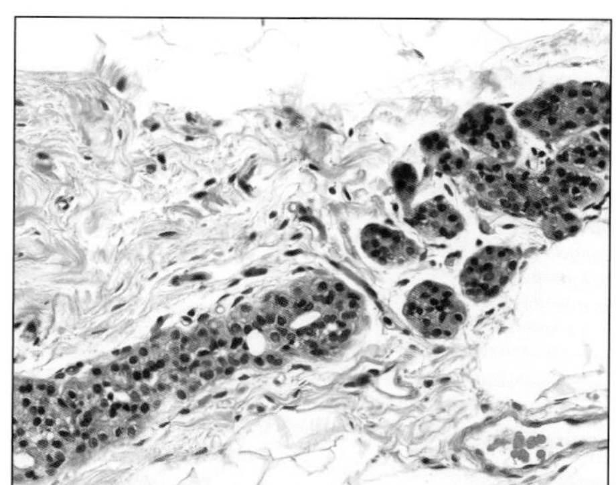

i4.42 A normal lobule of the breast in the upper right, consisting of 10-12 acini emptying into the intercalated duct on the left

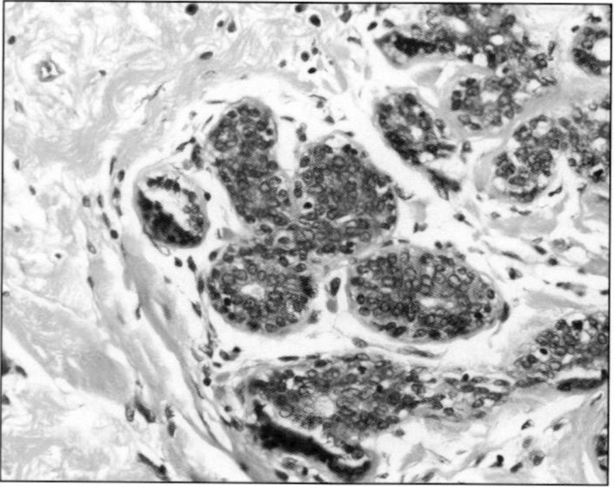

i4.43 Simple lobular hyperplasia (lobular neoplasia grade 1) with a mild increase in the number of cells lining some of the acini, but no complete filling and no significant expansion

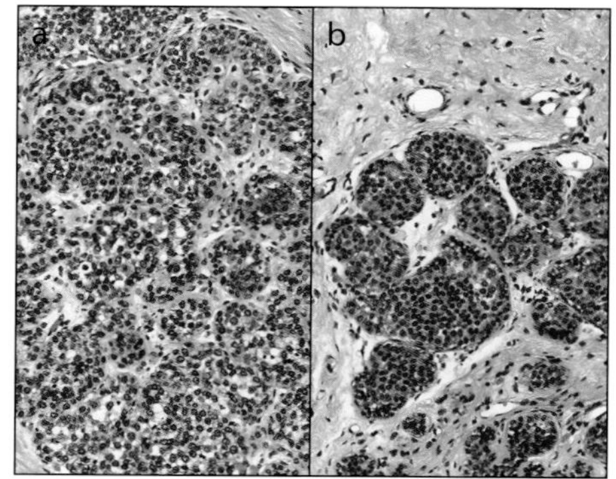

i4.44 **a** Atypical lobular hyperplasia (lobular neoplasia grade 2). The lobule is expanded but most acini are not completely filled. **b** An intralobular proliferation that some would interpret as atypical lobular hyperplasia (LN2) and others as LCIS (LN3). Acini are generally filled and expanded, but not markedly.

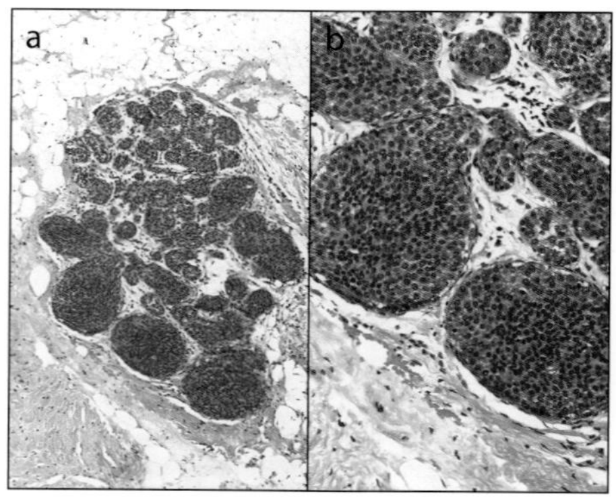

i4.45 **a** Obvious lobular carcinoma in situ (lobular neoplasia grade 3) with complete filling and distension of most of the acini and expansion of the lobule. Compare to normal lobule on the left. **b** Same case as in i4.45**a**, highlighting the complete filling and distention of the acini and the expansion of the lobule

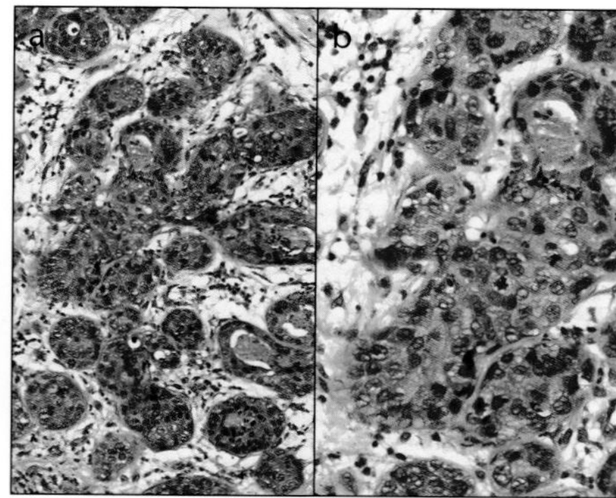

i4.46 **a** Lobular extension of DCIS with the acini filled and distended by cells that are more pleomorphic than in a lobular process. **b** A higher-power view of the same case as i4.46a, confirming the greater nuclear pleomorphism of a ductal process that extends into lobules

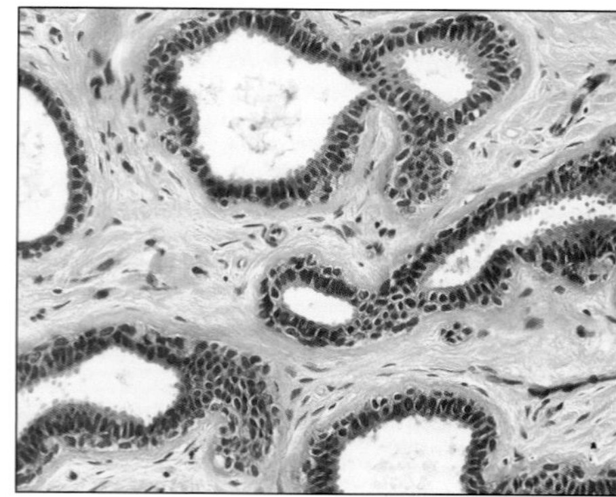

i4.47 Columnar cell change of the terminal duct/lobule. If there is multilayering or atypia, the significance is that of an in situ carcinoma.

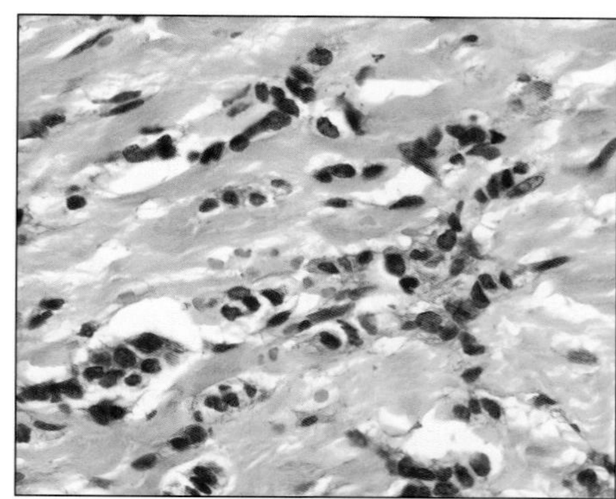

i4.48 Infiltrating lobular carcinoma demonstrating the relatively uniform nuclei, with minimal cytoplasm and no gland formation

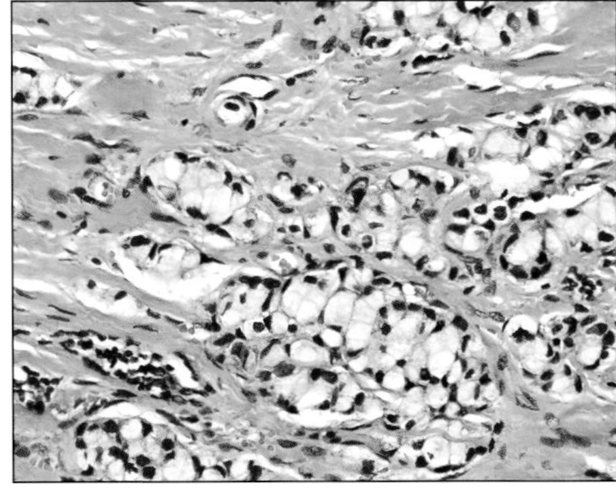

i4.49 The signet ring form of infiltrating lobular carcinoma with abundant mucinous cytoplasm and eccentric nuclei

i4.50 The single file infiltration ("Indian filing") pattern that is often seen in infiltrating lobular carcinoma

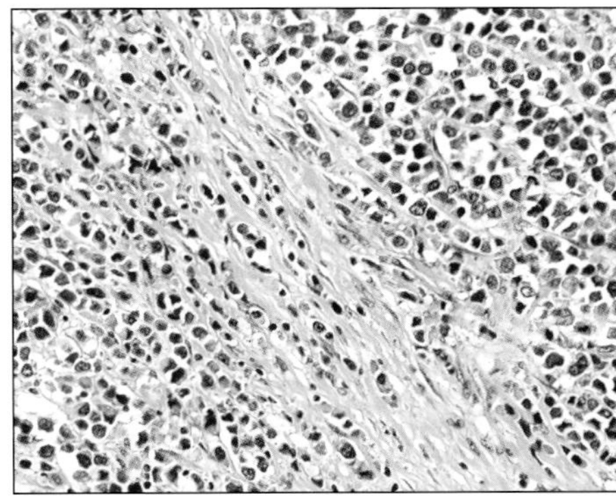

i4.51 The pleomorphic/solid variant of lobular carcinoma. In the center, there is a relatively classic infiltrating lobular carcinoma, with small nuclei, but on either side the neoplastic cells are much larger and more pleomorphic.

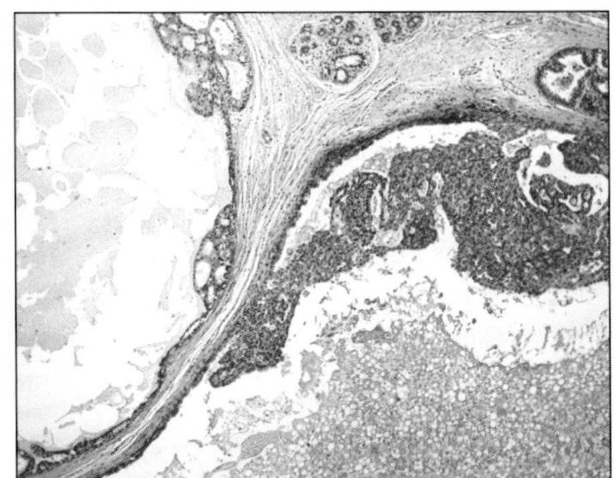

i4.52 Juvenile papillomatosis, with epithelial hyperplasia and distended ducts

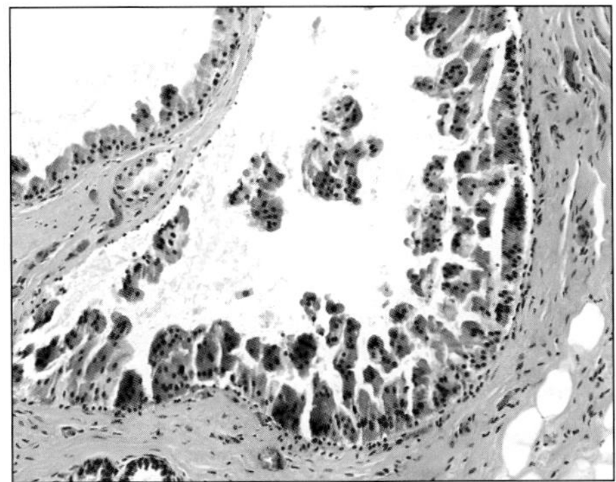

i4.53 Juvenile papillomatosis with epithelial hyperplasia and apocrine metaplasia

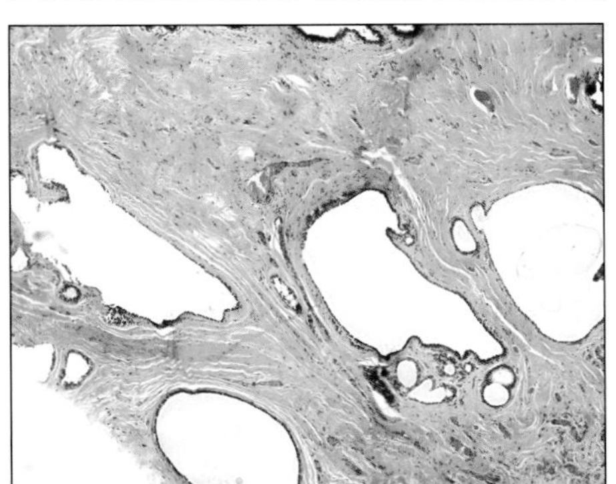

i4.54 Juvenile papillomatosis with predominance of dilated ducts (microcysts) and little epithelial hyperplasia

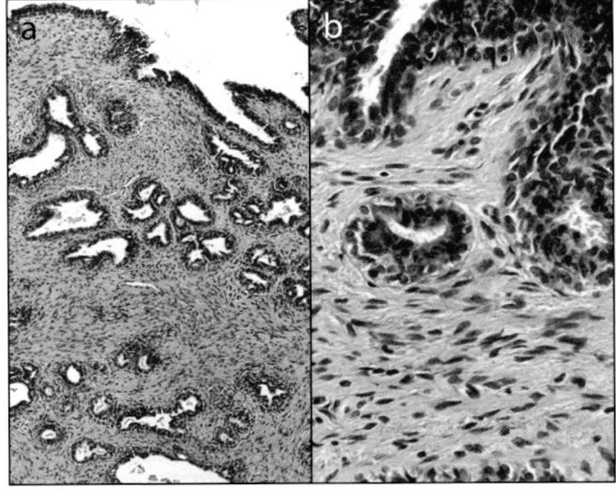

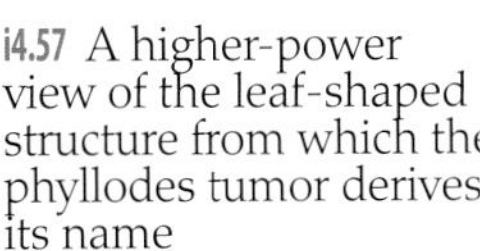

i4.55 **a** A juvenile fibroadenoma, characterized by slightly higher cellularity in both the stroma and in the epithelial component than a classic fibroadenoma. **b** A higher-power view of juvenile fibroadenoma, demonstrating the increased cellularity of both the epithelial and stromal components, but there is no significant atypia or mitotic activity of either component.

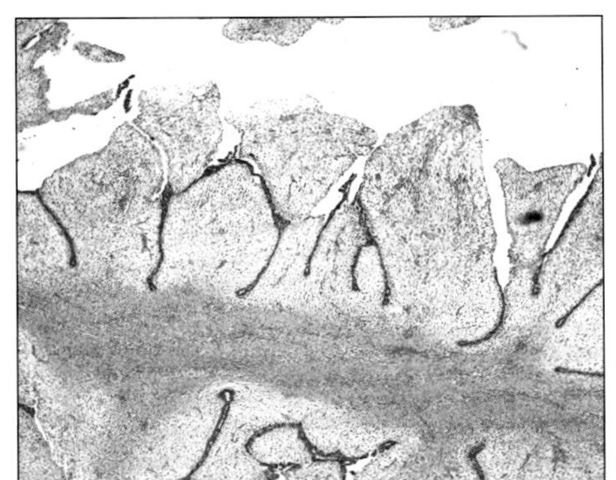

i4.56 A benign phyllodes tumor, with leaf-shaped structures

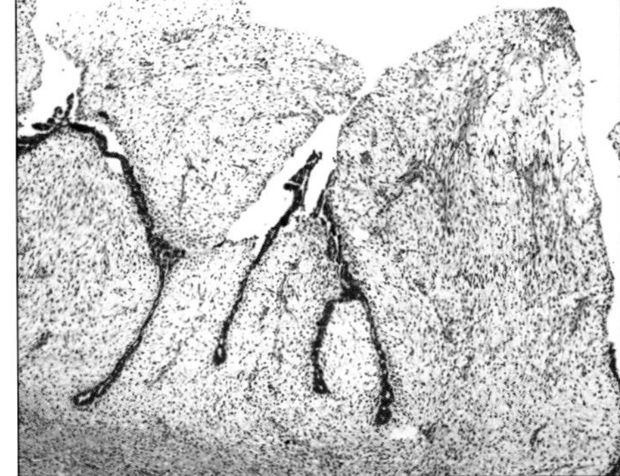

i4.57 A higher-power view of the leaf-shaped structure from which the phyllodes tumor derives its name

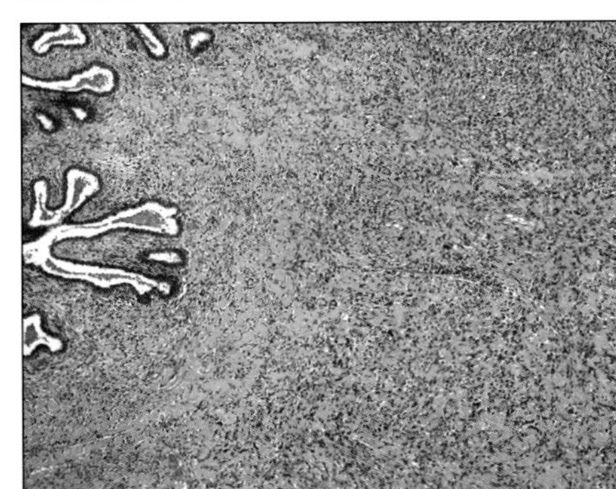

i4.58 While this phyllodes tumor has a normal mixture of epithelial and stromal components on the left, there is stromal overgrowth in the center and on the right, a sign of possible malignancy.

ISBN 978-089189-5886

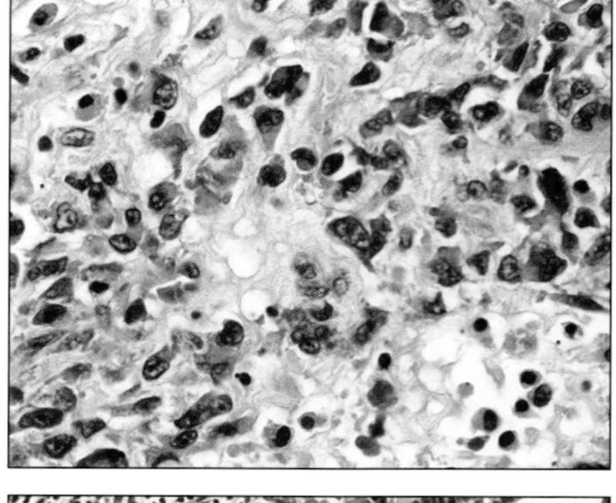

i4.59 A high-power view of the stromal cells of this phyllodes tumor identifies it as malignant.

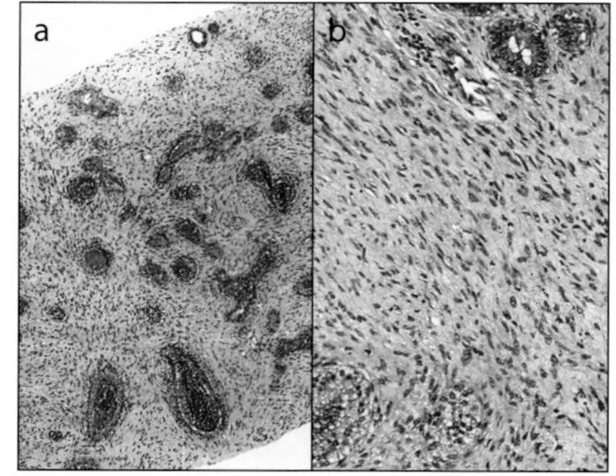

i4.60 **a** A biopsy illustrating a fibroepithelial lesion, which could be either a cellular fibroadenoma or a phyllodes tumor
b A higher-power view of the biopsy in i4.60a confirming stromal hypercellularity but demonstrating no significant atypia or mitotic activity of either the epithelial or the stromal component

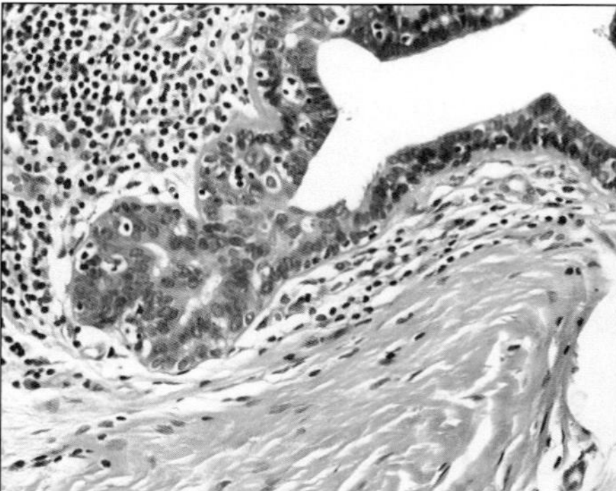

i4.61 Diabetic mastopathy, illustrating the periductal lymphocytes and stromal fibrosis

i4.62 Another example of diabetic mastopathy, again with periductal lymphocytes and fibrosis, but also with epithelioid stromal cells on the right. These stromal cells have enlarged nuclei and small nucleoli.

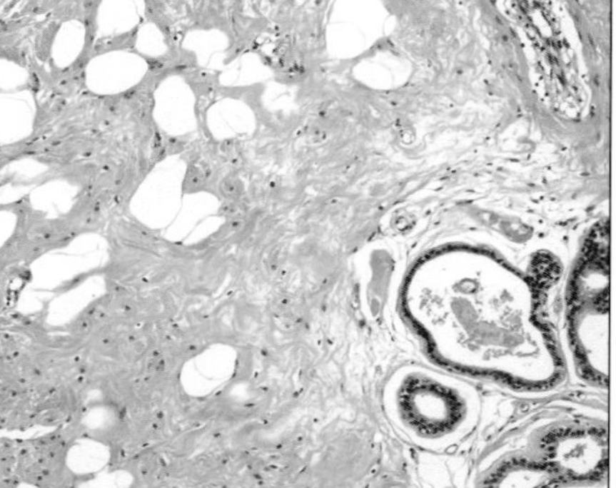

i4.63 A hamartoma of the breast (fibroadenolipoma), which presented as a distinct mass and which consists of epithelium, fibrous stroma, and adipose tissue

i4.64 A cellular example of a myofibroblastoma

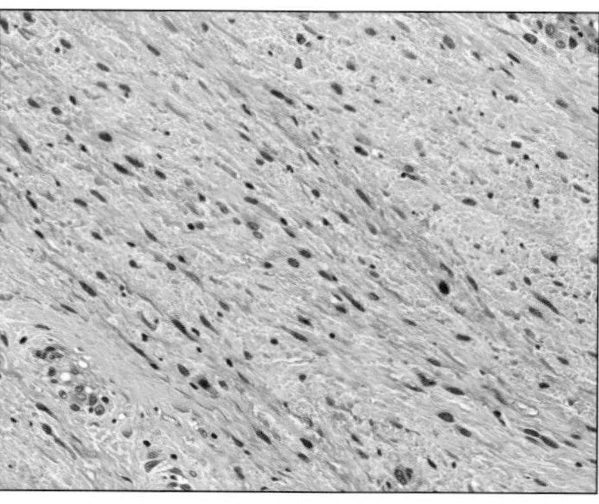

i4.65 A myofibroblastoma, which is less cellular and has a collagenous stroma

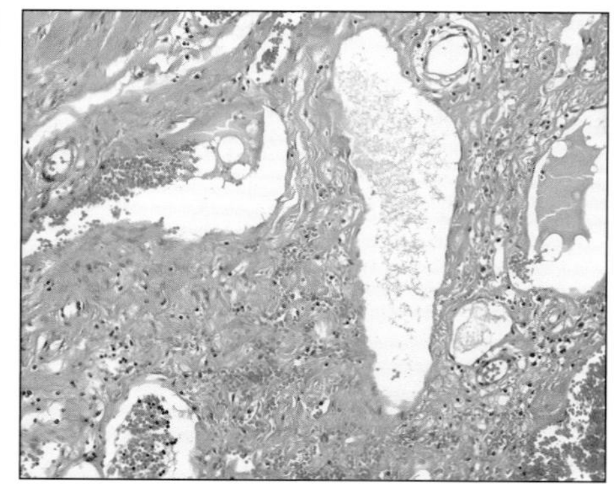

i4.66 A hemangioma of the breast in which there is no endothelial atypia or crowding. The vascular channels are well defined and do not dissect into the stroma.

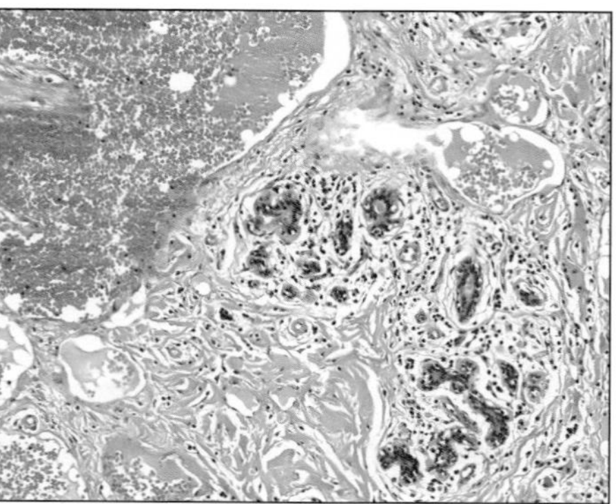

i4.67 A hemangioma of the breast in which the vascular channels do not invade or disturb the lobules

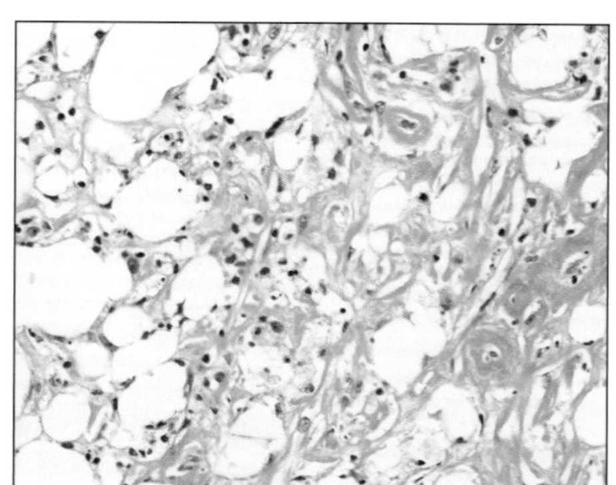

i4.68 A low-power view of fat necrosis, with necrotic adipocytes, fibrosis, and inflammation

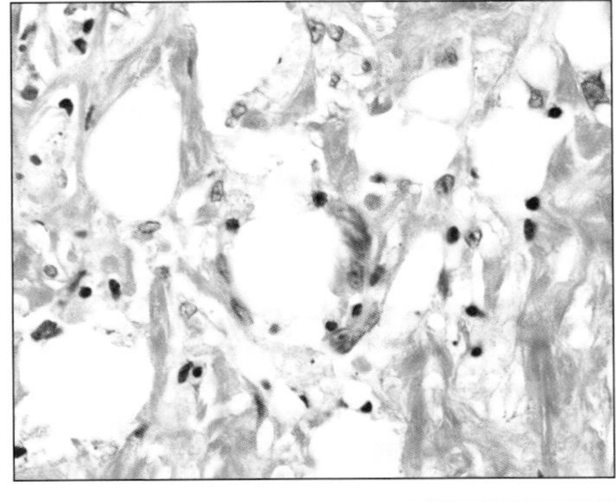

i4.69 A high-power view of fat necrosis, in which reactive fibroblasts and endothelial cells may be confused with carcinoma

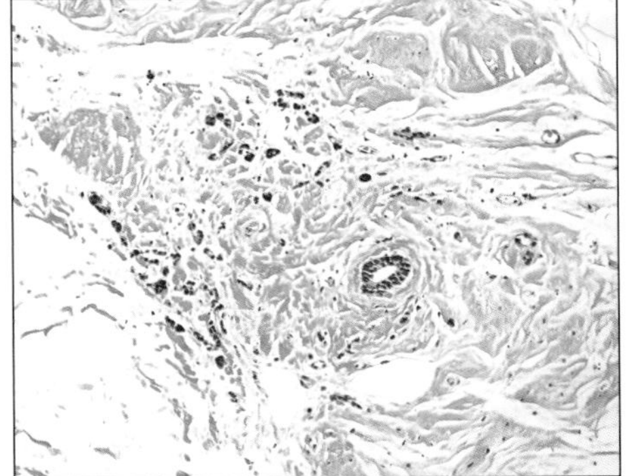

i4.70 Radiation change in a lobule. There is cellular atypia, but the focus is small (this is its entirety) and a lobular pattern is maintained. Most acini are atrophic.

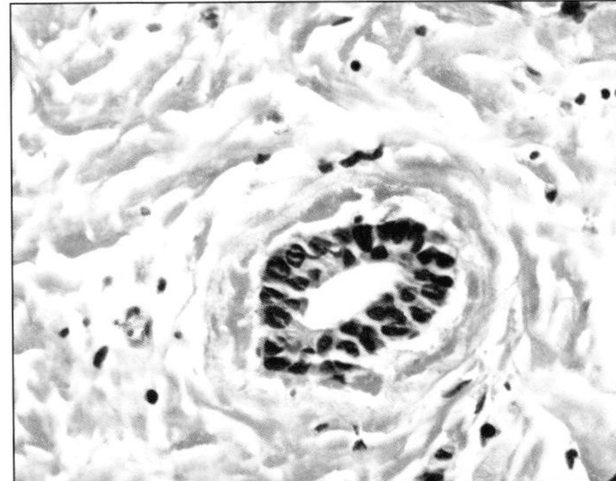

i4.71 Radiation change illustrating the concentric fibrosis that surrounds an acinus. Note the spindled myoepithelial cell at the bottom of the acinus.

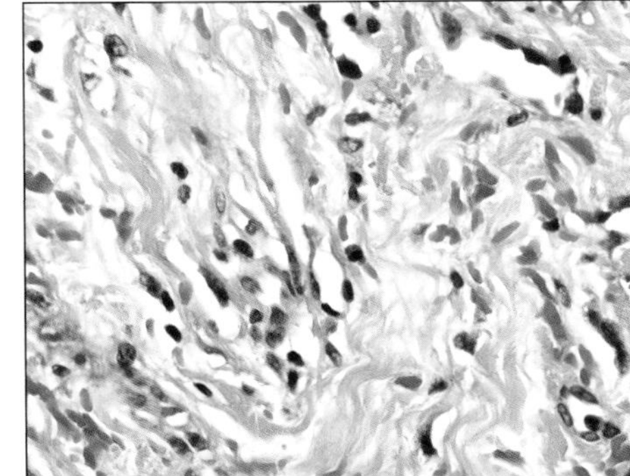

i4.72 Postirradiation vascular atypia in which there is mild, focal endothelial atypia and hypercellularity, but vascular channels remain well defined and there is no invasion into the stroma. This is a dermal lesion in a patient who received radiation therapy for breast carcinoma.

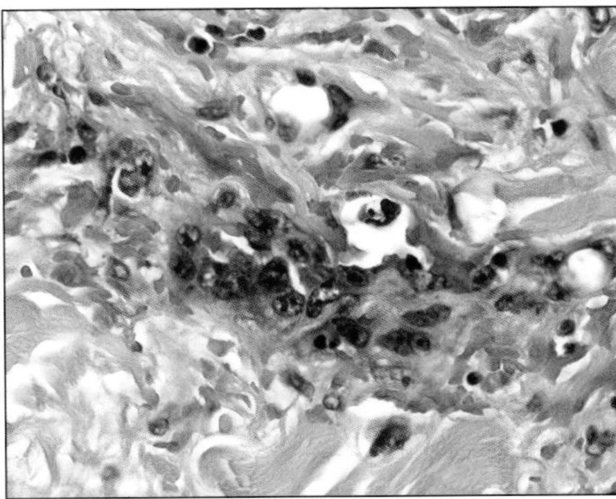

i4.73 A moderately differentiated angiosarcoma in which there is obvious nuclear atypia but the neoplastic cells form well defined vascular channels. This is a dermal lesion in a patient who received radiation therapy for breast carcinoma.

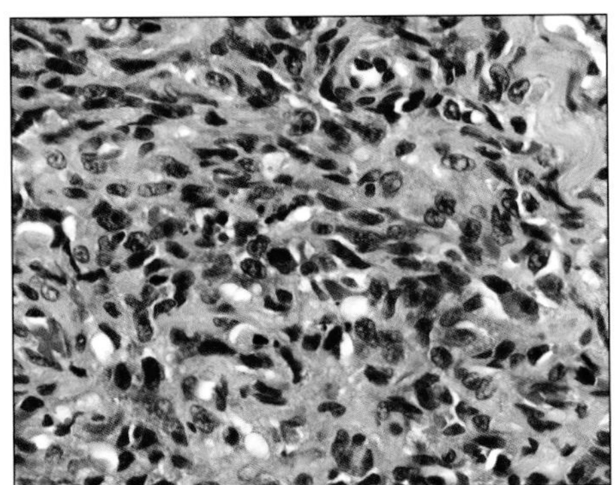

i4.74 A high-grade angiosarcoma with only minimal formation of vascular channels. Most of the neoplastic cells grow as diffuse clusters with no recognizable attempt to form blood vessels. This is a dermal lesion in a patient who received radiation therapy for breast carcinoma.

ISBN 978-089189-5886

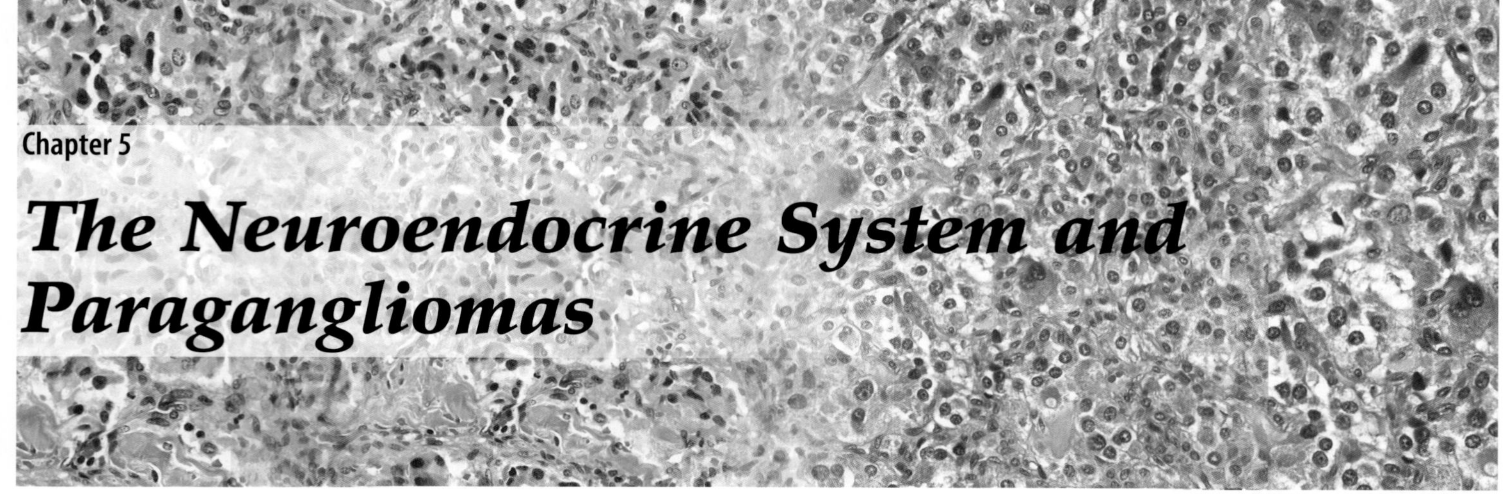

Chapter 5

The Neuroendocrine System and Paragangliomas

Dense core vesicles (also called neurosecretory vesicles) are intracellular structures found in many types of endocrine cells that store peptide hormones for eventual secretion i5.1. Many well-known hormones are stored in these vesicles in endocrine cells. Dense core vesicles may also store other locally acting products, such as amines and catecholamines.

Synaptic vesicles are specific to neurons and store neurotransmitters, while dense core vesicles are much more ubiquitous and store a variety of hormones, but there are appreciable similarities between these 2 types of vesicles, and neurons also contain dense core vesicles.

Other than recognized endocrine glands, dispersed cells found in many types of tissues may produce bioactive substances, store them in dense core vesicles, and release them as hormones. These dispersed endocrine cells are often called neuroendocrine cells because they have properties of both endocrine cells and neurons [PMID179139], and collectively, they form the dispersed neuroendocrine system (DNS). Cells of the DNS are currently identified by the H&E appearance in conjunction with ultrastructural, immunohistochemical, and molecular biological characteristics.

As might be expected from the hybrid epithelial/neural properties of the cells of the dispersed neuroendocrine system, they and the neuroendocrine neoplasms derived from them may be divided into 2 groups: epithelial and neural, depending on whether epithelial or neural properties predominate [PMID11993690]. Examples of the epithelial group of neuroendocrine neoplasms include carcinoid tumor, small cell carcinoma, medullary thyroid carcinoma, cutaneous neuroendocrine tumors (Merkel cell carcinomas), pancreatic islet cell tumor, some large cell lung carcinomas, and miscellaneous neuroendocrine neoplasms of a variety of tissues, all of which are discussed and illustrated elsewhere in this work. The important considerations here are nomenclature and the immunohistochemical stains that assist in the diagnosis of this group of neoplasms.

The terms "neuroendocrine neoplasia" or "neuroendocrine carcinoma" are now recognized and should be reported, with the degree of differentiation, together with the more conventional name. For example, a carcinoid tumor should also be called a grade 1 neuroendocrine carcinoma, an atypical carcinoid a grade 2 neuroendocrine carcinoma, and a small cell carcinoma a grade 3 neuroendocrine carcinoma [PMID10705811].

There are a number of proteins that are characteristic of all neuroendocrine cells and which can be demonstrated immunohistochemically. Chromogranin is a group of related proteins that are found inside the dense core vesicles. The major chromogranin proteins are chromogranin A, chromogranin B, and chromogranin C (also called secretogranin II). The unspecified term "chromogranin" usually refers to chromogranin A. The chromogranin proteins are associated with a group of proteins called secretogranins inside vesicles and are secreted with the other contents of the vesicle [PMID12646671]. Chromogranin is an excellent marker of neuroendocrine differentiation, but may be absent in poorly differentiated neuroendocrine tumors (eg, small cell carcinoma) because these tumors often have few dense core vesicles.

Synaptophysin was originally described as a glycoprotein in the synaptic vesicles of neurons. It was subsequently found to be a component of the membranes of dense core vesicles of neuroendocrine cells, rather that of the interior, as is the case for chromogranin [PMID3093369]. Synaptophysin is more likely to be positive in poorly differentiated neuroendocrine tumors, but it is also found in some tumors that are not of neuroendocrine origin, such as adrenal cortical tumors.

CD56 (neural cell adhesion molecule [NCAM]) is a cell surface glycoprotein expressed by neurons and glia, and also by natural killer cells, and more recently shown to be present in neuroendocrine cells [PMID12925986].

Many neuroendocrine neoplasms of the epithelial type express somatostatin receptors even if they do not make somatostatin, and somatostatin analogues are occasionally used in diagnosis and treatment [PMID18524947]. The octreotide scan uses a somatostatin analogue to detect neuroendocrine tumors of many types by binding to somatostatin receptors.

The second large group of tumors of the dispersed neuroendocrine system is those of the neural (or neuroectodermal) type, in which neural properties predominate over epithelial. The neural group of neuroendocrine tumors, in turn, can be divided into those tumors that are paragangliomas and those that are not.

Paraganglia are collections of cells of neuroectodermal origin (the neuroectoderm is a group of embryonic ectodermal cells that differentiate into neural tissues) that synthesize catecholamines and/or regulatory peptides. Because the adrenal medulla is a paraganglia, pheochromocytomas can be called called extraadrenal pheochromocytoma.

Extraadrenal paraganglia are symmetrically distributed from the base of the skull to the pelvic floor. They are usually found in association with either autonomic nerves or ganglia, or with vascular structures. Paraganglia in the head and neck (eg, the carotid, vagal, and jugulotympanic bodies) are aligned with the parasympathetic nervous system. Extraadrenal paraganglia below the neck tend to be aligned with the sympathetic nervous system. Other than the adrenal medulla, the only sympathetic paraganglia whose location is known and which has an individual name is the organ of Zuckerkandl, found near the bifurcation of the aorta. Because the organ of Zuckerkandl involutes after birth, paragangliomas associated with this body are rarely encountered.

A zellballen pattern, in which clusters of round cells are surrounded by delicate strands of fibrous tissue, resulting in an appearance of balls of cells, is characteristic of paragangliomas i5.2, but this appearance is not always seen. The cells may be spindled and the fibrous tissue may be dense, so the diagnosis depends on evidence of neuroendocrine differentiation. Paragangliomas will stain for the neuroendocrine markers discussed above, and these markers can be helpful in the diagnosis. The location of a tumor is a helpful clue to its possible neuroendocrine nature in many cases, such as the adrenal medulla and the carotid bifurcation, but because the locations of most of the sympathetic paraganglia are not known, paragangliomas can occur in unexpected places. Whereas neuroendocrine tumors of the epithelial type have well-developed desmosomes and claudins and occludins on electron microscopy (features associated with epithelial cells) [PMID9865821], these findings are rare in paraganglioma.

It is not possible to determine whether a paraganglioma will behave in a benign or malignant manner based on histology, though the usual red flags of pleomorphism, necrosis, invasion, and mitoses may arouse concern.

Gangliocytic paragangliomas are an unusual type of paraganglioma, often located around the duodenum, that has larger, ganglion-like cells and a schwannoma-like stroma, in addition to the characteristic paraganglioma cells i5.3 [PMID15740625]. This results in an appearance that is a mixture of a traditional paraganglioma and a ganglioneuroma.

Examples of tumors of the neural type of neuroendocrine neoplasms that are not paragangliomas include neuroblastoma, olfactory neuroblastoma, and the Ewing/PNET family (which includes medulloblastoma, retinoblastoma, and pineoblastoma), all of which are discussed elsewhere. Tumors in this group may express the neuroendocrine markers described above, but are generally less positive for them [PMID9646033], and other immunohistochemical stains are generally more useful in the diagnosis. These tumors are also discussed and illustrated elsewhere in this work.

At one time, it was thought that all neuroendocrine tumors were derived from the neural crest. The neural crest (not to be confused with the neural tube, which develops into the brain, spinal cord, and retina) is a transient ectodermal structure whose cells migrate widely during embryogenesis and give rise to an astonishing array of seemingly diverse and unrelated cells and tissues in the periphery, including ganglia, Schwann cells, melanocytes, and the adrenal medulla [Strachan ISBN978-0815341499]. Even now, some equate all neuroendocrine neoplasms with neural crest origin, but this is not correct. Paragangliomas (including adrenal pheochromocytomas), neuroblastomas, and medullary carcinomas of the thyroid are derived from the neural crest [PMID19377845], but other neuroendocrine tumors are now thought to arise from endodermic stem cells rather than from the neural crest [PMID6129173, PMID14713256]. Neuroendocrine tumors share biochemical features, not an embryological origin [PMID9924424].

There is a great diversity of tumors derived from the neural crest because of the great diversity of tissues derived from it. Just as some neuroendocrine tumors do not arise from the neural crest, so the neural crest gives rise to many tumors that are not neuroendocrine, including peripheral nerve sheath tumors and melanomas. Thus, the equation of neural crest-derived and neuroendocrine tumors is erroneous in both directions.

Core Points for the Neuroendocrine System and Paragangliomas

- Dispersed endocrine cells (neuroendocrine cells) have properties of both endocrine cells and neurons.
    - Found in many sites.
    - Have dense core vesicles, within which are peptide hormones, amines, or catecholamines.
- Epithelial group: carcinoid tumors, small cell carcinoma, medullary thyroid carcinoma, cutaneous neuroendocrine tumors, pancreatic islet cell tumors, and some large cell lung carcinomas.
- Neural group: paragangliomas (collections of cells of neuroectodermal origin that synthesize catecholamines or regulatory peptides), neuroblastoma, olfactory neuroblastoma, and the Ewing/PNET family.
- Most common neuroendocrine markers are chromogranin, synaptophysin, and CD56, though these are less useful in neuroendocrine neoplasms of the neural type that are not paragangliomas.

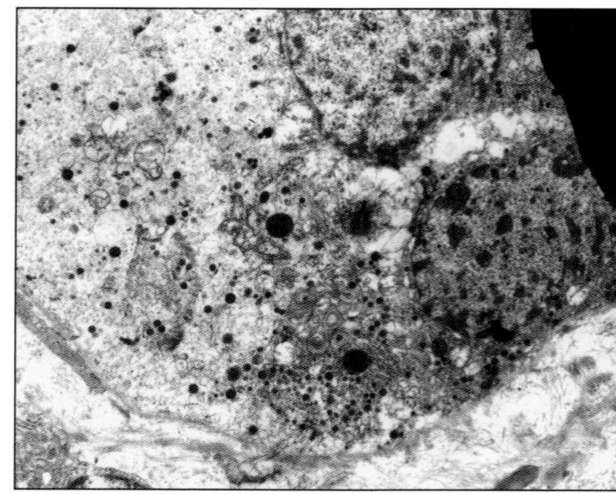

i5.1 Neurosecretory granules characteristic of neuroendocrine carcinoma.

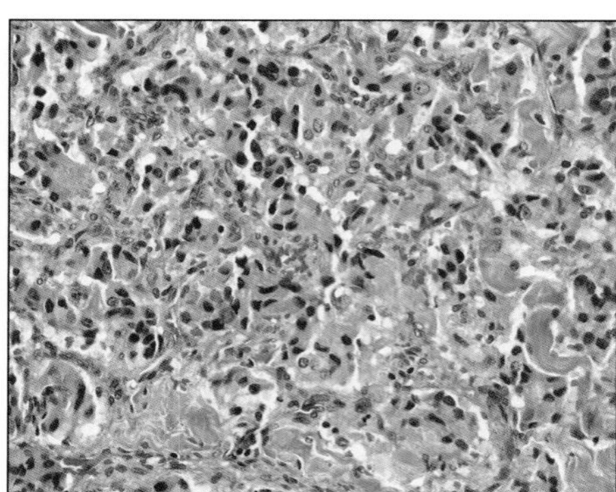

i5.2 A paraganglioma, illustrating the classic "zellballen" pattern, in which there are subtle clusters of tumor cells separated by fine fibrovascular septae

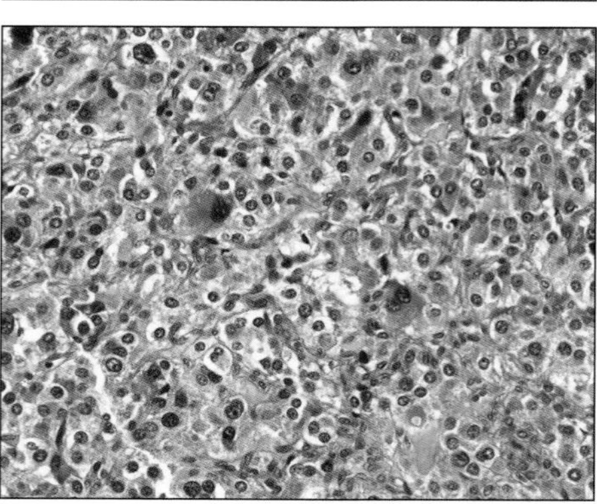

i5.3 A gangliocytic paraganglioma, in which large, ganglion-like cells are dispersed among the typical cell type

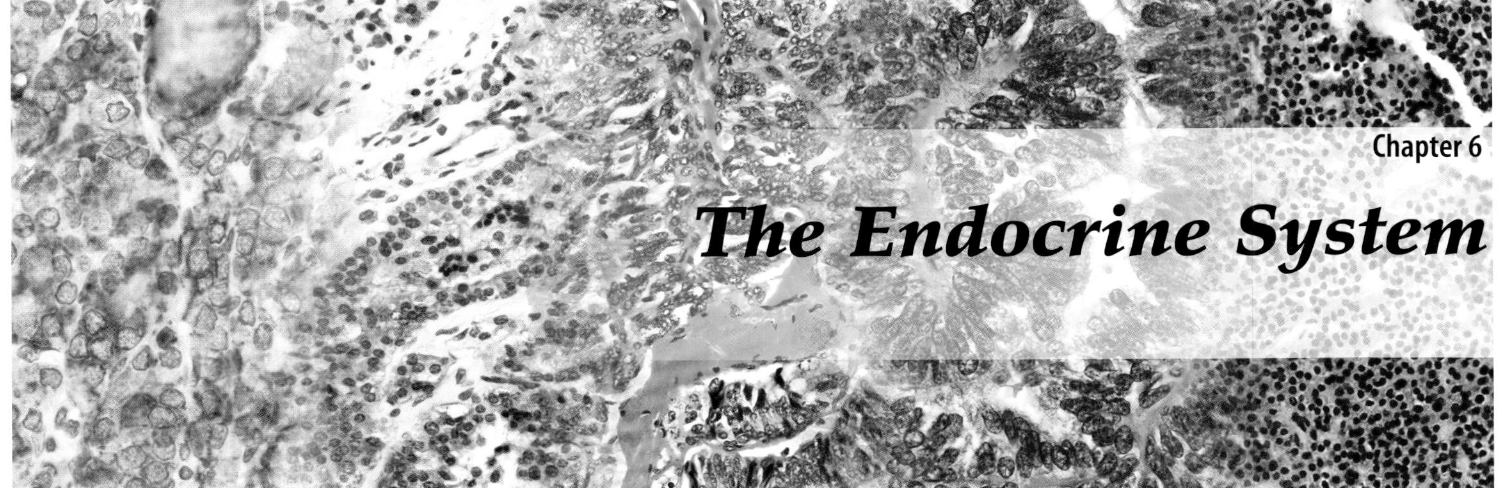

The pituitary gland is covered in Chapter 41 with the central nervous system. Here, we consider commonly encountered entities in the thyroid, the parathyroids, and the adrenals.

The Thyroid Gland

Inflammatory and Autoimmune Conditions of the Thyroid

Graves disease and Hashimoto thyroiditis are both autoimmune disorders characterized by autoantibodies to thyroid antigens. They may overlap clinically and histologically in their early stages, but patients with Graves disease become hyperthyroid, while those with Hashimoto thyroiditis become hypothyroid.

Untreated Graves disease is histologically characterized by hyperplasia of the thyroid epithelium, with infoldings of the epithelium into the follicles i6.1. Colloid may be pale and scalloped i6.2. Lymphocytes may be only an occasional finding, or there may be appreciable lymphocytic thyroiditis. However, most cases of Graves disease that the pathologist will encounter have been treated with propylthiouracil, so these classic histologic changes are likely to be attenuated.

Untreated Hashimoto is characterized histologically by an intense lymphoid infiltrate, often with germinal centers i6.3, and oncocytic epithelium (with densely pink cytoplasm because of large numbers of mitochondria) that may not form distinct follicles i6.4. Follicular atrophy may be seen i6.5. Some cases have extensive fibrosis that may result in a clinical nodularity that simulates a neoplasm i6.6. The distinction between nonspecific lymphocytic thyroiditis and Hashimoto thyroiditis is not based on histology, but rather on the presence or absence of hypothyroidism and autoantibodies to thyroid antigens, though the presence of oncocytic epithelium and lymphoid follicles with germinal centers suggests Hashimoto.

3 primary autoantibodies are found in autoimmune thyroid disease. The first of these is directed to the TSH receptor and is called TRAb (it was formerly called "long-acting thyroid stimulator [LATS]). The second is directed to thyroid peroxidase, the enzyme that oxidizes dietary iodide to iodine, making if available for the production of thyroid hormone, and is called TPOAb. TPOAb was previously called antimicrosomal antibodies (microsomes are vesicular structures created in the laboratory when the endoplasmic reticulum is broken up). The third autoantibody is directed to thyroglobulin (TgAb).

TRAb usually results in Graves disease by binding to the TSH receptor and activating it. Most cases of Graves disease are caused by this autoantibody, but it may rarely cause Hashimoto if it binds to and blocks the TSH receptor without stimulating it. TPOAb is associated primarily with Hashimoto or atrophic thyroiditis because it inhibits synthesis of the thyroid hormone. TgAb are also associated with Hashimoto, but testing for them adds little to testing for TRAb and TPOAb and the role of TgAb in autoimmune thyroid disease is unclear [PMID8466378].

At the DNA level, a number of genes have been associated with autoimmune thyroiditis. *HT-1* (on 13q32) and *HT-2* (on 12q22) have been linked to Hashimoto, while *GC-1* (on 14q31), *GD-2* (on 20q11.2), and *GD-3* (on Xq21) are linked to Graves disease [PMID9589659, PMID17824829], though the details of autoimmune thyroiditis at the molecular level have not yet been elucidated.

2 very rare inflammatory conditions involving the thyroid are granulomatous thyroiditis (also called De Quervain disease) and Riedel thyroiditis, which is not actually a thyroiditis, but a fibrosing condition that involves structures of the neck and secondarily affects the thyroid.

Mass Lesions of the Thyroid, Neoplastic and Nonneoplastic

Nodular and Multinodular Hyperplasia

While Graves disease and Hashimoto thyroiditis may occasionally present with a clinically evident mass, most thyroid masses are caused by hyperplasia (goiter) or neoplasia. Most cases of nodular or multinodular hyperplasia of the thyroid in developed countries, where iodine deficiency is rare, are likely caused by a differential response of thyrocytes to TSH. In developing countries, where iodine is not added to salt, hyperplasia may be caused by a diminished ability to synthesize thyroid hormone, called dyshormonogenetic hyperplasia.

In nodular hyperplasia, there are usually at least some follicles that are dilated i6.7 unless the cause is dyshormonogenetic hyperplasia. The stroma in nodular hyperplasia is often edematous or fibrotic, frequently with hemosiderin macrophages i6.8. Many cases of nodular hyperplasia have dilated follicles into which project pseudo-papillary structures that contain smaller follicles i6.9. Follicle-within-follicle formation is commonly seen in hyperplasia. This is in contrast to Graves disease, in which hyperplastic epithelium without follicle formation protrudes into the lumen, and is also in contrast with papillary carcinoma,

ISBN 978-089189-5886

in which the papillary structures do not contain follicles and do not protrude into the lumen of a follicle. Even if there is only 1 clinically evident mass, nodular hyperplasia is often multiple **i6.10**.

Papillary Carcinoma

The classic form of papillary carcinoma, with well developed fibrovascular cores **i6.11**, is rarely a diagnostic challenge, though the rare sclerosing form of classic papillary carcinoma may be momentarily perplexing. In contrast, there is perhaps no area in all of surgical pathology more subject to interobserver variation than the diagnosis of follicular variant of papillary carcinoma (FVPC). Even so-called "expert" thyroid pathologists exhibit very large variation in the diagnosis of problematic follicular masses [PMID18854266, PMID15371949]. One of these studies involved "6 thyroid experts." As we saw in problematic intraductal proliferations of the breast [PMID1847606], the belief that the community hospital pathologist should seek a consult from an "expert" appears flawed if the so-called "experts" cannot agree among themselves.

The diagnosis of FVPC hinges on 5 nuclear features that are also found in the classic form and that should be compelling before the diagnosis of FVPC is made [PMID602974, PMID6660353, PMID21169742]. These 5 features are as follows **i6.12a**, **i6.12b**:

1. Nuclear crowding
2. Nuclear enlargement
3. Peripheralized chromatin (so-called "ground glass nuclei")
4. Cytoplasmic invagination into the nuclei (so-called "orphan Annie" nucleus)
5. Nuclear grooves

In practice, it can be difficult to discern whether nuclear clearing is secondary to peripheralization of chromatin or cytoplasmic invagination. In addition, darker, denser colloid (occasionally described by the confusing terms "ropey" or "bubble gum" **i6.13** is often seen. Psammoma bodies and multinucleated macrophages may be helpful in the diagnosis. Psammoma bodies **i6.14** are generally thought to be caused by necrosis of cells at the tips of papillae, followed by dystrophic calcification, with lamellations resulting from successive cycles of this process. However, this theory has not been proven and has been challenged [PMID19373908]. FVPC may have a sclerotic stroma, particularly at the periphery. The diagnosis of the diffuse form of FVPC may be difficult because unlike the localized forms, no particular area stands out and there is no adjacent normal thyroid tissue with which to compare the problematic area, but the characteristic findings are the same.

Cellular hyperplasias may have occasional nuclei that share some features with those of FVPC, but the nuclear changes are not as widespread or compelling as in FVPC, and the other features of FVPC are not seen. Many cases of apparently diffuse, widespread FVPC are actually diffuse hyperplasia. Likewise, the presence of multiple masses is more suggestive of multinodular hyperplasia than multinodular FVPC.

There are 2 varieties of FVPC: encapsulated and diffuse (infiltrative or nonencapsulated). Encapsulated FVPC have a generally good prognosis, while the diffuse form of FVPC is often more aggressive [PMID16900519].

There is a tendency to overdiagnose the FVPC because of clear nuclei. Clear nuclei are not specific for papillary carcinoma, are seen in a variety of benign conditions, and, by themselves, do not make secure a diagnosis of FVPC. In questionable cases, it is reasonable and prudent to err on the side of a benign diagnosis, as long as the report discusses the histologic features, because most cases of FVPC that will metastasize distantly are either of the diffuse form or have vascular or capsular invasion at the time of diagnosis [PMID16900519, PMID19191744]. If the focus in question is small, encapsulated, and without capsular or vascular invasion, a benign diagnosis can be rendered with little fear that a clinically significant papillary carcinoma will be missed. While cases of FVPC that are diffuse or have invaded a capsule may require more aggressive treatment, simple lobectomy without a total thyroidectomy or subsequent radioactive iodine ablation appears adequate for an encapsulated FVPC if there is no vascular or capsular invasion [PMID19191744]. Indeed, all follicular lesions of the thyroid that are encapsulated and noninvasive, including FVPC, ultimately have a good prognosis [PMID20463572].

Cell membrane staining for HBME-1 is emerging as the most sensitive and specific marker for papillary carcinoma, with a reported sensitivity of 96% and a specificity of 93%. Cytokeratin 19 is not as specific as HBME-1 but has 96% sensitivity. The principal value of CK19 is that a negative result has good predictive value [PMID16998461]. The combination of HBME-1 and CK19 is excellent, and in most cases, staining with HBME-1 alone provides sufficient immunohistochemical confirmation of a FVPC **i6.15a**, **i6.15b** [PMID17050067].

Abnormalities in 3 genes may be found in papillary thyroid carcinoma: *BRAF*, *RET*, and *RAS*. Approximately 70% of papillary thyroid carcinomas will have 1 of these 3 mutations [PMID18437172]. While most clinically important kinases add a phosphate group to tyrosine residues in proteins, many kinases add the phosphate group to serine or threonine residues. The raf family of enzymes is a group of serine/threonine kinases important in cell signaling. A mutation in *BRAF*, which codes for one of the raf enzymes, is the most common mutation in thyroid papillary carcinoma. *RET* is a proto-oncogene (ie, a normal gene that becomes an oncogene when it undergoes a gain of function mutation) on chromosome 10q11.2 that codes for a cell membrane receptor tyrosine kinase. A variety of translocations have been found between *RET* and various partners, resulting in a variety of neoplasms, including papillary carcinoma if the translocation partner is the *PTC* gene [PMID16946010].

These mutations correlate with the histologic or clinical findings. *BRAF* mutations cause tumors of a papillary pattern in older patients, often with metastases to local lymph nodes, while tumors with rearrangements between the *RET* and the *PTC* genes also have a classic papillary pattern and metastases to local lymph nodes, but occur more commonly in younger patients. Papillary carcinomas with mutations in a ras protein are of the follicular variant and are less likely to have nodal metastases [PMID16434896].

At both the DNA and amino acid levels, mutations are denoted by the base or amino acid that should be present, followed by the position of the abnormality, followed by the base or amino acid that is actually present. In the *BRAF* mutation in papillary carcinoma, there should be a thymine base in the DNA at base position 1799, but instead there is an adenine. This is written as T1799A. The result of this is that there should be a valine at amino acid position 600, but instead there is a glutamate, denoted Val600Glu. There are single-letter abbreviations of amino acids, and Val600Glu can be written as V600E (E is the single-letter abbreviation for glutamate). While mutations in *BRAF* are found in many cancers, its identification in problematic thyroid lesions strongly suggests papillary carcinoma [PMID20230995].

There is no uniform consensus as to whether or not a total thyroidectomy is needed in small, incidentally discovered papillary carcinomas. The term "papillary microtumor" was advocated in 2003 for a focus of occult papillary carcinoma that is <1 cm [PMID14615819]. Since then, the term has gained increasing acceptance and its use appears prudent [PMID18611929], as such small tumors may be less aggressive.

Whereas the neoplastic cells of a typical papillary carcinoma are essentially cuboidal, those of the tall cell variant are distinctly columnar. Specifically, the cells should be at least 3 times as tall as they are wide and these cells should constitute >30% of the tumor for the final designation of tall cell variant of papillary carcinoma **i6.16**. The tall cell variant of papillary carcinoma has distinctly eosinophilic cytoplasm [PMID20174895].

The columnar cell variant has a papillary architecture **i6.17a** and is currently considered a type of papillary carcinoma, but its nuclei do not have the characteristics of papillary carcinoma. Whereas the nuclei of a typical papillary carcinoma are relatively round, those of the columnar variant are distinctly ovoid. They are also more hyperchromatic than those of the common type of papillary carcinoma, with punctate chromatin, scant cytoplasm, and often pseudostratification **i6.17b** [PMID7927316]. The columnar variant of papillary carcinoma roughly resembles a colonic adenomatous polyp. It has a poor prognosis, and it is likely that this variant will eventually be considered a neoplasm of a different type.

Follicular Neoplasms

Other than the diagnosis (and overdiagnosis) of FVPC, the most difficult problem in thyroid pathology is the distinction of follicular adenoma from well differentiated follicular carcinoma. A thyroid follicular neoplasm without the features of FVPC and without invasion of either vessels or a capsule is a follicular adenoma. Follicular adenomas generally have smaller follicles than hyperplasia **i6.18**. A number of types of follicular adenoma are recognized, but these have no clinical consequences. The distinction of an adenoma from the FVPC can be challenging and may require immunohistochemical stains **i6.19a**, **i6.19b**, **i6.19c**.

The diagnosis of follicular carcinoma requires either vascular invasion or complete invasion of the capsule (invasion into the capsule is not a sign of malignancy). In assessing vascular invasion, the involved vessel must be within or on the outside of the capsule. It cannot be within the tumor. Well differentiated follicular carcinoma of the thyroid may be widely invasive or minimally invasive. The former is rarely a diagnostic challenge, but the diagnosis of minimally invasive well differentiated thyroid follicular carcinoma can be difficult because both capsular and vascular invasion may be subtle.

Capsular invasion requires penetration of the entire thickness of the capsule **i6.20** [PMID11914475]. Serial levels are often needed to demonstrate complete capsular penetration. Because a tumor that has invaded through a capsule may engender the formation of a secondary capsule, encapsulation is not necessarily indicative of an adenoma. To prove benignity, one must show that the capsule is a single capsule surrounding the entire proliferation and that there has been no secondary capsule formation engendered by the tumor cells that pierced the original capsule. The clue to either complete penetration or secondary capsule formation is that there is an area of an otherwise encapsulated tumor that is not covered at all by a capsule, or if it is, a line extending the outer contour of the capsule of the main portion of the tumor transects the tumor at the suspicious focus. In the latter case, there should be discontinuity of the capsule at the problematic focus, suggesting secondary capsule formation. If there is no discontinuity, the tumor may simply be bulging into the capsule and pushing it outward, which is insufficient for the diagnosis of minimally invasive carcinoma.

Vascular invasion requires either that the tumor be attached to the wall (a tumor thrombus) or that it have penetrated the wall of an arteriole or venule and be covered only by that vessel's endothelium **i6.21a**, **i6.21b**, **i6.21c** [DeLellis ISBN978-9283224167]. The rationale for these requirements is to eliminate the artifactual appearance of tumor cells within a vessel secondary to fixation and processing. It can be argued that tumor in a vessel wall, but covered by endothelium, is not true vascular invasion because the tumor cells have not gained access to the lumen. However, the majority opinion is that in the absence of a tumor thrombus, this finding is both necessary and sufficient for vascular invasion because it proves that the tumor has invaded through the muscular wall of the vessel. After some initial misgivings, I have come to support this view, as an adenoma would not be expected to invade through the muscular wall of a vessel. If there is doubt, immunohistochemical stains may clarify the relationship between the neoplastic cells and the endothelial cells.

In the case of a well differentiated follicular carcinoma, the report should indicate whether it is invasion of the capsule or of the vessels therein that has merited the designation of carcinoma, and indicate whether it is focally or widely invasive. A single focus of capsular or vascular invasion, even if definitive, is not as prognostically unfavorable as wide invasion and is usually designated as minimally invasive. Follicular neoplasms with uncertain behavior regarding the vessels or the capsule can be designated "follicular tumors of uncertain malignant potential."

About 40% of follicular carcinomas of the thyroid have a translocation between the *PAX8* gene and the *PPARγ* gene. This translocation is much rarer in follicular adenomas and its presence suggests malignancy [PMID21455199]. Mutations in *RAS* also occur in follicular carcinoma [PMID18437172], and are mutually exclusive with *PAX8/PPARγ* translocations.

The criteria for malignancy for Hürthle tumors are the same as for any other follicular lesion, but they will be satisfied more often, and a higher percentage of Hürthle tumors are malignant. Once the diagnosis of follicular carcinoma of the Hürthle cell type is made, size >4 cm, a solid or trabecular growth pattern, mitoses, or >3 foci of vascular invasion suggest a more aggressive course [PMID16534796].

Although thyroid tissue within a lymph node is usually indicative of metastatic carcinoma, some believe that lymph nodes may occasionally contain benign thyroid tissue. This is a matter of controversy, in contrast to the acceptance of benign salivary gland tissue in lymph nodes. One argument for occasional benign thyroid inclusions in a lymph node is that such inclusions have been found in the absence of a thyroid tumor. Before even addressing that issue, however, one must be sure that the structure is truly a lymph node. The thyroid often contains lymphoid clusters that simulate a node, especially if the patient has lymphocytic thyroiditis.

Medullary Carcinoma

Although a component of multiple endocrine neoplasia type 2, only about 10-20% of medullary carcinomas are familial. The cells of medullary carcinomas may be round **i6.22** or spindled **i6.23** and may or may not have eccentric nuclei **i6.24**. The growth pattern may be solid **i6.25**, follicular, or papillary **i6.26**. This variety of appearances, the common absence of family history, and the frequent lack of amyloid can make the diagnosis of medullary carcinoma challenging. This entity should be considered in any situation where there is an odd-looking thyroid tumor that is not readily classified.

80% of thyroid medullary carcinomas produce amyloid, which is eosinophilic, amorphous, and somewhat "waxy" on H&E **i6.27**. Amyloid stains pink-orange on Congo red **i6.28** but is identified by its subtle yellow-green birefringence upon examination with polarized light after Congo red stain **i6.29**. Because medullary carcinomas arise from the thyroid C cells rather than from follicular epithelium, they will stain for calcitonin **i6.30** and will usually not stain for thyroglobulin. In addition, medullary carcinomas are often CEA positive [PMID360824], so if a medullary carcinoma is being considered, or if an unusual thyroid tumor is being immunostained, a stain for CEA should be included.

C cell hyperplasia and medullary adenoma (small and encapsulated) are occasionally diagnosed, but usually only in situations of familial medullary carcinoma. Both familial and sporadic cases of medullary thyroid carcinomas are associated with mutations in the *RET* proto-oncogene [PMID18437172, PMID19522831].

Unusual Forms of Thyroid Carcinoma

Insular carcinoma is a poorly differentiated follicular carcinoma that resembles a neuroendocrine carcinoma **i6.31** but is thyroglobulin positive and chromogranin negative [PMID16735986]. Necrosis and vascular invasion are common, with a relative nuclear uniformity **i6.32** that belies its aggressive behavior. The main entities in the differential diagnosis of an insular carcinoma are a neuroendocrine carcinoma and a medullary carcinoma.

True primary small cell carcinomas of the thyroid are very rare. Most such tumors are actually metastatic small cell carcinomas, insular carcinomas, or a small cell variant of medullary carcinoma. Clues to the diagnosis of a small cell variant of medullary carcinoma **i6.33** include high nuclear grade, histologically similar to small cell carcinoma of lung **i6.34**, thyroglobulin negativity, with immunohistochemical evidence of neuroendocrine differentiation, but also with calcitonin or CEA positivity.

Anaplastic thyroid carcinoma is often composed primarily of spindle cells with high-grade nuclei, with giant cells and numerous mitoses **i6.35**. These highly aggressive neoplasms are often negative for thyroglobulin, though liberal sampling may disclose areas of better differentiation that may be thyroglobulin positive. Vimentin positivity is characteristic, causing a diagnosis of sarcoma to be considered, but again, apparent sarcomas in organs are much more likely to be high-grade carcinomas with metaplasia.

In addition to the usual form of mucoepidermoid carcinoma, there is also a sclerosing mucoepidermoid carcinoma with eosinophilia in the thyroid that is characterized by sclerosis, a lymphoid infiltrate punctuated by eosinophils, often with focal squamous or glandular differentiation **i6.36**, **i6.37**. This may initially simulate metastatic carcinoma [PMID10912941].

Carcinoma showing thymus-like elements (CASTLE) is a rare thyroid neoplasm that resembles a nasopharyngeal or thymic squamous carcinoma of the lymphoepithelioma type, and may in fact arise from ectopic thymic tissue. There are usually islands of cells separated by dense fibrous tissue **i6.38**. The individual cells have prominent nucleoli **i6.39**. The H&E diagnosis of CASTLE is supported by demonstrating keratin positivity and thyroglobulin negativity, and by excluding a metastatic tumor [PMID2050369].

Nonepithelial Neoplasms of the Thyroid

Mesenchymal neoplasms are very rare. The most common lymphoma of the thyroid is an extranodal marginal zone lymphoma ("MALToma"), and most of the remaining lymphomas are of the diffuse large B-cell type. These are diagnosed as discussed elsewhere.

Fine Needle Aspiration of the Thyroid

On thyroid aspirations, the first priority is to comment on whether or not the smears are of sufficient cellularity to be of any assistance. If they are, one can then diagnose an obvious papillary carcinoma, if there are well developed fibrovascular cores, nuclear enlargement, and cytoplasmic invagination into the nucleus (the remaining nuclear features, such as chromatin peripheralization and nuclear grooves, require formalin fixation and paraffin processing and are not evident on smears). One can also diagnose a malignancy of another type, such as poorly differentiated follicular carcinoma or medullary carcinoma. Well differentiated follicular carcinoma will escape detection on smears, and FVPC is likely to do so as well.

If there is no obvious malignancy, the pathologist is limited in what he or she can say. Cases with abundant extrafollicular colloid and macrophages, preferably with hemosiderin, are highly likely to be hyperplasias and can be signed out as probable nonneoplastic processes, with the caveat that neoplasms may rarely undergo cystic degeneration.

Fine needle aspiration (FNA) cases with follicular epithelial cells primarily in a 2-dimensional arrangement, with minimal follicle formation, are more likely hyperplastic than neoplastic because 2-dimensional sheets of epithelial cells on an aspirate generally correspond to macrofollicles on a resection, and follicular neoplasms are more likely to be composed of microfollicles than macrofollicles. On the other hand, aspirates with follicles, especially with microfollicles, are of greater concern for follicular neoplasia [PMID8453583] and, in general, must be excised to distinguish between a follicular adenoma and a well differentiated follicular carcinoma, but even in these cases, many will be cellular hyperplasias. Some feel that these correlations are sufficiently strong that aspiration cases with 2-dimensional sheets of epithelial cells, extrafollicular colloid, or large numbers of macrophages can be diagnosed as probable hyperplasias and can be safely be followed if there is no other reason to excise, but to my mind, other than exclusion of classic papillary carcinoma and the rare cases that demonstrate an obvious malignancy of another type, most aspirates can only be classified as "follicular lesions," with a differential diagnosis of hyperplasia, follicular adenoma, well differentiated follicular carcinoma, and the FVPC.

A system based on the Bethesda system for Pap smears has been proposed for thyroid aspirates, stratifying them into 6 categories, ranging from nondiagnostic/unsatisfactory to clearly malignant [PMID19846805]. This system proposes 2 categories that are suspicious for malignancy and a third category that is of undetermined significance. With all due respect to the meticulous thinking that clearly went into this system, my experience has been that a simpler algorithm—unsatisfactory/nondiagnostic, follicular lesion (with differential diagnosis as discussed above), and malignant—suffices quite well. Any indication of uncertainty—be it phrased as "undetermined significance" or "suspicious"—will be followed by an additional procedure that is likely to supersede the cytology.

FNAs may be supplemented by molecular testing. Testing for Braf V600E, mutations in the RAS family, and rearrangements of RET/PTC and PAX8/PPARγ help identify the subset of follicular lesion patients that are more likely to have a benign process and that can be observed [PMID21880806].

A final comment on thyroid aspirates is that consideration should be given to the performance of a core biopsy in lieu of an aspirate because a biopsy offers 2 advantages over an aspirate. First, the cells are seen in their normal architectural context (ie, their relationship to each other). Second, immunohistochemical stains, though theoretically possible on Pap-stained slides that have been destained, are far easier on tissue that has not been previously stained in any way. The second advantage has assumed prominence now that immunohistochemistry—especially HBME-1—has proven helpful in the exclusion of FVPC. While some believe that a core biopsy does not add additional information to an aspiration and carries risks of hematoma and infection [PMID18558594], others have not experienced these problems and routinely perform biopsies, with excellent results [PMID12601219].

Frozen Sections of the Thyroid

To my mind, frozen section of thyroid masses should be discouraged because there is too little chance of a definitive frozen section diagnosis that will materially change intraoperative management or improve patient care and too much opportunity for error, even in experienced hands. The diagnosis of minimally invasive follicular carcinoma requires extensive study of multiple paraffin sections and cannot possibly be made on a frozen section [PMID12469789]. Likewise, the diagnosis of FVPC can be challenging enough on a full set of paraffin-processed sections that liberally sample the mass, and one of the key diagnostic features—peripheralization of chromatin (so-called ground glass nuclei)—will not be seen on frozen section because it requires formalin fixation and paraffin processing [PMID10792769, PMID7536449].

Moreover, cases of nodular hyperplasia may have papillations that can simulate those of papillary carcinoma on frozen section. In my experience, total thyroidectomy based on a frozen section diagnosis of papillary carcinoma is a cause of a disproportionate number of lawsuits. While frozen sections of thyroid masses may rarely be diagnostic, there will be many cases in which the frozen section diagnosis appears assured, but the paraffin sections provide a very unpleasant surprise. If used at all, frozen section should be preserved for those rare cases in which a technically excellent preoperative FNA or needle biopsy is not completely diagnostic and there is a *genuinely compelling need* for the surgeon to know at the time of surgery because the patient is high risk from a surgical or anesthesia standpoint and a second surgery is highly undesirable.

I do not recommend a frozen section to avoid a second surgery for a completion thyroidectomy in a healthy patient. Likewise, with all due respect to the likely anxiety of the patient and his or her family members, a frozen section of the thyroid (or of any tissue) should never be performed to get a diagnosis more rapidly. Indeed, it is *precisely because* there is anxiety for the diagnosis that 24 hours should be taken to get it right. To my mind, the best policy, with the best patient care and the least opportunity for error, is for the surgeon to excise any masses that are of clinical concern and then wait a day or two for the pathologist to do a good job. Any form of thyroid carcinoma is a serious enough matter that a wait of a day or two, and a possible second surgery is a small price to pay to work with the best material in the best circumstances.

The Parathyroid Gland

Normal parathyroid tissue has 3 types of parenchymal cells: chief, oxyphil, and clear cells. Normal parathyroid glands also have a considerable amount of adipose tissue, usually between 20% and 40% of the volume of the gland **i6.40**, **i6.41**.

Except for the very rare lipoadenoma, any parathyroid hyperplasia or adenoma should have a clear reduction of fat, and this reduction is a reliable way to recognize that one of these processes is present **i6.42**. Size is a secondary method of recognizing that a hyperplasia or adenoma is likely, as a normal parathyroid gland generally should not exceed 6 mm or 60 mg. In theory, parathyroid hyperplasia or adenoma should have only 1 of the 3 types of cells, but in practice, this is rarely a useful criterion.

Parathyroid adenoma and hyperplasia may have an identical appearance. There may be a rim of normal parathyroid in adenomas **i6.43**, but often there is not. There is no consensus as to whether or not a hypercellular gland, without fat, surrounded by a rim of normal-appearing gland, is sufficiently diagnostic of adenoma that no further sampling of another gland is needed. Some would answer this question in the affirmative, while others believe that the definitive distinction between an adenoma and hyperplasia rests on whether or not the other parathyroid glands are normal since hyperplasia should cause the enlargement of all glands. However, in hyperplasia, the parathyroid glands may have differing degrees of enlargement and there are difficult situations, such as where 2 glands are abnormal and 2 are normal. These situations have been regarded as a "double adenoma," but most now regard these cases as asymmetric hyperplasia because some of these patients have again developed hyperparathyroidism after excision of both "adenomas," which suggests the better diagnosis is hyperplasia that was unevenly apparent in the 4 glands at the time of surgery.

Because of the very short half-life of parathyroid hormone (about 4 minutes [PMID11485536]), it is possible to assess the effectiveness of surgery by intraoperative assay for the hormone in lieu of frozen section. With only a 10- to 15-minute wait after removal of the tissue, a drop of 50% or more relative to the preoperative parathyroid hormone level suggests successful removal of the responsible tissue [PMID7536449]. The sensitivity of intraoperative parathyroid hormone in determining that the necessary and appropriate tissue has been removed is 97%, and the specificity is 100%, equaling or exceeding frozen section [PMID8957480]. When specifically compared to frozen section, the superiority of intraoperative parathyroid hormone determination has been affirmed [PMID16360404]. Intraoperative assessment of parathyroid hormone can replace frozen section in any situation of primary hyperparathyroidism and is especially superior to frozen section in cases where >1 gland is involved [PMID15491966]. Such cases are very prone to error in frozen section because the surgeon will see an apparently enlarged gland and, after its identity as parathyroid is confirmed by frozen section, will assume that the problem has been corrected, whereas with intraoperative assay of the hormone, he or she will realize the need to continue the surgery when the hormone level fails to fall adequately.

As is the case for most endocrine neoplasias in general, the only definitive criterion for parathyroid carcinoma is the presence of metastatic disease. Malignancy is suggested by mitoses (>5/10 HPF), capsular and vascular invasion i6.44, necrosis, or generalized significant nuclear pleomorphism (localized pleomorphism is meaningless) [PMID20310041]. In questionable situations, a parathyroid neoplasm of uncertain malignant potential may be diagnosed.

The Adrenal Glands

The Normal Adrenal Cortex

From the outside in, the 3 layers of the adrenal cortex are the zona glomerulosa, the zona fasciculata, and the zona reticularis i6.45. The zona glomerulosa secretes aldosterone. Although there is some overlap, the fasciculata primarily secretes cortisol while the reticularis accounts for most of the production of sex steroids. Importantly, ACTH stimulates only the 2 inner zones, and does not affect the zona glomerulosa or aldosterone production. Thus, an ACTH-secreting tumor may cause hypersecretion of cortisol (Cushing syndrome), but will not cause hyperaldosteronism (Conn syndrome). Conn syndrome is usually caused by an aldosterone secreting adenoma of the zona glomerulosa.

Adrenal Cortical Masses

There may be nonneoplastic adrenal cortical masses in patients with congenital adrenal hyperplasia, which results from an enzyme deficiency that prevents biochemical reactions from going to completion, resulting in increased levels of ACTH from loss of negative feedback. Because sex steroid synthesis is impeded, there may also be testicular masses that strongly resemble Leydig cell tumors.

Although there is no uniformity of opinion, most feel that an adrenal cortical adenoma should be 1 cm or larger, and that smaller masses are hyperplastic nodule. H&E examination and immunohistochemical stains can usually differentiate a primary adrenal cortical mass from a metastatic lesion and provide information about the likely source of a metastasis, but if there is any question about the nature of an adrenal mass in an adult, it might be desirable to perform a chest CT to exclude a lung mass because lung carcinomas often metastasize to the adrenal cortex.

Adrenal cortical tumors are often keratin negative, and when they are positive, it is usually for low molecular weight keratin. These tumors are negative for chromogranin, but often stain for synaptophysin [PMID1735954]. Vimentin staining is commonly seen [PMID2418689]. Adrenal cortical tumors may also stain for Melan-A, inhibin, and calretinin [PMID12808065], and a mistake is easily made if immunohistochemical stains of an adrenal cortical tumor are evaluated out of context.

In adrenal cortical tumors, we again encounter the problem of determining which tumors are malignant. There are several algorithms in use to determine malignancy in adults, the most common of which remains that proposed by Weiss in 1984 [PMID6703192]. These algorithms are generally based on a combination of size, nuclear pleomorphism, mitoses, capsular or vascular invasion, and necrosis. In adults, cortical neoplasms >100 g are almost always malignant. Small neoplasms with uniform nuclei and no invasion are regarded as adenomas i6.46, while tumors that are large, have generalized nuclear atypia, or invasion are malignant i6.47, i6.48. It is important to note that while capsular or vascular invasion is one of the proposed criteria, it does not establish a malignant diagnosis by itself, in contrast to the thyroid gland. As is the case in other endocrine sites, the better part of valor in many cases may be a designation of uncertain malignant potential.

It is controversial whether cortical tumors in children should be assessed the same way, or predominantly on the basis of size. In children, large tumors may still be benign. In children, most tumors <400 g will behave in a benign fashion, though severe atypia, extensive necrosis, and abundant mitotic activity are still considerations [PMID12826878]. In an adult, a 200 g cortical neoplasm will almost always be malignant, but in a child, a 200 g cortical tumor, even if it fulfills the histologic criteria for malignancy by the commonly used systems, will engender different opinions on its biologic potential. Many would comment that there is uncertain malignant potential in many of these situations.

Neoplasms of the Adrenal Medulla

Neuroblastic tumors are considered on the basis of both the degree of ganglion differentiation and the amount and nature of the stroma. The stroma may be neuropil (neuronal processes only) in the less well differentiated tumors or schwannoma-like (ganglioneuromatous), with contribution from nonneuronal cells, in the better differentiated tumors. There are a number of grading systems, but the system advocated by the international neuroblastoma pathology committee, based on a combination of the presence or absence of neuropil and the degree of differentiation, is generally in favor [PMID10421272].

Neuroblastomas have <50% of the tumor in the form of any type of stroma. They are considered undifferentiated if there is no histologic evidence of differentiating neuroblasts. Differentiating neuroblasts are defined by a large, eccentric nucleus, with a vesicular chromatin pattern (ie, the chromatin is primarily on the nuclear periphery rather than being evenly distributed in the nucleus), a prominent nucleolus, with a cell diameter that is twice the nuclear diameter. Undifferentiated neuroblastomas have little or no stroma of any type, including neuropil. Therefore, they do not have Homer Wright pseudorosettes, which are concentric structures with cell bodies on the periphery and neuropil fibers projecting into a vaguely defined lumen that does not have a basement membrane. Undifferentiated neuroblastomas are simply sheets of small blue cells i6.49.

Poorly differentiated neuroblastomas have some neuropil stroma and rare differentiating neuroblasts (also called gangliocytic differentiation) that do not exceed 5% of cells. Because there is some neuropil stroma in poorly differentiated neuroblastomas, occasional Homer Wright pseudorosettes may be seen i6.50, but very little or no schwannian stroma.

Differentiating neuroblastomas have some schwannoma-like stroma i6.51, but this is <50% of the total stroma. If >1/2 of the tumor is schwannian stroma, it is a ganglioneuroblastoma.

In a differentiating neuroblastoma, >5% of cells will be differentiating i6.52.

In a ganglioneuroblastoma, gangliocytic cells and schwannoma-like stroma predominate i6.53, but there are nests of neuroblastoma cells i6.54. These nests may be in the form of demarcated nodules or intermingled with more mature elements. If neuroblastoma cells are absent, or only present as rare individual cells, amidst mature ganglion cells in a schwannoma-like stroma, the tumor is a ganglioneuroma i6.55. Neuroblastomas are neurofilament positive, neuroendocrine marker positive, CD99 negative, and muscle marker negative.

Neoadjuvant (ie, prior to resection) therapy effect in neuroblastomas may be evident as necrosis, inflammation, and fibrosis, but as is the case for sarcomas, it may also be manifest as increased differentiation i6.56.

The myc family (including N-myc, C-myc, and L-myc) is a family of transcription factors that are implicated in a number of neoplasms. C-myc is important in some lymphomas, but significant amplification of the *N-MYC* proto-oncogene (>10-fold normal) is present in about 30% of neuroblastomas and is associated with a more aggressive course [PMID15975048]. Loss of heterozygosity (ie, a microdeletion on one chromosome) of 1p36, 11q, or 14q is an unfavorable prognostic sign in neuroblastomas [PMID19192278].

Pheochromocytoma is an intraadrenal paraganglioma. Like any paraganglioma, pheochromocytomas often have a Zellballen pattern i6.57, but there are other patterns, including alveolar, trabecular, and solid. Most cases have large polygonal cells, but there are also spindle cell and small cell variants. A helpful diagnostic feature is that the cytoplasm is often amphophilic and granular i6.58. A diagnosis of pheochromocytoma should not be made solely on the basis of synaptophysin positivity, as adrenal cortical tumors may be positive for synaptophysin. Unlike cortical tumors, however, pheochromocytomas are positive for chromogranin [PMID19370504]. Most pheochromocytomas are positive for neurofilament proteins [PMID2159272] and vimentin [PMID10974931], but are usually negative for keratin [PMID11979086]. Most pheochromocytomas are negative for S100, but this may stain the sustentacular cells, a small, subtle second population of cells on the periphery of the clusters of tumor cells in paragangliomas. The diagnosis of pheochromocytoma has historically been established by 24-hour urine collection for metanephrines, but serum metanephrines are also a good test [PMID19152190, PMID20142367], and serum levels of chromogranin A can also be used [PMID20514823], though this may also be elevated in low-grade neuroendocrine carcinomas (carcinoid tumors).

Only about 10% of pheochromocytomas occur as part of a multiple endocrine neoplasia syndrome; the remaining 90% are sporadic or part of another syndrome (usually von Hippel-Lindau syndrome). It has long been known that about 10% of pheochromocytomas are malignant, but other than distant metastases, there are no absolute criteria to distinguish benign from malignant pheochromocytomas. Capsular and vascular invasion i6.59, necrosis, and increased mitoses are of concern [PMID10974931].

Composite pheochromocytoma, also called compound tumor of the adrenal medulla, is a tumor consisting of pheochromocytoma with foci of another tumor, such as neuroblastoma, ganglioneuroma, or malignant peripheral nerve sheath tumor.

Core Points for the Endocrine System

- 3 autoantibodies associated with autoimmune thyroid disease.
    - 2 most important are TRAb, usually found in Graves disease, and TPOAb, found in most cases of Hashimoto or atrophic thyroiditis.
- Most thyroid masses are nonneoplastic hyperplasias.
- DNA abnormalities in 3 genes—*BRAF*, *RET*, and *RAS*—may occur in papillary thyroid carcinoma.
- Papillary microtumor: <1 cm.
    - Significance is unclear.
- Follicular variant of papillary carcinoma (FVPC): can be localized and encapsulated, or diffuse and infiltrative.
    - Infiltrative form is more aggressive.
    - Most important changes are in the nuclei:
        - Crowding
        - Nuclear grooves
        - Chromatin peripheralization
        - Cytoplasmic invagination
    - Nuclear changes should be compelling before the diagnosis of FVPC is made.
    - Psammoma bodies, multinucleated macrophages, a sclerotic stroma, and denser colloid also found
    - In difficult cases, positivity for HBME-1 suggests FVPC.
- Diagnosis of thyroid follicular carcinoma requires demonstration of either vascular invasion or full thickness invasion of the capsule.
    - Vascular invasion can be diagnosed without penetration of endothelium.
    - A single focus of vascular or capsular invasion can be designated as "minimally invasive."
- Thyroid medullary carcinomas: variety of appearances
    - Should be considered in any thyroid neoplasm that is difficult to classify.
    - Typically calcitonin positive, thyroglobulin negative, and many will stain for CEA.
- Intraoperative parathyroid hormone determination: superior to frozen section identification of parathyroid tissue, especially if there are 2 culprit glands.
- Adrenal cortical tumors: Size is important.
    - 100 g likely malignant in adults.
    - In children, most tumors under 400 g will be benign.
    - Also nuclear atypia, necrosis, and mitoses.
- Tumors of the neuroblastoma/ganglioneuroma family are classified on their degree of ganglion differentiation and on the amount and type of stroma.
- Pheochromocytomas: intraadrenal paragangliomas.
    - Variety of patterns
    - Granular cytoplasm

ISBN 978-089189-5886

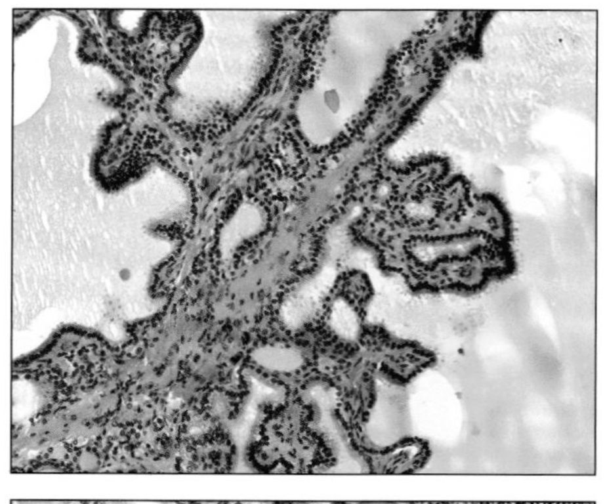

i6.1 Graves disease with hyperplasia of the thyroid epithelium infolding into the follicles

i6.2 Graves disease with epithelial hyperplasia, scalloped colloid, and a lymphoid infiltrate

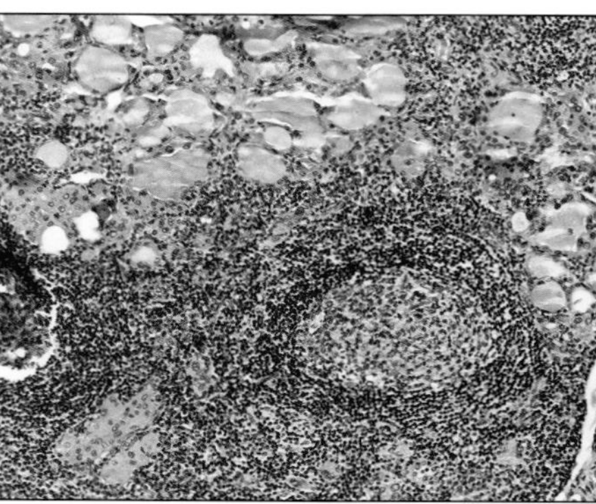

i6.3 Hashimoto thyroiditis with lymphoid nodules, including germinal centers

i6.4 Hashimoto thyroiditis with intense lymphoid infiltrate and oncocytic epithelium that does not form distinct follicles

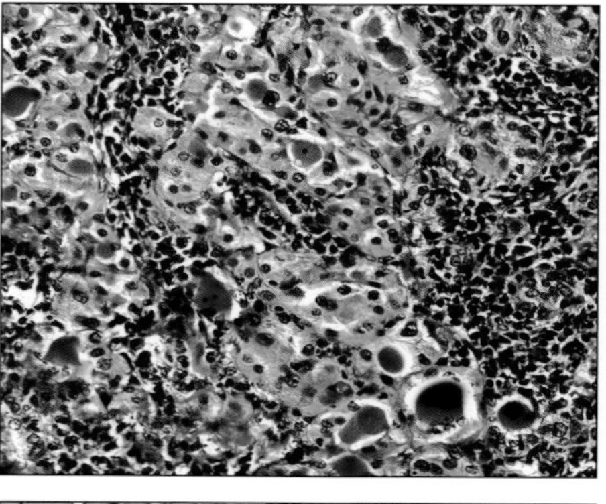

i6.5 Hashimoto thyroiditis with atrophic follicles

i6.6 Hashimoto thyroiditis with extensive fibrosis, resulting in multinodularity

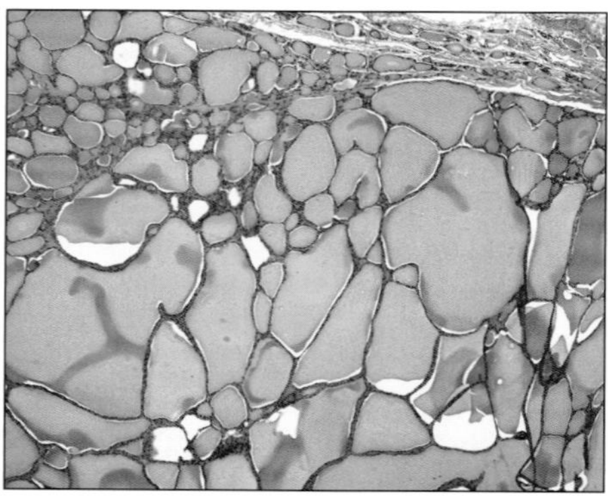

i6.7 Nodular hyperplasia with follicles that are generally dilated

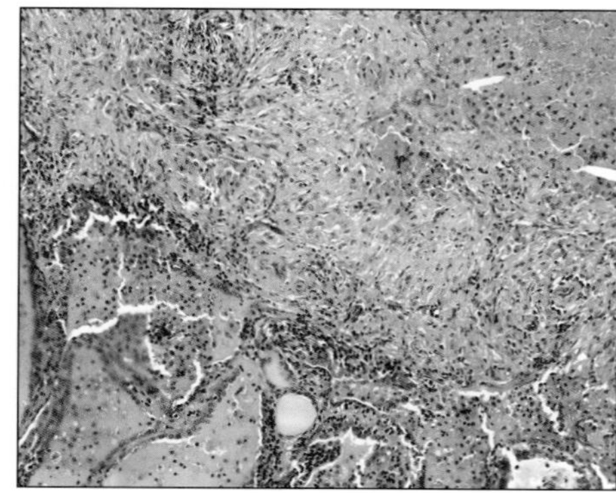

i6.8 Nodular hyperplasia with fibrotic stroma and hemosiderin macrophages, indicating previous hemorrhage

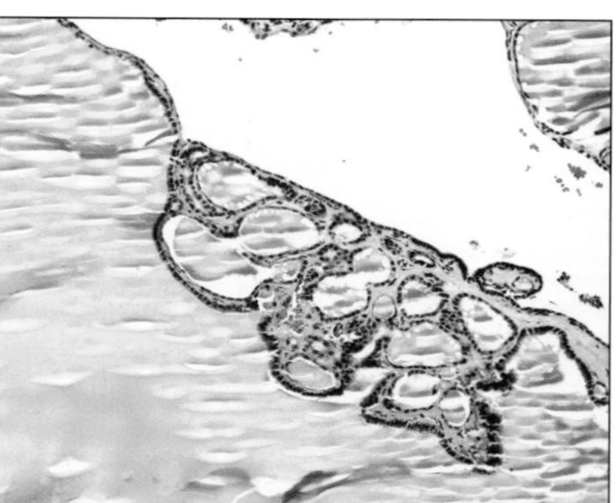

i6.9 Nodular hyperplasia with follicles projecting into the lumen of a dilated follicle. Compare to Graves disease i6.1 and i6.2 in which the epithelium that projects into follicles generally does not form secondary, smaller follicles, as shown here.

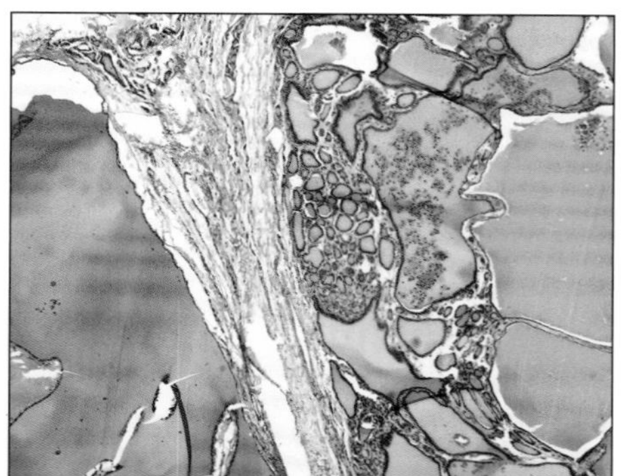

i6.10 Multinodular hyperplasia with distinct hyperplastic nodules on either side of the fibrous septa

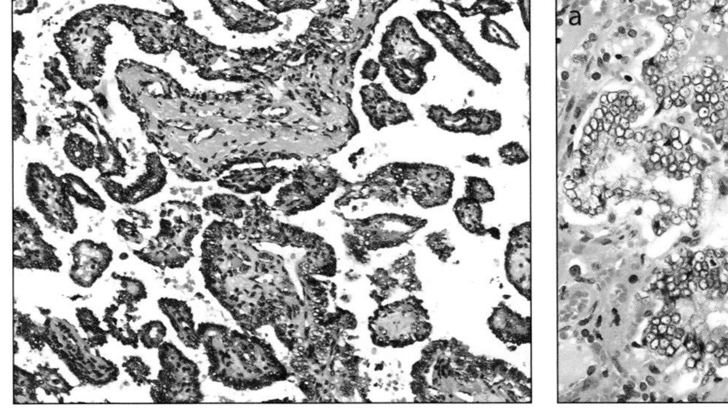

i6.11 Classic papillary carcinoma of the thyroid, with distinct fibrovascular cores

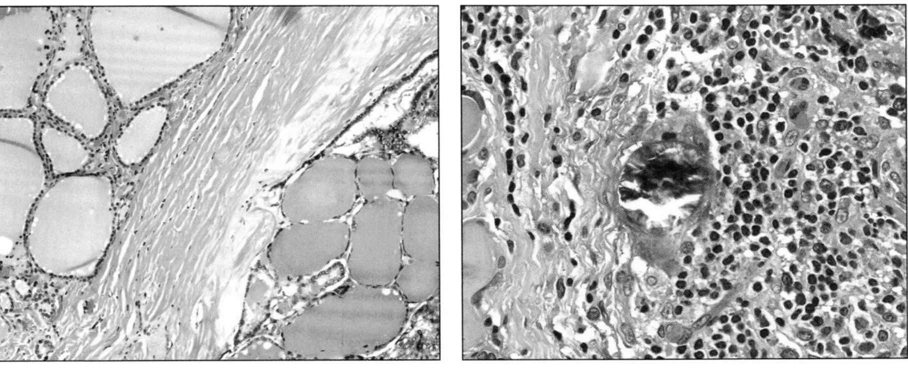

i6.12 **a** Follicular variant of papillary carcinoma demonstrating nuclear crowding and clearing **b** A high-power view demonstrating nuclear crowding, nuclear enlargement, peripheralized chromatin, cytoplasmic invagination into the nucleus, and uneven nuclear membrane (nuclear grooves)

i6.13 A focus of follicular variant of papillary carcinoma on the right shows somewhat darker colloid than the benign thyroid tissue on the left.

i6.14 A psammoma body, laminated concretions of calcium. They also contain iron.

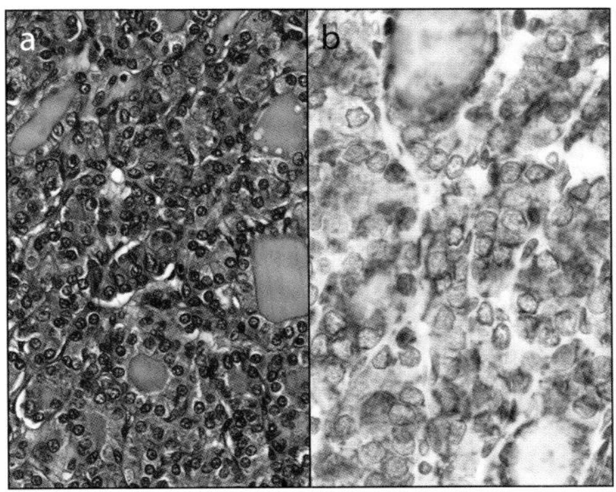

i6.15 **a** A problematic follicular process that is suspicious for follicular variant of papillary carcinoma. **b** Positive cell membrane staining for HBME-1, confirming the diagnosis of FVPC

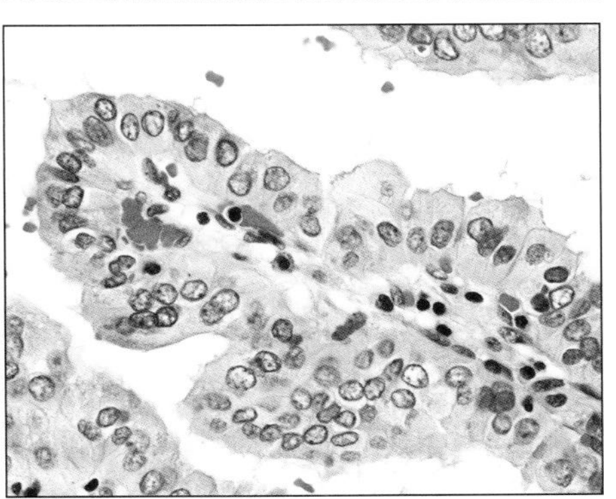

i6.16 The tall also variant of papillary carcinoma. Note the otherwise identical morphology of classic papillary carcinoma.

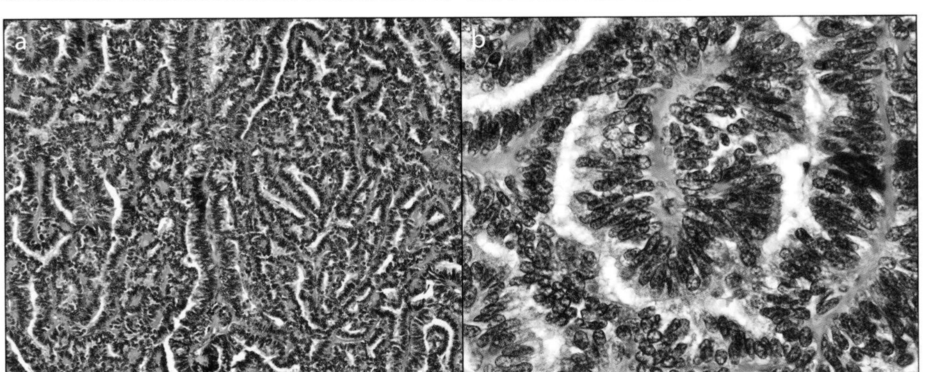

i6.17 **a** The so-called columnar cell variant of papillary thyroid carcinoma. At this low power, the papillary architecture is readily noted.

b A higher-power view of the columnar cell variant of papillary thyroid carcinoma demonstrating that the nuclei are fundamentally different in their appearance from either the classic or tall cell form of papillary carcinoma. They are more elongated, with much coarser cytoplasm, and are typically pseudostratified. Note the resemblance to a colonic adenomatous polyp.

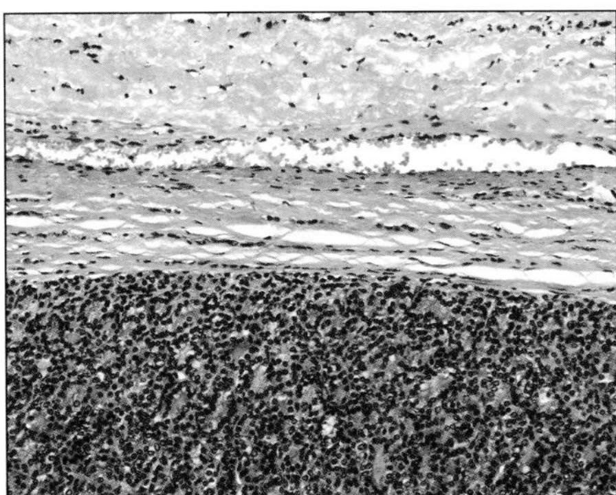

i6.18 A follicular adenoma. Although either hyperplasias or adenomas may have larger or small follicles, the follicles tend to be smaller and more uniform in follicular adenomas than in nodular hyperplasia. There is no invasion of the capsule of the blood vessels therein.

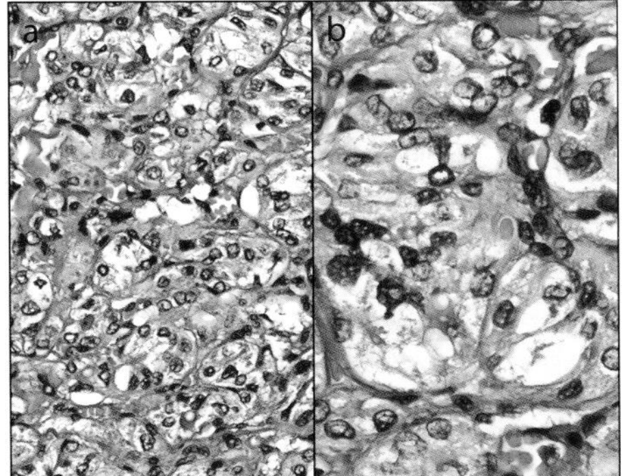

i6.19 **a** A problematic follicular process, which is suspicious for follicular variant of papillary carcinoma **b** A higher-power view demonstrating nuclear clearing, heightening that is suspicious for FVPC. A negative stain for HBME-1 would suggest a diagnosis of follicular adenoma rather than FVPC

ISBN 978-089189-5886

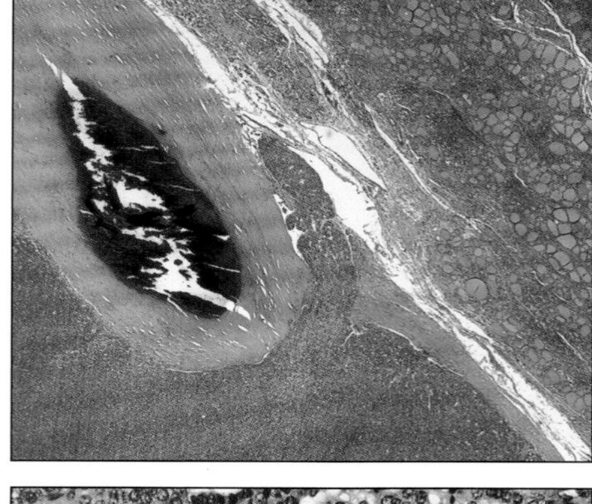

i6.20 Minimally invasive follicular carcinoma of the thyroid, with a focus of full thickness penetration of the capsule

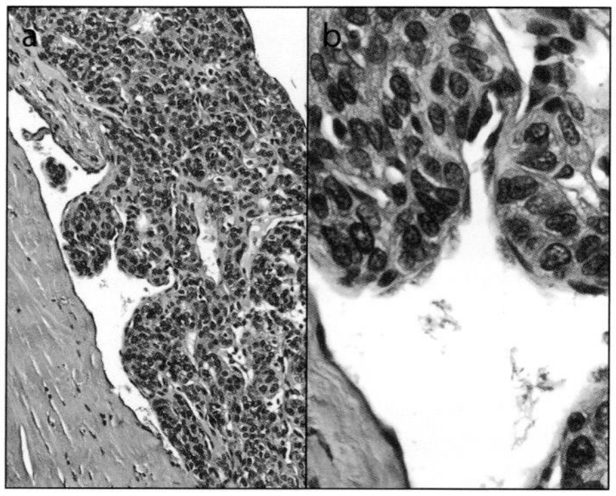

i6.21 **a** Vascular invasion in a well differentiated follicular carcinoma. **b** Higher-power view of i6.21a, confirming that the clusters of neoplastic cells are surrounded by endothelial cells and may or may not have actual access to the vascular space

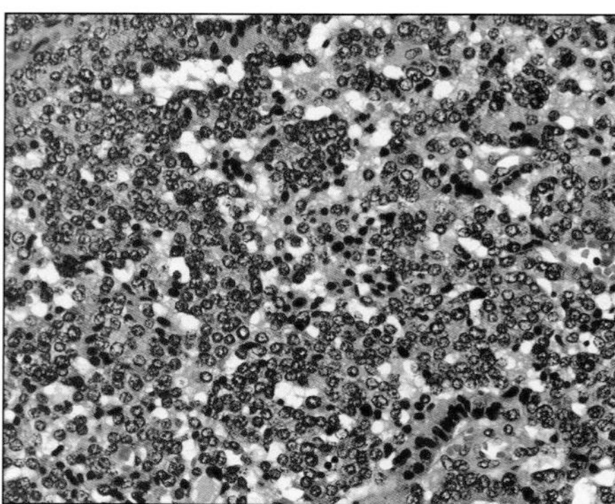

i6.22 Medullary carcinoma of the thyroid with round nuclei

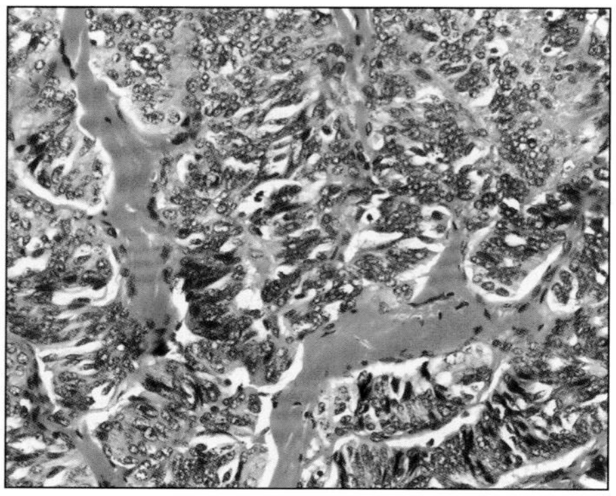

i6.23 Medullary carcinoma of the thyroid with spindled nuclei

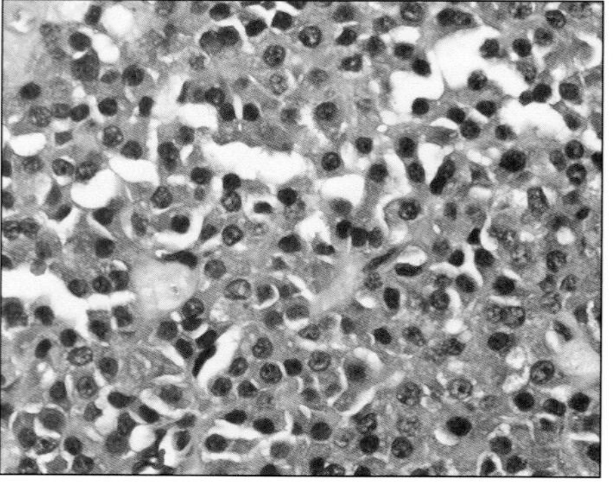

i6.24 Medullary carcinoma of the thyroid with eccentric nuclei

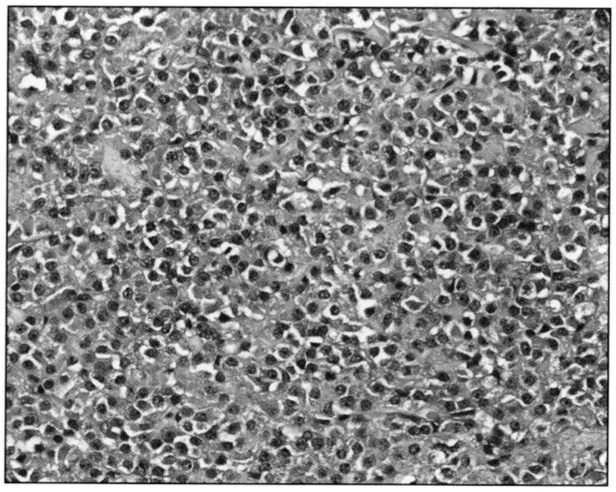

i6.25 Medullary carcinoma of the thyroid with a solid growth pattern

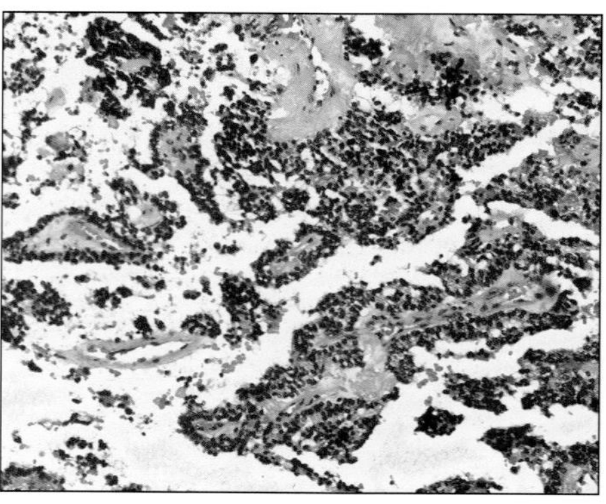

i6.26 Medullary carcinoma of the thyroid with a papillary growth pattern

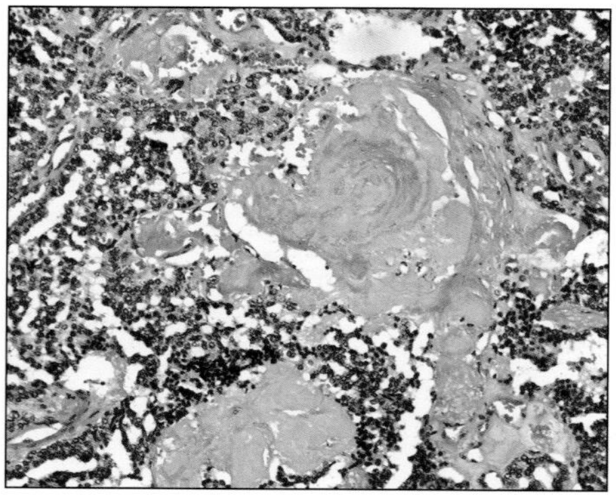

i6.27 Medullary carcinoma of the thyroid with amyloid deposition, seen on H&E as eosinophilic and amorphous

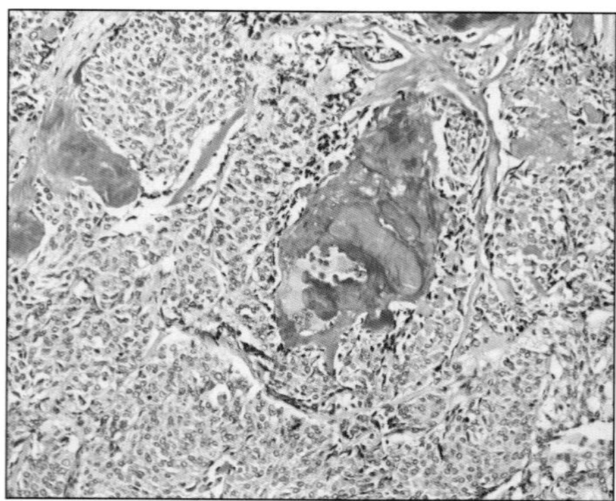

i6.28 The same case as in i6.27 stained with Congo red and viewed with ordinary light

i6.29 The same case as in i6.27 stained with Congo red and viewed with polarized light, demonstrating the classic "apple green" birefringence

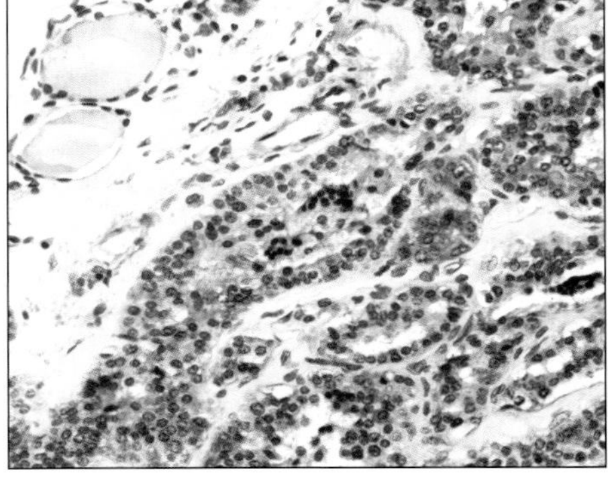

i6.30 Medullary carcinoma of the thyroid immunohistochemically stained for calcitonin. Note the negativity of the nonneoplastic thyroid tissue in the upper-left corner.

i6.31 Insular carcinoma of the thyroid with a trabecular growth pattern that resembles a low-grade neuroendocrine carcinoma (carcinoid tumor)

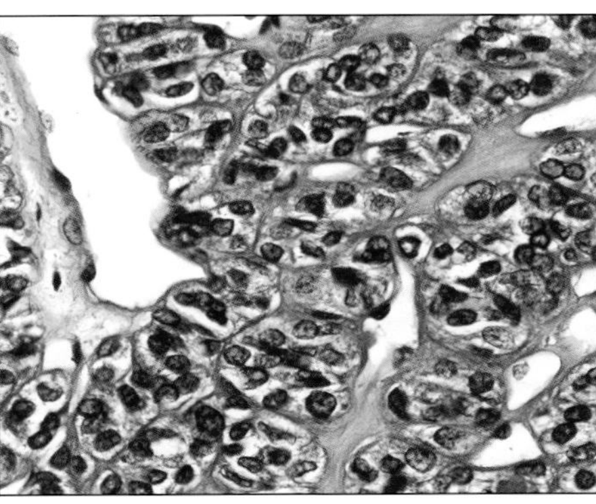

i6.32 Insular carcinoma of the thyroid with relative nuclear uniformity despite its aggressive behavior

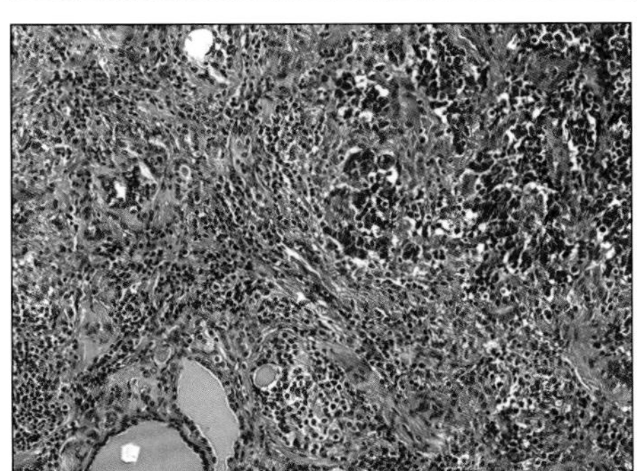

i6.33 Low-power view of small cell variant of medullary carcinoma of the thyroid

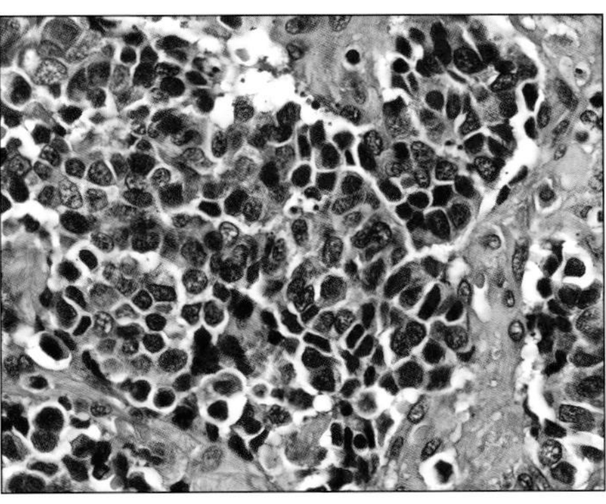

i6.34 High-power view of small cell variant of medullary carcinoma of the thyroid.

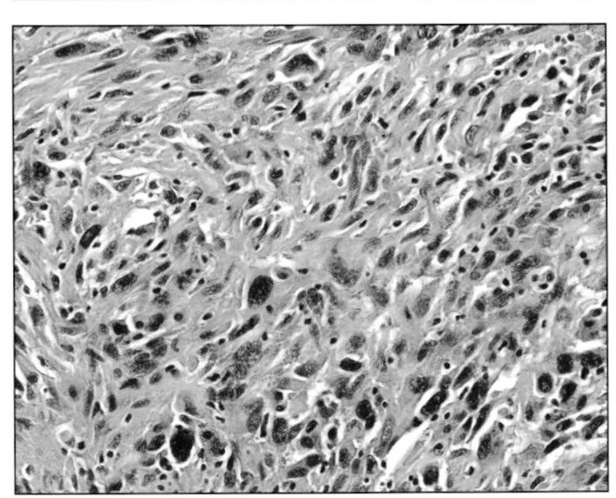

i6.35 Anaplastic carcinoma of the thyroid with giant cells and spindle cells, all with high-grade nuclei

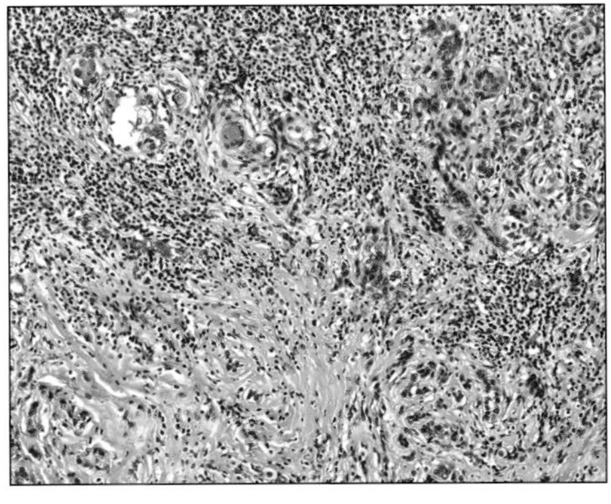

i6.36 Low-power view of sclerosing mucoepidermoid carcinoma with eosinophilia of the thyroid

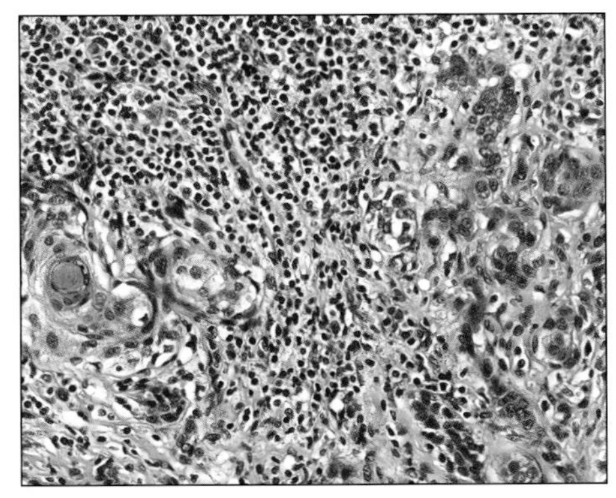

i6.37 High-power view of the same case in i6.36 demonstrating the fibrosis, lymphocytes, and eosinophils. There is a keratinizing cluster of tumor cells on the left and a cluster with glandular differentiation on the right.

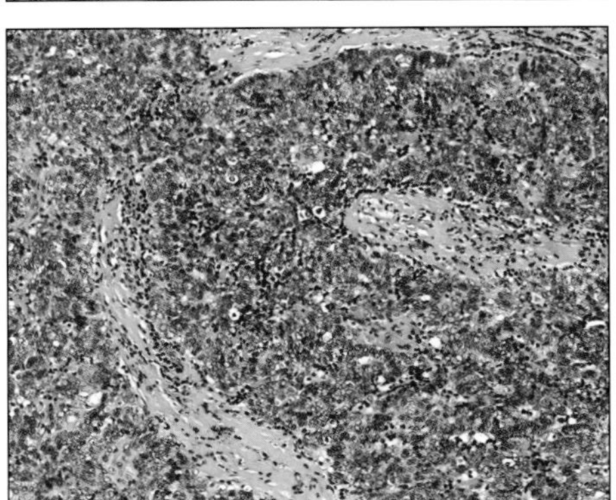

i6.38 Carcinoma showing thymus-like elements (CASTLE). This low-power view demonstrates sheets of tumor cells separated by dense fibrous tissue.

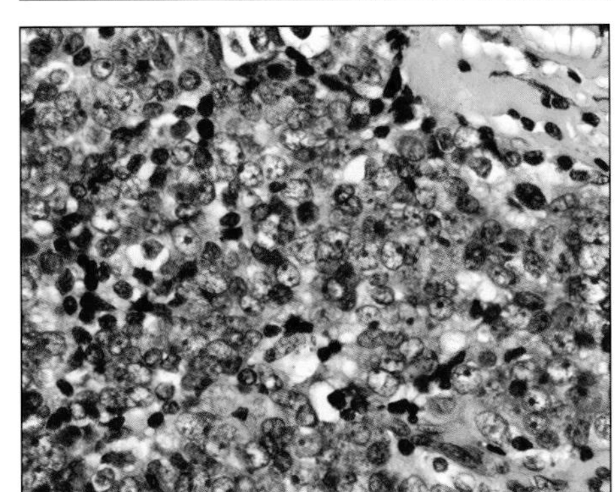

i6.39 High-power view of CASTLE demonstrating the lymphoepithelioma-like nuclei, with prominent nucleoli

ISBN 978-089189-5886

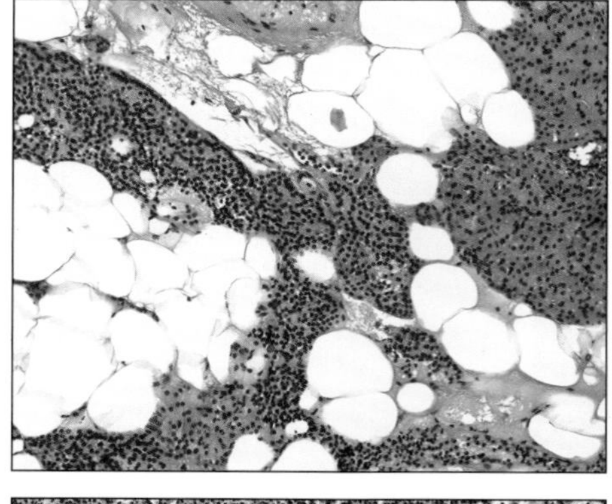

i6.40 A normal parathyroid gland. Note the abundance of adipose tissue. Clusters of oxyphil cells are seen on the right. Most of the remaining cells are chief cells.

i6.41 A higher-power view of another normal parathyroid gland showing adipose tissue and numerous clear cells, with a few oxyphil cells

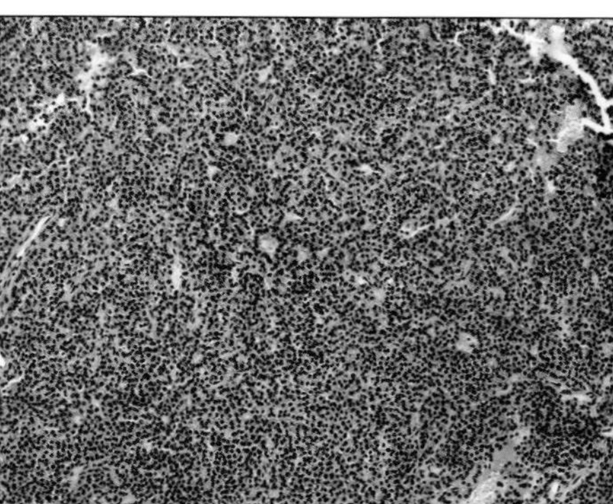

i6.42 Parathyroid hyperplasia or adenoma. Note the essential absence of adipose tissue.

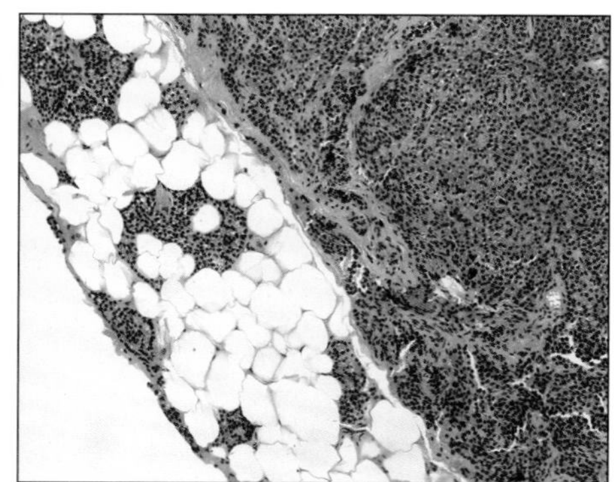

i6.43 Normal parathyroid tissue on the left, and a probable parathyroid adenoma on the right

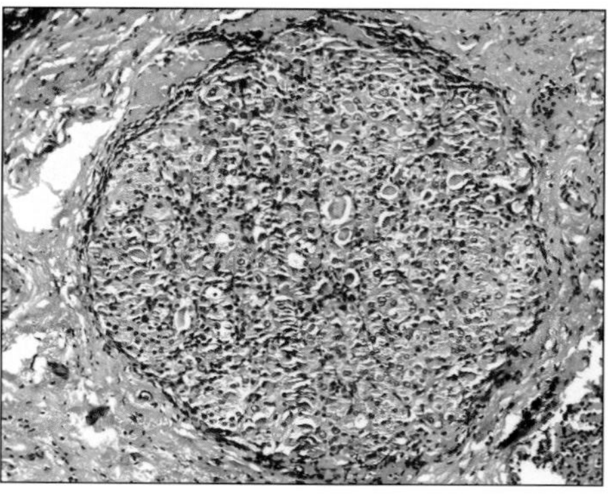

i6.44 Vascular invasion by a parathyroid carcinoma

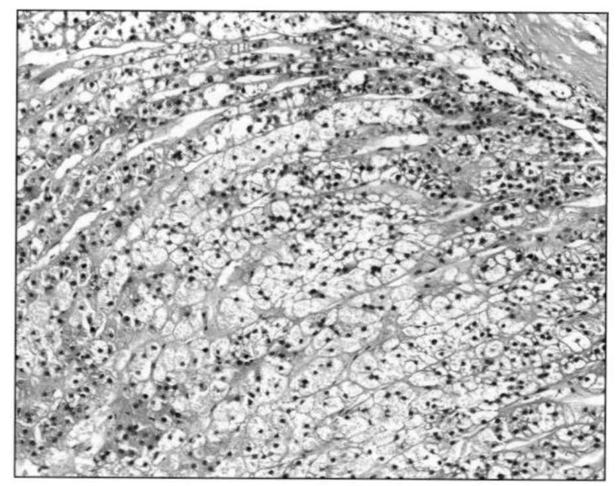

i6.45 A normal adrenal cortex. The capsule is seen in the upper right. Immediately beneath it is a small zone of cells with amphophilic cytoplasm, the zona glomerulosa. Most of the photograph is occupied by clear cells, the zona fasciculata. On the left are small clusters of cells with eosinophilic cytoplasm, the zona reticularis.

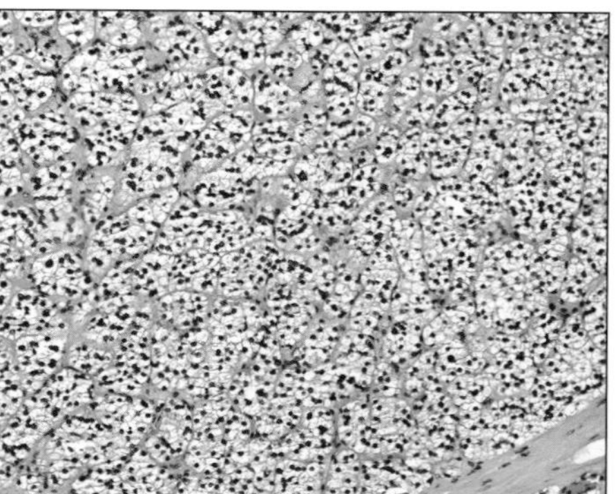

i6.46 An adrenocortical adenoma with uniform nuclei and no invasion of the capsule at the lower right

i6.47 An adrenocortical carcinoma with generalized nuclear atypia

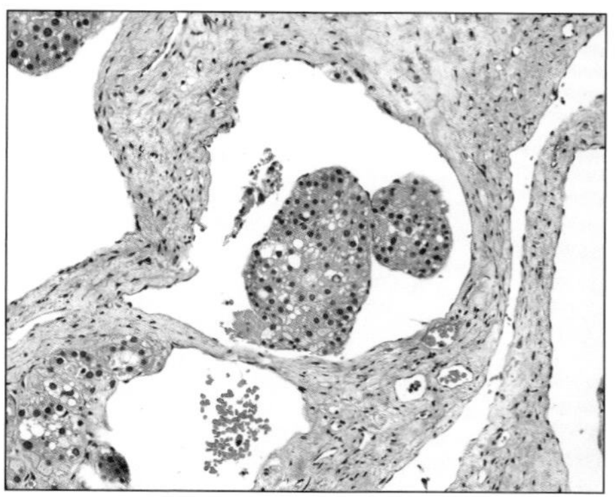

i6.48 An adrenocortical carcinoma with vascular invasion

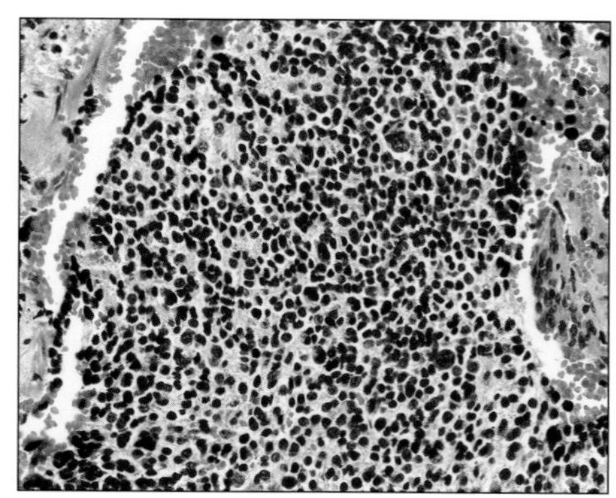

i6.49 An undifferentiated neuroblastoma with no neuropil stroma and no differentiating neuroblast

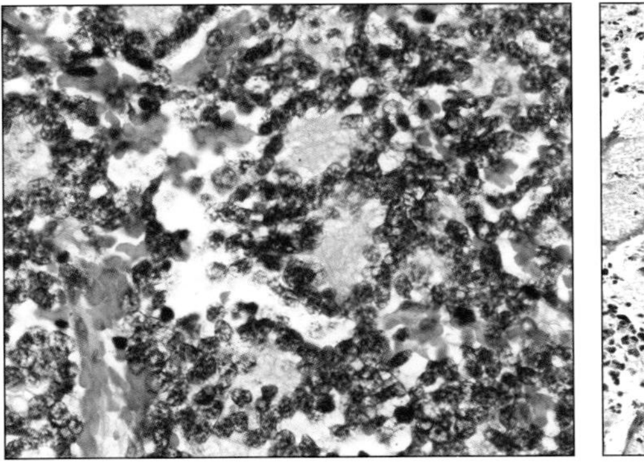

i6.50 A poorly differentiated neuroblastoma with Homer Wright pseudorosettes with neuropil stroma in the center. Note the absence of schwannian stroma and differentiating neuroblasts.

i6.51 A differentiating neuroblastoma with schwannian stroma

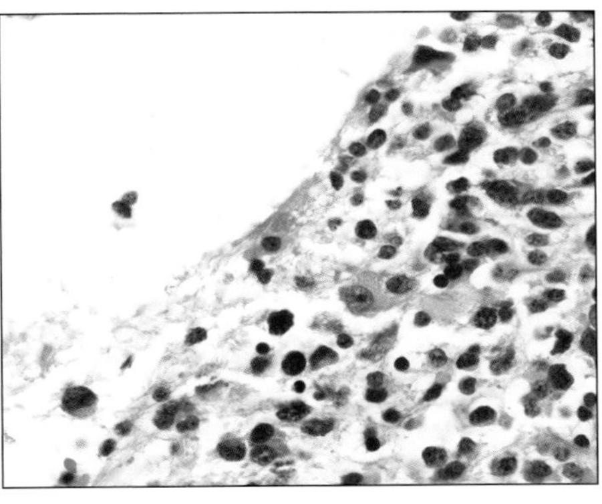

i6.52 A differentiating neuroblastoma with a differentiating neuroblast, containing a nucleolus, in the center

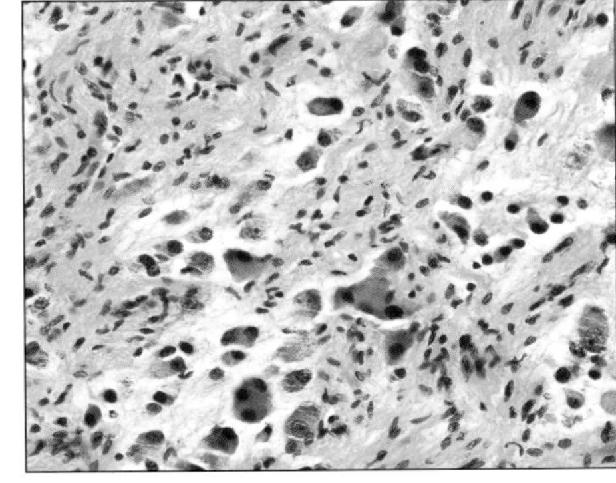

i6.53 Ganglioneuroblastoma with gangliocytic cells and schwannian stroma. There are no neuroblastoma cells in this field.

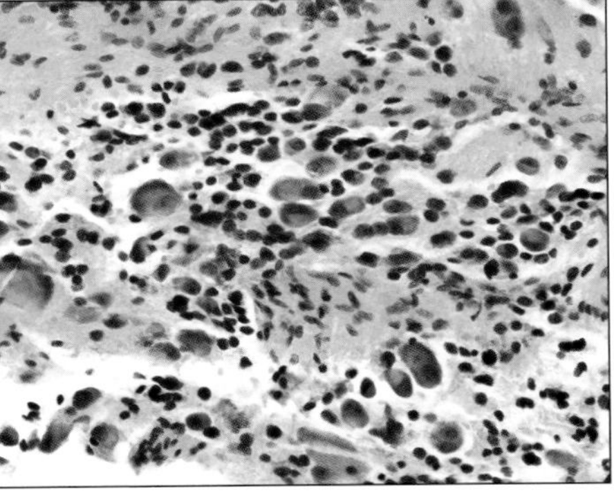

i6.54 The same case as in i6.53 showing occasional clusters of neuroblastoma cells

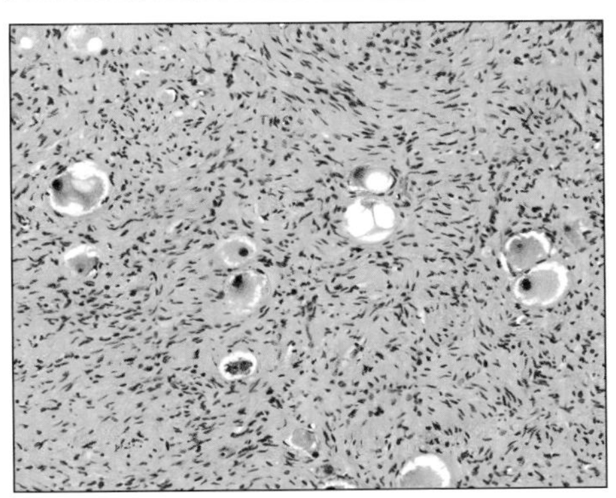

i6.55 A ganglioneuroma with no neuroblastoma cells

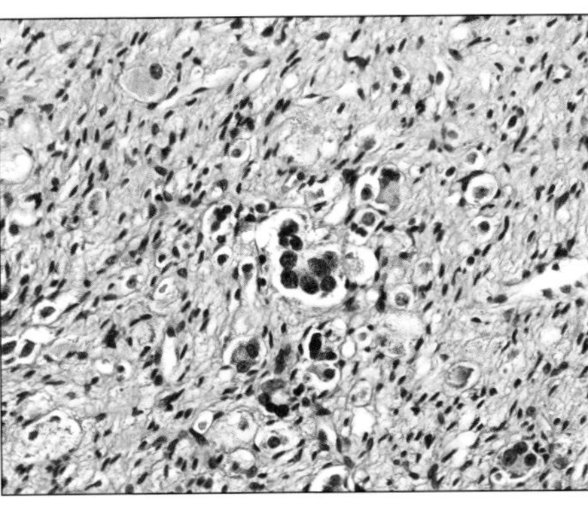

i6.56 A neuroblastoma, which has been treated with neoadjuvant therapy, resulting in appreciable differentiation

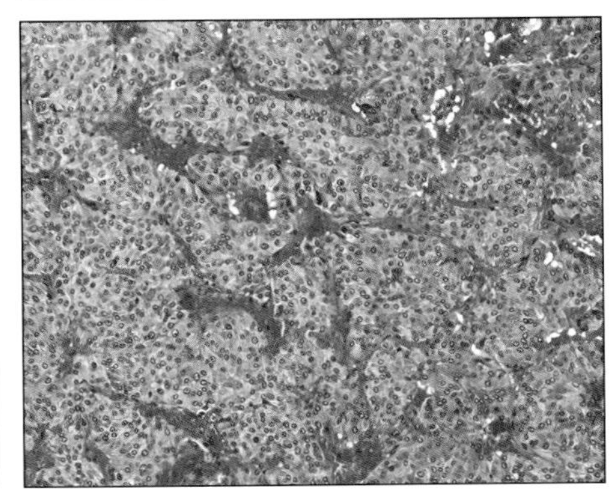

i6.57 A pheochromocytoma with a zellballen pattern

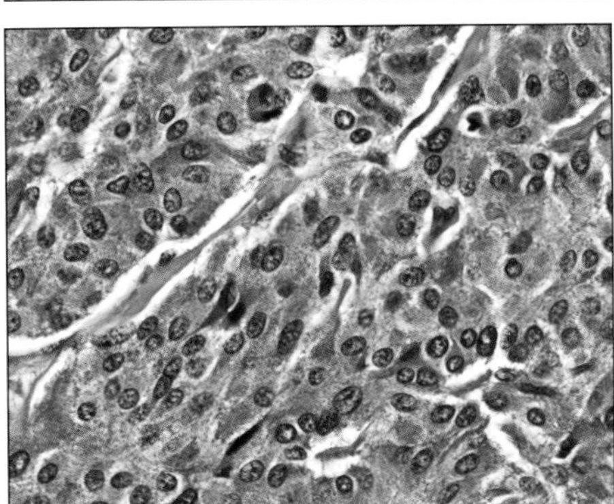

i6.58 A pheochromocytoma with distinctly amphophilic and granular cytoplasm

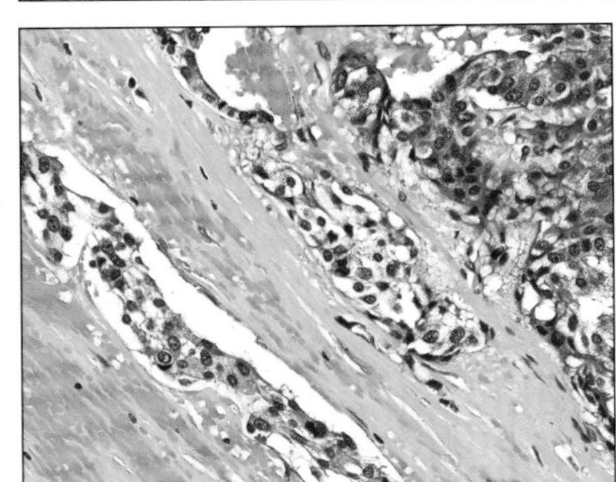

i6.59 A malignant pheochromocytoma with vascular invasion

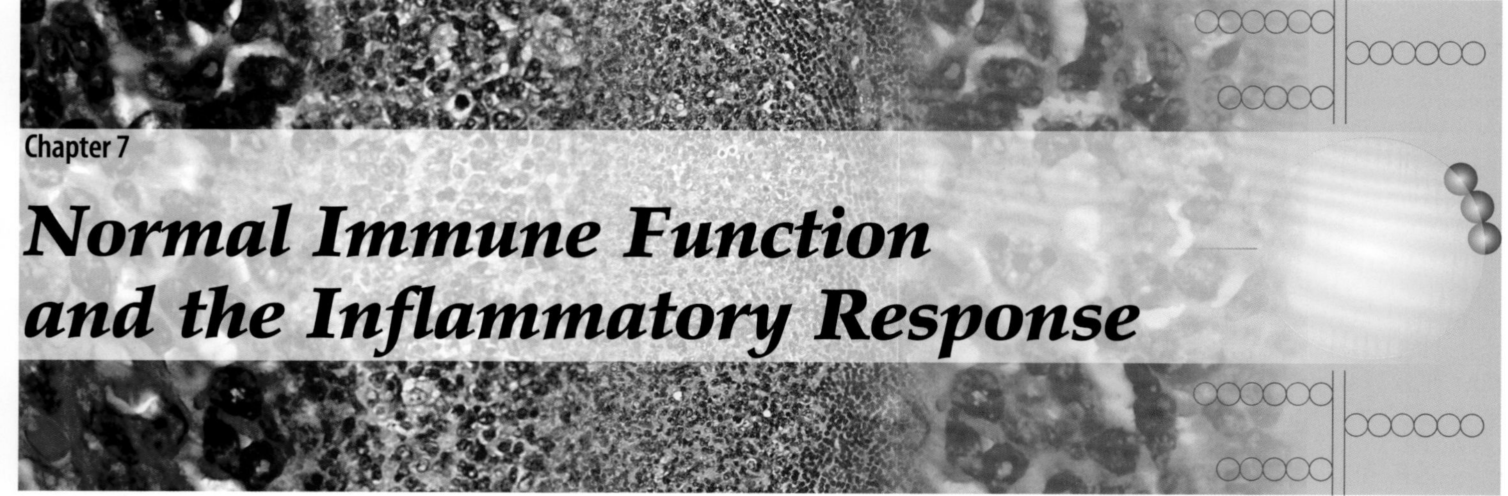

Chapter 7

Normal Immune Function and the Inflammatory Response

To enhance our understanding of lymph node pathology and lymphomas, we will first examine normal immune function. Excellent and comprehensive treatments of normal immune function can be found in major textbooks, such as those by Abbas et al [Abbas ISBN978-141603122] and Murphy et al [Murphy ISBN0-81534123-7]. A shorter, but still ample treatment is found in Coico and Sunshine [Coico ISBN978-0470081587]. The processes reviewed in this chapter are also discussed in *Robbins Pathology* [Kumar ISBN1-41603121-9].

The immune response has 2 components. The first component is innate immunity, which is a general defense against a range of pathogens. Innate immunity acts very quickly, but is nonspecific. Acute inflammation is part of the innate immune response.

The second component is adaptive immunity (also called acquired or specific immunity), which is slower, but is antigen-specific and results in immunologic memory. During vertebrate evolution, the innate response developed first and was followed by the adaptive response. Adaptive immunity consists of humoral and cell-mediated immunity and is more specific than innate immunity, both in regard to the nature of the response and to the site. Importantly, however, innate immunity continues to function after adaptive immunity has been called into play. Indeed, the 2 responses overlap and can be difficult to separate.

Innate Immunity Is Rapid but Nonspecific

The purpose of innate immunity is to elicit a very early response to an offending agent. But the price of such an early response is a lack of specificity. If the innate response is unable to take care of the problem, it will elicit the slower, but much more specific adaptive immune response.

Innate immunity consists of physical barriers as well as the acute inflammatory response. The cells of the skin, respiratory tract, and gastrointestinal tract are connected by tight junctions, which do not allow foreign material to pass between cells. Defensins are peptides with antimicrobial action that are produced by epithelia. The skin also has several additional barriers—keratin, an acidic pH of 3.5-4.0, and the presence of lysozymes in perspiration. The epithelium of the gastrointestinal tract secretes peptides called cryptocidins.

Acute Inflammation

Should physical barriers of epithelia fail, the acute inflammatory response—the second portion of innate immunity—occurs. Acute inflammation is the reaction of vascular tissue to injury, toxin, or an infectious agent. Acute inflammation is a rapid general response to an injurious agent, and occurs before there is a full antibody response.

Some 2,000 years ago, Celsus described these clinical signs as calor (heat), rubor (redness), dolor (pain), and tumor (swelling). We now know the microscopic correlates of what Celsus described.

The major participants in the acute inflammatory response are the leukocytes, connective tissue cells (such as mast cells, fibroblasts, endothelial cells, and tissue macrophages), the extracellular matrix (such as collagen and basement membranes), and plasma proteins (such as complement, proteins involving coagulation, and inhibitory proteins), and numerous molecular mediators, including histamine, some cytokines, arachidonic acid metabolites, nitric oxide, and the complement system.

Because many of the mediators in the acute inflammatory response are within the vascular space, much of acute inflammation involves getting those mediators into the tissue, to the precise site of the infection or injury, followed by their activation, interaction, and regulation.

The stages of acute inflammation are as follows:

1. An increase in blood flow
2. Increased vascular permeability
3. Slowing of the circulation in the affected area
4. Exit of white blood cells, especially neutrophils and monocytes, from the vascular space into the tissue
5. The migration of these white blood cells in tissue to the affected site
6. The activation of these white blood cells, so that the relevant biochemical pathways become activated
7. Phagocytosis of the offending organism
8. The killing of the offending organism

There is initially a vasodilatation, which brings more blood and consequently more participants in the inflammatory reaction, to the affected part of the body. There is then an increase in the permeability of the blood vessels, particularly the small venules immediately adjacent to the capillaries in the tissue bed. Normally, the balance between fluid in the vascular space and in the extravascular space is maintained by an interplay between the hydrostatic pressure within the vessels (which tends to force fluid out of the vascular space) and the oncotic pressure within the vessels (which tends to hold fluid back). The net effect of these 2 processes is a slight flow of fluid from the vascular space into the extravascular space. This fluid bathes the tissues in nutrients and is then collected by the lymphatic system, after which it is returned to the vascular space via the thoracic duct.

In acute inflammation, the increased permeability of blood vessels disturbs this normal balance and causes an increased flow into the extravascular space. This causes edema, which is the collection of fluid within tissue. Edema is the hallmark of acute inflammation, and its purpose is to achieve the relocation of vascular participants in inflammation (such as white blood cells and plasma proteins) into the tissue, where they are needed. There are several mechanisms involved in this increased permeability, but the most important is a contraction of the endothelial cells away from each other, thus greatly increasing the gap between adjacent cells.

Edema fluid, which is formed only from small gaps between endothelial cells and which has very few cells, is called a transudate. This has a low specific gravity (1.012 or less) and is essentially an ultra-filtrate of plasma. A transudate will have more proteins than are usually found in intercellular tissue, but it is cell-poor.

If this gap is sufficiently large, leukocytes are also able to leave the vascular space and enter the tissue. If edema fluid forms from large gaps between endothelial cells or from injury to those cells, it will contain many leukocytes and more protein. This form of edema is called an exudate. Exudates tend to a specific gravity >1.020. There are 4 types of exudates. A serous exudate is a watery, low-protein fluid derived from blood serum. This type of exudate is almost a transudate and can be hard to identify in tissue sections. A fibrinous exudation contains large amounts of fibrinogen and fibrin clot. This type is commonly found in inflammatory reactions that involve extensive endothelial tissue injury. A catarrhal exudate is characterized by the accumulation of mucus during inflammation. This type of exudate occurs only in inflammatory reactions that involve tissues with cells capable of mucus production. In this situation, the inflammatory process causes increased mucus secretion. An example is the common cold. A suppurative exudate, also known as a purulent exudate, occurs when pus (a fluid product of inflammation consisting of a viscous liquid containing copious neutrophils and the debris of dead cells and tissue elements that have been liquefied by proteolytic enzymes of the neutrophils) is produced and large numbers of neutrophils accumulate.

Because certain microbes routinely give rise to suppurative inflammations, they are routinely referred to as pyogenic (pus producing) bacteria. Common groups of pyogenic bacteria include the staphylococci, pneumococci, meningococci, gonococci, and some nonhemolytic strains of streptococci.

The migration of leukocytes out of the vascular compartment occurs in several stages. First, a gap is induced between endothelial cells. Second, the increased permeability lessens the velocity of blood flow in this area, just as water flowing down a garden hose will flow more slowly if the hose is perforated at many points along its length. This partial stagnation of the blood permits the leukocytes to more closely approach and to contact the endothelium. Third, inflammatory mediators to be described later greatly increase the number of adhesion molecules on the leukocytes and on the endothelial cells. The adhesion molecules on the endothelium and the leukocytes interact, causing the leukocytes to slow down and to eventually stop and bind to endothelial cells. The leukocytes then undergo the process of diapedesis, in which a rearrangement of the cytoskeleton allows them to squeeze between endothelial cells into the extravascular space.

The next stage is the migration of the leukocytes within the tissue to the relevant site, which is achieved by chemotaxis, the directed migration towards a gradient. The leukocytes that migrate to the affected area become activated by intensification of the biochemical pathways that are responsible for phagocytosis and killing. Phagocytosis is almost completely restricted to neutrophils and monocytes and involves 3 steps: recognition of the offending agent, attachment, and engulfment.

After phagocytosis, there are both oxygen-dependent and oxygen-independent pathways to killing. In the more important oxygen-dependent pathway, there is increased oxygen uptake, called the respiratory burst, during which the enzyme complex NADPH oxidase generates a free radical-containing oxygen. This free radical then combines with other substances to generate hydrogen peroxide, as well as a hydroxyl (OH–) radical and a singlet oxygen atom whose electrons are in an excited state. Under the action of the enzyme myeloperoxidase, hydrogen peroxide is converted to hypochlorite, the principal killing agent in the oxygen-dependent pathway.

Disease states can arise from any disruption in the oxygen-dependent killing pathway. Chronic granulomatous disease (CGD) is characterized by a defect in one of the subunits in the NADPH oxidase complex. The most common defect is the gp91 glycoprotein complex, encoded by the *CYBB* gene on the X chromosome, so most cases of CGD are X-linked. Less common, autosomal forms occur when there is a mutation in one of the other subunits of the NADPH complex. Patients with CGD cannot get a respiratory burst and therefore cannot utilize any part of the oxygen-dependent killing pathway. Genetic testing can determine a mutation in the *CYBB* gene [PMID20228266]. In contrast to CGD, patients with myeloperoxidase deficiency lack only one aspect of the oxygen-dependent pathway and have a much better prognosis.

There are also multiple oxygen-independent mechanisms of bacterial killing. Leukocytes, especially the granulocytes (neutrophils, basophils, and eosinophils), have primary (also called azurophilic) and secondary (or specific) granules. Myeloperoxidase is present in the primary granules, but there are many other proteins in both the primary and secondary granules that can kill bacteria by mechanisms that do not involve oxygen, including lysozyme, lactoferrin, bacterial permeability-increasing protein, major basic protein, and defensins. Both the oxygen-independent and oxygen-dependent pathways are inhibited by steroids via multiple mechanisms, one of which is the stabilization of the lysosomal membranes where bactericidal proteins are located.

ISBN 978-089189-5886

Types and Functions of Leukocytes

Neutrophils are the most common type of leukocyte in the blood under normal conditions and account for the majority of phagocytic activity in acute inflammation. The neutrophil is in the bloodstream for only a few hours before it migrates into the tissue, where it will perform its life's work by participating in the acute inflammatory reaction, largely through phagocytosis. Neutrophils only live 1 or 2 days in tissues. In severe infections, immature neutrophils (band forms, metamyelocytes, or even myelocytes) may be released from the bone marrow.

Eosinophils are rare leukocytes. Although they have long been associated with parasites and allergic reactions, many cases of eosinophilia cannot be linked to either of those etiologies. Eosinophils are generally found in the connective tissue just beneath the epithelium in a number of organs. They have minimal phagocytic ability, only about 10% that of a neutrophil, but their granules are toxic to pathogens that might enter through the epithelium—microorganisms, protozoa, or helminth—and they release cytokine molecules that can amplify the inflammatory response. They have a receptor for IgE and also for CCR3, which recognizes a variety of chemokines.

Basophils are the rarest of all leukocytes. Little is known about them, but they have the same receptor for IgE that is found on eosinophils, and like eosinophils, can respond to chemokines (chemotactic cytokines).

Lymphocytes are normally second in number to neutrophils in the blood. They are not phagocytic and unlike other leukocytes, their role is primarily in adaptive immunity, not innate immunity. Lymphocytes are divided into B cells, which make antibodies (humoral immunity) and T cells, which bring about cell-mediated immunity and facilitate humoral immunity. B lymphocytes secrete antibodies and both B and T lymphocytes may secrete cytokines, molecular mediators of inflammation (discussed subsequently). Antibodies are Y-shaped molecules. The 2 "arms" are the Fab regions. They contain the variable regions and react with the antigen, while the "base" of the molecule is the Fc portion that interacts with other cells of the immune system. Lymphocytes and monocytes are active participants in the chronic inflammatory process and tend to replace neutrophils in the tissues as the inflammatory process persists. Because lymphocyte function is nearly synonymous with adaptive immunity, we will study them much more closely in that section.

Monocytes are less common in the blood than neutrophils or lymphocytes, but they are crucial in innate immunity. Like neutrophils, monocytes leave the vascular space and migrate into the tissues, where they actively phagocytose. But unlike neutrophils, monocytes are not a terminal cell. Once they migrate into tissues, monocytes are transformed into macrophages (also called histiocytes) that may be active for up to 2 weeks and can even divide in tissues. Macrophages are part of the mononuclear phagocytic system, a collection of tissue-based monocyte-like cells that patrol body sites and phagocytose infectious agents (examples include the Kupffer cells in the sinusoids of the liver and the macrophages in the sinuses of lymph nodes).

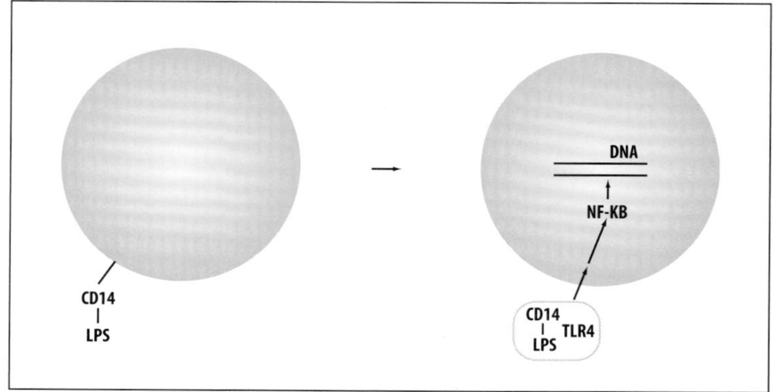

f7.1 The interaction of toll-like receptor 4 (TLR4) with the complex of CD14 and lipopolysaccharide (LPS). This interaction initiates a sequence of intracellular reactions terminating in the modification of DNA transcription.

Like neutrophils, monocytes and macrophages have primary and secondary granules that contain similar enzymes (even myeloperoxidase), but they are few in number, and macrophages do not appear granulated under normal microscopic observation. Like neutrophils, macrophages are phagocytic, and they also have receptors for complement components and for the Fc component of antibodies.

Innate immunity responds rapidly to certain antigens that are found only on pathogenic bacteria, fungi, viruses, and parasitic protozoa. Examples of these antigens include lipopolysaccharide (LPS), CpG sequences, and double-stranded RNA. LPS is a constituent of the outer membrane of gram-negative bacteria. CpG areas (referring to consecutive cytosine and guanine bases on a strand of DNA) are common in bacterial DNA but rare in eukaryotic DNA. Double-stranded RNA is characteristic of viruses but very rare in eukaryotes.

Special receptors called toll-like receptors (TLRs) on host phagocytic cells recognize these antigens. In mammals, the TLR family consists of 10 structurally similar proteins that are expressed on phagocytic cells. Most TLRs are transmembrane proteins, spanning the cell membrane, though a few are attached to the membranes of intracellular organelles, where they defend against intracellular pathogens.

Each TLR recognizes a particular foreign antigen. For example, TLR4 binds to LPS, TLR5 binds to flagellin, a protein that confers mobility to some bacteria, TLR3 binds to double-stranded RNA, and TLR9 binds to GpC residues. Binding of the TLR to antigen initiates a cascade of reactions, which eventuate in the activation of transcription factors such as NF-κB, which then enter the nucleus and instigate the transcription of cytokines and some of the proteins involved in adaptive immunity (this is one of a number of ways in which innate immunity activates adaptive immunity).

As an example, LPS is delivered to the cell membrane of the macrophage by a plasma protein called LPS-binding protein, after which LPS binds to a cell surface receptor called CD14. TLR4 then interacts with the CD14-LPS complex to set in motion the sequential reactions that activate NF-κB **f7.1**.

The response to some antigens recognized by phagocytes in the innate immune response is not mediated by TLRs. Phagocytic cells respond innately to carbohydrates or proteins that contain the sugar mannose, which is common in bacteria, but rare in eukaryotes. This response works through the complement system, as we will see in a moment. N-formyl-methionyl is common at the amino end of bacterial proteins, but not found in eukaryote proteins. The receptors on phagocytes that respond to N-formyl-methionyl peptides belong to a family of receptors called G-protein-coupled receptors, which we will examine shortly.

Like lymphocytes, macrophages are rare in acutely inflamed tissue, but become more conspicuous in chronic inflammation. If the acute inflammatory process is unsuccessful, so that a chronic inflammatory stage ensues, neutrophils secrete a cytokine that recruits macrophages to the site. Thus, in subacute inflammation (also called acute and chronic or chronic active inflammation), there is a mixture of neutrophils with macrophages and lymphocytes.

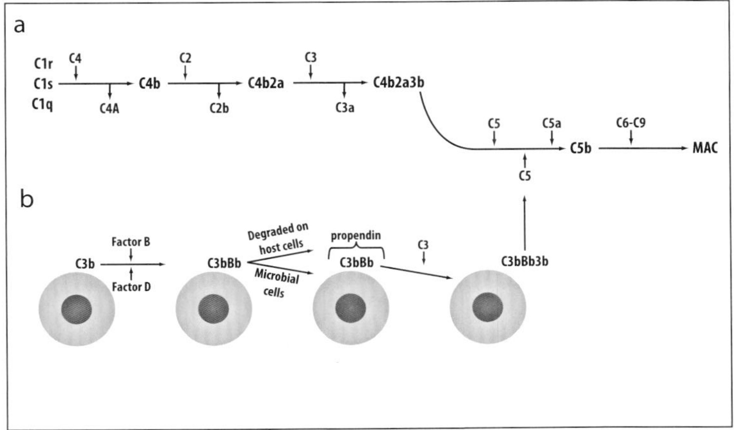

f7.2 **a** Activation of the complement cascade by the classical pathway. At the end, C5 is cleaved and C5b participates with C6-C9 in formation of a membrane attack complex (MAC).
b Activation of complement by the alternate pathway, which also eventuates in the cleavage of factor 5 and the formation of C5b. The final stages of the classical and alternate pathways are identical.

Molecular Mediators of Inflammation

In addition to leukocytes, there are molecular mediators of acute inflammation, which may be in the blood or secreted by cells. These molecules are instrumental in bringing about the stages of acute inflammation. In general, each of these mediators has a specific receptor, binding to which results in a specific action, and most of them have a very short lifetime. The advantage of a short lifetime is easier regulation. The major molecular mediators of inflammation are histamine, components of the complement system, components of the coagulation cascade, arachidonic acid metabolites, nitric oxide, cytokines, growth factors, and cell adhesion molecules.

Histamine is found in the granules of mast cells and basophils. Its main action is to facilitate the contraction of endothelial cells, thereby increasing vascular permeability. Other mediators are more effective in this regard, but they must be induced by the inflammatory response, whereas histamine is constitutive (present at all times) and is therefore the most important early mediator of increased vascular permeability.

The Complement is a system of approximately 30 proteins that are found in plasma. The activation of complement is an example of proteolytic cascade, wherein a protein is activated and, by cleaving off a few amino acids of another protein, activates it. The first protein in the sequence activates the second by cleaving a small portion from it, after which the activated second protein then activates the third protein by cleaving a small portion of it, etc. Because one protein molecule can potentially activate thousands of molecules in the subsequent step, enormous amplification is possible.

While much of the complement cascade involves adaptive immunity, there are components that are part of innate immunity, so it is discussed here. The principal components of the Complement system are numbered 1-9. Complement may be activated by 2 mechanisms: the classic pathway and the alternate (or properdin) pathway.

In the classical pathway, complement is activated by immune complexes, a product of adaptive immunity. In the classical pathway, the component C1 binds to immune complexes. C1 is a complex composed of 3 subunits—C1q, C1r, and C1s. C1q binds to the Fc region of IgM and IgG molecules if and only if the antibody has bound antigen on a foreign cell. C1r and C1s are proteases. After binding of C1q, C1r cleaves C1s, which then cleaves C4 to generate C4b and C4a. C4a diffuses away while C4b binds to the cell surface (after proteolytic cleavage, the fragment designated with a "b" generally binds to the cell membrane of the foreign cell and participates in further reactions by activating the next component, while the fragment designated with an "a" diffuses away and does not participate in any further activation of the sequence, though it may have proinflammatory activities of its own). C2 binds to C4b and is cleaved by C1s into C2a and C2b. C2a diffuses away, while C2b remains attached to C4b, resulting in a complex of C4b2b bound to the cell surface (an exception to the general rule that the "a" fragment diffuses way and the "b" fragment remains attached). This complex is the classical C3 convertase. It binds C3 and cleaves it into C3a and C3b. Again the C3a diffuses away, while some of the C3b binds to C4b2a to result in a C4b2a3b complex **f7.2a**. This complex then activates complement factor 5 to initiate the final stages of the cascade, to be described below.

The classical pathway is an integral part of adaptive immunity, but in a wonderful example of overlap between innate and adaptive immunity, the classical activation of complement may be initiated in innate immunity by a protein called mannose-binding lectin (MBL; also called mannose-binding protein). Lectins are proteins that contain sugar moieties. MBL is a serum protein that binds to mannose, a sugar found in cell membranes of bacteria but rare in eukaryotes. The complex of MBL and a mannose-containing portion of microorganisms then activates C1, resulting ultimately in activation of complement by the classical pathway, but without on immune complexes.

In addition to the classical pathway, complement can be activated by the alternate (or properdin) pathway, which is also part of innate immunity. In the alternate pathway of complement activation, the latter stages (those following the activation of C5) are the same as for the classical or lectin pathway, but C5 is activated by a slightly different mechanism. A small amount of C3 is always being activated by a low level of spontaneous cleavage, without antecedent activation of any other complement component. This results in a small amount of C3b adhering to the surface of all cells, both foreign and host.

In the alternate pathway, some of the small amount of C3b that is always present becomes attached to the surface of any cell, host or foreign. C3b then binds a plasma protein called factor B. After it is bound to C3b, factor B is cleaved by a plasma protein called factor D to generate a fragment called Bb, which remains attached to C3b. This complex of C3bBb is quickly degraded on the host cells before further activation of the cascade can occur, but microbial cells are unable to degrade C3bBb and are thereby exposed to further activation. In addition, a host protein called properdin (also called factor P) binds to C3bBb on microbes, stabilizing it and allowing it to activate the cascade. C3 binds to the C3bBb complex, after which C3a and C3b are generated in much larger amounts than is possible with spontaneous cleavage (for this reason, C3bBb is sometimes called the alternative pathway C3 convertase). Some of this C3b binds to C3bBb, forming C3bBbC3b, which can activate factor C5 just as C4b2a3b activates C5 in the classical pathway **f7.2b**. The advantage of the alternate pathway is that antigen-antibody complexes are not required, so the response can be rapid.

Once C5 is activated, there is no difference between the classical and alternative pathways. In fact, there is interaction of the 2 pathways. For example, C3b generated by the classical path can interact with Bb generated by the alternate pathway.

Regardless of which way the complement activation is initiated, the final 2/3 of the proteolytic cascade is the same. The final component of complement activation is a complex of C5-C9. This is known as the membrane attack complex, because it can kill bacteria by perforating its membrane.

Complement is important for much more than just the membrane attack complex. Many of the components of the complement cascade facilitate many steps in the inflammatory process. For example, C3b is an important opsonin (a compound which facilitates phagocytosis by binding to the infectious agent and furnishing a receptor for the phagocyte to bind to; an opsonin literally furnishes a handle for the phagocyte). C3a increases vascular permeability. C5a facilitates many stages in the inflammatory process. It increases vascular permeability, is a potent chemotactic agent, induces the formation of adhesion molecules, induces the oxidative respiratory burst in leukocytes, and mobilizes arachidonic acid, which is the precursor for other mediators of inflammation.

The other example of a proteolytic cascade that is relevant in acute inflammation is the clotting sequence. Clotting of blood has 2 principal components. The first is platelet aggregation, called primary hemostasis. In secondary hemostasis, a serum protein called fibrinogen is cleaved into a fibrin monomer. These fibrin monomers then polymerize into fibrin and are stabilized by the cross-linking of factor 13. A blood clot contains both cross-linked fibrin and aggregated platelets.

Like complement, secondary hemostasis involves a proteolytic cascade. As in the activation of complement, there are 2 proteolytic cascade pathways by which fibrin may be created, and as is the case for complement activation, these pathways differ only in their initial steps and employ a common final pathway. One pathway to fibrin, called the intrinsic pathway, begins when clotting factors are exposed to collagen, as occurs when there is injury to endothelial cells.

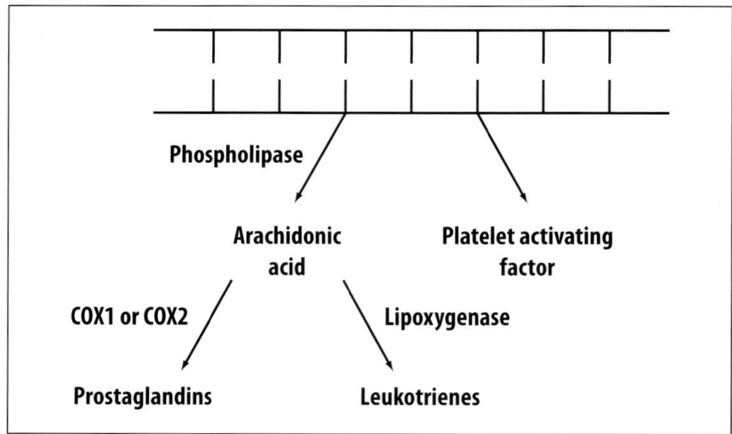

f7.3 Phospholipase acts on lipids in the cell membrane to generate both platelet-activating factor and arachidonic acid. Arachidonic acid is acted on by the enzyme cyclooxygenase (COX) to generate prostaglandins or by the enzyme lipoxygenase to generate leukotrienes.

The other pathway, called the extrinsic pathway, occurs when there is a more severe injury to tissue. In this case, the injured tissue liberates tissue factor, which initiates the clotting sequence by a different pathway. The intrinsic and extrinsic pathways converge and have a final common pathway.

The intrinsic pathway is relevant in acute inflammation. Activation of the first factor in the intrinsic pathway, factor 12, results in factor 12a. Factor 12a cleaves off a portion of the plasma protein prekallikrein, resulting in the active enzyme kallikrein, which, in turn, cleaves off a portion of high molecular kininogen, to make bradykinin. Bradykinin increases vascular permeability, furnishing a connection between acute inflammation and coagulation. The plasma enzyme plasmin cleaves the fibrin clot into fibrin degradation products (FDP; also called fibrin split products [FSPs]), which increase vascular permeability and are chemotactic.

Arachidonic acid is part of the phospholipids that are an integral part of the cell membranes of all cells. In acute inflammation, the enzyme phospholipase cleaves arachidonic acid from these phospholipids (as one of their many actions, steroids inhibit phospholipase). The free arachidonic acid can then enter a number of enzymatic pathways, to give a number of different products. Any product derived from arachidonic acid that is a mediator of acute inflammation is called an eicosanoid. The most important eicosanoids are the prostaglandins, which are derived from arachidonic acid by the enzyme cyclooxygenase **f7.3**. It is this enzyme that is inhibited by aspirin and other non-steroidal anti-inflammatory agents.

Cyclooxygenase (COX) exists in 2 forms. COX-1 is constitutive (always present) and found in many tissues, even those not inflamed. COX-1 is involved in "housekeeping" functions as well as in the inflammatory process. COX-2 is induced by the inflammatory process and therefore (at least theoretically) found primarily in inflamed tissues. Because traditional non-steroidal anti-inflammatory agents, such as aspirin, act on both isozymes (and hence have undesirable side effects because of their actions on COX-1), newer drugs supposedly act only on COX-2 and were initially thought to have fewer side effects.

Both COX-1 and COX-2 generate prostaglandin G2 (PGG2). From PGG2, other prostaglandins are derived from the action of other enzymes. Because these additional enzymes are somewhat tissue specific, the different cells involved in acute inflammation may have different types of prostaglandins. For example, mast cells contain prostaglandin D2, which causes vascular dilatation and increased permeability. Endothelial cells contain prostaglandin I2 (sometimes called prostacyclin). Prostaglandin E2 seems to be the primary prostaglandin involved in the generation of pain, but it also has a protective effect on gastric mucosa. This is why COX inhibitors can cause gastritis [PMID12646969]. COX-2 inhibitors, however, diminish prostaglandin I2 levels more than COX-1, which is a problem since prostaglandin I2 exerts a protective effect on endothelium. This is the likely mechanism for the increased cardiovascular events with COX-2 inhibitors that were first noticed in the early 2000s [PMID18030055].

Prostaglandins are also one cause of the hypercalcemia that is seen in many cases of bony metastases (other causes include bone breakdown and the secretion by the neoplastic cells of a protein that is similar to parathyroid hormone).

Thromboxane, though not referred to as a prostaglandin, is derived from cyclooxygenase pathway. It is found predominantly in platelets, where it facilitates aggregation.

The enzyme lipoxygenase is also active on arachidonic acid. The products of this enzyme are referred to as leukotrienes f7.3. Leukotriene B4 (LTB4) is chemotactic for leukocytes, while LTC4, LTD4, and LTE4 increase vascular permeability and cause bronchospasm. The latter 3 leukotrienes, before their nature was understood, were referred to as the slow-reacting substance of anaphylaxis.

In addition, by a separate enzymatic pathway not involving phospholipase, platelet activating factor is also derived from phospholipids. Originally thought to affect only platelet aggregation, platelet activating factor is now known to facilitate almost every step in acute inflammation [PMID18028783].

Nitric oxide (not to be confused with nitrous oxide, which is laughing gas) is a molecular mediator that is important in vasodilatation, and it also exerts a protective effect on endothelium by inhibiting platelet aggregation and thrombosis. A deficiency of nitric oxide leads to endothelial damage and an increased incidence of thrombosis [PMID21572574].

Cytokines

Cytokines are cell-signaling polypeptides that are active in intercellular communication and are secreted by many different cell types. In the context of the immune response, cytokines are important in both innate and adaptive immunity. Cytokines made by activated macrophages, natural killer (NK) cells, dendritic cells (a type of antigen-presenting cell [APC]), and some T lymphocytes are an important part of innate immunity, while cytokines important to adaptive immunity are mostly made by specific subsets of T lymphocyte. Cytokines work through specific receptors and modulate the function of other cells in the immune response and inflammatory process.

Cytokines have either an autocrine function (acting on the cell that produced them) or a paracrine function (acting on other cells in the immediate vicinity). Cytokines are one of the major groups of intercellular messengers, along with hormones, growth factors, and neurotransmittors. Unlike hormones, cytokines rarely act at distant sites. Cytokine actions are often pleiotrophic (meaning that one cytokine can affect a number of different cell types), redundant (meaning that multiple cytokines may have the same effect), or multifunctional (meaning that 1 cytokine can affect a number of different functions).

"Signal transduction" is the term used for the series of reactions that begins with the binding of an extracellular signal to a receptor and ends with a change in the metabolism, function, or differentiation of the cell. Signal transduction induced by cytokines begins with the binding of the cytokine to a specific transmembrane receptor, so we must digress a moment to review the types of receptors.

Roughly speaking, there are 2 basic types of receptors for extracellular signals. The first, used primarily by steroid messengers, such as estrogen and progesterone, is located in the nucleus. Steroid molecules can diffuse through the lipid bilayer of the cell membrane to the nucleus and require no elaborate mechanism or sequence of reactions to contact DNA and modulate its transcription. The second broad class of receptors is membrane or transmembrane proteins that bind to an extracellular messenger then set in motion a series of intracellular chemical reactions that open channels in the membrane, initiate important cytoplasmic enzymatic reactions, and/or modulate DNA transcription. The elucidation of these sequences of reactions, and the commonalities and differences in them among different receptors, has been a triumph of contemporary medicine.

More specifically, there are 4 superfamilies of receptors in eukaryotic cells (a gene superfamily is a collection of genes that have a related structure and function, caused by substantial evolutionary conservation). The first superfamily is the nuclear receptor superfamily, members of which receive extracellular signals via molecules that diffuse through the cell membrane and migrate to the nucleus. Steroid hormone receptors belong to this family. The other 3 receptor superfamilies are all membrane or transmembrane proteins. The second receptor superfamily consists of those receptors that are coupled to ion channels. Ion channel-coupled receptors are ubiquitous but are especially important in neurons and muscle cells.

Cytokine receptors belong to the third and fourth superfamily of receptors. The third receptor superfamily consists of single-pass transmembrane proteins that are coupled to enzymes. These receptors are single-pass transmembrane proteins. Transmembrane proteins are not to be confused with membrane-anchored proteins, which are simply attached to the cell membrane, usually via a fatty acid or glycosylphosphatidylinositol (GPI). Transmembrane proteins pass entirely through the cell membrane from the exterior surface to the cytoplasm. There are a number of classifications of transmembrane proteins, but the important point is that some transmembrane proteins cross the membrane only once and some cross multiple times. The former proteins, called single-pass transmembrane proteins, are divided into types I and II, which differ from each other in whether the amino terminus is on the exterior side and the carboxyl terminus on the interior (type I) or the reverse (type II). The extracellular portion of the receptor either has direct enzymatic activity or is coupled to an enzyme just inside the cell. Either way, binding of ligand activates an enzyme and initiates a series of reactions that eventually affect either DNA transcription or intracellular reactions. The first enzyme activated after receptor-ligand binding is often a kinase that adds a phosphate group to other proteins, usually to tyrosine residues, but

ISBN 978-089189-5886

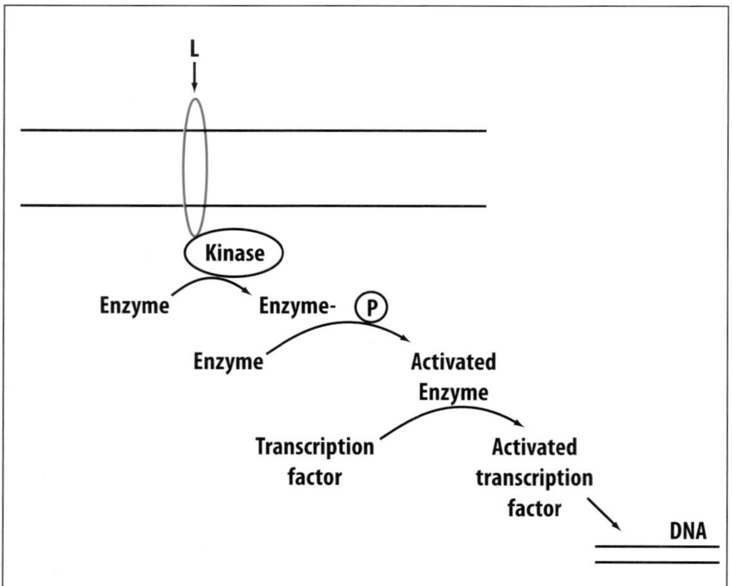

f7.4 An example of a single-path transmembrane receptor. After binding of the ligand (L), the intracellular portion of the receptor activates a kinase, initiating a cascade, often involving sequential phosphorylations, that terminates in the modification of DNA transcription.

sometimes to serine or threonine residues. Phosphorylation activates the next protein in the signaling cascade, and the reactions continue until the endpoint, often the activation of a transcription factor, is reached **f7.4**. Epidermal growth factor receptor, Her2, and the fibroblast growth factor receptors belong to this superfamily. Most toll-like receptors and most cytokine receptors are members of this family, though chemokines, a group of cytokines that cause chemotaxis, work through the fourth superfamily of receptors, G-protein-coupled receptors.

G-protein-coupled receptors are an example of transmembrane proteins that cross multiple times, called multipass transmembrane proteins. In particular, G-protein-coupled receptors are a family within the superfamily of 7-pass transmembrane proteins, serpiginous transmembrane proteins that weave back and forth from the cytoplasm to the extracellular space, crossing the cell membrane 7 times.

G-protein-coupled receptors are the largest family of cell surface receptors in eukaryotes and play an important role in the immune response. In addition, the action of many neurotransmitters, many nonsteroid hormones, and about half of drugs are mediated by G-protein-coupled receptors. While the innate immune response often uses TLRs, the innate response to N-formyl-methionyl peptides (characteristic of bacteria) is mediated by G-protein-coupled receptors. Chemokines—those cytokines that induce chemotaxis—also work through G-protein-coupled receptors.

When a chemokine binds to its receptor, the receptor molecules cluster, bringing their cytoplasmic portions into proximity with each other. This proximity allows additional enzymatic reactions to occur and is critical to the initiation of a cascade of enzymatic reactions (clustering of receptors upon binding of ligand is a common mechanism for cellular responses to extracellular signals).

When stimulated by an external signal, the internal portion of a G-protein-coupled receptor stimulates a G protein (guanine nucleotide-binding protein). G-proteins consist of α, β, and γ subunits. For this reason, they are sometimes called trimeric

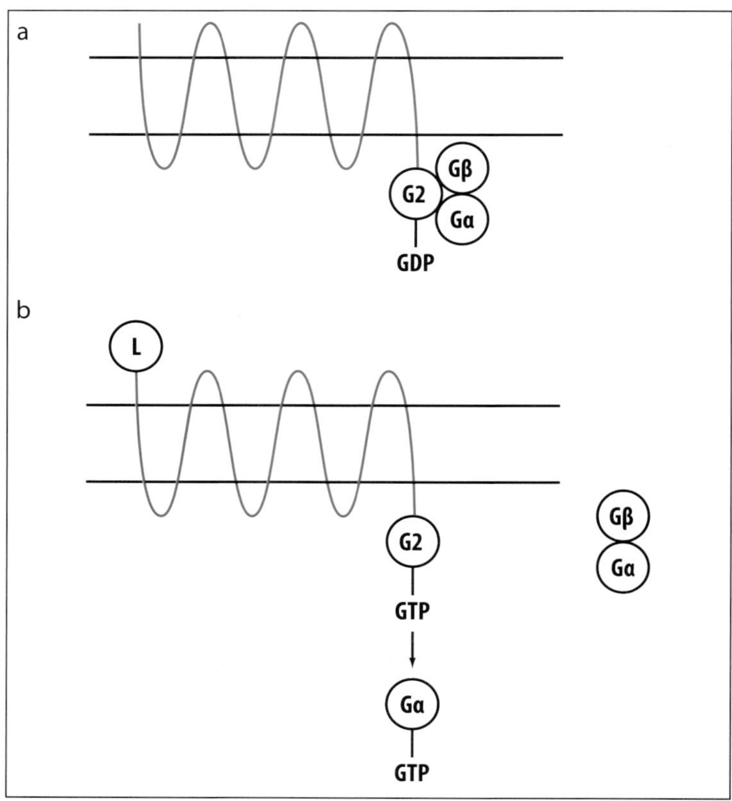

f7.5 **a** A G-protein-coupled receptor. In the inactive state, without bound ligand, the α, β, and γ portions of the G-protein are complexed to each other and to GDP.
b In the active state, with bound ligand, the α subunit of the G-protein has dissociated from the β and γ subunits and has bound GTP rather than GDP.

G-proteins, to differentiate them from the smaller, monomeric G proteins that are of a different family and which do not work through G-protein-coupled receptors. In the resting state, G-proteins form a stable complex in which GDP is bound to the α subunit **f7.5a**. This complex is inactive. When the G-protein-coupled *receptor* is occupied, GTP replaces GDP on the α subunit of the G *protein*. In addition, there is dissociation of the protein, so that the α subunit/GTP is separated from the β/γ subunits of the G-protein **f7.5b**. Both of these components then activate a number of enzymes.

In general, the actions of cytokines ultimately result from modulation of transcription. Some of the more important classes of cytokines are as follows:

- Tumor necrosis factor (TNF)
- Interleukins (ILs)
- The interferons (IFNs)
- Chemokines (cytokines with chemotactic activity)

Occasionally, growth factors such as epidermal growth factor, fibroblast growth factor, transforming growth factor-β, insulin-like growth factor, nerve growth factor, platelet-derived growth factor, hematopoietic colony stimulating factors (CSFs), vascular endothelial growth factor, etc. are considered to be types of cytokines, but others regard them as a separate class of molecular mediators.

Cytokines important for innate immunity include interleukin 1 (IL-1; throughout this chapter IL will indicate an interleukin), IL-6, the interferons, chemokines, and the TNF family (primarily TNF-α). An important function of some of these cytokines is to activate and recruit neutrophils and macrophages to the site of infection, in large part by increasing the expression of endothelial adhesion molecules (primarily integrins). Macrophages are the primary source of many of these cytokines, and they and other cells secrete the chemokine CXCL8 (previously called IL-8), which attracts neutrophils.

Tumor necrosis factor (TNF) is primarily secreted by macrophages and some T lymphocytes and is a major cytokine concerned with innate immunity, particularly with regard to gram-negative organisms. Unless specified otherwise, TNF refers to TNF-α. TNF-β, now more often called lymphotoxin, has considerable homology to TNF-α, binds to the same receptor, and has many of the same actions. The most potent stimulus for tumor necrosis factor is lipopolysaccharide, which is part of the cell wall of gram-negative organisms (also called endotoxin).

There are many receptors for TNF. These receptors are divided into subgroups depending on precisely how the binding of TNF is translated into an intracellular signal [PMID19851428], but all TNF receptors initiate an intracellular signal via coupling proteins. Many of these coupling proteins are members of the TRAF (*t*umor necrosis factor *r*eceptor *a*ssociated *f*actor) family. There are 6 members of the TRAF family, some of which modulate DNA expression by activating the transcription factor NFκB [PMID11607847]. The major action of tumor necrosis factor is to activate phagocytes (neutrophils and monocytes) and bring them to the site of action. To do this, they exert several effects, including increasing the expression of adhesion molecules on endothelial cells, increasing the production of other chemokines, and increasing the expression of both class 1 and class 2 human leukocyte antigen (HLA) molecules, which, as we will see, are critical in adaptive immunity.

TNF, IL-1, and IL-6 act on the hypothalamus to induce the fever that is characteristic of the acute inflammatory response, probably by working through prostaglandins. Before their nature was understood, these 3 cytokines were collectively referred to as endogenous pyrogen. In addition, these 3 cytokines induce the formation of acute phase reactants, which are serum proteins that are greatly increased in concentration during acute inflammation. There are many acute phase reactants, but some prominent examples include the complement proteins and C reactive protein (CRP). CRP is important in the inflammatory response because it acts as an opsonin, and it can also activate complement by the classic pathway. CRP levels are occasionally used in the diagnosis of an acute inflammatory condition, especially as a possible early indicator of coronary artery atherosclerosis, and sequential CRP levels are used to monitor the effectiveness of treatment.

Excessive levels of TNF may be produced in response to severe infection by gram-negative bacteria (specifically to the lipopolysaccharide component). If this happens, TNF may have systemic effects, which is unusual for cytokines. Mild systemic effects of TNF include fever and an increase in acute phase reactants, as discussed above. More severe systemic effects include the following:

1. Suppression of appetite, and to inhibition of the enzyme lipoprotein lipase, which is needed to release fatty acids from circulating lipoproteins so that they can be used by tissues. These effects lead to cachexia.
2. Suppression of myocardial contractility and vascular smooth muscle tone, resulting in hypotension.
3. Metabolic disturbances, such as a fall in blood glucose.
4. Intravascular thrombosis, primarily through a reduction in endothelial cell synthesis of thrombomodulin (a suppressor of thrombosis) and an increase in endothelial synthesis of tissue factor. TNF may also activate neutrophils prematurely, before they leave the vascular space, damaging endothelial cells and further facilitating intravascular thrombosis. These actions also potentially lead to diffuse intravascular coagulation (DIC). The ability of TNF to cause tumor necrosis—the reason for its name—is due to these actions on the vasculature, which deprived tumors of their blood supply in initial studies.

These effects become clinically evident as septic shock. While TNF is the major cytokine implicated in septic shock, other cytokines, such as IL-1 and INF-γ may also contribute, as serum levels of these cytokines are also increased in severe gram-negative infections (the term "cytokine storm" has been used to describe these increased levels). Serum levels of tumor necrosis factor have prognostic value in severe gram-negative bacterial infections. Some use the terminology of systemic inflammatory response syndrome (SIRS). In this terminology, a mild case of SIRS would be manifested by mild fever, leucocytosis, and a rise in acute phase reactants. These patients are commonly seen. But a severe case would have the symptoms of septic shock.

There are 2 drugs that antagonize the action of TNF by binding to it before it can bind to its receptor. These are etanercept (trade names Enbrel or Immunex) and infliximab (trade name Remicade). These drugs are actually soluble TNF receptors that bind TNF before it can bind to the "real" receptors on the cell membrane. Remicaid has been used effectively in rheumatoid arthritis and Crohn disease.

As their name implies, the ILs are cytokines secreted by one type of leukocyte to modulate the action of another. While some ILs, such as IL-1 and IL-6, are active in innate immunity, most are active in adaptive immunity and are therefore considered in that section.

The IFNs can be divided into 2 groups, type I and type II. Type II IFN is synonymous with IFN-γ (γ interferon). It is made by CD8 cytotoxic T cells and a type of activated T-lymphocyte called TH-1 cells, and functions in both innate and adaptive immunity. It activates macrophages by increasing the synthesis of reactive oxygen intermediates and nitric oxide, making them more effective against intracellular microbes. IFN-γ also has a number of actions that are important in adaptive immunity, such as increasing the expression of class I and class II HLA molecules, increasing the expression of costimulator molecules on APCs, and facilitating the switching from IgM to IgG antibodies in B lymphocytes.

In contrast, α and β IFNs (IFN-α and IFN-β) are collectively called type 1 IFNs and function in innate immunity. They are induced by double-stranded RNA, which is characteristic of many viruses, and increase resistance to viral replication by acting through the JAK tyrosine kinase signal transduction pathways to increase the production of proteins that either degrade viral RNA or inhibit viral replication. Type I IFNs also activate NK cells which selectively kill viral infected cells. Type I interferons increase TH-1 cells. Because TH-1 cells are a major

ISBN 978-089189-5886

source of IFN-γ, IFN-α and IFN-β increase the level of IFN-γ. Recently, a third group of interferons, called either type III IFNs or λ IFN, has been recognized, and also has antiviral properties [PMID20624172].

Chemokines are chemotactic cytokines (the name comes from "*chemo*tactic cyto*kines*"). There are 4 classes of chemokines, depending on how many cysteine amino acids there are at the N-terminal region of the peptide (the amino terminus) and how they are positioned. C chemokines have a single cysteine amino acid in their N terminus. CC chemokines have 2 adjacent cysteine residues in the amino terminus. CXC chemokines have 2 cysteine amino acids in the amino terminus, but there is a third amino acid between them. CX3C chemokines have 2 cysteine amino acids in the amino terminus, with 3 interposed amino acids between them.

Chemokine receptors are G-protein-coupled receptors, and are therefore members of the 7-pass transmembrane receptor superfamily. At this writing, there are 10 separate receptors for the CC chemokine family, designated CCR1 through CCR10, and there are 6 known receptors for the CXC family, designated CXCR1 through CXCR6. 2 chemokine receptors, CCR5 and CXCR4, have been found to be a required coreceptor for HIV.

Not all of the cytokines are stimulatory. IL-10 inhibits the production of IL-12 and tumor necrosis factor by activated macrophages. Transforming growth factor-β (TGF-β), a family or 30-40 related proteins, all of which are dimeric, inhibits the proliferation and differentiation of T cells and the activation of macrophages. IL-13 antagonizes IFN-γ and stimulates B cells, favoring adaptive immunity over innate immunity.

In addition, the suppressor of cytokine signaling (SOCS) proteins antagonize cytokines in a variety of ways, ranging from blocking receptors to degrading intermediate signaling proteins. SOCS are not general suppressors of all cytokine function. To understand their function, it is important to note that the actions of many cytokines oppose the actions of other cytokines. By preferentially antagonizing some cytokines, SOCS augment the effects of others by allowing their actions to be unopposed [PMID19755183].

The DNA coding for cytokines is polymorphic (ie, there are multiple alleles for each individual cytokine) and genetic research has characterized mutations that lead to aberrant cytokines that can compromise the immune response.

Growth factors that stimulate hematopoiesis include erythropoietin, stem cell factor (also known as c-Kit ligand), IL-7, IL-9, IL-11, and leukocyte CSFs. The 2 most common leukocyte CSFs are granulocyte CSF (G-CSF) and granulocyte-monocyte CSF (GM-CSF). There is also a monocyte stimulating factor. IL-3 stimulates multiple lines of leukocytes and is also called multi-CSF.

Erythropoietin is a growth factor that facilitates erythroid maturation by decreasing apoptosis of erythroid precursors [PMID15243580]. The erythropoietin receptor engages the intracellular tyrosine kinases of the JAK family. Erythropoietin, G-CSF, and GM-CSF can all be used therapeutically. A marrow sample taken soon after therapy with G-CSF or GM-CSF may have myeloid cells that have not have progressed past the promyelocyte stage and can resemble residual acute myelogenous leukemia, especially if the initial type was M3, acute promyelocytic leukemia. Immunophenotyping may be needed to distinguish between therapy effect and residual leukemia. After treatment with G-CSF or GM-CSF, there may also be morphologic abnormalities of the mature myeloid cells, such as bilobed nuclei and hypergranular cytoplasm, which should not be mistaken for a primary myelodysplasia.

Cell Adhesion Molecules

Cell adhesion molecules are part of the cell membrane and have the capacity to interact with components of other cells or the extracellular matrix. Commonly, one end of the molecule interacts with an extracellular moiety while the other end influences proteins of the cytoskeleton. Some cell adhesion molecules are important in acute inflammation because they permit leukocytes to slow done, adhere to the endothelium, and exit the vascular space.

Families of cell adhesion molecules include the selectins, integrins, the cadherins, and the cell adhesion molecules of the immunoglobulin superfamily. Selectins are expressed largely by endothelial cells and primarily bind leukocytes with weak affinity, causing them to "roll" slowly along the vascular endothelium. IL-1 and TNF-α induce some selectins.

Integrins are a large family of proteins and have a broader scope than the selectins. They are transmembrane proteins that are expressed by many cell types, including leukocytes. Integrins are composed of an α chain and a β chain that are noncovalently linked. The integrins permit phagocytes to bind to endothelial cells with greater affinity, so that they are brought to a complete stop and can pass out of the vascular space and into the tissue space. Integrins also bind to proteins in the extracellular matrix, such as fibronectin. They also function in adaptive immunity by stabilizing contact between of T lymphocytes and APCs, permitting their interaction to be completed.

The cadherins are calcium-dependent transmembrane proteins that bind to other cadherins from other cells. Of the approximately 20 cadherins, the most important are those in epithelial (E-cadherin) and neural cells (N-cadherin; not to be confused with NCAM).

The cell adhesion molecules of the immunoglobulin superfamily include vascular cell adhesion molecule (VCAM), platelet-endothelial cell adhesion molecule (PECAM), neural cell adhesion molecule (NCAM), and the intercellular adhesion molecules (ICAMs). There are several types of ICAMs, expressed by a variety of cells. A common pattern in acute inflammation is that integrins on leukocytes bind to ICAMs on the surface of endothelial cells.

In addition to their role in acute inflammation, cell adhesion molecules may also control the type of junction between adjacent cells. Tight junctions form when transmembrane proteins between adjacent cells bind to each other, sealing the space between cells and preventing any passage between them **f7.6a**. Though many proteins may be involved, the most common proteins in tight junctions are claudins and occludins.

An adherens junction is slightly more porous than a tight junction and consists of intracellular binding of actin microfilaments to cadherins (via a group of proteins called catenins), in conjunction with intercellular binding of cadherinproteins from different cells **f7.6b**.

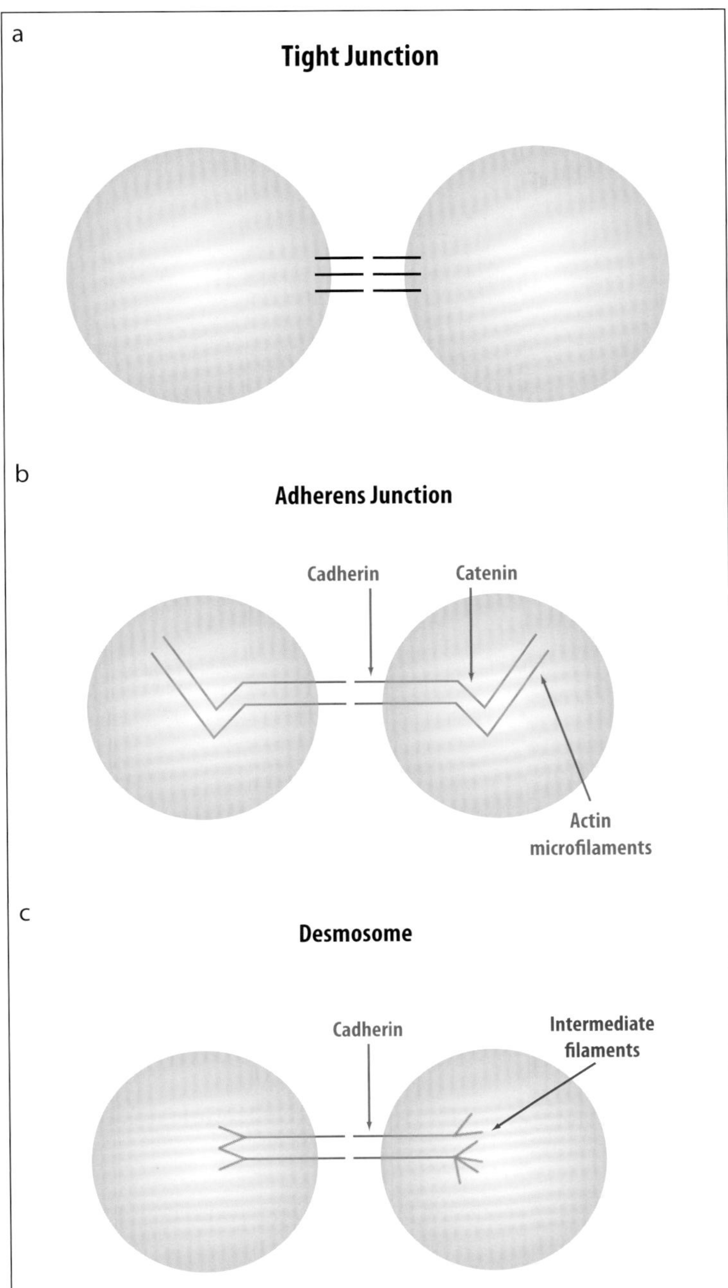

f7.6 a A tight junction forms by the binding of the extracellular portions of transmembrane proteins from two adjacent cells.
b An adherens junction forms from the intercellular binding of cadherin proteins between adjacent cells. Intracellularly, the cadherins bind to actin microfilaments.
c A desmosome forms in the same manner as an adherens junction except that intracellularly, the cadherins are bound to intermediate filaments, not to actin microfilaments.

The intracellular linking of intermediate filaments to cadherins, coupled with intercellular cadherin-cadherin binding (ie, substituting the thicker intermediate filaments for the thinner actin microfilaments) results in a desmosome, a junctional complex typically found in squamous epithelium **f7.6c**. Cadherin binding between adjacent cells underlies both adherens junctions and desmosomes, depending on whether actin microfilaments or intermediate filaments bind to the cadherins intracellularly.

The intracellular linking of intermediate filaments to integrins, in conjunction with linking of the extracellular portion of the integrin molecule to the basement membrane, results in a hemidesmosome, a structure that anchors epithelial cells to basement membranes. Adherens junctions, desmosomes, and hemidesmosomes all result in the anchoring of the cell, either to another cell or to the extracellular matrix.

Gap junctions are a unique form of intercellular junction. They form from small channels in the cell membrane, each of which is composed of 6 connexin proteins in a concentric arrangement. Channels between adjacent cells are juxtaposed and in continuity, permitting ions and small molecules to pass directly between adjacent cells, effectively coupling them into a single metabolic and electrical unit.

A summary of the mediators of the acute inflammatory response is as follows:

- Vasodilatation: prostaglandins, nitric oxide
- Increased vascular permeability: histamine, C3a, C5a, LTC4, LTD4, LTE4, platelet activating factor, bradykinin, prostaglandins
- Neutrophil and macrophage recruitment and chemotaxis: IL-1, IL-6, type 1 TNF, the chemokine CXCL8, the complement byproduct C5a, leukotriene B4, bacterial products, platelet activating factor, N-formyl-methionyl peptides, and the interaction of cell adhesion molecules
- Induction of fever: IL-1, IL-6, and TNF
- Production of pain: prostaglandins and bradykinin
- Tissue damage: products of leukocytes involving killing, such as oxygen metabolites and lysosomal enzymes
- Opsonization: the Fc receptor on antibodies and C3b

This bewildering array of inflammatory mediators serves both to amplify the response, and because their effects are sometimes antagonistic, to regulate it. Such a large number of short lived and locally acting mediators serves to make the acute inflammatory response one of the most effective and well-regulated cellular processes in nature.

There can be numerous outcomes to acute inflammation, including resolution, ulcer formation, abscess formation, cellulitis, and chronic inflammation. Total resolution occurs when the normal architecture of the tissue is restored. This is the most common outcome in minor inflammation, and it occurs when the offending agent is removed without permanent damage to tissue.

An ulcer is a form of acute inflammation that involves the loss of an epithelial covering, such as the skin, the lining of the GI tract, etc. Sometimes, malignant tumors may ulcerate, so malignancy should be excluded whenever there is an ulcer.

Pseudomembranous inflammation is a type of ulcer found on mucous membranes, primarily on the intestinal tract. It is a response to bacterial toxins or ischemia that results in necrosis and shedding of epithelial cells and copious amounts of fibrinosuppurative exudate, resulting in the formation of a covering (pseudomembrane) composed of fibrin, necrotic epithelium, and leukocytes. An example is pseudomembranous enterocolitis, caused by *Clostridium difficile*.

An abscess is a collection of neutrophils in tissue which destroys or displaces normal tissue elements and is well demarcated or "walled off" (in contrast to a cellulitis). Because abscesses are isolated from the vascular system, antibiotics are unlikely to help. Small abscesses may heal by resorption, though this may result in some fibrosis, but large abscesses must often be drained. Acne lesions are small microabscesses of hair follicles.

A cellulitis is a diffuse acute inflammation occurring within solid tissues. In contrast to an abscess, it is not circumscribed or confined and tends to spread through tissue spaces and along fascial planes. Highly invasive bacteria that produce large amounts of hyaluronidases and fibrinolysins, such as the β hemolytic streptococci, are the most common initiators of a cellulitis (the so-called flesh-eating strep). These can be difficult to treat because the inflammatory process may destroy the small blood vessels in the area, compromising the ability of antibiotics to get to the site, and because its poorly circumscribed nature precludes drainage, the common surgical treatment for an abscess.

If the acute inflammatory response is unable to resolve the problem or demarcate it into an abscess, then the inflammation moves into a chronic stage. In general, neutrophils are replaced by macrophages, lymphocytes, and plasma cells. Indeed, neutrophils may secrete a protein that causes other neutrophils to leave the area and is chemotactic for macrophages. In chronic inflammation, adaptive immunity, which we will consider when we examine normal lymph node function, becomes operative, though innate immunity continues. Generally speaking, any process that does not quickly resolve with innate immunity, including acute inflammation, will proceed into chronic inflammation, involving adaptive immunity in the process.

Chronic inflammation can be defined as inflammation of duration greater than a few days, in which the battle against the offending agent proceeds simultaneously with attempts to heal and restore damaged tissue. Chronic inflammation may follow acute inflammation, or it may arise without a well defined acute stage, such as in autoimmune disorders and inflammatory bowel disease (ulcerative colitis and Crohn disease).

Chronic inflammation is generally characterized by fewer neutrophils in the tissue than in acute inflammation, and more mononuclear cells (macrophages, lymphocytes, and plasma cells). However, the differential in the blood is usually unchanged, with neutrophils continuing to predominate (but in some viral infections, the blood differential may be shifted towards lymphocytes from the beginning).

Chronic inflammation also differs from acute inflammation in that there is a simultaneous attempt to repair the damage done by the inflammatory process. Many of the steps in the reparative process are initiated by molecular mediators secreted by macrophages. If the inflammation is severe or prolonged, complete restoration of normal tissue architecture may not be possible, in which case healing may consiss largely of fibrosis.

A granuloma is a focus of chronic inflammation characterized by a peculiar type of activated macrophage, called an epithelioid macrophage because it has more cytoplasm than usual and somewhat resembles an epithelial cell. Epithelioid macrophages are often accompanied by giant cells (formed from the aggregation of individual epithelioid macrophages) and large numbers of lymphocytes, but granulomas are defined by epithelioid macrophages, not by giant cells. The purpose of a granuloma is to isolate an infectious organism, or a foreign substance, that the body is unable to completely eliminate. Thus, a granuloma represents a sort of "stalemate" in the inflammatory battle. With time, the granuloma may become fibrotic, with loss of the epithelioid macrophages, and may calcify.

Classic examples of granulomatous inflammation include tuberculosis, many fungal infections, sarcoidosis (a disease of unknown etiology), and reactions to certain inanimate materials such as silicon and beryllium. There are 3 types of granulomas: noncaseating, caseating, and necrotizing. A noncaseating granuloma does not have any necrosis or acute inflammation. A caseating granuloma has necrosis of the central portion, without significant numbers of neutrophils, while a necrotizing granuloma has central necrosis with neutrophils.

Healing and Repair

Healing is the attempt to expunge any offending material, repair damage, and reconstitute normal structure and function of the tissue. Healing proceeds concurrently with chronic inflammation, but also requires 2 additional components: the extracellular matrix and new blood vessels.

The extracellular matrix consists of proteins and soluble molecules and has 4 major components: collagen, elastin, glycosaminoglycans, and fibronectins.

Collagen

The collagens are a group of proteins involved in the support of tissues and in interactions with cells. There are over 20 different kinds of collagen, but only 4 types are common.

Collagen is the major extracellular protein. The polypeptide chains are made on ribosomes, like any protein. The amino acid proline is hydroxylated, which permits 3 chains to come together and form procollagen. The hydroxylation of proline depends upon ascorbic acid (vitamin C), and this is why vitamin C is necessary to proper wound healing. The procollagen molecule is secreted from the cell. In the extracellular space, a portion of the procollagen molecule is cleaved, and the remainder is crosslinked to form the mature collagen matrix. Like bone, collagen appears at first glance to be an impregnable material, but both bone and collagen can be extensively remodeled by resorption and resynthesis. In fact, the healing process involves active remodeling of collagen.

Many of the molecular mediators of coagulation, inflammation, and repair interact with collagen, so it provides much more than physical support. Collagen also performs a very specific role as the principal component of basement membranes. Basement membranes occur at the interface of epithelial or endothelial cells and the underlying stroma, and are made by the cells that rest on the stroma. These cells secrete a thin layer of type 4 collagen called the basal lamina, which can only be seen with the electron microscope, but the adherence of glycoproteins dramatically increases the thickness of the basal layer to a structure that can be with the light microscope. This thicker structure is called the basement membrane. The function of the basement membrane is attachment of the cells to the underlying stroma, and frequently, the basement membrane assists in filtration (such as in capillaries and the glomerulus).

Elastin

Elastic fibers have the capacity to stretch and then return to their original position. They are composed of a central core, made from the protein elastin, surrounded by microfibrils that are composed of the proteins from the fibrillin family. Mutations in the *FIBRILLIN 1* gene on chromosome 15 cause Marfan syndrome [PMID12082143].

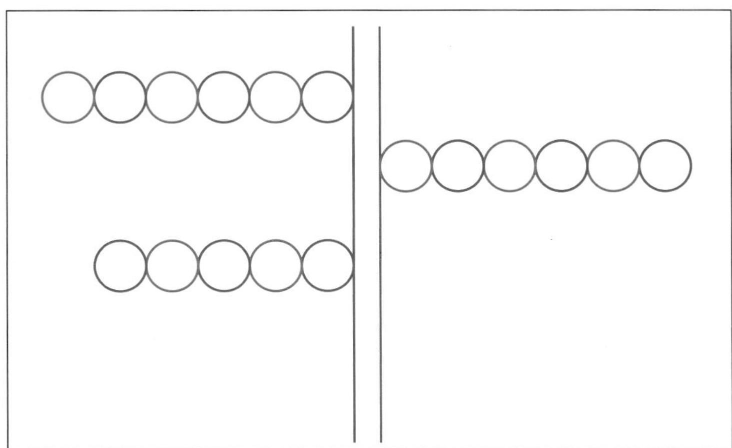

f7.7 A proteoglycan, consisting of a protein core from which extends glycosaminoglycans, each of which consists of alternating disaccharide units.

Glycosaminoglycans (GAGs)

GAGs are long unbranched polysaccharides containing repeating disaccharide units (usually 2 different units that alternate). The GAGs of physiological significance are hyaluronic acid, dermatan sulfate, chondroitin sulfate, heparin, heparan sulfate, and keratan sulfate. These are often tissue specific. For example, chondroitin sulfate is found in cartilage and dermatan sulfate is found in skin. Most GAGs have a combination of high viscosity, structural rigidity, and high oncotic pressure that permits them to function in support and lubrication of tissues. In addition, because they are negatively charged, GAGs exert an influence on the passage of molecules into and out of the healing site. Except for hyaluronic acid, GAGs are linked to core proteins, forming proteoglycans (also called mucopolysaccharides f7.7). In proteoglycans, the sugar moieties can be as much as 95% of the total weight of the molecule. GAGs also bind to collagen and fibronectin and can therefore facilitate wound healing.

Fibronectins

The fibronectins are a family of proteins that bind to GAGs, collagen, fibrinogen, fibrin, and proteoglycans. Because they bind to all of these molecules, as well as to cell membranes, they are important in early crosslinking and help provide temporary structural support. They are also chemotactic for macrophages and fibroblasts, thus helping to facilitate final wound healing. In normal tissue that is not undergoing healing or repair, fibronectin is critical in the attachment of cells to the matrix, largely through binding to integrins. Osteonectin is a related protein found in bone.

If the acute inflammatory process destroys only parenchymal cells and leaves intact a stromal framework, it is likely that there will be complete restoration of the normal tissue, by building on the stromal framework. On the other hand, if the collagenases and elastases of the inflammatory process destroy the stromal framework, then there is no foundation upon which to repair the tissue, fibrosis results, and a scar is likely. The process of fibrosis begins with angiogenesis, the formation of new blood vessels. Then fibroblasts proliferate and migrate into the area. These fibroblasts lay down new extracellular matrix, principally collagen. Finally, there is some remodeling of this fibrous tissue in very much the same way that a broken bone is remodeled during healing.

The phenomenon of angiogenesis is important not only in fibrosis but is also important in certain malignant tumors. There is compelling evidence that no neoplasm can grow to an appreciable size or metastasize unless it induces the formation of new blood vessels within it [PMID20563532]. Every malignant neoplasm is now thought to secrete molecular factors that facilitate the formation of new blood vessels. Macrophages secrete angiogenesis factors, cytokines that induce the proliferation and activation of fibroblasts, and collagenases and elastases that participate in the remodeling of connective tissue.

The fibrotic tissue becomes more collagenous and less cellular with time. It also becomes less vascular with time. In the early stages, very little actual collagen is deposited. The damaged area is filled with young fibroblasts that have not yet secreted much collagen, and also contains acute and chronic inflammatory cells and new blood vessels. This very early scar tissue is sometimes called granulation tissue. With the passage of a few weeks, the fibroblasts will secrete abundant extracellular collagen, the inflammatory cells will dissipate, and the blood vessels will become rare, so that the process eventuates in a thick collagenous scar which contains very few cells and very few blood vessels. This process, for the most part, is initiated and guided by secretory products of macrophages.

Sequence of Events in Wound Healing

1. The cavity fills with blood. This blood clots and adheres to the tissue—largely through fibronectin—providing some minimal closure and support.
2. Epidermal cells adjacent to the wound undergo mitosis. The trigger for this mitosis is apparently loss of contact with other epithelial cells, as most dividing cells cease to divide when they contact cells like themselves (contact inhibition).
3. There is migration of epithelial cells across the wound to provide a very thin covering to the wound. The breakdown products of the injured cells attract white blood cells, fibroblasts, myofibroblasts (cells with properties of both fibroblasts and muscle cells), and stimulate the proliferation of endothelial cells
4. Phagocytic cells, in conjunction with the plasmin system, begin to break down and remove the clot. Fibroblasts and myofibroblasts lay down new extracellular matrix. Vascularity increases. Histologic examination of the healing wound at this time demonstrates large numbers of fibroblasts, large numbers of inflammatory cells, large numbers of capillaries, but little collagen. This is granulation tissue, the hallmark of early wound healing.
5. As epithelial continuity is restored on the surface of the wound, the new epithelial cells lay down a basement membrane between themselves and the stroma. The interior of the wound becomes less cellular as fibroblasts and myofibroblasts secrete abundant amounts of extracellular matrix (principally collagen). The number of inflammatory cells diminishes, as does the vascularity. The healing wound becomes much more collagenous, and greatly increases in tensile strength. There is remodeling of the collagen and usually a change in the type of collagen (from type 3 to type 1). A number of growth factors come into play, including epidermal growth factor and fibroblast growth factor.

ISBN 978-089189-5886

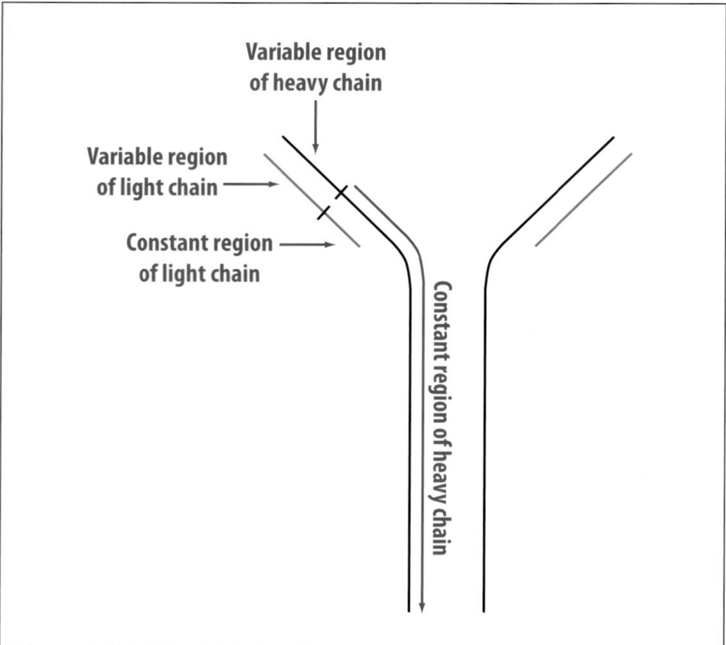

f7.8 The basic structure of an antibody molecule. 2 heavy chains in a "Y" configuration face each other. The apical portions of these heavy chains are loosely bound to light chains. Both the heavy and light chains consist primarily of constant regions, but have variable regions near the apices.

For a noninfected wound, the ends of which are in contact, healing will be the least complicated, with little or no scar formation. This is often called primary union, or healing by first intention. An example of this is a surgical incision. Secondary union, or healing by second intention, occurs in situations where the gap to be bridged is larger. The large gap is bridged by a large amount of granulation tissue. Although more scar tissue is laid down than in primary union, the amount of scar tissue that is finally required will be less than one might think because of the phenomenon of wound contraction, brought about by myofibroblasts. Because of wound contraction, large defects may, over a period of weeks, be reduced to appreciably less than half their original size. The resulting scar will be smaller than expected, but still larger than in primary healing. In addition to the size of the injury, infection and ischemia are major clinical causes of prolonged or poor wound healing.

Adaptive Immunity and Normal Lymph Node Function

Now that we have examined innate immunity, including the acute inflammatory response, we will look at adaptive immunity, normal lymph node function, and the role of the HLA system in the immune response, after which we will be ready to examine lymph node pathology. If innate immunity is unable to resolve the problem, it elicits the more specific, but slower adaptive immunity. Whereas some form of innate immunity is found in invertebrates (indeed, the restriction enzymes found in bacteria are a form of innate immunity), for all practical purposes, adaptive immunity is unique to vertebrates. Adaptive immunity consists of humoral (antibody mediated) and cell-mediated immunity, both of which depend on lymphocytes.

B-lymphocytes make antibodies, each of which consists of a combination of heavy chains and light chains. For IgG, the antibody molecule consists of 2 heavy chains and 2 light chains and has a "Y" structure, with the 2 heavy chains spanning the entire length of the "Y" and the 2 light chains spanning only the upper portion f7.8. Within these molecules, there is an antigen binding site at each of the 2 "tips," where a light chain and a heavy chain face each other, because these are the variable regions that can recognize different antigens. The base of the "Y," consisting entirely of 2 heavy chains, forms the Fc portion, which does not recognize antigen, but is vital in other immune functions. All antibody molecules have this same basic structure, but IgA is usually a dimer of the basic unit, especially if it is in its secretory form (sIgA), which is made in the gastrointestinal tract and secreted into the lumen, and IgM is usually a pentamer.

The word antigen is short for "antibody generator." The specific region of the antigen that elicits the response and to which the antibody binds is called the epitope. Affinity refers to the binding force of 1 antibody to 1 epitope of 1 antigen. When an antigen has multiple identical epitopes, each "tip" of the Y-shaped structure of the antibody can bind 1 epitope. This means that IgG, IgD, and IgE antibodies can each bind 2 epitopes, IgA can bind as many as 4, and IgM antibodies can bind up to 10 epitopes.

Although the binding force to each individual epitope is unchanged, the antibody as a whole—particularly if it is an IgM—can bind to the antigen with greater force than is obtained from the binding to 1 epitope. The overall binding capacity of an antibody to the antigen as a whole is called avidity and will be as strong or stronger than its affinity to a single epitope.

Adaptive immunity involves the maturation of B and T lymphocytes, followed by their activation and interaction. These activities are largely controlled by ILs. IL-2 is the principal inducer of the proliferation and differentiation of T cells. IL-2 is predominantly produced by CD4 helper T lymphocytes after they have recognized an antigen, and it has multiple actions, chief of which is to increase the proliferation of other CD4 cells. In effect, IL-2 is a growth factor for T lymphocytes that have already been antigen stimulated. IL-2 also increases the production of other cytokines, such as IFN-γ.

IL-2 works through the IL-2 receptor, which is composed of 3 transmembrane proteins (α, β, and γ) that are noncovalently linked. The α and β chains bind extracellular IL-2, while signal transduction occurs via the β and γ chains. The γ chain of the IL-2 receptor is also found in a number of other interleukin receptors, such as those for IL-4, IL-7, IL-9 and IL-15, and is sometimes called the common γ chain. The β chain interacts with the tyrosine kinase JAK1, while the γ chain interacts with JAK3. Phosphorylation through the JAKs ultimately leads to increased transcription of cyclin D, which regulates entry into the cell cycle, thus inducing cell proliferation. Most cases of severe combined immunodeficiency (SCID) are X-linked and are caused by defects in this shared γ chain.

Adaptive immunity—both cellular and humoral—is entirely dependent on antigen presentation. Unlike innate immunity, adaptive immunity is not capable of responding to offending organisms in their native state. There must be some breakdown and processing of the organism before adaptive immunity can begin. This breakdown and processing is one of the reasons that adaptive immunity is more specific than innate immunity. It also furnishes the critical connection between innate and adaptive immunity because innate immunity presents antigens to cells that trigger the adaptive immune response, and it does so in conjunction with molecules of the Human Leukocyte Antigen system, to which we now turn.

The Human Leukocyte Antigen (HLA) System

The HLA system is an incredibly complex collection of well over 2,500 alleles on over 200 genes on the short arm of chromosome 6 (6p). This huge complex is itself a subdivision of an even larger collection of related genes, the immunoglobulin superfamily. The HLA system is critical in the adaptive immune response because it participates in the presentation of antigens to lymphocytes. Proper presentation of antigens, and thus proper lymphocyte response, is impossible without the HLA system.

The "major histocompatibility complex" (MHC) is a general term applied to a large collection of alleles that all mammals have. Most workers in the field consider the HLA system to be the human counterpart to the MHC system in other animals, but a few use the term a little differently. The HLA system consists of 3 major regions or classes. HLA class 1 molecules are expressed all the time on virtually all nucleated cells. Only very rare cell types, such as mature red blood cells, do not have these molecules. On the other hand, HLA class 2 molecules are much more restricted in their expression. They are found only on some cells of the immune system, including B lymphocytes, macrophages, and dendritic cells (which we will discuss later), collectively known as professional antigen presenting cells (APCs). The class 2 HLA genes were formerly called the immune response (Ir) genes. All cells that have class 2 HLA antigens also have class 1 antigens.

Classes I and II encode for membrane proteins that are important in antigen presentation to cells of the immune system. The HLA class III genes encode for genes that are important in the immune response, but not in antigen presentation, and they are secreted rather than bound to cell membranes (examples include some complement proteins). Some workers, therefore, restrict the term "HLA" to those genes of the human MHC that encode for membrane proteins important in antigen presentation (ie, they do not consider HLA class III genes to be a true part of the HLA system). Whatever the preferred nomenclature, it is the class I and II genes that are primarily of concern in organ transplantation and we will focus on these genes. This work will use the term "HLA" rather than "MHC."

The HLA class I genes are found primarily on 3 loci—A, B, and C—on chromosome 6. There are several other minor class 1 loci, such as the E, F, and G genes. Class II genes are primarily found on 3 loci—HLA-DR, HLA-DP, and HLA-DQ—with a smaller contribution from DM and DO. All protein products of the HLA class I and II genes are glycoproteins that consist of 2 chains, an α and a β chain, which are noncovalently joined. All class I proteins have the same β chain—β2 microglobulin, a small protein encoded by a gene on chromosome 15. In class I proteins, only the α chain is a transmembrane protein. β2 microglobulin is entirely exterior. In addition to the intra-membranous and cytoplasmic portions, the α chain of HLA class I proteins has 3 extracellular domains. The

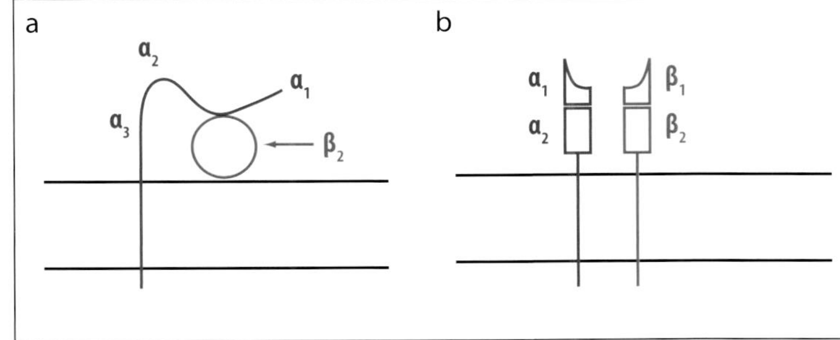

f7.9 **a** A class I HLA molecule with a single transmembrane α chain, consisting of 3 extracellular domains, complexed to β-2 microglobulin. Note the U-shaped configuration created by the folding of the α chain.
b A class II HLA molecule, consisting of an α chain and a β chain, both of which are transmembrane and both of which have 2 extracellular domains. Note the U-shaped space created by the juxtaposition of the 2 terminal extracellular domains of the 2 proteins.

extracellular portion of the α chain of HLA class I proteins loops around and forms a U-shaped structure that binds the antigen that the cell will present to lymphocytes **f7.9a**.

In the case of class II proteins, the α and β chains are both encoded on chromosome 6p and are approximately equal in size. Both chains are transmembrane molecules, and both chains have 2 extracellular domains. The tips of the α and β chains form a U-shaped indentation where they face each other **f7.9b**. This is where the antigens that the cell will present to lymphocytes are bound. In both class I and class II proteins, the similarity to the double-chain structure of antibody molecules reflects a common origin within the immunoglobulin superfamily.

HLA loci have 2 important properties. First, they demonstrate enormous polymorphism (a polymorphism is a genetic variant that is found in 1% or more of the population and therefore, often considered a variant of normal). Second, they are codominantly expressed (ie, a protein product is made from both alleles). In class I alleles, the polymorphism stems from the α chain, since the β chain is constant (β2 microglobulin). In class II alleles, the polymorphism is primarily a function of the β chain, as the α chain has much less variation. Because of the enormous polymorphism at each of the many HLA loci, the cumulative polymorphism at this region of chromosome 6 within the human species is colossal, even though each individual has only 2 alleles at each focus. A haplotype (short for "haploid genotype") is a set of alleles on a single chromosome that tend to be inherited together. In the current context, a haplotype is the set of all HLA genes on 1 chromosome.

As part of their central role in adaptive immunity, HLA molecules are critical in transplantation, and the system was first understood by transplant biologists. HLA antigens were originally identified serologically by testing for the protein products of the HLA genes. Antiserum specific for a particular HLA antigen was mixed with the cells to be tested, after which complement was added. Cell death implied the presence of the particular HLA antigen because there must have been an antigen-antibody reaction for complement to have been activated and to have destroyed the cell. Nomenclature for the protein antigens identified in this manner simply listed the HLA locus and a number indicating the antigen variant, such as HLA-A32 or HLA-DR8, etc. This worked reasonably well for the class I gene products, but less well for class II proteins.

A set of cell culture methods, based on the principle that a mismatch of class II proteins would elicit an immunological reaction, was then developed for better classification of class II antigens. This aided greatly in the identification of class II proteins and permitted HLA typing to become practical in some cases of solid organ transplantation. However, identification was still not good enough for effective bone marrow transplantation, which had to await DNA work.

Initial DNA work greatly expanded the number of known HLA alleles and indicated that in many cases, what had been thought to be a single HLA protein could be the product of 2 or more separate alleles, differing by only a few nucleotides, with the antigens differing by only 1 or 2 amino acids. For example, DNA work done on HLA alleles has shown that there are some 31 slightly different forms of the HLA-A24 gene. The nomenclature was modified to reflect this increased understanding.

In testing for HLA alleles, the gene for the β chain of the class I molecules need not be tested for since it is always the same (β2-microglobulin). In class I molecules, only the α chain, or the proteins it codes for, are tested. In class II molecules, because there is much more polymorphism in the alleles for β chains than in those for α chains, typically only the β chain alleles are examined.

In addressing the nomenclature of HLA alleles, we must first realize that naming can occur at 3 levels: there is a general name for the gene, a name for the specific allele, and a name for the protein product of the allele. We must also realize that with the increasing characterization at the DNA level, newer alleles may not have a serological description or fit well into existing serological groups.

The nomenclature for an HLA allele begins with the locus, followed by asterisk, followed by the allele family, and finally followed by the specific allele (the variant of the allele based on the time of its discovery). For example, HLA-B*2712 refers to the B locus (one of the class I loci), allele family 27, and the 12th specific variant of that allele. In this example, DNA methods have identified a 12th allele in the HLA-B27 family. Allele families were often initially defined serologically and have since been expanded by DNA methods. For example, a zero is used before the family name if the designation is for 1 of the first 9 families of a locus (eg, HLA-A*05 refers to the fifth family of alleles in the HLA-A locus). Likewise, if less than 10 allelic variants are described, the specific allele will start with a zero (ie, if only 9 variants have been described in HLA-A*24 family, the ninth variant is denoted as HLA-A*2409), so there were always at least 4 digits to the right of the asterisk [PMID15935895].

One occasionally encounters additional digits at the end, referring to nucleic acid variations that do not result in amino acid changes (silent mutations). For example, HLA-A*241203 is the third described variation of the 12th allele whose amino acid sequence is unchanged relative to 2 previously described variants of the 12th allele. If there had been a change in the amino acid sequence, it would be a new allele, such as HLA-A*2413.

The letter or letters before the asterisk denotes the locus, such as the A, B, C, or DR. In any notation of a class I HLA gene, it is understood that only the α chain is described, while any notation of a class II HLA gene, such as DR, DP, or DQ, is very likely to be followed by a "B," indicating testing for β chain, resulting in DRB, DPB, or DQB. HLA-DRA*XXYY would be a description of an allele YY in the XX family that codes for the α chain of the DR locus. In practice, since the α chain has little current clinical utility in class II alleles, an allele description beginning with HLA-DRA would be unusual.

HLA-DRB*1115 refers to the B gene (ie, encoding for the β chain) of the DR locus, 11th allele family, and the 15th described variant of that family (in actuality, this is more likely to be written as HLA-DRB1*1115, because the β chain of the DR locus contains 5 gene families, of which the first, B1, is the most common and is present in all individuals, while the others are present only in certain haplotypes, and the designation is likely to indicate the first gene family of the β chain of the DR locus to the left of the asterisk).

In 2010, HLA nomenclature was modified slightly, as has been described by Marsh et al [PMID20356336]. The huge and growing number of HLA alleles led to the decision to use a colon (:) to separate the different parts of an allele's name. There may be a moment of confusion as to whether HLA-A*2409 denotes the 9th variant of the 24th family, or perhaps the 409th variant of the second family, or perhaps the 9th variant of the 240th family. In the 2010 nomenclature, this possible confusion is avoided by using the designation HLA-A*24:09. In HLA-A*241203, there may be a brief period of uncertainty as to whether this is the third silent variation of the 12th allele in the 24th family, or perhaps the 203rd allele in the 241st family. In the 2010 nomenclature, this would be designated as HLAA*24:12:03. The 2010 nomenclature stipulates that there must be at least 2 numbers preceding and following colons (eg, one should not write HLAA*24:12:3).

In the 2010 nomenclature, the numbers between the colons are called fields. The first field, between the asterisk and the first colon, is the allele family. The second field is the specific allele in that family. The third field denotes an allele with a synonymous (ie, coding for the same amino acid) substitution. A fourth field indicates a difference in a noncoding region of the DNA. A suffix may be used at the end to denote some information about the protein product. For example, the suffix N (for null) indicates that there is no known protein product. The suffix L indicates low levels of expression, the suffix S indicates that the protein is secreted, while the suffix C indicates that the protein is cytoplasmic. Thankfully, there are computer programs that will assist in the conversion from the older nomenclature to the newer.

While the 2010 nomenclature modification is helpful, we are still left with a combination of traditional serological/cell culture methods and DNA typing methods. Depending on the choice of methods and the degree to which they are employed, HLA typing is considered to be low, medium, or high resolution. Low-resolution typing is more or less equivalent to the traditional purely serological methods, targeted at the protein products and often leaving considerable ambiguity with regard to the precise allele at a given locus. In the above example, a result for low-resolution testing of the HLAA*2412 allele might simply render a result of A2.

An example of low-resolution testing for anti-HLA antibodies is panel reactive antibody screening (also called percent reactive antibody, and abbreviated PRA). The PRA test is a serological test that checks for preformed antibodies to HLA antigens and is performed by mixing the patient's serum with a panel of donor lymphocytes. The PRA score represents the percentage of people to whom the potential recipient has formed anti-HLA antibodies, and is expressed as a percentage from 0 to 99. A high PRA score suggests a higher probability of rejection. PRA is performed in any patient who is awaiting a renal transplant to assess the odds of rejection. In addition, PRA may be used in the workup of any possible reaction to HLA antigens in other clinical situations.

High-resolution typing relies primarily on DNA work. Early DNA work used restriction fragment length polymorphism (RFLP), which relied on restriction endonucleases to cut DNA. Depending on where the precise cutting point was, HLA typing by RFLP generated only marginal improvement over purely serological methods. Later DNA work, based on techniques we will encounter in Chapter 45, such as polymerase chain reaction, sequence-specific primers, and sequence-specific oligonucleotide probes, is often able to pinpoint the precise variant of an allele. Medium resolution provides partial resolution. An example of a medium-resolution report might be HLAA*2401/2402/2403, meaning that the actual variant of allele 24 is one of several possibilities.

Transplantation testing for solid organs can be reasonably effective with low-resolution testing and, in fact, did well before the advent of DNA HLA testing. On the other hand, bone marrow transplantation requires more precise matching and higher resolution testing. For most transplants, and certainly for bone marrow transplants, HLA loci A, B, and DR are of prime importance [PMID16790851], and currently, the National Marrow Donor Program focuses on these 3 loci. Because each of these loci has 2 alleles, there are a total of 6 alleles. The National Marrow Donor Program currently requires that 5 of the 6 alleles be matched (this means the α chains of HLA A and B and the β chain of HLA DR). For this reason, it is critical to detect heterozygosity in testing.

There is a general trend toward exclusively high resolution typing by DNA techniques, not only because of its greater precision, but also because DNA is stable and one no longer needs to worry about the viability of the cells or the preservation of protein antigens. However, DNA techniques are not perfect or foolproof. One area in which DNA identification of HLA antigens has proven imperfect is in dealing with the massive polymorphism of these alleles. Many of these polymorphisms are only a few nucleotides in length and are shared among different variants of an allele. As a hypothetical example, if HLAA*2412 differs from HLAA*2413 by 6 base pairs, 4 of those 6 base pair differences may also be found in HLAA*2414. Even with DNA techniques, it may be impossible to differentiate these alleles. One approach to this problem is sequential testing, in which an initial test may narrow down a locus to within a few possible alleles, after which a second round of testing targeted at those alleles may reveal the precise identity.

Another difficulty in HLA testing by DNA methods is pseudogenes. Pseudogenes are DNA sequences that nearly match the normal sequence, but are nonfunctional because of a slight error, such as a premature stop codon, a flawed promoter, or an erroneous base pair at a critical position. Because the base pair sequence of a pseudogene is so close to that of the normal gene, even meticulous DNA work may indicate what appears to be a well-identified, functional allele, when in fact, there is no functional protein product from that gene. In these situations, we are ironically better served by the old serological testing for protein products of the genes, which will reveal the absence of a protein.

Once direct DNA sequencing becomes the rule, as it surely will, these problems will be eliminated, but even here, the sequencing will have to annotated, meaning that we will need to understand "punctuation," such as start and stop codons, intron/exon boundaries, and an understanding the function of the genes and their products. Such complete and annotated sequencing is currently prohibitive from a time and labor standpoint, though in many cases, a definitive identification can be made by sequencing only a portion of an allele.

A final point on HLA testing before we investigate its applications in immunology is that because of the great degree of polymorphism in these genes and the fact that many new alleles are being discovered, there are databases that can help keep track of what is known and how that knowledge is changing. One such database can be found at www.ebi.ac.uk/imgt/hla.

Synthesis of the B Cell Antigen Receptor—Immunoglobulin Gene Rearrangement

We begin our discussion of the maturation of B and T lymphocytes with a consideration of an amazing process that is nearly unique to lymphoid tissue—the breaking and rearrangement of DNA.

Not so long ago, it was thought that at least 50% of the genome must be reserved for immunoglobulin and T-cell receptor synthesis, because this was felt to be the only way that such an enormous diversity of antigen recognition could be achieved, and that so many different proteins could be made. We now know that this is not the case. Rather, the DNA involved in the synthesis of these proteins is actually cut and pieces of DNA from different locations are used to assemble these unique antigen receptor proteins very much the same way that letters are combined to make words. The phenomenon by which antibodies (both circulating and on the B cell surface for use as a receptor) and the T-cell receptor are created is called gene rearrangement. Gene rearrangement is not completely specific for lymphoid cells and may be seen in some cases of AML and myelodysplastic syndromes, but lymphocytes are the only cells that do this to any significant extent, and they only do it for antibodies and proteins involved in antigen recognition.

Both the heavy and light immunoglobulin genes undergo rearrangement, but only the variable regions of each are rearranged at the DNA level in the initial production of an IgM molecule. The constant region will be modified at the RNA level. The heavy chain locus contains about 45 variable gene segments (V), about 23 diversity gene segments (D), 6 joining gene segments (J), and about 9 constant region gene segments (C; 1 for each class and subtype of antibody, such as IgG1, IgG2, etc.). These segments are arranged on the

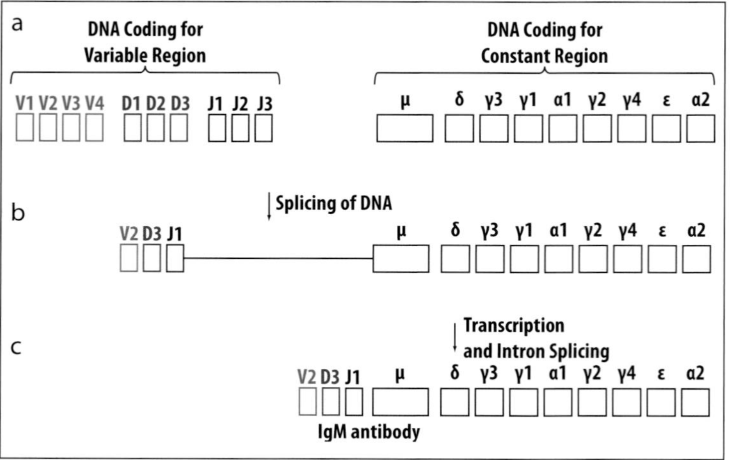

f7.10 **a** The germline configuration of the DNA for the heavy chain of an immunoglobulin molecule. On the left, there are many variable (V), diversity (D), and joining (J) regions. On the right is the DNA coding for the constant region.
b After splicing of the DNA, one variable region, one diversity region, and one joining region come together and are joined to the still-unmodified DNA of the constant region. Light chains are rearranged in the same manner except that they do not have diversity regions.
c After transcription and intron splicing, the RNA for the selected variable, diversity and joining regions remains attached to the RNA for the constant region. Only the μ, and perhaps some of the δ region, will be translated, resulting in an IgM antibody, perhaps with some co-expression of IgD. The B cell has not yet been stimulated.

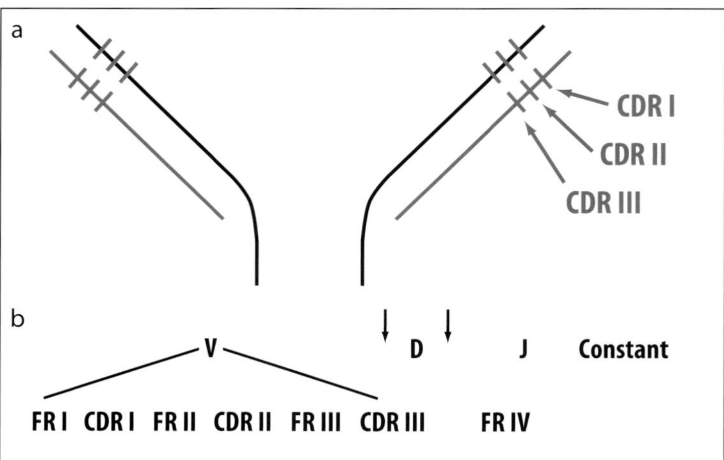

f7.11 **a** The complementarity determining regions (CDRs) of an antibody molecule. There are 3 such regions in the variable region of each light chain and each heavy chain.
b CDR3 is situated primarily inside the diversity region and is therefore subjected to gene rearrangement on both sides. In addition, the arrows indicate the site of action of the enzyme terminal deoxynucleotidyl transferase (TdT), further increasing the diversity of CDR3.

chromosome in the order (left to right) of variable, diversity, joining, and constant **f7.10a**.

The one constant region gene segment that is operative will code for more amino acids than all of the V, D, and J regions combined, but antigen specificity comes from the small amount of DNA that undergoes rearrangement. The κ and λ genes have a similar structure, except that they do not have any diversity regions. The κ light chain contains only one constant region, while the λ light chain contains 4 constant regions. It is now understood that immunoglobulin gene rearrangement in B cells and T-cell receptor gene rearrangement in T cells are completely antigen independent and occur before any antigen exposure. The synthesis of both chains in the T-cell receptor, and of both the heavy chain and light chains in immunoglobulin molecules, demonstrates a phenomenon called allelic exclusion (or monoallelic expression), wherein only 1 strand of DNA is used (normally, both chains of DNA are used in transcribing a protein, unless there is an autosomal recessive gene). In immunoglobulin synthesis, heavy chain rearrangement begins with 1 D segment joining with 1 J segment, after which a V segment is added, forming a VDJ sequence. This rearranged VDJ DNA, which will form the variable region of the heavy chain, is attached to the entire constant region DNA, which has not yet been modified **f7.10b**.

The rearranged VDJ segments form one exon that encodes for the variable region of the heavy chain. The constant region has not yet been modified and consists of multiple exons. In the constant region, the μ portion of the constant region is the closest to the rearranged VDJ DNA. After transcription, intron regions of the DNA between the J segment and the μ portion of the constant region are spliced from the RNA. Because translation stops after the RNA of one constant region exon is translated, an IgM molecule is made **f7.10c**. In actuality, a small amount of the δ heavy chain exon is translated in many young B cells, resulting in expression of both IgM and IgD, the only exception to the rule that individual B cells make antibodies of only one type. All antibodies begin as IgM because the μ gene of the constant region is closest to the variable region that was generated by DNA splicing. Later, after antigen stimulation, antibodies of other classes can be made (this is called class switching and will be discussed momentarily).

Both immunoglobulin and TCR gene rearrangement are mediated by a stretch of noncoding DNA called a recombination signal sequence (RSS). An RSS contains a sequence, consisting of either 12 or 23 base pairs, that is attached to the ends of the V, D, and J segments. The key concept in RSS is that an RSS with a 12 base pair spacer can only join to an RSS with a 23 base pair spacer. This is called the 12/23 rule, and it prevents direct joining of a V to a J region, as both of these have 23 base pair spacers. On the other hand, the D region between the V and the J regions is flanked by a 12 base pair region on both its ends and can therefore join to both a V region and a J region.

Immunoglobulin gene rearrangement is carried out by a complex of enzymes called the V(D)J recombinases. Some components of this complex are found in other cells, but the primary components are unique to lymphocytes and are called recombination activating proteins 1 and 2, the products of recombination activating genes 1 and 2 (RAG-1 and RAG-2).

Both the immunoglobulin genes and the T-cell receptor genes may undergo additional diversification by the addition or deletion of single nucleotides at the V-D junctions or the D-J junctions after recombination by the action of the enzyme terminal deoxynucleotidyl transferase (TdT). TdT adds or subtracts nucleotides without a template. The action of TdT causes small changes in the variable region and therefore results in groups of related clones, not in markedly different B cells. Roughly, gene rearrangement result in about 10^6 different possible combinations of DNA sequences, and TdT adds another 10^6, so that the total number of DNA constructs is about 10^{11}-10^{12}.

The rearranged DNA sequence in both the light and heavy chains contains hypervariable regions called complementarity determining regions (CDRs). There are 6 CDRs in each arm, 3 in the heavy chain and 3 in the light chain. The regions between the CDRs are called framework regions (FRs) and have less diversity than the CDRs. CDR3 is particularly diverse because it occurs at the junction of the V-D-J region where both gene rearrangement and TdT are active **f7.11a** and **f7.11b**.

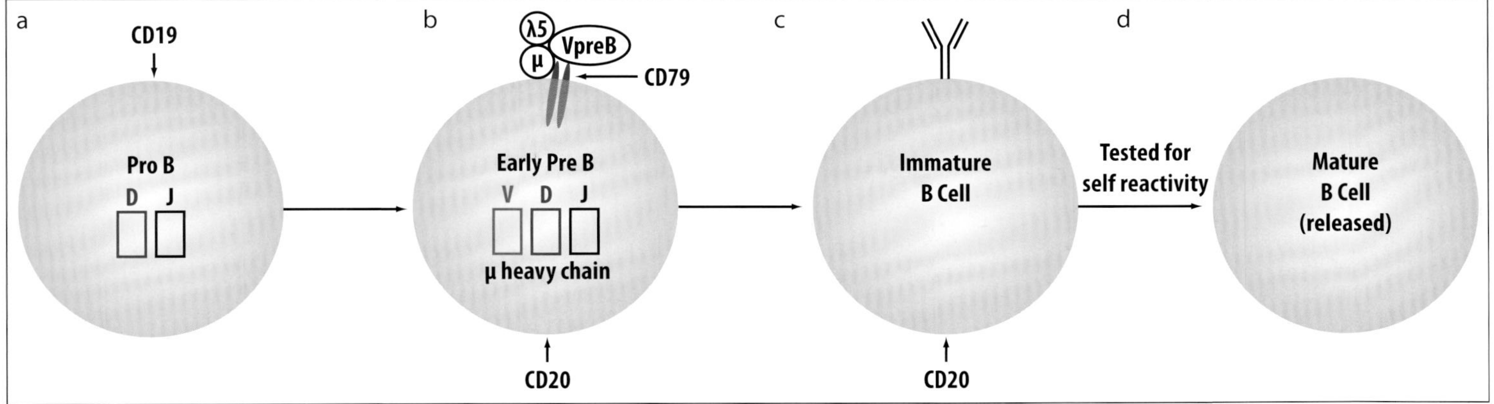

f7.12 Maturation of B cells.
a The pro-B cell, has rearranged the diversity and joining region and may express CD19.
b The pre-B cell as rearranged the variable, diversity, and joining regions, expresses CD20, and expresses the pre-B-cell receptor, which consists of a μ heavy chain and the protein λ5, VpreB, and CD79.
c The immature B cell expresses a fully formed immunoglobulin molecule on the surface and is tested for self-reactivity. If it passes, it is released from the thymus into the periphery for further maturation.
d The released cell, still not yet antigenically stimulated, is called a mature B cell.

Light chains are generated by the same process, except there are no D regions. Again, a variable portion is made by splicing DNA, resulting in a VJ region separated from a C κ or λ region by intronic DNA, which is removed from the RNA transcript. As is the case for the initial heavy chain, the constant region does not participate in splicing at the DNA level. Light chain synthesis is attempted first on one of the κ chains. If the light chain V-J rearrangement is not productive (ie, an out of frame rearrangement occurs), another such rearrangement is attempted on the other κ light chain gene. If both of these are nonproductive, the process starts over on the λ light chain gene. Neither λ chain is attempted unless there has been failure of both κ chains. This accounts for the 2:1 ratio of κ to λ light chains. If the attempt on the first λ chain is unsuccessful, the other λ gene is employed. If all 4 attempts at light chain rearrangement fail, the cell dies in the bone marrow. If one of these attempts is successful, the enzyme TdT adds and subtracts nucleotides, as it does with heavy chain synthesis.

Unlike the T-cell receptor, immunoglobulins can be either membrane-bound or free. This distinction is accomplished by the differential splicing of the heavy chain RNA. In a molecule that is destined to be membrane-bound, the portion of RNA, which, if translated, would confer secretory properties, is spliced out. If the molecule is destined to be a free antibody, the portion of RNA, which, if translated, would permit attachment to the cell membrane, is spliced out [PMID6771019, PMID6771020].

Maturation of B Lymphocytes

During fetal development, B lymphocytes mature in the liver, and after birth, in the bone marrow. The earliest bone marrow cell that is committed to become a B lymphocyte is called a pro-B-cell. These do not produce immunoglobulin, although D-J immunoglobulin gene rearrangement of the heavy chain has been detected, and these cells have TdT. Pro-B cell also express some proteins that identify them as early B cells, such as CD19 **f7.12a** and occasionally (though not always) CD10. CD19 is a very early B marker [PMID19798033], even earlier than CD79, but is also found in some cases of acute myeloid leukemia.

The next stage is the pre-B cell. V-D-J rearrangement occurs and this is the first stage at which a detectable immunoglobulin heavy chain—μ heavy chain—can be found. The pre-B cell expresses μ heavy chains primarily in the cytoplasm but also on the cell surface. Light chains are not made yet, and the μ heavy chains are expressed in conjunction with 2 chains, λ5 and VpreB, that function as substitutes for light chains. This is also the stage during which the 2 important molecules Igα (CD79a) and Igβ (CD79b), members of the immunoglobulin superfamily which we will discuss in a moment, appear. This complex of proteins— μ heavy chain, λ5, VpreB, Igα, and Igβ—forms the pre-B-cell receptor **f7.12b**.

The pre-B cell is also the first stage that consistently expresses CD20. Immature B cells are capable of light chain rearrangement and therefore of placing a fully formed immunoglobulin molecule (an IgM) on the cell surface by replacing λ5 and VpreB with rearranged light chains **f7.12b**.

Immature B cells are tested for reactivity to self-antigens, and if they pass this test (ie, do not react with self-antigens), they are released into the periphery to undergo further maturation in the periphery, usually in lymph nodes or the spleen **f7.12d**. Any B lymphocyte precursor that is found in the bone marrow, such as the pro-B lymphocyte, the pre-B lymphocyte and early stages of the immature B cell, can be lumped together under the term "lymphoblast."

After the immature stage is reached, alternative splicing of heterogeneous RNA will permit the synthesis of δ heavy chains and the attachment of IgD immunoglobulin molecules on the cell surface, at which time the cell coexpresses both IgM and IgD and is called a mature B cell (the terms "mature" and "naïve" are used generally synonymously in B-cell development and refer to a B cell that is able to receive and respond to antigenic stimulation, but has not yet done so).

The stimulation of pro-B and pre-B cells is driven by antigen-independent stimuli, such as IL-7. The maturation and survival of immature B cells is dependent on a successful challenge (non-reactive) to self-antigen. On the other hand, the stimulation and maturation of mature B cells are dependent on foreign antigen stimulation and interaction with T cells. This stimulation results in an activated B lymphocyte. Because activation of a mature B cell requires T cell assistance, we will pause and review the maturation and activation of T cells, after which we will examine the interaction of these 2 types of lymphocytes, once they have both matured.

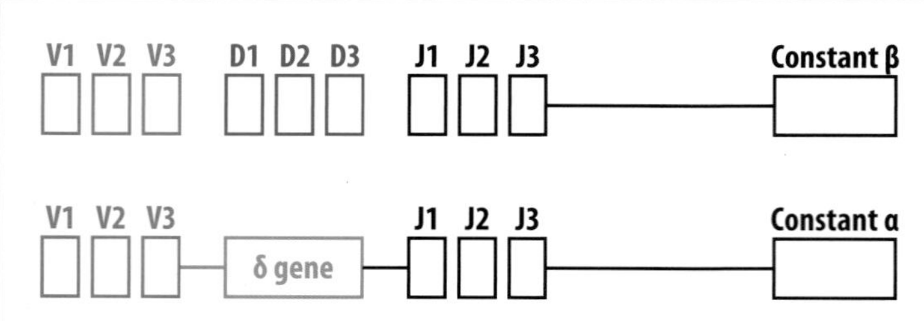

f7.13 The α and β chains of the T-cell receptor are rearranged in a very similar manner to the immunoglobulin chain. The α chain lacks diversity regions, but contains the entirety of the δ gene. Gene rearrangement of the α chain generally deletes the entire δ region.

T-cell Receptor Gene Rearrangement

The T-cell receptor (TCR) undergoes gene rearrangement in a manner that is very similar to that used for immunoglobulin gene rearrangement, using the same enzymes, but the process is simpler. The reason for the greater simplicity in TCR gene rearrangement is that the product of immunoglobulin gene rearrangements—antibody molecules—must function both in antigen recognition and as the effector molecules that are responsible for the B cell's actions. Consequently, profound diversity is required to both recognize and respond to the myriad antigens that might be encountered. In contrast, the TCR functions only in antigen recognition. Effector functions in T cells result from the secretion of cytokines rather than antibodies.

There are 2 types of TCRs, the α-β and the γ-δ. α-β receptors are much more prevalent. γ-δ TCRs are rare, largely found in epithelial locations, and are of unclear function. The β and δ genes consist of V, D, J, and C regions, as do immunoglobulin heavy chains, but the α and γ genes consist of V, J, and C regions, without D regions. Interestingly, the δ gene is entirely contained within the α gene f7.13.

The α and β chains each have 3 hypervariable, complementarity-determining regions, and the same principles apply in DNA rearrangement in the synthesis of the α-β receptor as for the immunoglobulin receptor in B cells. There are again recombination signal sequences (RSS) and recombination activating genes 1 and 2 (RAG-1 and RAG-2) are active in the rearrangement of the TCR, as they are in the rearrangement of immunoglobulin molecules.

Because the δ gene is located entirely within the α gene, between the variable and joining regions, V-J rearrangement of the α gene will completely delete the δ gene. Like the α and β chains, the γ and δ chains form from DNA rearrangement, but the number of variable segments is much less, so the diversity that is finally achieved with the γ-δ receptor is less than with the α-β receptor. This is important in assessing clonality of γ-δ lymphoid proliferations, as this limited diversity may give the impression that there is clonality when there actually is not.

Maturation of T Lymphocytes

T lymphocytes develop in the thymus gland, though the stem cell precursors arise in the fetal liver. In adults, precursors may arise in the bone marrow. Young T cells in the thymus are called thymocytes (a thymocyte is an immature T cell in the thymus, but a thymoma is an epithelial neoplasm). As the T cell matures in the thymus, it migrates from the cortex to the medulla.

The first stage of the T cell in the thymus is called the pro-T cell. This cell does not express any part of the TCR, nor does it express any of the proteins that are associated with the TCR, including CD4 and CD8. Because neither CD4 nor CD8 is expressed, pro-T cells are also called double negative thymocytes f7.14a.

The next stage in the development of the much more common α-β T cell is the pre-T cell, which is characterized by rearrangement of the β chain gene. The pre-T cell expresses the β chain of the TCR, and also 2 proteins that are associated with the receptor, CD3 and the ζ protein f7.14b.

This is followed by expression of the α chain of the TCR and the expression of both CD4 and CD8. Because both CD4 and CD8 are expressed, the young T cell at this stage is sometimes called a double-positive thymocyte f7.14c. In addition, the full TCR complex is now synthesized. Up to this stage, development has taken place in the thymic cortex.

There are 2 final stages of T-cell development in the thymus. One of these is the generation of a single positive (also called immature) thymocyte, which expresses either CD4 or CD8 f7.14d. Selection for CD4 or CD8 occurs in the medulla of the thymus.

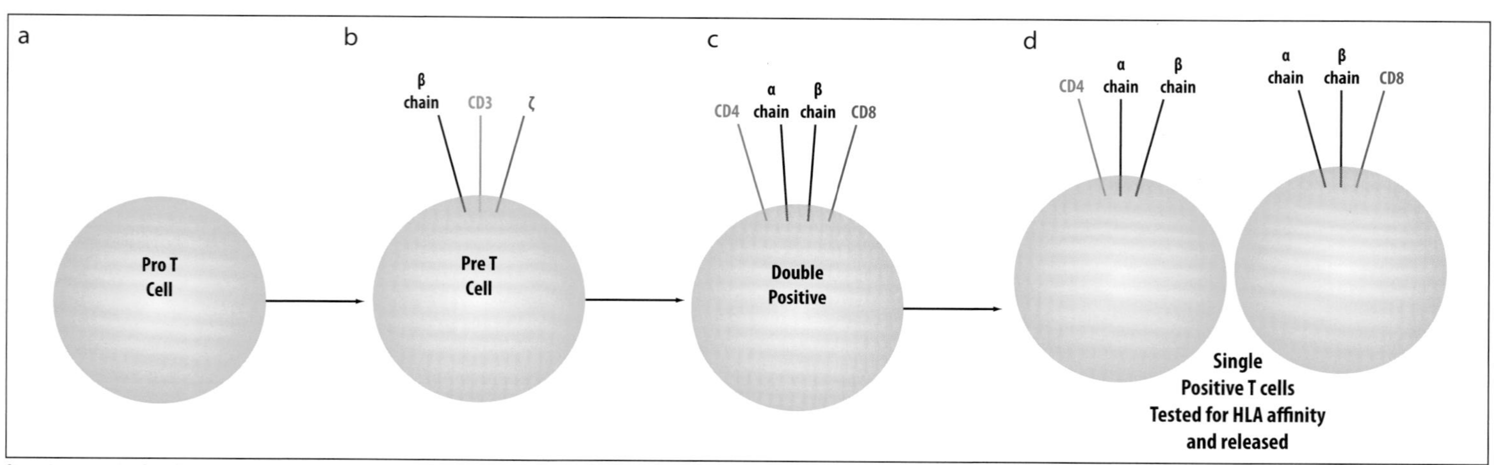

f7.14 Maturation of T cells (thymocytes).
a The pro-T cell is a double-negative thymocyte because it does not express either CD4 or CD8.
b The pre-T cell expresses the β chain of the T-cell receptor, along with CD3 and the ζ protein. These proteins, along with pre-Tα, constitute the pre-T-cell receptor.
c The double-positive stage of thymocyte development expresses a complete α and β chain as well as both CD4 and CD8.
d The single-positive stage of development expresses either CD4 or CD8.

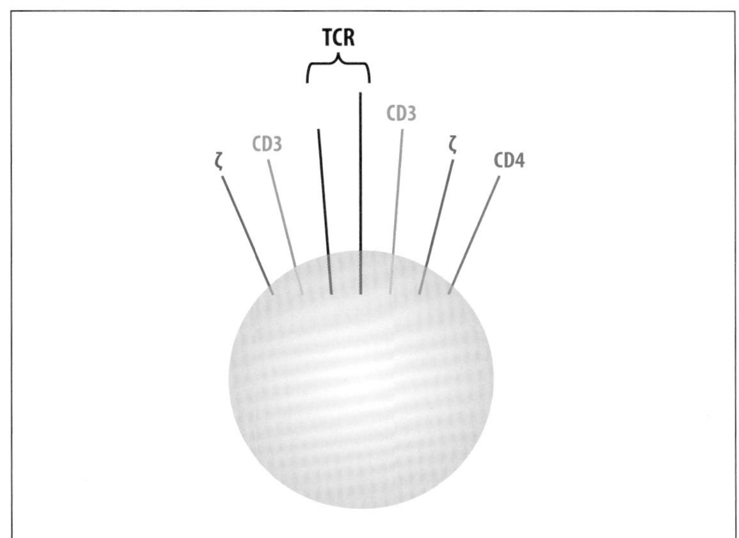

f7.15 The T-cell receptor complex consisting of the α and β chains of the T-cell receptor (TCR), 2 CD3 molecules, 2 ζ chains, and a CD4 or CD8 molecule.

The other final act of maturation is called thymic selection, in which young T cells that do not have exactly the right interaction with HLA molecules die. Thymic selection, which begins in the cortex and is completed in the medulla, consists of 2 phases. In the first phase, there is positive selection, in which only those T cells that have an affinity with HLA molecules (with which they will have to interact) survive. In the second phase, negative selection (also called central tolerance), those T cells whose affinity for HLA molecules is too high (such that an autoimmune reaction is likely) will not survive.

The essence of central tolerance is that those immature lymphocytes—B or T—that recognize self-antigens with high affinity are killed. This illustrates the general principle in development that much of the precision of the final product comes from the selective killing of certain cells. The end result is that in a finely tuned process, young T cells that recognize self peptide-HLA antigens with low affinity survive, but those that recognize self peptide-HLA antigens with high affinity are destroyed.

The mature (also called naïve) T cell emerging from the thymus not only has a receptor, but it also has 2 associated proteins, CD3 and 2 ζ chains. The combination of the TCR, CD3, and the ζ chains is called the TCR complex. The TCR *complex* consists of the following **f7.15**:

1. The α and β chains of the TCR itself. These chains are similar in structure to an antibody molecule, with a constant and a variable region. The constant regions of these chains are anchored in the cell membrane, and the variable regions protrude into the extracellular space. Because the ends of the α and β chains of the TCR are variable, like the Fab portion on an antibody molecule, each TCR recognizes a specific complex of antigens. However, unlike an antibody molecule, a TCR does not recognize or react to antigen by itself. The antigen must be presented in conjunction with HLA molecules.
2. 2 ζ chains, which are primarily intramembranous and cytoplasmic. These are situated between the α and β chains of the TCR.
3. 2 CD3 molecules, one on each side of the α and β chains of the TCR, which have extracellular, membranous, and cytoplasmic domains.
4. The CD4 or CD8 molecule that is characteristic of the mature T cell and which recognizes class II or class I HLA antigens, respectively.

The α and β chains of the TCR, CD3, CD4, and CD8 are all members of the immunoglobulin superfamily, the giant collection of structurally related molecules that are constantly encountered in the study of the immune response.

The very rare TCR that is composed of a γ chain and a δ chain function very much like those composed of α and β chains. They also have a variable region, undergo gene rearrangement, and generate a response in conjunction with CD3 and the ζ protein. Unlike TCR of the α-β type, those of the enigmatic γ-δ type are not generally associated with CD4 or CD8, and unlike TCRs of the α-β type, they do not recognize HLA-associated antigens.

NK cells also develop in the thymus, probably from the same multipotent progenitor cell as the T lymphocyte, but after the early lymphocyte progenitor developmental stage, T cells and NK cells diverge into separate developmental pathways. As we will see, NK cells are part of innate immunity and have a very specific function. They do not express a TCR

Activation of T Cells

Naïve T cells usually complete their maturation in lymph nodes or in the spleen. T cell must be brought to a stop as they circulate so that chemotaxis can bring them to the specific site where their maturation is completed. T cells express adhesion molecules, just as phagocytes do, and migration of a T cell into lymph nodes is governed by these molecules, as is the case for other types of leukocytes. Selectins and integrins work together to slow down the desired circulating cell, bring it to a stop, and cause it to adhere to the endothelium. T cells express a selectin called L-selectin (CD62L) and an integrin called α 4 β 7 (α4β7). The former adhesion molecule appears more important in homing T cells to lymph nodes, while α4β7 seems critical in causing T cells to come to rest in extranodal sites, such as the gastrointestinal tract [PMID8674147].

In addition, naïve T cells also express the chemokine receptor CCR7 (the CC chemokine family has 10 separate receptors, numbered CCR1 through CCR10), which binds to binds to the chemokines CCL19 and CCL21 that are present on endothelial cells and stromal cells in T zone areas of lymph nodes. These bindings facilitate the expression of the integrin LFA-1 on T cells, which interacts with intercellular adhesion molecule 1 (ICAM-1; also called CD54) on endothelial cells in lymph nodes. Once a naïve T cell is activated, it becomes either an effector T cell or a memory T cell. Memory T cells maintain the same pattern of adhesion molecules as naïve T cells and continue to home in on lymphoid tissue, but effector T cells turn off these adhesion molecules and switch to a new set that enables them to enter other tissues.

T lymphocytes cannot respond to antigens by themselves, but require that antigens be broken down and portions of them be presented to them by APCs. These APCs include macrophages, B cells, and dendritic cells. There are several types of dendritic cells. One of these, called a *follicular* dendritic cell, stimulates

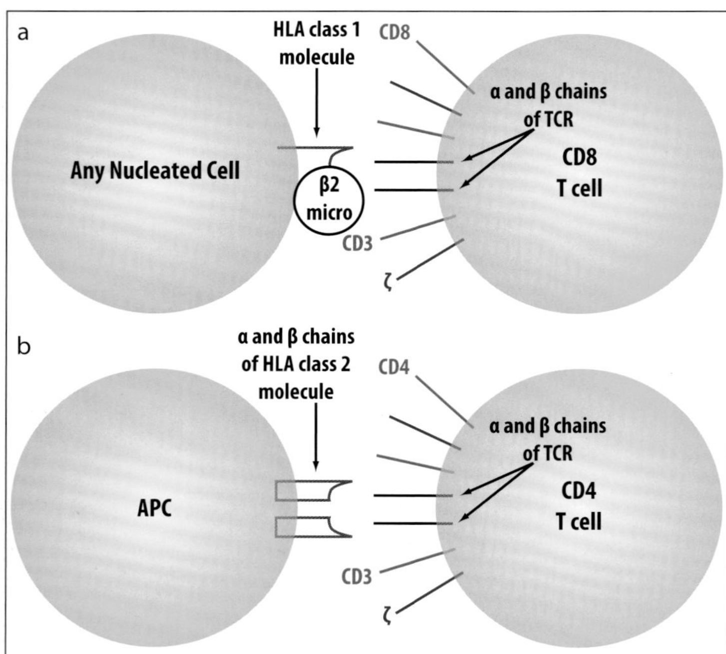

f7.16 a The receptor complex of a CD8 T cell interacts with HLA class 1 molecules on any nucleated cell. **b** The receptor complex of a CD4 T cell interacts with an HLA class 2 molecule on an antigen presenting cell (APC).

B cells in lymph nodes and is discussed later. The 2 types of dendritic cells that act as APC to T cells are called *conventional and plasmacytoid* dendritic cells. Plasmacytoid dendritic cells are rare cells found in the blood and respond primarily to viruses. Upon stimulation, they migrate to lymph nodes and secrete large amount of type 1 (ie, α and β) interferons. We will not further consider plasmacytoid dendritic cells.

Conventional dendritic cells are important in antigen presentation to naïve CD4 helper T cells. They are derived from bone marrow and express class 2 HLA proteins. The most important conventional dendritic cell is the immature dendritic cell. Immature dendritic cells are found in sites that make "first contact" with the environment, such as the skin and the gastrointestinal and respiratory tracts. For example, Langerhans cells in the skin are phagocytic and present antigens in association with class 2 HLA molecules.

After internalizing foreign antigens, immature dendritic cells migrate to regional nodes, where they mature, break down the antigens, and display fragments from them on their surface in conjunction with class 2 HLA molecules. The mature dendritic cell comes to rest in the T cell areas of lymph nodes where it displays antigen in conjunction with class II HLA molecules and activates naïve T cells in the node. In the node, the mature dendritic cell may also be called an interdigitating dendritic cell because its processes intermingle with T cells and to distinguish it from the follicular dendritic cell, which is not an APC.

The other 2 types of APCs are found primarily in lymph nodes rather than in the periphery. The macrophage is found predominantly in the sinuses of the node and the B lymphocyte is found in lymph node follicles. All of these APCs work in conjunction with HLA molecules. HLA class 1 molecules are expressed all the time on virtually all cells that have a nucleus, while HLA class 2 molecules are restricted to APCs, such as B-lymphocytes, macrophages, and conventional dendritic cells. CD4 helper T cells recognize and respond to the bound complex of the antigen and class 2 HLA molecules on the surface of APCs **f7.16a**. CD8 cytotoxic T cells recognize the combination of bound peptide and class 1 HLA molecules **f7.16b**.

Each APC has hundreds or thousands of HLA antigens on its surface, some of which will be coupled to an antigen that the cell is presenting and some of which will not be. These HLA antigens are genetically fixed and of limited variability in one individual since there is a maximum of 2 alleles per locus, but individual HLA molecules may present different antigens, so there may be dozens of different HLA-antigen complexes on the surface of an APC. Consider for a moment the surface of a macrophage. As an APC, it has class 2 HLA molecules on its surface, but as a nucleated cell, it also has class 1 HLA molecules. Over the course of its lifetime, it has encountered and phagocytized many different cells. Proteins from each of these encounters will be displayed on its surface in association with both HLA class 1 and class 2 molecules. An individual T cell can react to only one combination of HLA molecule and antigen, and because there are many such combinations on the surface of the macrophage, it can stimulate many different T cells. Even after a T cell is committed to particular type, such as CD8 or CD4, and is therefore restricted in the HLA class that it recognizes, it still may or may not react with a given APC since that cell will express both HLA class 1-antigen complexes and HLA class 2-antigen complexes. A lymphocyte needs only 1 occurrence of the HLA-antigen combination that it seeks, and will ignore all other HLA-antigen combinations on the APC.

CD4 class 2 restricted T cells recognize peptides that derive mainly from extracellular proteins, such as those produced by microbes. These proteins are ingested by APCs via endocytic vesicles, which are then acidified to activate proteases that fragment the antigens. The endocytic vesicles then fuse with vesicles containing HLA class 2 proteins. The antigen fragments are bound between the α and β chains of the HLA proteins, after which they are transported to and presented on the exterior surface of cell.

The pathway of antigen presentation is somewhat different for CD8 cytotoxic T lymphocytes. Although the antigens that stimulate CD8 cells may derive from extracellular fluid, as is the case for CD4 helper T lymphocytes, more commonly they derive from the cytosol of any nucleated cell that is infected by a pathogen. These antigens are broken down by the proteasome, an organelle that is concerned with the breakdown and recycling of intracellular proteins that are no longer needed. Proteasomes break down proteins that have been tagged for destruction by having multiple small protein molecules called ubiquitin attached to them. Ubiquitin is a small protein (76 amino acids) that is attached to senescent proteins by ubiquitin ligase. The attachment of multiple ubiquitin molecules to a protein directs it to the proteasome for degradation.

Interferons, especially IFN-γ, stimulate genes that modify the proteasome, producing an immunoproteasome. The immunoproteasome breaks down proteins in a different way from the normal proteasome, one that allows the fragments to be taken up and displayed by cells of the immune system. Antigens derived from the immunoproteasome are transported to the endoplasmic reticulum by 2 proteins called transporters associated with antigen processing (TAP1 and TAP2; members of a family called ATP-binding cassette [ABC]). In the endoplasmic reticulum, these peptides are attached to proteins of HLA class 1. The

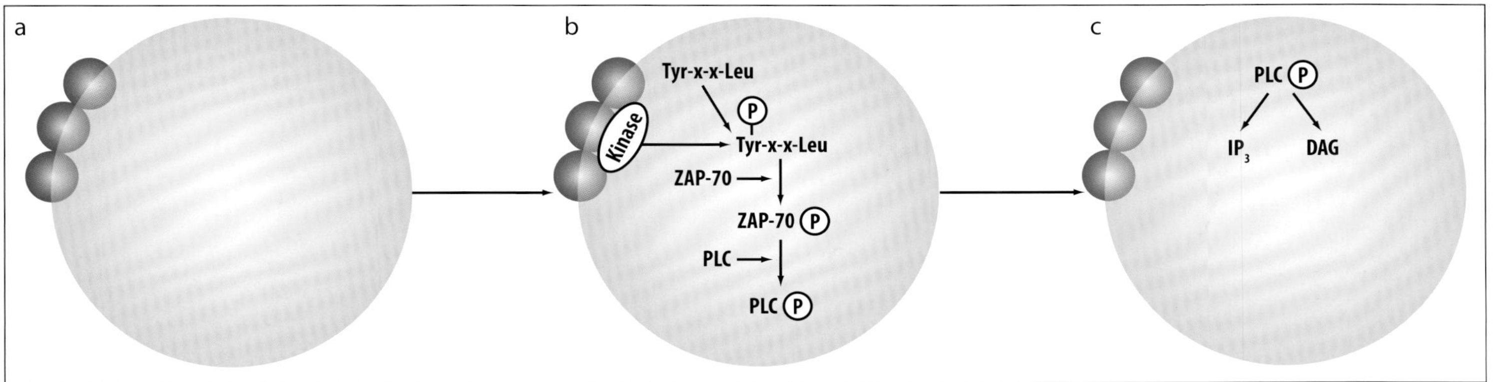

f7.17 After interaction with another cell, a clustering of the T-cell receptor complex leads to activation of an intracellular kinase that b initiates a chain of phosphorylations eventuating in the phosphorylation and activation of phospholipase C (PLC). c Activated PLC then cleaves phosphatidylinositol bisphosphate (PIP_2) from the cell membrane into inositol triphosphate (IP_3) and diacylglycerol (DAG).

complex then leaves the endoplasmic reticulum and is transported to the cell membrane, where they are displayed on the surface of the cell. The antigen that has been processed by the immunoproteasome is held between the loops in the α chain of the class 1 HLA molecule, since the small β chain (β-2 microglobulin) cannot effectively participate in the grasping of an antigen. This complex of antigen and HLA class 1 molecules is then recognized by CD8 lymphocytes. The end result is that intracellular proteins that are made by microbes (for example, from a virus which has integrated its DNA into that of the host cell) trigger a response from CD8 cytotoxic T cells, often resulting in eradication of the entire cell.

The fact that CD4 helper T cells recognize the restricted class 2 HLA antigens while CD8 cytotoxic T cells recognize the ubiquitous class 1 HLA antigens is very important. CD4 helper T lymphocytes work in conjunction with other cells of the immune system and therefore need to communicate only with these cells. That is why they respond only to class 2 HLA molecules, whose expression is restricted to cells of the immune system. On the other hand, CD8 cytotoxic T lymphocytes have a somewhat different function. Their job is to destroy any cell expressing foreign antigens in its cytoplasm. They must therefore be able to interact with and destroy *any* cell, even if it is not part of the immune system. This is why they interact with the more generalized class 1 HLA molecules, whose expression is universal. CD4 helper T lymphocytes respond to individual proteins of foreign origin, while CD8 cytotoxic T lymphocytes respond to whole cells that have been infected. The effect of this is that adaptive immunity can result in 2 very different outcomes—either CD4 T cell interaction with HLA class 2 antigens on APCs, eventuating in an antibody response from B cells or CD8 interaction with HLA class 1 antigens on APCs, eventuating in cellular destruction.

Cells of the immune system often touch each other during an immune response and form connections similar to neural synapses. These connections are sometimes called an immunological synapse. After binding antigen and stimulatory molecules on the APC, the TCR complex sets in motion the biochemical reaction to that lead to the T-cell response after stimulation.

Lymphocyte activation follows the general principles of signal transduction, and to understand these, we must briefly review the structure of the cell (or plasma) membrane. The cell membrane consists of a lipid bilayer composed of complex lipids (often phospholipids) that have polar, hydrophilic heads and nonpolar, hydrophobic chains. The polar heads are oriented outwards, towards either the interior or exterior (both of which are aqueous), while the hydrocarbon tails are oriented towards the interior of the bilayer. The lipid bilayer contains many proteins, some of which are transmembrane, spanning it entirely, some of which protrude only from one side, and some of which are completely embedded within the bilayer. Some proteins can diffuse within the cell membrane. Lipid bilayer cell membranes have 2 beautiful properties. First, they are intrinsically impermeable to water and ions, a must for the homeostasis of the cell, but second, the proteins in them can form selective channels for the passage of ions, another must for life. The combination and interaction of these properties allows for exquisite control of the cell interior.

The cell membrane contains minute areas called lipid rafts, which are regions in which protein diffusion is particularly prominent and which function in transport and signaling. The molecules in lipid rafts are reorganized in response to stimuli, and this reorganization allows them to participate in further reactions [PMID11739628].

The cytoplasmic portions of the ζ chains and the CD3 chains on T lymphocytes both contain immunoreceptor tyrosine-based activation motif (ITAM). Each ITAM contains 2 copies of a motif that is composed of tyrosine-X-X-leucine (where X is another amino acid). After the TCR complex binds its target antigen, in association with CD4 or CD8 and an HLA antigen coreceptor, lipid rafts permit clustering of the receptor complex. As is typical for signal transduction, clustering of the receptor complex initiates downstream reactions that bring about the ultimate effect.

The less adventurous need only remember that the end result of T lymphocyte activation is that antigen binding initiates a phosphorylation cascade that, in part due to release of calcium, activates 3 transcription factors—NFAT, the NFκB family, and activator protein 1 (AP-1), but for the bolder, the following 4 paragraphs provide some details.

Clustering of the TCR complex activates the CD4-associated kinase Lck and kinases associated with the TCR complex itself, such as Fyn. These kinases then phosphorylate tyrosine residues on ITAM moieties. This sets in motion a cascade of events, beginning with the phosphorylation of the tyrosine kinase ZAP-70 (ζ-associated protein 70). Through intermediate molecules, ZAP-70 leads to the phosphorylation of phospholipase C (PLC), a family of enzymes that cleave phospholipids. Phosphorylated PLC then cleaves phosphatidylinositol bisphosphate (PIP2), found in the cell membrane, into inositol triphosphate (IP3) and diacylglycerol (DAG) f7.17.

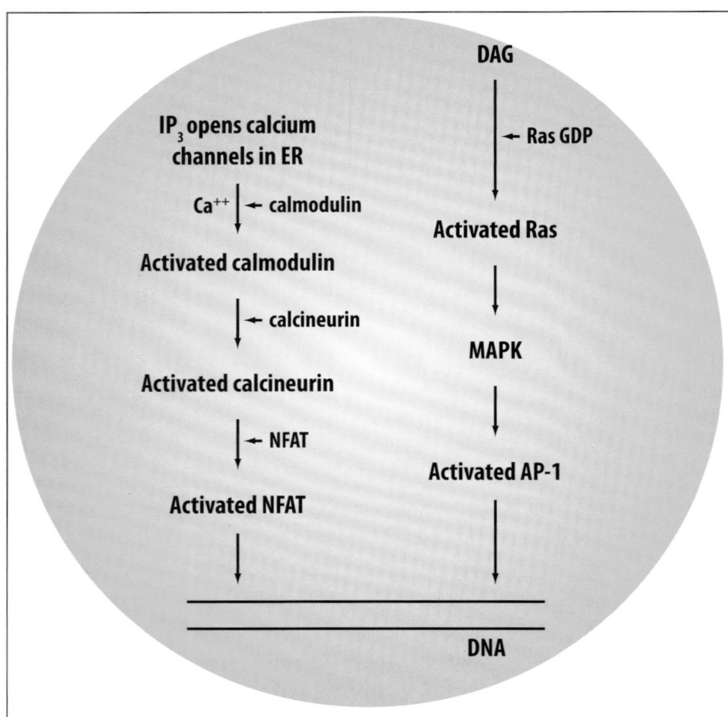

f7.18 IP_3 opens calcium channels in the endoplasmic reticulum (ER) to initiate a sequence, involving calmodulin and calcineurin, that ultimately activates the transcription factor NFAT (image A). DAG stays in the membranes and initiates a sequence of events, involving Ras and mitogen activated protein kinases (MAPK) that activates the transcription factor AP-1 (image B).

We will consider IP3 first. IP3 moves from the cell membrane, into the cytoplasm and to the endoplasmic reticulum, where intracellular calcium is stored. IP3 opens calcium channels, causing entry of calcium into the cytoplasm. In large part, lymphocyte activation involves the entry of calcium into the cytoplasm. Calcium binds to the protein calmodulin, changing its conformation so that it can bind to and activate the enzyme calcineurin. Calcineurin then dephosphorylates nuclear activator of activated T cells (NFAT), a transcription factor that then enters the nucleus **f7.18**. The antirejection drugs cyclosporine and tacrolimus that are used in organ and bone marrow transplantation inhibit the enzyme calcineurin, so that NFAT is never dephosphorylated and therefore cannot enter the nucleus and modulate transcription.

DAG, the other product obtained from the cleavage of phosphatidylinositol bisphosphate, stays in the cell membrane, but diffuses within it. DAG recruits additional signaling molecules. One of these is the protein RasGDP, which activates the protein ras by binding it to GTP instead of GDP. Ras is a G-protein, but it is a monomeric G protein rather than a trimeric G-protein; monomeric G-proteins are similar to the α subunit of trimeric G-proteins, and they work through receptors, but not through a 7-pass receptor. Activated ras then activates MAP (mitogen-activated protein) kinases, which then activate the transcription factor AP-1 **f7.18**.

DAG also activates protein kinase C (PKC), which participates in the activation of a third family of transcription factors, the rel/nuclear factor-κB (NFκB) family. There are 5 members of this family: NF-κB1, NF-κB2, RelA, RelB, and c-rel. In their inactive state, the proteins of the NFκB family are in the cytoplasm and are bound to and inhibited by members of the NFκB inhibitor (I-κ-B) family. During activation, I-κ-B is phosphorylated by

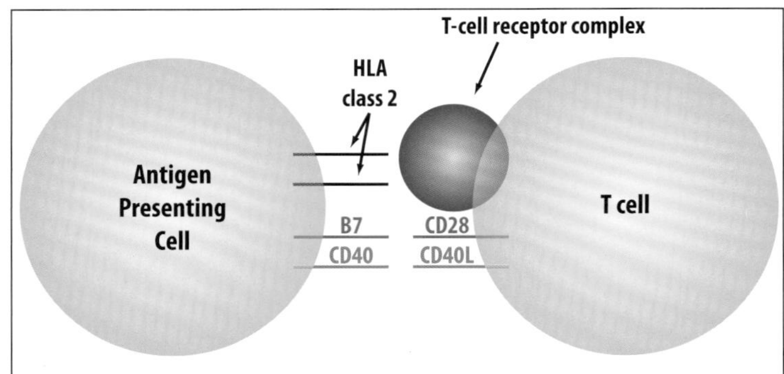

f7.19 In addition to the interaction between the T-cell receptor complex and class II HLA molecules, CD4 T cells also express CD28 and CD40 ligand, which interact with B7 and CD40 on the antigen presenting cell, respectively.

I-κ-B kinases (IKKs). This phosphorylation degrades I-κ-B, thus liberating the active NFκB complex, which then translocates to the nucleus and modulates transcription [PMID9299584]. Calcineurin, important in the activation of the NFAT family of transcription factors, is also important in activating the NFκB family. It and protein kinase C, activated by DAG, work together to activate the IKK complex, which then phosphorylates and degrades I-κ-B, the inhibitor of the NFκB family, permitting the latter proteins to become active transcription factors [PMID10438457]. Members of the NFκB family are normal proteins, but if present in abnormal amounts or refractory to normal regulation, can facilitate tumors.

T cells in their naïve state require additional signals to induce their proliferation and activity. The second additional signal is an interaction involving the costimulatory receptor CD28 on the T cell and its interaction with B7 on APCs. In this interaction, CD28 is phosphorylated at tyrosine residues, but not in an ITAM manner. Phosphorylated CD28 has a number of actions, one of which is to modulate the activities of the transcription factors of the NFκB family and of AP-1, so as to increase the production of IL-2. Another action of phosphorylated CD28 is to activate phosphoinositol 3-kinase, which then produces phosphatidylinositol triphosphate (PIP3). PIP3 activates a kinase called Akt (which is of the serine/threonine type, not the tyrosine type). Through a continuation of a phosphorylation cascade, Akt inhibits the programmed cell death pathway (in which the T cell will automatically die unless this pathway is operative), thus facilitating the survival of the cell. This is the pathway that is blocked by the immunosuppressive drug rapamycin (ie, rapamycin allows the T cell to die a natural death). For this CD28 phosphorylation cascade to occur, a T cell must bind multiple copies of the antigen molecule that it recognizes.

A third signal between an antigen-presenting cell and a T cell occurs between CD40 on the APC and the CD40 ligand (CD40L) on the T cell, which we will re-visit in our discussion of B cell activation **f7.19**.

CD8 T cells are activated by pathways that are very similar to those used by CD4 cells. However, CD8 cytotoxicity often requires concomitant recognition of the target cell by CD4 T cells in conjunction with HLA class 2 molecules. The reason for this requirement is not completely clear, but since the consequence of CD8 T cell action is destruction of the target, it makes sense that there would be an additional requirement to modulate the process.

Yet another signal between the APC and the naïve T cell is the cytokines secreted by the APC. The cytokines secreted by the APC determine which type of effector T cell results. This is the ultimate connection between the innate and adaptive immune systems—the products of the cells of the innate system influence the differentiation of cells of the adaptive system. It is becoming clear that the precise function of a lymphocyte is not so much dependent on its CD4 or CD8 expression as on a combination of signals, especially on the cytokines it is exposed to when it moves from a naïve to an effector T cell.

There are 2 primary subsets of CD4+ cells—TH-1 and TH-2—which have different effector functions. Secretion of IL-12 by an APC favors differentiation of T cells toward TH-1 cells, which secrete both IFN-γ, an activator of macrophages, and IL-2, an activator of T cells, making TH-1 cells integral to both innate and adaptive immunity.

TH-2 cells facilitate adaptive immunity. Secretion of IL-4 by the APC favors development of a TH-2 T cell, which then secretes a number of cytokines, such as IL-10, which inhibit macrophages and facilitate humoral immunity by several mechanisms, one of which is to increase the expression of HLA class 2 molecules. TH-2 cells secrete a number of cytokines, including IL-4, IL-5, IL-9, and IL-13, that activate B cells and stimulate the production of antibodies. They also promote the switching of the type of heavy chain type, which results in the making of a different class of antibody (eg, IgM to IgG). This is class switching, to be discussed in a moment). In addition, IL-4 also increases IgE and IL-5 also activates eosinophils, making TH-2 cells a leading defense mechanism against allergens and helminths.

In addition, there are 2 other subsets of CD4 T cells whose development and function are not as well described as TH-1 and TH-2 cells. Regulatory T cells (T-regs), formerly called suppressor T cells, and formerly thought to predominantly express CD8, is a subset of T cells that produce cytokines that inhibit both TH-1 and TH-2 cells. T-regs are a heterogeneous group of T cells that are usually CD4 positive. T-regs may be natural (central) or adaptive (made in the periphery). Natural T-regs are made in the thymus and escape negative selection there. Adaptive T-regs are made in peripheral sites in response to cytokines. T-regs produce FoxP3, a transcription factor that interferes with the transcription of IL-2, perhaps the single most important stimulator of T cells in general.

Another unusual regulatory T-cell subgroup is TH-3, which is a type of adaptive T-reg that regulates the immune response in mucosal sites. Lack of or dysfunction of these cells may be a factor in gastrointestinal autoimmune disorders and inflammatory bowel disease. TH-3 cells produce IL-4, IL-10, and transforming growth factor β (TGF-β) [PMID19210347].

A recently described subset of CD4 T cells is the TH-17 group. TH-17 cells are among the first T cells to be generated in the adaptive response, but their primary function is to enhance innate immunity, illustrating the temporal overlap between these phases of the immune response. TH-17 cells stimulate neutrophils, primarily through the production of IL-17, and also facilitate the production of antimicrobials from epithelia (such as β-defensins from keratinocytes). The cytokines IL-6 and transforming growth factor β (TGF-β) favor the development of TH-17 cells and are typically made before the cytokines that favor the development of other types of T cells. TH-17 cells have been implicated in graft vs host disease (GVH) after bone marrow transplantation [PMID18957685].

Once a naïve T cell has been fully stimulated, it is called an effector T cell. If a naïve T cell is not exposed to the required set of stimuli in a lymph node, it may exit and return to the circulation, to reenter a node later. But if a naïve T cell is stimulated into an effector T cell in a node or in the spleen, it is likely to leave the node (in contrast, activated B lymphocytes are more likely to remain in lymphoid organs or in the bone marrow). Importantly, effector T cells no longer require the above mentioned multiple stimulations to act, though they still require that the antigens be presented with appropriate HLA molecules. Contact with the specific antigen for which it is primed, in conjunction with HLA molecules, is all that is needed. In this manner, effector T cells—able to respond to their antigen without costimuli—constantly "patrol" the periphery for foreign or damaged antigens.

This is why a PPD is positive in patients who have been exposed to TB, but negative in patients who have not been. In the latter group of patients, the naïve T cells in the skin cannot respond to antigen presentation by APC in the skin. In a positive test, previous exposure has resulted in the presence of mature effector T cells that can respond to antigen presentation in the skin, after which there is a delayed-type hypersensitivity reaction (a form of cell-mediated immunity, which we will consider shortly) mediated by mature TH-1 cells.

The adaptive immune response begins with the creation of effector T cells from naïve T cells. After activation, CD4 helper T cells of the TH-1 type focus on macrophage activation and intracellular pathogens. They activate phagocytosis by secreting the cytokines IFN-γ and TNF-β (also called lymphotoxin), which stimulate macrophages. They also secrete IL-2, an activator of T cells, IL-3, and granulocyte/monocyte CSF (GM-CSF), which induces macrophage differentiation in the bone marrow. Finally, they secrete IFN-α and the chemokine CXCL2. The action of the last 2 cytokines is to recruit macrophages and allow them to pass out of the vascular space and to accumulate at the relevant site.

The principal cytokine product of CD8 cytotoxic T cells is IFN-γ, which activates macrophages and inhibits viral replication (CD8 T cytotoxic cells and TH-1 cells are the principal sources of IFN-γ). CD8 cells also secrete IFN α and β, additional activators of macrophages. Moreover, as we will see, CD8 cytotoxic T cells, after activation, can destroy entire cells if they carry an unwanted antigen, by secreting molecules that directly damage the cell membranes of target cells.

Like B cells, some antigen-stimulated effector T cells will respond to the immediate problem, while others will develop into memory cells that are specific for that antigen, though the precise nature of memory T cells is not as well understood as for memory B cells.

Activation of B Cells

We have seen that the stages in the maturation of a B cell in the bone marrow are the pro-B, pre-B, which can synthesize μ heavy chains, and the immature B cell, which can synthesize light chains and place a complete IgM molecule on the cell surface. Immature B cells leave the bone marrow to undergo further development in the periphery, especially in lymph nodes and the spleen. Once an immature B cell acquires the ability to synthesize a δ heavy chain, it displays IgD on the surface as well as IgM. The cell is now called a mature (of naïve) B cell.

Initially, there is a recognition phase in which antigen is bound to membrane immunoglobulin molecules (IgM and IgD) on the mature B cell. The antigen receptor is an antibody that is antigen-specific. The antigen specificity of the antibody is determined by the variable region, while the constant region of the antibody determines the class of the antibody (ie, IgM, IgD, IgG, IgA or IgG) and interacts with other cells of the immune system. Though the class of antibody expressed by the lymphocyte's progeny may change during the course of the immune response (typically there is a change from IgM to IgG or IgA), all of the progeny of the original cell are committed to the recognition of the same antigen.

Most of the initial stages of adaptive immunity take place in lymph nodes. APCs, B cells, and helper T cells all come together in the lymph node. Some of the APCs, such as conventional dendritic cells, have been transported in their entirety from peripheral sites. Naïve T cells use a combination of molecules to come to rest in lymph nodes or extranodal lymphoid nodules. Mature B cells use an almost identical set of molecules to home in on the areas of the lymph node that will become B cells areas. These young B cells, like their T counterparts, also employ molecules such as L-selectin (CD62L) and the integrin α4β7, but whereas T cells often preferentially express one or the other, depending on whether their destination is a lymph node or a nonnodal site, naïve B cells tend to express both, so that some of them will settle down in both nodal and nonnodal lymphoid tissue. Like naïve T cells, mature B cells express the chemokine receptor CCR7.

At this point, there are T and B areas in this region of the node, but no distinct germinal centers. Both naïve T and mature B lymphocytes, as they circulate, pass through lymph nodes. Naïve CD4 helper T cells recognize antigen in T-cell rich zones of lymphoid organs, while mature B-lymphocytes recognize antigens in B-cell rich zones.

These B-cell areas are called primary follicles, but do not yet have distinct germinal centers and mantle zones. Histologically, they are indistinct tiny nodules. Circulating mature B cells enter the node and come to rest in a primary follicle if they recognize an antigen there. Although B cells require T-cell activation for a full response or antibody production, there may be an initial activation of B cells without T-cell participation in a primary follicle. If this does not happen, the mature B cell simply passes through the follicle and on to another node, and the follicle is not transformed. But if a mature B cell is antigen stimulated in a primary follicle, it then moves toward the T-cell area of the node and encounters T cells. If it then encounters a T cell that recognizes the same antigen (called a cognate T cell) from its prior contact with an APC, it becomes further activated and goes on to further development. For a B cell to be fully activated, it must undergo a 2-stage stimulation—the mature B cell must recognize an antigen in a primary follicle and then the partially stimulated B cell must find and interact with a cognate T cell, which has been activated by contact with the same antigen, in a T-cell area of a node. The initial interaction between B and T lymphocytes that have been stimulated by the same antigen occurs at the interface of the B cell zone (the primary follicle) and the T-cell zone. Here, the B cell and the T cell exchange mutually stimulating signals—the B cell may present antigen to the T cell, but the primary effect is maturation of the B cell by the T cell. At this time, there is still no sharply defined germinal center or mantle zone.

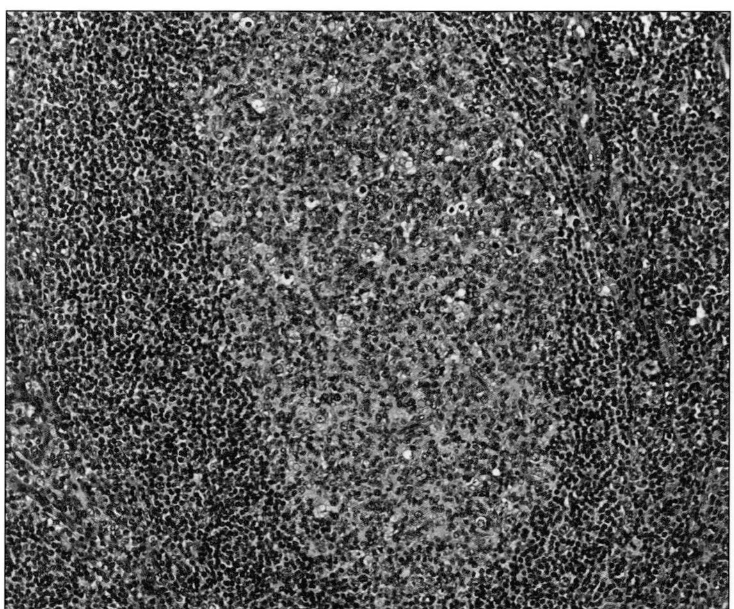

f7.20 A germinal center and mantle zone of a lymph node. These are both B cell areas of the node and together constitute a follicle.

Within 4-7 days after antigen exposure, some of the activated B cells that have encountered cognate T cells migrate back into the primary follicle and begin to proliferate, initiating a second phase of B-cell activation. These areas are the *secondary* follicles, each of which consists of a germinal center and an associated mantle zone, both B-cell areas **f7.20**. The terms "cortex" and "paracortex" are somewhat confusing in lymph nodes, but roughly speaking, the cortex consists of the B-cell areas and the paracortex consists of the T-cell areas. In a lymph node that has seen many antigenic stimulations, the cortical region consists of the germinal centers and their associated mantle zones, while the paracortical region consists of the T-cell rich areas between the follicles.

In the germinal center, the mature B cell undergoes yet another process that leads to diversity—somatic hypermutation. In somatic hypermutation, some cytosine bases are changed to uracil, a base that is not normally found in DNA, in a process mediated by the enzyme activation-induced deaminase (AID). The uracils are then removed by repair endonucleases, after which the resulting gaps are filled in, by a variety of enzymes, some of which are error-prone, introducing mutations and further increasing diversity **f7.21**. Rarely, there will be insertions or deletions instead of simple base replacement. Somatic hypermutation primarily occurs in complementarity determining region III, but also to some extent in framework region III, the adjacent portion of the Variable region. For some B cells, somatic hypermutation results in a B cell that has greater affinity and an enhanced ability to survive. This is called affinity maturation.

There are 5 classes of antibodies in humans—IgM, IgG, IgA, IgD, and IgE, depending on differences between their heavy chains. Some isotypes have subclasses. For example, there are 4 types of IgG and 2 types of IgA (there are no subclasses for IgM, IgD, and IgE). Thus, IgG1 is a different subclass of IgG than IgG2. This results in 9 subclasses of antibody molecules. The slightly different heavy chains that are found in classes and subclasses

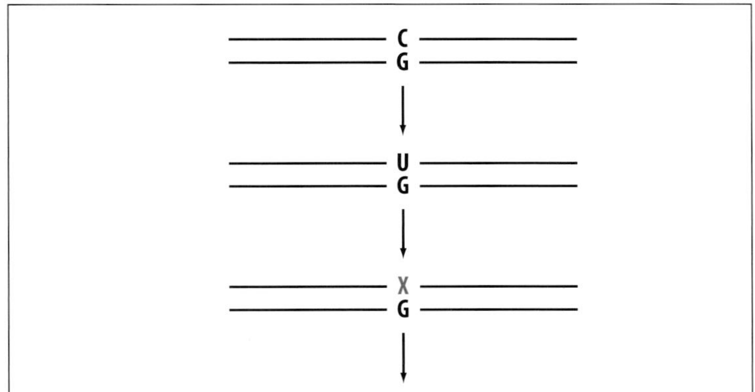

f7.21 After antigenic stimulation, the process of somatic hypermutation occurs. Cytosine bases are changed into uracils, after which they are excised and replaced by a variety of enzymes, resulting in additional diversity.

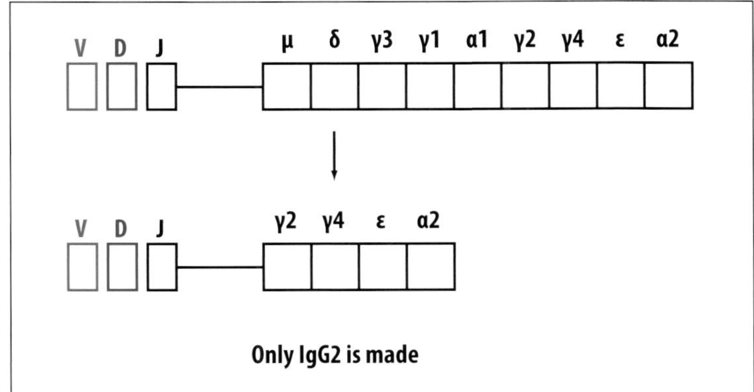

f7.22 Class switching occurs in the germinal center after antigenic stimulation and after somatic hypermutation. In class switching, DNA of the constant region is deleted, but in a simple cut and paste manner. There is no complex rearrangement of DNA in the constant region as there is in the variable region. In this example, there is deletion of the μ, δ, γ3, γ1 and α1 regions, resulting in fusion of the rearranged variable-diversity-joining regions to a portion of the constant region that begins with the γ2 gene. Only the γ2 gene is fully transcribed and translated, the result being an IgG2 molecule.

are called isotypes. For example, γ1 and γ2, the heavy chains of IgG1 and IgG2, are different isotypes.

There are 2 other terms used in reference to antibodies. The term "allotypes" refers to differences in antigenicity caused by simple allelic variation in the constant regions of the immunoglobulin chains. Allotypes are not related to gene rearrangement or to antigenic stimulation, but simply represent differences between the same proteins in any 2 individuals. For example, if 2 people have both been vaccinated against hepatitis B by exposure to the surface antigen, the antibodies they make will be very similar, but not identical because there will be minor allelic differences between the genes coding for the constant regions of their antibodies. The term "idiotype" refers to unique sequences of amino acids at the antigen binding sites. The complementarity determining regions (CDRs) are hypervariable regions of DNA that add greatly to antibody diversity. Because of CDRs, the antibodies made by different people, even if to the same antigen, will differ slightly at the actual antigen binding site. Whereas isotypes and allotypes refer to differences in constant regions, idiotypes refer to differences in the variable region.

IgM is the original immunoglobulin product, but the other classes may be synthesized in the process of class switching. Class switching is often accompanied by isotype switching, via the same mechanism, so that there is a change, for example, not just from IgM to IgG, but specifically to IgG2 or IgG3, etc. Class switching of the B cell occurs in the germinal center after antigen stimulation and somatic hypermutation. Class switching involves the Constant regions only. In class switching, there is deletion of the DNA, at the germline level, of all of the constant regions of the heavy chain between the VDJ construct that was previously created and the portion of the constant (C) gene that is to be transcribed. Because the order of heavy chain regions of the C gene is μ, δ, γ 3, γ 1, α1, γ 2, γ 4, ε, and α 2, the μ and δ regions of the C gene are deleted to make an IgG3 antibody and the μ, δ, all of the γ, α 1, and the ε regions are deleted to make an IgA2 transcript. After this DNA is deleted, subsequent transcription and translation produces an antibody of a new class or isotype **f8.22**. Other than the simultaneous production of IgM and IgD before antigenic stimulation, a B cell can make only one class of antibody. Hence, translation terminates after the first heavy chain region to be encountered.

Unlike the immunoglobulin gene rearrangement described earlier, class switching is a simple 2-point breakage and reconnection of DNA rather than a complex, multicentered rearrangement. Remarkably, class switching is mediated by the same enzyme—activation-induced deaminase—that catalyzes somatic hypermutation. In general, both somatic hypermutation and class switching occur only after antigen stimulation and interaction with T cells, whereas the initial V-D-J rearrangement occurs before antigen stimulation [PMID14724175].

In general, antigens that enter the blood or the skin eventually lead to antibodies of multiple isotypes through class switching, whereas antigens that enter through the respiratory or GI tract and then enter lymph node tissue in those areas undergo a more limited form of class switching that results in antibodies of the IgA variety (secretory IgA).

The constant region of an antibody molecule, though not used in antigen recognition, is vital in effector functions. The Fc portion of an antibody molecule, consisting entirely of a C region, defines the class of antibody (IgG, IgM, IgA, etc.) and is important as an opsonin for phagocytes and in fixing complement. It also serves to provide a receptor in the transportation of the antibody molecule to extravascular spaces, such as into breast milk or across the placenta. Because of different C regions, IgG crosses the placenta while IgM does not. IgM remains in the intravascular space, while IgG and IgA can exit the vascular space and enter into tissues.

We thus have 4 mechanisms by which enormous diversity of immunoglobulins can arise from DNA. These are gene rearrangement, the action of TdT, somatic hypermutation, and class/isotype switching. The first 2 mechanisms occur in the bone marrow, before antigen stimulation, while the last 2 occur in the germinal center, after antigen stimulation. Gene conversion is another process that occurs in the germinal center in some animals (it does not appear to occur to any extent in humans). Gene conversion modifies the variable regions by replacing whole blocks of DNA with pseudogenes, sequences of DNA that are derived from functional genes and closely resemble them, but which are not functional.

Most B cells that have undergone class switching and activation are recognizable as plasma cells, but some activated B lymphocytes do not secrete immunoglobulin at all, and become memory cells, which are important in secondary antibody responses. Indeed, the capacity to retain a "memory" of the antigen is a feature unique to adaptive immunity (both humoral

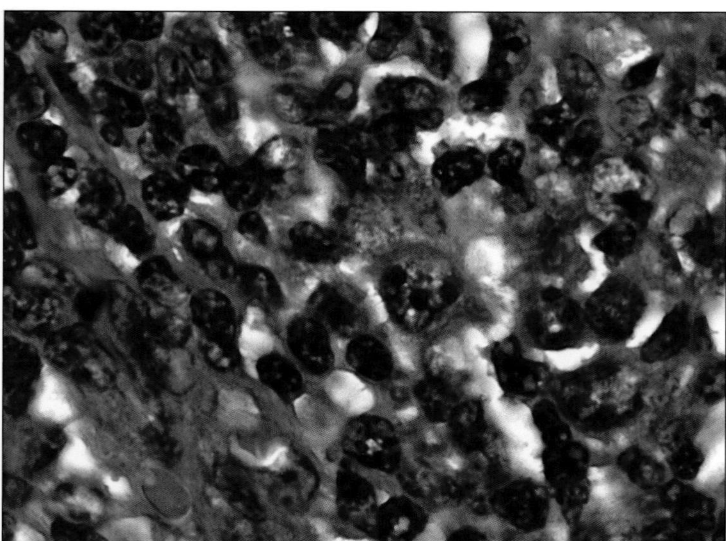

f7.23 The large cell in the center, with vesicular chromatin and multiple nucleoli is a centroblast. The smaller cells around it, with inconspicuous nucleoli, more coarsely clumped chromatin, and often with cleaved nuclear membranes, are centrocytes.

and cellular) that is not shared by innate immunity. Usually, though not always, a B cell must transit a germinal center to receive the necessary stimuli to form memory cells.

Most people now endorse the Kiel conception of the formation of germinal centers, proposed by Karl Lennert, whereby centroblasts, cells with noncleaved nuclei, divide and give rise to centrocytes, smaller cells with cleaved (ie, indented) nuclei. After years of debate, there is now a general consensus that the noncleaved centroblasts are the rapidly dividing fraction. Centroblasts have a vesicular nucleus (with peripheralized chromatin), several nucleoli, and a moderate amount of cytoplasm. Centroblasts express both CD10 and bcl-6, 2 markers of follicular center origin. It is thought that somatic hypermutation takes place in centroblasts. Centroblasts are sometimes referred to as "activated lymphocytes." The term "activated lymphocyte" is not a specific term, but generally refers to a more mature cell that has left the germinal center, such as an immunoblast. Specifically, the term "activated lymphocyte," if it is to be used at all, should be restricted to B cells that have lost bcl-6 and which express MUM1.

Centrocytes are smaller than centroblasts, with smaller nuclei, very small or absent nucleoli, and little cytoplasm. In contrast to centroblasts, they often have a cleaved nuclear membrane f7.23. Antigen exposure and T cell contact transform mature B cells into a centroblasts, which then enter or form a germinal center and divide to become centrocytes. Centrocytes go on to either mature plasma cells or death if they do not correctly navigate the many steps to maturity.

Each germinal center contains cells derived from only one, or perhaps a few, B-cell clones. Normal germinal centers are very mitotically active, as shown by immunohistochemical staining for the proliferation marker Ki-67. This gives them an overall lighter staining than the surrounding mantle zone. Close examination of a germinal center shows that it has a darker zone and a lighter zone. The darker zone is where the centroblasts, once stimulated by interaction with T cells, initially reside and where most mitoses occur. In contrast, the follicles in follicular lymphomas are not zones of B-cell maturation. Therefore, they are not as mitotically active and mitoses are evenly distributed throughout the follicle.

The progeny of centroblasts are called centrocytes. Centrocytes migrate to the light area of the germinal center, where they can continue dividing to a reduced extent. The light area of the germinal center has fewer mitoses, but more follicular dendritic cells. The follicular dendritic cell (also called a dendritic reticulum cell) is different from the conventional, or interdigitating dendritic cell. The latter cell type is important in antigen presentation to naïve T cells, but the follicular dendritic cell is found in the germinal center, which is a B-cell area of lymphoid follicles. The follicular dendritic cell, in contrast to the interdigitating dendritic cell, does not express HLA molecule, and is not clearly derived from the bone marrow. The follicular dendritic cell presents antigens to B cells, whereas the interdigitating dendritic cell presents antigens to T cells. Follicular dendritic cells also seem to play a role in which B cells are selected for survival and which will undergo programmed death.

In the lighter area, centrocytes come into contact with the processes of the many follicular dendritic cells that are present there. B cells that bind to epitopes on follicular dendritic cells with high affinity will survive. The others undergo apoptosis. Because of this, many of the centrocytes in the germinal centers will not survive, and it is their death that leads to the characteristic presence of many macrophages, who remove the centrocytes that do not have sufficient affinity. However, the centrocytes that do survive will become plasma cells that produce antibodies of higher affinity. It is generally believed that heavy chain class switching occurs in centrocytes.

The mantle zone surrounds the germinal center in a secondary follicle. In a normal lymph node, the mantle zone asymmetrically surrounds the germinal center, with a more cellular area adjacent to the lighter zone of the germinal center i8.42a. The precise function of the mantle zone in B-cell maturation is not completely clear, but it is established that the mantle zone consists of mature B cells that have not yet been stimulated. It may be that the lymphocytes of the mantle zone are the cells of the primary follicle after the formation of the secondary follicles.

The B-cell receptor itself is an immunoglobulin molecule, but as is the case for T cells, the B-cell receptor does not function alone, but rather is part of a receptor complex. The companion molecules that complete the B-cell receptor complex are called CD79a (Igα) and CD79b (Igβ). These 2 molecules together form CD79, a marker of B cells that is clinically useful for 3 reasons. First, it precedes the presence of CD20 and is more likely to be found on young B cells. Second, is more likely to be found on plasma cells, which often lose CD20 expression. Third, rituximab (Rituxan; a monoclonal antibody directed to the CD20 antigen, used to treat some B-cell lymphomas) may cause loss of that antigen, in which case CD79 is an important indication of B-cell differentiation [PMID11396639]. CD79a and CD79b serve the same function that CD3 and the ζ protein do in T-lymphocyte activation. They are transmembrane, with extracellular, membranous, and cytoplasmic portions, and their cytoplasmic domains contain immunoreceptor tyrosine-based activation motif (ITAM), as is the case for the ζ and CD3 chains in the TCR complex. The immunoglobulin molecule, with CD79a and CD79b, form the *receptor complex* of a B cell.

Also like T cells, the B-cell receptor complex is associated with coreceptors. In the case of the T cell, the coreceptor was a CD4 or a CD8 molecule. In the case of a B cell, the coreceptors are the transmembrane proteins CD21, CD19, and CD81. Collectively, these 3 proteins are often called the B-cell *coreceptor complex*. The B-cell

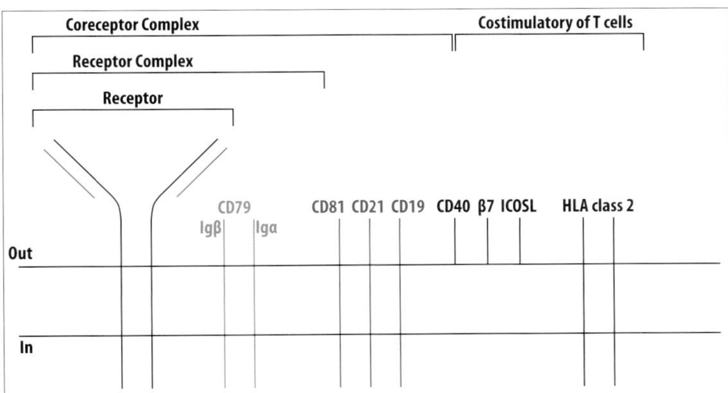

f7.24 The important proteins expressed by a mature B cell. A fully-formed immunoglobulin molecule, identical to the one expressed by the cell, constitutes the receptor. The receptor complex consists of the receptor and CD79. The addition of CD19, CD21, and CD81 constitutes the co-receptor complex. In addition to HLA class II molecules, the B cell also expresses 3 molecules—CD40, B7, and ICOSL—that stimulate T cells.

coreceptor complex markedly lowers the threshold for an intracellular response from the B cell upon binding to antigen.

In addition, B cells express several molecules that are costimulatory with HLA receptor molecules in their interactions with T cells of either the CD4 or CD8 type, but are not part of a receptor or coreceptor because they do not bind antigen. These molecules include B7, CD40, and inducible costimulatory ligand (ICOSL). During the mutually activating interactions between B and T cells, the B7 proteins bind with CD28 on the T cell, while CD40 binds to the CD40 ligand (CD40L) on the T cell, and ICOSL binds to the inducible costimulatory molecule (ICOS) on the T cell **f7.19, f7.24**. The CD40-CD40L interaction appears critical in immunoglobulin class switching.

There are remarkable parallels between T-cell and B-cell activation. Crosslinking of the surface immunoglobulin by antigen leads to clustering of the CD79a and CD79b molecules, which in turn leads to phosphorylation of the tyrosine residues on the ITAMs by receptor-associated kinases, thus setting in motion the activation cascade that is very similar to what we encountered in T-cell stimulation. Unlike T cells, however, normal B cells do not express ZAP-70 (ZAP-70 is of importance in T-cell activation and is found in developing B cells and also in some cases of B-cell chronic lymphoid leukemia, but it plays no significant role in the activation of normal B cells). Instead, B lymphocytes have a related tyrosine kinase called Syk, which functions in the B cell in a similar manner to ZAP-70 in the T cell. Through intermediate molecules, Syk leads to the phosphorylation of PLC. Phosphorylated PLC then cleaves phosphatidylinositol bisphosphate (PIP2) into inositol triphosphate (IP3) and diacylglycerol (DAG). As is the case for T cell activation, DAG recruits protein kinase C and IP3 releases calcium from the endoplasmic reticulum. The eventual result of ITAM activation is an increase in a number of transcription factors, many of which, such as NFAT, NF-κβ, and AP-1, are also increased in T-cell activation. Proteins of the myc family are additional transcription factors in B cell activation [PMID19607732].

As is the case for T cells, there is an additional signaling pathway in B cells, stemming from DAG, and involving the activation of small proteins that bind to monomeric G-proteins. As is the case in T cells, ras is one of these proteins and becomes activated by binding GTP instead of GDP. Activated ras switches on the MAP kinases, leading to increased activity of transcription factors.

There is an alternative pathway for activation of B cells. CD21, part of the B cell coreceptor complex, is a complement receptor that binds to the C3d component of complement and was formerly called complement receptor 2. If a microbial antigen has bound C3d, it may also simultaneously bind to the B-cell receptor and to CD21, then recruit CD19 and initiate a series of reactions that eventuate in the activation of ITAMs of both CD79a and CD79b [PMID15778510]. This pathway may be very significant and may allow complement to participate in humoral immunity [PMID12149415]. Often, both the classical B-cell receptor pathway and the alternative, CD21-mediated receptor signaling proceed simultaneously.

CD21 is also the receptor for the Epstein-Barr virus (EBV), a rare cause of T cell-independent B-cell proliferation. This virus causes mononucleosis by infecting B cells by binding to CD21 (complement receptor 2) and HLA class 2 antigens. This causes a proliferation of B cells that does not require T-cell stimulation, though it is eventually reined in by cytotoxic T cells. A latent form of EBV infection does not cause clinical manifestations because there is no replication of the virus. EBV may also induce B-cell lymphomas by producing proteins that inappropriately simulate T-cell activation of B cells.

No biologic process is complete without some means of regulation. In the B cell, the action of ITAM is opposed by immunoreceptor tyrosine-based inhibition motif (ITIM), a motif consisting of a 6 amino acid sequence of isoleucine-X-tyrosine-X-X-leucine, which sets in motion an inhibitory chain of events via phosphorylation of its tyrosine residues. In addition, CD22 furnishes negative feedback by inhibiting the coreceptor, and CD32 works with antibodies to inhibit the production of more immunoglobulin molecules.

Fully developed plasma cells are made mostly in bone marrow, although some may be made in the medullary cords of the lymph node, the collections of lymphocytes that are between the sinuses in the central and hilar areas of the node. Many mature plasma cells will leave the node to settle in virtually every site in the body. The gastrointestinal tract is particularly rich in plasma cells. In the process of becoming fully mature plasma cells, some of the mature B cells become memory cells, capable of quickly differentiating into plasma cells upon subsequent contact with the antigen. Some of these memory cells remain in the lymph node, while others do not. Memory B cells still interact with T cells in a manner similar to that for mature B cells, but move more rapidly through the T cell interaction process because they already have high affinity receptors for the antigen.

There are 4 major exceptions to the previous discussion of the activation and interaction of T cells and B lymphocytes. The first 2 exceptions concern unusual T cell responses, while the last 2 concern the B cell response. The first exception concerns superantigens. Very rare molecules, called superantigens, can simultaneously bind to the variable region of the β chain of the TCR and to an HLA class II molecule, directly stimulating the cell without breakdown or antigen presentation by HLA molecules. Such binding causes an outpouring of cytokines (similar to the cytokine storm seen in some severe gram-negative infections), but contrary to what one might suspect, this does not enhance adaptive immunity. To the contrary, superantigens do us no favor. The effect of superantigens is to contribute to systemic toxicity and to suppress adaptive immunity. Some of these superantigens are of viral origin, but the most clinically significant ones are exotoxins from bacteria. Toxic shock syndrome and the staphylococcal entertoxins that cause food poisoning are examples of superantigens.

The second exception concerns a response to lipids and glycolipids by an unusual group of T cells that have α-β receptors, but do not express either CD4 or CD8. The CD1 family is a group of 4 proteins (CD1a, CD1b, CD1c, and CD1d), very similar to HLA class 1 molecules in their structure, that are expressed on the surface of APCs in association with β2 microglobulin, just as class 1 HLA molecules are. The CD1 proteins on APCs bind lipid or glycolipid antigens and present them directly to the TCR of these unusual T cells without either internal processing or HLA molecules. The CD1d protein presents lipid antigens to a special type of T cell called the NKT cell, which has features of both T cells and NK cells (unlike other NK cells, NKT cells do express a TCR).

The third exception is the antibody response to T cell-independent antigens. Antibody responses to protein antigens require helper T-cell assistance, but antibody responses to polysaccharide and lipid antigens do not. These are called T cell-independent antigens. T cell-independent antibodies are not class switched, so they are IgM only. They are of lower affinity, there are no memory cells, and they usually do not cause follicular hyperplasia in lymph nodes. Lipopolysaccharides of gram-negative bacteria are important T cell-independent antigens. Lipids and glycolipids may therefore cause both an unusual T cell response via the CD1 family and T-independent B-cell antibody production.

The fourth exception concerns B-1 cells. B-1 cells develop initially in the fetal or neonatal period, and do not express TdT during their development. B-1 cells are found in the periphery, not in lymph nodes or in the marrow. They are especially prevalent in the peritoneal and pleural cavities. Whereas conventional B cells (called B-2 cells) divide only in response to antigenic stimuli and only in marrow or a lymph node, B-1 cells can self-renew without stimulation and they do so in the periphery. B-1 cells demonstrate limited immunoglobulin gene rearrangement and express IgM without class switching. They react mostly with other immunoglobulin molecules, self-antigens (they are often increased in autoimmune disorders), and polysaccharides in bacterial cell walls. B-1 cells can produce these antibodies without T cell help and are therefore part of innate immunity. B-1 cells rarely form memory cells [PMID16920907].

There are similarities between the immunohistochemical profiles of B-1 cells and those of mantle cell lymphoma and chronic lymphoid leukemia/small lymphocytic lymphoma (particularly the expression of CD5), and there is long been thought that some mantle cell lymphomas, particularly of the blastic type, and chronic lymphoid leukemia/small lymphocytic lymphoma originate from B-1 cells [PMID9753060], but a direct connection has not been established.

Assessment of Clonality

PCR is the most common method of assessing clonality of lymphocyte proliferations. The primers are usually directed to the V and J regions. If there has been no rearrangement, the primers are too far apart and there is no amplification **f7.25a**, but if there has been gene rearrangement, the primers are close enough that amplification is possible **f7.25b**. Most procedures are directed at amplifying complementarity determining region (CDR) III on the heavy chain. Typically, such assays employ a primer for the framework regions FR1, FR2, or FR3 on the variable chain on one side of CDR3 and a primer for the FR4 region, on the J chain, on the other side of CDR3, so that amplification is carried out across the entire CDR3 region. Somatic hypermutation occurs primarily in CDR3, but also to some extent in FR3. For this reason, clonality tests by PCR that use primers directed only at FR3 can give misleading results, and primers directed at FR1 and FR2 are often used. Primers that bind to the CDR3 region are avoided because somatic hypermutation may cause sufficient variability that the primers will not bind. For most TCR studies, unless a γ-δ process is suspected, the β chain is targeted, and probes that will hybridize to the β chain J regions are used **f7.25c**.

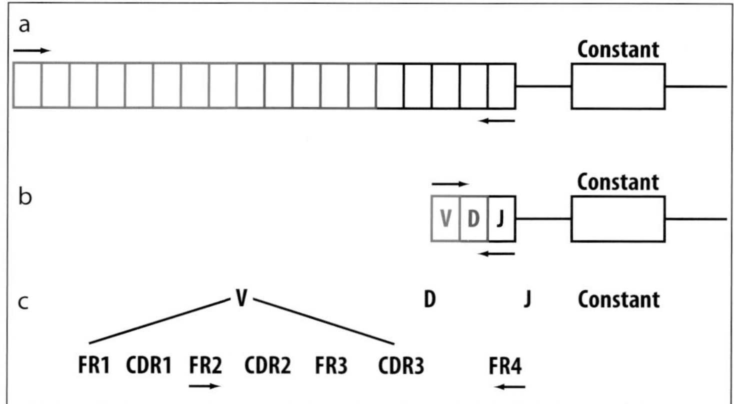

f7.25 Assessment of clonality by PCR with primers to the V region on the left and the J region on the right.
a Without gene rearrangement, the two primers are too far apart for PCR to occur and there is no amplification.
b If there had been gene rearrangement, the primers are close enough together to permit PCR and amplification to occur, resulting in a noticeable band.
c At a more detailed level, the specific target of most immunoglobulin heavy chain gene rearrangement studies is CDR3, and typically, primers are designed to bind to the regions around FR2 and FR4.

Because lymphomas are often accompanied by large numbers of nonneoplastic lymphocytes, most studies of immunoglobulin or TCR gene rearrangement require that 5% or more of the cells be of monoclonal origin for the process to be assumed to be neoplastic. In any molecular study performed on paraffin-embedded tissue, it is prudent to examine an H&E stained section on either side of the tissue taken for molecular analysis, so that one can be sure that the submitted tissue corresponds to the histologically abnormal tissue.

A potential pitfall in clonality studies is a false positive caused by a paucity of lymphocytes, such that the fortuitous amplification of a small area of DNA stands out. This risk can be minimized by testing only tissue that has good numbers of lymphocytes. Also, benign lymphoid proliferations in some autoimmune disorders and in *Helicobacter pylori* can simulate a clonal lymphoproliferative process and a firm determination of a clonal process should be made with caution in these cases.

Peripheral Tolerance

Both T and B lymphocytes become tolerant to self-antigens. The biochemical mechanisms of tolerance are not as well understood as those of activation. Apparently, APCs play a major role in this area as well. This process can take place at the site of maturation (in the bone marrow for B lymphocytes and in the thymus for T lymphocytes) or in the peripheral tissues after maturation. The former process is called central tolerance, and is largely synonymous with negative selection in the site of lymphocyte development. An example of central tolerance is negative selection of thymocytes in the thymus in the maturation of T lymphocytes.

Not all self-antigens are present in the locations where lymphocytes develop, so there is also a mechanism for inducing tolerance in mature lymphocytes in peripheral tissues. This is called peripheral tolerance. Peripheral tolerance may work along the same lines as central tolerance—killing of cells which recognize self-antigens with high affinity—but it may also take 2 forms that are not found in central tolerance. In one of these forms, lymphocytes that recognize the self-antigen, but do not have the required costimulators, will not be able to respond to that antigen in the future, even if the appropriate costimulators are present.

A second mechanism of peripheral tolerance involves the death of lymphocytes that repeatedly respond to the same antigen. Many cells, including T lymphocytes, express Fas, a receptor which is a member of the TNF receptor superfamily. Repeated stimulation leads to the expression of Fas ligand (FasL). Binding of Fas and FasL (either on the same cell or on different cells) leads to the clustering of 3 Fas molecules which then bind a cytosolic protein called Fas-associated death domain (FADD). FADD binds to and activates caspase 8 (the caspases are a group of proteins involved in apoptosis, or programmed cell death). Caspases 8 and 9 both initiate a proteolytic cascade directed at several key cellular targets. Because Fas and FasL are host proteins, excessive Fas-FasL interaction can only occur in repeated self-recognition. This is an example of extrinsic apoptosis, cell death that occurs by an external stimulus that binds to the cell surface. Extrinsic apoptosis always involves some form of a so-called "death receptor" on the cell surface that triggers a sequence of events eventuating in activation of the caspase cascade. Defects in FAS-FASL interactions play a role in some autoimmune disorders.

On the other hand, lymphocytes that fail to respond to appropriate stimuli are equally valueless. Periodic stimuli are required to sustain the lymphocyte. Permanent loss of stimuli leads to diffusion of cytochrome C out of the mitochondria. Cytochrome C then combines with apoptosis activating factor-1, and that complex activates caspase-9, leading to apoptosis. This is an example of intrinsic apoptosis, cell death that occurs without an external stimulus. Intrinsic apoptosis begins in mitochondria, when cytochrome C, which normally functions in electron transport, enters the cytosol and takes on a very different role by initiating the caspase cascade.

Mechanisms of Cell-Mediated Immunity

Cell-mediated immunity is an immune response to *intracellular* microbes and antigens. There are 2 main forms of cell-mediated immunity, depending on whether the antigens are in phagocytes or nonphagocytic cells. In the first form, CD4 TH-1 cells recognize intracellular antigens inside phagocytes via their presentation on the surface and then activate those phagocytes by releasing cytokines, primarily IFN-γ and tumor necrosis factor. In this form of cell-mediated immunity, TH-1 cells that have previously recognized an antigen and undergone proliferation and differentiation, respond to the same antigen if it is displayed by an APC in conjunction with class 2 HLA molecules. The APC is not killed, but activated. A useful way to think of this form of cell-mediated immunity is that a macrophage signals that it needs help to destroy the internalized material.

In the second type of cell-mediated immunity, CD8 cytotoxic T cells kill any nucleated cell that contains foreign antigens. For microbes or antigens that are in the cytoplasm of nonphagocytic cells, the mechanism of cell-mediated immunity is CD8 cytotoxic T-cell lysis of the cell. Because the infected cells do not have the capacity to kill the microbes, even if stimulated by T cells, the entire cell must be eradicated. This is the primary mechanism of action against viruses. The cytoplasmic proteins that elicit the CD8 cytotoxic response are degraded and presented on the surface of the doomed cell in association with class 1 HLA molecules. HLA class 1 is used instead of class 2 because the response must be able to destroy any infected cell (which will surely express HLA class 1 molecules), and not just cells of the immune system (which are the only cells that express HLA class 2 molecules). For example, a respiratory epithelial cell that contains a virus expresses class 1 HLA molecules but not class 2. If the CD8 cytotoxic cell recognized only class 2 HLA molecules, as does the CD4 TH-1 cell, there would be no way for it to destroy the infected epithelial cell. While "professional" APCs include macrophages, dendritic cells, and B lymphocytes, almost any cell can be an APC if it is infected with a virus. But a cell that presents foreign antigens in conjunction with only class 1 HLA molecules and not with HLA class 2 molecules or coreceptors is unlikely to survive the presentation.

CD8 cytotoxic T cells deliver cytotoxic granules into the target cell. The 3 most important of these are perforin, granzymes, and granulysin. The details of how these molecules induce cellular death are not clear, but it is thought that cytochrome C and enzymes of the caspase family are involved.

Mechanisms of Humoral Immunity

Humoral immunity is the portion of adaptive immunity that is responsible for *extracellular* microbes and antigens. Humoral immunity works in conjunction with cell-mediated immunity and innate immunity. For example, both humoral and cell-mediated immunity are important in the adaptive response to viruses. Antibodies block virus binding and entry, while cytotoxic T cells eliminate infected cells. In addition to physically blocking the binding of toxins and microbes to cell receptors, antibodies also often bring about effector functions, such as opsonization, activation of the complement system, and activation of mast cells. These effector functions are mediated by the constant region of the heavy chain, but are not operative until the variable region has bound to the antigen. For example, once an antibody binds to an antigen,

ISBN 978-089189-5886

the Fc receptor on phagocytes binds to the Fc region of the heavy chain, thus facilitating phagocytosis.

There is a classical and an alternate pathway of complement activation. The classical pathway is activated by either immune complexes (in adaptive immunity) or by mannose-binding lectin (in innate immunity). The alternate or properdin pathway is set in motion by the direct activation of C3b. Activation of complement by any mechanism sets in motion a proteolytic cascade that does 2 things. First, it eventuates in a membrane attack complex that literally puts a lethal hole in the cell wall of an offending organism. Second, during that process, there are "spinoff" molecules that have a variety of stimulatory effects on the inflammatory process.

The Type 1 complement receptor on B cells and follicular dendritic cells binds C3b, and is important in opsonization. The Type 2 complement receptor (CD21), which is the same receptor that the EBV uses, binds C3d and enhances antigen-mediated B cell activation.

In the gastrointestinal tract and the respiratory tract, B lymphocytes make antibodies in the lamina propria, primarily of the IgA type. The Fc portion of these antibodies binds to leukocytes, as would be expected, but also facilitates transport of the antibody molecule across the epithelium to protect the mucosal barrier [PMID9467977]. Oral vaccines generally work in part by stimulating this secretory antibody production.

The Immune Response to Viruses

Viruses have several mechanisms for foiling the immune response. First, some viruses produce proteins called immunoevasins that impede the presentation of class 1 HLA complexes on the cell surface. Because the viral antigens must be presented in concert with HLA class 1 molecules to trigger a CD8 cytotoxic T-cell response, a decreased presentation of class 1 HLA molecules attenuates the CD8 response. It is thought that NK cells evolved specifically to deal with this issue. The NK cell is an unusual type of lymphocyte that is neither T nor B, and unlike T and B cells, can kill without being activated. NK cells share some cell membrane proteins with T cells, but except for the very rare NKT cell, do not express a TCR or undergo the gene rearrangement. NK cells are inhibited by cells that express class I HLA molecules, and therefore, they do not kill host cells unless they are infected by viruses which have inhibited the expression of class I HLA molecules.

The Fc receptor of NK cells, CD16, works in a different way from the Fc receptor on phagocytes. The NK cell Fc receptor binds to the Fc portion of IgG1 and IgG3 antibodies that are attached to cells, resulting in the release of granules such as perforin and granzymes from the NK cells. These granules lyse the antibody-coated cells via a mechanism that is essentially identical to that employed by CD8 cytotoxic T cells and similar to the membrane attack complex of complement. This is called antibody dependent cell-mediated cytotoxicity (ADCC). NK cells also secrete cytokines, principally IFN-γ.

A second mechanism that viruses use to escape CD8 T cell-mediated destruction of the cells they have commandeered is to alter their antigens, so that the immune system is trying to hit a "moving target." A third mechanism that allows some viruses to evade the cellular immune response is that they can produce molecules that inhibit innate or adaptive immunity (for example, pox virus can make molecules that are similar to the receptors for several cytokines, so the cytokines bind to these molecules without effect). Because innate and adaptive immunity are intimately intertwined, the inhibition of the former invariably impedes the latter.

The Immune Response to Parasites

The major innate response to parasites is phagocytosis, but this is often not effective. The primary adaptive response to intracellular parasites is cell-mediated immunity, as is the case for intracellular bacteria and viruses. In contrast, helminths are extracellular, and the adaptive response to them is primarily humoral, mediated by TH-2 cells. A component of this humoral response is the binding of IgE molecules to the helminth. Eosinophils then bind to IgE molecules. This binding triggers the release of proteins present in the granules of eosinophils, such as eosinophil cationic protein, eosinophil major basic protein, eosinophil myeloperoxidase, and eosinophil-derived neurotoxin, which can kill the helminth by disrupting its cell membranes.

Hypersensitivity Reactions

There are 4 types of hypersensitivity reactions, the first 3 of which are mediated directly or indirectly through antibodies and take place very quickly after exposure. Type I hypersensitivity is mediated through IgE antibodies and histamine. It is the common allergic reaction, though it can be serious if it progresses to anaphylaxis, a sudden dramatic increase in vascular permeability and airway constriction caused primarily by a surge of histamine. Many allergens that cause type I hypersensitivity reactions are enzymes that can penetrate an epithelial barrier, after which they engender a TH-2 response. Type II hypersensitivity reactions involve the direct targeting of a cell by an antibody, such as in hemolytic disease of the newborn. Type III hypersensitivity is mediated through immune complexes (antibodies and complement) and is characteristic of many autoimmune disorders, such as lupus.

Type IV hypersensitivity reactions are the only type that do not involve antibodies. Type IV hypersensitivity is cell mediated and therefore much slower in its evolution than the first 3 types. It is in fact called delayed type hypersensitivity. We have already met the basic concepts of type IV hypersensitivity when we examined cell-mediated immunity because this form of hypersensitivity involves a TH-1-mediated reaction to a protein in tissues (a positive PPD is the classic example), but other types of type IV hypersensitivity include contact hypersensitivity (eg, poison ivy) and gluten-sensitive enteropathy (celiac disease).

Vaccines and DNA Vaccines

Vaccines based on killed pathogens or isolated antigens primarily give rise to humoral, rather than cellular immunity, because the antigens do not enter cells and exogenous proteins are not well recognized by the class 1 HLA CD8 pathway. A humoral response to antigen vaccines is effective in preventing disease produced by a toxin because the antibodies neutralize the toxin by preventing it from binding to its normal site of action. A type of vaccine that is related to purified antigen vaccine is the synthetic antigen vaccine. This offers the potential advantage of being more immunogenic, especially if epitopes of different antigens can be combined into 1 molecule. The proteins for many antigen-based vaccines are now made by recombinant or cloning technologies, as will be discussed in Chapters 45 and 46. Additional considerations in vaccine manufacture and use include the size of the dose, mode of administration, and the use of adjuvants.

Attenuated live vaccines do enter cells and therefore give rise to both humoral and cellular immunity. They are generally made by repeated culture on an unfavorable medium, which prevents full virulence. Not only is the immune response from live viruses more complete, but it also lasts longer. A potential problem with attenuated live vaccines is that vaccinated people may temporarily shed virus into the environment. This is not a problem unless the shed virus has reverted to its wild-type, which may occasionally happen if the attenuation resulted from a point mutation. Genetic engineering of the viral nucleic acid minimizes this risk by introducing changes that are unlikely to revert to the wild-type. Genes conferring virulence or controlling crucial metabolic pathways can be removed or disabled. A currently insurmountable difficulty with live vaccines, however, is that they are unsuitable for anyone who is unable to mount a cell-mediated response (eg, an HIV+ patient). In addition, any vaccine that has extraneous substances involved in its manufacturing (eg, eggs) can cause allergies, which is a contraindication to its use.

DNA vaccines work along a different principle. A fragment of DNA encoding for a protein from the organism to be vaccinated against is inserted into a bacterial plasmid. After the introduction of the plasmid into the target cells, the stimulating antigen is produced inside the cell. Even RNA viruses such as hepatitis C and HIV should prove amenable to DNA vaccines because the nucleic acid that is inserted into the host genome is DNA encoding for viral proteins. As is the case for the live virus vector, DNA vaccines provide for a complete response, including cell-mediated immunity, because the immunogenic proteins that are encoded by the bacterial plasmid are synthesized in the cytoplasm of the patient's own cells, just as viral proteins would be. This means that they will have the complete posttranslational modification and 3-dimensional conformation to engender a maximal response.

In addition, the relevant DNA can be surrounded by DNA that enhances the body's reaction to the foreign DNA. For example, CD4 TH-1 lymphocytes secrete cytokines that favor cellular immunity at the expense of humoral immunity, whereas the converse is true of CD4 TH-2 cells. In dealing with HIV, for example, where a cellular response is needed, the portion of HIV RNA can be packaged with DNA from TH-1 lymphocytes, or with DNA encoding for interleuken12, which is one of the cytokines that stimulates cellular immunity. In addition, the plasmid itself has a considerable amount of unmethylated CpG nucleotides, characteristic of bacteria, and therefore serves as an excellent adjuvant. It is possible that with right "packaging" of DNA, a DNA vaccine could obviate the need for APCs or traditional adjuvants. Another advantage of DNA vaccines is that they do not require refrigeration and can be used more easily in underdeveloped regions.

A related approach is to introduce genes that encode for the antigens of interest into an attenuated virus and introducing this into patients. In this case, the virus is used as a vector. The intent is to induce a response to the proteins encoded by the new DNA it carries, not to the virus itself. Because viruses induce the full complement of immune responses, this procedure also induces a full humoral and cellular response.

Before we leave the immune response, we will have a final word on its possible applications in tumor biology. Many attempts have been made to battle neoplasms with immune therapy. These have generally been disappointing, undoubtedly because the body has already been exposed to and reacted to the tumor antigens that are administered iatrogenically. However, there is hope that a deliberate modification of the immune response, taking advantage of what has been learned in immunology, will permit us to engender a more effective immune response to tumor cells than nature is able to do. This, however, is a tall order, as nature has had many millions of years of experience and we have only a very incomplete picture assembled from a few generations of research.

Core Points for Normal Immune Function and the Inflammatory Response

- Innate immunity: early, but nonspecific response
  - o Physical barriers
  - o Acute inflammation
- Acute inflammation:
  - o Increase in blood flow
  - o Increased vascular permeability
  - o Adherence of leukocytes to the endothelium via cell adhesion molecules
  - o Diapedesis, chemotaxis, and activation of leukocytes
- Molecular mediators of acute inflammation:
  - o Those derived from arachidonic acid (prostaglandins and leukotrienes)
  - o Cytokines.
- If the outcome of acute inflammation is not favorable, chronic inflammation and/or scarring may result.
  - o Adaptive immunity: much more complex process that takes time, but the response is specific.
  - o Requires HLA molecules.
  - o HLA class 1 molecules are expressed on all nucleated cells, but class 2 HLA molecules are found only on some cells of the immune system.
- Both T and B lymphocytes undergo gene rearrangement in early development.
  - o B cells: rearrangement of the DNA that will form the immunoglobulin (Ig) molecule.
  - o T cells: DNA of the receptor is rearranged
- After gene rearrangement, additional diversification by addition or deletion of single nucleotides by the enzyme terminal deoxynucleotidyl transferase (TdT).
- In both T and B lymphocytes, the receptor is part of a much larger receptor complex.
- B and T cells then go through a series of additional maturational steps.
  - o The development of self-tolerance is an important part of maturation.
  - o Once mature, T and B cells must be activated by a series of interactions in lymph nodes or in the spleen.
- Product of B cell is Ig. Product of the T cell is a cytokine.
- Humoral immunity: portion of adaptive immunity that addresses *extracellular* microbes and antigens.
- Cell mediated immunity addresses *intracellular* microbes and antigens.
  - o CD8 cytotoxic T cells recognize antigen that is presented in conjunction with HLA class I molecules, permitting them to destroy any infected cell
  - o CD4 helper T cells recognize antigen that is presented in conjunction with HLA class 2 molecules, permitting them to work with other cells of the immune system.

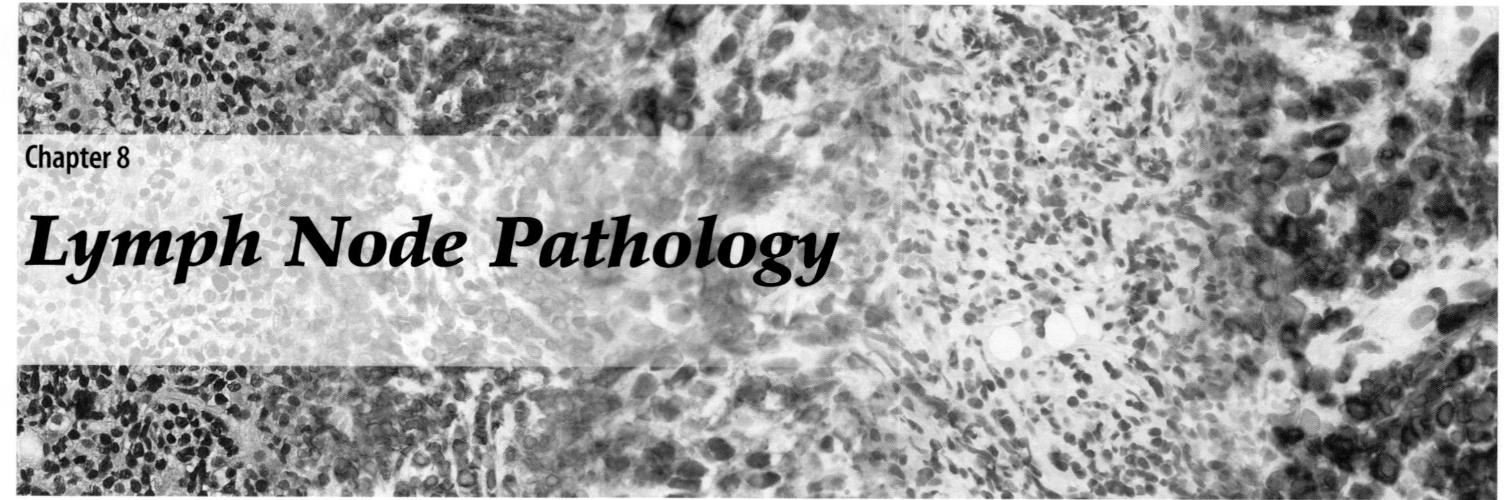

Chapter 8

Lymph Node Pathology

Benign Causes of Lymphadenopathy

Lymphadenopathy is a common presentation in medical practice, but over 80% of cases are caused by a benign process, a consequence of 1 or more lymph nodes reacting to antigenic stimulation [PMID15266094]. Benign lymphoid hyperplasia may be follicular or paracortical. The former primarily involves B cells, while the latter primarily involves T cells.

Follicular hyperplasia i8.1 is the most common form and is not discussed here, but its distinction from follicular lymphoma will be considered subsequently. Paracortical hyperplasia (also called interfollicular hyperplasia and sometimes called by the less appropriate term "diffuse hyperplasia") is often caused by a reaction to viruses or drugs. In paracortical hyperplasia, the normal lymph node architecture may be partially obscured and follicles may be indistinct i8.2a, i8.2b, i8.2c. Although the familiar follicular pattern may be vague, there is still a mixture of cell types, with numerous reactive T and B lymphocytes, and smaller lymphocytes dispersed throughout the node, imparting a "mottled" or "speckled" appearance i8.2d, i8.2e. Accentuation of sinuses ("sinus histiocytosis") is also sometimes considered a form of reactive hyperplasia, but is often associated with 1 of the other 2 forms i8.3.

A particularly troubling virus is the Epstein-Barr virus (EBV), which causes almost all cases of infectious mononucleosis, though other agents, such as toxoplasma, are rare causes of clinically similar findings. Mononucleosis is self-limiting but is of great importance in surgical pathology because tonsils or cervical lymph nodes involved by EBV, in addition to the loss of normal follicular architecture, may often have many very atypical immunoblasts that perfectly simulate large cell lymphoma. Nowhere is caution more needed than in the diagnosis of large cell lymphoma in the tonsillar/nasopharyngeal/cervical area in a young person for whom mononucleosis has not yet been excluded. The clue that mononucleosis should be considered is the mixture of cell types in addition to the putative large neoplastic lymphocytes i8.4a, i8.4b, but immunohistochemical stains are often needed to avoid an inappropriate diagnosis.

Drugs may cause a paracortical hyperplasia similar to that of viruses. The time-honored example is dilantin, but with the enormous expansion of our pharmaceutical arsenal and the great variety of idiosyncratic reactions, the list of exogenous agents that can cause a paracortical hyperplasia is nearly endless.

Dermatopathic lymphadenitis is characterized by paracortical hyperplasia caused by the arrival in the node of many interdigitating dendritic cells, such as Langerhans cells, which then elicit an immune response i8.5a. Melanin from the skin may be seen in paracortical areas i8.5b.

Kikuchi disease (also called Kikuchi-Fujimoto disease or histiocytic necrotizing lymphadenitis) is a self-limiting disorder, usually affecting cervical nodes in young Asian women, characterized by areas of necrosis with abundant neutrophilic karyorrhectic debris, but few intact neutrophils i8.6a. Histiocytes may be prominent in the areas that are not necrotic i8.6b.

Lymph nodes in any autoimmune disorder usually have follicular hyperplasia with essential architectural preservation, but plasma cells and immunoblasts can usually be found between the follicles, and there may be areas of paracortical necrosis and karyorrhectic debris.

Vascular transformation of lymph node sinuses involves the capsule and subcapsular sinuses. It resembles a diffuse hemangioma spreading throughout the sinuses and perhaps focally disrupting the architecture. It differs from Kaposi by sparing the parenchyma, having focal fibrosis, lacking spindle cell fascicles, and having better defined vessels i8.7.

Early lymph node involvement with HIV is characterized by follicular hyperplasia with unusually shaped follicles. This may be followed by hyperplasia of monocytoid B cells in paracortical areas, but the eventual result is follicular lysis i8.8 and follicular involution i8.9. Finally, there is lymphoid depletion of the node, as cell mediated immunity fades away [PMID8081317, PMID16341147].

Each of the 3 types of granulomas described in Chapter 7—caseating i8.10, necrotizing i8.11, and noncaseating, nonnecrotizing i8.12—can be found in lymph nodes, and each is theoretically associated with a relatively specific set of causes (eg, mycobacteria with caseating granulomas, cat-scratch disease with necrotizing granulomas, etc), but in practice, there is overlap and a frustrating inability to identify the cause of the process. Special stains are almost always negative unless the patient is immunocompromised, and most cases are either attributed to sarcoid or simply labeled as idiopathic. Nucleic acid amplification tests are becoming available for many causative organisms and might be undertaken in addition to or instead of the traditional acid fast and fungal stains [PMID21704272].

Progressive transformation of germinal centers is characterized by the entry of small lymphocytes into the germinal centers, such that the demarcation between the germinal center ıd a mantle zone is indistinct. The result is that some germinal nters are larger and darker than normal i8.13. The primary nportance of progressive transformation is the similarity of s appearance to that of nodular lymphocyte predominant odgkin disease (NLPHD), discussed momentarily.

There are 2 types of Castleman disease (angiofollicular yperplasia): the hyaline vascular type and the plasma cell type. he hyaline vascular variant of Castleman disease usually presıts as a single lymph node or a small group of adjacent lymph odes. This type has small germinal centers which have fewer mphocytes and relatively more follicular dendritic cells i8.14a, .14b. Immunohistochemical staining for follicular dendritic ells (CD21, CD35, clusterin, fascin) may help to highlight gerıinal centers and to identify the relative increase in follicular endritic cells. The mantle zones may have an "onion skin" ppearance i8.15. The interfollicular areas have increased vascurity but indistinct sinuses. Some apparent follicles may appear) have >1 germinal center and there may be some progressive ansformation of the atrophic germinal centers, rendering them ven less distinct. Some germinal centers will contain a hyalinzed vessel i8.16. The atrophic germinal centers may initially esemble granulomas.

The plasma cell variant of Castleman disease has fewer bnormalities of the follicles and is primarily characterized y large numbers of plasma cells between follicles i8.17a, i8.17b, ıough there may be some attenuation of sinuses. Unlike the yaline vascular type, the plasma cell type of Castleman may e either unicentric or multicentric, and is often accompanied y systemic symptoms, such as cytopenias, adenopathy, spleomegaly, night sweats, and hypergammaglobulinemia. In he unicentric presentation of this type of Castleman disease, ystemic symptoms may reverse after excision. The multicentric orm of the plasma cell type of Castleman disease may be assoiated with human herpesvirus-8 (HHV-8), in which case there s an association with HIV and the plasma cells are more likely o be plasmablastic. Multicentric Castleman disease almost nvariably has systemic symptoms as described above and is ggressive [PMID20461118, PMID19546611].

An important consideration in the diagnosis of the plasma ell variant of Castleman disease is IgG4-associated lymphdenopathy. Lymph nodes may be involved in the IgG4 disorders [PMID20403026], and if they are, there may be substantial imilarities to the plasma cell variant of Castleman disease PMID19270642]. Lymph nodes in IgG4 lymphadenopathy also have nany plasma cells, and these patients may also have anemia ınd hypergammaglobulinemia, but unlike Castleman disease, here will often also be numerous eosinophils in the node n IgG4-associated adenopathy, and there is often peripheral eosinophilia. Serum IgG4 will be elevated and immunohistochemistry will demonstrate that the plasma cells in the tissue express IgG4. It is prudent to measure serum IgG4, perform an mmunohistochemical stain for IgG4 on the lymph node tissue, and exclude fibroinflammatory conditions at other sites before making the diagnosis of the plasma cell form of Castleman disease. Because the pancreas is the most common site of the IgG4-related sclerosing disorders, this entity is discussed in detail in Chapter 24.

Metastatic Neoplasms in Lymph Nodes

Little will be said of metastatic malignancies to lymph nodes, as these are seldom diagnostically difficult, except to point out that some malignancies, such as lymphoepithelial carcinoma, lobular carcinoma of the breast, melanoma, and seminoma, may resemble a lymphoma in a metastasis.

Immunohistochemistry in Lymphomas

Because immunohistochemistry is essential in the diagnosis of hematopoietic neoplasms, we must be aware of potential difficulties in the interpretation of these stains. In Chapter 1, we encountered some of the potential pitfalls in the interpretation of immunohistochemical stains. In hematopathology, there are 3 additional hazards. First, some antigens may have more than 1 name. These include CD10 (=CALLA), CD20 (=L26), CD15 (=LeuM1), CD30 (=Ber-H2), cyclin D1 (=bcl-1), and CD45RO (UCHL1, a T-cell antigen). CD45 (=leukocyte common antigen [LCA]) is a family of related antigens, 1 or more of which is found on all nonerythroid hematopoietic cells.

Second, as discussed in Chapter 1, before interpreting immunohistochemical stains, one should be certain where in the cell the target protein should be found. Subcellular localization of staining can be important in many types of tumors, but is especially important in hematopoietic tumors. Many of these stains, such as CD3, CD4, CD5, CD8, CD10, CD20, CD23, CD30, CD43, CD45, CD45RO, CD56, CD99, and CD138, are cell membrane stains. CD15 staining is predominantly membranous, though there is some staining of the Golgi zone, which imparts a cytoplasmic component. Bcl-2 is a perinuclear stain (it is on the outer membrane of mitochondria), though admittedly in a small lymphocytes, the distinction between perinuclear, cytoplasmic, and cell membrane staining is difficult. Transcription factors, proliferation factors, TdT, cyclin D1 (bcl-1), and bcl-6 are nuclear stains. CD79 is cytoplasmic. General background staining is more likely to be interpreted as a false positive with nuclear staining than with positivity in other locations, so one should compare possible positive nuclear staining with the control and with background in cells believed to be negative. Also, nuclear antigens are more sensitive to artifactual negativity from degeneration than those in the cytoplasm.

Third, many B-cell lymphoid proliferations have a population of benign T cells, and CD5 and CD43 stain normal T cells as well as some neoplastic B cells (CD43 also stains some myeloid cells). Therefore, in interpreting these 2 immunohistochemical stains in B-cell lymphomas, it is essential to compare any positivity to the number and distribution of T cells, as seen by the CD3 stain. Only if the CD5 and CD43 show clearly more positivity than CD3 can it be concluded that the stain is in a B-cell population of interest.

Hodgkin Disease

The WHO classification of Hodgkin disease [Swerdlow ISBN978-9283224310] has largely replaced the older Rye system and recognizes classical Hodgkin disease (HD) and nodular (not diffuse) lymphocyte predominant (NLPHD) types. The classical type is further broken down into nodular sclerosing, mixed cellularity, lymphocyte rich, and lymphocyte depleted.

ISBN 978-089189-5886

Classical Hodgkin Disease

Classical HD is a lymphoproliferative disorder characterized by enigmatic lymphocytes called Reed-Sternberg cells (R-S cells), which are the only neoplastic cells. There are a number of morphologic variants of R-S cells, but all have some expression of B-cell antigens and may have immunoglobulin gene rearrangement. For years, the nature of the R-S cell was unclear, and while its precise nature has still not been fully clarified, they occasionally react with the postgerminal center marker MUM1, suggesting that they are crippled germinal center or late germinal center B cells that cannot express antigen receptor. B cell transcription factors are expressed, but in diminished amounts in classical HD [PMID12118370].

The 2 immunohistochemical stains that are associated with R-S cells are CD15 and CD30, and the cells are generally negative for CD20. However, about 20% of R-S cells in classical Hodgkin may be CD20 positive and about 40% may be negative for CD15. CD30 is much more commonly positive and is virtually required for the diagnosis of classical HD, but CD30 is not specific for R-S cells, and may also stain the neoplastic cells in anaplastic lymphoma, T-cell rich B-cell lymphoma (TCRBCL), rare cases of diffuse large cell B lymphoma that are not anaplastic, and benign T and B immunoblasts. In addition to CD30 positivity, the putative R-S cells should also be either CD15 positive or CD45 negative. CD45 negativity is more important than CD15 positivity. The 3 most important stains in the workup of a possible case of classical HD are CD15, CD30, and CD45. CD30 positivity and CD45 negativity in the putative R-S cells are essentially required for the diagnosis of classical HD. There is some association of HD with EBV, but only in about 50% of cases [PMID20008234].

Nodular sclerosing Hodgkin disease (NSHD) is characterized by fibrous bands that anastomose and divide the tissue into lobules i8.18, but the critical criterion is the nature of the R-S variant. While all forms of the R-S cell can be found in any form of Hodgkin disease i8.19, in NSHD, the most common form is called a lacunar cell and consists of an atypical nucleus that is surrounded by a clear area i8.20. This clear area is actually an artifact, but it is useful and reproducible. Like all forms of R-S cells, the lacunar cell is negative for CD45 i8.21a, positive for CD15 i8.21b, and positive for CD30 i8.21c.

Cellular forms of NSHD may resemble mixed cellularity HD because the fibrous bands are less prominent, but the predominant R-S type is still the lacunar cell, and the diagnosis of NSHD takes precedent over other types, even if it is only present focally.

NSHD has been subclassified into lymphocyte predominant, mixed cellularity, and lymphocyte depleted subtypes, but this subclassification is unlikely to be clinically useful, and it runs the risk of obscuring the fundamental diagnosis of NSHD, perhaps causing the reader to believe that the fundamental diagnosis is classical HD of another type or NLPHD, a very different entity. If any subclassification of NSHD is helpful, it is a 2-tiered system, wherein grade 2 NSHD occurs if any of the following are found [PMID11896065]:

1. >25% of nodules show lymphocyte depletion or increased numbers of R-S cells. These 2 features occur together because the large number of R-S cells results in fewer lymphocytes. Confluent sheets of R-S cells simulate a syncytium, accounting for the designation of the syncytial variant of NSHD i8.22.
2. >25% of nodules have bizarre R-S cells i8.23.
3. >80% of nodules have a fibrohistiocytic reaction.

More than the other forms of classical HD, the mixed cellularity type (MCHD) typically has the classic, mirror-image form of the R-S cell i8.24a, i8.24b. The background cells are a mixture of inflammatory cell types, with eosinophils being occasionally prominent, along with neutrophils, plasma cells, and macrophages. Fibrosis may be present, but not to the extent that is seen in NSHD. Some cases of MCHD have an interfollicular growth pattern that leaves the nodal architecture partially intact.

Lymphocyte-rich classical HD is a new category of the WHO system. It is characterized by minimal fibrosis, a growth pattern that is generally at least partially nodular i8.25a, minimal numbers of nonlymphoid background cells, and R-S cells that can have several appearances, including classical, lacunar, or the LP cell that is found in NLPHD.

The subtle nodular pattern and the occasional morphologic similarity of the R-S cells in lymphocyte-rich classical HD with the LP cells in NLPHD may cause these 2 lymphomas to appear similar. The similarity of these 2 entities is heightened by the fact that most cases of classical HD have a predominance of T lymphocytes in the background, but B lymphocytes predominate in NLPHD [PMID19605845] and in lymphocyte-rich classical HD [Swerdlow ISBN978-9283224310]. However, the atypical cells in lymphocyte-rich classical HD have all the immunohistochemical features of the R-S cells in other forms of classical HD. Specifically they are positive for CD15 and CD30 i8.25b, i8.25c, and negative for CD45, whereas the reverse is true for the LP cells in NLPHD (see below).

Lymphocyte-depleted HD is a high-grade form that is rarely specifically diagnosed [PMID19455461]. Almost all of these cases are a lymphocyte depleted form of NSHD i8.26a, i8.26b, i8.26c or they are non-Hodgkin lymphoma (NHL), and in fact, lymphocyte-depleted HD may not be a distinct entity. Lymphocyte depleted Hodgkin disease is associated with greatly diminished cell mediated immunity. The lymphocyte depleted and syncytial variants of Hodgkin disease are the major high-grade forms.

The differential diagnosis of HD is wide and includes a number of entities, depending on the location and type of HD under consideration. Carcinoma is a possibility in cases of the syncytial form. Nasopharyngeal carcinoma, with its many "passenger" lymphocytes, can be confused with HD. Progressive transformation of germinal centers, granulomatous lymphadenitis, germ cell tumors, reactive immunoblastic proliferations, and sarcoma (if there is a fibrohistiocytic reaction) must all be excluded. Once the diagnosis of lymphoma has been secured, a NHL must be excluded, especially such entities as TCRBCL, large cell lymphoma, and anaplastic lymphoma (because the atypical nuclei in anaplastic lymphoma are also CD30 positive). A useful algorithm is to ask a series of questions in succession: Is the process fundamentally lymphoid, or are the lymphocytes incidental? If the process is fundamentally lymphoid, is it malignant or reactive? If it is the former, is it HD or a NHL?

In a patient with known Hodgkin disease, a problematic uation may arise in regard to what constitutes sufficient teria for involvement by Hodgkin of secondary sites, such marrow and spleen. One can be suspicious of bone marrow volvement if there are such findings as fibrosis, necrosis, sinophilia, architectural distortion, or aggregates of lym- ocytes or macrophages, but these are not diagnostic. Some m of R-S cells is required for the diagnosis of classical HD any site at any time i8.27, but if the diagnosis of Hodgkin sease has already been documented, atypical mononuclear ls in an additional site, if they are CD15 or CD30 positive pecially CD30) and CD45 negative, can be regarded as R-S ls and the diagnosis of an additional focus of classical HD n be made, even if the atypical cells do not manifest the ssic H&E morphologic features of a R-S cell variant.

odular Lymphocyte Predominant Hodgkin isease (NLPHD)

NLPHD is a lymphoproliferative disorder characterized a vaguely nodular proliferation i8.28. The vast majority of nphocytes are small and benign, but within the nodules, e neoplastic cells are large lymphocytes i8.29 that often ve lobated nuclei i8.30. These cells have been called L&H mphocytic and histiocytic) cells. Because of the frequently bated nucleus, they have also been called popcorn cells. The rrently preferred term is "LP cell" [PMID20029973].

LP cells were thought to be a type of R-S cell, but in con- st to classical HD, the atypical cells in NLPHD are negative CD15 i8.31 and CD30 i8.32, and are positive for CD45 i8.33. ey demonstrate greater staining for CD20 and CD79 than e neoplastic cells of classical HD. The neoplastic cells in LPHD are positive for bcl-6, a marker for follicular center cells [PMID12579988]. Classic R-S cells or atypical cells that stain sitively for CD15 or CD30 are very rare in NLPHD, and e diagnosis should be questioned if such cells are found. hereas a minority of cases of classical HD is positive for 3V, NLPHD is uniformly negative for this virus [PMID20063524].

This combination of immunohistochemical staining and formation from molecular biology studies distinguishes LPHD from classical HD, and satisfies most investigators at NLPHD is in fact a type of NHL or an initial stage of HL. There is evidence that both NLPHD and classical HD e neoplasms of germinal center B cells, the difference being at there are ongoing somatic mutations in NLPHD, whereas e cells in classical HD are crippled and do not undergo addi- nal mutations [PMID20008234].

The diagnosis of NLPHD requires a nodular architecture roughout the node. The existence of a diffuse form of lym- ocyte predominant Hodgkin disease is questioned and the HO does not currently recognize such a variant. However, e nodules are subtle. In NLPHD, the atypical cells should essentially completely restricted to the nodules. CD20 will ghlight the nodules i8.34 and should confirm that the atypi- l cells are essentially found only within them. CD21, which ains follicular dendritic cells, highlights follicles even better 35. If lymphoid tissue has a distinct nodular architecture, it not NLPHD and the diagnosis is more likely either follicu- r hyperplasia or follicular lymphoma.

Although there may be more B cells in the background in NLPHD than in classical HD, CD3 staining will also show that the atypical cells are surrounded by a collarette of T cells i8.36 [PMID12579988].

The differential diagnosis of NLPHD includes classical HD of the lymphocyte-rich type, NHL with a follicular pattern, TCRBCL, and progressive transformation of germinal centers [PMID19605845]. Differentiation of NLPHD from lymphocyte-rich classical HD is accomplished by immunohistochemistry, as the atypical cells of the latter entity have classic R-S staining characteristics.

The immunohistochemical profile of NLPHD substantially overlaps that of NHL, but 4 findings are helpful in distinguishing NLPHD from follicular NHLs. First, there may be as many as 15-20 atypical cells per high-power field (HPF) in the nodular areas in NLPHD i8.37, but an appreciably larger number is suggestive of a NHL. Second, in NLPHD, the atypical cells are confined to the nodules. Any significant number of atypical cells between the nodules warrants a consideration of a NHL rather than NLPHD. Third, focal staining of the atypical cells for epithelial membrane antigen (EMA) suggests NLPHD i8.38, but only 21% of NLPHD will have any such staining [PMID12579988]. Fourth, follicular lymphomas with a follicular pattern are generally positive for bcl-2, whereas only 5% of NLPHD will express this protein [PMID12579988].

NLPHD may resemble TCRBCL, and immunohistochemically, no single marker separates these 2 entities. But a panel, exploiting differences in the probability that a given marker will be positive, is effective, and even on H&E, TCRBCL differs from NLPHD in being diffuse and having higher grade nuclei [PMID20063524].

Progressive transformation of germinal centers causes an appearance similar to NLPHD because it partially obscures the germinal centers, and NLPHD must be excluded before a diagnosis of progressive transformation is made. Progressive transformation of germinal centers, NLPHD, and TCRBCL may be related entities [PMID19918327]. Activated lymphocytes from the germinal center in progressive transformation may resemble the LP cells of NLPHD and may be CD20 positive, but immunohistochemical staining will not show rosetting by T lymphocytes, which is occasionally seen in NLPHD.

Non-Hodgkin Lymphomas (NHLs)

The NHLs and sarcomas are the 2 groups for which the greatest progress is being made in understanding pathogenesis through cytogenetic abnormalities. In the case of NHLs, many of these abnormalities are translocations that result in proto-oncogenes coming to rest next to the regulatory portion of immunoglobulin genes. This leads to high levels of gene expression and/or gene expression at inappropriate times, and transforms the proto-oncogene into an oncogene. The clinical presentation of B-cell lymphomas varies greatly, but patients often have classic "B symptoms": fever, weight loss, and night sweats.

The REAL classification system, published in 1994, takes into account immunohistochemical and genotypic information in addition to morphology. The WHO classification of systemic NHLs [Swerdlow ISBN978-9283224310] is based on the REAL system and is presented below, after which each entity will

ISBN 978-089189-5886

be discussed separately. For lymphomas confined to the skin, the joint WHO/European Organization for the Research and Treatment of Cancer (EORTC) classification [PMID16293178, PMID15692063] is recommended and is discussed in Chapter 40.

The diagnosis of hematopoietic neoplasms requires either flow cytometry or an extensive panel of immunohistochemical stains. Flow cytometry passes cells past a laser. The scattering of the light in the forward direction, parallel to the laser light, provides information on the size of the cell (specifically on the cell surface area). Side-scattered light, at right angles to the laser light, provides information about the granularity of the cytoplasm, including the number and distribution of organelles and the nature and number of leukocyte granules.

Flow cytometric light scattering is used in many automated hematology analyzers, but is rarely used in the diagnosis of hematopoietic neoplasms. In these neoplasms, the tissue is disaggregated and the cells are exposed to monoclonal antibodies that bind both to individual proteins and to a fluorescent dye. As the cells pass a laser, the intensity of fluorescence permits a determination of the number of cells that express that protein and the degree of expression, permitting the classification of the cell [PMID21204710]. Current antigen retrieval and immunohistochemical techniques can almost always substitute for flow cytometry, thus bringing the diagnosis of hematopoietic neoplasms into the purview of the community hospital laboratory.

While clonality is the essence of neoplasia, it is fortunately not necessary in most cases to demonstrate clonal origin to diagnose and characterize a lymphoma. The H&E appearance, in conjunction with the immunohistochemical/flow cytometric profile establishes the diagnosis of lymphoma in the vast majority of cases. In the rare cases in which clonality must be shown, a ratio of kappa to λ light chains of 16:1 or more is suggestive of clonality, but definitive proof requires demonstration of immunoglobulin gene rearrangement, the details of which were discussed in Chapter 7.

Although a lymphoid mass that is composed only of B cells or T cells is suspicious for a lymphoma, as normal or hyperplastic nodes generally contain both cell types, malignancy must be proven by a combination of morphology of individual cells, architectural distortion, and immunophenotyping. In benign effusions with lymphocytes, the lymphocytes tend to be T cells [PMID3087054], and a large number of B lymphocytes in an effusion is suspicious, but confirmation is necessary. Because there is no opportunity to assess architecture in effusions, the appearance of the cells and their immunohistochemical characteristics are used.

Unlike carcinomas and melanomas, an in situ stage is not readily recognized or employed in lymphomas or sarcoma, but the concept of in situ lymphoma is gaining acceptance and is characterized by lymph nodes in which lymphocytes remain in their normal intranodal compartments, such that the histologic appearance is unaltered, but express aberrant antigens [PMID21224472]. Specifically, convincing positivity of B lymphocytes in germinal centers for bcl-2 is an indication of probable in situ follicular lymphoma [PMID21771030].

World Health Organization Classification of B-Cell Neoplasms

I. Precursor B-cell neoplasms:

Because precursor B-lymphoblastic leukemia/lymphoma (the cells are identical in the leukemic and solid tissue manifestations) usually presents as a leukemia, it is discussed in Chapter 10, as are the numerous genetic abnormalities that have been described for this group of neoplasms.

II. Mature (peripheral) B-cell neoplasms

- a. B-cell chronic lymphocytic leukemia/small lymphocytic lymphoma
- b. B-cell prolymphocytic leukemia
- c. Lymphoplasmacytic lymphoma
- d. Splenic marginal zone B-cell lymphoma (+/– villous lymphocytes), discussed in Chapter 9
- e. Hairy cell leukemia
- f. Plasma cell neoplasms: myeloma, plasmacytoma, Ig deposition disease, heavy chain disease, discussed in Chapter 10
- g. Extranodal marginal zone B-cell lymphoma of mucosa-associated lymphoid tissue type
- h. Nodal marginal zone lymphoma (+/– monocytoid B cells)
- i. Follicle center lymphoma, follicular, grades 1-3
- j. Mantle cell lymphoma
- k. Diffuse large cell B-cell lymphoma, with numerous variants, including:
    1. Centroblastic (usual type). Mixture of cleaved and noncleaved cells, despite the fact that the normal centroblast is noncleaved.
    2. Immunoblastic
    3. T cell/histiocyte rich
    4. Anaplastic (very rare; most anaplastic lymphomas are of T origin)
    5. Mediastinal large B-cell lymphoma
    6. Primary effusion lymphoma
    7. Intravascular
    8. Plasmablastic
- l. Burkitt lymphoma/Burkitt cell leukemia and Burkitt-like lymphoma

The "Small Cell" Lymphomas

We first consider lymphomas in which the neoplastic cells are only slightly larger than normal lymphocytes, as opposed to the significantly larger lymphocytes of the diffuse large cell group. The "small cell" group consists primarily of lymphomas that arise from the follicular center (ie, from cells in the germinal center itself), the mantle zone, the marginal zone, small lymphocytic lymphoma (SLL; tissue counterpart to chronic lymphoid leukemia [CLL]), and the lymphoplasmacytic lymphoma.

Follicular Lymphomas

Even with immunohistochemical and DNA studies, the differentiation of follicular hyperplasia from follicular lymphoma remains difficult, and H&E examination remains a mainstay in this distinction. Because follicles in follicular mphomas no longer contain the admixed benign cells (such macrophages with tingible bodies) that are seen in normal rminal centers, and because they no longer perform the nctions of a normal germinal center, they are often referred as nodules rather than follicles. These 2 terms are used nonymously when referring to lymphomas, but the term erminal center" is not appropriate in lymphomas. Although e WHO specifically uses the term "follicular lymphoma," I commend the designation of "nodular lymphoma" because ollicle is a normal structure (consisting of a germinal center d a mantle zone), whereas the term "nodule," which is not ed in referring to normal lymph nodes, ensures that there is misunderstanding that the clusters are abnormal. In defer-ce to the WHO, however, one could say "follicular (nodular) mphoma."

Follicular lymphomas usually have more follicles than fol-ular hyperplasia, and they are more uniform in size and ape i8.39, but the most important feature of follicular lym-oma on H&E is the lack of the normal mixed population of lls in the putative germinal center i8.40. Because the normal chitecture of the node is largely lost and there are no sinuses demarcation of cortical and paracortical areas, the follicles e found throughout the node, in areas where normal germi-l centers would not be expected.

In a benign follicle, the mantle zone is asymmetric and more cellular adjacent to the lighter zone of the germinal nter i8.41a. In follicular lymphomas, since the follicles are normal and not places of B-cell maturation, this polariza-n is not seen. Instead, mantle zones are less prominent d surround the follicle with evenly distributed cellularity 41b. Mitoses in benign follicles are predominantly in the rk area of the germinal center, away from the more cel-lar area of the mantle zone. There are fewer mitoses in fol-ular center lymphomas than in benign follicles i8.42a, i8.42b, though the number of mitoses increases as the number of rge cells increases, and mitoses in neoplastic follicles tend be evenly distributed (this is best shown with Ki-67 stain-g). These changes result in follicles that do not have the tricate internal structure of normal follicles, but rather are ore homogeneous in size, shape, distribution, composition, d mitotic activity.

CD21, which stains the follicular dendritic cells (not lym-ocytes) in the follicles can highlight subtle follicles and monstrate that a lymphoma is not diffuse i8.43a, i8.43b. mphomas of follicular center origin are negative for CD5, sitive for bcl-6 i8.44, and usually (but not always) positive r CD10 i8.45. In general, the presence of CD10 or bcl-6 has significant role in the diagnosis of lymphoma, but rather restricted to the subtyping of a lymphoma. However, the esence of CD10 or bcl-6—markers for follicular center lls—between follicles is an indication of neoplasia because demonstrates that follicle center cells are in an abnormal cation [PMID10843287].

BCL-2 is a normal gene whose protein product, bcl-2, otects the cell from intrinsic apoptosis. Following conven-n, *BCL-2* (italicized capital letters) refers to the gene, while l-2 (small letters) refers to the protein product of the gene nall-case letters are used for most proteins in this work, ough geneticists use unitalicized capital letters for proteins). eterodimers of bcl-2-bax lead to a normal state of balance between apoptosis and survival. Bax-bax homodimers lead to early apoptosis, while bcl-2 homodimers prevent apoptosis, and facilitate cell survival [PMID21056595]. *BCL-2* is an example of a normal gene that functions as an oncogene when overex-pressed. 85% of follicular lymphomas have t(14;18)(q32.3;q21) i8.46. This number rises to essentially 100% if it is a grade 1 fol-licular center cell lymphoma. This translocation results in the juxtaposition of the *BCL-2* gene (normally on chromosome 18) to the J region of immunoglobulin heavy chain gene on chro-mosome 14, resulting in overexpression of the bcl-2 protein and diminished apoptosis. The presence of this translocation is essentially diagnostic of follicular center cell lymphoma in the presence of a compatible histologic picture. This transloca-tion is usually demonstrated by fluorescent in situ hybridiza-tion (FISH), though PCR can be used.

Rarely, a lymphoma will be positive for the t(14;18), but neg-ative for the bcl-2 protein by immunohistochemistry. These cases are thought to be point mutations in the translocated *BCL-2* gene that do not change the FISH results, since FISH probes are large and usually will hybridize even in the pres-ence of a point mutation, but result in a slightly altered bcl-2 protein that is not detected by available antibodies.

Because bcl-2 is a normal product that can be detected by immunohistochemistry even without overexpression, its presence does not necessarily imply lymphoma or, if lym-phoma has been proven, the finding of bcl-2 does not neces-sarily imply follicular center origin. This is why the t(14;18) is essentially specific for follicular center lymphoma if the histologic appearance is supportive, but the presence of bcl-2 is not, and can be found in benign lymphoid tissue, marginal zone lymphomas, mantle cell lymphomas, and even T-cell lymphomas. Because the bcl-2 protein is found in many different situations, it is one of the less important markers obtained in lymph node immunophenotyping studies. Bcl-2 protein expression is an indication of malignancy only in the restricted situation of follicular hyperplasia vs follicular lym-phoma, and only if it is positive throughout the follicle i8.47. A normal follicle may have bcl-2 positivity in the mantle zone, but not in the germinal center (the reason for this is that clonal selection via apoptosis is an important event in the germinal center, and the protective presence of excess bcl-2 there would undermine this important occurrence), whereas this matura-tional process does not occur in neoplastic follicles.

Although there are rare exceptions, lymphomas that have a distinct follicular (nodular) pattern will generally be of B-cell origin and will generally be derived from germinal center lymphocytes. In the WHO system, follicular (nodular) lymphomas are graded 1, 2, or 3 depending on the number of large cells (centroblasts) *in the follicles*. As discussed in Chapter 7, centroblasts are the precursor cells of centrocytes and are generally larger, with peripheralized chromatin, 1 or more nucleoli, and more cytoplasm than is present in a centrocyte. Those follicular lymphomas with 5 large cells or less per HPF are grade 1 i8.48. Some might use the term "cen-trocytic lymphoma" for these lymphomas because they are composed almost entirely of centrocytes. Follicular lympho-mas with between 6-15 large cells per HPF are grade 2 i8.49, and those with >15 are grade 3 i8.50 [PMID17616995], following the general principle that higher-grade neoplasms are composed of less mature cells.

ISBN 978-089189-5886

This raises the difficult and unsettled question of how centroblasts should be identified. Some believe that centroblasts should be identified on the basis of the physical size of the cell. The initial definition of a large cell, still used by some, is that it is 3 times the size of a centrocyte. Others believe that the chromatin pattern and presence of nucleoli is the deciding factor. There are occasional cases in the size of the cells suggests 1 grade while the chromatin pattern suggests another i8.51. In these cases, it may be helpful to consider the proliferation as assessed by Ki-67. A grade 1 or 2 follicular lymphoma usually does not have a Ki-67 in excess of 10%, and certainly not in excess of 20%. In a borderline case, if the proliferation is in excess of 20%, it might be prudent to lean toward a higher grade i8.52 [PMID16224216].

Grade 1 follicular lymphomas are indolent, though about a third may transform into a large cell lymphoma, and they are actually more difficult to cure than high-grade follicular or diffuse large cell lymphomas. The prognostic breakpoint in follicular lymphomas is between a grade 2 and a grade 3, as the latter tends to behave like a diffuse large cell lymphoma. Grade 3a lymphomas still have some small cells, while 3b lymphomas are essentially a pure large cell neoplasm and differ from diffuse large cell lymphoma only in the presence of discernible follicles. Any lymphoma that has been treated will likely have a higher percentage of small cells than it had in its original state, as these are more resistant to therapy than larger cells. In a patient who has been treated, a grade 1 follicular lymphoma may have originally been a grade 2 or grade 3.

In any lymphoma with any follicular architecture, there should be an estimation of the percentage of diffuse areas. A lymphoma should be specifically called "follicular and diffuse" if the follicular areas are between 25% and 75%.

A grade 1 follicular lymphoma with *only* small lymphocytes and with a *completely* diffuse pattern is not specifically recognized in the WHO system, and most of these lymphomas will be of another type, such as mantle cell. A lymphoma of follicular center origin, even if low-grade, virtually always has a few centroblasts.

Mantle Cell Lymphoma

Mantle cell lymphomas are thought to arise from lymphocytes that are prefollicular and not yet exposed to antigen stimulation [PMID19880776]. When a mature B cell is stimulated, it becomes a larger dividing cell called a centroblast, which after division becomes a small centrocyte. Because the lymphocytes in a mantle cell lymphoma have not been antigenically stimulated, they have not been transformed into a larger centroblast, and are essentially indistinguishable from lymphocytes of follicular center origin that have been transformed into larger cells, but have divided and returned to their original size. Because they have never been exposed to antigen, they do not form follicles. The result is a diffuse growth of small lymphocytes i8.53, but there may be a faint nodularity i8.54, especially if there is growth around residual, naked germinal centers i8.55. For this reason, the presence of occasional normal germinal centers does not exclude a mantle cell lymphoma. Residual normal germinal centers may cause an erroneous diagnosis of benign lymph node or result in an inappropriate diagnosis of follicular lymphoma, implying follicular center origin. In mantle cell lymphoma, neoplastic cells may also enter normal germinal centers, and obliterate them or render them indistinct i8.56. This is called follicular colonization and can cause the lymphoma to appear follicular.

The bcl-1/cyclin D1 positivity that is characteristic and nearly diagnostic of mantle cell lymphomas stems from a t(11;14)(q13:q32.3) that places the *BCL-1* gene (also called *CCND1*), normally present on chromosome 11, adjacent to the gene coding for immunoglobulin heavy chain on chromosome 14. The product of *BCL-1* is a protein called bcl-1, or cyclin D1, which regulates entry into the cell cycle. Like *BCL-2*, *BCL-1* is a normal gene that functions as an oncogene if it is overexpressed.

Cyclins are considered in detail in Chapter 46, but overexpression of cyclin D1 causes the retinoblastoma tumor suppressor protein to be phosphorylated and to lose its ability to regulate transcription factor E2F. The demonstration of bcl-1/cyclin D1 by immunohistochemistry in a lymphoproliferative disorder i8.57 is essentially diagnostic of mantle cell lymphoma in most cases.

The rare cases of mantle cell lymphomas that do not have demonstrable bcl-1 protein by immunohistochemistry can be diagnosed by demonstrating translocation of the *BCL-1* gene by FISH i8.58. PCR is not a good method of detecting t(11;14)(q13:q32.3) because there are multiple breakpoints, each requiring a different set of primers, whereas a FISH probe is large enough to sit atop any of these breakpoints and still give a positive reading. Exceptionally rare cases of mantle cell lymphomas do not have t(11;14)(q13:q32.3) and are thought to involve other cyclins that are also involved in regulation of the cell cycle.

In addition to bcl-1, CD5 and CD10 are also useful in the diagnosis of mantle cell lymphoma, as these lymphomas stain in a reverse pattern from those of germinal center origin—mantle cell lymphomas are usually positive for CD5 and negative for CD10. The difficulty here, however, is that not all lymphomas of germinal center origin are positive for CD10, and CD5 also stains T cells (for this reason, it is wise to compare CD5 positivity with any CD3 staining in the evaluation of a B-cell lymphoma; if the 2 stains are similar, the population is of T-cell origin and should not be considered in evaluating the lymphoma).

CD43 may help in the distinction of mantle cell lymphoma from lymphomas of germinal center origin, as it is positive in 90% of the former [PMID10095879] and is rare in the latter [PMID18359244]. Most mantle cell lymphomas are positive for FMC7, a particular conformation of CD20 [PMID14608903]. Bcl-6 may help, as it stains follicular center cells, benign or malignant, but not mantle cells i8.59. Bcl-6 expression, if any, should be restricted to residual germinal centers, whereas much greater and more widespread expression is to be expected in lymphomas of follicular center origin. But bcl-1 expression by immunohistochemistry or identification of t(11;14)(q13:q32.3) is by far the sentinel characteristic of mantle cell lymphoma.

Mantle cell lymphoma may also resemble CLL/SLL, as both of these consist of small lymphocytes with a diffuse growth pattern. Because both mantle cell lymphoma and CLL/SLL are positive for CD5 and CD43, and negative for CD10, their immunohistochemical separation relies primarily on the bcl-1 positivity in mantle cell lymphoma. CD23 (mantle cell lymphoma negative, CLL/SLL positive) and FMC7 (mantle ll lymphomas positive, CLL/SLL negative) can also be helpl [PMID14608903]. Also helpful is that in the absence of residual rminal centers and follicular colonization, there should be rtually no large cells in a mantle cell lymphoma, whereas rger cells are routinely seen in SLL around vaguely defined dules called proliferation centers.

While mantle cell lymphoma is nearly always a uniform pulation of small lymphocytes, a rare blastic form has been scribed i8.60a, i8.60b, i8.60c [PMID9753060].

rginal Zone Lymphoma

WHO recognizes 3 varieties of marginal zone lymphoma: dal, splenic, and extranodal [Swerdlow ISBN978-9283224310]. The tranodal form is often clinically manifest as a proliferation of mucosa-associated lymphoid tissue (the so-called ALToma). Marginal zone lymphomas have a monocytoid cell morphology (ie, a moderate amount of clear cytoplasm) 61a, i8.61b about half of the time, and can also be plasmacyd i8.62 or simply small lymphocytic in their appearance. oreover, a monocytoid morphology does not guarantee arginal zone lineage. Consequently, the term "monocytoid mphoma" is now discouraged.

To my mind, the term "MALToma" is no longer appropri- because mucosa-associated lymphoid infiltrates are a terogeneous and diagnostically challenging collection of tities that must be individually evaluated. Not all clini- "MALTomas" will be of marginal zone origin (eg, many strointestinal lymphoid polyps are of mantle cell origin). e only way to properly work through such a situation is employ the same step-by-step algorithm that should be ed elsewhere. Is it lymphoid? Is it benign or malignant? me mucosa associated lymphoid infiltrates are benign and active. The best known example of this is gastric reactive mphoid infiltrates—simulating a lymphoma to perfecn on H&E—caused by *Helicobacter pylori*, but there is also inking that some mucosa-associated lymphoid infiltrates the eye may be secondary to *Chlamydia psittaci* [PMID20574170]. a mucosa-associated lymphoid proliferation is neoplastic, hat is the specific type of lymphoma? Some are marginal ne lymphomas and some are lymphomas of another type. ucosa-associated lymphoid proliferations are immunohischemically evaluated as in other sites to reach a specific agnosis. The use of the word "MALToma" short-circuits this ethodical thought process.

The growth pattern of marginal zone lymphomas is difse, but like mantle cell lymphomas, they may grow between rmal germinal centers i8.63, creating the illusion of a nodu- lymphoma or even of a benign process because the idenication of germinal centers is reassuring. Consequently, the ne-honored concept that germinal centers indicate a benign ocess, while fundamentally sound, is not airtight. Germinal nters that are polarized into centroblastic and centrocytic eas, that are surrounded by asymmetric mantle zones, and at are part of an overall architecture that includes paracortil areas and sinuses, are the true key to a benign process.

Also like mantle cell lymphomas, marginal zone lymomas may exhibit follicular colonization i8.64, leading to a guely nodular architecture and diminished demarcation tween the neoplastic and nonneoplastic zones. Not all noral germinal center cells are positive for CD10, but a large number of CD10– cells in a vaguely defined apparent follicle suggests that follicular colonization by a mantle cell or marginal zone lymphoma should be excluded. In follicular colonization by either a mantle cell or a marginal zone lymphoma, immunohistochemical staining for bcl-6 may help identify germinal centers, as it stains lymphocytes of germinal center origin. CD21, CD35, clusterin, and fascin highlight follicular dendritic cells and can also assist in recognizing subtle or colonized germinal centers.

Many marginal zone lymphomas have trisomies of 3, 12, or 18, though none of these are specific. Marginal zone lymphomas are generally negative for both CD5 and CD10. About 30% express CD43 [PMID12945935], a significantly lower number than in mantle cell or SLL, but higher than in follicular center lymphomas. The monocytoid morphology, with clear cytoplasm, may simulate hairy cell leukemia, angioimmunoblastic lymphadenopathy with dysproteinemia (AILD), or mastocytosis. The plasmacytoid morphology may greatly resemble lymphoplasmacytic lymphoma (see below) and the small cell type simulates lymphomas of follicular center origin or SLL.

Several translocations have been described in extranodal marginal zone lymphomas, all activating the transcription factor NFκB [PMID21261681]. One of these is t(11;18)(q21:q21) that fuses the *MALT1* gene on 18q21 and the *AP12* gene on chromosome 11. This translocation is prevalent in extranodal marginal zone lymphomas of the stomach and lung. *MALT1* codes for a caspase-like protein that facilitates apoptosis, but *AP12* is an inhibitor of apoptosis [PMID11736940]. The fusion product does not have the action of *MALT1*, so apoptosis is diminished and cell survival is increased. Neoplastic gastric "MALTomas" usually have this translocation, whereas those caused by *H pylori* usually do not [PMID15577674]. While extranodal marginal zone lymphoma can occur in many sites, the most common site is the stomach and a significant minority of patients who appear to have an isolated lymphoma of this type in another location will also have gastric involvement. For this reason, esophagogastroduodenoscopy is reasonable in any patient with an extranodal marginal zone lymphoma in any location [PMID21157949].

Small Lymphocytic Lymphoma

"Small lymphocytic lymphoma" (SLL) is the new term for well differentiated lymphoma and represents the lymphoma manifestation of CLL. Because almost all cases of CLL have a marrow manifestation, the leukemic and lymphoma phases coexist in most patients, and the diagnosis is often written as CLL/SLL. In the lymph node, the morphology of the individual cells is the same as in the marrow, but there will be areas of slightly diminished cellular density, where the cells have more cytoplasm. These areas are called proliferation centers (or pseudofollicles). These proliferation centers are subtle, but can be detected on routine H&E examination i8.65a, i8.65b. Their presence should not be confused with a nodular component to the process, nor should the larger cells in them lead to a diagnosis of mixed large and small cell lymphoma. SLL is positive for CD5 and CD23, and is negative for CD10. It is positive for CD20 in 95% of cases [PMID14608903]. In addition to these markers, CD43 may assist in the diagnosis, as it is positive in about 80% of cases [PMID20408870]. The principal mimic of CLL/SLL is mantle cell lymphoma and the primary means of distinction is the positive bcl-1 in mantle cell lymphoma, and the presence of proliferation centers and positivity for CD23 **i8.66** in CLL/SLL.

CLL/SLL had been thought to be a proliferation of mature (naïve) B cells, but it is now known that about half of these cases have undergone somatic hypermutation, and therefore must have been antigenically stimulated and transited the germinal center of a lymph node. Indeed, those cases that have evidence of somatic hypermutation of the immunoglobulin heavy chain gene appear less aggressive [PMID16075892].

Several cytogenetic abnormalities have been associated with CLL, and preliminary data suggests that these have different clinical courses. These cytogenetic studies in CLL/SLL have traditionally been performed by FISH, but microarray technology (discussed in Chapter 45) is increasingly being used [PMID20075210]. Cytogenetic information will likely eventuate in the identification of subtypes of CLL/SLL.

Lymphoplasmacytic Lymphoma/Immunocytoma

"Lymphoplasmacytic lymphoma/immunocytoma" (LLI) is a term generally used for lymphomas that have some plasmacytic differentiation and that make immunoglobulin, but which do not have as well developed plasma cell morphology as a plasmacytoma **i8.67a**, **i8.67b**. Many lymphoplasmacytic lymphomas are CLL/SLL, follicular center cell lymphomas, or marginal zone type, because all of these may have plasmacytic differentiation and all may make immunoglobulin. For this reason, some have historically believed that the term "lymphoplasmacytic lymphoma" is inappropriate, and that these are lymphomas of another type, while others feel there is a small group that is distinct from other lymphomas, particularly if IgM is made, or if the patient clinically has Waldenström macroglobulinemia. However, Waldenström is *defined* by IgM monoclonality, often with hyperviscosity, and not by the presence of any particular type of lymphoma. Most patients with Waldenström macroglobulinemia will have LLI, but there are exceptions in both directions. Some LLI patients will not have Waldenström, and some Waldenström patients may have lymphomas of a different type [PMID11395551]. The diagnosis of LLI hinges on the exclusion of other types of lymphoma, and is easier if there is an IgM paraprotein. Approximately half of LLI cases exhibit a deletion of 6q23, but this finding is not specific for LLI, and is also occasionally found in CLL/SLL [PMID22156831]. Nonsecretory cases (without Waldenström features) have been reported to be associated with a t(9;14)(p13;q32.3)(*PAX-5/IgH*) [PMID17672883]. The association of these cytogenetic abnormalities with LLI suggests that it is a distinct entity.

LLI and marginal zone lymphoma share many morphologic and immunohistochemical characteristics. Both are low-grade and diffuse, and both are usually negative for CD5 and CD10 [PMID22156831]. Both are usually negative for CD23 and CD43, though LLI can be positive for CD23 in up to 40% of cases [PMID11395551]. The most difficult differential diagnosis for LLI is marginal zone lymphoma with a plasmacytoid appearance. Areas with a monocytoid morphology favor marginal zone lymphoma, while cytoplasmic or surface IgM favors lymphoplasmacytic lymphoma, especially if the patient clinically has Waldenström. Patients with paraprotein secondary to other types of lymphomas usually have IgG or IgA monoclonality rather than IgM. At this writing, the diagnosis of LLI is a diagnosis of exclusion in the presence of an appropriate clinical picture.

The following chart may help in separating small cell lymphomas (these staining patterns are generally valid in extranodal sites as well):

	CD5	CD10	CD23	CD43 bcl-1
Follicular center	–	+	–	rare –
Mantle	+	–	94% –	+
CLL	+	–	+	80% –
Marginal	–	–	+/–	30% –
LLI	–	–	–	rare –

Diffuse Large Cell B-Cell Lymphomas

The diffuse large cell B-cell lymphomas (DLBCLs) are a collection of related entities, with essentially similar behaviors, on which new work in immunohistochemistry and molecular pathology has shed considerable light. The common denominator for this group of neoplasms is a diffuse growth pattern, without follicles **i8.68a**, **i8.68b**, and a neoplastic cell whose nucleus is twice the size of a normal lymphocyte **i8.68c**. In addition to the centroblastic (usual) type, the WHO recognizes the entities of immunoblastic, T cell or histiocytic rich B-cell lymphoma, anaplastic lymphoma, mediastinal large cell lymphoma, primary effusion lymphoma, intravascular lymphoma, and plasmablastic lymphoma, but recommends that these terms be used only within the context of a DLBCL. These entities are distinct enough in their behavior and characteristics that the use of the terms is encouraged *concurrent* with the diagnosis of DLBCL. For example, a diagnosis should be "diffuse large cell B lymphoma, immunoblastic type" rather than "immunoblastic lymphoma."

Gene expression studies have shown at least 2 major types of DLBCL—centroblastic (germinal center) and postgerminal center [PMID15816558, PMID19097355]. Centroblastic large cell lymphomas seem to be of germinal center origin because they express bcl-6, which is restricted to B cells in germinal centers. They often express CD10 and appear to be composed of the neoplastic counterpart to the centroblast. The diffuse large cell lymphomas that are composed of larger, immunoblastic-like cells appear to be of postgerminal center origin because they express MUM1 (IRF4), a transcription factor that is associated with activated lymphocytes that have been stimulated and have left or are about to leave the germinal center (the term "activated lymphocyte" is a loose one, but generally refers to a cell that has moved out of the germinal center and has lost bcl-6). Although CD10 is usually positive in centroblastic lymphomas, true postgerminal center lymphomas are usually CD10–.

The phenotype of most follicular center cell lymphomas, of either follicular or diffuse architecture, is CD10+, bcl-6+/MUM1–. Most DLBCLs are negative for CD138, a plasmacytic marker. Many cases of postgerminal center lymphoma, such as diffuse large cell lymphomas of the so-called immunoblastic type, are bcl-6–, MUM1+, and CD138–. In general, expression of bcl-6 and MUM1 is mutually exclusive in normal B cells, but there may be overlap in lymphomas **i8.69a**, **i8.69b**, **i8.69c** [PMID12393466]. CD138 is generally expressed in postgerminal center diffuse large cell lymphomas only if they have taken an additional step in differentiation towards plasma cells. Prior to routine therapy with rituximab, postgerminal center lymphomas, as indicated by the expression of MUM1 or CD138, even in e continued presence of CD10 or bcl-6, were more aggressive ˈIID15087665], but currently, differences in germinal center vs post-rminal center immunophenotype are of minimal prognostic gnificance [PMID21536860].

TCRBCL is a type of DLBCL in which small, bland, nonneo-astic T cells, sometimes accompanied by histiocytes, greatly tnumber the larger, neoplastic B cells i8.70. Because of the rela-e paucity of neoplastic cells, this lymphoma may resemble a D. The neoplastic B cells are positive for CD20 and sometimes so for epithelial membrane antigen, as in NLPHD [PMID16545182], d there has been speculation that NLPHD and TCRBCL may related [PMID18784812].

Primary mediastinal large B-cell lymphoma is a distinct type DLBCL that usually occurs in the mediastinum of younger omen and is characterized by sclerosis. The sclerosis may ini-lly mask the neoplastic nature of the process i8.71a, but closer ıdy will disclose malignant lymphocytes i8.71b. Primary ediastinal large B-cell lymphoma may demonstrate focal munohistochemical characteristics of Hodgkin disease, such focal or weak expression of CD30 in 70-80% of cases [Swerdlow N978-9283224310]. MAL, a family of proteins that is important in organization of lipid rafts (regions of the cell membrane in hich proteins can more readily diffuse, important in cell sig-lling) is present in the cytoplasm in 54% of mediastinal large cell lymphomas, but only 3% of the usual DLBCL [PMID16707382]. terestingly, MAL is also present in 19% of Hodgkin lympho-as, primarily of the nodular sclerosing type [PMID12429796], sug-sting a possible relationship of these 2 entities.

There are other immunohistochemical differences between imary mediastinal large B-cell lymphoma and the usual LBCL, and the former neoplasm has several molecular prop-ties in addition to MAL expression that are nearly unique nong NHLs and closer to the expression profile of Hodgkin mphomas [PMID18774728]. Perhaps the most interesting of the olecular features of the primary mediastinal large B-cell lym-ioma is that 65% of them express c-rel, a member of the Rel/ FκB family of transcription factors, in contrast to only 18% ordinary DLBCL, and 62% of them stain for TRAF1 (*t*umor crosis factor *r*eceptor *a*ssociated *f*actor), in contrast to only % of the usual variety of DLBCL. Expression of both c-Rel d TRAF1 has 98% specificity for primary mediastinal large cell lymphoma [PMID17197926]. The primary mediastinal large cell lymphoma is further discussed in Chapter 18 and further ustrated in i18.23 and i18.24.

Primary effusion lymphoma almost always occurs in immu-compromised patients—specifically in HIV/AIDS patients— d is associated with HHV-8 (other neoplasms associated with HV-8 include some cases of the plasma cell type of Castleman sease, some cases of Kaposi sarcoma, some cases of multiple yeloma, and some cases of the angioimmunoblastic lymph-lenopathy group of disorders) [PMID20461118]. In primary effu-on lymphoma, the tumor cells are usually of immunoblastic orphology. However, most effusions that are positive for mphoma are not of this entity, but simply reflect the spread of other type of lymphoma into pleural or peritoneal fluid. Even cases where the diagnosis of lymphoma has not been made, ost lymphomatous effusions will turn out to be secondary to other type of lymphoma that has not yet been detected.

In addition to effusion lymphomas, DLBCLs may occur in a background of chronic inflammation. These lymphomas are recognized as a specific group by WHO [Swerdlow ISBN978-9283224310] and tend to be associated with EBV [PMID20062008].

Intravascular lymphoma is a rare form of DLBCL in which the neoplastic cells are found predominantly in small blood vessels, creating the illusion that they have originated from the endothelium i8.72. Clinical symptoms are related primarily to the skin and the central nervous system [PMID19055170]. Because other lymphomas may have a leukemic phase, the diagnosis of intravascular lymphoma is generally not made if there has been a previous diagnosis of another lymphoma or if there is a lymphoid mass.

Plasmablastic lymphoma is an exceptionally rare DLBCL that occurs primarily in the oral cavity of HIV-positive patients i8.73a, i8.73b. This is an aggressive lymphoma that may be associated with EBV [PMID18939960]. While the clinical presentations of plas-mablastic lymphoma and the plasmablastic form of myeloma are quite different, there is overlap in the immunohistochemical profiles of the 2 entities, and the existence of a plasmablastic lymphoma as a separate and distinct entity has been challenged [PMID15578069].

Microvillous lymphoma is a rare diffuse large cell B lym-phoma that is not specifically recognized in the WHO system. Electron microscopy is required to see the microvilli, which have no known clinical significance. This entity is distinct from splenic lymphoma with villous lymphocytes (now considered by many to be synonymous with splenic marginal zone lym-phoma; see Chapter 9).

Burkitt and Burkitt-Like Lymphomas

Few lymphomas have perennially caused as much confusion as the Burkitt group, which has historically consisted of true Burkitt lymphoma and Burkitt-like lymphoma. Both are charac-terized by a diffuse proliferation of medium-sized lymphocytes with prominent nucleoli, very large numbers of mitoses, and admixed histiocytes with tingible bodies, accounting for the so-called "starry sky" appearance i8.74a, i8.74b.

The first difficulty is distinguishing the true Burkitt lympho-mas and the Burkitt-like lymphomas, on the one hand, from other types of lymphoma on the other. The differential diagno-sis of Burkitt and Burkitt-like lymphoma includes lymphoblastic lymphoma, the blastic variant of mantle cell lymphoma, and dif-fuse large cell B lymphoma of follicular center origin (especially immunoblastic type).

The immunohistochemical profiles of lymphoblastic lym-phoma and the blastic variant of mantle cell lymphoma differ sufficiently from that of the Burkitt group and DLBCL (eg, bcl-1 positivity in mantle cell lymphoma and tdt positivity in lymphoblastic lymphoma) that these entities can usually be rela-tively quickly eliminated from further diagnostic consideration, but the distinction of the Burkitt group from DLBCL of follicular center origin can be challenging, as the immunophenotype of the two is similar. Indeed, Burkitt lymphoma is thought to be of follicular center origin.

Burkitt lymphoma has a diffuse growth pattern and is CD10 positive, CD20 positive, bcl-6 positive, MUM1 negative, CD138 negative, CD5 negative, and CD23 negative in almost all cases, making a strong point for follicular center origin [PMID18519409].

But in contrast to the typical DLBCL, Burkitt lymphomas are usually bcl-2 negative (80-90% of cases) and CD43 positive, and they generally have a Ki-67 proliferation index of 95% or greater (100% is not uncommon) [PMID18519409], while Ki-67 in most common DLBCLs will not exceed 80%. While Ki-67 proliferations of 60% sound (and are) high, they are too low for Burkitt. However, the immunophenotypes are similar enough to cause confusion. Indeed, the WHO recognizes a category of "B-cell lymphoma, unclassifiable, with features intermediate between diffuse large B-cell lymphoma and Burkitt lymphoma." For example, one will rarely encounter a Burkitt that expresses bcl-2, and approximately 10% of non-Burkitt diffuse large cell B lymphomas will have a Ki-67 in excess of 90%, simulating a Burkitt lymphoma **i8.75a**, **i8.75b**, **i8.75c**. EBV is also helpful if present, but whereas it is found in nearly 100% of endemic cases, it is present in only 20-25% of sporadic cases. Moreover, about 1/4 of lymphomas that appear morphologically to be more consistent with DLBCL than with the Burkitt group have been shown to have molecular features of the latter type. For this reason, it is worthwhile to exclude the Burkitt group before making the diagnosis of an "ordinary" DLBCL.

If immunohistochemical studies do not provide this distinction, a FISH study for *C-MYC* translocation may be necessary **i8.76**, **i8.77**. Burkitt lymphoma is essentially defined by a t(8;14)(q24;q32.3), which results in the juxtaposition of the *C-MYC* gene and the immunoglobulin heavy chain locus, resulting in overexpression of *C-MYC* (many translocations in hematopathology place a proto-oncogene adjacent to an immunoglobulin gene). In a minority of cases of lymphomas of the Burkitt group, the *C-MYC* is translocated next to an immunoglobulin light chain. Although the *C-MYC* oncogene can also be present in a small percentage of diffuse large B-cell lymphoma, a translocation that places *C-MYC* adjacent an immunoglobulin gene (heavy or light chain) seems to be essentially specific for Burkitt leukemia/lymphoma [PMID16760442, PMID16760443].

Gene expression work is clarifying lymphoma classification, and a 58 gene expression profile has been offered to distinguish the Burkitt group from DLBCL [PMID16760442].

After the distinction from other types of lymphoma is made, and the process is placed in the Burkitt group, the second difficulty is the difference, if any, of the "true" Burkitt from so-called Burkitt-like lymphoma. This is a long-running controversy, with some observers ("splitters") believing that a Burkitt lymphoma has more nuclear uniformity and multiple nucleoli, while a Burkitt-like lymphoma has more nuclear pleomorphism and a single nucleolus, while others ("lumpers") have not found significant morphological or immunophenotypic differences within this group. The WHO has placed many of the Burkitt-like lymphoma into the overlap category of "B-cell lymphoma, unclassifiable, with features intermediate between diffuse large B-cell lymphoma and Burkitt lymphoma." As gene expression studies of the DLBCL and Burkitt continue, definitive clarification may emerge, but at this writing, I do not believe the "splitters" have proven their case, and I believe it is much more important to thoroughly characterize a DLBCL, including a FISH study for t(8;14) in those cases that are unclear, than it is to create and defend a category of "Burkitt-like." Much more important than distinguishing Burkitt from Burkitt-like lymphomas is to distinguish the Burkitt group, which is more aggressive, from a typical DLBCL.

Lymphoproliferative Disorders in Immunocompromised Patients

Lymphoproliferative disorders in immunocompromised patients is a family of entities, one example of which is post-transplant lymphoproliferative disorders (PTLDs), a spectrum of lymphoproliferative disorders ranging from benign to lymphoma. Most cases of PTLD are B cell proliferations, though there are a few cases are of T-cell origin. Most, but not all, cases are associated with EBV, a double-stranded DNA virus of the herpes family [Swerdlow ISBN978-9283224310]. The *primary* EBV syndromes are infectious mononucleosis, chronic EBV infection, and X-linked lymphoproliferative disorder (patients develop a fatal primary infection with EBV). The *reactivation* syndromes are lymphoproliferative disorders in the immunocompromised, Burkitt lymphoma, and nasopharyngeal carcinoma. There are a number of other disorders linked to EBV, such as oral hairy leukoplakia, Hemophagocytic lymphohistiocytosis, and some cases of Hodgkin disease.

The benign expressions of PTLD often have a paracortical expansion of plasma cells and immunoblasts. The benignity of these situations has been clearly established by their regression upon reduction of immunosuppression. The clearly malignant cases of PTLD are usually diffuse large B-cell lymphomas, often of the so-called immunoblastic type, although rarely, they may be a plasmacytic **i8.78a**, **i8.78b**, or a Burkitt lymphoma. Plasmablastic lymphoma may also occur in this population, especially in the oral cavity, and any DLBCL in an immunocompromised patient should receive a CD138 to confirm or exclude plasmacytic differentiation. Because PTLDs are a heterogeneous group, demonstration of immunoglobulin gene rearrangement may be necessary to determine if a particular case is a true neoplasm.

In addition to PTLD, lymphoproliferative disorders in immunocompromised patients include those in patients with HIV/AIDS, who may develop both benign and neoplastic lymphoid proliferations that are similar to those seen in transplant patients. AIDS patients are prone to large B-cell lymphomas, often associated with EBV, and 2 lymphomas—primary effusion lymphoma and plasmablastic lymphoma of the oral cavity—are almost unique to AIDS patients. Patients with congenital immunodeficiencies are also at risk for a variety for both reactive and neoplastic lymphoid proliferations.

B-cell Lymphomas Are Often Treated with a Monoclonal Antibody to CD20

A final point before we complete our discussion of B-cell lymphomas is that if they are CD20 positive, they are often treated with Rituxan (rituximab; a monoclonal antibody to CD20) in combination with CHOP chemotherapy (cyclophosphamide, doxorubicin, vincristine, and prednisone). However, about half of CD20 positive cases that initially respond to this treatment will not respond to a second course of Rituxan, often because of a loss of CD20 expression [PMID21385115]. Therefore, a recurrent lymphoid mass should be tested for CD20, even if the original tumor was shown to be positive for this marker, both to ensure B lineage and to verify the continued efficacy of Rituxan (this situation is analogous to that of *HER2* and ER, whose status in a recurrence or metastasis of breast carcinoma may differ from the primary).

'-Cell and Natural Killer Cell Neoplasms

Before considering T-cell lymphomas, 3 general points should e made. First, as is the case for B cells, there is no one antigen iat is expressed by all T cells at all stages of development. ven CD3 does not stain all T cells. The percentage of positive aining increases if we realize that early T cells may have cyto-lasmic rather than cell membrane CD3, but is still not 100%, nd the antigen can also be expressed by natural killer (NK) ells. Coexpression of both CD4 and CD8, failure to express ther CD4 or CD8, or inappropriate expression of an immature ntigen (such as CD1a) in a T cell population are also associated 'ith malignancy, but none of these is perfect.

More recent work has focused on CD2, CD5, CD7, and βF1 he T-cell receptor β chain). CD2 is the first to appear during -cell development. CD2, CD3, CD5, and CD7 are called the an-T antigens, and virtually all normal and neoplastic T cells ill stain with at least 1 of these markers. These 4 markers not nly identify T cells, but the failure of a T cell to express any f them suggests that it may be abnormal. This is called loss of an-T cell expression. The principal caveat here is that CD5 also ains mantle cell lymphomas, the cells of CLL/SLL, and a rare -cell lymphoma of follicular center origin. It should also be emembered that about 20-40% of T-cell lymphomas will stain r CD15 or CD30. This is why the diagnosis of HD requires a egative CD45 and a compatible H&E morphology in addition) a positive CD15 and/or CD30.

A second general point is that unless T-cell receptor gene rear-angement has been shown, proof of T origin requires not only iat the target lymphocytes be shown to stain for T markers, but lso that they do not stain for B markers. CD20 is the most com-ionly used stain to verify B lineage, but early B cells may not yet xpress CD20, and some B-cell lymphomas may be CD20 negative r they may have lost their initial CD20 expression after the use f the anti-CD20 drug rituximab. For this reason, before turning way from a B-cell origin and toward a T lineage, additional mark-rs of B lineage should be performed and shown to be negative. In iost situations, CD79a is an excellent additional marker of B-cell ifferentiation. Pax5, a transcription factor, also stains B cells at iore stages than CD20, and is an excellent stain, but will also tain most atypical cells in Hodgkin disease, either of the classic ype or of the nodular lymphocyte predominant type [PMID17529924]. D19 and CD22 both stain B cells at an earlier stage than CD20, ut CD19 is found in some cases of acute myeloid leukemia.

Third, as is the case for B-cell neoplasms, proof of clonality is eldom necessary in the diagnosis of T-cell lymphomas. This is good thing because clonality is notoriously difficult to demon-trate in T-cell proliferations, and can only be done by proving '-cell receptor gene rearrangement. A set of antibodies to dif-erent families of the variable region of the β chain of the T-cell eceptor β chain gene is available. If immunohistochemistry an show that most of the T cells express antigens of the same ene family in the variable region of the β chain of the receptor, lonality can be suspected [PMID15023042].

Young T cells go first into the cortex of the thymus, and hen migrate into the medulla before leaving the thymus. '-cell lymphomas are divided into precursor (immature) and eripheral (phenotypically mature or postthymic) categories. '-lymphoblastic lymphoma is an example of a precursor T-cell ymphoma. The term "peripheral" refers to occurrence outside f the thymus/mediastinum, though a thymic T-cell lymphoma, if it has a mature immunophenotype, would still be considered "peripheral," and a systemic lymphoma may have an immature phenotype. The important concept is not the physical location, but the degree of maturity. Some peripheral T-cell lymphomas occur in the skin (this group was formerly called mycosis fungoides and is now called peripheral cutaneous T-cell lymphoma [PCTCL]). As is the case for B-cell neoplasms without systemic manifestations, the joint WHO/EORTC system is recommended for primary cutaneous T-cell lymphoproliferative disorders.

WHO Classification of T-cell Neoplasms

I. Precursor T-cell neoplasm:
   a. Precursor T-lymphoblastic lymphoma/leukemia
II. Mature (peripheral) T-cell and NK-cell neoplasms
   a. T-cell prolymphocytic leukemia
   b. T-cell granular lymphocytic leukemia
   c. Chronic lymphoproliferative disorder of NK cells
   d. Aggressive NK-cell leukemia
   e. EBV+ T-cell lymphoproliferative disorders of childhood
   f. Adult T-cell lymphoma/leukemia (HTLV1+)
   g. Extranodal NK/T-cell lymphoma, nasal type
   h. Enteropathy-type T-cell lymphoma
   i. Hepatosplenic γ-δ T-cell lymphoma
   j. Subcutaneous panniculitis-like T-cell lymphoma
   k. Peripheral cutaneous T-cell lymphoma (mycosis fungoides/ Sézary syndrome)
   l. Anaplastic large cell lymphoma, T/null-cell, primary cutaneous type
   m. Primary cutaneous γ-δ T-cell lymphomas
   n. Peripheral T-cell lymphoma, not otherwise characterized
   o. Angioimmunoblastic T-cell lymphoma
   p. Anaplastic large cell lymphoma, T/null-cell, primary systemic type

Precursor T-lymphoblastic Lymphoma

Almost all lymphoblastic lymphomas are of T-cell origin and are terminal deoxynucleotidyl transferase (TdT) positive. Almost all cases of what initially appear to be a B-lymphoblastic lymphoma or actually T-lymphoblastic lymphomas or, if B lineage is confirmed, are the blastic variant of mantle cell lymphoma, and both of these entities must be excluded before the diagnosis of B-lymphoblastic lymphoma is made. In addition to the previously discussed immunohistochemical stains that characterize mantle cell lymphomas (bcl-1 and CD5 positive, CD10 and CD23 negative), blastic mantle cell lymphomas are also distinguished from true lymphoblastic lymphomas by absence of TdT.

The cells of a precursor T-cell acute lymphoid leukemia are morphologically and phenotypically identical to those of a T-lymphoblastic lymphoma, and blood, bone marrow, and the mediastinum are usually examined when either T-lymphoblastic lymphoma or leukemia is diagnosed. The cells in either entity have minimal cytoplasm, fine chromatin, and small nucleoli i8.79. They will express CD3 (usually in the cytoplasm, but occasionally on the surface), as well as CD2, CD5, CD7, and TdT. TdT and cytoplasmic CD3 are the most useful markers. CD4 and CD8 may or may not be expressed, and there may be double positivity for these 2 markers [PMID6784790]. Lymphoblastic lymphomas occur primarily in the mediastinum and are further discussed in Chapter 18 and illustrated in i18.25 and i18.26.

ISBN 978-089189-5886

Mature (Peripheral) T-Cell and Natural Killer Cell Neoplasms

The clinical presentation is also variable. Some patients may have symptoms associated with B-cell lymphomas (fever, weight loss, and night sweats). The individual cells vary greatly in peripheral (mature) T-cell lymphomas, but a diffuse growth pattern is the rule i8.80a. To secure a diagnosis of peripheral T-cell lymphoma, multiple T markers should be positive and multiple B markers should be negative. Lineage should not be established on a single marker. In the case illustrated in i8.80, for example, both CD3 and CD2 (another T marker) are positive i8.80b, i8.80c. It is also wise to verify absence of B-cell differentiation before T lineage is assumed. In this case, CD20 is negative i8.80d. Once T lineage is demonstrated, the next task is to exclude a specific kind of T-cell lymphoma. In the case in i8.80, the lymphoma was negative for tdt, indicating it is not a lymphoblastic lymphoma. It was negative for CD30 and ALK, suggesting it is not an anaplastic T-cell lymphoma, and it was negative for CD56 and EBV, excluding a NK-cell lymphoma. This T-cell lymphoma was also positive for bcl-2 i8.80e, illustrating that the bcl-2 protein is not specific for B cell processes.

The differential diagnosis of peripheral T-cell lymphoma includes a B-cell lymphoma, Hodgkin disease, and a benign paracortical reactive process (which usually has some residual follicular architecture, a mixture of cell types, and a "mottled" appearance).

As is the case for B-cell lymphomas, there is often a leukemic phase in T-cell lymphomas, and there is clinical, pathologic, and immunophenotypic overlap between a lymphoma and a leukemia. T-cell prolymphocytic leukemia (T-PLL), T-cell large granular lymphocytic leukemia, and aggressive NK-cell leukemia are mature T-cell neoplasms that tend to present as leukemias.

T-PLL is a rare leukemia that morphologically resembles the prolymphocytic phase of B-cell CLL. It is associated with inv(14q). It is TdT negative and usually positive for CD4, though it may express CD8, or both Cd4 and CD8. T-cell large granular lymphocytic leukemia is usually CD3 and CD8 positive.

The NK-cell lymphoproliferative disorders are NK lymphoma, aggressive NK leukemia, and a provisionally recognized chronic NK condition of uncertain malignant potential. NK lymphomas are rare outside of Asia. They are aggressive, often angiocentric, and often begin in the sino-nasal area, though disseminated disease is common. Pure nodal NK-cell lymphoma is very rare and almost all cases are extranodal.

EBV is important in the pathogenesis of NK lymphoma and aggressive NK leukemia, but the mechanism is unknown [PMID21541194]. Detectable EBV DNA in blood by PCR portends a more aggressive course of NK/T-cell lymphoma [PMID21984805].

NK-cell lymphomas i8.81a, i8.81b have features of T-cell lymphoma. They are generally negative for cell surface CD3, but may express cytoplasmic CD3 i8.81c, and also express other T-cell antigens, such as CD2 i8.81d and CD7 i8.81e [PMID21628857], and absence of B lineage must also be shown i8.81f. Because of these shared features, NK-cell lymphomas are often called NK/T-cell lymphomas, but true NK-cell lymphomas do not have the usual T-cell receptor and do not rearrange their receptor [PMID19593607]. The presence of CD56 i8.81g and EBV i8.81h, and cytoplasmic staining for CD3, are most helpful in identifying an NK lymphoma and excluding a "simple" T-cell lymphoma. Demonstration of the cytotoxic granules granzyme B i8.81i and TIA-1 i8.81j are also highly supportive of a diagnosis of NK-cell lymphoma [PMID21867533].

Aggressive NK-cell leukemia may be a leukemic counterpart to NK-cell lymphomas, though this has not been definitively settled [PMID10389582]. The chronic lymphoproliferative disorder of NK cells has similar morphologic and immunophenotypic properties to aggressive NK-cell leukemia, but lacks an association with EBV and is less aggressive. It is unclear if this indolent process is neoplastic or reactive [PMID20425414].

Hepatosplenic γ-δ T-cell lymphoma, enteropathy-associated T-cell lymphoma, subcutaneous panniculitis-like T-cell lymphoma are discussed in Chapters 9, 23, and 40, respectively.

Anaplastic lymphomas are divided into systemic and cutaneous forms. The systemic type often expresses a translocation between chromosomes 2 and 5 t(2;5)(p23;q35) which results in fusion of the *ALK* (anaplastic lymphoma kinase) gene on chromosome 2p with the *NPM1* (nucleophosmin) gene on chromosome 5q [PMID11266530]. After transcription and translation, the resulting novel protein consists of the *ALK* gene product, a tyrosine kinase, fused to *NPM1* gene product, a phosphoprotein that shuttles proteins from the nucleus to the cytoplasm and is needed for centrosome and ribosome synthesis. This translocation causes the *ALK* gene product to be found in both the nucleus and the cytoplasm.

The neoplastic cell in anaplastic lymphoma is generally large and pleomorphic i8.82a, i8.82b, but small cell i8.83a, i8.83b, monomorphic, and lymphohistiocytic forms are recognized. Although anaplastic lymphoma is a T-cell neoplasm and may be positive for CD3 i8.84a, many cases are negative for CD3. All cases should be CD30 positive i8.84b. Negativity for CD30 essentially rules out this entity, but a number of other neoplasms are also positive for CD30, and additional evidence is required for the diagnosis of anaplastic lymphoma. The immunohistochemical demonstration of the ALK protein i8.84c or of t(2;5) by FISH is sufficient additional evidence, and the presence of either of those in conjunction with CD30 secures the diagnosis even without proof of T-cell origin, provided that there is no indication of B-cell differentiation (this is the null cell immunophenotypic variant of anaplastic lymphoma). However, if CD30 is unaccompanied by either ALK positivity or demonstration of t(2;5), then proof of T lineage is needed (the T-cell immunophenotypic variant) [PMID11266530]. The WHO does not recognize a B-cell form of this entity. Unlike most T-cell lymphomas, the anaplastic lymphoma often does not show any TCR gene rearrangement.

The presence of the ALK protein is a good prognostic sign in the systemic form. The cutaneous form does well even without ALK, and the monomorphic, small cell, and lymphohistiocytic subtypes of systemic anaplastic lymphoma are aggressive even if ALK positive.

Because of the morphologic variants of anaplastic lymphoma and the possibility of a null immunophenotype, it is generally prudent to stain unusual hematopoietic neoplasms for ALK and CD30 if they cannot be precisely classified. Many cases formerly thought to be true histiocytic lymphomas are now known to be anaplastic lymphomas. Because anaplastic lymphomas are often EMA positive and CD45 negative, an EMA positive, CD45 negative tumor should not be accepted as a carcinoma without excluding anaplastic lymphoma and demonstrating keratin positivity.

Adult T-cell leukemia/lymphoma is caused by human :ell lymphotropic virus type 1 (HTLV1). The cells have high- convoluted nuclei and usually infiltrate lymph nodes and gans. The skin may or may not be involved, but if it is, there ll also be other sites, and this is not a cutaneous lymphoma.

munoblastic Lymphadenopathy (IBL) and gioimmunoblastic Lymphadenopathy with Dysproteinemia

Historically, immunoblastic lymphadenopathy (IBL) and gioimmunoblastic lymphadenopathy with dysproteinemia ILD) were considered to be abnormal immune reactions. tients are often anemic, with Coombs-positive erythrocytes, d many will have a polyclonal hypergammaglobulinemia. me patients are immunodeficient.

Most now consider IBL and AILD to be peripheral T-cell nphomas. A polymorphous cell population, accompanied small blood vessels, usually distorts the nodal architecture d effaces all germinal centers i8.85a, i8.85b. This polymor- ous cellular composition obscured the true nature of this ocess for many years. Even today, because of the large mixture of benign cells, the neoplastic nature of the process ay not be initially clear. The neoplastic cell is a T lymphocyte at is usually CD4 positive, CD8 negative (rarely, it may show reverse staining, be double negative, or double positive). It ay be small or large, often has clear cytoplasm, and tend to ister around vessels i8.86a, i8.86b. One should look for arbo- ing venules with hyalinized walls that stain with periodic id-Schiff. Follicular dendritic cells (positive for CD21, CD35, isterin, fascin, and occasionally for CD23) are seen outside their normal follicular location, often surrounding the borizing vessels. The neoplastic cells often express CD10, a arker more often seen in some B-cell neoplasms, and have en lost 1 or more pan-T markers, such as CD2, CD3, CD5, or)7. EBV may be present.

tramedullary Myeloid Tumors

Extramedullary myeloid tumor (also called granulocytic rcoma or myeloid sarcoma; formerly called chloroma) is a lid tissue manifestation of acute myelogenous leukemia. ie morphology of an extramedullary myeloid tumor will pend on the nature of the underlying AML. There are istic, immature, and differentiated types of extramedullary yeloid tumor, corresponding to the degree of differentiation the AML i8.87a, i8.87b, i8.87c. Myeloid sarcomas derived from nonoblastic AML whose leukemic phase was not apparent count for a number of cases of what had been called true stiocytic lymphomas.

The differential diagnosis of extramedullary myeloid mor includes lymphoblastic lymphoma and blastic variants other lymphomas. The most difficult part of the diagnosis extramedullary myeloid tumor is to think of the possibil- . The clues that a "lymphoma" may be an extramedullary yeloid tumor are:

Odd-looking and difficult to classify lymphoma.

Cells with eosinophilic cytoplasm.

Large numbers of eosinophils in a NHL and, especially, eosinophilic myelocytes, though these may be rare in the blastic form of extramedullary myeloid tumor.

4. CD43 or CD45 positivity in the absence of other markers of lymphoid differentiation, such as CD20 or CD79a (B cells), or CD3 or CD2 (T cells). A neoplasm should not be accepted as a lymphoma based only on a positive CD43 or CD45 without additional lymphoid markers. Indeed, 10% of extramedullary myeloid tumors are TdT positive, potentially causing a false diagnosis of lymphoblastic lymphoma if T-cell markers are not performed.
5. In addition to myeloperoxidase, CD117 stains extramedullary myeloid tumors. Lysozyme and CD68 also stain extramedullary myeloid tumors, but are nonspecific (CD68 also stains mature neutrophils, macrophages, and normal developing myeloid cells). A panel of lysozyme, CD68, CD3, CD20, CD43, myeloperoxidase, and CD117 is very sensitive for extramedullary myeloid tumor, with the latter 2 having the best specificity vs lymphoid lesions [PMID17974004].

It is wise to exclude an extramedullary myeloid tumor if an apparent lymphoma cannot be precisely classified. A bone marrow can be suggested if there is any question, but rarely, an extramedullary myeloid tumor may occur in the absence of leukemia or a demonstrably abnormal bone marrow.

Mastocytosis can look very much like an extramedullary myeloid tumor and should be excluded whenever the latter entity is considered. Clues to mastocytosis include occasional recognizable mast cells i8.88a, clear cytoplasm i8.88b, and fibrosis i8.88c. Mastocytosis may also be positive for CD43, CD117, and CD68, but differs from extramedullary myeloid tumor in its positivity for tryptase.

Very Rare Neoplasms of Lymph Nodes

Primary sarcomas of lymph nodes are quite rare and consist of 2 types: follicular dendritic cell sarcomas and interdigitating dendritic cell sarcomas. Both are largely diagnoses of exclusion, but there is a set of immunohistochemical characteristics for follicular dendritic cells, which includes CD21, CD35 (C3d complement receptor), and fascin [PMID19391666]. Clusterin is perhaps the most specific marker for follicular dendritic cells [PMID15252304]. Follicular dendritic cell sarcomas also stain for vimentin and are negative for CD45, confirming that they are true sarcomas and not lymphomas. Morphologically, they may have several patterns, but usually demonstrate ovoid to spindled nuclei, with a moderate amount of eosinophilic cytoplasm and indistinct cell borders i8.89a, i8.89b. Interdigitating dendritic cell sarcomas are very rare and may require electron microscopy for diagnosis. They will lack follicular dendritic cell markers and will be positive for CD1a and S100, simulating a Langerhans proliferation. They are also positive for CD68 and CD163 [PMID19845032].

The palisaded myofibroblastoma (also called hemorrhagic spindle cell tumor with amianthoid fibers) occurs in lymph nodes and is characterized by a bland spindle cell proliferation i8.90a, aggregates of collagen i8.90b, and extravasated red cells i8.90c [PMID2712187]. This can resemble a follicular dendritic cell sarcoma, Kaposi sarcoma, or an intranodal nerve sheath tumor.

ISBN 978-089189-5886

Core Points for Lymph Node Pathology

- Lymphadenopathy: common and usually benign.
- Diagnosis of Hodgkin disease (HD) requires the demonstration of Reed-Sternberg (R-S) cells or their variants.
  - o R-S cells: CD15+ and CD30+, CD45–.
  - o Lymphocyte-rich HD: a new category in the WHO system.
- Nodular lymphocyte predominant HD: likely a form of NHL
  - o Greater staining for CD20 and CD79 than in classical HD disease and positive for bcl-6.
- Cytogenetic abnormalities in NHL: often translocations that juxtapose oncogenes with regulatory portion of immunoglobulin gene.
- Majority of follicular center cell lymphomas have t(14;18) but usually not necessary to demonstrate this
- Mantle cell lymphoma: essentially defined by a t(11;14)
  - o But a compatible H&E appearance with the IHC demonstration of bcl-1 almost always sufficient.
- 3 varieties of marginal zone lymphoma: nodal, splenic, and extranodal.
- Small lymphocytic lymphoma is the tissue counterpart to CLL
  - o Positivity for CD5 and CD23, with negativity for CD10.
- Diffuse large B-cell lymphomas: heterogeneous group of entities.
  - o Usually CD10+, bcl-6+ negative for post-germinal center markers MUM1 and CD138.
  - o Some cases bcl-6– and MUM1+ or CD138+.
- Unusual forms of B-cell lymphoma: T-cell rich B-cell lymphoma, primary mediastinal large B-cell lymphoma, and Burkitt/Burkitt-like lymphoma.
  - o Burkitt group: CD10+, CD20+, and bcl-6+.
  - o Essentially defined by a t(8;14), but H&E and immunohistochemical characteristics, with a proliferation rate in excess of 90%, usually secures diagnosis.
- Many NHLs will express CD20 and are amenable to treatment with rituximab, though this marker may be lost in clinical recurrence.
- Posttransplant lymphoproliferative disorders: spectrum, some reactive and some neoplastic.
- WHO has also applied immunohistochemical and cytogenetic information to the classification of T-cell lymphomas.
- Lymphoblastic lymphoma: central (thymus), immature phenotype.
- Mature (peripheral) T-cell proliferations: anaplastic lymphoma and peripheral cutaneous T-cell lymphoma.
  - o Other forms of mature T-cell and NK-cell lymphoma are rare.
- Prudent to demonstrate specific B- or T-cell markers before making a diagnosis of lymphoma, as extramedullary myeloid tumor is positive for the general lymphoid marker CD45.

Follicular hyperplasia a lymph node. Note at the follicles are of fering sizes and that rminal centers are adily noted.

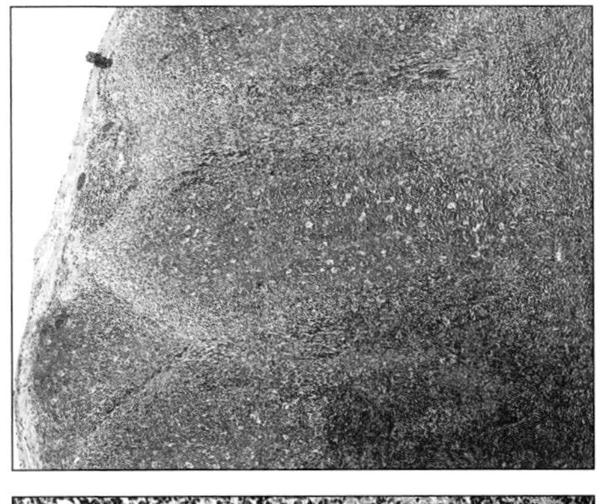

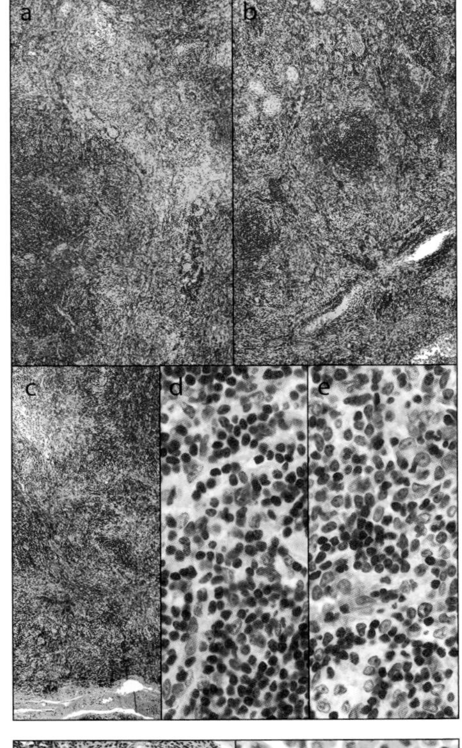

i8.2 Paracortical or interfollicular (so-called diffuse) hyperplasia. Normal lymph node architecture is difficult to recognize, but it is present and the lymph node is not effaced.
In **a**, a normal follicle is seen in the lower left.
b and **c** illustrate hyperplasia of the paracortical area.
d and **e** illustrate the mixed population of cells, including lymphocytes, plasma cells, and rare eosinophils. This is not the monomorphic population that would be expected in a lymphoma.

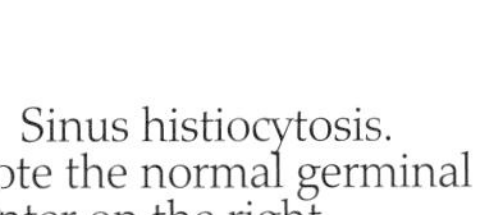

Sinus histiocytosis. ote the normal germinal nter on the right.

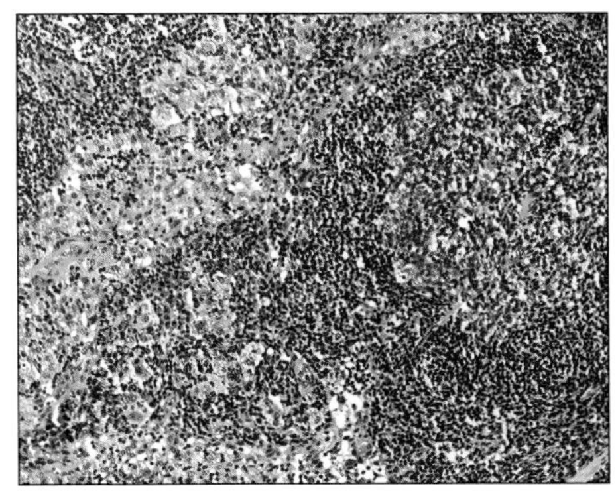

a Epstein-Barr infection a cervical lymph node in ononucleosis. The larger lls suggest a lymphoma. A higher-power view of e same case as in i8.4a, nderscoring the similarity a large cell lymphoma. ne scattered plasma cells ggests that this may be hyperplastic process, but ten, immunohistochemi- l stains are necessary secure the proper agnosis.

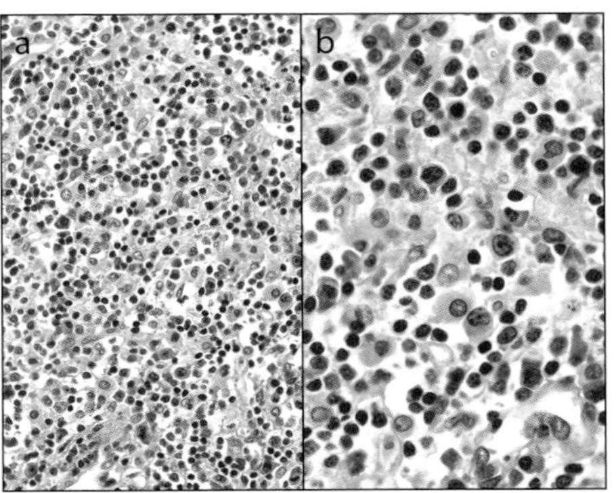

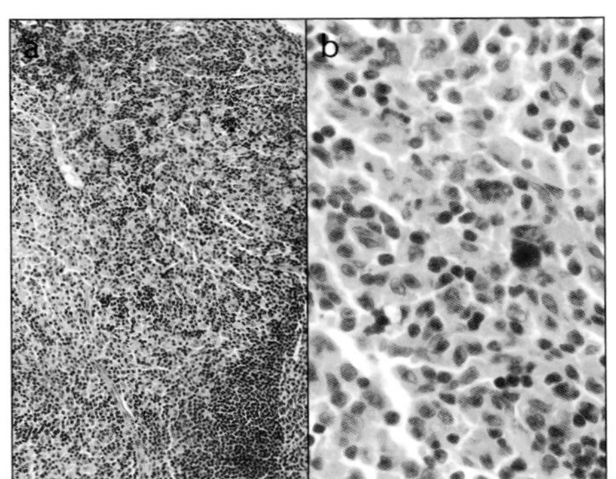

i8.5 **a** Dermatopathic lymphadenitis, with paracortical hyperplasia in the central and left portions of the photograph
b The same case as in i8.5a, illustrating the pigmented Langerhans cells in the paracortical area

a Kikuchi disease illus- ating the karyorrhectic eutrophils and necrosis. hile this has some milarity to a necrotizing anuloma, the differences e that the neutrophils e not intact in Kiku- ni disease and they are n the periphery of the ecrotic area rather than ithin it. **b** Histiocytic yperplasia is often seen Kikuchi disease.

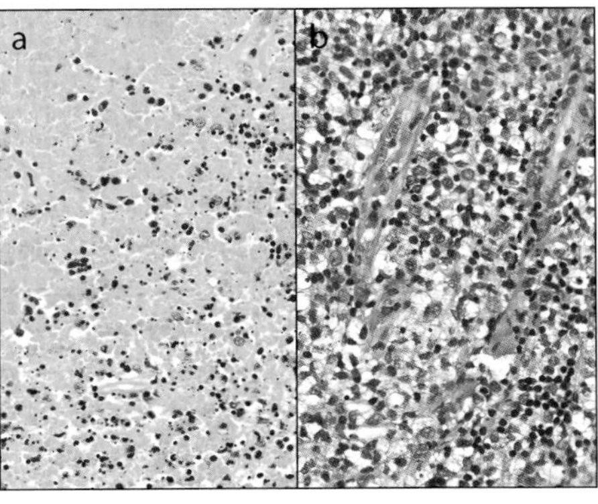

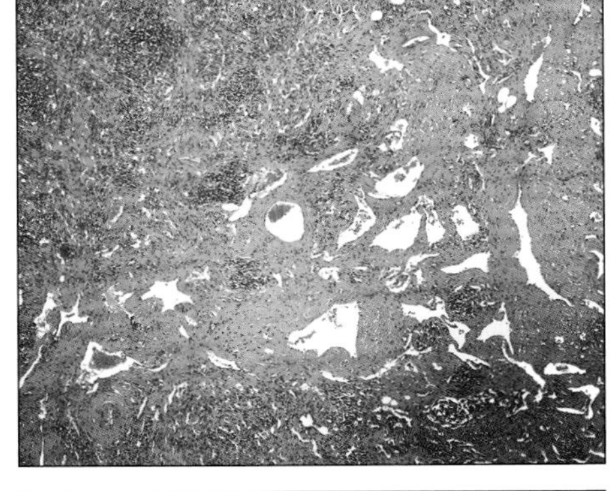

i8.7 Vascular transfor- mation of lymph node sinuses. This process in- volves the sinuses within the lymph node and the capsule of the lymph node but generally not the fol- licles or the interfollicular region.

8 A lymph node in a atient with AIDS. There follicular hyperplasia, ut the germinal center beginning to break up ollicular lysis).

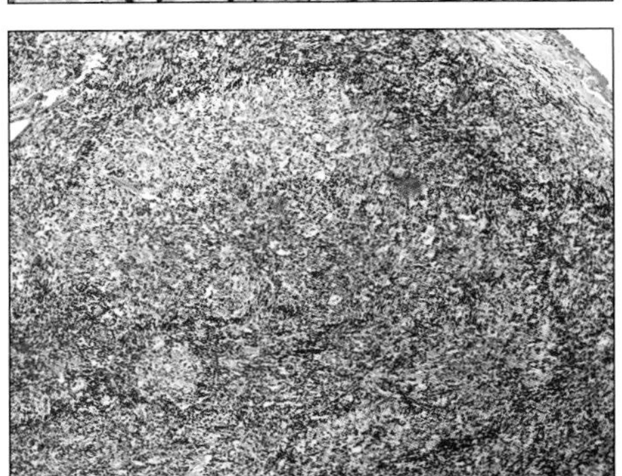

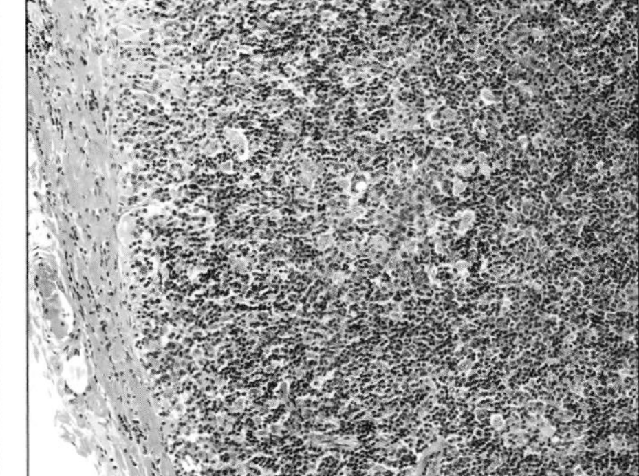

i8.9 Follicular involution in a patient with AIDS. This is a barely recognizable germinal center.

ISBN 978-089189-5886

i8.10 A caseating granuloma. Epithelioid histiocytes surround a necrotic central area within which there are few inflammatory cells.

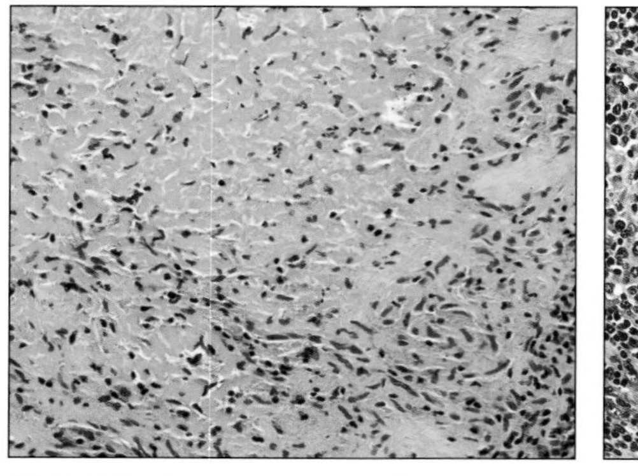

i8.11 A necrotizing granuloma in a patient with cat scratch disease. Neutrophils are found within the necrotic area.

i8.12 A nonnecrotizing, noncaseating granuloma in a patient with sarcoidosis

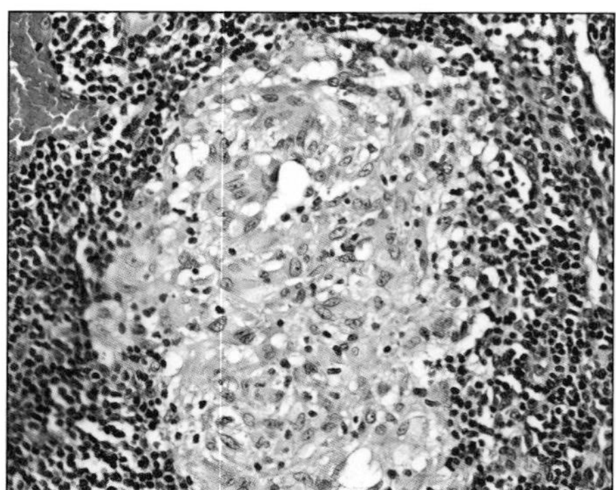

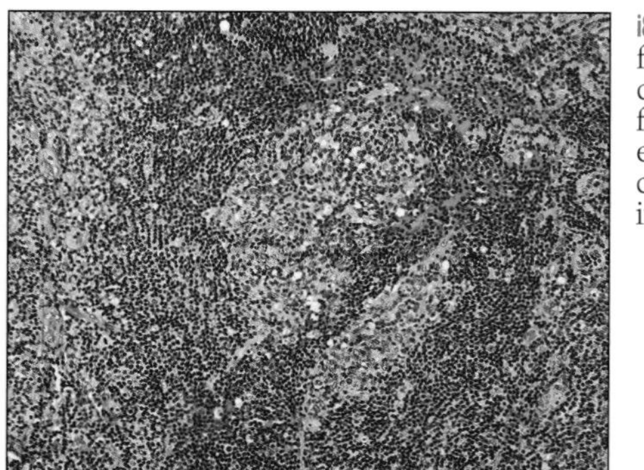

i8.13 **3**. Progressive transformation of germinal centers. Lymphocytes from the mantle zone are entering the germinal center and have divided it into 2 sections.

i8.14 **a** The hyaline vascular type of Castleman disease. These 2 germinal centers are atrophic. **b** Another example of the hyaline vascular form of Castleman disease with pronounced atrophy of the germinal center

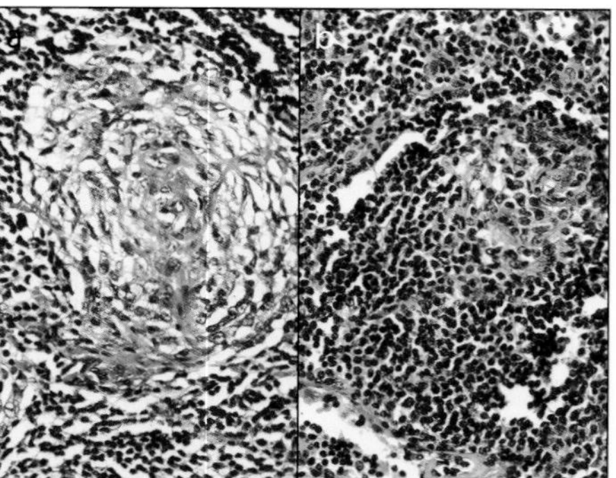

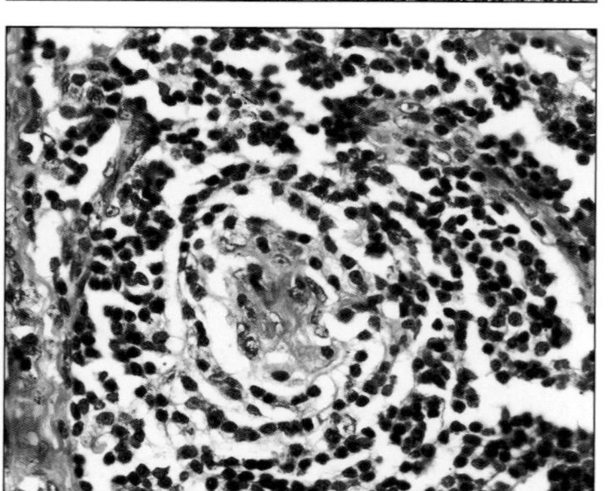

i8.15 The hyaline vascular form of Castleman disease with nearly-complete atrophy of the germinal center and an "onion ring" pattern of the lymphocytes in the surrounding mantle zone

i8.16 A blood vessel with a hyalinized wall entering an atrophic germinal center in the hyaline vascular form of Castleman disease

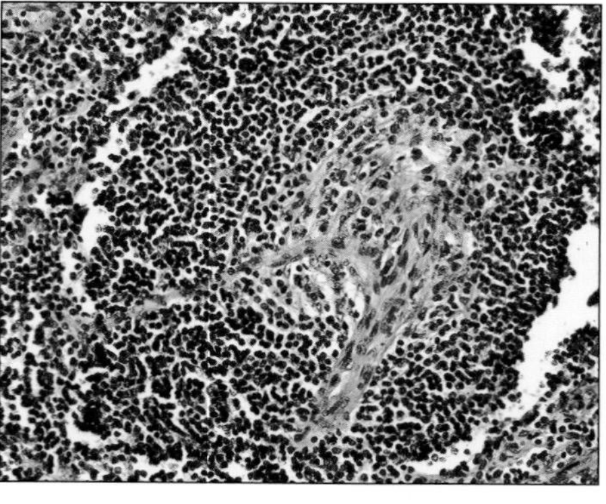

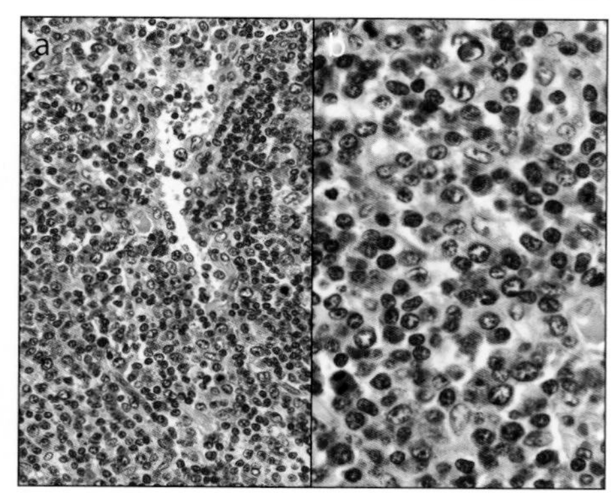

i8.17 **a** The plasma cell form of Castleman disease with numerous plasma cells between germinal centers. A normal germinal center is seen on the right while numerous interfollicular plasma cells are seen in the center and on the left. **b** The same case as in i8.17a, highlighting interfollicular plasma cells.

i8.18 Nodular sclerosing Hodgkin disease. This low-power view illustrates the anastomosing bands of collagen that divide the lymph node into lobules.

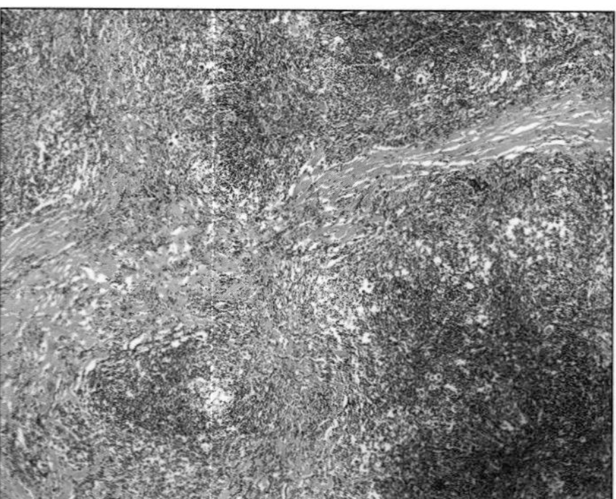

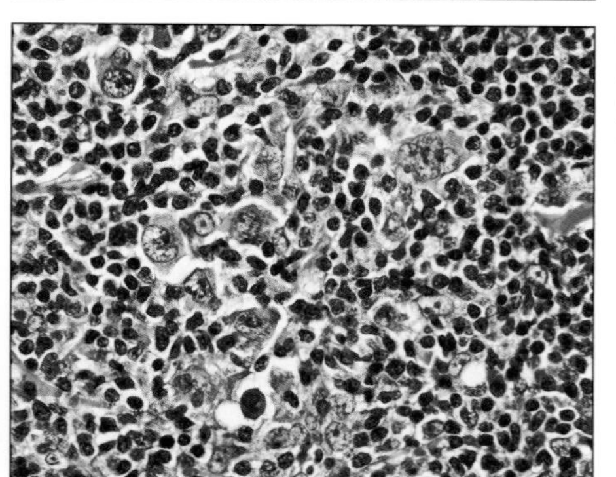

i8.19 Several different forms of Reed-Sternberg cells in nodular sclerosing Hodgkin disease

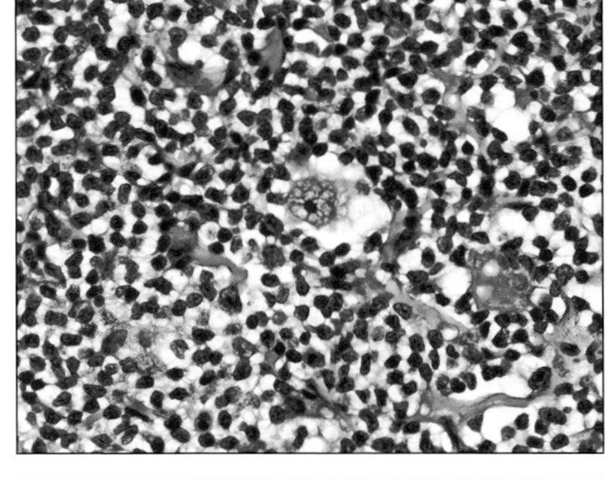

0 The lacunar cell, with
e characteristic clear
ace surrounding the
cleus

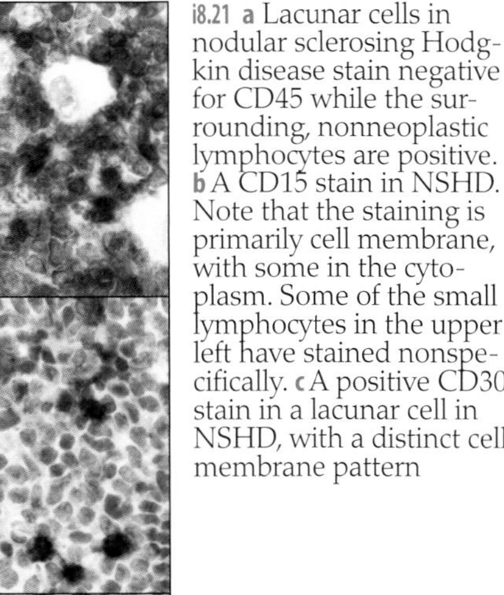

i8.21 **a** Lacunar cells in nodular sclerosing Hodgkin disease stain negative for CD45 while the surrounding, nonneoplastic lymphocytes are positive. **b** A CD15 stain in NSHD. Note that the staining is primarily cell membrane, with some in the cytoplasm. Some of the small lymphocytes in the upper left have stained nonspecifically. **c** A positive CD30 stain in a lacunar cell in NSHD, with a distinct cell membrane pattern

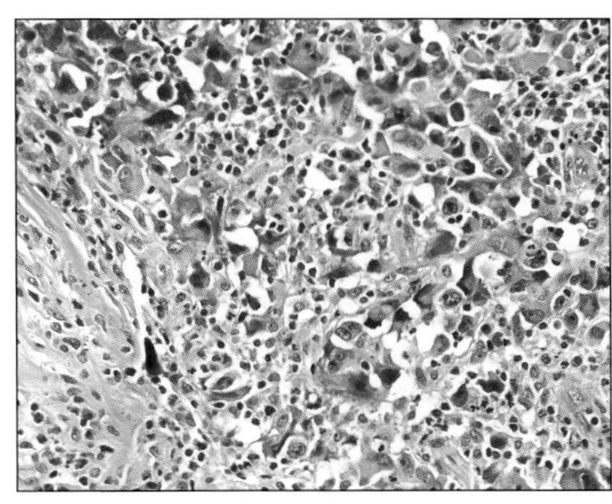

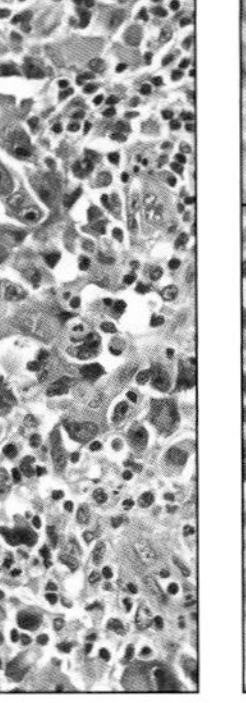

2 The syncytial form
NSHD, in which the
ed-Sternberg cells form
arly confluent sheets.
ote the fibrous septa in
e lower left and the eo-
nophils, which are often
en in Hodgkin disease.
is is a high-grade form
Hodgkin disease.

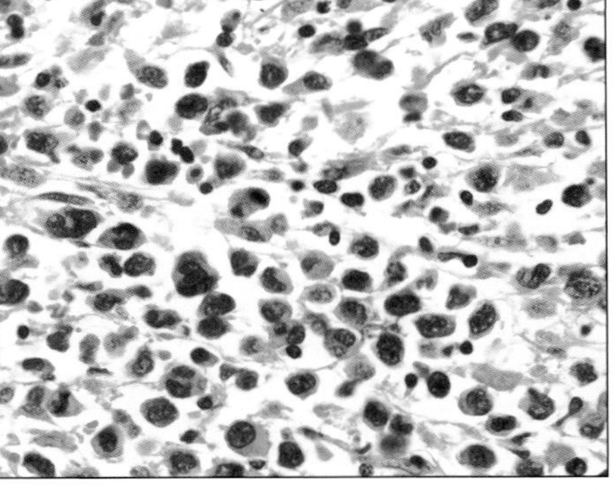

3 An example of high-
ade Hodgkin disease
cause of the bizarre
ed-Sternberg cells that
e present

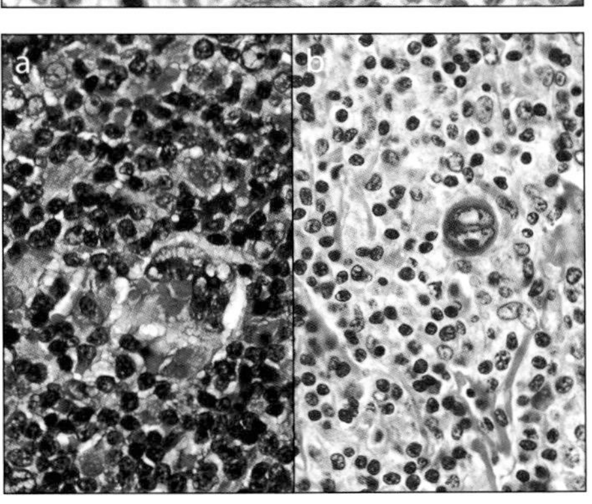

i8.24 **a, b** Classic Reed-Sternberg cells in cases of mixed cellularity Hodgkin disease

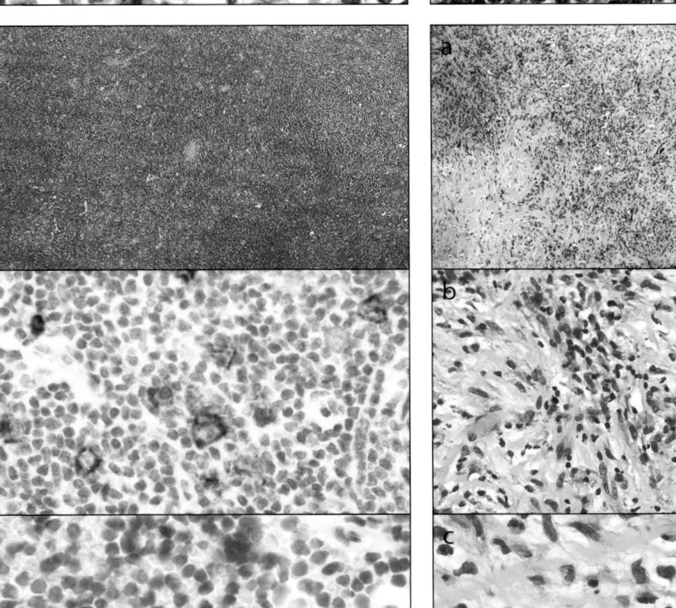

5 **a** Lymphocyte-rich
assical Hodgkin disease.
this low-power H&E
ew, there is a faint
odularity that initially
ggests either a nodular
ollicular) non-Hodgkin
mphoma or NLPHD.

The same case as
i8.25a, with positive
aining for the large
ypical cells for CD15

he same case as in i8.25a
ith positive staining
r CD30. The CD15 and
D30 stains identify the
se as a lymphocyte-
ch classical Hodgkin
sease rather than a
on-Hodgkin lymphoma
NLPHD.

i8.26 **a** An example of the so-called lymphocyte depleted form of Hodgkin disease. Note the extensive fibrosis.

b The same case as in i8.26a, highlighting the almost complete absence of lymphocytes and the extensive fibrosis. There are numerous eosinophils, left over from an earlier stage.

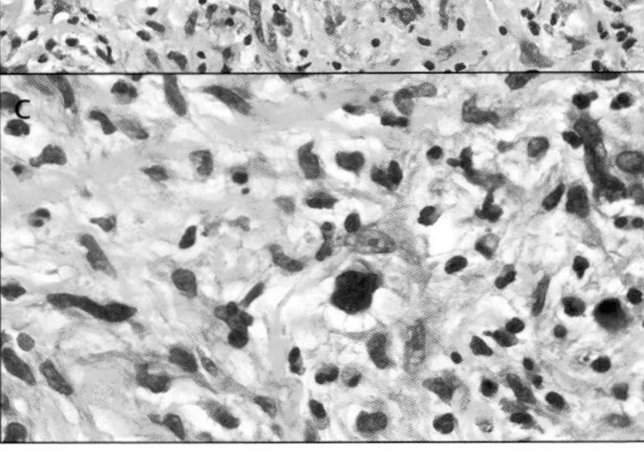

c The same case as in i8.26a, illustrating a rare residual lacunar cell, now pyknotic

ISBN 978-089189-5886

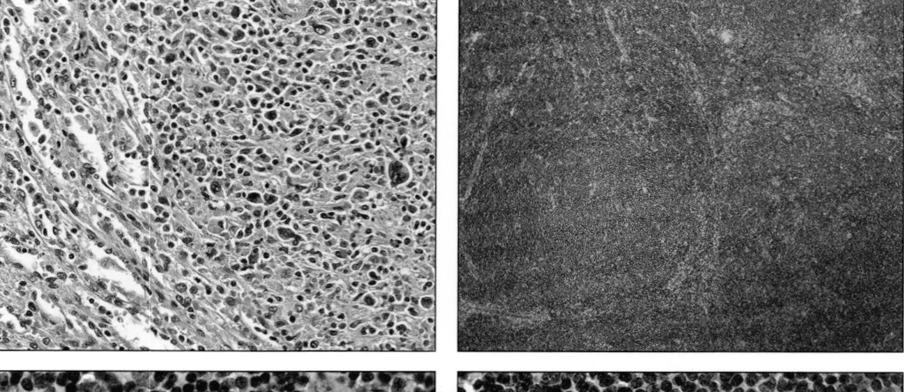

i8.27 Hodgkin disease of the spleen. Note the residual splenic tissue on the left and the Reed-Sternberg cells on the right.

i8.28 A low-power view of NLPHD, illustrating the faint nodularity

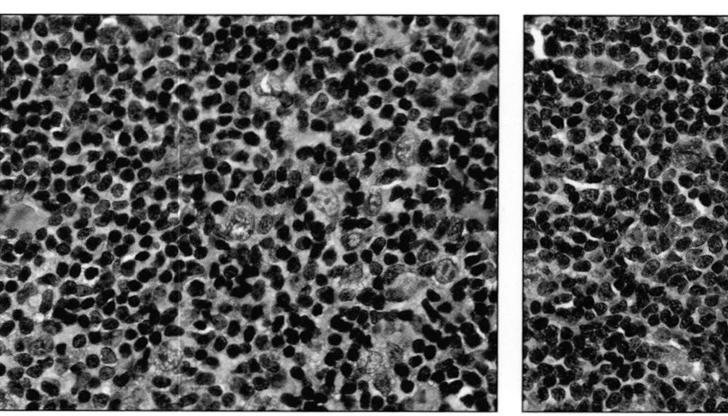

i8.29 A higher-power view of the same case as in i8.28, illustrating LP cells

i8.30 An LP cell, with a lobated nucleus, in NLPHD

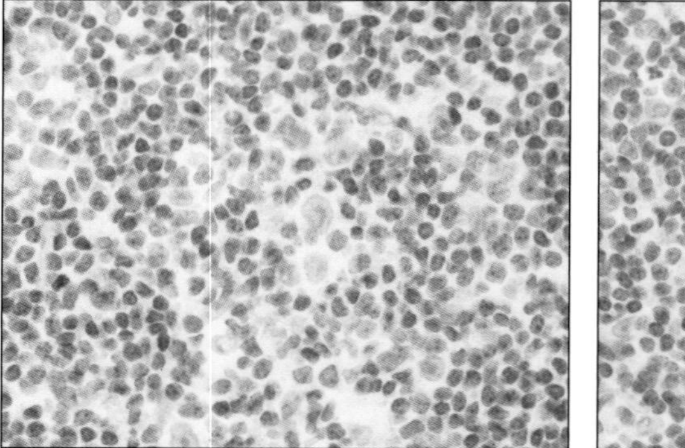

i8.31 Negative staining of an LP cell for CD15

i8.32 Negative staining of an LP cell for CD30. Note the faint positivity of some of the associated, nonneoplastic lymphocytes, illustrating that CD30 may be positive in an "activated" lymphocyte.

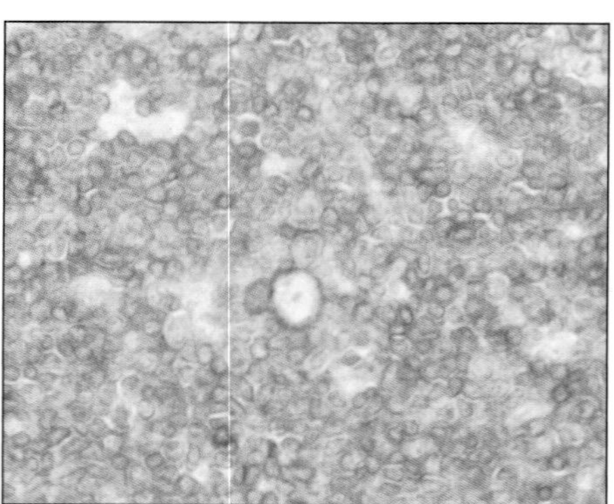

i8.33 Positive staining for an LP cell in NLPHD for CD45 (center), which is not seen in a true R-S cell

i8.34 A case of NLPHD stained with CD20 to highlight the subtle nodular architecture

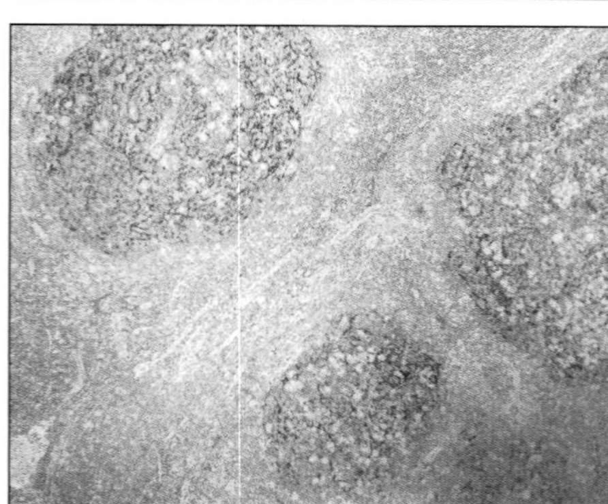

i8.35 The same case as in i8.34 stained for CD21, which highlights nodules by staining follicular dendritic cells. CD21 is always a very helpful stain to demonstrate nodules that are inconspicuous on H&E.

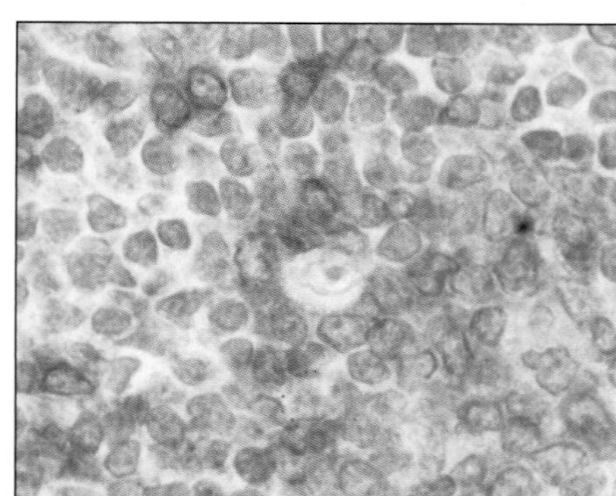

i8.36 A case of NLPHD, stained with CD3, in which the LP cell is surrounded by T cells. Note that while many of the background lymphocytes are negative for CD3 (indicating B-cell origin), those lymphocytes that surround the LP cell are T cells.

A case of NLPHD strating that the mber of LP cells in a dule may be more than ially suspected, but will ely equal that in a non- dgkin lymphoma

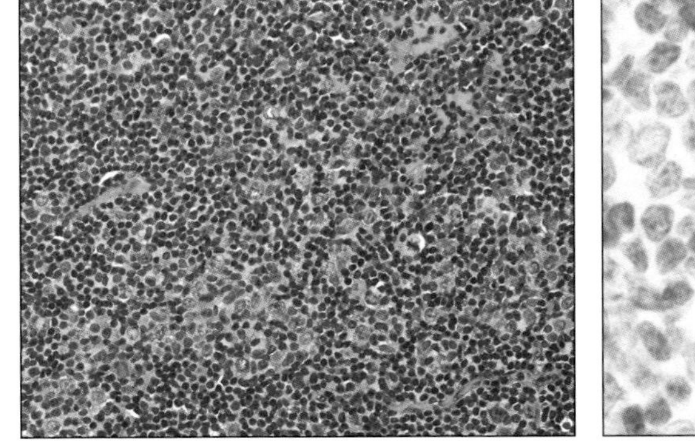

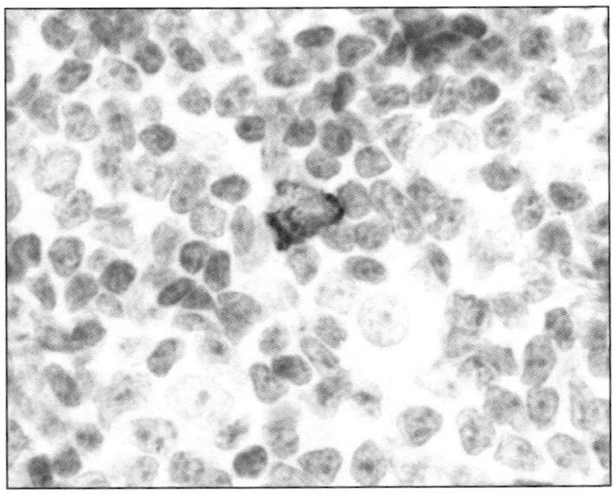

i8.38 An LP cell that stains for epithelial membrane antigen

A follicular lymphoma strating the widespread tribution of follicles dules)

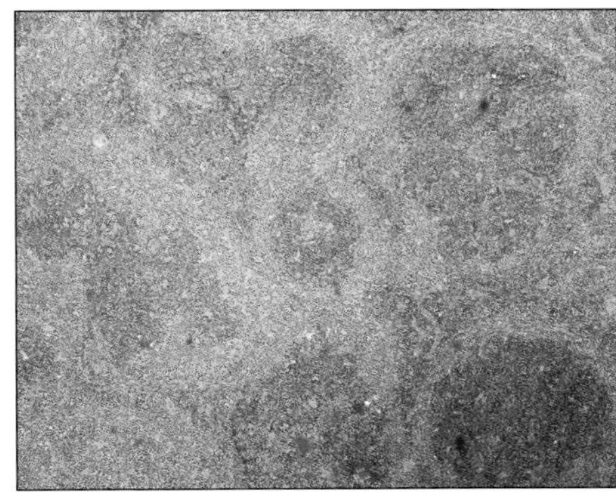

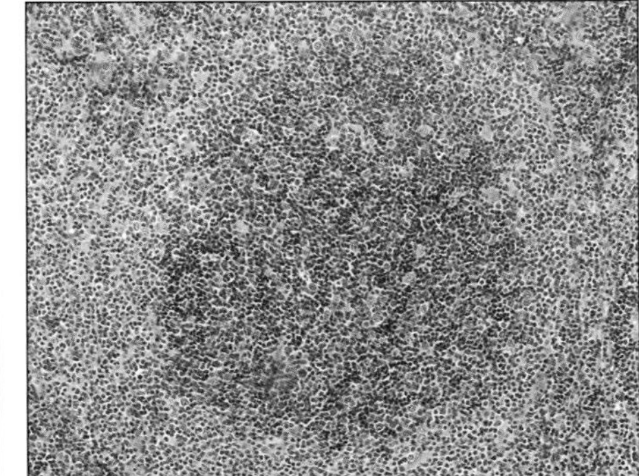

i8.40 The same case as in i8.39, illustrating that the putative follicles do not have a normal population of cells and they do not contain germinal centers

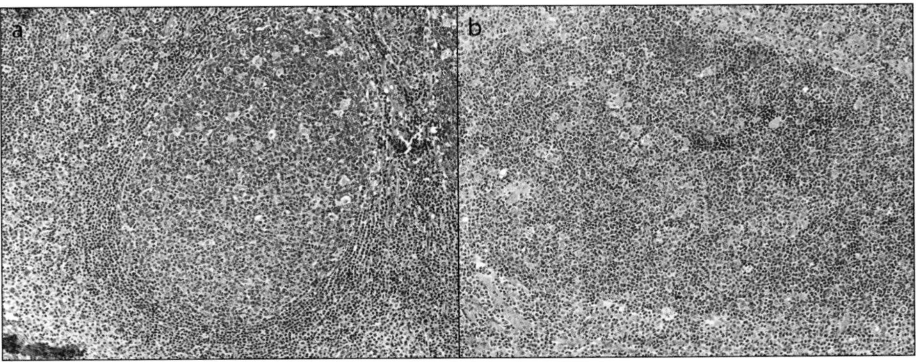

a A normal lymphoid licle. The mantle zone more cellular at the ttom of the photograph n at the top. The ttom of the germinal nter, abutting the more lular area of the mantle ne, is lighter and has ver centroblasts and ver mitoses than the rtion of the germinal nter that faces away m the more cellular a of the mantle zone.

b A neoplastic lymphoid follicle. The demarcation between the apparent mantle zone and the interior portion is indistinct and there is no area of greater cellularity in the outermost portion, unlike a normal mantle zone.

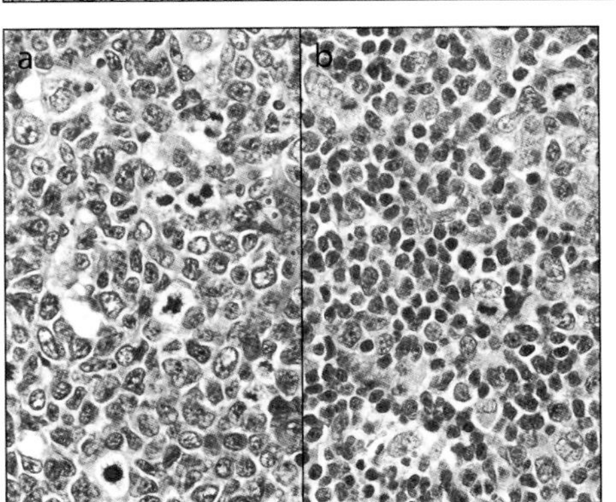

2 a The centroblastic a of a normal germinal nter, showing numerous ntroblasts and merous mitotic figures he interior portion of a oplastic follicle. There is s of demarcation of the ntroblastic/centrocytic eas, mitoses are fewer, d they are evenly stributed throughout the licle.

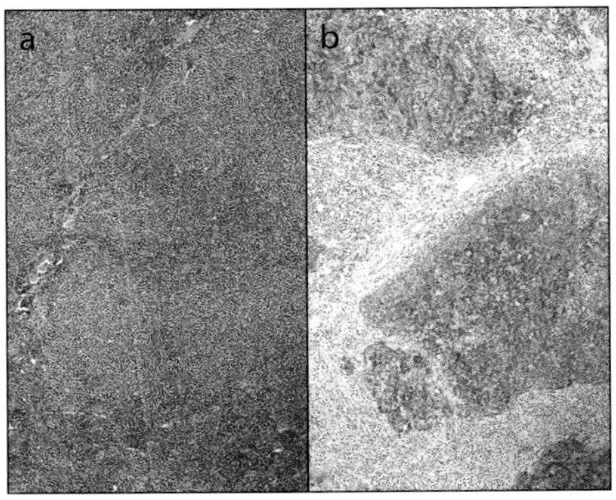

i8.43 a A follicular lymphoma with subtle nodularity b A CD21 immunohistochemical stain highlighting the follicular dendritic cells, and thus highlighting the follicles

4 A follicular lymphoma ined for bcl-6, nfirming the nodularity the process

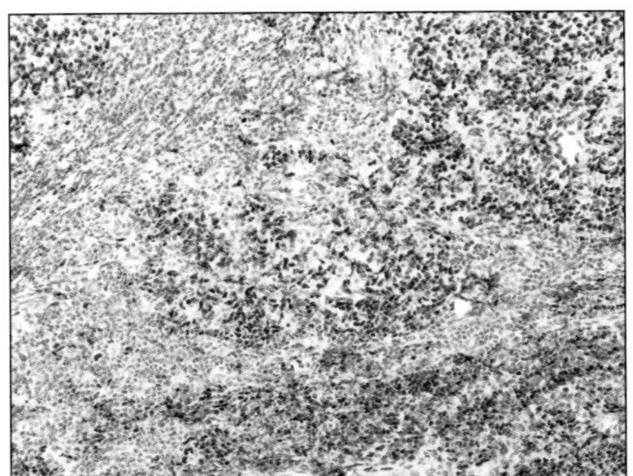

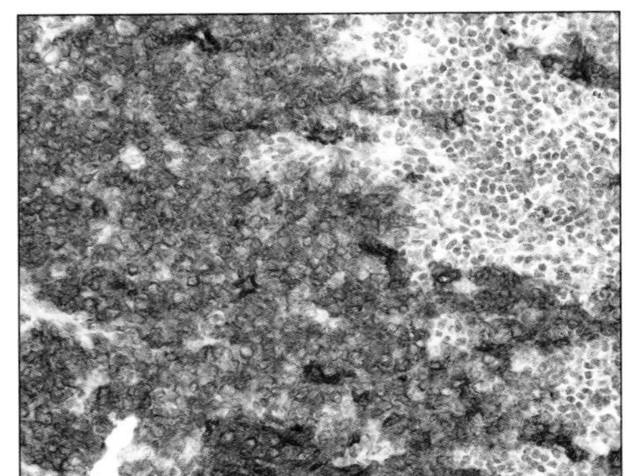

i8.45 The same case as in i8.44 stained for CD10, again highlighting a neoplastic follicle

ISBN 978-089189-5886

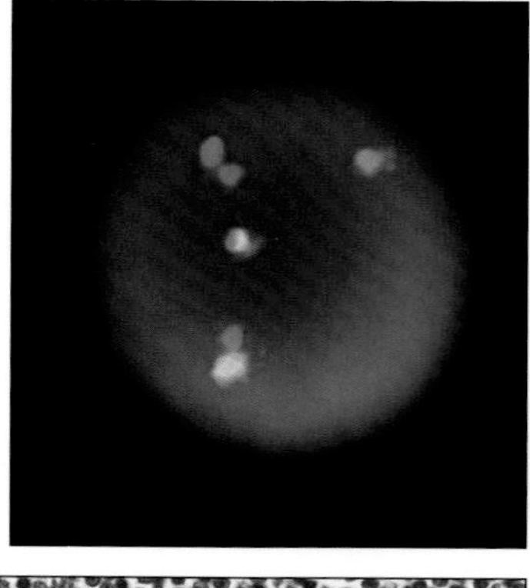

i8.46 Dual-fusion FISH of the t(14;18) that is found in most cases of follicular lymphoma in which separate red and green probes are used for the *BCL-2* gene on chromosome 18 and the J region of immunoglobulin heavy chain gene on chromosome 14. In the normal situation, these signals remain separate, but in the center and lower portion of this cell, the yellow signal indicates that the red and green signals have been juxtaposed by a translocation, causing them to blend into a single yellow color.

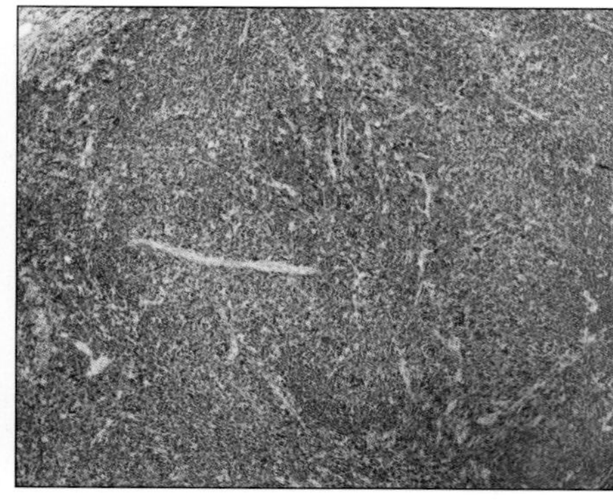

i8.47 A follicular lymphoma stained for bcl-2. Note the diffuse positivity, including within the follicles. Normal germinal centers are not positive for bcl-2.

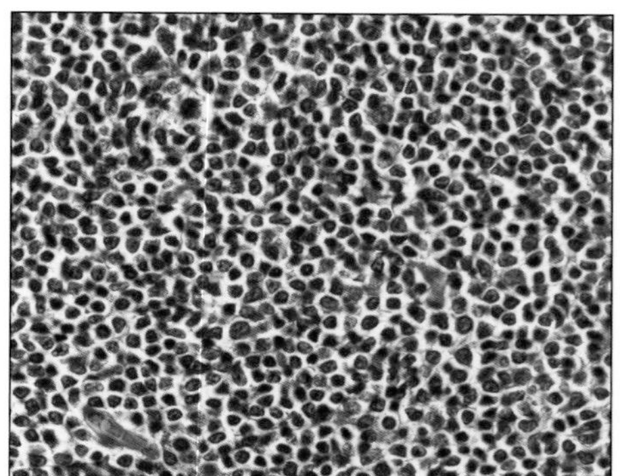

i8.48 A high-power view of a follicle in a grade 1 follicular lymphoma. There is a nearly uniform population of centrocytic cells with very few centroblasts.

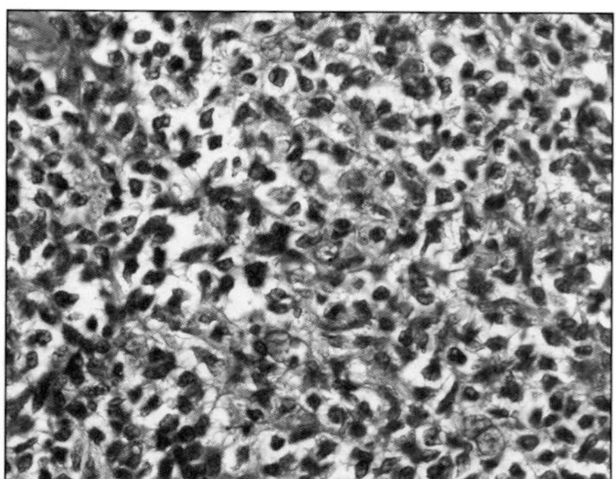

i8.49 A high-power view of a follicle in a grade 2 follicular lymphoma. Small centrocytic cells predominate, but larger centroblasts are readily noted.

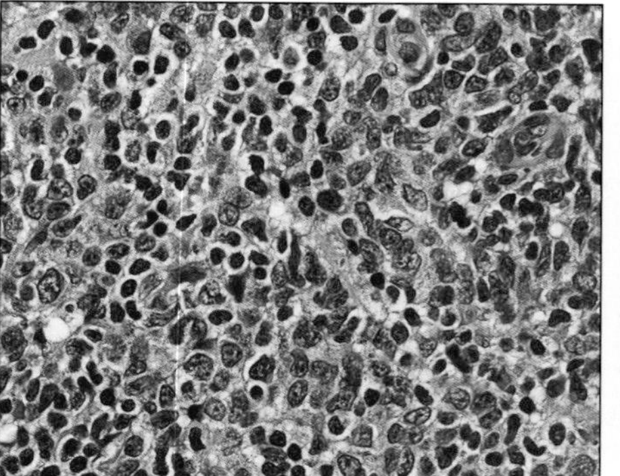

i8.50 In a grade 3 follicular lymphoma, centroblasts exceed 15 per high-power field in the follicles.

i8.51 A follicular lymphoma in which H&E examination of the follicles is somewhat equivocal as to grade. There are only a small number of large cells in this photograph, but there are numerous cells that are smaller but have vesicular chromatin and nucleoli.

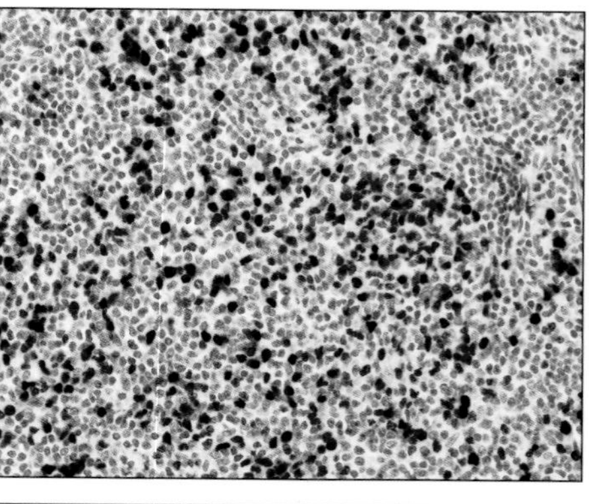

i8.52 The same case as in i8.51, stained for Ki-67. Approximately 30% of cells stain, a higher number than would be expected in a grade 2 follicular lymphoma, suggesting this may be best regarded as a grade 3 follicular lymphoma.

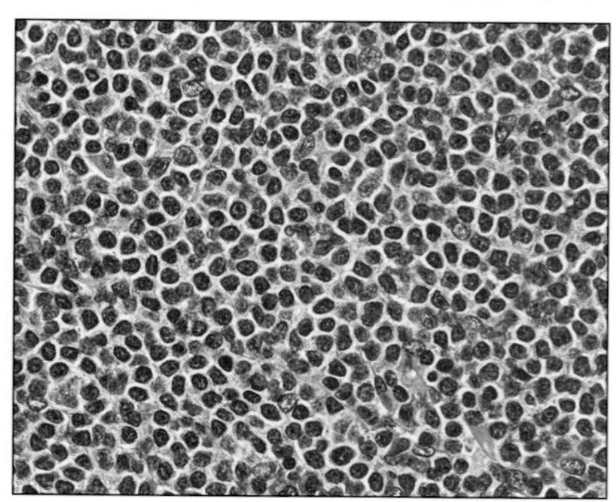

i8.53 Mantle cell lymphoma. Note the uniform population of small cells with essentially no large cells whatsoever. A diffuse pattern and an absence of large cells suggest a mantle cell lymphoma.

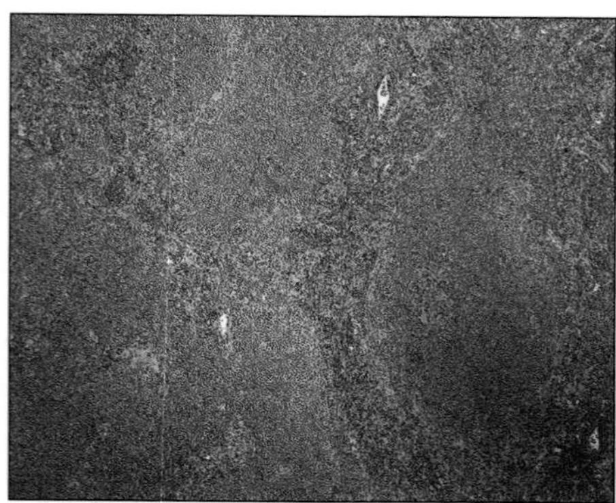

i8.54 A mantle cell lymphoma with a faint nodularity

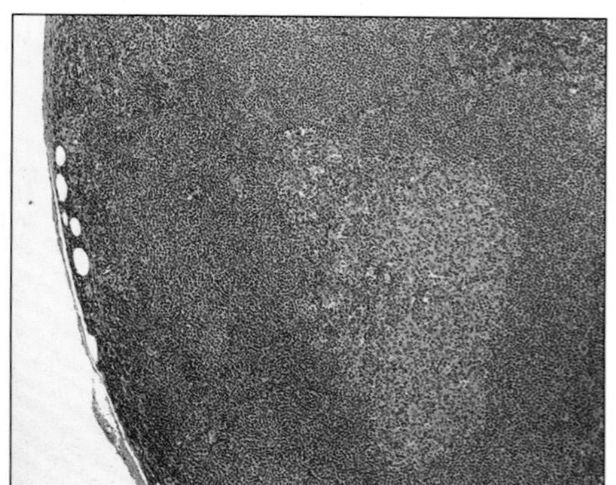

i8.55 A mantle cell lymphoma with growth around a residual germinal center. The mantle zone around this germinal center is composed of neoplastic cells that merge with the neoplastic cells throughout the lymph node.

6 Follicular colonization
a mantle cell
nphoma. This germinal
nter has been heavily
onized and is barely
cognizable.

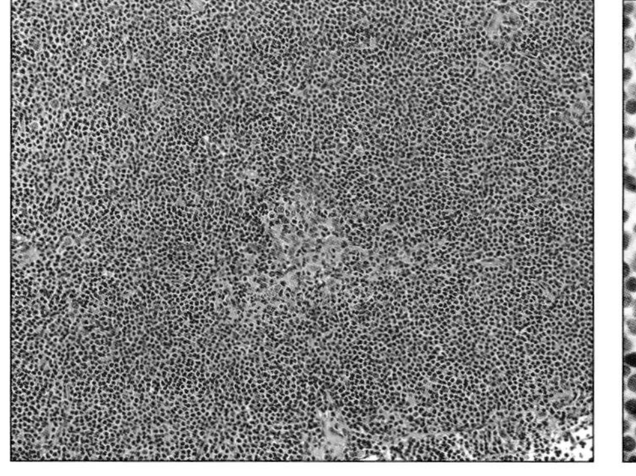

i8.57 Positive bcl-1 staining in a mantle cell lymphoma.

8 Dual-fusion FISH
dy confirming the
1;14), between
BCL-1 gene and
immunoglobulin
avy chain gene. The
nslocation is essentially
ique to mantle cell
nphoma.

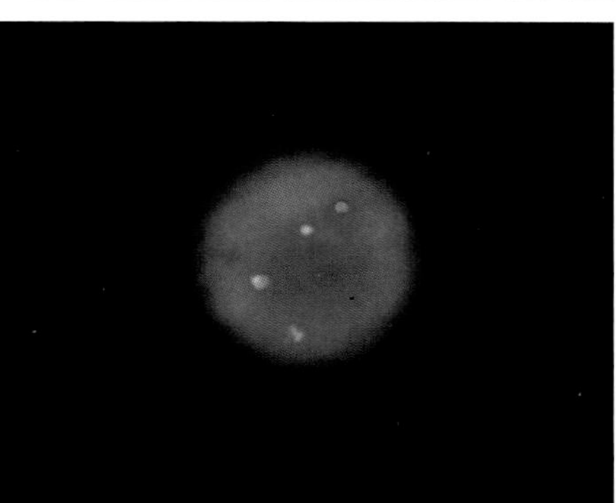

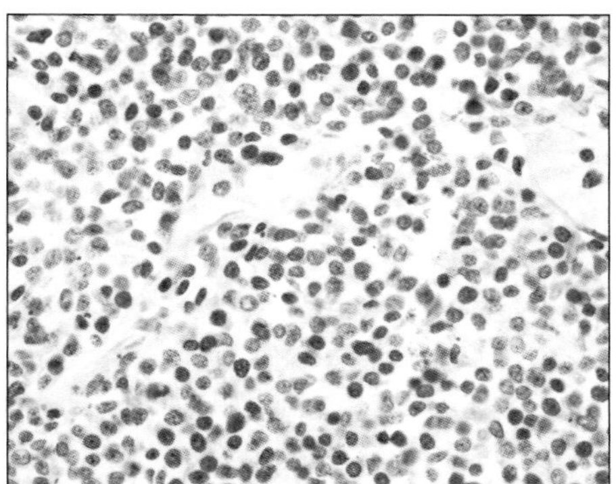

i8.59 The same case as in i8.57, with uniformly negative staining for bcl-6, indicating these cells are not of germinal center origin

0 **a** The rare blastic form
mantle cell lymphoma
he same case as in
0a, illustrating larger
ls with more variability
an in the typical mantle
l lymphoma. Note the
merous mitotic figures,
t usually seen in most
ntle cell lymphomas.
he same case as in i8.60a,
ined for bcl-1

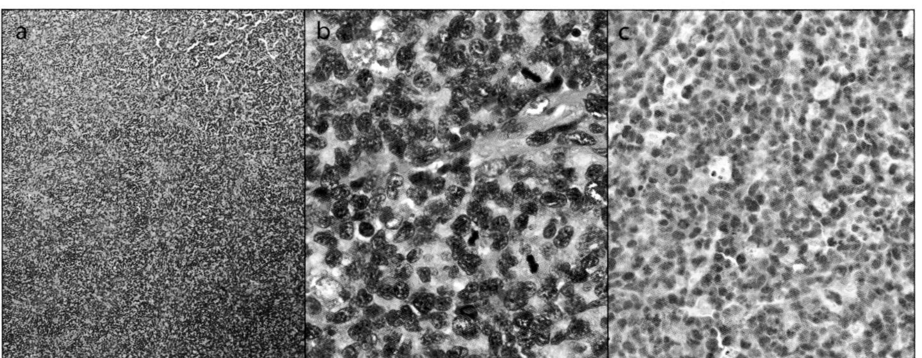

1 **a** A marginal zone
nphoma with a so
led "monocytoid"
pearance caused by
ar cytoplasm **b** A
gh-power view of the
me case as in i8.61a,
ghlighting the large
nount of faintly staining
toplasm

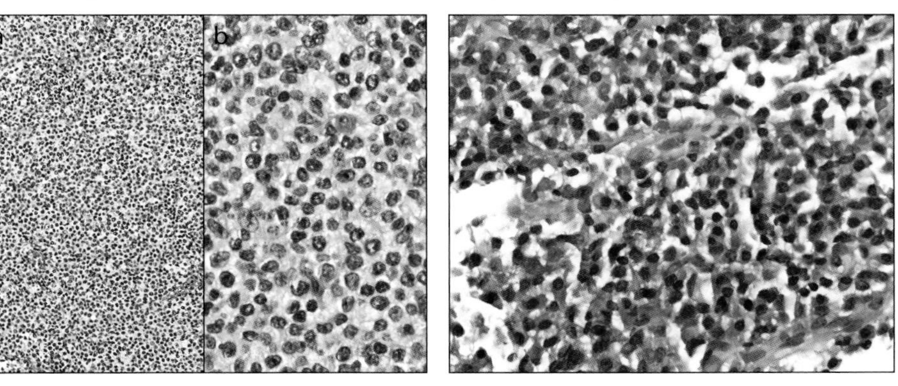

i8.62 Another example of marginal zone lymphoma with a plasmacytoid appearance

3 A marginal zone
nphoma growing
ound a residual benign
rminal center

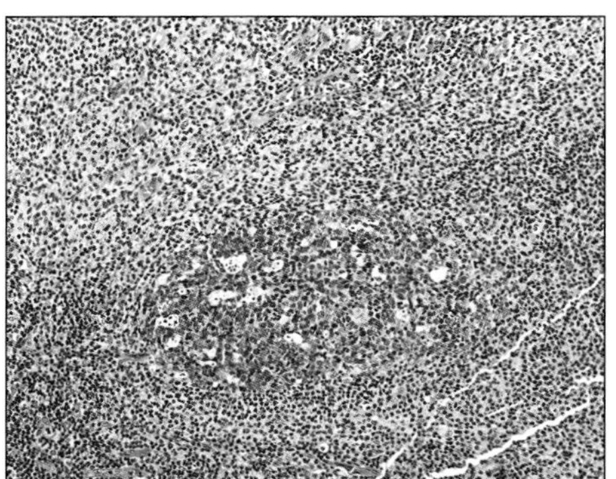

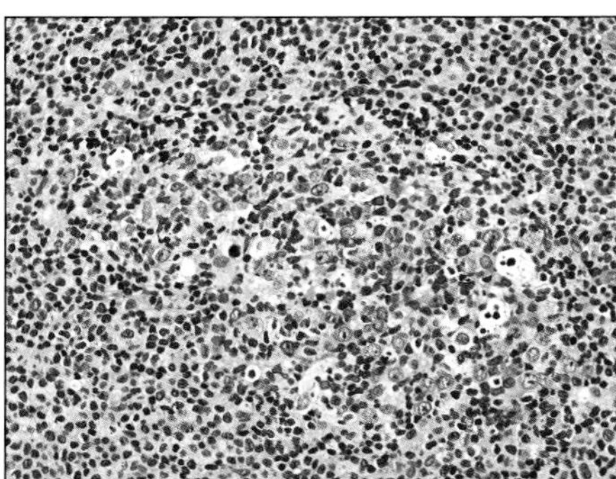

i8.64 Follicular colonization in a marginal zone lymphoma

ISBN 978-089189-5886

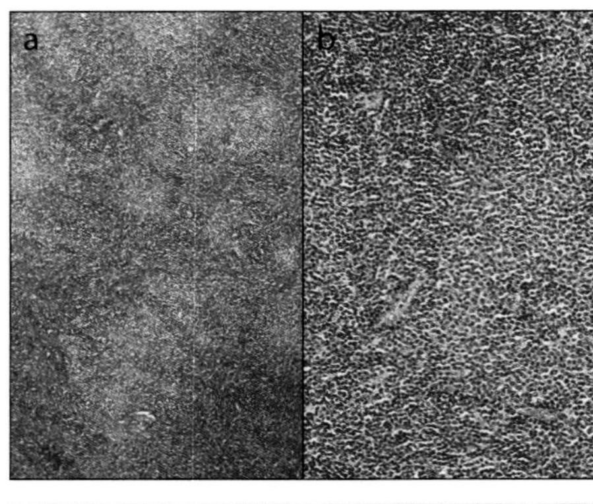

i8.65 **a** Small lymphocytic lymphoma at low power, demonstrating lighter areas that are proliferation centers **b** A higher-power view of the same case as in i8.65a, illustrating a proliferation center in the lower right that is lighter staining and of lower cellular density than in the upper left

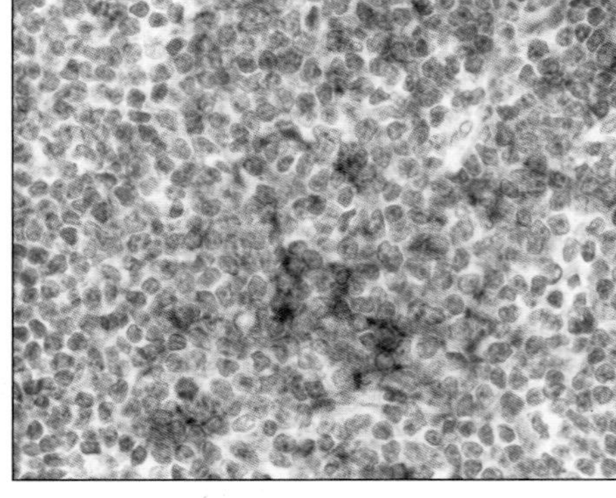

i8.66 Small lymphocytic lymphoma staining positively for CD23

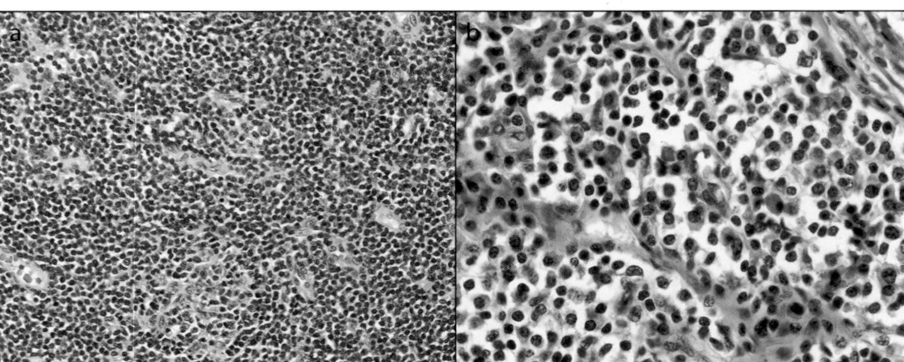

i8.67 **a** Lymphoplasmacytic lymphoma at low power demonstrating a diffuse proliferation of small lymphocytes **b** The same case as in i8.67a, illustrating the eccentric nuclei and occasional plasmacytoid morphology of the neoplastic cells

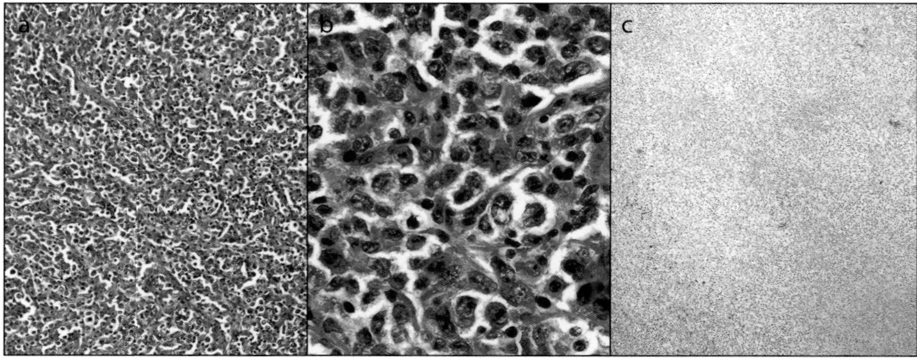

i8.68 **a** A diffuse large B-cell lymphoma illustrating the diffuse architecture **b** A higher-power view of the same case as in i8.68a illustrating the large size of the cells compared to the few small lymphocytes in the field **c** The same case as in i8.68a. This CD21 stain for follicular dendritic cells highlights the absence of follicles.

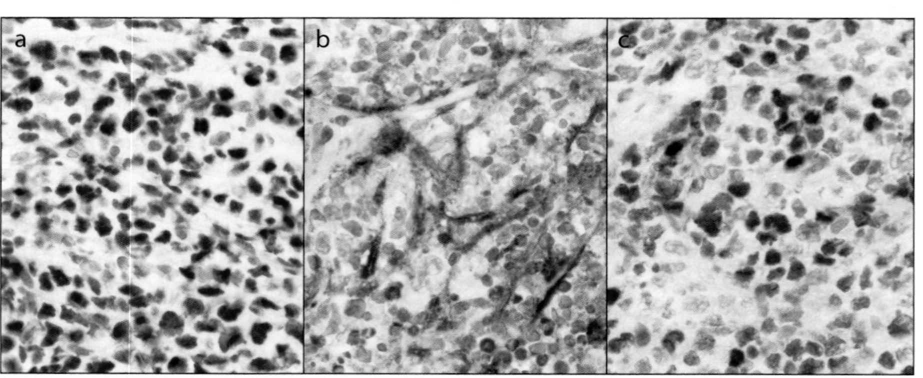

i8.69 A diffuse large B-cell lymphoma simultaneously expressing **a** bcl-6, **b** CD10, and **c** MUM1, a staining pattern not usually seen in benign lymphocytes. Note the nuclear staining for bcl-6 and MUM1, and the cell membrane staining for CD10.

i8.70 A T-cell-rich B-cell lymphoma. Note the small number of large neoplastic B cells surrounded by larger numbers of nonneoplastic T cells and histiocytes.

i8.71 **a** A primary mediastinal large B-cell lymphoma. At this low-power view, neoplastic cells are difficult to identify. **b** A higher-power view of the same case as in i8.71a, illustrating the neoplastic cells.

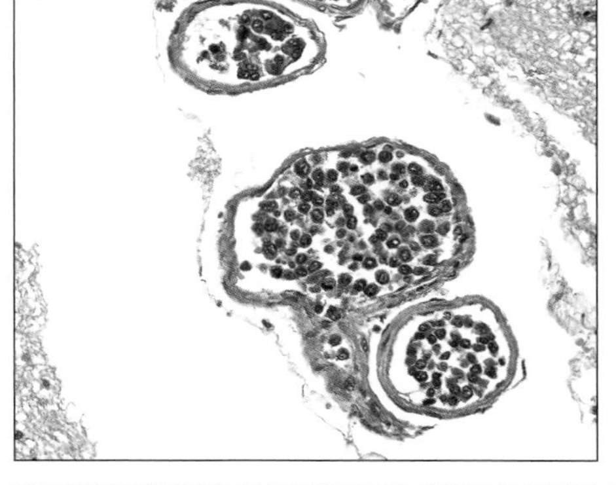

: An intravascular nphoma occurring in blood vessels in the ain

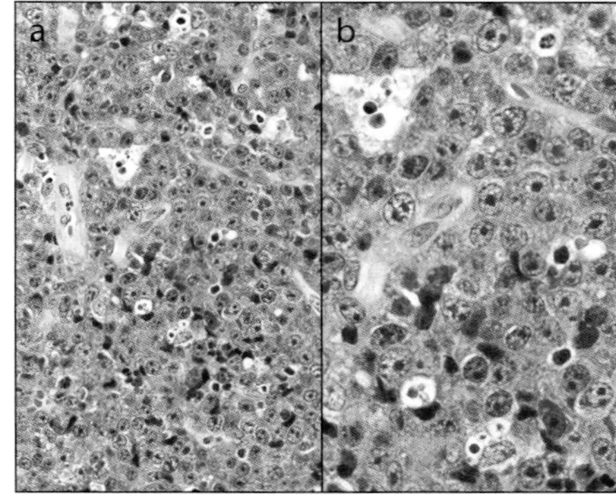

i8.73 **a** A plasmablastic lymphoma occurring in the oral cavity of an HIV-positive patient **b** A higher-power view of the same case as in i8.73a, illustrating the plasmablastic morphology

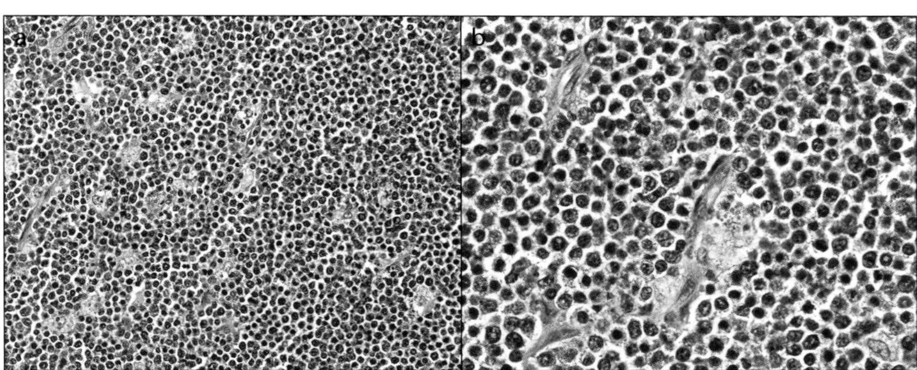

a A low-power view Burkitt lymphoma istrating the numerous icrophages mixed h the neoplastic cells, counting for the "starry " appearance **b** The same case as in i8.74a, highlighting a macrophage in the center

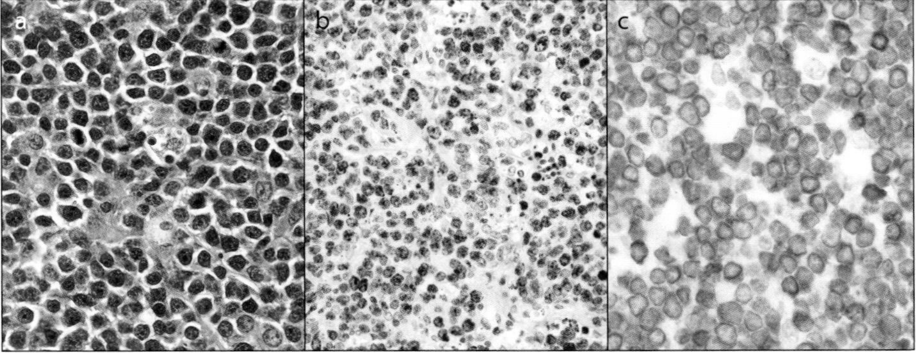

a A diffuse large B-cell nphoma that has very nilar to appearance to a rkitt lymphoma, even th macrophages **b** A -67 stain on the same se as in i8.75a, illustrating ery high proliferation e (in excess of 90%), ain suggesting a Burkitt nphoma **c** The same se as i8.75a stained bcl-2. The positivity ggests this may not be a rkitt lymphoma as most Burkitt are negative for bcl-2. Because the bcl-2 protein is on the outer mitochondrial membrane, and the neoplastic cells are relatively small, note that this stain, while perinuclear, appears cytoplasmic or even membranous. This case was studied for the t(8; 14) translocation that is characteristic of Burkitt lymphoma and found to be negative.

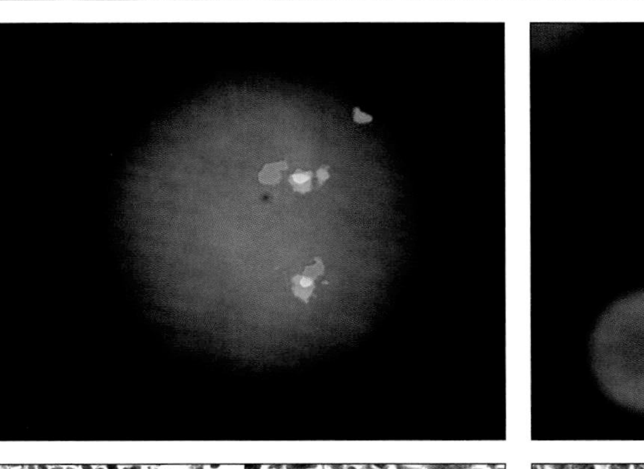

6 Dual-fusion FISH dy for the t(8;14) that characteristic of Burkitt nphoma. The t(8;14) 24;q32.3) translocation sults in the juxtaposi- n of the *C-MYC* gene d the immunoglobulin avy chain locus, result- in overexpression of *MYC* (many transloca- ns in hematopathology ice a proto-oncogene jacent to an immuno- bulin gene).

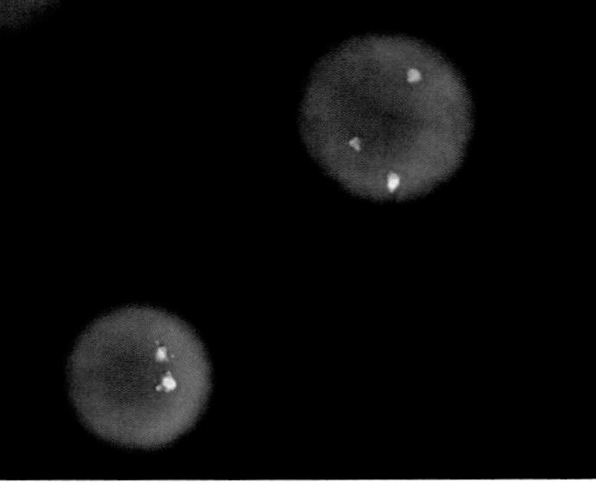

i8.77 Break apart FISH study for the t(8;14) that is characteristic of Burkitt lymphoma. In this break apart study, the 2 signals for *C-MYC* gene and the immunoglobulin heavy chain remain together in the normal cell, but are separated in a translocation. The cell in the upper right most clearly shows the separate red and green signals.

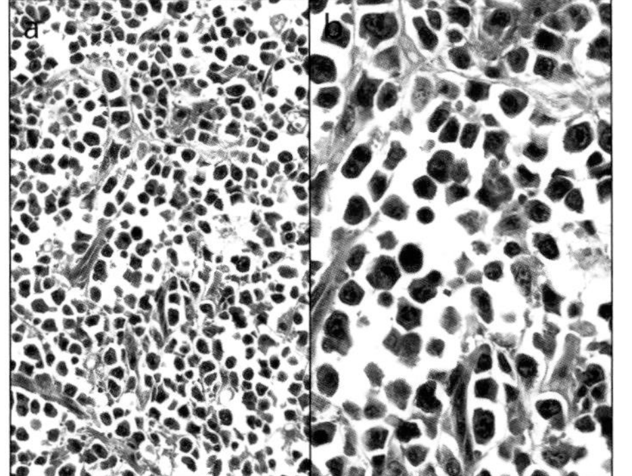

8 **a** A posttransplant nphoproliferative sorder with a ismacytic morphology he same case as in 8a, highlighting the ismacytic appearance

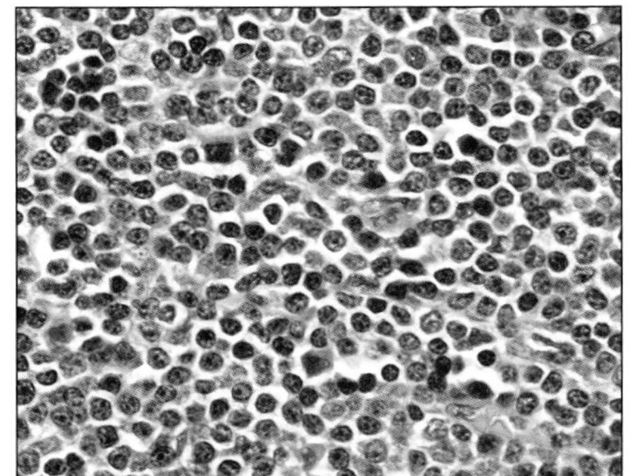

i8.79 A T-lymphoblastic lymphoma, illustrating the fine chromatin, small nucleoli, and minimal cytoplasm of the lymphoblasts. T-lymphoblastic lymphomas are also illustrated in i18.25 and i18.26.

ISBN 978-089189-5886

i8.80 **a** A T-cell lymphoma with a diffuse growth pattern. **b,c** The same case as in i8.80a stained for **b** CD3 and **c** CD2. Note the positive cell membrane staining for both T-cell antigens.

d The same case as in i8.80a, stained for CD20. This case has positive staining for 2 T-cell markers and was negative for CD20 and other -cell markers, confirming T-cell lineage.
e The same case as in i8.80a, stained for bcl-2, illustrating that bcl-2 staining is not specific for B-cell processes

i8.81 An NK-cell lymphoma.
a illustrates the diffuse architecture, as is the case for virtually all T-cell lymphomas.
b highlights the generally large nature of the neoplastic cells.
c illustrates expression of CD3 in the cytoplasm rather than in the usual cell membrane location.

d and **e** are CD2 and CD7, respectively. These additional T-cell stains, in conjunction with the negative CD20 stain in **f** confirm the T-cell origin.

g is a positive CD56 stain, separating this lymphoma from other T-cell lymphomas and suggesting it is likely of natural killer origin.
h is a positive in situ hybridization stain for EBV, which is very characteristic of NK-cell lymphomas.

i and **j** illustrate cytoplasmic staining for granzyme B and TIA-1, respectively, also very supportive of a diagnosis of natural killer cell lymphoma.

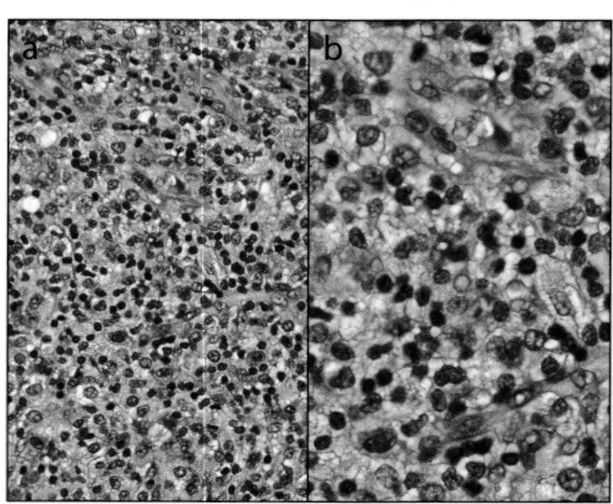

i8.82 **a** A low-power view of the large cell variant of anaplastic lymphoma **b** The same case as in i8.82a, illustrating the large size of neoplastic cells and the admixture of nonneoplastic smaller lymphocytes

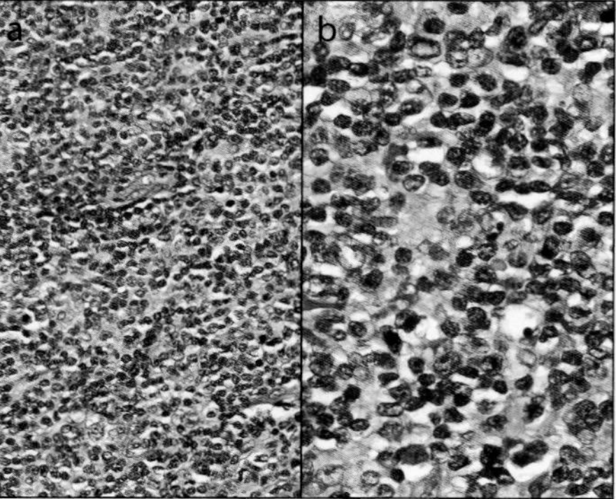

i8.83 **a** The small cell variant of anaplastic lymphoma illustrating the diffuse architecture **b** The same case as in i8.83a, confirming the smaller size of the neoplastic cells relative to the case in i8.83

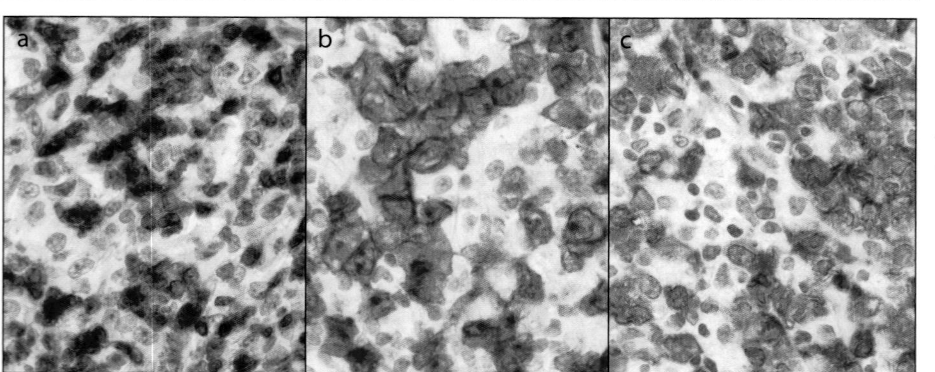

i8.84 **a** The same case as in i8.82, demonstrating positive staining for CD3 **b** The same case as in i8.82, illustrating positive staining for CD30

c An anaplastic lymphoma (the same case as in i8.82, illustrating positive staining for the ALK protein. Note that the staining is both cytoplasmic and cell membrane, a consequence of translocation between chromosomes 2 and 5.

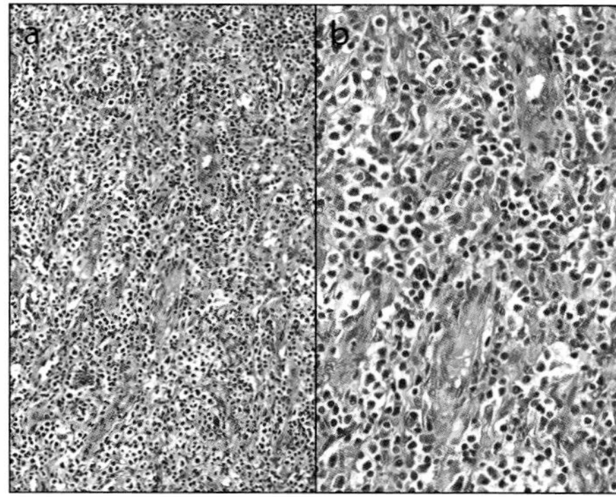

a Angioimmuno- stic lymphadenopathy strating the diffuse hitecture and the ef- ement of normal lymph de structures he same case as in 5a, highlighting the ensive vascularity

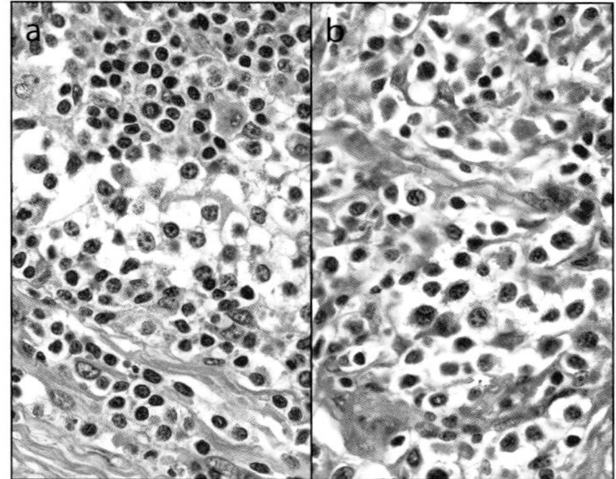

i8.86 The same case as in i8.85, highlighting that the neoplastic cells often have clear cytoplasm and are generally found adjacent to or between blood vessels

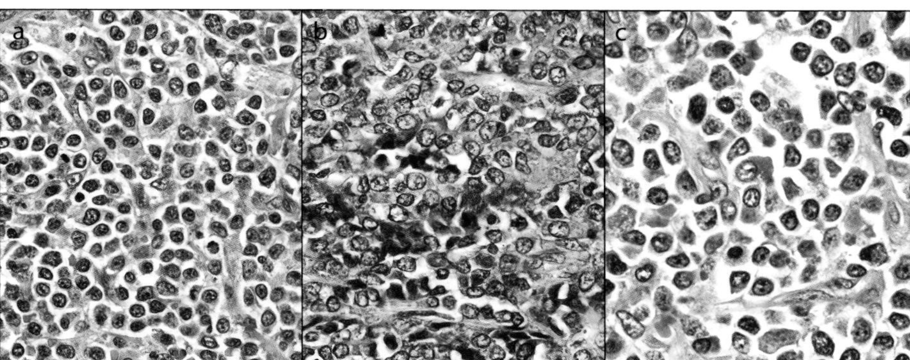

a,b Extramedullary eloid tumors of blastic tures. Note that the oplastic cells have nost no clumping of omatin and that there no differentiation.

c Another example of extramedullary myeloid tumor with minimal differentiation, as indicated by the eosinophilic myelocyte in the center

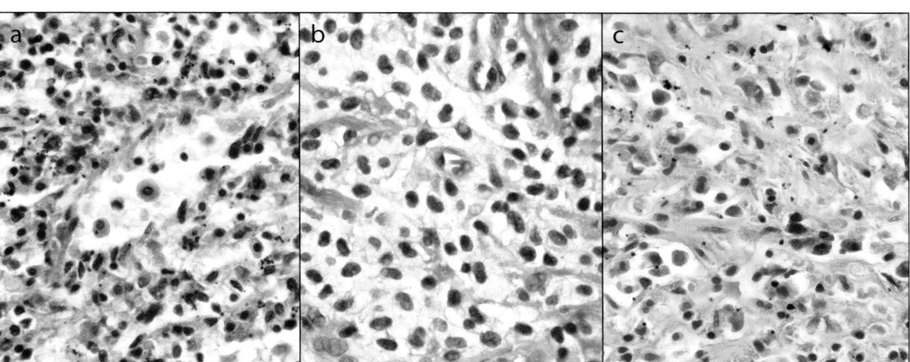

a Mastocytosis with ognizable mast cells, ch as the one in the nter lastocytosis with oplastic cells that have ar cytoplasm

c Mastocytosis with fibrosis

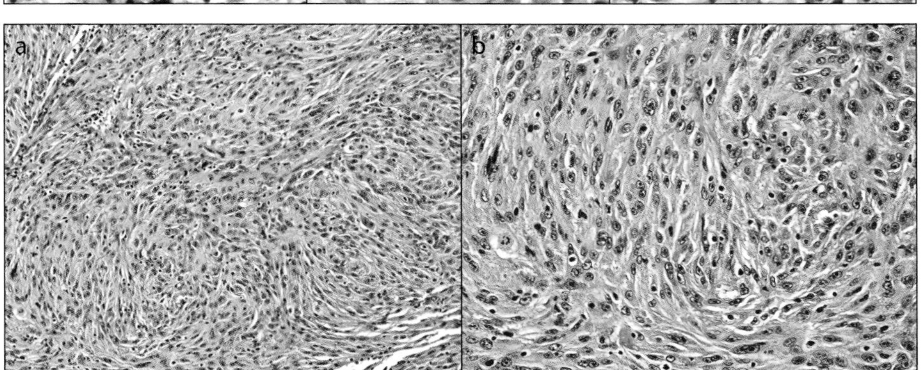

a A primary follicular ndritic cell sarcoma strating the spindle l morphology and appearance that is ferent from most matopoietic processes

b The same case as in i8.89a, highlighting the spindle cell appearance. This case was positive for both CD21 and CD35.

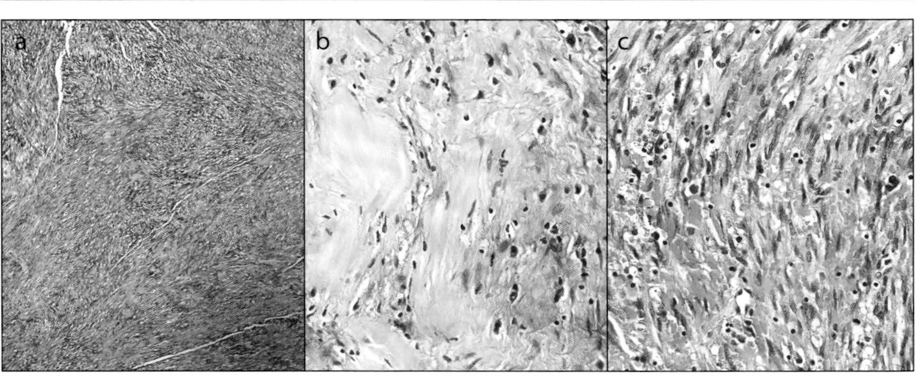

a A low-power w of a palisaded ofibroblastoma strating the spindle cell pearance. At this power, process could be nfused with a follicular ndritic cell sarcoma. he same case as in 0a, illustrating areas of lagen deposition that uld not be expected in ollicular dendritic cell coma

c The same case as in i8.90a, illustrating the extravasated erythrocytes intermingled with the spindle cell proliferation, which can cause confusion with Kaposi sarcoma

ISBN 978-089189-5886

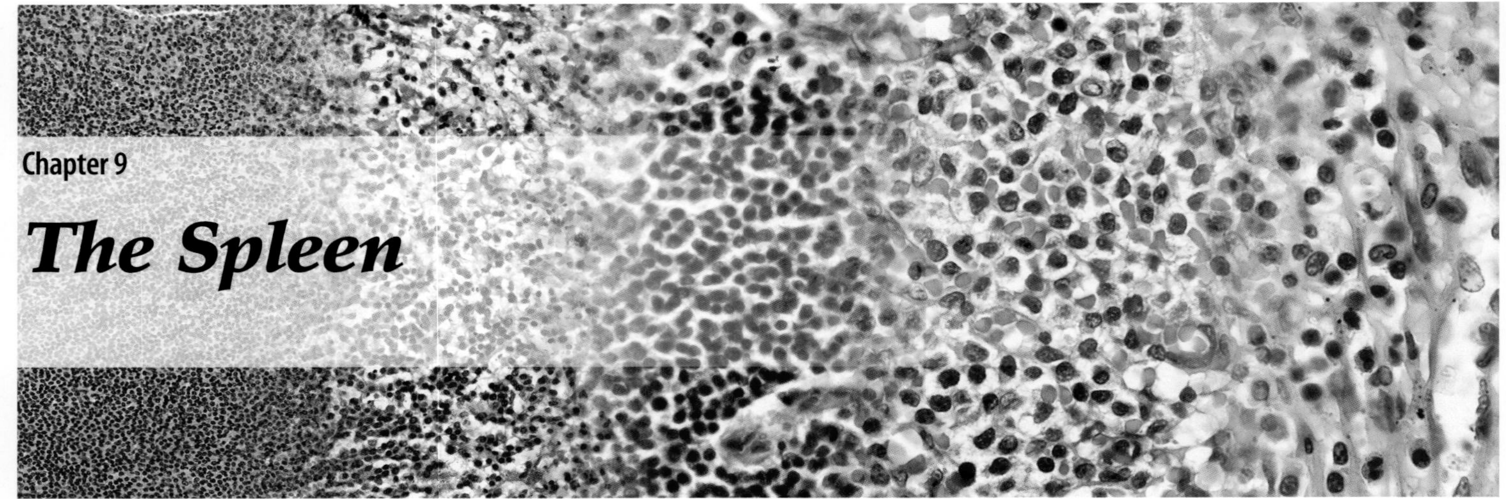

The spleen consists of red and white pulp i9.1. The white pulp of the spleen is essentially a large lymph node. The basic unit of the white pulp is the Malpighian corpuscle, an aggregate of B cells around an arteriole i9.2. The Malpighian corpuscle may consist of a germinal center and a mantle zone, as in a lymph node, but germinal centers in the splenic white pulp are less common in adults than in children. Another difference between splenic lymphoid tissue and lymph nodes is that the marginal zone, an area of noncirculating B cells external to the mantle zone, is more developed in the spleen. The marginal zone is important in the production of T cell-independent IgM. This is not an especially important function in adults, but in young children, these antibodies are important in defense against bacteria that have large amounts of polysaccharides in their capsules, such as Haemophilus influenzae b [PMID2478621]. This is why splenectomy is harmless in adults and older children, but should be undertaken with caution in the very young child.

The red pulp consists of trabecular cords of cells and sinuses, both readily seen on light microscopy i9.3. The red pulp contains macrophages and primarily functions to destroy senescent erythrocytes. Any lymphoid aggregate in the red pulp is suspicious for lymphoma.

The spleen has one of the more complicated vascular patterns of any organ. The white pulp lacks the normal afferent lymphatic channels that would normally bring fluid and antigens into contact with the lymphocytes. Instead, it relies on branches of the splenic artery to receive antigens. The arterial tree in the spleen does not branch into capillaries in the usual manner. Most of the ultimate divisions of the splenic artery terminate in or near the marginal zone, fulfilling the role of afferent lymphatic vessels. This blood, after contacting white pulp, works its way into the sinuses of the red pulp. A minority of the final branches of the arterial tree terminate directly in the red pulp [PMID17067945], then percolates through the endothelium into the sinuses, so that the sinuses of the red pulp are the final pathway for all blood that enters the spleen. The sinuses are lined by macrophages and littoral cells that have characteristics of both endothelial cells and macrophages, and coalesce into venules, allowing the blood to exit the spleen.

Benign Lesions of the Spleen

Splenic hamartomas can be single or multiple. They are usually nodules of pure red pulp, and the absence of well defined white pulp i9.4 is an important low-power clue to the diagnosis [PMID2759557]. Architecture is disorganized, and the sinuses are haphazard. Fibrosis and extramedullary hematopoiesis i9.5 may be found. If there is extramedullary hematopoiesis that is restricted to only a portion of the spleen, a hamartoma should be suspected, especially if the area lacks the normal red pulp/white pulp architecture.

Immunocompromised patients may get a mycobacterial-associated spindle cell pseudotumor in the spleen or in lymph nodes that resembles an inflammatory myofibroblastic tumor. To make the diagnosis of mycobacterial-associated spindle cell tumor, the organisms must be demonstrated because the ordinary inflammatory myofibroblastic tumor also occurs in the spleen. The corollary of this is that if the patient is immunocompromised, a mycobacterial-associated spindle cell tumor should be excluded before the diagnosis of inflammatory myofibroblastic tumor is made in the spleen.

Splenic cysts are common and are usually pseudocysts, without an epithelial lining, surrounded by fibrous tissue. These are usually caused by trauma. True splenic cysts, with an epithelial lining, are less common and may be lined by squamous, cuboidal, or columnar epithelium. These are likely primarily developmental in nature.

Hemangiomas are relatively common in the spleen and are generally encapsulated. Rarely, they will be multifocal, resulting in nodularity. The littoral cell angioma i9.6 has morphologic and immunohistochemical characteristics that differ from a hemangioma and reflect its hybrid endothelial/macrophage origin [PMID1928554]. It has larger lining cells with cuboidal cytoplasm, often with micropapillae i9.7 and focal desquamation i9.8. It demonstrates positivity for all vascular antigens except CD34 [PMID12945936], but it is also positive for CD68 and CD21 [PMID9236839].

The spleen is the primarily affected organ in many metabolic storage diseases, where macrophages sharply distend the red pulp. Examples include Niemann-Pick i9.9 and Gaucher disease i9.10. In general, the histologic features in the spleen are nonspecific, and additional techniques and clinical correlation are needed to distinguish between the different storage diseases.

Like any lymphoid tissue, the spleen may undergo reactive ʻperplasia, and as is the case for other lymphoid organs, this ay be nodular or diffuse. The diagnostic criteria for distin-ıishing a hyperplasia from a lymphoma, and for classifying mphomas, parallel those used in other lymphoid tissue.

Ialignant Lesions of the Spleen

As in the bone marrow, one can be suspicious of splenic volvement by classical Hodgkin disease if there is a history Hodgkin disease and there is fibrosis or necrosis i9.11, but e definite diagnosis requires Reed-Sternberg cells (R-S cells) 12, or at least atypical mononuclear cells which are positive for D15 or CD30 and negative for CD45. The same type of R-S cell in the initial tissue is not required.

Most of the common non-Hodgkin lymphomas in the spleen imarily involve the white pulp and are diagnosed as described other sites. Here, we will consider only those entities that eferentially involve the spleen.

Splenic marginal zone lymphoma (SMZL) affects the white ılp i9.13a, i9.13b, i9.13c and is probably of the same lineage as ›dal marginal zone lymphoma, but there is no universal ;reement on this [PMID17325486]. Almost 1/2 of SMZLs are associ-ed with del(7q) [PMID15998972].

Splenic lymphoma with villous lymphocytes (SLVL) affects der men and leads to massive splenomegaly, circulating oplastic cells, and bone marrow involvement. Many feel that VL is a form of SMZL with leukemic involvement [PMID12945935, N978-9283224310], but others believe they are different entities, ting different behaviors and pointing out that rare patients ill have peripheral villous lymphocytes with another kind of lenic lymphoma. 1/3 of these patients will have a monoclonal otein [PMID16007426]. "Lumpers" believe that extranodal marginal ll lymphoma, splenic marginal cell lymphoma, and SLVL are l essentially the same entity, while "splitters" believe they are parate, and we may need to for wait more definitive charac-rization of these neoplasms at the DNA level before passing dgment on this matter.

The γ-δ T-cell receptor precedes and is usually replaced by e α-β receptor in development, but there will normally be a w persistent γ-δ T cells, which have a cytotoxic effect. Normal δ T cells are CD4 negative and usually CD8 negative, though casional CD8 expression may be seen [PMID17509984]. The hepa-splenic γ-δ T-cell lymphoma primarily affects the liver and leen. In the spleen, it is one of the lymphomas that have a edilection for red pulp i9.14, causing splenomegaly without rming a discrete mass. In the liver, there will be a sinusoidal volvement, with relative sparing of portal areas, analogous the red pulp involvement of the spleen. The bone marrow frequently involved in addition to the liver and spleen, but mph node involvement is rare. γ-δ T-cell lymphomas may also volve the skin and may be associated with hemophagocytic ndrome. The hepatosplenic γ-δ T-cell lymphoma is found sproportionately in young men and those who are immuno-ppressed, including those who receive immunosuppressive erapy for inflammatory bowel disease.

70% of patients with hepatosplenic γ-δ T-cell lymphoma ıve isochromosome 7q, denoted i(7q) [PMID17509984]. Despite the latively small cells with minimal pleomorphism, this is a gh-grade lymphoma with a poor prognosis. While generally negative for both CD4 and CD8, these lymphomas may express other T-cell antigens and are often positive for CD56, so care must be taken not to confuse these with T-cell lymphomas or NK/T-cell lymphomas. NK/T-cell lymphomas usually express Epstein-Barr virus, whereas γ-δ T-cell lymphomas do not. One can also show the some degree of gene rearrangement of the γ chain, but this gene rearrangement is more limited than that seen in α-β rearrangement. The acid test is the demonstration of the γ-δ receptor by immunohistochemical stains, which at this writing, requires fresh or frozen tissue.

Other such processes that are primarily in the red pulp include chronic myelogenous leukemia, acute leukemia, hairy cell leukemia, myelofibrosis, myelodysplastic syndromes, lymphoproliferative disorder of granular lymphocytes, storage diseases, and Langerhans cell histiocytoses. All of these processes can appear similar on H&E and can be diagnostically challenging.

Chronic myelogenous leukemia (CML) is the prototype for a process that mainly affects the red pulp i9.15a, i9.15b. In a spleen that is involved with CML, there may be some immature erythroid or megakaryocytic cells, but significant numbers of such cells are more consistent with splenic involvement by idiopathic myelofibrosis.

Hairy cell leukemia diffusely infiltrates the spleen, primarily the red pulp i9.16a, i9.16b. The neoplastic cells often have clear cytoplasm i9.16c, simulating a marginal zone lymphoma. Occasionally, blood vessels are dilated i9.16d, simulating a cavernous hemangioma, and tumor cells may infiltrate the vessel wall i9.16e.

Systemic mastocytosis affecting the spleen may diffusely infiltrate the red pulp i9.17a. The cells may be recognizable as mast cells i9.17b or may have clear cytoplasm i9.17c, in which case the process may resemble marginal zone lymphoma, hairy cell leukemia, or γ-δ lymphoma. More commonly, however, it forms nodular aggregates with fibrous tissue i9.17d and occasional eosinophils i9.17e. Smaller numbers of mast cells may be missed amidst the fibrosis and other cells types. Mast cells are CD68 (KP1) positive, and usually also positive for CD43, CD117, and tryptase. The main obstacle to the correct diagnosis of systemic mastocytosis is to think of it. It is the "forgotten" chronic myeloproliferative neoplasm. Because the actual neoplastic cells may be relatively rare, mastocytosis can be a subtle process that often can only be diagnosed by additional testing after it is suspected by the milieu in which it is found. Mastocytosis should be considered whenever there are nodules of fibrous tissue that contain eosinophils.

Core Points for the Spleen

- Hamartomas, hemangiomas, and cysts are common in the spleen.
- Lymphoproliferative disorders: diagnosed as elsewhere, but note if process is centered primarily in red pulp or white pulp.
- Spleen is also the site of red pulp processes that can cause extreme splenomegaly, including chronic myelogenous leukemia, hairy cell leukemia, and storage diseases.

ISBN 978-089189-5886

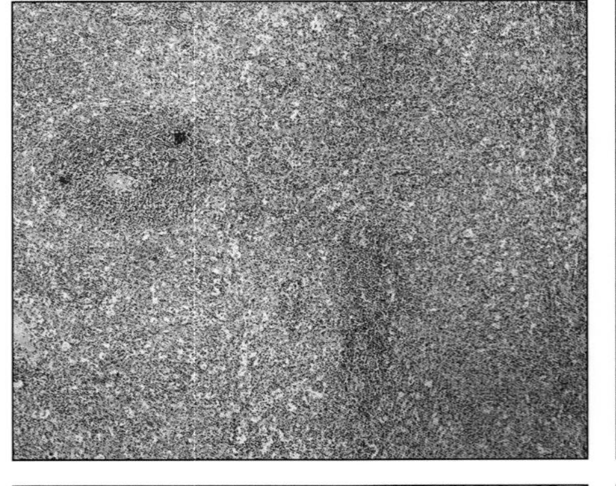

i9.1 Normal splenic tissue illustrating the demarcation of the white pulp and the red pulp

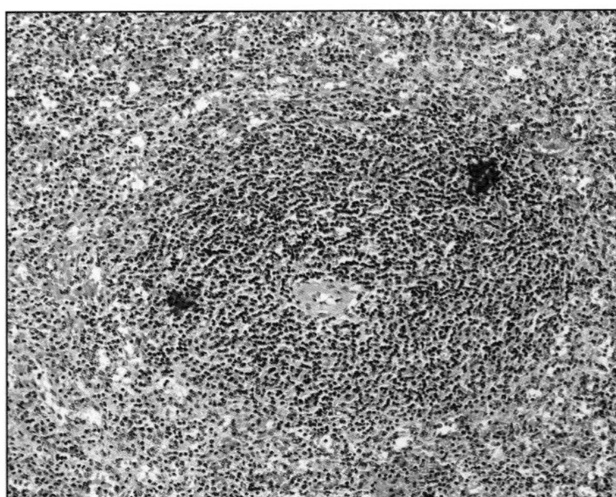

i9.2 A Malpighian corpuscle consisting of a small arteriole surrounded by lymphocytes. Note the absence of a germinal center, which are uncommon in splenic white pulp in adults.

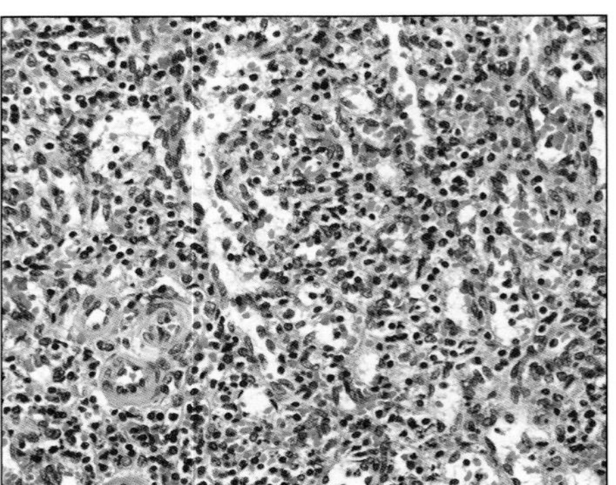

i9.3 The red pulp of a normal spleen, illustrating the sinusoidal architecture. Although difficult to visualize, the sinusoids are lined by macrophages that phagocytize senescent erythrocytes.

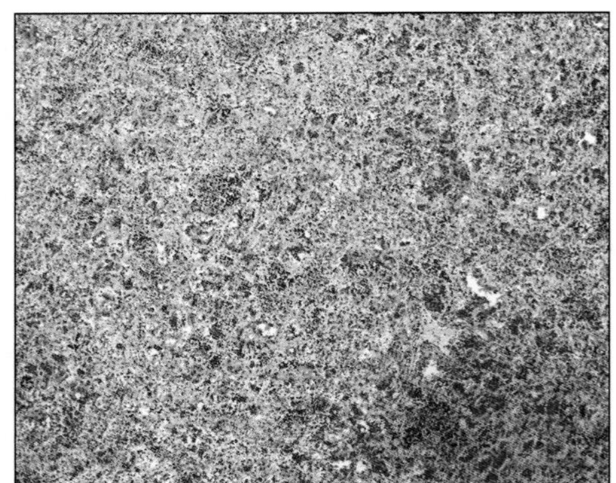

i9.4 A splenic hamartoma. There are small clusters of lymphocytes, but the normal white pulp/red pulp architecture is disrupted.

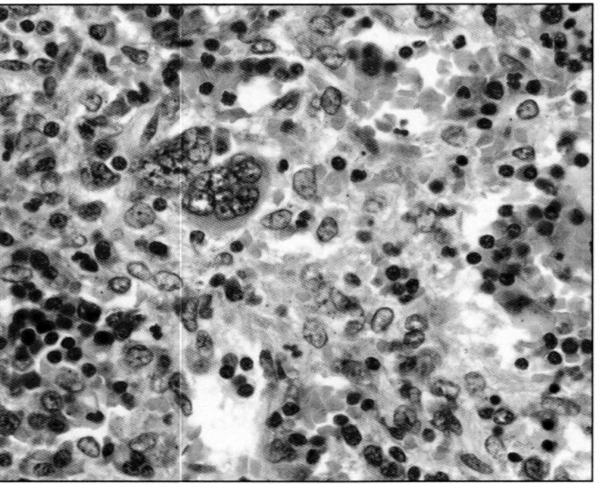

i9.5 A higher-power view of the same case as in i9.4, illustrating extramedullary hematopoiesis in a hamartoma. 2 megakaryocytes are noted in the upper left, and there are also nucleated erythrocytes.

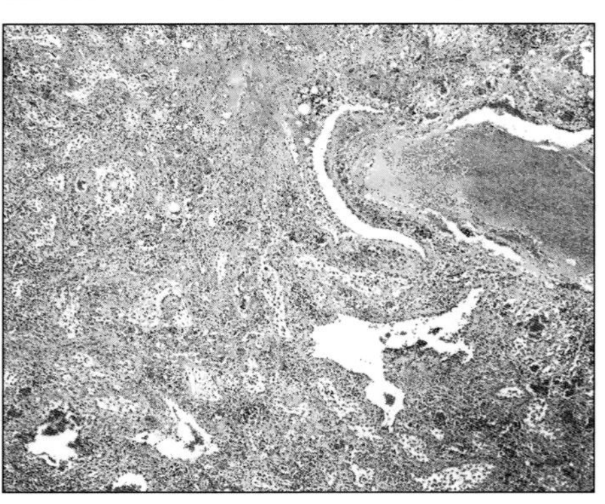

i9.6 A littoral cell angioma illustrating disruption of the splenic architecture and dilated blood vessels

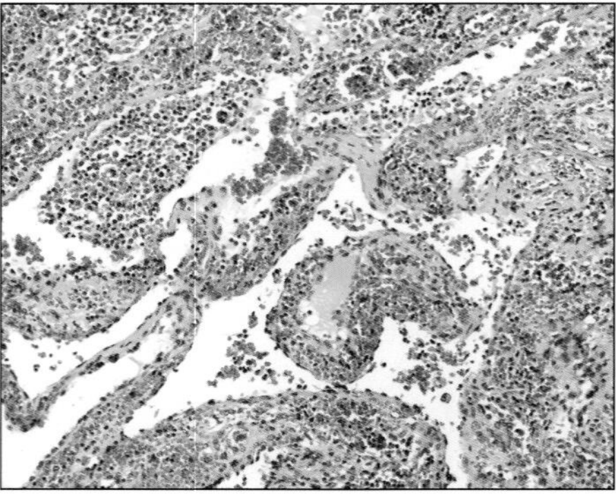

i9.7 The same case as in i9.6 illustrating micropapillae

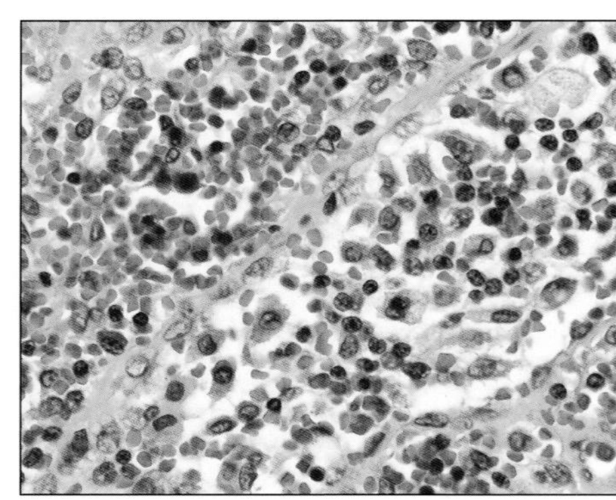

i9.8 A littoral cell angioma illustrating the desquamation of the neoplastic cells into the vascular lumen. Note that the cells are larger, with more rounded nuclei, than typical endothelial cells, a reflection of their hybrid endothelial/macrophage properties.

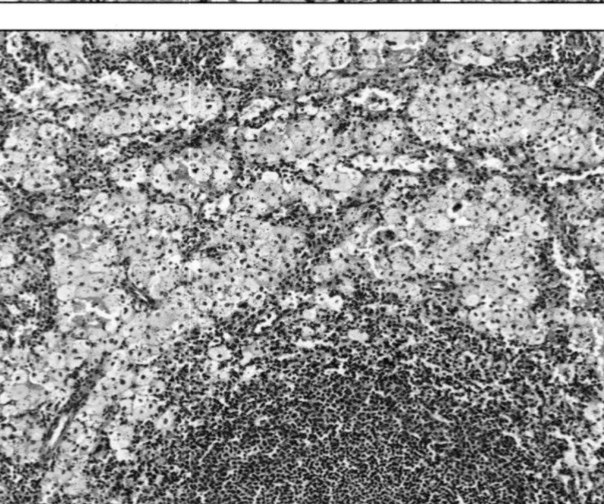

i9.9 Niemann-Pick disease with abundant numbers of distended macrophages in the red pulp. Normal white pulp is seen at the bottom.

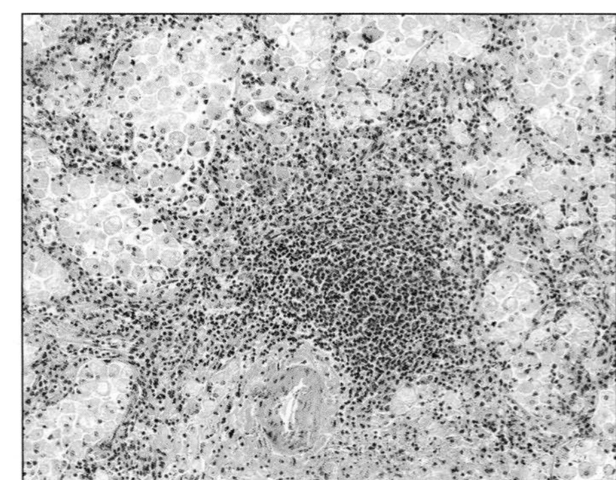

i9.10 Gaucher disease. As is the case for Niemann-Pick disease, the red pulp is effaced by distended macrophages.

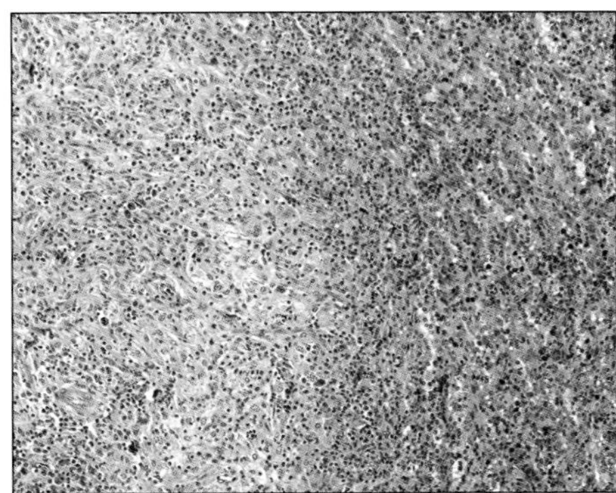

Hodgkin disease
the spleen. There is
rmal splenic tissue on
right and a fibrotic
dule on the left.

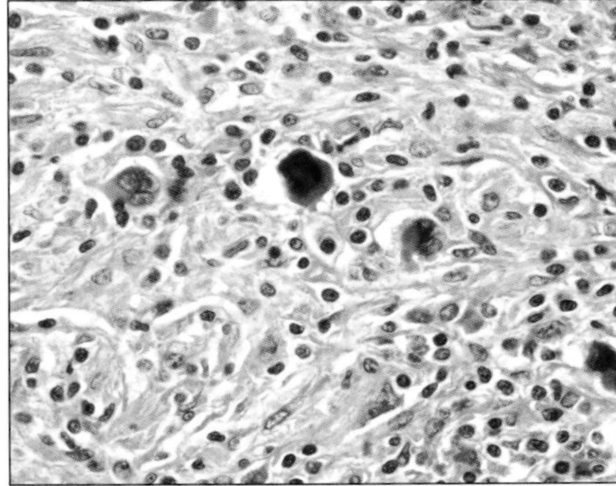

i9.12 The same case as in i9.11, illustrating Reed-Sternberg cells

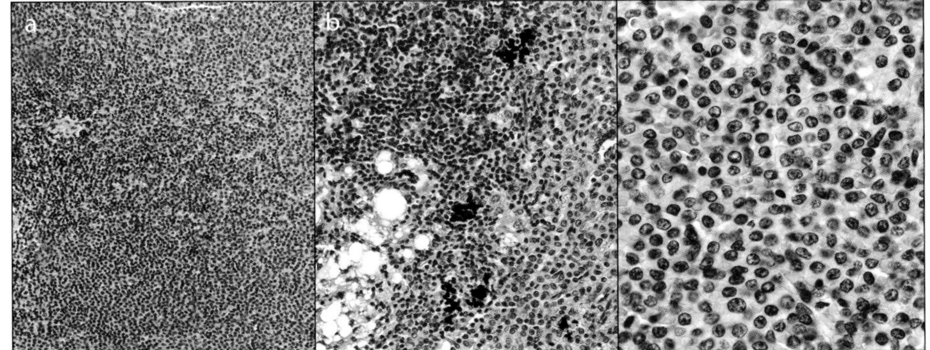

3 **a** Splenic marginal
ne lymphoma. There
sharp expansion of the
ite pulp. The sheath of
arteriole in the center
the white pulp is visible
the lower left. **b** Splenic
arginal zone lymphoma.
the central and left
rtion of the photograph
ere is normal splenic
ite pulp. On the right is
lymphoma, consisting
slightly larger cells with
ore cytoplasm and less
clumped chromatin than in the normal white pulp. **c** A higher-power view of the neoplastic cells in a splenic marginal zone lymphoma. As is the case in other body sites, splenic marginal zone lymphomas may have several appearances but typically have a "monocytoid" appearance with clear cytoplasm, as is the case here.

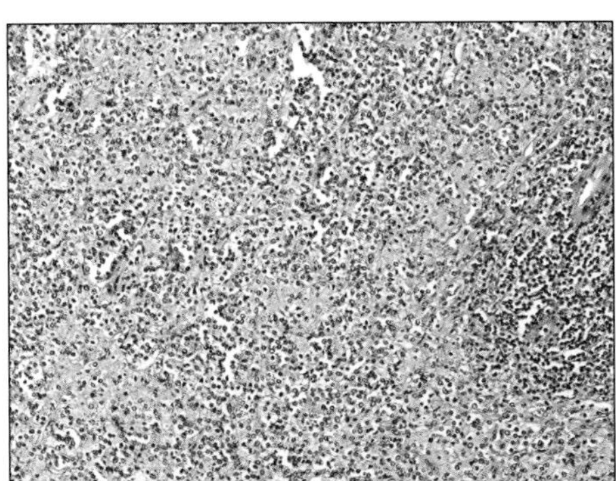

4 A γ-δ T-cell
nphoma of the spleen
ustrating effacement of
e red pulp in the central
d left portions of the
otograph. Normal
ite pulp is seen on the
ght.

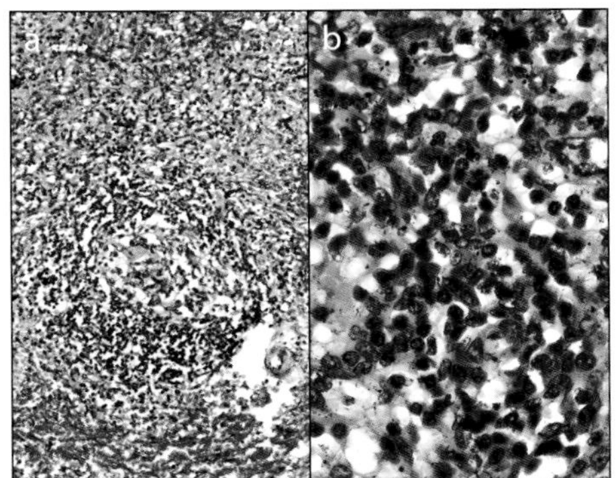

i9.15 a Chronic myelogenous leukemia in the spleen. In the center there is normal white pulp. To the right there is fibrosis, and to the left there is red pulp with increased cellularity and loss of normal architecture. **b** A higher-power view of the same case as in i9.15a illustrating the hypercellularity of the red pulp

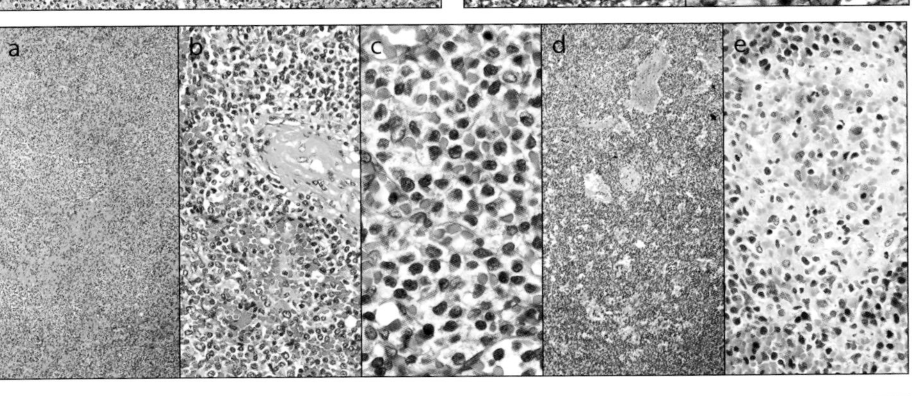

6 **a** Hairy cell leukemia
the spleen diffusely
filtrating the red pulp
The same case as in
16a. Although the neo-
astic cells have prob-
ly infiltrated the white
lp to some extent, the
hite pulp continues to
monstrate numerous
nall, normal lympho-
tes, while the red pulp is
mpletely effaced by the
oplastic cells.
c A higher-power view of hairy cell leukemia of the spleen illustrating the clear cytoplasm that is characteristic of this entity **d** Hairy cell leukemia in the spleen with dilated, thin-walled blood vessels **e** Hairy cell leukemia of the spleen with infiltration of the neoplastic cells into the wall of an arteriole.

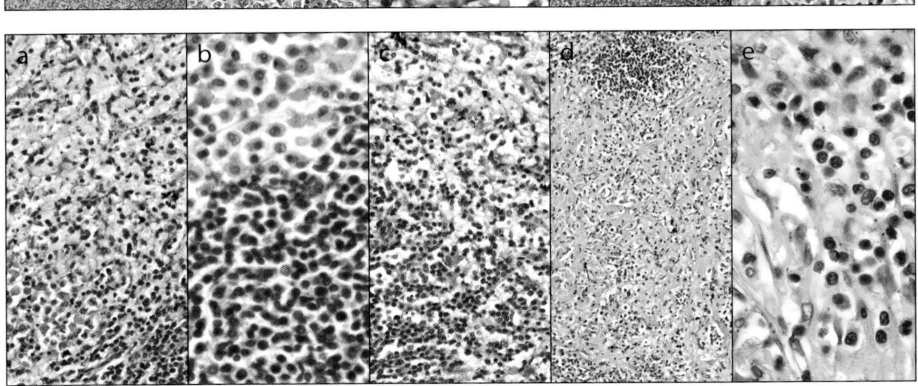

17 **a** Systemic mastocy-
sis affecting the spleen.
ormal splenic white
lp is visible in the lower
ght corner. The red pulp
effaced. **b** The same
se as in i9.17a, illustrat-
g recognizable mast
lls adjacent to a normal
alpighian corpuscle.
Splenic mastocytosis in
hich the neoplastic cells
ave clear cytoplasm and
nerally do not resemble
ormal mast cells.
d Systemic mastocytosis with a fibrotic nodule. **e** Systemic mastocytosis in the spleen with eosinophils in a fibrotic nodule.

ISBN 978-089189-5886

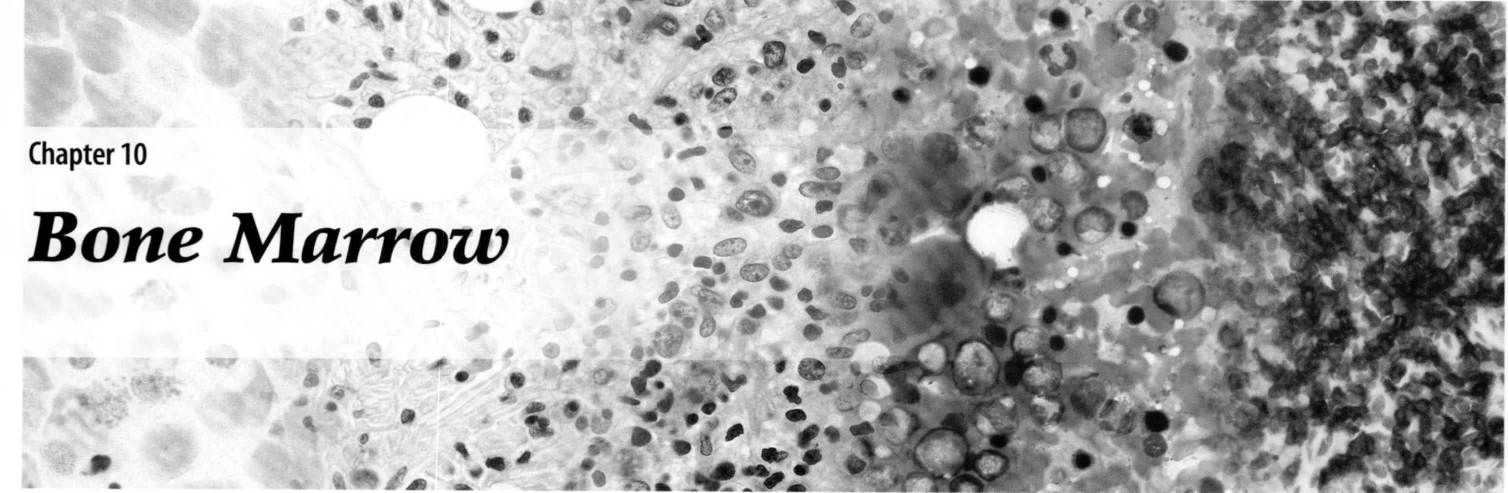

Chapter 10

Bone Marrow

The normal hematopoietic bone marrow elements are megakaryocytes, erythrocytes, granulocytes (neutrophils, eosinophils, and basophils), lymphocytes, and their precursors. These elements are mixed with adipose tissue in an environment with appreciable microvascularity i10.1a, i10.1b. The percentage of bone marrow that is the actual hematopoietic component decreases with age, but roughly ranges from about 70% in youth to about 30% in older patients. Because marrow just under the cortical bone is usually hypocellular and not reflective of the general marrow i10.2, cellularity should not be assessed there. Likewise, cellularity should not be assessed in areas of aspiration artifact, which differ from hypocellular marrow in the absence of fat i10.3. Normally, 10-15% of nucleated cells in the marrow are lymphocytes. The T:B lymphocyte ratio in marrow is about 3, and the CD4:CD8 ratio of the T lymphocytes is about 2 [PMID2499393].

The normal bone marrow often has benign lymphoid nodules that simulate lymphoma. Immunohistochemical characterization of these nodules may clarify their nature, but it is generally wise not to make an initial diagnosis of lymphoma from a small lymphoid nodule in the marrow. Even in staging marrows where the diagnosis of lymphoma has already been established, lymphoid nodules must be interpreted conservatively, as benign nodules may be misconstrued as evidence of marrow involvement by the lymphoma. Caution is especially warranted if the patient has been treated with rituximab (anti-CD20), as this drug can cause reactive T cell nodules i10.4a, i10.4b, i10.4c [PMID17949786].

Most benign follicles in bone marrow are composed of T cells, with or without Rituxan use, but only if a panel of B markers (including CD20, CD79a, and Pax-5) is negative and at least 2 T markers (CD2, CD3, CD5, and CD7) are positive, should T-cell origin (and clinical insignificance in a staging marrow in a patient with a history of a B-cell lymphoma) be assumed for these bone marrow lymphoid aggregates. A paratrabecular location is a point for lymphoma, but immunohistochemical confirmation is essential.

Nonneoplastic Processes in the Marrow

Nonneoplastic processes in the bone marrow include reactive hyperplasia, in which the marrow is hypercellular i10.5, and inflammatory/infectious processes such as sarcoidosis i10.6 and herpes i10.7. The marrow may also be affected in storage disorders such as Gaucher disease i10.8. These are not discussed because they are diagnosed as in other sites and are rarely a diagnostic problem. The major exceptions are that a recovering marrow may simulate acute myeloid leukemia with its large number of young cells and severe megaloblastic anemia may resemble an acute leukemia.

Metastatic Carcinoma, Hodgkin Disease, and Lymphomas

Metastases to bone marrow i10.9 are not discussed here because the workup of an unknown metastatic tumor by immunohistochemical stains is as described elsewhere. Antigen retrieval techniques have largely eliminated the former problem of the decalcification process rendering some antigens undetectable in bone marrow specimens. The only comment is that it is wise to consider keratin immunohistochemical stain when the suspected primary is lobular carcinoma of the breast, as this type of carcinoma can be quite subtle in a bone marrow biopsy, as it can be in a lymph node.

Metastatic malignancy is a myelophthisic process. Myelophthisis refers to the destruction of hematopoietic precursor cells or their nurturing microenvironment by nonhematopoietic elements ("phthisis" is Latin for "declining" or "wasting away"). The most common causes of myelophthisis are metastatic tumors and idiopathic fibrosis. The myelophthisic destruction of the microenvironment prevents normal maturation, so that immature forms in both the erythroid and myeloid lines are prematurely released into the blood (leukoerythroblastotic reaction).

Likewise, Hodgkin disease i10.10a, i10.10b and most lymphomas i10.11 are not discussed because they are diagnosed as in other sites. The discussion here is limited to those processes that primarily involve the marrow.

The Myelodysplastic Syndromes (MDSs)

The myelodysplastic syndromes (MDSs) are a group of disorders of development and function of erythrocytes, leukocytes, or platelets. They have colloquially been called "preleukemia" conditions because a high percentage of MDS patients will go on to develop acute myelogenous leukemia (AML). The term "MDS" is conventionally applied to acquired disorders and not to congenital disorders of bone marrow or e production of blood cells (eg, there are several types of ngenital dyserythropoietic anemia that are not included in e MDS).

There is evidence of clonal origin in many MDSs [PMID15051892], ggesting that they are neoplasms whose nature has been asked by the prominent ineffective poiesis and morphologic normalities that characterize these syndromes.

While the findings in the blood and bone marrow of MDS tients depend on the type of MDS, the general rule is a mac-cytic anemia, often accompanied by morphologic abnor-alities of the erythrocytes and leukocytes. The marrow is ually hypercellular in MDS, but hypocellular MDS occurs d may even be a distinct entity. Some cases of MDS have normal location of precursors in the marrow, away from the ual paratrabecular location.

Defects at many stages of neutrophil function—adhesion, otility, phagocytosis, killing, etc—have been shown in the DS. The original French-American-British (FAB) classifica-on of MDS rested on the blast count in the blood and bone arrow, as well as morphologic abnormalities of bone mar-w precursor cells that were not completely specified. These nsiderations remain paramount in the WHO classification, hich more specifically defines morphologic abnormalities of ecursor cells, but the newer classification also assigns a cen-al role to cytogenetic findings [Swerdlow ISBN978-9283224310], which often as important as the blast count.

Half of MDS patients have cytogenetic abnormalities, and contrast to other hematologic disorders, translocations are re. Instead, deletions are the rule. Many cytogenetic abnor-alities have been found and often, there are multiple simul-neous abnormalities. Normal cytogenetics is considered vorable, as are del(5q), –Y, and del(20q), provided that they e the sole abnormalities (some older men will lose some of eir Y chromosomes, so one must be sure there is a true clon-loss of Y in abnormal cells before advocating this as a favor-ble sign). Additional favorable cytogenetic prognostic factors clude –X, +1, +1q, t(1q), t(7q), del(9q), del(12p), t(17q), mono-my 21, trisomy 21, and any abnormalities of chromosome 5 [PMID17726160]. Abnormalities of chromosome 7, as well as 4 more abnormalities (called complex chromosomal abnor-alities), are considered unfavorable. All other cytogenetic normalities have an intermediate prognosis [PMID9058730]. In ntrast to other hematologic disorders, the mechanisms of tion of the large number of cytogenetic abnormalities that e found in MDS are not understood.

The World Health Organization (WHO) classification of DSs builds on the older FAB classification and is as follows:

Refractory anemia is largely a diagnosis of exclusion, ased on a persistent, unexplained anemia. The blast count ould not exceed 5% in the marrow or 1% in the peripheral ood. There are no specific findings, but some of the erythroid ecursors in the marrow have an abnormal appearance, such s nuclei with budding, multinucleation, karyorrhexis, or elayed maturation relative to the cytoplasm (megaloblastic anges). The marrow often has an erythroid hyperplasia.

Refractory anemia with ringed sideroblasts; a sideroblast a normoblast that contains iron and is a normal stage in the aturation of red cells. In a normal sideroblast, an iron stain ill demonstrate granules that are dispersed throughout the ytoplasm. A ringed sideroblast contains iron granules in the mitochondria, and because these tend to be juxtanuclear in the normoblast, the iron stain will demonstrate granules hugging the nuclear membrane. A ringed sideroblast is morphologically defined by juxtanuclear iron, but it is really a normoblast in which iron has been inappropriately deposited in mitochondria. To be a ringed sideroblast, a normoblast must have at least 5 iron granules in a juxtanuclear location, and the granules must extent at least 1/3 of the way around the circumference of the nucleus i10.12a, i10.12b. The diagnosis of sideroblastic anemia requires that 15% of normoblasts be ringed sideroblasts. There is usually an erythroid hyperplasia and a marked increase in storage iron. In a pure case, the marrow blast count does not exceed 5%.

Refractory anemia with excess blasts (RAEB) has 5-9% myeloblasts i10.13a, i10.13b in the marrow or 2-19% blasts in the blood. This form of MDS takes diagnostic priority over all other types because the blast count conveys significantly increased potential to develop into acute leukemia.

The above 3 types of MDS are little changed from the FAB system. The following 3 types of MDS are new in the WHO classification:

Refractory cytopenia with multilineage dysplasia, a form of MDS, has dysplasia in 10% or more of cells from at least 2 lines. In the marrow, erythroid cells have abnormal nuclei or nuclear-cytoplasmic dyssynchrony i10.14a, i10.14b. Myeloid cells have poor nuclear maturation or abnormal granulation i10.15. Megakaryocyte nuclei are abnormally lobated, their nuclear lobes are not connected, or the cytoplasm is poorly granulated i10.16a, i10.16b. In the blood, there are a variety of abnormal erythroid forms. Neutrophils have incomplete nuclear segmentation and either poor granulation or large primary granules. Circulating blasts do not exceed 1%, and those in the marrow do not exceed 5% (otherwise, it would be RAEB, which would preempt the diagnosis of refractory cytopenia with multilineage dysplasia).

MDS associated with isolated del(5q) i10.17, i10.18, which is the most common single cytogenetic abnormality in MDS, occurring in about 30% of patients, and the only one of many to be specifically enumerated as a category of MDS. The responsible gene(s) on the long arm of chromosome 5 has not yet been identified. In addition to the characteristic chromosomal abnormality, blasts must not exceed 5% in blood or marrow (otherwise, it would be RAEB because that diagnosis takes priority). Although cases of MDS with deletion of 5q tend to have megakaryocytes with hypolobated nuclei i10.19a, i10.19b, there are no specific morphologic features. The diagnosis of this form of MDS is made only from the demonstration of the cytogenetic abnormality and the absence of excess blasts.

MDS, unclassifiable is clinically and morphologically recognizable as an MDS, but it does not fit precisely into one of the above categories. This form of MDS has a marrow blast count that does not exceed 5% (otherwise, it would be RAEB), and dysplasia that is confined to only 1 line (otherwise, it would be MDS with multilineage dysplasia). Neutropenia or thrombocytopenia is the rule.

2 subtypes of MDS are particularly challenging. The first of these is MDSs that are associated with fibrosis i10.20a, i10.20b, i10.20c, i10.20d, as it can be confused with primary idiopathic myelofibrosis or with variants of acute myeloid leukemia that

have fibrosis, such as acute panmyelosis with myelofibrosis (see following discussion of AML). The second diagnostically difficult form of MDS is the hypocellular subtype, especially in regards to its relationship to aplastic anemia [PMID19605823].

After the adoption of the WHO classification system of MDS, the International Prognostic Scoring System (IPSS) was adopted. This system was used only at diagnosis and was not used to restage patients during the course of their disease or treatment, but the Prognostic Scoring System (WPSS) was created to permit serial assessment of patients [PMID18813205, PMID21594886]. Also important in the diagnosis and prognosis of some cases of MDS are abnormal antigens as identified by flow cytometry [PMID17971483] though abnormal antigen expression on a myeloblast does not by itself establish a diagnosis of either MDS or a myeloproliferative neoplasm [PMID20959658].

At this writing, there are 3 drugs specifically for MDS: azacitidine, lenalidomide, and decitabine. Tentatively, it appears that the choice and effectiveness of these drugs depends more on cytogenetics, specifically on the presence or absence of del(5q), than on the blast count [PMID20486832].

Acute Myelogenous Leukemia (AML)

Before we consider AML, it is wise to remember that a "recovering" bone marrow may have large numbers of early cells that can simulate an acute leukemia, particularly if the patient has been treated with a hematopoietic growth factor **i10.21**.

Prior to the publication of the WHO classification of AML, some cytogenetic abnormalities were recognized and were beginning to be integrated into the older FAB system. For example, a subtype of AML-M2 with t(8;21), large salmon-colored granules, and aberrant expression of CD34 and the B marker CD19 was recognized. But it was not until the WHO classification system of AML that cytogenetic abnormalities became central to categorization.

A myeloblast is the earliest recognizable cell that is committed to myeloid differentiation. It is characterized by fine chromatin, 1 or more nucleoli, and minimal cytoplasm **i10.13a**, **i10.13b**. The WHO system has defined AML as occurring when 20% of nucleated cells in the marrow are myeloblasts, replacing the previously required number of 30% **i10.22** [PMID10697278]. This is true for any AML, including those with monocytic differentiation. In effect, this removes the FAB category of RAEB in transformation (RAEBIT).

There are 5 broad categories in the WHO classification of AML. The first is AML associated with cytogenetic abnormalities. There are a few cytogenetic abnormalities which, if present, take precedence over other features in the classification of AML. In these cases, the karyotype is sufficiently specific for AML that the definitive diagnosis does not even require 20% blasts [Swerdlow ISBN978-9283224310].

This first category initially consisted of 4 subtypes of AML that are defined solely by cytogenetic abnormalities. The first of these subtypes is acute promyelocytic leukemia (APL) **i10.23**. Almost all patients with APL have t(15;17)(q22;q21.1), which juxtaposes the retinoic acid receptor α gene (*RARA*) on chromosome 17 to the *PML* gene on chromosome 15 **i10.24**, **i10.25**. The normal function of the *PML* gene is not known, but the translocation results in the novel protein PML-RARA, which functions as an oncoprotein [PMID17217040]. There are several possible breakpoints of the *PML* gene on chromosome 15, necessitating different sets of primers in PCR testing. Very rarely in APL, the translocation partner for *RARA* will not be *PML*. All-trans retinoic acid is a specific and effective treatment for APL [PMID20929432], but it is unlikely to work in the rare cases in which the translocation is not the classic *PML/RARA*. There are 2 morphologic variants of APL—hypergranular and hypogranular (also called microgranular).

The blasts in APL, including these variant forms, have absent expression of CD11b and CD11c by flow cytometry, a finding that is nearly specific for this form of acute myeloid leukemia [PMID21173127] and which may become a standard method of diagnosis.

In addition to the t(15;17)(q22;q21.1) that characterizes APL (FAB-M3), 3 additional subtypes of acute myeloid leukemia (AML) were defined early on in the WHO system solely by specific karyotypes.

The first of these additional specific karyotypes is t(8;21)(q22;q22), resulting in the molecular construct *RUNX1/RUNX1T1* at the genomic level. The protein RUNX1 is a transcription factor whose function is diminished by this translocation [PMID17934489]. While the precise pathogenesis of this translocation is unclear, it appears to result in decreased transcription of the tumor suppressor gene p14ARF [PMID12732181]. t(8;21)(q22;q22) is generally favorable and often results in an M2 immunophenotype. *RUNX1* was formerly called *AML1* and *RUNX1T1* was formerly called *ETO*, so many of the papers describing this translocation use the terminology *AML1/ETO* [PMID11869944].

The second additional specific cytogenetic abnormality in AML is inv(16)(p13.1q22) **i10.26**, **i10.27** or t(16;16)(p13.1;q22), either of which results in fusion of the core binding factor β gene (*CBFB*) to the smooth muscle myosin-heavy chain gene (*MYH11*). The first case is a pericentric inversion (an inversion in which the 2 breakpoints are on different sides of the centromere) of 1 chromosome, while the second involves transfer of DNA from 1 chromosome 16 to the other. This fusion product, *CBFB/MYH11*, encodes for a novel protein and is associated with most cases of M4E, a form of AML with many eosinophils [PMID15044690], though 1/3 of cases of AML with inv(16) will not have increased eosinophils.

The third additional specific cytogenetic abnormality in AML is abnormalities in 11q23. A number of breakpoints and translocations have been described in the 11q23 region, all involving the *MLL* (mixed lineage leukemia) gene **i10.28**. Different breakpoints are associated with different types of leukemia and different patient ages [PMID16158928]. In addition to translocations with other genes, *MLL* may also undergo intragenic rearrangements because it has a region of partial tandem repeats (MLL-PTD) [PMID20805748]. When implicated in pure AML, the *MLL* gene is associated with monoblastic differentiation and an intermediate prognosis [PMID12139726].

By 2009, additional categories of AML were recognized solely by karyotype. These include t(9;11), t(1;22), t(6;9), inv(3), +8, +21, –5, –7, and abnormalities of 3q. Of these new categories, t(9;11) is favorable, +8 and +21 convey an intermediate prognosis, while abnormalities of 5, 7, and 3q are unfavorable [PMID21239770]. These new categories increase to about 60% the number of cases of AML that are sufficiently associated with ɜpecific cytogenetic abnormality as to be essentially defined ʼ it rather than by blast count [PMID21034669].

10% or more of cases with any of the aforementioned ·togenetic abnormalities will be missed with conventional ɪryotyping, so FISH or PCR must be performed in all cases suspected AML.

In addition to prognoses conveyed by cytogenetic abnor-alities, there are 2 proteins, mutations of which are prog-ɔstically important: FLT3 (FMS-like tyrosine kinase 3) and ɪcleophosmin (NPM1) [PMID19557552]. The FLT3 protein is trans-embrane, with a tyrosine kinase in the cytoplasmic portion. ɔout 30% of cases of acute myeloid leukemias either have ndem duplications or point mutations of the *FLT3* gene, and .ch mutations are among the most important single prog-ɔstic indicators in cases of AML that are cytogenetically nor-al [PMID19671038]. Tandem duplications change the length of the ·ne and are called *FLT3-ITD* or *FLT3-LM* (length mutations), hile point mutations in the portion of the gene that codes for e tyrosine kinase moiety are called *FLT3-TYR*. Either type abnormality conveys constitutive activity to the kinase and ɔrtends a more aggressive course [PMID20923295].

Mutations in the *NPM1* gene on 5q35, are also found in ɔout 30% of AML patients [PMID20616361]. Most such mutations e an insertion of 4 base pairs. Expression of the protein PM1 is associated with *FLT3-ITD* at the genomic level and erefore associated with a more aggressive course, but if PM1 expression is found alone, it is a favorable prognostic dicator [PMID16109776]. NPM1 is a shuttle protein that is gener-ly found only in the nucleus in the normal cell but often in e cytoplasm in the abnormal cell. While DNA techniques e superior to immunohistochemistry in the identification of is subset of patients, the finding of the protein in the cyto-asm by immunohistochemistry suggests an abnormality.

Patients with mutations in either *FLT3* or *NPM1* will usu-ly be normal on all cytogenetic studies and are not included the group of AML patients with cytogenetic abnormalities, ıderscoring that even in the so-called normal cytogenetic ·oup, there may be important mutations.

The second broad category is AML with multilineage dys-asia, in which there are dysplastic features in 50% or more the nonblast cells in 2 or more cell lines **i10.29a**, **i10.29b**, **i10.29c**, **).29d**, **i10.29e**, **i10.29f**.

The third category is therapy-related myeloid neoplasms, which some, but not all, are AML. WHO originally spe-fically identified therapy-related AML, but in 2008, placed l therapy-related myeloid disorders in 1 category because was clear that therapy can cause MDS features, with cyto-ɜnias and dysplastic cells, as well as overt AML. Attempts identify specific morphologic or cytogenetic features of ɪerapy-related myeloid disorders have been elusive and the ɪagnosis can only be made by a history of radiation therapy chemotherapy [PMID21039422]. Alkylating agents and topoi-ɔmerase inhibitors given for another hematologic disorder ·e the primary culprits [PMID19860183].

The fourth category is AML of ambiguous lineage. There ·e 3 categories of ambiguous lineage. The first is an acute ukemia with completely undifferentiated blasts that can-ɔt be classified as either AML or acute lymphoid (lympho-astic) leukemia (ALL). The second is bilineal acute leuke-ɪia, in which there are 2 separate blast populations. Some believe these 2 populations should be distinctly lymphoid and myeloid, while others feel that only 1 of the populations should be clearly lymphoid or myeloid, and that the other can be mixed lymphoid/myeloid. The third type of acute leu-kemia of ambiguous lineage is biphenotypic, in which there is a population of blasts that has mixed immunophenotypic characteristics and expresses both myeloid and lymphoid markers. The most important markers for separating AML from ALL are CD13, CD33, and CD117 for myeloid lineage, and CD79a, CD10, CD2, and CD3 for lymphoid lineage (CD79a and CD10 indicate B cell lineage, while CD2 and CD3 suggest T-cell origin). There are some differences of opinion on the precise definition of mixed in biphenotypic acute leukemia. All investigators require at least 2 lymphoid or myeloid mark-ers before such a component is considered present, but some require more evidence. There is general agreement that both precursor T and B-ALL may express 1 or both of the myeloid antigens CD13 and CD33, and this is not interpreted as a true biphenotypic leukemia.

The fifth category is AML, NOS (not otherwise specified). AML, NOS is subdivided into 10 subgroups. In contrast to the first 4 categories of AML under the WHO system, most of the subgroups of AML, NOS roughly correspond to the old FAB classification. Some cases of AML, NOS are associated with mutations in CCAAT enhancer binding protein α (CEBPA), a transcription factor that is critical in normal myeloid develop-ment. CEBPA is mutated in 13-19% of AML patients with a normal karyotype [PMID21354046], and such cases tend to be less aggressive [PMID19525338].

The 10 subgroups of AML, NOS are as follows:

1. AML, minimally differentiated. Myeloid differentiation is evident only by immunophenotype. This is roughly comparable to FAB M0.
2. AML without maturation. Blasts must account for >90% of nucleated nonerythroid cells (ie, promyelocytes will be <10% of all nucleated cells), but unlike AML, minimally differentiated, individual blasts will show myeloid maturation by morphology or cytochemical stains, and there may be Auer rods **i10.30** or promyelocytic differentiation. This is essentially FAB M1.
3. AML with maturation. Promyelocytes or more differentiated myeloid cells comprise 10% or more of all nucleated bone marrow cells. This is roughly comparable to FAB M2.
4. Acute myelomonocytic leukemia (AMML), similar to FAB M4, with differentiation towards both granulocytic and monocytic lines **i10.31a**, **i10.31b**. However, most cases of AMML with eosinophilia (the old FAB M4E) **i10.32** do have a specific chromosomal abnormality, either inv(16) (p13.1q22) or t(16;16)(p13.1;q22), and therefore fall under the WHO category of AML with cytogenetic abnormalities.
5. AML, monoblastic, as in FAB M5.
6. AML, monocytic. This differs from AML, monoblastic, in that the immature cells are promonocytes rather than monoblasts (ie, the characteristic nuclear folding of a monocyte is typically present) **i10.33**.

7. Acute erythroid leukemia. Like the FAB system, the WHO system recognizes 2 forms of erythroid leukemia. The usual and more common type requires that erythroid cells must constitute 50% of nucleated cells and at least 20% of nonerythroid cells must be myeloblasts. This was M6A in the FAB system. There is also a pure erythroid leukemia, in which there is no myeloblastic component, and all of the neoplastic cells are erythroid. This has been called Di Guglielmo disease, or M6B, in the FAB system **i10.34a**. Either form is often has associated with multilineage myelodysplasia and myelofibrosis **i10.34b**. If immature cells that are committed to the erythroid line, as opposed to the myeloid or lymphoid lines, are difficult to identify, staining for aldehyde dehydrogenase may help, as this highlights early erythroid cells [PMID22180476].
8. Acute megakaryoblastic leukemia (AMKL). This is often associated with myelofibrosis. Down syndrome patients may get, in the neonatal period, a transient myeloproliferative neoplasm resembling AMKL, but it resolves spontaneously in 2 weeks to several months (although 30% of these patients will subsequently develop AMKL).
9. Acute basophilic leukemia.
10. Acute panmyelosis with myelofibrosis. This is a rare form of AML that has a bone marrow blast count in excess of 20%, but also has marrow fibrosis and myeloid dysplasia. Acute panmyelosis with myelofibrosis morphologically overlaps with and may be hard to distinguish from acute megakaryoblastic leukemia, AML with multilineage dysplasia, idiopathic myelofibrosis, or MDS with a fibrotic component.

In addition, there are 2 unusual forms of AML. The first of these is the extramedullary myeloid tumor (also called granulocytic sarcoma or myeloid sarcoma), a solid tissue manifestation of AML. The second of these unusual forms of AML is hypocellular (or hypoplastic) AML, a rare form of AML that occurs primarily in elderly patients and must be distinguished from hypocellular MDS and aplastic anemia [PMID19144661].

A bone marrow is seldom performed to verify a diagnosis of megaloblastic anemia, but this condition may be unexpectedly encountered in a bone marrow examination and may simulate an MDS or an AML, in which case a mistaken diagnosis is avoided by recognizing the following attributes of megaloblastic change:

- Nuclear maturation lags behind cytoplasmic maturation in all cell lines, most noticeably in the erythroid line. In the erythroid line, there is persistence of the chromatin/parachromatin demarcation in the nucleus even after hemoglobinization of the cytoplasm rather than the expected nuclear pyknosis **i10.35a**, **i10.35b**.
- The marrow has an increased number of early normoblasts, young cells committed to erythroid maturation, but not of true, uncommitted myeloblasts **i10.36**.
- These early normoblasts do not mature well, and the ineffective erythropoiesis results in an unexpectedly diminished number of mature normoblasts. In severe cases, the abundant early normoblasts with minimal maturation may simulate an acute myeloid leukemia **i10.37**.
- There are large metamyelocytes.
- The blood demonstrates pancytopenia with an increased MCV, but without significant erythroid morphologic abnormalities.
- Serum B_{12} or folate levels are low.

We close our discussion of AML with the concept of the assessment of treatment and residual disease. Although the time-honored morphologic examination of posttreatment bone marrows remains essential in the care of patients with acute leukemia, there are numerous cases in which there is residual disease that is detectable only by special techniques, such as PCR for genetic abnormalities or by flow cytometry for aberrant expression of antigens. This is called minimal residual disease (MRD). MRD casts the concepts of remission and relapse in a new light and is changing the way new therapeutic agents are evaluated [PMID19778853]. In evaluating for MRD by assessing the level of residual cytogenetic abnormalities, it should be remembered that many of the important abnormalities found in hematopoietic processes, such as *PML/RARA*, *MLL*, *RUNX1/RUNX1T1*, *CBFB/MYH11*, and *BCR/ABL* can be found in very low levels in normal patients [PMID21354057].

Chronic Myeloproliferative Neoplasms

The chronic myeloproliferative disorders or diseases are now called chronic myeloproliferative neoplasms, reflecting the general acceptance of clonal origin, even when a neoplastic cell is not readily identified. Relative to the MDS, the myeloproliferative neoplasms have more effective poiesis, so that the blood has more cells with fewer morphologic abnormalities. The WHO classification of chronic myeloproliferative neoplasms [Swerdlow ISBN978-9283224310] recognizes and provides diagnostic criteria for the following 8 chronic myeloproliferative neoplasms:

1. Chronic myelogenous leukemia (CML)
2. Chronic neutrophilic leukemia
3. Chronic eosinophilic leukemia/hypereosinophilic syndrome
4. Chronic idiopathic myelofibrosis (CIMF), also called myelofibrosis with myeloid metaplasia.
5. Polycythemia vera (PV)
6. Essential thrombocythemia (ET)
7. Systemic mastocytosis
8. Chronic myeloproliferative neoplasm, unclassifiable

The disorders in the chronic myeloproliferative group have overlapping features and individual cases may be difficult to definitively classify. This is particularly true since these disorders evolve, and as they do so, their clinical and morphologic features may change. Some degree of panhyperplasia of the marrow is the general rule in all of these entities. There are a riety of cytogenetic abnormalities in the chronic myelopro- ›rative neoplasms [PMID20231614], but except for the *BCR/ABL* in ⁄IL, they are not currently used for diagnosis.

In CML, the classic Philadelphia chromosome, initially fined as a shortened chromosome 22, has now been solved as a rearrangement involving the *ABL* gene on chro- ›some 9, and *BCR* (breakpoint cluster) gene on chromosome . This is t(9;22)(q34;q11.2) i10.38, 10.39. The product of the *ABL* ne is a receptor tyrosine kinase (ie, part of a transmembrane otein) that functions in cell signaling. In CML, the break- ints on chromosome 22 are usually around exons 13 and . This is called the major breakpoint cluster region (M-bcr, th an uppercase M). The protein product that results from is translocation consists of the N-terminal portion of the CR protein and the C-terminal portion of the ABL protein. cause this novel protein has a molecular weight of 210,000 ltons, it is called p210.

The ABL protein retains its tyrosine kinase activity even nen its N-terminal region is replaced by the N-terminal gion of the BCR protein (not all of a gene must be translo- ted for it to retain full activity or be augmented by its new ighbors). In fact, the substitution of the BCR N-terminal gion makes the ABL protein constitutively active, and the creased activity of tyrosine kinase is the foundation of CML thogenesis and the basis of the drug imatinib (Gleevec or ivec), which inhibits tyrosine kinase.

Like all chronic myeloproliferative neoplasms, CML can olve and change its features. In its classic form, the blood ntains copious myeloid forms at all stages of maturation, ough myelocytes and metamyelocytes are more common an blasts i10.40. Nucleated erythrocytes may be seen, but e also much less common than myelocytes and metamyelo- tes. Eosinophilia and basophilia are common.

Both an accelerated phase and a blast crisis phase of CML ay occur. Although the precise criteria are not always uni- rmly agreed upon [PMID20592475], an accelerated phase is gener- ly diagnosed when the number of blasts in either the blood marrow reaches 10%. However, there are additional, less ten used criteria, any one of which is sufficient for the diag- osis of an accelerated phase. These are >20% basophils in the ood, persistent thrombocytopenia (<100,000) unrelated to erapy, persistent thrombocytosis (>1,000,000) unresponsive therapy, increasing white count or splenomegaly unrespon- ve to therapy, and cytogenetic evidence of clonality.

Blast crisis occurs when there are 20% blasts in either the ood or the marrow. Depending on the individual case, it ay be desirable to count promyelocytes in these determina- ons. Because 20% blasts is the definition of acute leukemia, ML patients who are in blast crisis can be regarded as hav- ıg AML. Interestingly, the blast crisis phase of CML may ccasionally demonstrate lymphoid blasts, effectively causing transition from CML to ALL.

The *BCR/ABL* translocation product in CML can be detect- d by PCR or FISH, either of which is a more sensitive test ıan conventional cytogenetics. Reverse transcriptase quanti- ative PCR for the transcript is emerging as the most common echnique [PMID19959086]. The reason reverse transcriptase PCR is sed (ie, the reason mRNA is investigated instead of DNA) is hat for *BCR/ABL* (and for som other fusion genes), the break- oints are somewhat variable, making a DNA-based PCR difficult because the breakpoints are always precisely known. Even if they are, separate sets of primers would be needed for each breakpoint (in practice, virtually a separate set for each patient). However, after RNA splicing, there are many fewer breakpoints. Compare i10.41a a negative PCR result for *BCR/ABL*, i10.41b a positive, and i10.41c a weak positive.

The conventional demonstration of the Philadelphia chromosome will substitute for the demonstration of *BCR/ABL* in the diagnosis, but is more labor-intensive and only 95% sensitive, so in practice, the role for traditional cytogenetics in suspected cases of CML is diminished, though some feel that a karyogram should still be performed in *BCR/ABL* proven CML to exclude additional abnormalities that may have prognostic significance or may portend blast crisis (at this writing, there is no molecular test that can predict acute transformation). The difficulty with obtaining a karyogram is that a bone marrow is required to obtain a sufficient number of proliferating cells, whereas molecular techniques can be applied to circulating tumor cells.

Molecular testing in CML also has a role in monitoring response and resistance to therapy, and in the assessment of MRD i10.42. Even if a laboratory has chosen FISH over PCR as the method of initial diagnosis, PCR is superior to FISH in monitoring response to therapy or assessing MRD because of its quantitative nature.

Molecular testing in CML illustrates several important points about preferred techniques. More often than not, in most diseases for which there is a molecular correlate, either FISH or PCR can be used as an initial diagnostic technique, and the choice is dependent on the individual laboratory's experience and preference. FISH is often better for numeric abnormalities, but in most cases, either technique can be used for translocations. FISH probes are usually larger than PCR primers and may therefore offer fewer false negatives (ie, greater sensitivity) because the longer probes bind with less selectivity. On the other hand, PCR may sometimes by more specific because shorter probes are more fastidious in seeking a specific area with which to hybridize. However, after the diagnosis, in matters such as assessing MRD or response to therapy, PCR is generally preferred because it is quantitative.

While primary resistance to imatinib may rarely occur, after 5 years of imatinib therapy, about 98% of patients will have achieved and maintained a clinical remission, about 85% will have reverted to a normal karyogram, about 75% will have a sharp drop in the number of *BCR/ABL* transcripts detected, and about 10% will have no *BCR/ABL* transcripts by conventional PCR.

Many patients who initially respond to imatinib will subsequently become refractory. Secondary resistance after an initial response is much more common and is seen in 10-15% of patients in the chronic phase, in a higher number in an accelerated phase, and in up to about 90% in patients in blast crisis. There are numerous reasons for resistance, including multidrug resistance (MDR) mediated by the protein P-glycoprotein (Pgp, which pumps the drug out of the cell), mutations in the tyrosine kinase, and overexpression of other tyrosine kinases [PMID21505592].

Mutations in the tyrosine kinase are not caused by the drug but are selected for by its use, very much the way that antibiotics may select for resistant organisms. Over 100 point mutations have been described in the tyrosine kinase domain of the *BCR/ABL* transcript, any of which can cause secondary resistance. Fortunately, 6 of these account for 2/3 of cases. Patients suspected of having secondary resistance to imatinib because of point mutations can be tested by several techniques. Direct DNA sequencing appears to be the most clinically useful test at this time. Allele-specific PCR is more sensitive, but there are many tyrosine kinase domains that would have to be tested for, and a PCR method runs the risk of detecting a small number of clones that may not have clinical significance [PMID19095773]. Second-generation tyrosine kinase inhibitors, including dasatinib, nilotinib, and bosutinib, are available for these patients, but bone marrow transplant still has a role in the treatment of CML for those patients who have failed both imatinib and second-generation tyrosine kinase inhibitors **i10.42**.

In older days, Philadelphia chromosome-negative CML was controversial. Many people classified such cases as atypical CML. Today, however, CML is *defined* by a *BCR/ABL* translocation, so there should be no diagnosis of CML, even with the qualifier "atypical" without demonstrating either a Philadelphia chromosome on classical karyogram, or *BCR/ABL* by a molecular technique. Cases that resemble CML clinically, but for which neither the Philadelphia chromosome nor *BCR/ABL* can be shown should be classified as chronic myelomonocytic leukemia (CMML) or chronic myeloproliferative neoplasm, unclassifiable (see below).

Chronic neutrophilic leukemia is characterized by sustained neutrophil counts in excess of 25,000 without clinical explanation. Chronic neutrophilic leukemia is occasionally considered to be a variant of CML, but is better regarded as distinct from CML because it has a better prognosis, without blast crisis, and is not associated with a specific cytogenetic abnormality.

Chronic eosinophilic leukemia is defined as sustained peripheral eosinophil counts of 1,500 or greater without explanation. There must also be proof of clonality or another indication of a chronic myeloproliferative neoplasm, such as an accompanying increase in other cell types or an increase in blasts. If these are not present, and there is only an eosinophilia, the diagnosis is hypereosinophilic syndrome. Before making either of these diagnoses, it is imperative to exclude secondary causes, such as reactions to drugs, parasites, and eosinophilia secondary to another proliferative disorder.

There is another group of disorders of eosinophils that is distinct from either eosinophilic leukemia or hypereosinophilic syndrome, and classed separately by WHO. This group has defects in platelet derived growth factor receptor A or B (PDGFRA or PDGFRB) or in fibroblast growth factor receptor 1 (FGFR1). PDGFRA and PDGFRB are both tyrosine kinases and patients with eosinophilic proliferations that have abnormalities in 1 of these 2 kinases will respond to imatinib [PMID15667033]. Patients with abnormalities of FGFR1 may have a variety of disorders in addition to those involving eosinophils.

Bone marrow fibrosis may be seen in a variety of situations, such as metastatic carcinoma, but CIMF, also called myelofibrosis with myeloid metaplasia (MMM), and formerly called agnogenic metaplasia, is bone marrow fibrosis without a preceding event. CIMF demonstrates distinct stages, both clinically and morphologically. There is initially a hypercellular phase in CIMF. Increased numbers of megakaryocytes, usually in clusters, are typically found in this early stage **i10.43**. In contrast to ET, the megakaryocytes in early CIMF often have morphologic abnormalities, furnishing a clue to the diagnosis before the advent of fibrosis [PMID21447832]. In the early stage of CIMF, reticulin fibrosis, as shown by a reticulin stain, may be surprisingly well developed or relatively minimal. A clue that a reticulin stain is needed is aspirate smears of low cellularity in the face of a cellular biopsy.

In the intermediate stage, a reticulin stain discloses a well developed meshwork of reticulin fibers **i10.44**. The caveat here is that focal reticulin fibrosis is typically seen in a variety of conditions, such as MDSs. In the well developed stage of CIMF, fibrosis is so well established that it is easily seen on H&E examination and can be confirmed by trichrome stain. Large numbers of abnormal megakaryocytes continue to be seen. CIMF is associated with splenomegaly, a peripheral leukoerythroblastotic reaction (the presence of immature cells from both the erythroid and leukocyte cell lines in the blood), and interestingly, with teardrop cells in the blood **i10.45**. Along with metastatic carcinoma, CIMF is a leading myelophthisic disorder. Both should be excluded when a leukoerythroblastotic reaction is identified in the blood.

As the disease progresses, the fibrosis of the marrow becomes obvious on H&E examination **i10.46**, with no need for a reticulin stain. The marrow becomes unable to perform effective hematopoiesis, and extramedullary hematopoiesis occurs, primarily in the spleen **i10.47**, accounting for the splenomegaly that is typical of CIMF.

Approximately 60% of CIMF patients have a cytogenetic abnormality, but there are none that are specific to that diagnosis, and by definition, the *BCR/ABL* translocation must be absent. Before making the diagnosis of CIMF, a PV that has entered a phase of bleeding and anemia should be excluded, as should other fibrosing conditions, such as mastocytosis, metastatic carcinoma with stromal desmoplasia, acute panmyelosis with myelofibrosis, and an MDS with fibrosis.

The chronic myeloproliferative neoplasms have evolutionary stages and overlapping features, but more than any other of these conditions, the evolution of PV causes it to resemble other conditions as it progresses. PV often has 2 stages, a proliferative stage, followed by a "spent" phase, in which the increased red cell mass is less evident because of bleeding or iron deficiency. The diagnosis of the proliferative phase of PV requires an increased hemoglobin without apparent cause and must be distinguished from secondary hypercythemia. Oxygen saturation must be normal and erythropoietin must not be elevated. Relative to secondary hypercythemia, the proliferative phase of PV usually has increases in other cell types in the marrow, especially in megakaryocytes **i10.48**. There is usually a reticulin fibrosis and greater marrow cellularity than in secondary polycythemia. In addition, splenomegaly is required for the diagnosis. CML must be excluded by a negative *BCR/ABL* study.

Because of the accompanying increase in megakaryocytes, PV may be difficult to distinguish from ET, especially as the patient approaches the "spent" phase, or if a superimposed iron deficiency masks or dilutes the polycythemia. Detailed studies of red cell mass may be needed, and even these may ve to be repeated after iron therapy to exclude the possibil- that a PV is obscured by superimposed bleeding and iron ficiency. Patients who appear to have ET should be given ery chance to demonstrate an increase in red cell mass to oid missing a correct diagnosis of PV.

In the "spent" phase, PV may have deceptively low hemo- obin levels and considerable marrow fibrosis, allowing it masquerade as CIMF. The marrow fibrosis causes a shift wards extramedullary hematopoiesis, resulting in spleno- egaly and leukoerythroblastosis, further simulating CIMF. deed, at this stage of PV, the distinction between this entity d CIMF may be impossible without knowledge of an earlier oliferative phase.

Essential thrombocytosis (ET) is a diagnosis of exclusion, sed on a persistent platelet count of 450,000 or more without her explanation. In addition, for the diagnosis of ET, all of e following must be met:

Exclusion of other entities by demonstration of negative *BCR/ABL*, normal or low hemoglobin (to exclude PV), and no significant marrow fibrosis (to exclude CIMF).

Increased and atypical megakaryocytes in the marrow **i10.49a**, **i10.49b** in the absence of significant abnormalities in number or morphology of the erythroid or granulocytic lines.

Exclusion of reactive thrombocytosis. This last criterion is usually fulfilled by the exclusion of conditions that are known to cause secondary thombocytosis, such as iron deficiency or inflammatory states. With the identification of mutations in the Janus kinase (JAK) family (see below), the demonstration of a mutation in the *JAK2* gene serves as an indication of clonality and excludes a reactive thrombocytosis.

Reactive thrombocytosis and PV are the major entities in e differential diagnosis of ET. The exclusion of PV is partic- arly important, as ET and PV can be strikingly similar. The agnosis of ET requires that the hemoglobin is not increased. addition, there must also be a demonstration of normal iron vels, to exclude a PV which has entered a chronic or "spent" ase, where superimposed iron deficiency from bleeding ten results in a normal or low hemoglobin. The demon- ation of normal iron is best done by preferably by finding rmal amounts of stainable iron on a marrow smear. A nor- al serum ferritin level is also helpful in excluding iron defi- ency, but less so than an iron stain of the marrow because rritin is an acute phase reactant and may be artifactually thin the normal range in iron deficiency patients if there is inflammatory condition or if there is hepatocyte necrosis at releases ferritin from the liver. As mentioned, iron thera- may be needed to exclude the "spent" phase of PV.

Systemic mastocytosis/mast cell leukemia is also a chronic yeloproliferative neoplasm, often missed because it was not ought of. Because accumulations of mast cells are relatively mmon in the skin, the major criterion for the diagnosis of stemic mastocytosis is multiple aggregates of mast cells in tracutaneous sites, where an aggregate is defined as 15 or ore mast cells whose identity has been confirmed by immu- histochemistry [PMID20684189]. The bone marrow is the most mmon extracutaneous site, but is not specifically required r the diagnosis. As is the case in other sites (eg, the spleen, **i9.17a**, **i9.17b**, **i9.17c**, **i9.17d**, **i9.17e**, mast cells in the marrow may be difficult to recognize and mastocytosis may be accompanied by fibrosis. While metachromatic cytochemical stains, such as toluidine blue, that target the granules of mast cells, may assist in the diagnosis, immunohistochemistry has largely supplanted these techniques. Mastocytomas are generally positive for CD43, CD117, and CD68, but so also are other myeloproliferative processes. While CD117 is certainly not specific for mastocytoma, its presence can be a strong diagnostic point in problematic cases for which extramedullary myeloid tumors or gastrointestinal stromal tumors have been excluded. A stain for tryptase is helpful.

CD117 is a receptor tyrosine kinase, meaning that it is a transmembrane protein whose extracellular domain binds signal molecules and whose internal domain contains a tyrosine kinase whose phosphorylation of other proteins initiates the intracellular response [PMID20533592]. Many mastocytomas have a D816V mutation (change of aspartate to valine) in the tyrosine kinase domain of CD117, corresponding to A2648T (thymine instead of adenine at nucleotide position 2648) at the DNA level. This mutation renders the neoplasm resistant to imatinib, but the rare cases of mastocytosis that have another activating mutation may respond to this drug. The presence of such a mutation is one of the minor criteria for the diagnosis of systemic mastocytosis [PMID20684189].

Chronic myeloproliferative neoplasm, unclassifiable, has increased peripheral leukocytes and platelets, with a hypercellular marrow and splenomegaly, but does not fit into an established category.

An exciting new development in the chronic myeloproliferative neoplasms is their frequent association with an abnormality in one of the enzymes of the JAK family. The JAK family consists of 4 enzymes, JAK1, JAK2, JAK3, and tyrosine kinase 2 (TYK 2). Unlike most growth factor receptors, such as Her2 and EGFR, which are transmembrane proteins, the JAKs are entirely intracellular and do not function as receptors for extracellular signals. JAK enzymes are cytoplasmic tyrosine kinases with the unusual property that they have 2 tandem tyrosine kinase domains, one of which is an inactive pseudokinase that serves a regulatory role. Enzymes of the JAK family bind the cytoplasmic portion of some of the transmembrane cytokine receptors, such as the β and γ chains of the Il-2 receptor, erythropoietin, and thrombopoietin [PMID15575979].

After the cytokine binds its receptor, the receptor undergoes a conformational change that results in the phosphorylation of the JAK. The phosphorylated JAKs then use their tyrosine kinase function to phosphorylate and activate enzymes called signal transducers and activators of transcription (STATs), which migrate to the nucleus and modulate transcription [PMID15575979].

The pseudokinase region contains the mutations that confer constitutive activity. Normal JAK2 has an autoregulatory domain in the pseudokinase region. The V617F mutation (valine to phenylalanine substitution at position 617) in exon 14 of this region negates the activity of this autoregulation, causing JAK2 to be constitutively active [PMID12686600]. This mutation keeps the cell constantly activated, even without cytokine binding [PMID16912229]. If present, JAK2 V617F can be identified in either blood or bone marrow [PMID21723416].

Abnormalities of one of the JAK enzymes are associated with various chronic myeloproliferative neoplasms, and can be assayed in either blood or bone marrow. Approximately 90-95% of PV patients, 50% of CIMF patients, and 40% of ET patients express JAK2 V617F. Although not specific for PV or even for a chronic myeloproliferative neoplasm, the incidence of JAK2 V617F is sufficiently high that some have proposed making it a major criterion for the diagnosis.

2 additional genetic abnormalities have been associated with some cases of myeloproliferative neoplasms. Rare patients with PV who do not have JAK2 V617F will have an abnormality in exon 12 of the *JAK2* gene and a minority of such patients may have a mutation at codon 515 in the gene for thrombopoietin receptor [PMID18754026].

JAK mutations have been reported in rare neoplasms that are not myeloproliferative, but at this time, they are of primary importance in myeloproliferative neoplasms and especially in PV. Although the official governing bodies have not yet passed definitive guidelines, for all practical purposes, the traditional criteria for PV have been replaced by these molecular criteria or at least supplemented by them to the point that the diagnosis of PV should be made with caution without a mutation in a JAK2 enzyme.

The tyrosine kinase activity of the JAK enzymes does not respond to existing tyrosine kinase inhibitors like imatinib, but a search is underway for effective antagonists of this activity. In the meantime, interferon remains a primary therapy for myeloproliferative neoplasms that are not CML.

Myelodysplastic/Myeloproliferative Neoplasms

The WHO classification now recognizes 4 conditions that have features of an MDS (cytopenias, abnormal morphology) and a chronic myeloproliferative neoplasm (elevated peripheral counts, hypercellular marrow, marrow fibrosis, and organomegaly). These are atypical CML, CMML, juvenile myelomonocytic leukemia (JMML), and myelodysplastic/myeloproliferative neoplasm, unclassifiable. At this writing, there have been no significant advances in the understanding of the molecular biology of these disorders since the 2008 WHO classification, and their diagnosis remains dependent on a combination of clinical/laboratory findings in the absence of any findings that would point to another diagnosis (ie, the presence of *BCR/ABL* fusion, an abnormality of JAK2, or of PDGFRA or PDGFRB) [PMID19605822].

Atypical CML closely resembles CML, except it lacks the *BCR/ABL* fusion product. Also, it often has less basophilia and more dysplasia (often trilineage). There is sometimes, but not always, a history of MDS prior to presentation of the CML-like illness.

CMML has a monocyte count of 1,000 or greater, often with dysplasia and splenomegaly. The monocytes may be abnormal, and promonocytes are often found in the blood, but individual monocytes may be relatively unremarkable **i10.50**. Immature monocytes in CMML may resemble the neoplastic cells in the monoblastic or monocytic forms of AML, so AML should be excluded by either a bone marrow examination or peripheral blood flow cytometry when a diagnosis of CMML is made. If there is an extensive concomitant myeloid hyperplasia in the blood, CMML can resemble atypical CML, but it usually has a higher monocyte count and fewer immature myeloid cells in the blood.

JMML is unique among the myelodysplastic/myeloproliferative neoplasms in affecting children. Like CMML, JMML requires a monocyte count of >1,000, but is more aggressive than CMML. Other distinguishing features include fever, rash, and hepatosplenomegaly. There is often marrow dysplasia. Many JMML patients have monosomy 7 and there is an association with neurofibromatosis type 1 [PMID19605822].

Myelodysplastic/myeloproliferative neoplasm, unclassifiable, has features of both an MDS and a myeloproliferative neoplasm, but cannot be classified as CMML, JMML, or atypical CML.

In addition to the above 4 neoplasms, refractory anemia with ringed sideroblasts and thrombocytosis is an entity that has been proposed for this category [PMID19692701].

Acute Lymphoid (Lymphoblastic) Leukemia (ALL)

While any lymphoma may be associated with a leukemic manifestation, in which case the leukemia and the lymphoma are considered different manifestations of the same entity and the circulating cells will be morphologically and immunophenotypically essentially identical to those in the lymphoma, the term "acute lymphoid leukemia" is used here to refer to those processes that primarily present in the blood rather than as a mass.

Blasts in ALL are usually smaller than those of AML and often have less distinct nucleoli **i10.51**, but immunophenotyping, or at least a cytochemical stain such as myeloperoxidase, is essential to differentiate ALL from AML. After the diagnosis of ALL is secured, subclassification is obtained.

The FAB classification of ALL was L1 (smaller blasts, little cytoplasm, small nucleoli, uniform cells, round nuclear membranes), L2 (larger cells, more cytoplasm, larger nucleoli, indented nuclear membranes), and L3 (large cells, basophilic cytoplasm with lipid vacuoles, multiple nucleoli). L3 was Burkitt leukemia, usually accompanied by a solid tissue manifestation, Burkitt lymphoma. L2 was thought to be more aggressive than L1, and L3 was more aggressive than either.

The WHO classification of ALL dispenses with the L1, L2, and L3 morphologies, and also dispenses with the previous terms of pro-B and pre-B leukemias (the former having a particularly immature phenotype). The WHO classification system is based on immunohistochemistry and cytogenetics and recognizes 2 categories of lymphoid malignancies that typically present as a leukemia: precursor B-cell lymphoma/leukemia (precursor B-ALL) and precursor T-cell lymphoma/leukemia (precursor T-ALL). Precursor B-ALL and precursor T-ALL are morphologically identical and may be of the old L1 or L2 morphology. Immunophenotyping is required to differentiate B- and T-cell acute leukemias.

The precursor B-cell leukemias are divided into those with recurrent cytogenetic abnormalities and those which are not otherwise specified. Precursor B-ALLs have well defined cytogenetic abnormalities in 80-90% of cases. Cytogenetic studies are needed to obtain the precise subtype and are also useful in tracking minimal residual disease (MRD) or response to therapy.

6 major recurrent cytogenetic abnormalities have been iden- ied, 4 of which involve translocations, and 2 of which involve oidy. One of the translocations is a t(9;22) (q34;q11). This sults in *BCR/ABL*, (Philadelphia chromosome, as in CML), it the precise breakpoint is different from that in CML. The eakpoint in most cases of ALL with t(9;22) is in intron 1, des- nated m-bcr (lowercase m, as opposed to the M-bcr in CML). iis results in a 190,000 Dalton fusion product, called p190, most cases of ALL that have t(9;22), instead of the p210 that found in CML. This is the most common translocation in lult ALL patients and has an unfavorable prognosis (a useful nemonic is that most translocations in ALL are unfavorable hile those in AML are favorable). ALL patients with t(9;22) do ot respond to imatinib. The blasts of ALL patients with t(9;22) ay express CD13 and CD33 (normally myeloid markers), so re must be taken not to inappropriately class these patients having a biphenotypic leukemia.

The second of the 4 groups based on translocations has a 12,21)(p13;q22), detectable by FISH. This is the most common anslocation in noninfant childhood ALL and one of the very w that usually conveys a favorable prognosis. Most of the asts in this group express CD10.

A third cytogenetic abnormality in precursor B-cell leu- mia is t(1;19)(q23;p13.3), which is intrinsically unfavorable, it which if recognized early, can be specifically treated, with bstantial improvement in prognosis.

A fourth well defined cytogenetic abnormality, and the last ie to involve a translocation, is t(5;14)(q31;q32). This is quite re and results from a translocation between the interleu- n-3 gene and the immunoglobulin heavy chain gene, with nsequent constitutive expression of interleukin-3.

A fifth group of ALL with recurrent cytogenetic abnormali- es, comprising about 25% of cases, is hyperdiploid (with >50 iromosomes) i10.52, and often does well. Hyperdiploid ALL ways has extra copies of chromosome 21, and usually other onormalities. A sixth group is hypodiploid (43 or fewer chro- osomes). Hypodiploidy suggests a more aggressive course adults, but is of relatively minimal significance in children.

Mixed lineage leukemia (MLL), with features of AML and LL, is associated with a variety of translocations involv- g the *MLL* gene at 11q23. It is more common in children MID19535349] and in patients who have been treated with topoi- merase inhibitors. The *MLL* gene has over 200,000 base iirs and a number of partners have been identified for *MLL* anslocations [PMID20539022]. Over 80 translocations involv- g MLL have been described, most in a breakpoint cluster gion between the 8th and 14th of its 37 exons, but 5 of them count for about 80% of all leukemias associated with the *LL* gene. Depending on the specific partner, the resulting ute leukemia may be predominantly lymphoid, predomi- intly myeloid, or mixed. t(4;11)(q21;q23) involving *AF4/MLL* the most common karyotype in infant ALL, and often has a ery immature pro-B immunophenotype that is negative for D10 and often classed as a B-lymphoblastic leukemia. Other anslocation partners with *MLL* result in AML, often myelo- onoblastic or monoblastic. In general, *MLL* acute leukemias nd to have a poorer prognosis.

The immunohistochemistry of precursor B-ALL is some- hat variable, but many blasts are positive for CD19, CD22, D79a, and TdT. The blasts in precursor B-ALL may be positive for CD5 and CD10, and are usually negative for CD20 and surface immunoglobulin [PMID21273093].

Cytogenetic abnormalities occur in a smaller percentage of precursor T-ALL than in B, about 50-60%, and cytogenetic classes are not as well defined as they are in precursor B-ALL. Classification of precursor T-ALL is currently by immunophenotype only. There is considerable clinical and immunophenotypic overlap between T-ALL and T-lymphoblastic lymphoma, and a lymphoblastic lymphoma should be excluded in any case of T-ALL just as a blood and bone marrow examination is typically performed upon the diagnosis of lymphoblastic lymphoma. The cells in acute T-cell leukemia/lymphoma cells generally express CD3 (usually cytoplasmic, occasionally on the surface) and CD2, CD5, and CD7 [PMID21273093]. TdT is usually found and CD10 is expressed in a minority of cases [PMID17708784]. The cells in acute T-cell leukemia/lymphoma may express CD4, CD8, both, or neither.

Special mention should be made of Burkitt leukemia, which consists of mature B cells that are indistinguishable from those of Burkitt lymphoma. Because Burkitt leukemia consists of mature B cells and because the WHO classification of ALL recognizes precursor B-cell leukemia and precursor T-cell leukemia, we do not usually speak of Burkitt leukemia specifically, but rather of Burkitt lymphoma, which is especially prone to a leukemic phase and is in fact likely to present as leukemia. Burkitt cells are larger than precursor B and T cells (the old FAB L3) and express fully formed surface immunoglobulin, CD10, and CD20, and are negative for TdT. Although a "starry sky" pattern (so named because there are numerous macrophages interspersed among the neoplastic cells) is characteristic of this entity in lymph nodes, it may not be seen in the bone marrow. Burkitt lymphoma is discussed in more detail in Chapter 8.

An important differential diagnosis in any ALL is hematogones. Hematogones are benign lymphocyte progenitor cells that have minimal cytoplasm, incompletely clumped chromatin, often with indented nuclei, and can therefore resemble neoplastic lymphoblasts [PMID20001239]. Nucleoli are unusual in hematogones, but may also be indistinct in lymphoid blasts. Hematogones are found mostly in infants and young children, but may be seen in older children in a variety of conditions, especially regeneration after chemotherapy. In some children, hematogones may be as much as 50% of bone marrow cells. When evaluating a bone marrow for acute leukemia or lymphoblastic lymphoma, immunophenotyping is needed to properly differentiate hematogones from blasts. Because of overlap in the antigen profiles of hematogones and lymphoid blasts (eg, both may be positive for TdT), conventional immunophenotyping may occasionally fail to make this distinction, and either multiparameter flow cytometry or PCR for antigen receptor gene rearrangement may be required [PMID10361511].

The Bone Marrow in Chronic Lymphoid Leukemia

The bone marrow may be involved in any lymphoma, but the diagnostic criteria are as described in lymph nodes, so the only 2 lymphomas discussed here are those associated with chronic lymphoid leukemia and multiple myeloma.

ISBN 978-089189-5886

Chronic lymphoid leukemia (CLL) is historically defined by a persistent lymphocyte count of 5,000/µL, with lymphocytes that are generally relatively bland in their appearance **i10.53**. But it is now understood that the immunophenotype is of equal or greater importance than the number of lymphocytes or their morphology in the diagnosis. The CD5 and CD10 pattern of CLL is the same as mantle cell lymphoma—CD5 positive and CD10 negative. However, CLL is CD23 positive, while mantle cell lymphoma is CD23 negative. The prevailing view is that CLL is a neoplasm of CD5 positive cells that have not been antigenically stimulated. Rare asymptomatic patients will have a small number of circulating B cells that are CD5 and CD23 positive, but any significant number of such lymphocytes is of concern for developing CLL, and 15% of these patients will go on to develop CLL [PMID18687638]. In addition to CD5 and CD23, CLL cells express surface immunoglobulin, CD19, CD79a, and CD20, and are positive for CD43 in 80% of cases. If a putative CLL does not have this immunohistochemical profile, it is likely to be a leukemic phase of another type of lymphoma.

Those cases that express CD38 in >30% of cells seem to do less well [PMID10477712]. Even if CD38 is low, a high CD31 (which is the ligand for CD38) appears to confer a more aggressive course [PMID12673718]. Those cases that have evidence of somatic hypermutation of the immunoglobulin heavy chain gene appear less aggressive [PMID10477713]. Expression of the tyrosine kinase ZAP-70 is associated with unmutated heavy chains (ie, those that have not undergone somatic hypermutation) in 70% of cases, and its expression in >20% of neoplastic cells is an unfavorable sign. Interestingly, ZAP-70 expression remains an indication of aggressiveness even in the 30% of cases in which it is not associated with unmutated heavy chains [PMID20008228]. Elevated serum β2 microglobulin is also a poor prognostic sign.

CLL is not uniformly associated with any particular cytogenetic aberration, and most patients have a normal karyotype. However, are a variety of abnormalities that may be present, of which del(13q14) is the most common, usually suggesting a less aggressive course. Del(17p13) and del(11q22) are associated with more aggressive forms of the disease, especially the former, which appears to be a deletion of the important tumor suppressor gene *P53*. For these prognostic reasons, karyotyping is recommended in CLL. FISH is the preferred method for detecting these abnormalities at this writing, as it is more sensitive than traditional karyotyping, but microarrays may also be used [PMID19074592].

In CLL, the marrow is invariably involved with small lymphocytic lymphoma (SLL; formerly called well differentiated lymphoma), and the entity is usually called CLL/SLL. The diagnosis of CLL should be questioned if the marrow is not involved. Most cases of CLL/SLL will express CD20, but only weakly and rituximab is often of marginal value. However, those cases that have trisomy 12 often exhibit greater cell membrane CD20 expression and therefore are more likely to benefit from rituximab [PMID18324964].

The lymphoma in the marrow may be nodular **i10.54**, diffuse **i10.55**, interstitial (intermingled with normal bone marrow cells without disturbance of the architecture) **i10.56** or mixed interstitial and nodular. The diffuse type has a poorer prognosis, while the nodular type of infiltration appears to be less aggressive [PMID21776871]. In CLL/SLL, the extent and nature of bone marrow involvement are important and should be mentioned. If only 1 or 2 nodules of lymphocytes are found, they should be immunohistochemically characterized to exclude benign lymphoid nodules that are occasionally found in normal marrow.

There are 2 aggressive manifestations of CLL. The first is Richter syndrome, which is a lymphoma is of the large cell type **i10.57**, rather than the usual and expected SLL. The second is CLL of the prolymphocytic type (or prolymphocytic leukemia). Whereas the lymphocytes in typical CLL have a reasonably mature appearance, prolymphocytes have a single prominent nucleolus **i10.58**, and in prolymphocytic leukemia, the peripheral lymphocyte count tends to be very elevated. The diagnosis of prolymphocytic leukemia requires that prolymphocytes account for 55% or more of the total lymphocytes in the blood. If prolymphocytes constitute between 10% and 55% of the total lymphocyte count, the leukemia is called mixed CLL/PLL, and up to 10% prolymphocytes are accepted into routine CLL.

Multiple Myeloma and Other Immunosecretory Disorders

Multiple myeloma is the prototype of a group of disorders that are immunosecretory (ie, characterized by the inappropriate secretion of immunoglobulins). Other examples of immunosecretory disorders include the lymphoplasmacytic lymphoma/immunocytoma that is associated with Waldenström macroglobulinemia, some cases of CLL/SLL, some cases of marginal zone lymphoma, monoclonal gammopathy of undetermined significance (MGUS), and µ and α heavy chain diseases [PMID18580096, PMID15842043].

Historically, the major criteria for myeloma are a distinct plasmacytoma, a bone marrow with >30% plasma cells, or a significant monoclonal protein (>3.5g/dL for IgG and IgM, >2.0 g/dL for IgA, or >1.0 g κ or λ light chain/dL on a 24-hour urine collection). The minor criteria are a bone marrow with between 10% and 30% plasma cells, a smaller monoclonal protein than is required for a major criterion, reduced antibody levels apart from a possible paraprotein, and lytic bone lesions. The diagnosis is then based on at least 1 major and 1 minor criterion or 3 minor criteria. However, the WHO classification relaxes these specific numbers and defines myeloma as damage to organs caused by a plasma cell proliferation or its immunoglobulin products [Swerdlow ISBN978-9283224310]. This concept has been generally adopted, and today, the key concept of multiple myeloma, as opposed to a simple proliferation of plasma cells and a monoclonal protein, is damage to organs, such as kidneys, bone marrow (such that there is an insufficient production of normal blood elements), and bones (lytic bone lesions) [PMID18580096]. Indeed, if the associated findings are clearly present, a marrow is unlikely to be needed for the diagnosis, but will be obtained in any case, not only to secure the diagnosis, but also to provide a baseline against which to monitor therapy.

MGUS is defined as <3 g/dL of serum paraprotein, <1g/24 hours of Bence Jones protein in the urine, and <10% bone marrow plasma cells. MGUS is quite common, occurring in

% of patients over the age of 70. 1% per year will progress to noldering or overt myeloma.

Smoldering multiple myeloma is defined by >3 g/dL of rum paraprotein, 1 g or more per 24 hours of urine Bence nes protein, or >10% bone marrow plasma cells. Smoldering ultiple myeloma has a 10% progression rate to overt myeloa. Indolent myeloma is defined as 30% or more bone marw plasma cells, but with no systemic symptoms or evidence organ involvement [PMID12057049].

By definition, MGUS, smoldering myeloma, and indolent yeloma do not have lytic bone lesions, hypercalcemia, renal sufficiency, or anemia. Any of these signs in conjunction ith a paraprotein or a plasma cell proliferation mandate e diagnosis of overt multiple myeloma. Serial measureents of the paraprotein in patients with any of these entis are important, and an increase is associated with a more gressive course. In equivocal situations, where the degree organ damage cannot be determined, strong expression CD56 favors smoldering or overt myeloma, while weak aining favors MGUS, and strong expression of CD19 favors GUS, while weak staining favors myeloma [PMID19728762]. CD19 sitivity, in conjunction with absence of microRNA 223 nicroRNAs are discussed in Chapter 44) suggest an isolated tramedullary plasmacytoma rather than an extramedullary anifestation of myeloma, a distinction that is important in erapy [PMID21401705].

Myeloma may be of the plasmablastic type, which has blas morphology with a large nucleolus and no perinuclear hof, e immature type with transitional differentiation **i10.59**, or the plasmacytic type, which has relatively mature plasma lls **i10.60** and a better prognosis [PMID10613359]. Plasma cell ukemia occurs when 20% of blood leukocytes are plasma lls. In contrast to common myeloma, plasma cell leukemia associated with thrombocytopenia.

Plasma cells are often negative for CD20. Most myelomas press CD56, and those that do not tend to be more aggresve [PMID15061198]. Myeloma cells tend to be negative for CD19, hich is often expressed by B-cell lymphomas that have plasacytic differentiation. A panel of CD19 and CD56 can help differentiate a true myeloma from a B-cell lymphoma of nother type with a plasmacytoid appearance [PMID17210522], and CD138 may also help in these situations. Again, however, e acid test for the confirmation of myeloma is the presence absence of ancillary findings, especially organ damage.

Although bone marrow smears are generally the best mateals for counting plasma cells, the number of plasma cells on e smears may vary greatly from field to field and there may so interobserver variation in the precise count. Therefore, in quivocal cases, it may be desirable to perform a CD138 stain the biopsy. Determination of residual myeloma is best done ith routine H&E morphology supplemented by immunohischemistry (using heat retrieval on paraffin for CD138, κ and . This technique was superior to conventional cytogenetics, w cytometry, molecular studies for immunoglobulin gene arrangements, and fluorescence in situ hybridization (FISH) MID16690489]. CD56 is also useful in morphologically subtle ses of myeloma or in assessing residual disease [PMID19864234]. D27, CD28, CD45, and CD117 are additional markers that are lpful in assessing the nature of plasma cell proliferations MID20201947].

About 90% of patients with myeloma have a cytogenetic abnormality [PMID9558394]. Because plasma cells are difficult to grow in culture and therefore, good metaphases are rare, it has only been with FISH that these cytogenetic abnormalities have come to light. About half of cases have hyperdiploidy of many of the odd-numbered chromosomes, which appears to be a favorable prognostic sign [PMID19798094]. The other half has a translocation involving the immunoglobulin heavy chain on chromosome 14. The 2 most common of these are t(4;14)(p16.3;q32), and t(11;14)(q13;q32). The former is unfavorable and the latter is neutral in prognostication. The t(11;14)(q13;q32) disrupts the *BCL-1* (*CCND1*) gene that codes for cyclin D1, as is the case in mantle cell lymphoma, illustrating that this translocation is not specific for mantle cell origin of a lymphoma. Unlike other lymphoid proliferations that have translocations involving the immunoglobulin heavy chain, those in myeloma occur later, at the time of class switching, not at the time of VDJ recombination. Almost half of myeloma patients will have del(13q), but this is of unclear clinical significance. Abnormalities of chromosomes 1 and 17 may also be found [PMID19798094].

A final comment on myeloma is that, rarely, free light chains will precipitate in either the marrow or the kidney, imbuing the tissue with crystals **i10.61**.

Waldenström macroglobulinemia is an immunosecretory disorder characterized by IgM monoclonality, often with hyperviscosity. Most patients with Waldenström macroglobulinemia will have will have a lymphoplasmacytic lymphoma/immunocytoma **i10.62**, but other lymphoproliferative disorders may give rise to a similar clinical picture.

Unusual Conditions Found in the Marrow or Blood

The cytoplasmic projections that furnish the name hairy cell leukemia may be subtle **i10.63a**. The chromatin in hairy cell leukemia is less clumped chromatin than CLL, and this finding in a marrow infiltrate **i10.63b**, in conjunction with the almost certain splenomegaly, may suggest the diagnosis. Hairy cells are negative for CD5 and CD10, and positive for surface immunoglobulin, CD11c, CD20, CD25, DBA44, FMC7, and CD103. The major entities in the differential diagnosis are splenic lymphoma with villous lymphocytes and systemic mastocytosis.

There is a rare T-cell prolymphocytic leukemia that is morphologically identical to the B cell counterpart that may be seen in progression of CLL. Before such a diagnosis is made, a leukemic manifestation of a T-cell lymphoma should be excluded. Some cases of apparent T-CLL are now classed as large granular lymphocytosis (LGL), which may be of either T cell or natural killer (NK) cell phenotype. LGL leukemias of either type may be either indolent or aggressive and therefore, 4 such leukemias are recognized: indolent or chronic T-cell LGL leukemia, aggressive T-cell LGL leukemia, indolent or chronic NK-cell leukemia, and aggressive NK-cell leukemia [PMID20425381]. The indolent forms are often treated with immunosuppressive therapy rather than traditional induction therapy.

μ chain disease is characterized by a paraprotein consisting only of the μ heavy chain, not by a complete immunoglobulin molecule. About 1/3 of μ chain patients have CLL, while 10% have myeloma. About 20% have no associated condition. α chain disease is usually associated with an extranodal marginal zone lymphoma, often of the gastrointestinal tract [PMID16026747].

Hemophagocytic syndromes are characterized by fever, cytopenias, and infections. In the marrow, spleen, or nodes, there is histiocytic hyperplasia with phagocytosis of erythrocytes or hematopoietic cells i10.64. Hemophagocytic syndromes may be primary (in which case they affect infants and are usually fatal) or secondary (to infection, malignancy, or compromised immune status) [PMID20383897]. Many cases of hemophagocytic syndrome in adults are secondary to a lymphoma, often of T cell lineage. The underlying problem seems to be a defective immune response. The differential diagnosis includes a reactive histiocytosis and a lymphoma. Epstein Barr virus (EBV) is often present in hemophagocytic syndromes [PMID22169321].

Paroxysmal nocturnal hemoglobinuria (PNH) is now recognized as a mutation in a hematopoietic stem cell, usually in an X-linked gene called *PIG-A*, that results in a defect in the protein glycosylphosphatidylinositol (GPI). GPI is important as an anchor for many other proteins, foremost among which are the proteins CD55 and CD59, which confer resistance to lysis by complement. In the presence of defective GPI, CD55 and CD59 cannot bind to and protect the red cell, resulting in spontaneous hemolysis. The diagnosis of PNH is now by the flow cytometric detection of diminished amounts of CD55 and CD59 on erythrocytes. These 2 proteins may also be diminished on lymphocytes, and there may also be a reduction of CD14 on monocytes in PNH, resulting in pancytopenia [PMID19080854, PMID19686268, PMID20498998]. More recently, direct detection of GPI on granulocytes by flow cytometry with fluorescent aerolysin has been shown to be more sensitive than detection of CD55 or CD59 [PMID20533382].

Core Points for Bone Marrow

- Myelodysplastic syndromes (MDS): group of disorders, often leading to acute leukemia.
  - Abnormal development and function of erythrocytes, leukocytes, and platelets.
  - Evidence for clonal origin, and these disorders may soon be considered neoplasms.
  - Cytogenetics has often replaced the blast count as the most important diagnostic criterion.
  - 3 new categories of MDS:
    - Refractory cytopenia with multilineage dysplasia
    - MDS associated with isolated del(5q)
    - MDS, unclassifiable
  - May be associated with fibrosis and may be hypocellular, causing resemblance to primary idiopathic myelofibrosis and aplastic anemia, respectively.
- Acute myeloid leukemia (AML): cytogenetic information important.
  - In addition to AML associated with cytogenetic abnormalities, 5 other broad categories of AML
  - The last of these, AML not otherwise specified, has numerous subgroups.
- Demonstration of characteristic cytogenetic abnormalities and the concept of minimal residual disease have redefined the conception of remission and relapse.
- 8 categories of chronic myeloproliferative neoplasms (CMN; formerly called chronic myeloproliferative disorders)
  - Most common are chronic myelogenous leukemia (CML), polycythemia vera, and chronic idiopathic myelofibrosis.
  - CML: Philadelphia chromosome is translocation between the *ABL* gene on chromosome 9 and the *BCR* gene on chromosome 22.
  - PCR is useful in CML in establishing the diagnosis and also in monitoring effectiveness of therapy.
- 4 conditions have features of both a myelodysplastic syndrome and a myeloproliferative neoplasm:
  - Chronic myelomonocytic leukemia
  - Juvenile myelomonocytic leukemia
  - Atypical chronic myelogenous leukemia
  - Myelodysplastic/myeloproliferative neoplasm
- 2 lymphoproliferative processes primarily present as leukemia: precursor B-cell acute leukemia and precursor T-cell acute leukemia.
- Precursor B-cell acute leukemias are subdivided into those that have reproducible cytogenetic abnormalities and those that do not.
- Cytogenetic abnormalities are not as well defined in precursor T-cell acute leukemia, and their subclassification is by immunophenotype only.
- CLL: Defined by immunophenotype as much as by absolute number of lymphocytes in the blood.
  - Cells of CLL are negative for CD10 and positive for CD5 and CD23.
  - Lymphoma counterpart to CLL is small lymphocytic lymphoma, which is almost always found in the bone marrow in patients with CLL.
  - CLL may become more aggressive by Richter syndrome (large cell lymphoma) or transformation to prolymphocytic leukemia.
- Diagnosis of myeloma now centers more on damage to organs than absolute numbers of plasma cells.
- Monoclonal gammopathy of uncertain significance replaces older term benign monoclonal gammopathy.
  - Many will progress to overt myeloma.

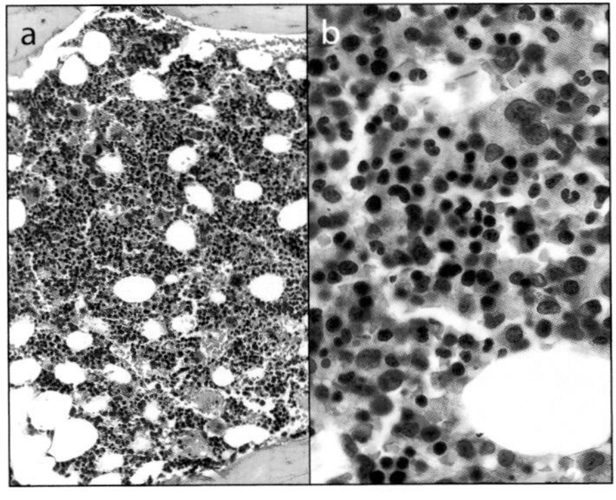

1 **a** Normal bone arrow with admixed fat The component lls of normal bone arrow, including lls of the erythroid, yeloid, lymphoid, and egakaryocytic lines

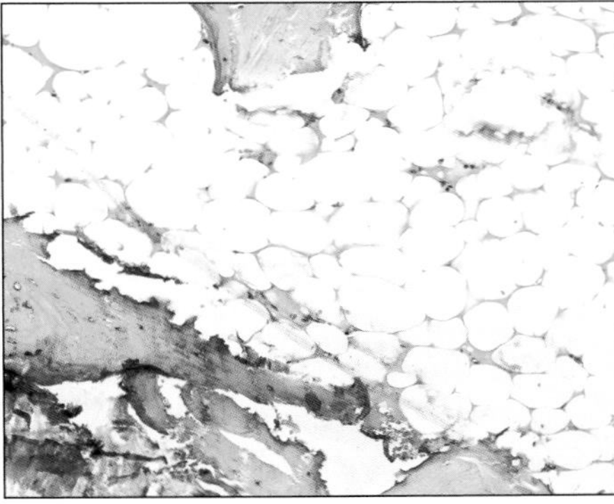

i10.2 The very hypocellular bone marrow that is typically found just underneath the cortex

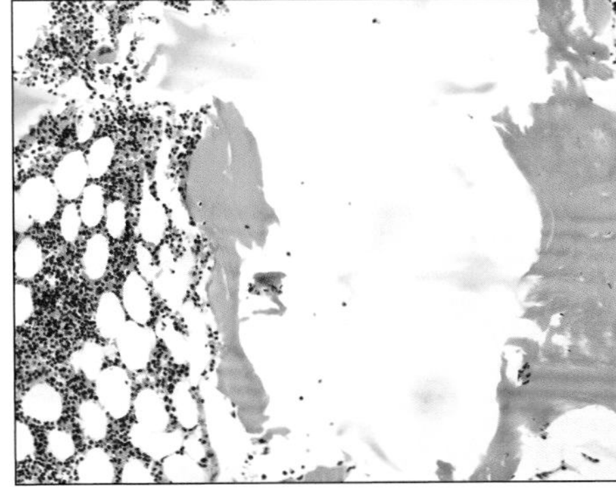

.3 Aspiration artifact. ypocellular bone arrow still has adipose ssue, but aspiration tifact is evident by the sence of both bone arrow elements and lipose tissue.

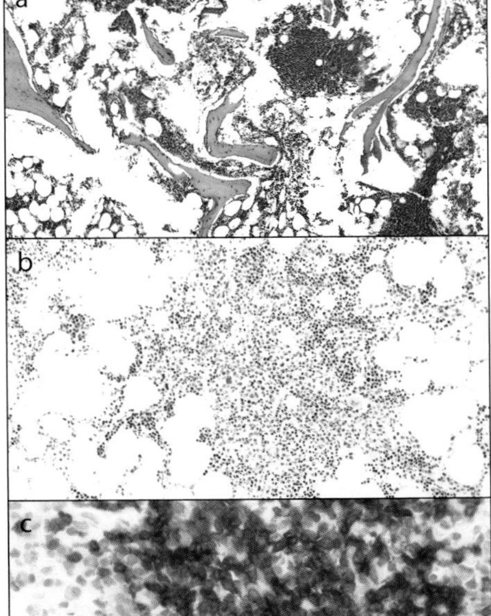

i10.4 **a** Lymphoid nodules in the bone marrow of a patient with a history of B-cell lymphoma. **b** A negative CD20 stain on 1 of these nodules. **c** Because not all B-cell lymphomas are positive for CD20, and because even if a lymphoma in a single site at one time is positive for CD20, it may not necessarily be positive at all times in all sites, the negative CD20 stain illustrated in i10.4b is insufficient to definitively exclude bone marrow involvement by the lymphoma. However, this CD3 stain clearly demonstrates that the lymphoid nodule is of T-cell origin, and not bone marrow involvement by the B-cell lymphoma.

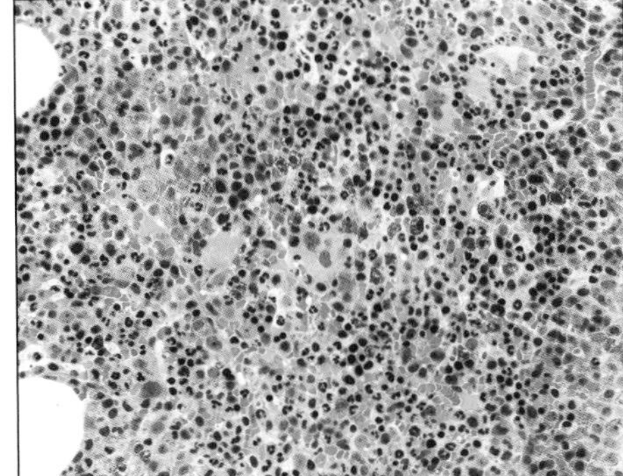

.5 Hypercellular bone arrow in reactive yperplasia

0.6 A noncaseating, onnecrotizing granuloma the bone marrow in arcoidosis

i10.7 Herpetic inclusions in the bone marrow in an AIDS patient

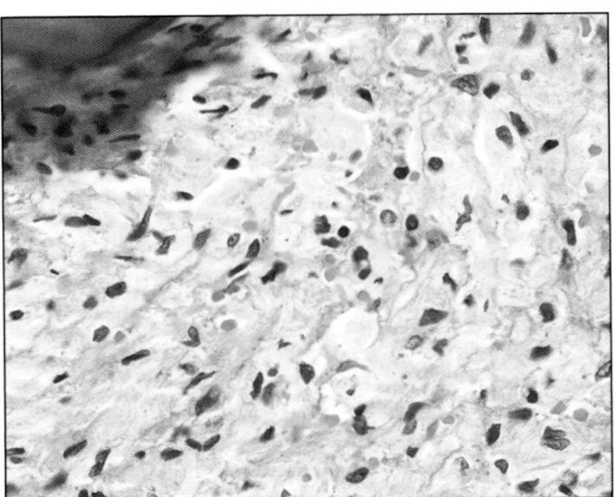

0.8 The bone marrow in patient with Gaucher isease, in which lipid-aden macrophages are nterspersed with fibrous issue to the exclusion f normal bone marrow lements

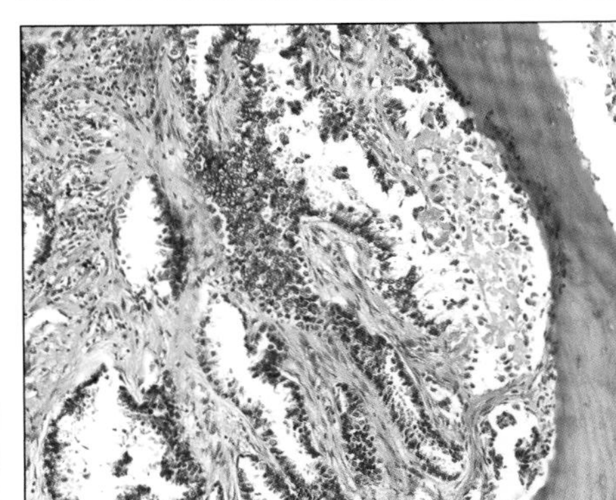

i10.9 Metastatic adenocarcinoma to the bone marrow. Immunohistochemical stains revealed this to be a lung primary.

ISBN 978-089189-5886

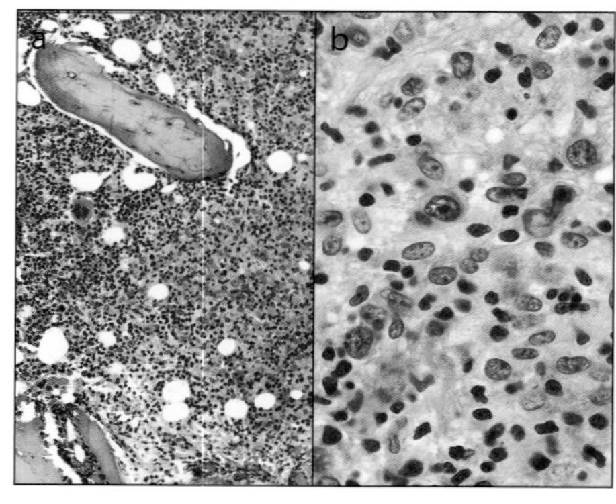

i10.10 a Hodgkin disease involving the bone marrow. There is normal bone marrow on the left but a fibrotic nodule, with abnormal cells, on the right. **b** A high-power view of the nodule depicted in i10.10a. The large cells with nucleoli stained as Reed-Sternberg cells.

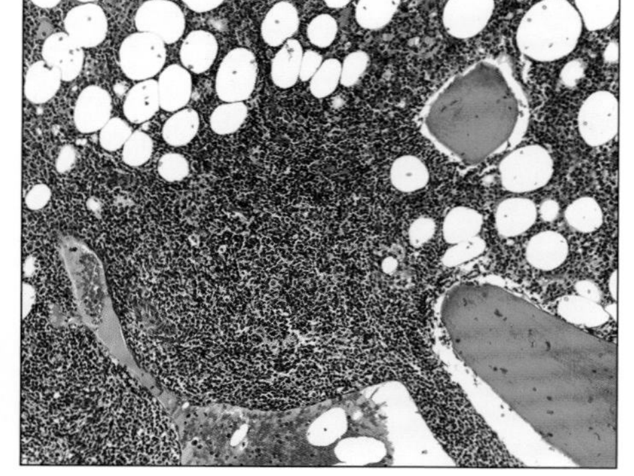

i10.11 A bone marrow biopsy with a lymphoid nodule whose immunohistochemical characterization showed it to be a manifestation of a follicular lymphoma. While of limited diagnostic utility, bone marrow involvement by follicular lymphoma tends to have a paratrabecular location, as shown here.

i10.12 a A ringed sideroblast is evident in the center. Note that the iron granules are immediately adjacent to a nucleus and largely encircle it. **b** The cell in the center is a sideroblast, but it is unlikely to be a true ringed sideroblast because the iron granules are not immediately adjacent to the nucleus (ie, they are not in mitochondria).

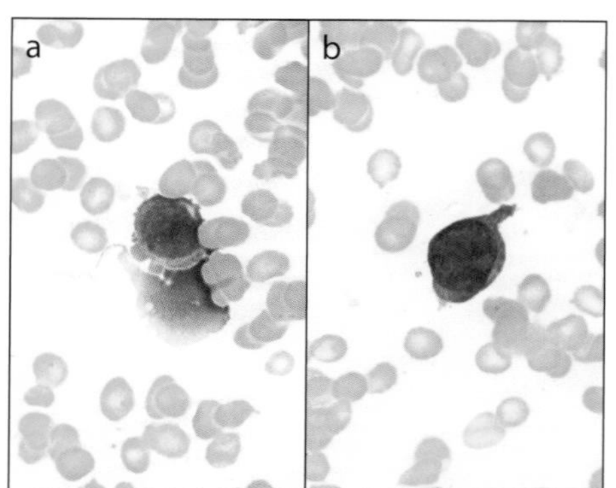

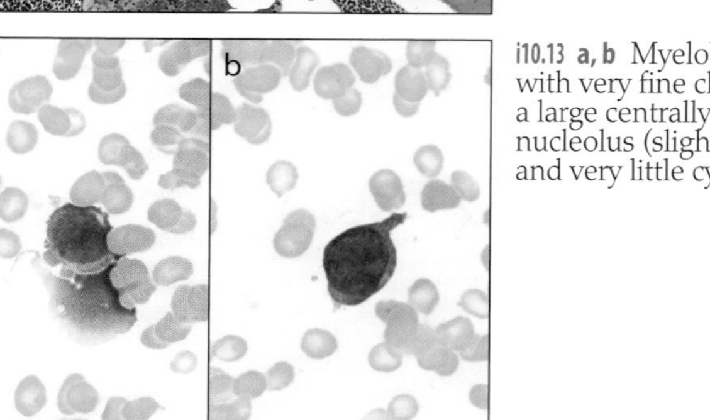

i10.13 a, b Myeloblasts, with very fine chromatin, a large centrally placed nucleolus (slightly purple) and very little cytoplasm

i10.14 a, b Refractory cytopenia with multilineage dysplasia illustrating abnormal erythroid forms

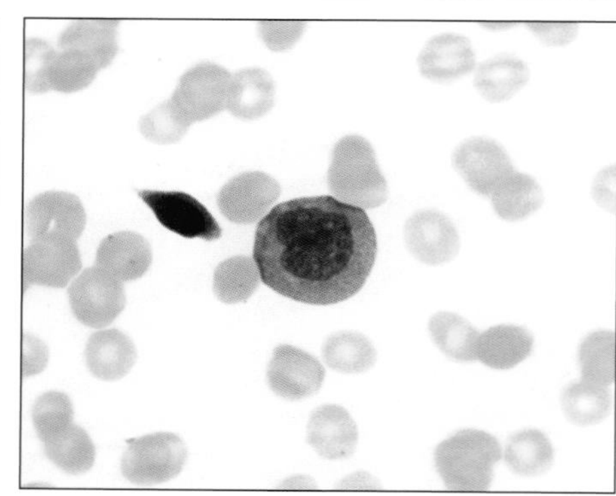

i10.15 Refractory cytopenia with multilineage dysplasia illustrating an abnormal myeloid cell with poor granulation

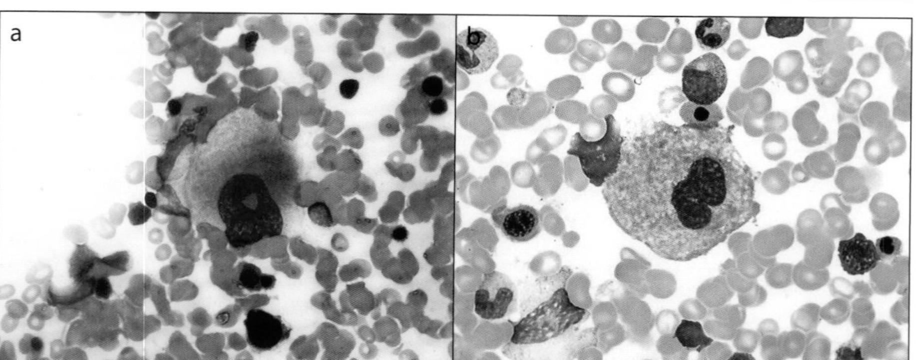

i10.16 a Refractory cytopenia with multilineage dysplasia illustrating a megakaryocyte with only 1 nuclear lobe **b** The same case as in i10.16a, illustrating a megakaryocyte with poorly granulated cytoplasm that cannot give rise to normally functioning platelets

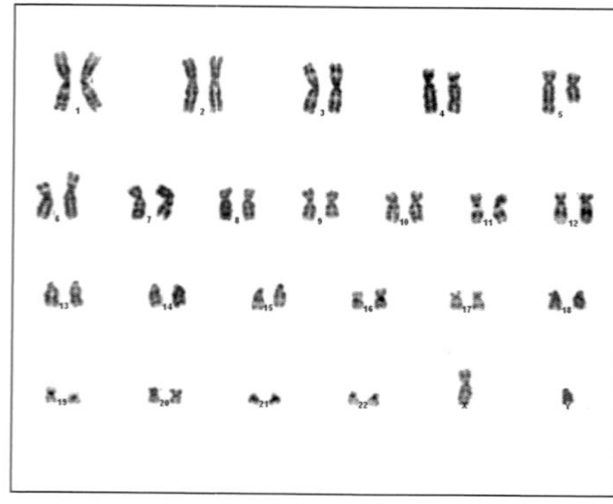

i10.17 del(5q) karyogram

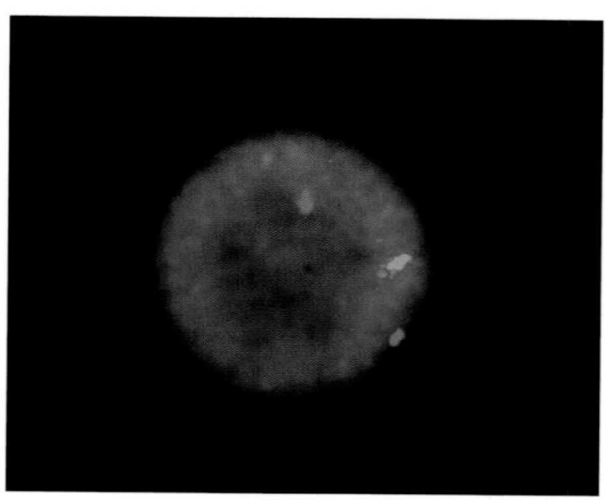

i10.18 FISH study confirming the del(5q) seen in the karyogram. The red probe hybridizes to the 5q region. There should be 2 signals in the cell (only 1 red signal is visible).

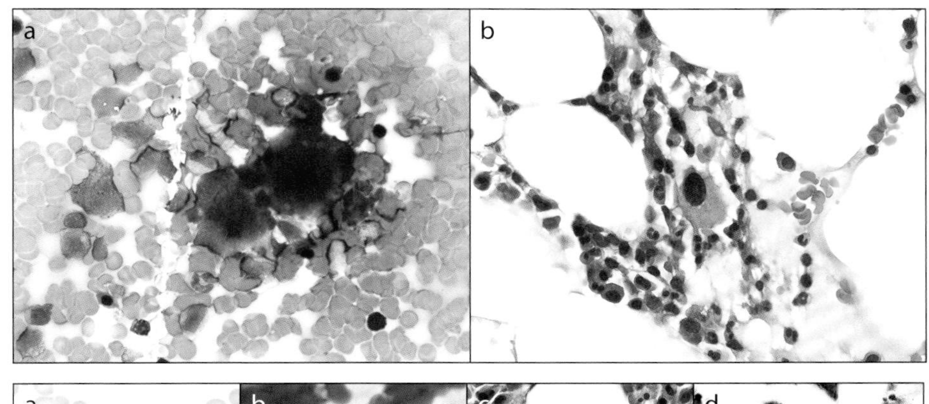

i10.19 **a, b** MDS associated with del(5q). Although there are no specific morphologic features of this form of MDS, megakaryocyte nuclei tend to be hypolobated, as shown here.

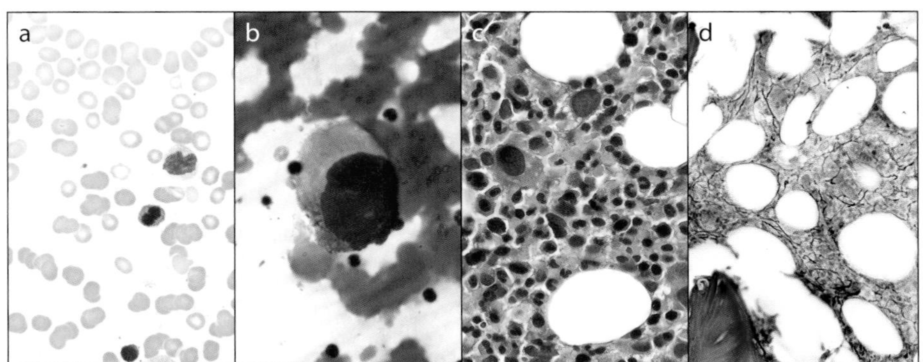

i10.20 MDS associated with myelofibrosis. **a** illustrates an abnormal erythroid form, **b** and **c** illustrate abnormal megakaryocytes, with monolobated nuclei, and **d** illustrates the myelofibrosis.

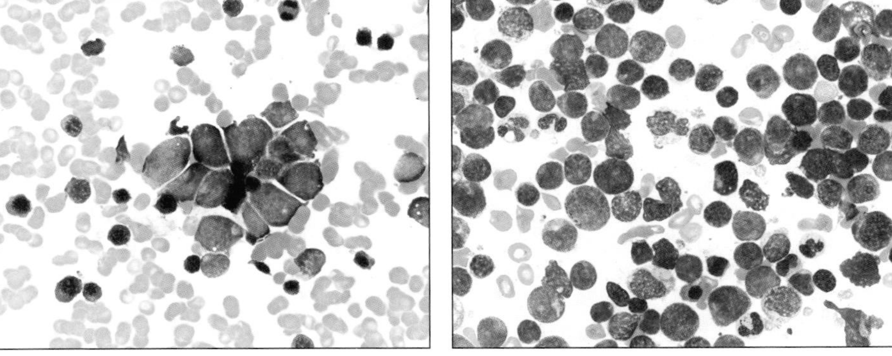

21 A "recovering" bone ırrow taken 2 days er the patient received ınulocyte colony mulating factor. While s collection of immature ls, out of context and thout the history, might ggest a possible acute ıkemia, they are benign d represent a response the colony stimulating tor.

i10.22 AML with >20% of the nucleated cells in the marrow being myeloblasts

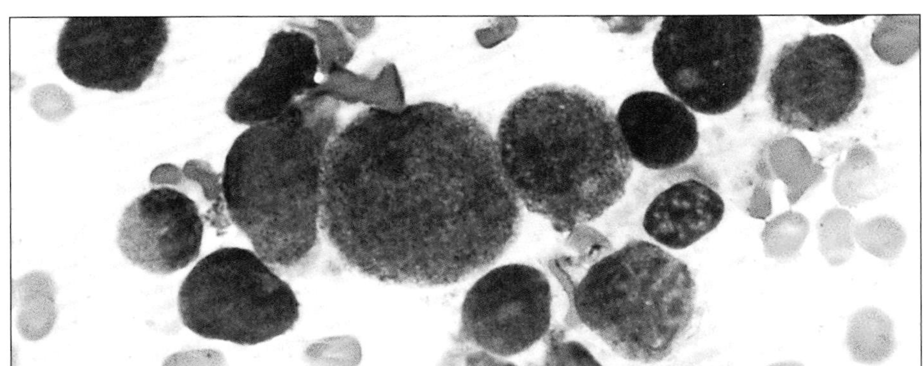

i10.23 Acute promyelocytic leukemia, with a mixture of classic blasts and blasts with copious primary granules, indicative of differentiation towards promyelocytes

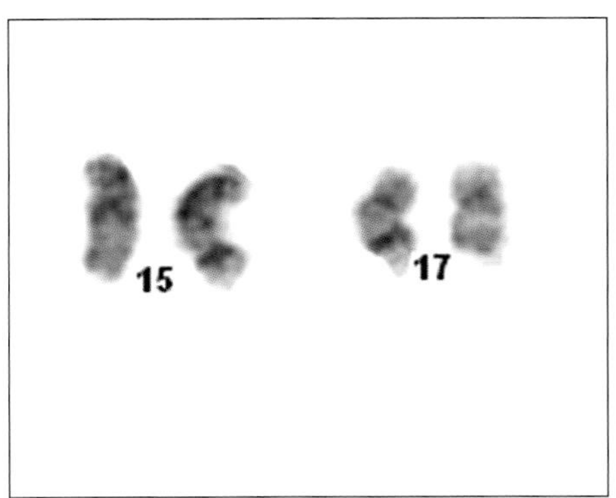

24 t(15;17) partial ryogram in a patient th APL.

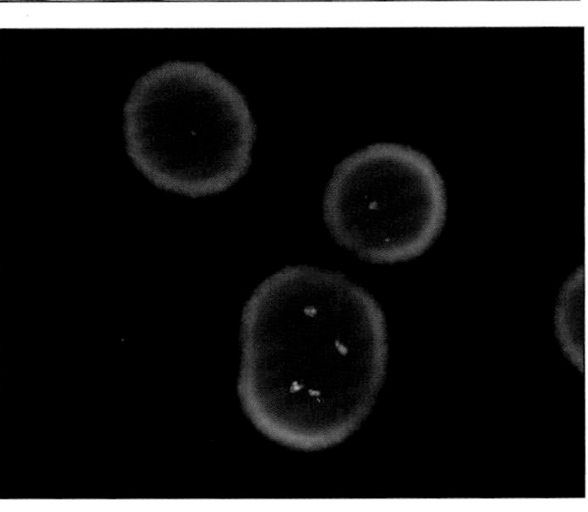

i10.25 t(15;17) FISH study in a patient with APL, confirming the t(15;17).

ISBN 978-089189-5886

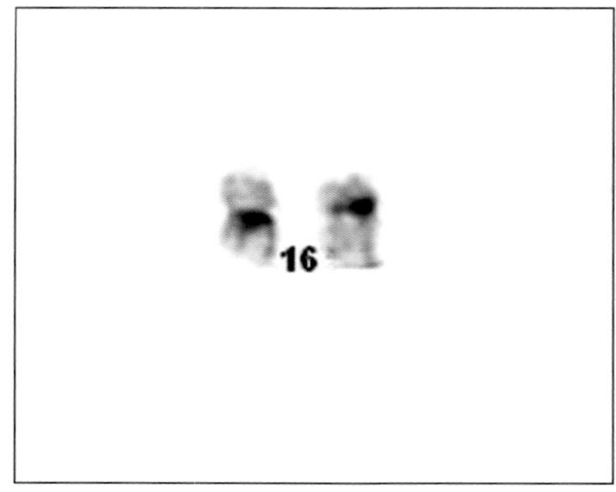

i10.26 AML. inv(16) partial karyogram. Note the prominent G band. This patient also had 3 copies of chromosomes 8 and 22 as well

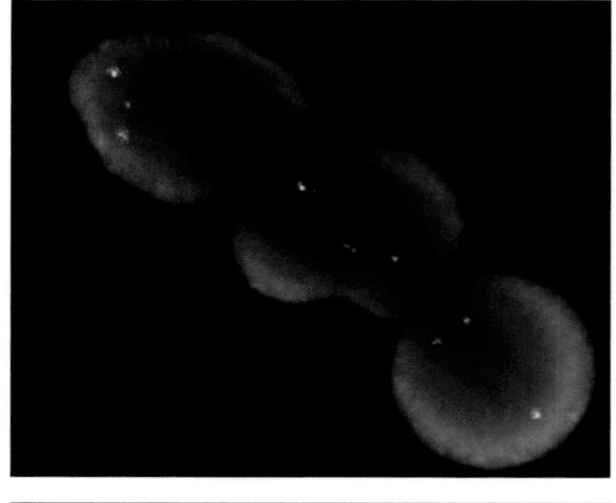

i10.27 AML. Break apart FISH study confirming the inv(16) shown in i10.26. Red and green signals that are adjacent (perhaps with an area of yellow between them) indicate retention of normal position and no inversion. But separation of red and green signals indicate an inversion.

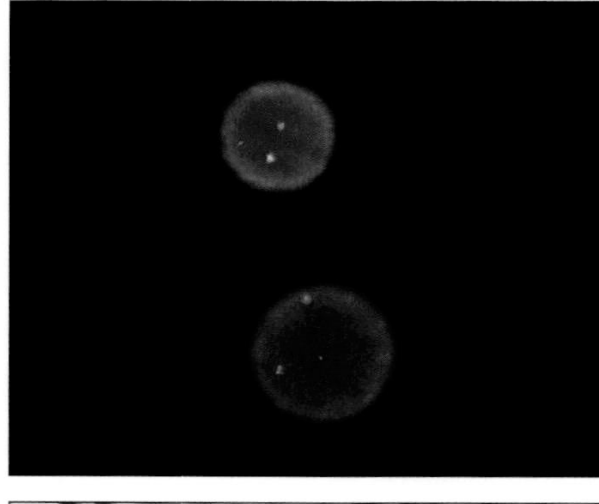

i10.28 MLL. Break apart FISH study confirming the presence of translocations within the MLL gene. Multiple breakpoints have been shown in this gene. Juxtaposed red and green signals, or a yellow signal, indicate absence of translocation, while separate red and green signals indicate a translocation.

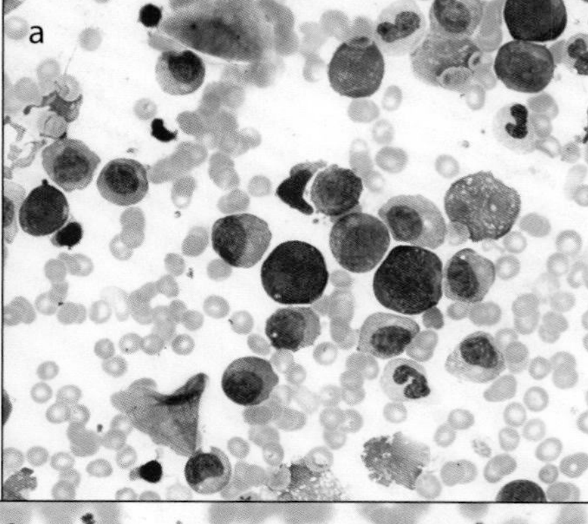

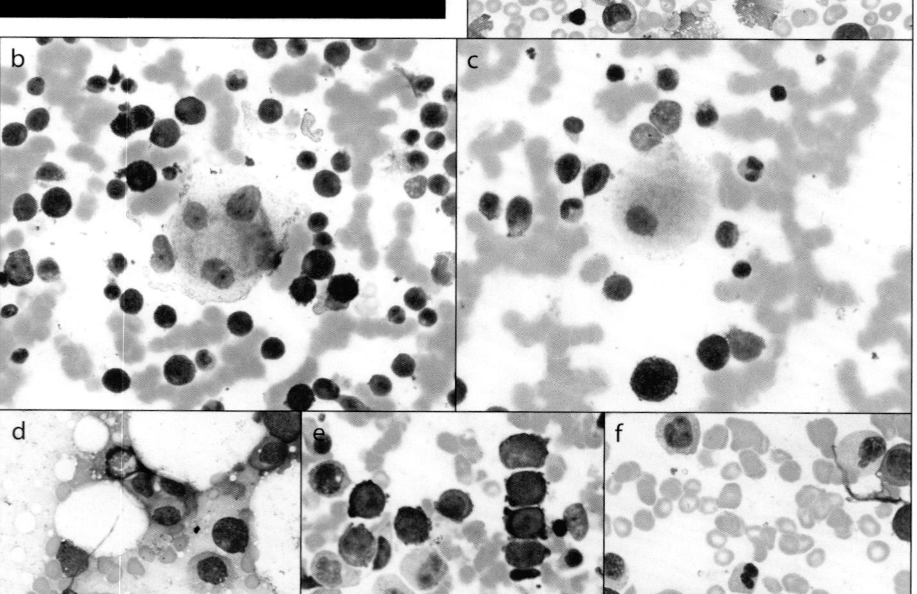

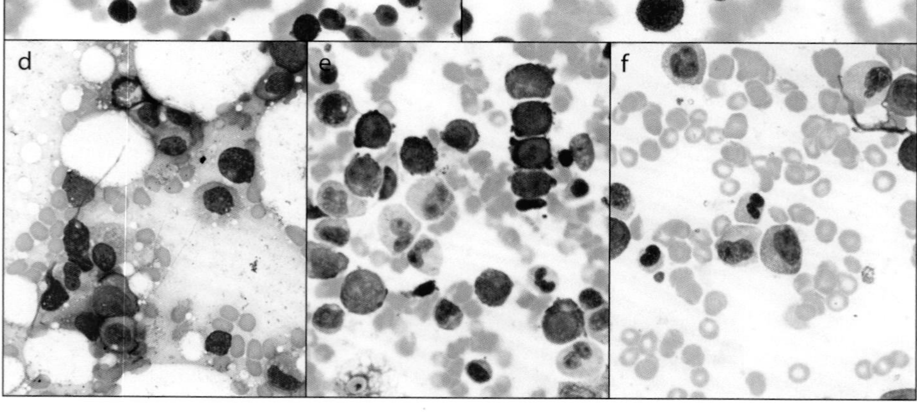

i10.29 AML with multilineage dysplasia. **a** illustrates the increased myeloblasts. **b, c, d, e** and **f** all come from the same case.

b illustrates a megakaryocyte with multiple, unconnected nuclei and cytoplasmic hypogranulation.

c illustrates a megakaryocyte with a monolobated nucleus.

d illustrates, in the center and at the approximate 7:00 position, myeloid cells with poor granulation cytoplasm.

e additionally illustrates, just to the left of center, myeloid cells with poor cytoplasmic granulation. **f** illustrates an abnormal erythroid precursor in the center.

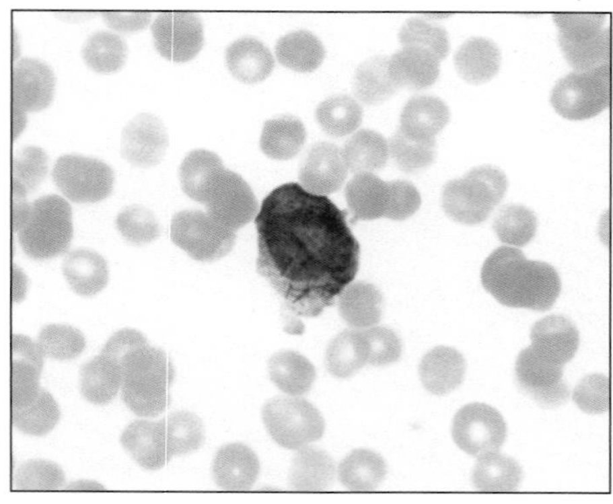

i10.30 A myeloblast with an Auer rod. Auer rods are needle-shaped collections of primary (also called azurophilic) granules.

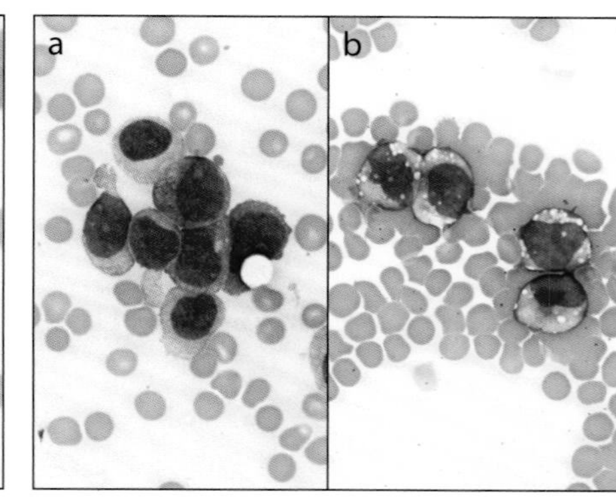

i10.31 **a** A cluster of myeloblasts in acute myelomonocytic leukemia with myeloid differentiation. Note the granulation in the blast at the top of the photograph. **b** The same case as in i10.31a with blasts showing cytoplasmic vacuolization, an indication of differentiation towards monocytes

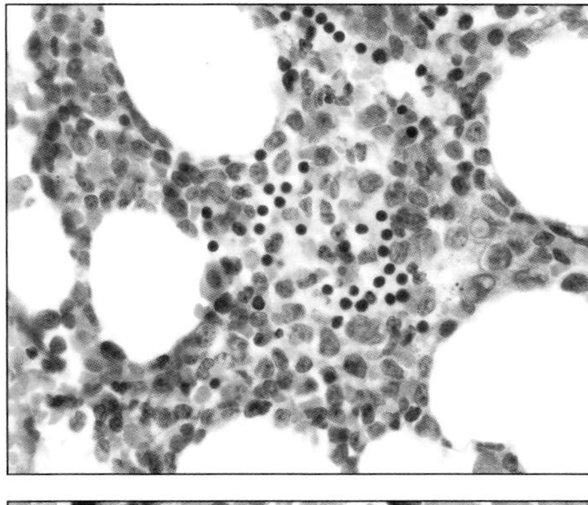

2 Acute
elomonocytic leukemia
h eosinophilia
merly called M4E).
en in this paraffin
tion, one can see
nerous eosinophils
ermingled with cells
h blasts that have
y fine chromatin and
cleoli.

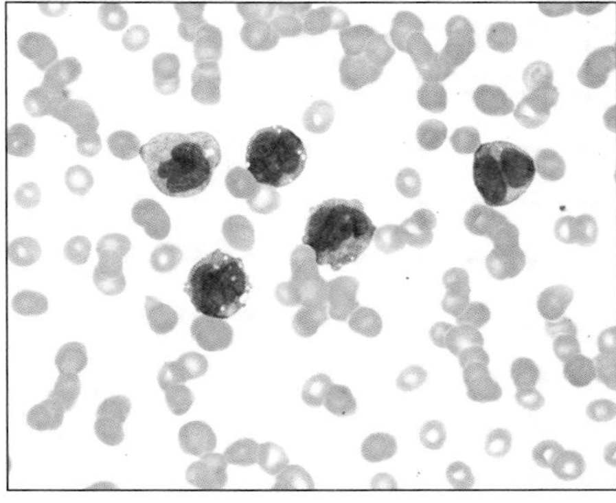

i10.33 The blasts in AML, monocytic, in which the cells have matured to the point of achieving nuclear folding

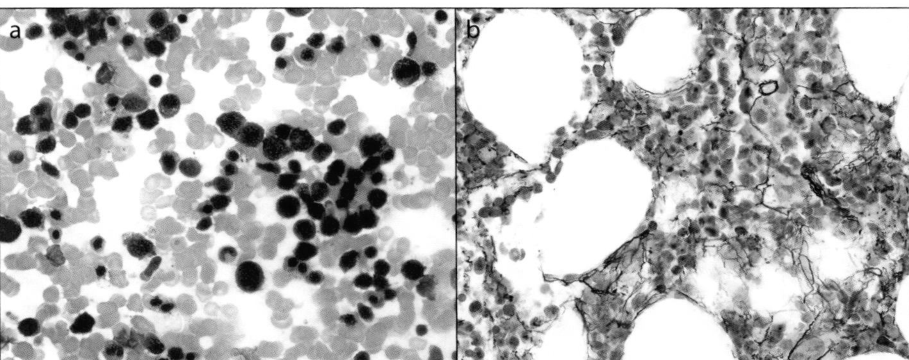

4 **a** Pure erythroid
kemia in which the vast
jority of the nucleated
s are of erythroid
eage and are neoplastic

b The same case as in i10.34a illustrating the myelofibrosis that is characteristic of erythroid leukemia

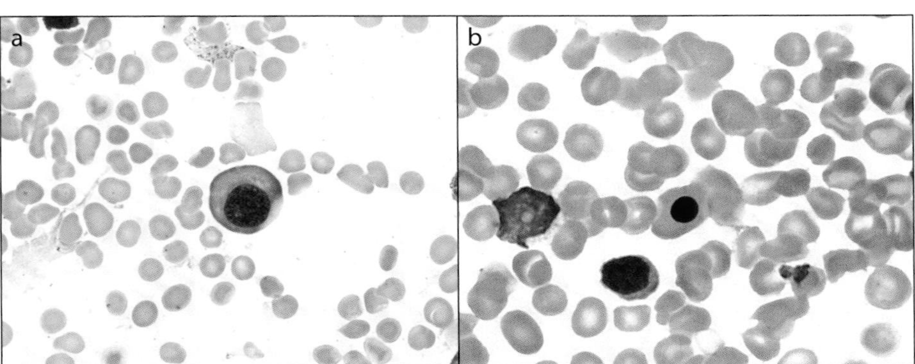

5 **a** A normoblast
a case of severe
galoblastic anemia.
hough the cytoplasm
vell hemoglobinized,
nucleus remains large
d immature rather
n pyknotic. There is a
marcation of chromatin
d parachromatin, which
ould not be apparent
h hemoglobinized
oplasm.

b For comparison a normal normoblast indicating a pyknotic nucleus, without discernible chromatin/parachromatin, in a normoblast whose cytoplasm is hemoglobinized

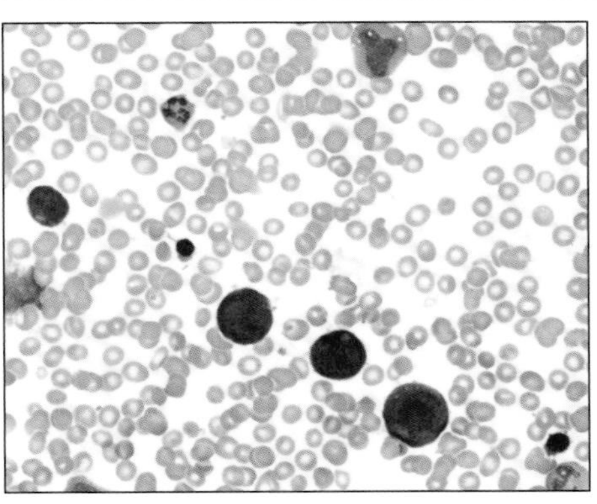

36 Early normoblasts
a case of megaloblastic
kemia

i10.37 A case of severe megaloblastic anemia with numerous early normoblasts and very little maturation because of ineffective erythropoiesis, simulating AML

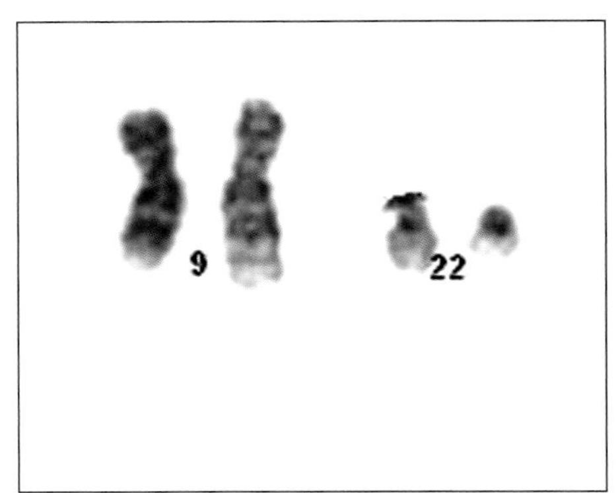

38 38 Partial karyogram
a patient with CML
owing the 2 relevant
romosomes. Note
e slightly lengthened
romosome 9 (right
nd member of the
ir) and the shortened
romosome 22 (right
nd member of the pair)

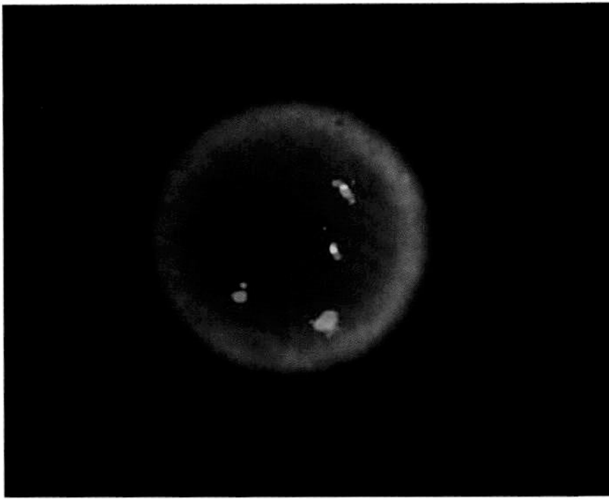

i10.39 CML. Dual-fusion FISH study confirming the t(9;22) in the case shown in i10.38. In the normal case, the red and green signals remain separate, but in a translocation, they are fused, as is seen in the 2 upper signals.

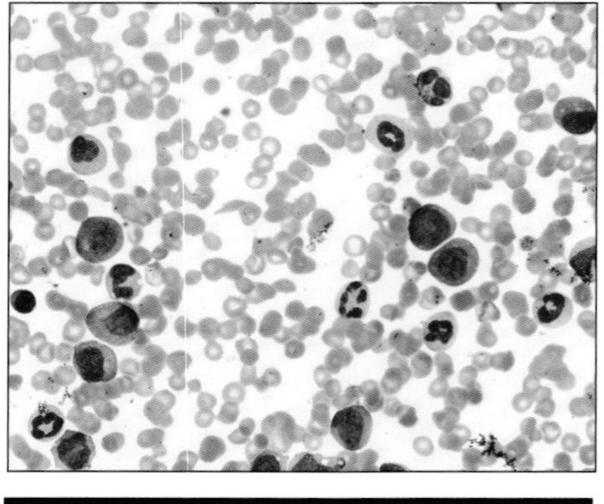

i10.40 The blood in a patient with CML illustrating numerous immature myeloid forms

i10.41 RT-PCR results for patients under investigation for possible CML. There will always be some ABL transcript in negative or positive cases, and amplification of ABL RNA is an internal control. **a** negative result on 2 different patients.

b positive result

c weak positive result, taking many cycles to be evident, but can still indicate CML in appropriate clinical context.

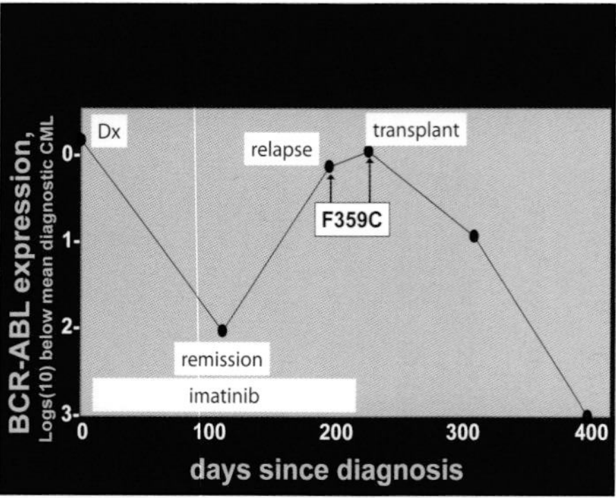

i10.42 Quantitation of BCR/ABL transcripts can monitor the effectiveness of therapy. This patient attained remission with Gleevec, but subsequently relapsed and was found to have an unusual mutation (F359C) in the tyrosine kinase that is the target of Gleevec. He then underwent a bone marrow transplant and did well.

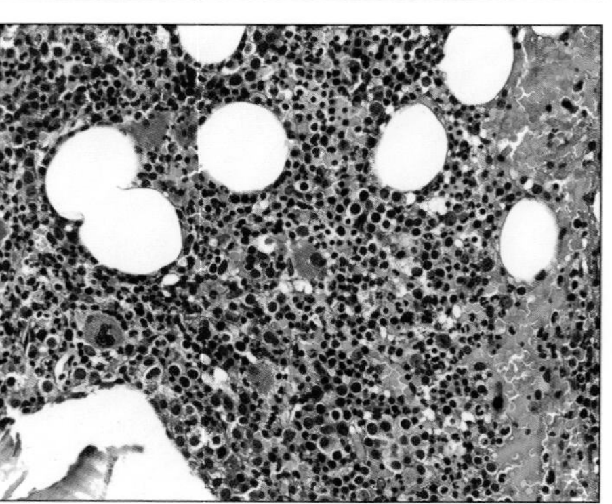

i10.43 The early stage of chronic idiopathic myelofibrosis (CIMF) illustrating hypercellularity and numerous megakaryocytes

i10.44 The intermediate stage of CIMF in which a reticulin stain demonstrates copious reticulin fibrosis

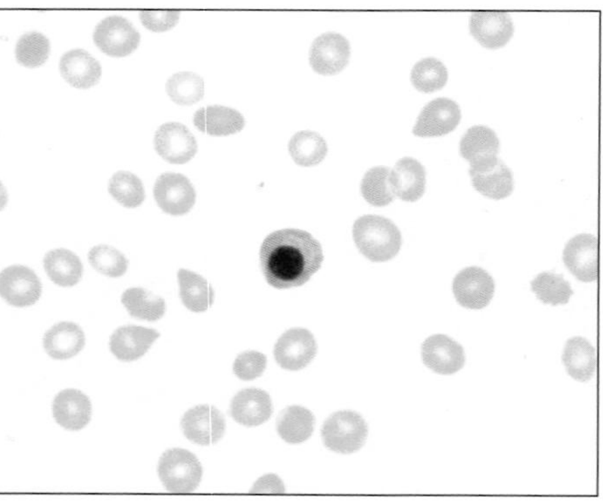

i10.45 The blood in a patient with well developed CIMF illustrating a nucleated erythrocyte next to 2 teardrop cells on the left

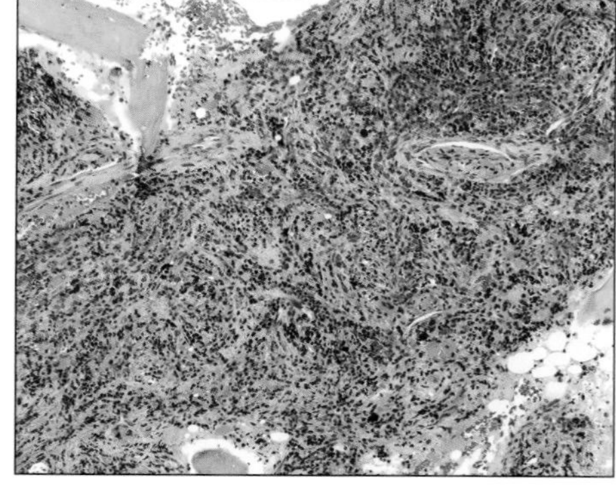

i10.46 A late stage of CIMF illustrating severe fibrosis of the bone marrow readily apparent on H&E

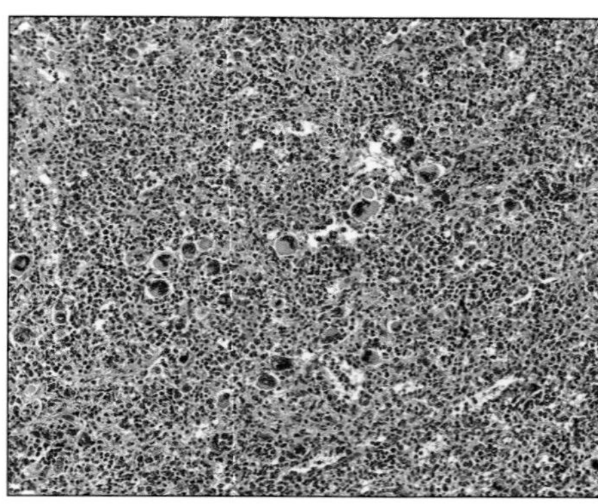

i10.47 Late stage CIMF with extensive extramedullary hematopoiesis in the spleen, readily apparent by the numerous megakaryocytes

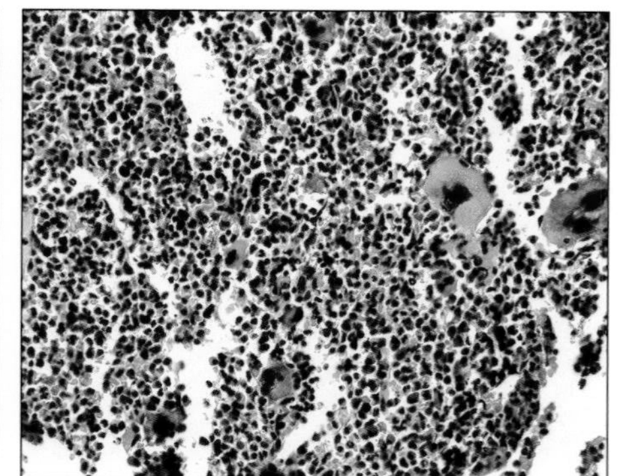

i10.48 The proliferative or early stage of polycythemia vera, illustrating hypercellularity and numerous megakaryocytes

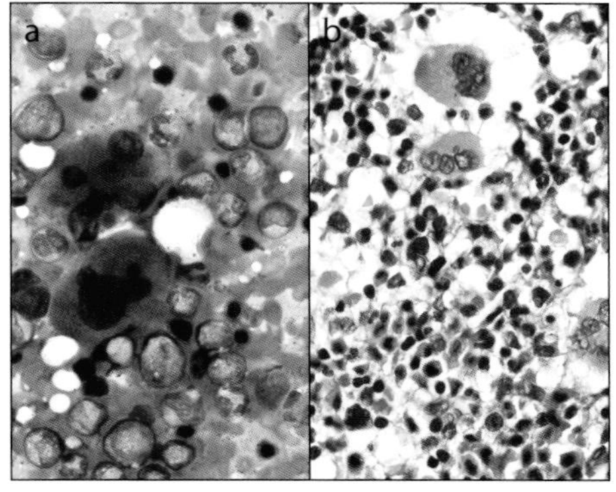

9 **a** A bone marrow
ear of essential throm-
ythemia illustrating
merous megakaryocytes
h abnormal nuclear
ation **b** A bone mar-
v section of essential
ombocythemia, again
strating increased and
normal megakaryocytes.
te the great similarity
early polycythemia vera
48. These 2 entities can
nearly indistinguish-
e morphologically.

i10.50 Chronic myelomonocytic leukemia. This blood smear demonstrates a mixture of mature neutrophils and slightly abnormal, early monocytes.

1 A lymphoblast.
mpared to
eloblasts i10.13a, i10.13b,
nphoblasts tend to be
newhat smaller, with
s conspicuous nucleoli,
there is appreciable
rphologic overlap.

i10.52 ALL hyperdiploid karyo

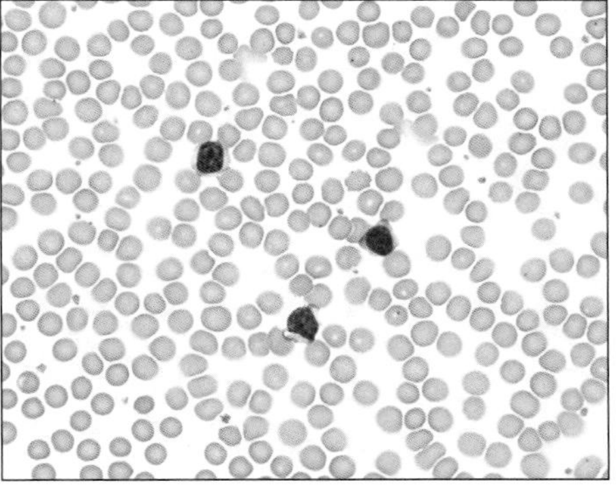

3 Chronic lymphoid
kemia. This blood
ear demonstrates
mphocytes that
nnot be discerned
neoplastic without
munohistochemical
aracterization.

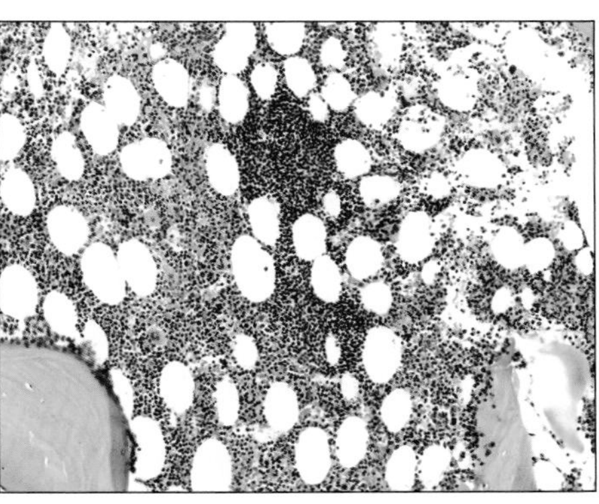

i10.54 Small lymphocytic lymphoma (involvement by CLL) of bone marrow with a nodular pattern

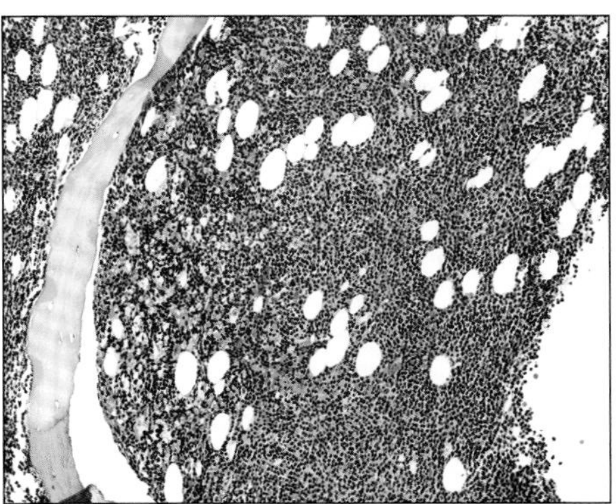

55 Diffuse involvement
the bone marrow
small lymphocytic
nphoma

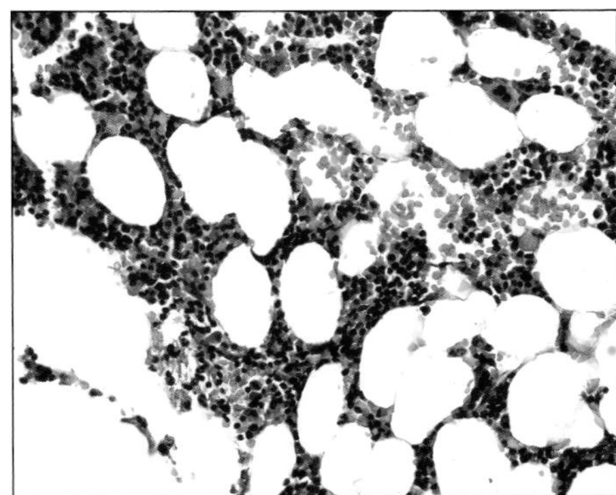

i10.56 Interstitial involvement of the bone marrow by small lymphocytic lymphoma. The neoplastic lymphocytes are insinuated without disruption of the architecture.

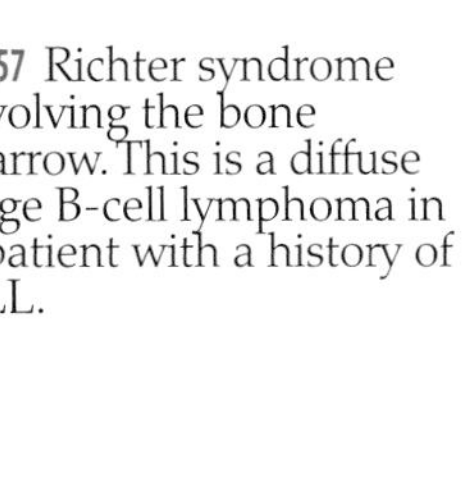

57 Richter syndrome
volving the bone
arrow. This is a diffuse
ge B-cell lymphoma in
patient with a history of
L.

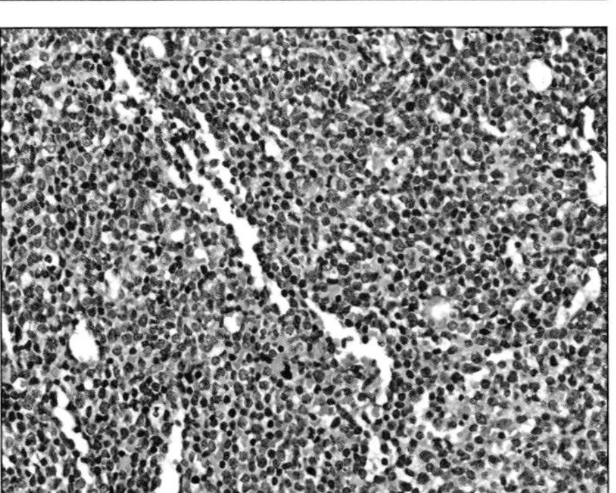

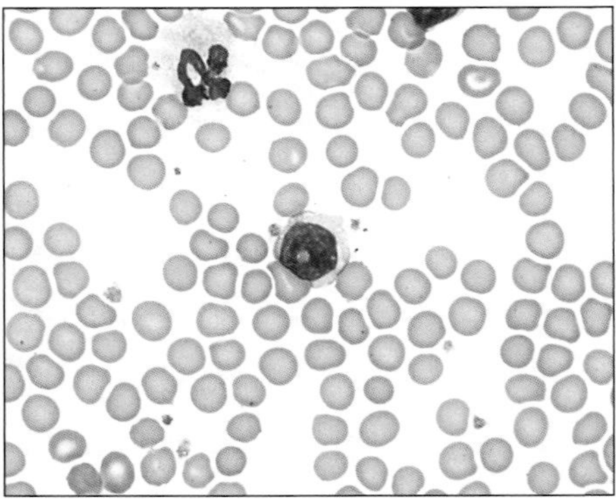

i10.58 A prolymphocyte, which is larger than a typical CLL cell and which has a prominent nucleolus

ISBN 978-089189-5886

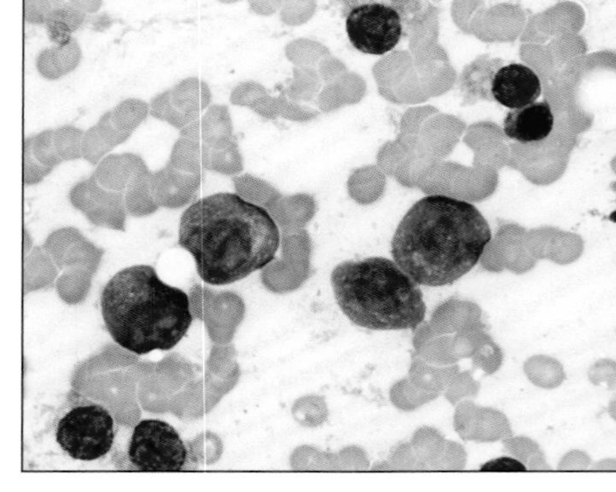

i10.59 The immature type of multiple myeloma. These plasma cells have nucleoli and fine chromatin, in contrast to mature plasma cells. Although very faint perinuclear hofs (Golgi zones) can be discerned, these are very indistinct relative to mature plasma cells.

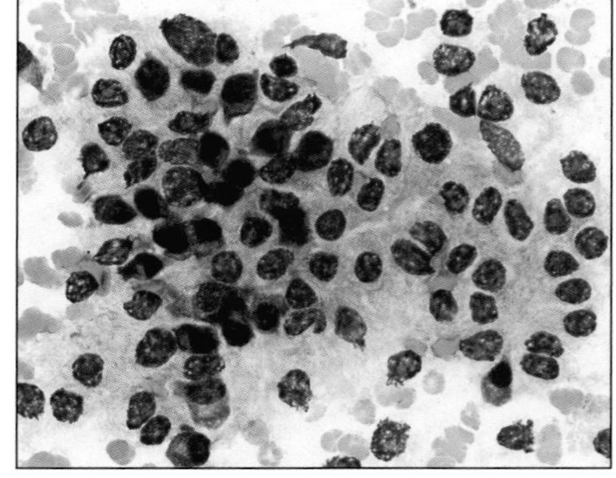

i10.60 The plasmacytic type of myeloma consisting of clusters of relatively mature-appearing plasma cells. Clinical correlation and evidence of organ damage are required for any diagnosis of myeloma, but is particularly required in a plasmacytic type, so as to differentiate between a simple plasmacytoma and myeloma.

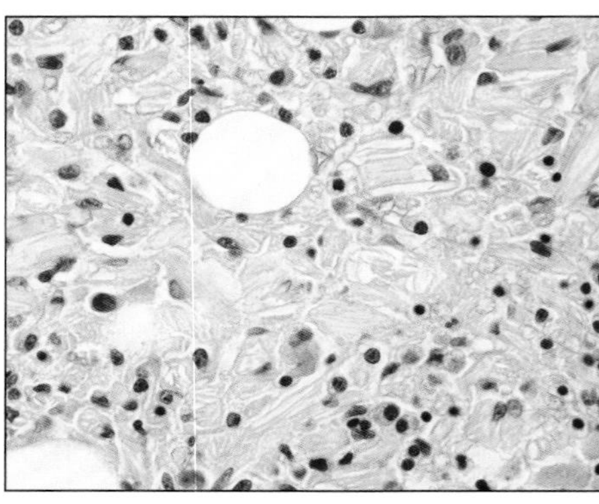

i10.61 Light chain disease with precipitation of light chains in the bone marrow, forming crystals. The crystals are faintly stained, needle-shaped, and best seen in the upper right portion of the photograph.

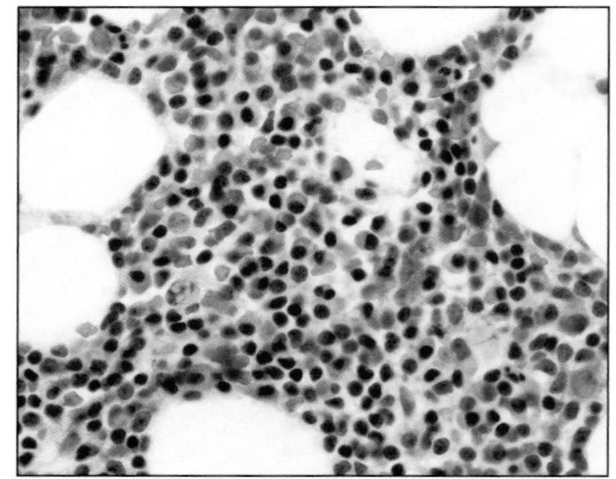

i10.62 The bone marrow in Waldenström macroglobulinemia. Like most Waldenström patients, this patient had a lymphoplasmacytic lymphoma.

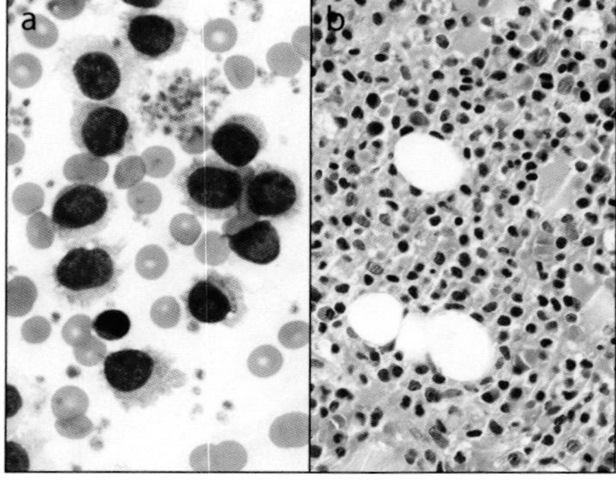

i10.63 **a** Hairy cell leukemia. These cells were obtained from a buffy coat of peripheral blood. Note the very subtle cytoplasmic projections with chromatin that is significantly less clumped than a mature lymphocyte. **b** The bone marrow in hairy cell leukemia. The marrow is filled with lymphoid forms that are slightly larger and have less clumped chromatin than mature lymphocytes.

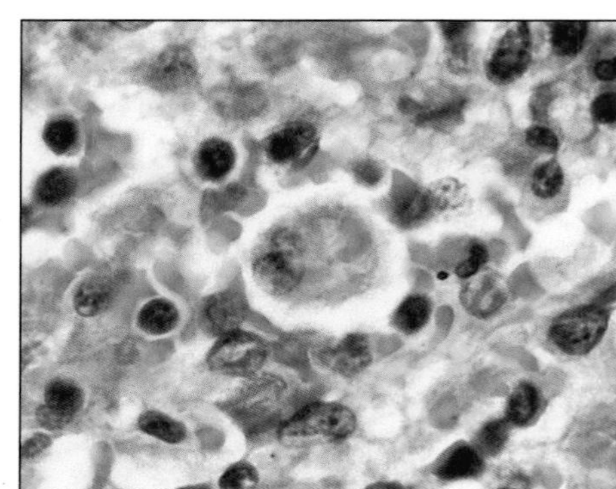

i10.64 A hemophagocytic syndrome with phagocytosis of erythrocytes by a macrophage

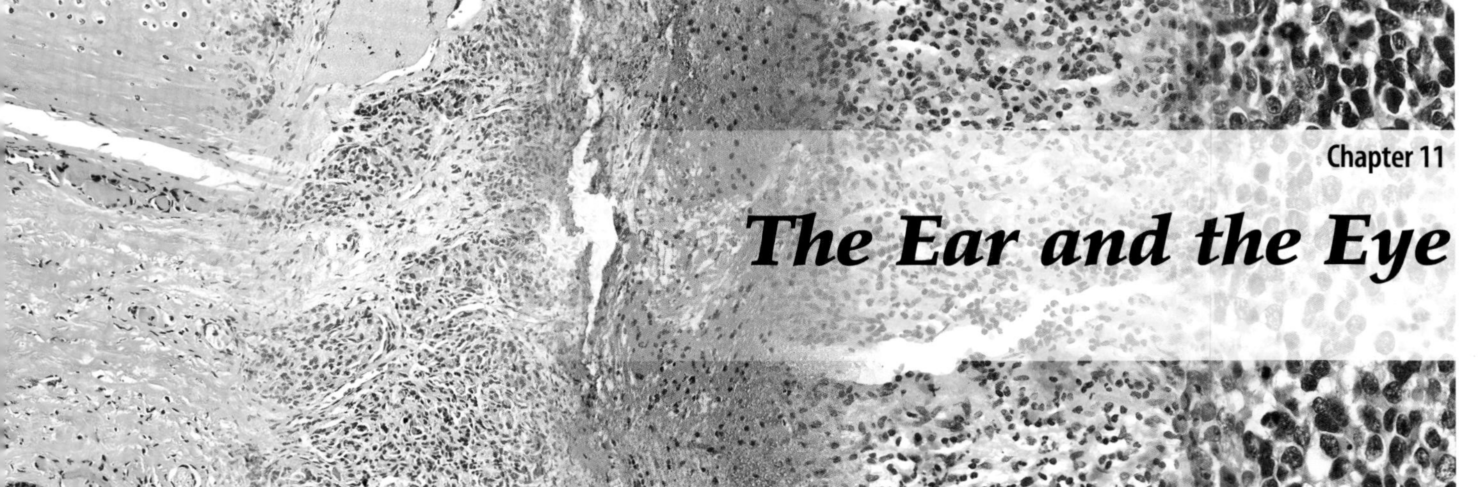

Chapter 11

The Ear and the Eye

ne Ear

ıe External Ear

The 2 common congenital anomalies of the external ear are :essory tragus and masses or cysts derived from branchial ·ft abnormalities. The accessory tragus is simply a well devel- ·ed preauricular skin tag with adnexal structures (which are t usually seen in a simple skin tag).

The external ear is the site of 3 nonneoplastic conditions: ondrodermatitis nodularis helicis, relapsing polychondri- . and idiopathic cystic chondromalacia. Chondrodermatitis dularis helicis (Winkler disease) is by far the most com- ɔn of these and is characterized in its most severe form by :eration, with inflammation and granulation tissue that may tend deeply into the dermis, but the cartilage is spared or only ınimally involved. In less severe chondrodermatitis, there is rmal inflammation and prominent capillaries i11.1, often with generation of collagen i11.2. Chondrodermatitis may be of hemic origin.

Relapsing polychondritis is a rare autoimmune disorder aracterized by recurring inflammation of cartilaginous struc- res, such as the ear, the joints, the respiratory tract, and the ·ynx. Involvement of the latter 2 sites can be life threaten- g. Other tissues, such as the eye and the myocardium, may secondarily damaged, but cartilage is the target and the ɔst usual clinical presentation is the external ear [PMID21246361]. ıondromalacia is an idiopathic cystic degeneration of cartilage ith little inflammation.

ıe Ear Canal

Other than the common squamous and basal cell carcino- as, frequently encountered conditions of the ear canal include ·crotizing external otitis, keratosis obturans, and the exter- l ear adenoma. Necrotizing external otitis is an ulcer of the ternal canal, sometimes with underlying osteomyelitis, often used by *Pseudomonas aeruginosa* and often occurring in older abetic or immunocompromised patients.

Keratosis obturans is a hyperkeratotic condition in which the ·ratin produced by cells in the canal is retained and eventually rms a solid plug. The external ear adenoma is usually a ceru- inoma that has decapitation secretion, reflecting the apocrine ture of the ceruminous glands. There is a rare malignant unterpart, the ceruminous gland adenocarcinoma.

The Middle Ear

A cholesteotoma is the presence of squamous epithelium, often with hyperkeratosis and sometimes with cholesterol clefts, in the middle ear. Most cholesteotomas are acquired and appear to arise from the entry of epithelium into the middle ear through a perforation in the tympanic membrane, usually secondary to otitis media. A minority are congenital and apparently result from embryologic rests in the middle ear. Either type can be locally destructive. Epithelium is required for the definitive diagnosis (in fact, cholesteotomas are perhaps more properly referred to as keratomas), though a diagnosis of consistent with cholesteotoma can be made if only keratin or cholesterol clefts are found i11.3. Chronic otitis media may also cause tympanosclerosis and dystrophic calcification of the tympanic membrane or the middle ear that can result in conductive hearing loss.

Otosclerosis is another cause of hearing loss that is of unclear etiology, but is not linked to chronic otitis media and is distinct from tympanosclerosis. Otosclerosis is abnormal bone remodeling, usually involving either the footplate of the stapes or the otic capsule (the bone that surrounds the cochlea) [PMID20513039]. While otosclerosis of the otic capsule causes a sensory hearing loss that is not amenable to surgical correction, if the process occurs in the stapes, the result is a conductive hearing loss that can be largely corrected by surgery. In these cases, the histologic appearance of otosclerosis, if fully studied, is the presence of new bone, mostly woven, with extensive vascularity, reminiscent of Paget disease of bone. The eventual result of this process is sclerotic bone that prevents the stapes from moving. The surgeons usually remove only a portion of the stapes i11.4 so pathologists do not see the complete pathologic process.

Neoplasms of the middle ear are rare. The most common of these is the paraganglioma i11.5. Middle ear adenomas are controversial and may be low-grade neuroendocrine neoplasms. These are not to be confused with the so-called Heffner tumor (also called endolymphatic sac papillary tumor, low-grade adenocarcinoma of endolymphatic sac origin, middle ear papillary tumor, or papillary tumor of temporal bone), described in 1989 [PMID2804921]. The Heffner tumor arises from the endolymphatic duct or endolymphatic sac, a structure of unknown function in the posterior petrous temporal bone. Heffner tumors have extensive papillarity and may resemble papillary carcinoma of the thyroid i11.6, i11.7. These may be associated with von Hippel-Lindau syndrome and may be locally destructive, requiring extensive surgery for cure. Heffner tumors are occasionally grouped with middle ear adenomas, but their more aggressive clinical course, distinctive morphology, and frequent association with von Hippel-Lindau syndrome suggests that they are distinct entities [PMID8352492].

Glial tissue i11.8, i11.9 and meningiomas may infrequently be found in the middle ear, usually as an extension from the brain, though rarely arising either from ectopic arachnoid cells.

The Inner Ear

The primary tumor of the inner ear region is a schwannoma arising from the 8th cranial nerve in the internal auditory canal i11.10. These are often inappropriately called acoustic neuromas, but are in fact benign peripheral nerve sheath neoplasms whose morphology is discussed in Chapter 2 (neuromas are nonneoplastic, disorganized collections of axons). Very rarely, a Heffner tumor of the middle ear may extend into the inner ear.

The Eye

Lesions of the Conjunctiva, Cornea, and Eyelids

Both benign squamous papillomas and squamous cell carcinomas occur on the conjunctiva, but these are very rare in comparison to benign conjunctival lesions. A pingueculum arises from solar elastosis of the conjunctiva. It is essentially an actinic keratosis of the conjunctiva. These are often not removed, but if examined, may contain mild epithelial atypia and a foreign body reaction to damaged collagen (so-called actinic granuloma). If the epithelial atypia is more than mild, an in situ or invasive squamous cell carcinoma should be excluded. A pterygium is essentially the same as a pingueculum except that it has grown over a portion of the cornea i11.11, i11.12.

The meibomian glands are sebaceous glands that directly convey their contents to the conjunctival surface without emptying into a hair follicle [PMID19856010]. A chalazion results from an obstruction of the meibomian ducts and consists of mixed inflammation that is often granulomatous i11.13 and may be suppurative if there has been a superimposed infection.

A hordeolum is a primary acute suppurative inflammation of the meibomian glands or of glands that drain into the follicles of the eyelid, often from staphylococcus. An internal hordeolum affects the meibomian glands and differs from a chalazion in having a significant neutrophilic component, reflecting a bacterial infection, as opposed to simple obstruction. An external hordeolum (stye) involves glands that drain into hair follicles, either the glands of Moll (apocrine glands which drain into hair follicles) or the glands of Zeis (sebaceous glands which empty into hair follicles).

Dermoid cysts of the skin occur predominantly on the eyelids. They differ from ordinary inclusion cysts in that adnexal structures are in the wall and are considered an integral part of the lesion.

A lacrimal caruncle is a small mass in the nasal portion of the interpalprebral fissure, at the entrance of the lacrimal duct. It is a nonneoplastic prominence of normal structures, such as sebaceous glands.

In the normal eye, the lens and the cornea both refract light to focus it sharply onto the retina. The lens, because of its proteins (called crystallins) and it ability to change shape, completes a fine focus after the cornea performs the first refraction. A cataract is a loss of the crystalline structure of the lens by a change in shape of the crystallin proteins or a disruption of the relationship of these proteins to each other, such that light can no longer be focused or even transmitted. While techniques in protein chemistry have provided considerable understanding of cataracts, the histologic changes in a cataract are subtle in ordinary light microscopy, with perhaps only stromal breakup, edema, and deposition of eosinophilic globules. Since there is almost never a clinical doubt as to the correct diagnosis, there is rarely a need for the pathologist to examine lenses removed as cataracts.

In contrast, the changes in corneal pathology are readily identifiable by the pathologist and examination of corneas removed by ophthalmic surgery can confirm or emend a clinical diagnosis. The normal cornea is lined on its anterior surface by an epithelium that sits on a basement membrane, beneath which is Bowman membrane, a collection of fine collagen fibers that merge with the corneal stroma i11.14. In sections, the stroma has clefts that are artifacts of fixation and processing i11.14. The most posterior portion of the cornea is a single layer of thin cells called the endothelium, sitting on a basement membrane called Descemet membrane i11.15. The term "endothelium" is a misnomer since it does not line a vascular channel. Rather, this layer of cells, forming the anterior boundary of the anterior aqueous chamber, is more epithelial in nature and is thought to pump excess water from the corneal stroma. Unlike the surface epithelium, the corneal "endothelium" does not regenerate well.

There are 3 common corneal conditions that will be briefly considered. Fuch corneal dystrophy is an idiopathic condition that results in injury to the "endothelium." This "endothelial" damage leads to corneal edema, with thickening of Descemet membrane i11.16. This thickening is often accompanied by the formation of nodules, called guttae, in Descemet membrane.

Bullous keratopathy refers to corneal edema secondary to "endothelial" damage from any etiology, but most often from cataract extraction and intraocular lens implantation. The damaged "endothelium" can no longer pump excess water from the cornea, resulting in edema and loss of transparency. The name is derived from the presence of bullae under the epithelium on the anterior surface i11.17. Bullae are not to be confused with guttae, which are excrescences of Descemet membrane, on the posterior surface of the cornea in Fuch dystrophy. Keratoconus is a thinning of the central cornea i11.18, often with deformation in its shape, preventing normal refraction. Keratoconus is often accompanied by stromal fibrosis i11.19 and disruption of Bowman layer, but unlike Fuch dystrophy and bullous keratopathy, the primary problem is not a general loss of transparency.

Neoplasms of the Eye

There are 3 terms referring to ophthalmic surgical procedures that the pathologist should be familiar with, though most lesions can be removed without resorting to any of these procedures. Evisceration is the removal of the contents the eye, while leaving the sclera and the extraocular ıscles. Enucleation removes the entire eye, including the era and extraocular muscles, but preserves the orbit itself. enteration, the most radical of the 3 procedures, removes e entire eye, along with the muscles, adnexa, and part of the ny orbit.

Lymphomas of the conjunctiva and orbit are diagnosed described in Chapter 8. Most of these are low-grade and e commonly considered to be of the so-called MALT type. any cases will be marginal zone lymphomas, but as is the se in all sites, they must be individually immunopheno-ped. As is the case for the stomach and bowel, some orbital v-grade lymphomas will respond to antibiotic therapy and erefore may not be true neoplasms [PMID17018784].

Melanocytic lesions of the conjunctiva include ephelis, nevi, ıtigo, and melanoma, all of which can be diagnosed as else-ıere. Primary acquired melanosis histologically resembles ıtigo maligna, a dysplastic nevus, or melanoma in situ, and essentially the ophthalmic term to encompass these prein-sive lesions, with diagnostic criteria fundamentally as in her sites [PMID3972395]. Complete removal of primary acquired elanosis prevents progression, but if this is not achieved, edictors of transformation into invasive melanoma are the ze of the lesion and the presence of nuclear atypia. In addi-on, epithelioid cells appear to indicate a greater propensity evolve into invasive melanomas [PMID18427595].

The melanocytoma is a benign, heavily pigmented mela-ocytic tumor of the optic disk, uveal tract (iris, ciliary body, d choroid), or the meninges [PMID17621182]. Although they are avily pigmented and may consist of large cells, they differ om melanomas in having small and uniform nuclei with ıall nucleoli [PMID16500211].

Uveal melanomas have traditionally been classified as indle A (smaller cells, better differentiated), spindle B ırger cells, less differentiated), and epithelioid [Schwent ISBN978-9398162], but these types often occur together i11.20, and as is e case for melanomas of the skin, prognostic factors other an depth of invasion, if any, have not been conclusively tablished [PMID15327098].

Retinoblastomas with some differentiation have Flexner-'intersteiner rosettes, which have a well defined central men lined by basement membrane i11.21a, i11.21b, in contrast the Homer Wright rosettes of neuroblastoma, which have ss defined lumens and little or no basement membrane aterial [PMID5357720]. Some use the term "florette" (also spelled leurette") for Flexner-Wintersteiner rosettes to underscore ıis difference. A Flexner-Wintersteiner rosette may have inimal photoreceptor differentiation. Undifferentiated reti-oblastomas either form solid clusters i11.22 or may form osettes of the Homer Wright type (ie, without a central base-ent membrane) instead of the Flexner-Wintersteiner type.

Treatment of retinoblastoma has historically been by enucleation, though attempts are being made to substitute chemotherapy and radiation therapy for this surgery. Retinoblastomas may invade the optic nerve, and in an enucleation, the nerve constitutes an important resection margin.

Other Pathologic Processes of the Eye

Age-related macular degeneration is a condition of unknown etiology that occurs in both a "wet" form (ie, with excessive vascularization) and a "dry" form. The disorder is linked to the presence of drusen, deposits of extracellular material in the choroid (the vascular layer between the retina and the sclera). The nature of drusen has not been clarified, but it is known to consist of protein and lipids.

Phthisis bulbi ("phthisis" is Latin for "declining" or "wasting away") is the endpoint of many processes, including trauma and severe inflammation of any etiology. The result is an atrophic disorganized eye, with fibrosis, often with calcification or even ossification i11.23, and without fluid production.

Core Points for the Ear and the Eye

- Actinic keratosis and chondrodermatitis nodularis helicis: most common benign processes of the external ear.
- Common middle ear processes: otitis media, cholesteotomas, and otosclerosis.
- Primary process in the inner ear is a benign peripheral nerve sheath tumor arising from the 8th cranial nerve.
- Pingueculum: actinic keratosis of the conjunctiva.
    - Pterygium is a similar process involving the cornea.
- Hordeolum: an acute suppurative inflammation of the glands of the eyelid.
- Cataract: loss of crystalline structure in lens from disruption of crystallin proteins.
- Most common corneal processes: Fuch corneal dystrophy, bullous keratopathy, and keratoconus.
- Retinoblastoma: most common malignant neoplasm of the eye in young children.
- In adults, most common eye neoplasms are lymphomas, often of the so-called MALT variety, and melanocytic processes.
- Age-related macular degeneration: "wet" form, with excessive vascularization, and a "dry" form.

ISBN 978-089189-5886

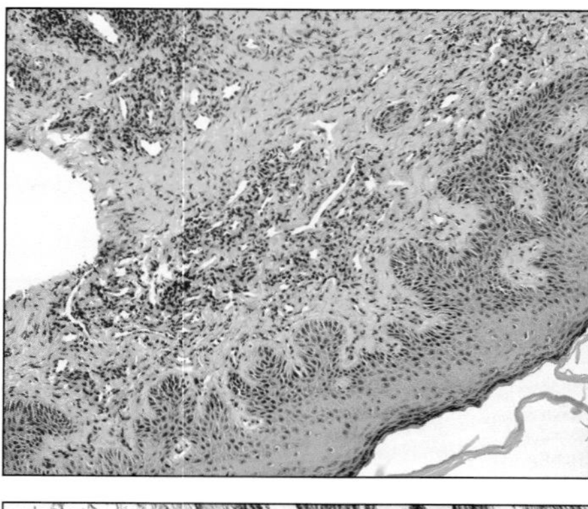

i11.1 Chondrodermatitis with dermal chronic inflammation and prominent capillaries

i11.2 Chondrodermatitis with degeneration of dermal collagen and sparing of the cartilage

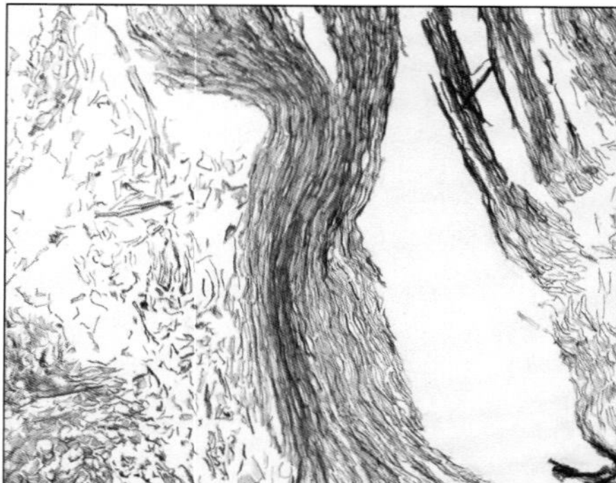

i11.3 Fragments of keratin, often the only specimen in a cholesteotoma

i11.4 The stapes, removed in a case of otosclerosis

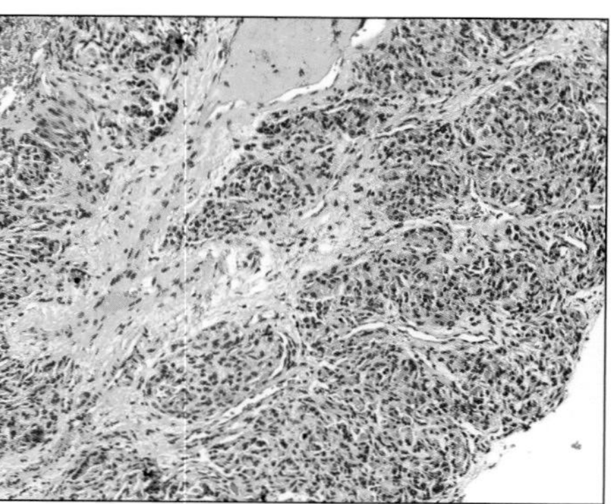

i11.5 Paraganglioma of the middle ear, with zellballen pattern

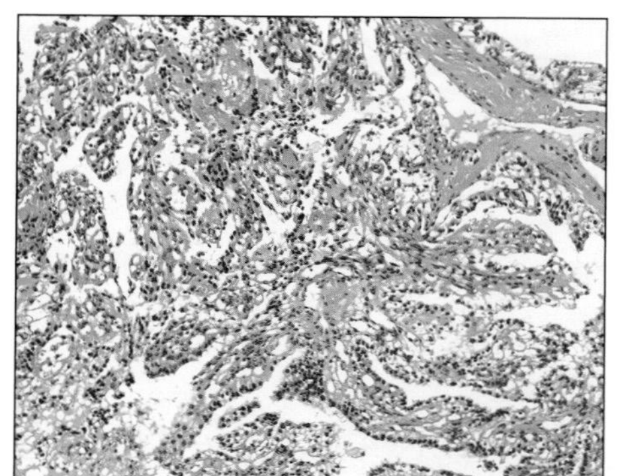

i11.6 Low-power view of a Heffner tumor of the middle ear, illustrating the papillary architecture and resemblance to papillary carcinoma of the thyroid

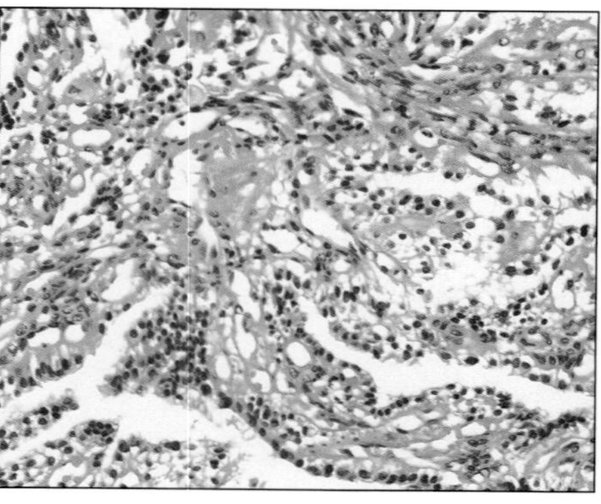

i11.7 High-power view of a Heffner tumor illustrating the nuclear uniformity

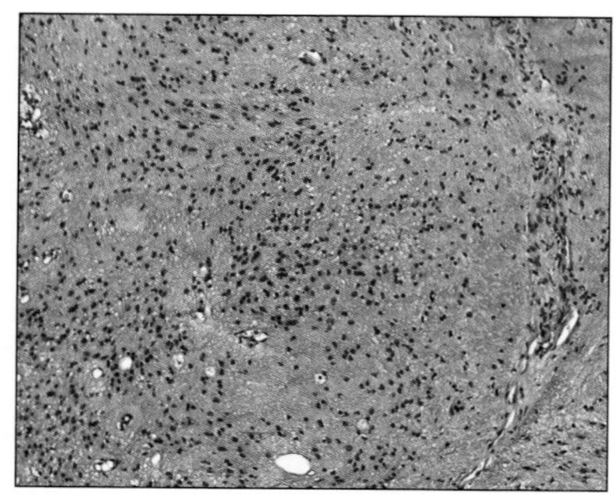

i11.8 Ectopic glial in the middle ear

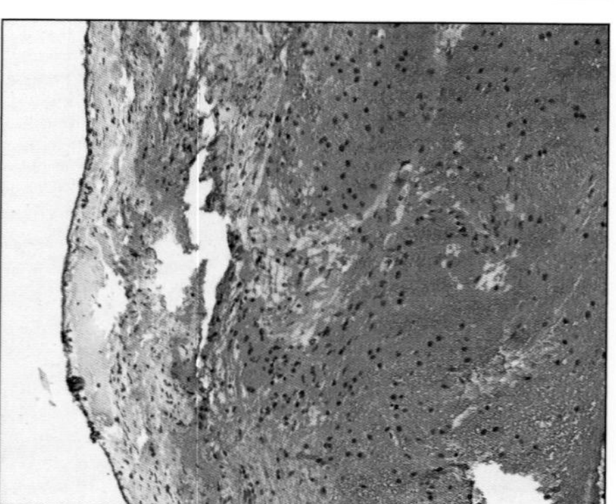

i11.9 Glial fibrillary acidic protein immunohistochemical stain on the same case as i11.8, confirming the diagnosis

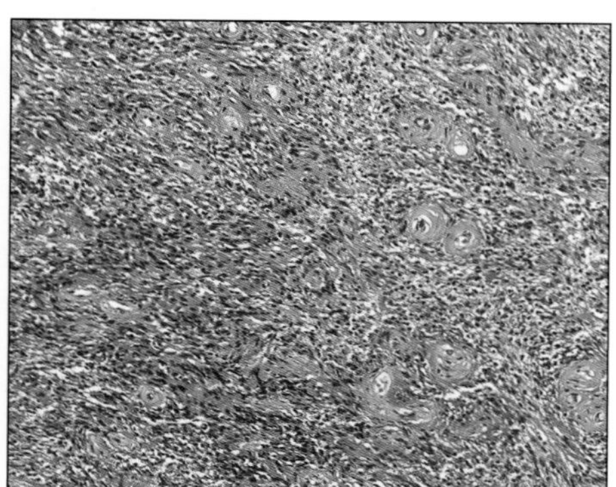

i11.10 Schwannoma in the inner ear, arising from the 8th cranial nerve ("acoustic neuroma")

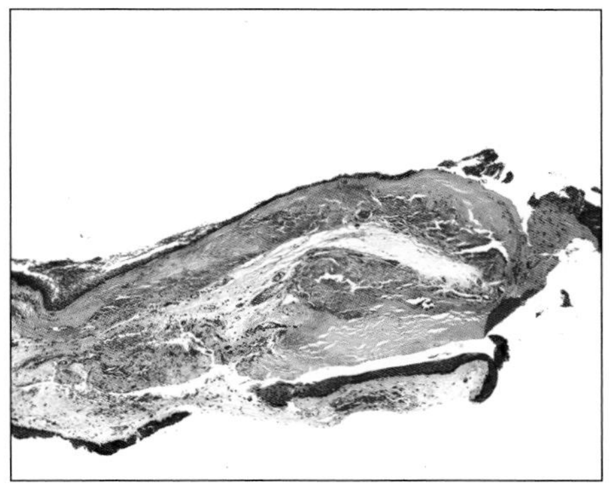

1 A low-power view of
terygium

i11.12 Higher-power view of the same case as i11.11, illustrating damaged collagen

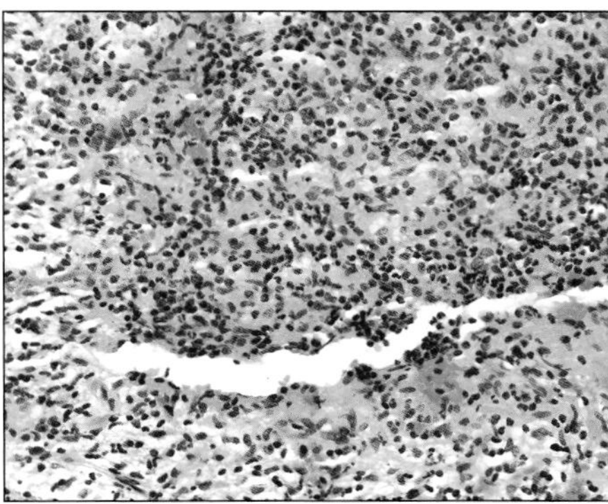

3 A chalazion,
h granulomatous
lammation, as indicated
the epithelioid
tiocytes

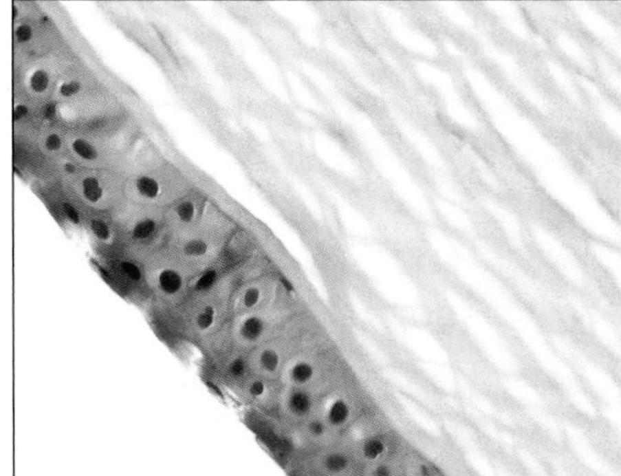

i11.14 The anterior surface of the cornea. The basement membrane is immediately beneath the epithelium and is very thin and difficult to see. Bowman membrane is readily noted and appears as a thickened basement membrane. It merges with the corneal stroma, which has artifactual clefts.

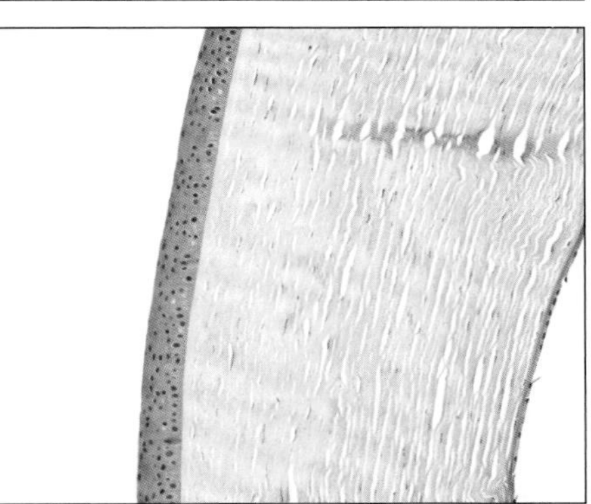

15 A full-thickness view
the cornea, with the
terior surface on the left
d the posterior surface
the right. Note the
gle layer of flattened
ing of Descemet
mbrane on the right
d its resemblance to
dothelium.

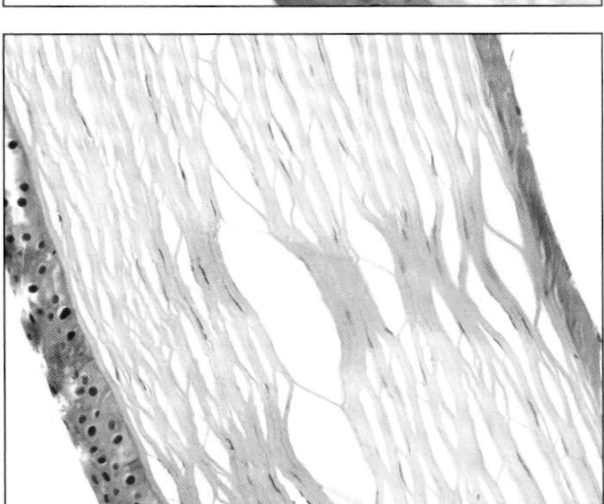

i11.16 Fuch dystrophy with marked thickening of Descemet membrane

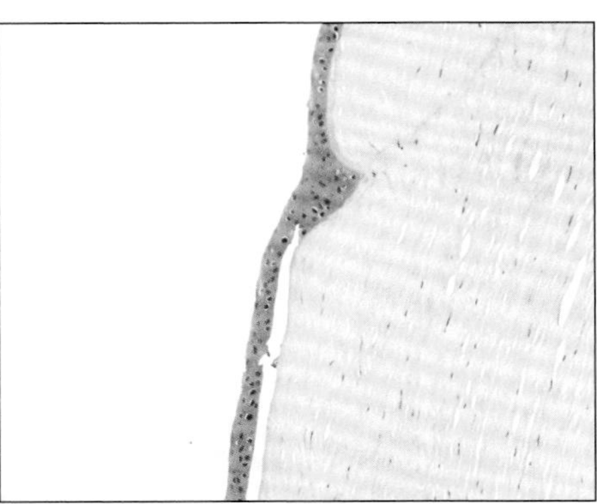

17 Bullous keratopathy,
th separation of the
ithelium on the anterior
rface from the stroma

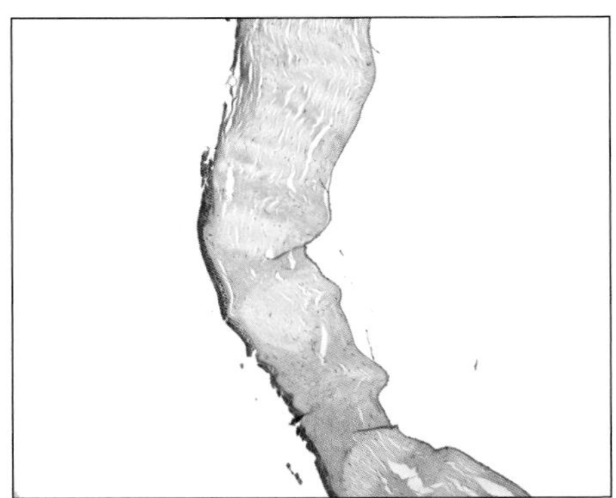

i11.18 Keratoconus, with thinning of the central portion of the cornea relative to the periphery (seen at the top and bottom)

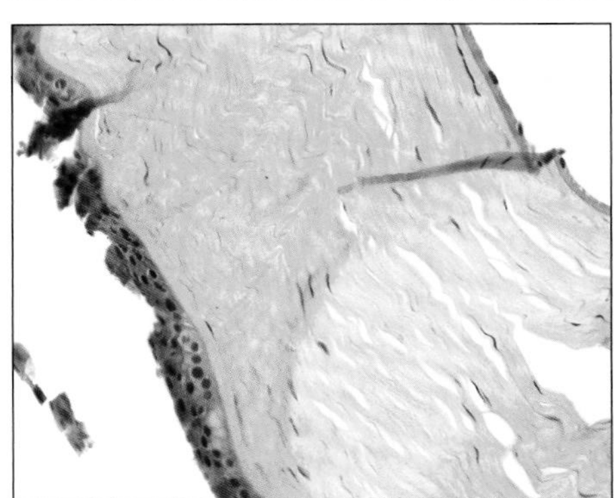

19 Higher-power view
keratoconus illustrating
e fibrosis of the corneal
oma in the upper
rtion of the photograph
ative to the normal
oma in the lower
rtion

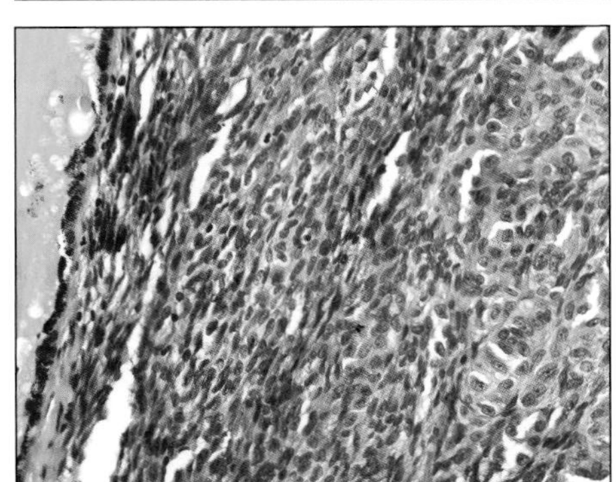

i11.20 Uveal melanoma, with smaller spindle cells (spindle A) in the upper portion and larger spindled cells (spindle B) in the lower portion

ISBN 978-089189-5886

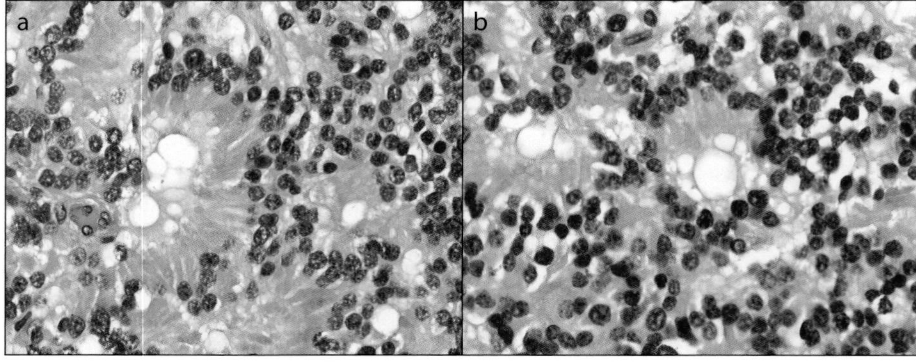

i11.21 **a** Retinoblastoma, with Flexner-Wintersteiner rosettes. Note that the central lumens of these rosettes are sharply defined relative to the Homer Wright rosettes of neuroblastoma i6.50.

b A higher-power view of Flexner-Wintersteiner rosettes. Note the thin, slightly amphophilic basement membrane in several rosettes, most notably in the central rosette.

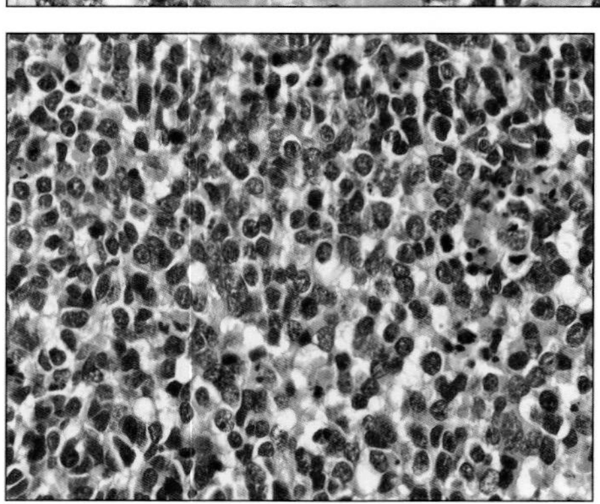

i11.22 Undifferentiated retinoblastoma without Flexner-Wintersteiner rosettes. Note the great resemblance to an undifferentiated neuroblastoma i6.49.

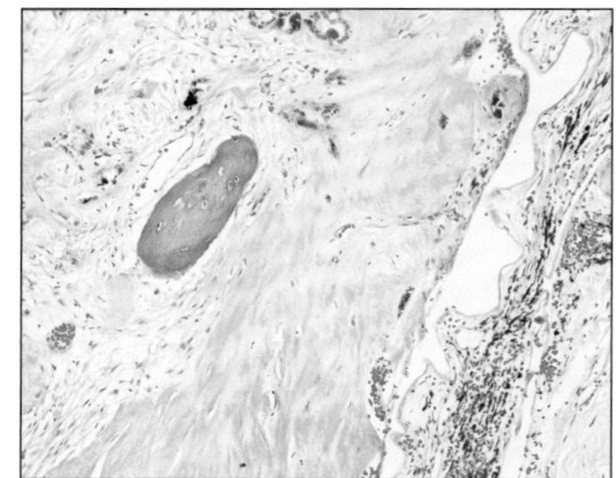

i11.23 Phthisis bulbi with ectopic bone formation, resulting from severe trauma

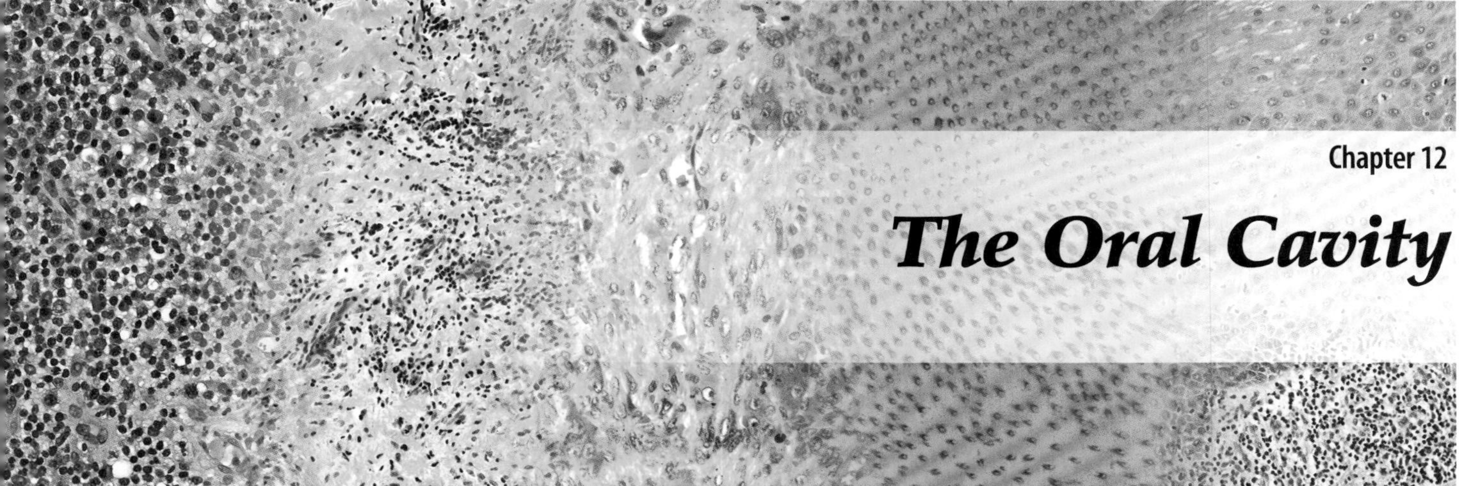

Chapter 12

The Oral Cavity

ıflammatory Lesions

Although candida is a normal oral flora, it is still the one of ɜ most common causes of infection in the oral cavity. Unlike ɑmmensal candida, pathogenic candidiasis is likely to be accom-ɴnied by neutrophils, to be largely in pseudohyphal form (as posed to yeast form) and to invade the epithelium.

Gingivitis, if severe or chronic, may ultimately cause periodon-ɪs and affect alveolar bone. Acute necrotizing gingivitis (trench ɔuth) is caused by a fusospirochetal group of bacteria.

Other common inflammatory conditions in the oral cavity :lude herpes, pemphigus, pemphigoid, and lichen planus, all of ıich are diagnosed as in the skin. As in the skin, direct immuno-orescence is occasionally required to determine the nature and :ation of immunoglobulins and complement components that ve been deposited in these conditions. Lichenoid mucositis (or ɔmatitis) is a diagnosis rendered in situations in which there is a ronic inflammatory infiltrate at the epithelial-stromal junction, t the clinical criteria for lichen planus are not fulfilled.

Geographic tongue occurs in 1-3% of people, primarily in ildren. Clinically, there is an area of erythema, with atrophy the filiform papillae. Surrounding this is a white, hyper-ratotic border. Individual lesions may spontaneously regress, ıt there is often recurrence in another site, accounting for the ernative name "benign migratory glossitis." The etiology and thogenesis are unclear. Most patients are asymptomatic, but ɪme experience sensitivity to hot or spicy foods. Geographic ngue is rarely biopsied because of its characteristic clinical pearance, but when it is, the histologic findings are similar to ɔse in cutaneous psoriasis.

dontogenic Cysts

Tooth formation is a complicated process, well covered in stan-ɪrd oral histology and embryology texts [Bhaskar ISBN978-0801602399, ɛry ISBN978-0323033398], but briefly, during embryogenesis, clusters of ithelial cells, called dental laminae, invaginate from the alveo-: mucosa and give rise to bell-shaped structures called enamel gans (or tooth buds). Filling the central portion of an enamel gan is the dental papilla, which is primarily derived from ɛsoderm, but also partly from the neural crest, an ectodermal ·ucture. Cells in the dental papilla differentiate into odontoblasts, ıich make dentin, the primary structural material of a tooth. lontoblasts also cause cells in the overlying enamel organ, called ıeloblasts, to produce enamel, the hard covering of a tooth. The amel is composed of enamel rods, which are attached to the dentin so vigorously that separation of enamel and dentin does not occur except in very severe trauma.

In a fully formed tooth, the crown is the visible portion above the gum line. The unseen portion below the gum line is the apex. The pulp chamber (colloquially called the root canal) is a narrow channel in the center of the tooth, containing the neurovascular supply. The crown is covered by enamel, but dentin devoid of an enamel covering is found below the gum line. In the apex, the dentin is covered by cementum, a bony material that connects the dentin to the periodontal ligaments. The periodontal ligaments are not macroscopically evident, but are microscopic filaments in a connective tissue matrix that is between the cementum and the bone.

There are a variety of odontogenic cysts ("odontogenic" refers to teeth or tooth formation), and these are divided into inflammatory and developmental. The most common inflammatory odontogenic cyst is the periapical (radicular) cyst, which results from severe inflammation of the pulp caused by caries (cavities) and is found in the apex of the tooth. The epithelium of periapical cyst is usually stratified squamous and sits on a chronically inflamed stroma i12.1. While there are often no specific histologic features, the epithelium may contain extracellular hyaline bodies called Rushton bodies.

As is always the case when epithelial cells migrate during development, some cells may be left behind or may not participate in the formation of the final product. In tooth formation, the result is remnants of epithelium near the tooth that can give rise to a number of developmental odontogenic cysts, the 3 most common of which are the dentigerous cyst, the lateral periodontal cyst, and the odontogenic keratocyst (OKC).

The dentigerous cyst surrounds the crown of an unerupted permanent tooth (since the tooth has not erupted, the word "crown" refers to the part that would be above the gum line had eruption occurred). Histologic findings are nonspecific, with either cuboidal or squamous epithelium, or a combination of the two. The stroma is chronically inflamed, sometimes with hemosiderin macrophages i12.2. Often, the epithelium is indistinct, leaving only an inflamed stroma i12.3, in which case the contribution of the pathologist is to enumerate pertinent negative finings, such as the absence of neoplasia, ameloblastic change, or evidence of an OKC.

The lateral periodontal cyst occurs adjacent to the lateral root surfaces, primarily in premolar and cuspid teeth. The lining is cuboidal to squamous. While the diagnosis is made by the location and clinical findings, a characteristic histologic feature is multiple minute areas of thickening of the epithelium.

The most clinically significant type of odontogenic cyst is the OKC. Although lacking metastatic potential, the OKC often recurs and can be clinically troublesome. It is important to diagnose this entity initially, in case the oral surgeon wishes to perform a wider excision to obviate the need for intervention later. The OKC is lined by bland stratified squamous epithelium but has several features not found in other odontogenic cysts. First, there is parakeratosis of an unusual type, resembling the teeth of a saw, often called corrugated parakeratosis i12.4. Second, the epithelium in an OKC often detaches from the stroma i12.5, whereas the epithelium remains attached in other types of cysts. Third, rete pegs are absent. In questionable cases, cytokeratin 10 and cytokeratin 17 tend to stain OKC, while CK19 does not i12.6. In a small series, cytokeratin 17 stained 93% of OKCs but only 35% of dentigerous or radicular cysts. Even more important, cytokeratin 19 was not found in any OKCs, making staining for CK19 essentially exclusive of the diagnosis [PMID16138895].

Fissural cysts are developmental but not odontogenic. They are found at points of junction in development, and they result from the trapping of epithelial tissue, usually in an inflammatory background. Fissural cysts are histologically nonspecific and indistinguishable from odontogenic cysts. Examples, depending on location, include nasopalatine i12.7, median palatal, median mandibular, nasolabial, and globulomaxillary.

Other Nonneoplastic Mass Lesions of the Oral Cavity

The central giant cell granuloma (also called central giant cell reparative granuloma) is an intraosseous entity of unclear nature that is usually found in the bones of the jaw. It is characterized by numerous innocuous-appearing giant cells in a cellular fibrous stroma with uniform nuclei and minimal mitoses i12.8, often with hemosiderin macrophages i12.9. Some regard the central giant cell granuloma as reparative, while others favor neoplasia. Some believe that the central giant cell granuloma is basically the same as an aneurysmal bone cyst, while others favor a relationship to the giant cell tumor of bone, and still others feel it is distinct from either of these entities [PMID18807393]. Those who favor a relationship to the giant cell tumor of bone believe that the central form of reparative granuloma may be a form of that neoplasm that does not metastasize [PMID19011995]. Although incapable of metastasis, the central giant cell granuloma may be locally aggressive and invade through bone into surrounding soft tissue [PMID16762013].

Other entities in the differential diagnosis of central giant cell granuloma include hyperparathyroidism i12.10 and, rarely, osteosarcoma. Because of its unclear etiology and histologic similarity to other entities, the central giant cell granuloma is a diagnosis of exclusion, based on clinical correlation.

"Epulis" is a clinical term referring to a swelling on the gingiva. There are 3 histologic types of epulis. The first type is the giant cell epulis, also called giant cell reparative granuloma or *peripheral* giant cell granuloma. The peripheral giant cell granuloma is histologically similar to the central giant cell granuloma i12.11, i12.12 and may erode into bone, but it is a different entity because it is based in the soft tissues adjacent to the bone [PMID18807393]. The second type is a fibrosing epulis, characterized by epithelial hyperplasia and fibrous stroma i12.13, often with metaplastic bone i12.14. This type is often associated with trauma, especially ill-fitting dentures, and is often clinically referred to as epulis fissuratum. The third type of epulis is a vascular type that can be regarded as a pyogenic granuloma i12.15.

Fibrous dysplasia is caused by a mutation in a gene in the *GNAS* gene on 20q13 that leads to an activating mutation in a G protein [PMID16085630]. The disorder is characterized by irregularly shaped bony trabeculae in a fibrous background. The bone is deposited on a collagenous matrix in a disorderly manner (woven bone), and the trabeculae are colloquially said to have a resemblance to fishhooks or Chinese characters i3.25. Fibrous dysplasia may affect one bone (monostotic) or more than 1 (polyostotic). About 3% of patients with fibrous dysplasia will have McCune-Albright syndrome, which is associated with endocrine abnormalities and skin pigmentation, and this syndrome should be suggested whenever this diagnosis is made [PMID18328981].

The ossifying fibroma is a related entity, with a similar appearance, and is regarded as synonymous with fibrous dysplasia by some observers. Even those who feel these entities are different acknowledge sufficient similarity in clinical behavior and histologic appearance that they are often grouped together as benign fibro-osseous lesion i12.16. These entities cannot be reliably separated by histology in the absence of McCune-Albright syndrome, but the *GNAS* mutation is specific for fibrous dysplasia [PMID21354047].

Periapical cemental dysplasia, cemento-ossifying fibroma, focal cemento-osseous dysplasia, and florid osseous dysplasia are related entities that are often grouped under the heading of osseous dysplasia. These entities have a similar histologic appearance not only to each other, but also to the benign fibro-osseous conditions described above, and a precise diagnosis rests largely on the clinical and radiographic findings. It is wise to include the entities of the osseous dysplasia group of benign fibro-osseous lesions [PMID18480400]. In most cases, a diagnosis of benign fibro-osseous lesion is sufficient, but if McCune-Albright syndrome is a clinical consideration, such that fibrous dysplasia needs to be differentiated from other benign fibro-osseous lesions, the demonstration of a mutation in GNAS may be beneficial and can be performed in formalin-fixed, paraffin-embedded tissue [PMID21354047].

Benign Odontogenic Neoplasms

Epithelial cells left behind in tooth development may also give rise to odontogenic neoplasms as well as to developmental odontogenic cysts. The ameloblastoma is the most common odontogenic tumor of significance. While lacking metastatic potential, it can recur and be locally destructive. As is the case for the OKC, the identification and complete removal of an ameloblastoma can prevent local recurrence and damage. Ameloblastomas are not encapsulated and may have many appearances, the most common of which is a follicular type, characterized by islands of epithelium in a fibrous stroma. These islands resemble the enamel organ, meaning that the interior consists of cells with a moderate amount of cytoplasm in a somewhat loose stroma, while the periphery is composed of cells that are more basaloid, with less cytoplasm, and often with peripheral palisading i12.17. These islands resemble a cutaneous basal cell carcinoma i12.18. Other types of ameloblastoma, with a less distinct dimorphic population of cells, include desmoplastic, plexiform, squamous i12.19, granular cell, and basaloid types. Most variations retain some degree of peripheral palisading. Cyst formation is common in ameloblastomas. Although a fibrous stroma is characteristic of an ameloblastoma, this stroma is considered to be a reaction to the neoplasm and not an integral part of it. The ameloblastoma does not have a true mesenchymal component.

Like the ameloblastoma, the adenomatoid odontogenic tumor is aracterized by bland epithelial cells in a loose spindle cell back-ound. The epithelial cells are cuboidal and usually are found in ncentric arrangements with circular lumens i12.20. These micro-sts may contain eosinophilic homogeneous material. The distin-uishing histologic features from an ameloblastoma are its orderly chitecture vs the irregularly shaped and unevenly distributed ithelial islands in an ameloblastoma, its central lumens, and the esence of a fibrous capsule around the tumor.

An odontogenic myxoma is a locally invasive tumor that looks uch like the mesenchymal component of an ameloblastic fibro-a. It is distinguished from the latter tumor by the absence of epi-elium (unless a little has been trapped) and a looser, more myx-d stroma, with small vessels i12.21. The odontogenic myxoma has oderate local aggressiveness that belies its innocent histology. ie primary differential diagnosis for the odontogenic myxoma is ntal papillae of undeveloped and unsuspected supernumerary eth. In tooth formation, the dental papilla produces odontoblasts, t if the papillae are not developed, their myxoid stroma will ve little epithelium and few odontoblasts. The clinical and radio-aphic findings are central to the distinction of an odontogenic yxoma from supernumerary teeth, though circumscription vors a supernumerary tooth, while the absence of this feature pports a diagnosis of odontogenic myxoma. Also, because an lontogenic myxoma is a locally invasive neoplasm, entrapped ne or epithelial cells may be present, a finding that is unlikely in supernumerary tooth.

The ameloblastic fibroma consists of thin, delicate (often ly 2 layers) strands of odontogenic epithelial, surrounded by basement membrane, in a fibromyxoid matrix that resembles e dental papilla i12.22. Occasionally, there may be small islands cells in which odontogenic epithelium surrounds less cel-lar areas composed of epithelial cells that resemble a part of e enamel organ called the stellate reticulum. In these cases, e islands resemble the enamel organ i12.23. The ameloblastic proma is regarded as a type of ameloblastoma by some but ot by others because it is usually less aggressive. A myxoid "tissue culture" background suggests ameloblastic fibroma er ameloblastoma. Also, the ameloblastic fibroma occurs in unger people than the ameloblastoma (average age 15 vs 20-40 r an ameloblastoma). In contrast to an ameloblastoma, both the ithelial and stromal components of the ameloblastic fibroma e considered to be neoplastic.

The odontogenic fibroma is a rare intraosseous mesenchymal oplasm that is also characterized by fibrous tissue containing usters of epithelial cells, but the epithelium is less conspicuous an in an ameloblastoma or an adenomatoid odontogenic tumor.

The squamous odontogenic tumor is a benign intraosseous ass, found in the jaw, which consists of clusters of benign uamous cells in a spindle cell stroma. Distinction from squa-ous carcinoma is made by the innocuous appearance of the uamous cells.

The odontomas are benign mesenchymal neoplasms character-ed by both ameloblasts (enamel-making cells) and odontoblasts vhich produce dentin), making these tumors unusual in that both iamel and dentin are present. Because both enamel and dentin e present, there is the production of a more complex structure at is in fact an attempt at tooth formation. A recognizable but isshapen tooth may be present (compound odontoma) i12.24, 2.25, or the elements may not form anything that can be identi-ed as a tooth (complex odontoma) i12.26, i12.27, though in practice, e distinction of these 2 kinds of odontomas is not helpful. In the identification of an odontoma, it is helpful to look for bone-like material that has a heterogeneous appearance or a mixture of enamel and dentin. A helpful feature in diagnosing odontomas is that the enamel rods in enamel appear as tiny channels i12.28. Dentin also contains tiny parallel tubules i12.29. The presence of such minute channels—the smallest channels likely to be seen in surgical pathology—suggests an odontogenic process.

"The cementoma" is a generic term for at least 4 cementum-forming mesenchymal lesions, some neoplastic and some not. The most common is the periapical cementoma (also called periapical cemental dysplasia), which is often multiple, occurs in the tooth apex and is thought to be a nonneoplastic deposi-tion of cementum around the periodontal ligament [PMID20614314]. The cementoblastoma is thought to be a true neoplasm and occurs primarily in the mandible of young people. It demon-strates nonspecific histologic features, including disorganized bone-like material and numerous giant cells in a fibrovascular stroma i12.30 [PMID22144847].

Proliferations of Squamous Epithelium

Squamous cell carcinoma of the oral cavity is diagnosed by the same criteria as are employed in other locations and is not discussed here, but brief mention will be made of 4 conditions that can mimic squamous carcinoma. Necrotizing sialometapla-sia is a squamous metaplasia of minor salivary glands, probably caused by ischemia, often occurring in an inflammatory back-ground. The keys to avoiding a diagnosis of squamous cell car-cinoma are the location, the lobular pattern, and the innocuous nuclear appearance i12.31 [PMID19415943]. Palatal papillomatosis (also called papillary hyperplasia) is usually secondary to ill-fitting dentures and is characterized by hyperplastic epithelium, a pap-illary architecture i12.32, and a fibrotic stroma i12.33 [PMID2197660]. Sialadenoma papilliferum is a simple squamous papilloma. The fourth condition that may mimic squamous cell carcinoma is epithelial hyperplasia secondary to a stromal granular cell tumor. Granular cell tumors most often occur on the dorsal sur-face of the tongue and should be specifically excluded before a squamous carcinoma is diagnosed in this site.

As is the case for other locations, and as pioneered in the uterine cervix, oral squamous carcinoma arises from dysplasia, which is now called oral intraepithelial neoplasia (OIN). OIN is diagnosed and graded on a scale of 1-3 as in other sites [PMID21234636]. If it is difficult to distinguish between reactive atypia and OIN, Ki-67 expression (an immunohistochemical stain that is associated with mitoses) above the basal layer is a point for OIN.

"Leukoplakia" is a clinical term, referring to a white patch that cannot be scraped off. The histologic diagnosis in these cases is epithelial hyperplasia and/or hyperkeratosis, with or without a verrucous architecture and with or without OIN. There are many types of leukoplakia, based on the clinical appearance. Most do not have OIN i12.34, but those that do or that have a verrucous architec-ture are predisposed to the development of carcinoma and should therefore be specifically mentioned [PMID21342275].

Verrucous lesions of the oral cavity are particularly challenging. Proliferative verrucous leukoplakia (PVL) is a clinicopathologic entity, occurring primarily in middle-aged and older women, char-acterized by histologically innocuous epithelial hyperplasia with hyperkeratosis that is clinically recurrent [PMID17448134]. The role of the pathologist in PVL, as in all leukoplakias, is to report epithe-lial hyperplasia/hyperkeratosis, and comment on the presence or absence of OIN and a verrucous architecture.

ISBN 978-089189-5886

There are 2 verrucous lesions that have special significance. The first is oral hairy leukoplakia, a painless verrucous lesion on the lateral aspect of the tongue. Although it is found in increased frequency in patients with HIV [PMID18417029], it is actually caused by Epstein Barr virus (EBV) [PMID16827715]. There is hyperkeratosis of an unusual type—discrete mounds of keratin separated by areas of minimal keratinization—accompanied by ballooning of the upper keratinocytes. Immunohistochemical stains will usually demonstrate EBV.

The second verrucous lesion of great importance is the verrucous carcinoma, first described by Ackerman in 1948 [PMID18907508]. The verrucous carcinoma often has verrucous epithelial hyperplasia on the surface i12.35, but the imperative histologic feature is broad rete pegs that push into the stroma while maintaining rounded contours i12.36. Special attention should be given to the interface of the epithelium and stroma in any verrucous lesion. The stroma in a verrucous carcinoma often contains a significant number of lymphocytes and plasma cells i12.37, but these are commonly seen in any lesion of the oral area because the oral mucosa often reacts to stimuli, with an initial plasmacytic response, just as the skin often reacts with an initial lymphocytic response.

The differential diagnosis of verrucous carcinoma includes reactive epithelial (pseudoepitheliomatous) hyperplasia, PVL, and verrucous hyperplasia. Reactive epithelial hyperplasia is unlikely to recur and usually has thinner rete pegs that do not push against the basement membrane and which may fuse at their base in a manner similar to that seen in psoriasis [Luna ISBN978-0721668567]. PVL also lacks the broad, pushing rete pegs that characterized verrucous carcinoma.

The distinction of verrucous carcinoma from verrucous hyperplasia is especially challenging and subject to substantial interobserver variation since both entities have broad epithelial hyperplasia in the lower portion, with pushing into the stroma. Fortunately, this differentiation is not usually clinically critical, as both verrucous hyperplasia and verrucous carcinoma are locally recurring, but nonmetastasizing processes with substantial clinical and histologic overlap. In verrucous carcinoma, the rete pegs are slightly broader and have pushed slightly more deeply into the stroma than in verrucous hyperplasia, but the 2 entities form a continuum and need not be differentiated from each other as long as they are distinguished from reactive epithelial hyperplasia. I recommend that the diagnosis of verrucous carcinoma be favored if the clinical impression is worrisome, because the clinical appearance is often more compelling that the histologic appearance.

A major problem in coming to terms with verrucous carcinoma is its frequent association with microinvasion [PMID6732584]. This has prevented a universal consensus as to whether or not verrucous carcinoma is by definition an in situ process. However one might regard a verrucous carcinoma, microinvasion should be excluded in any possible case, and if any is found, the diagnosis must either be verrucous carcinoma with focal microinvasion or simply focally microinvasive squamous carcinoma. A type 4 collagen or laminin immunohistochemical stains, or a simple periodic acid-Schiff stain, may identify a minute focus of basement membrane penetration.

Given that the verrucous carcinoma cannot metastasize or recur if there is complete excision, one can argue that the term is no longer needed. The imperatives are to exclude any degree of invasion and comment on resection margins. If invasion is excluded and the margins are negative, the verrucous architecture is irrelevant.

I recommend diagnoses and comments such as:

1. "squamous cell carcinoma in situ, verrucous pattern (also called verrucous carcinoma), negative margins"
2. "squamous cell carcinoma in situ, verrucous pattern (also called verrucous carcinoma), with focal microinvasion, negative margins," with a comment that there is local recurrence potential and minimal metastatic potential
3. "squamous cell carcinoma in situ, verrucous pattern (also called verrucous carcinoma), extending to a margin, with local recurrence potential, but no significant metastatic potential"
4. "squamous hyperplasia with a verrucous pattern (also called verrucous hyperplasia), cannot exclude squamous cell carcinoma in situ of the verrucous type (also called verrucous carcinoma), no invasive carcinoma seen, margins negative.

Core Points for The Oral Cavity

- Common inflammatory conditions of the oral cavity:
    - Herpes
    - Pemphigus
    - Pemphigoid
    - Lichen planus
    - Geographic tongue
    - Gingivitis
  - Pathologist often cannot provide a specific diagnosis
- Odontogenic cysts: inflammatory or developmental.
  - Periapical (radicular) cyst: most common inflammatory odontogenic cyst.
  - Common developmental cysts: dentigerous cyst, which surrounds the crown of an unerupted permanent tooth, and the odontogenic keratocyst, which has local recurrence potential.
- *Central* giant cell granuloma: within the bones of the jaw and is of unclear nature.
- Epulis: localized soft tissue enlargement of the gingival.
  - 3 forms:
    - Fibrosing (epulis fissuratum)
    - Vascular type
    - Giant cell epulis (giant cell reparative granuloma or *peripheral* giant cell granuloma).
- Benign fibro-ossifying lesions: cannot be definitively distinguished histologically.
  - Association of fibrous dysplasia with a mutation in the *GNAS* gene may permit a precise diagnosis.
  - McCune-Albright syndrome: associated with fibrous dysplasia
- Ameloblastoma: most common significant odontogenic tumor
  - Can be locally aggressive.
- Oral intraepithelial neoplasia (dysplasia) and squamous cell carcinoma are diagnosed and graded as in other sites.
- Oral hairy leukoplakia: lateral aspect of the tongue
  - May be associated with HIV.
- Verrucous hyperplasia/verrucous carcinoma group: diagnostically challenging, local recurrence potential, but no metastatic potential.
  - Essential comments concern the presence or absence of invasion and the status of margins.

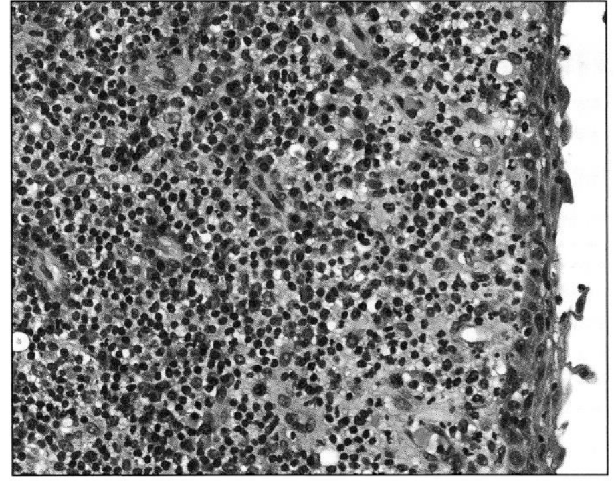

1 A periapical dicular) cyst, lined stratified squamous ithelium with severe ronic inflammation in e stroma

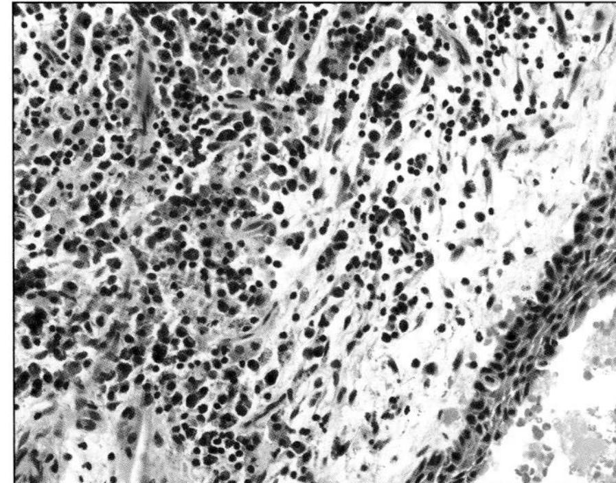

i12.2 A dentigerous cyst, lined by stratified squamous epithelium, with chronic inflammation and hemosiderin macrophages in the stroma

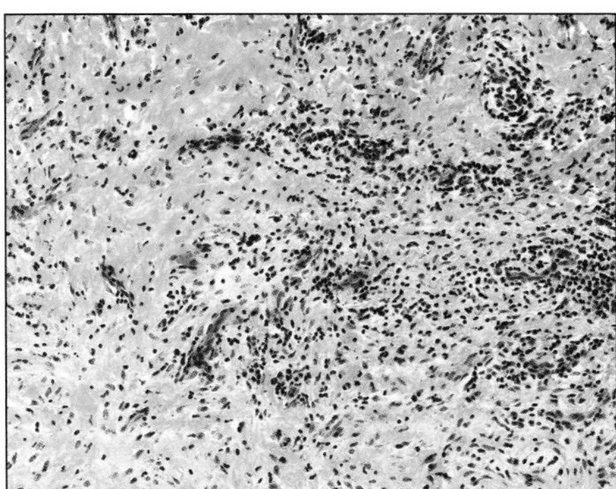

3 A dentigerous cyst th an indistinct lining, ident only as chronically lamed stroma

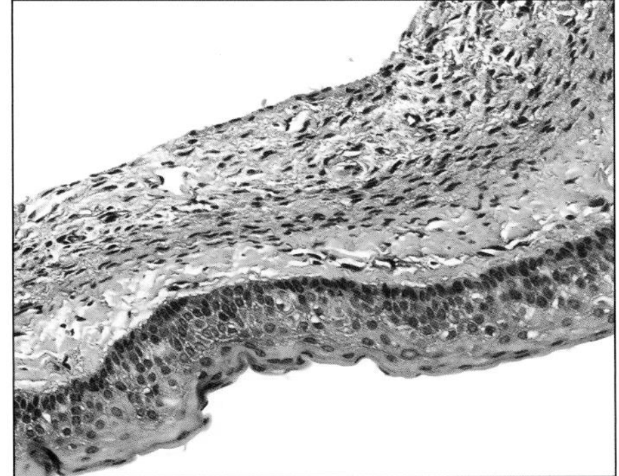

i12.4 An odontogenic keratocyst demonstrating parakeratosis in a "corrugated" pattern. Note absence of rete pegs.

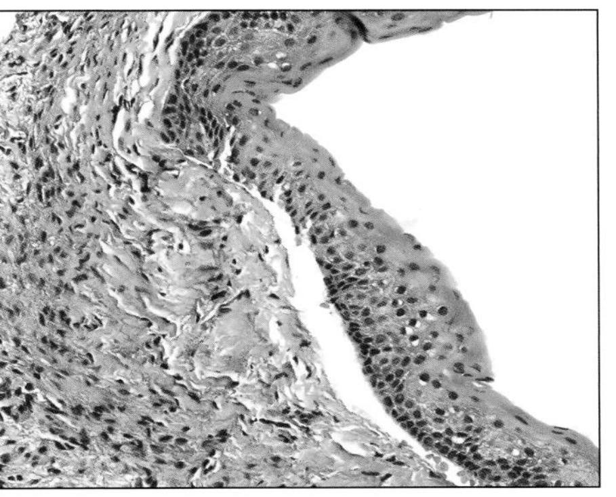

5 The same case as i12.4, which the epithelium s become detached m the stroma, another aracteristic of the ontogenic keratocyst

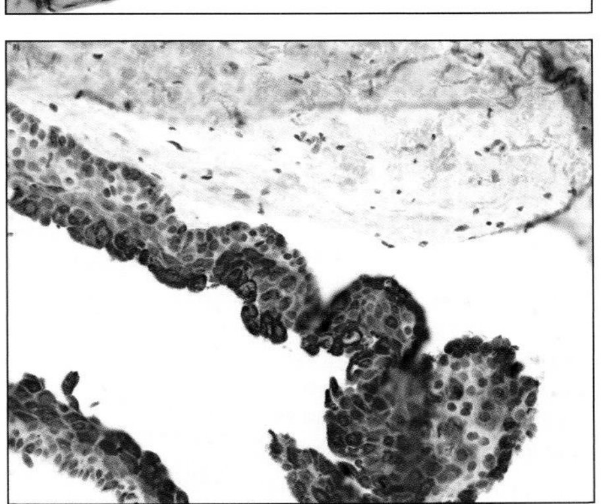

i12.6 Positive staining of a problematic odontogenic cyst with cytokeratin 19, essentially excluding an odontogenic keratocyst

CK17 is ⊕ in OKC

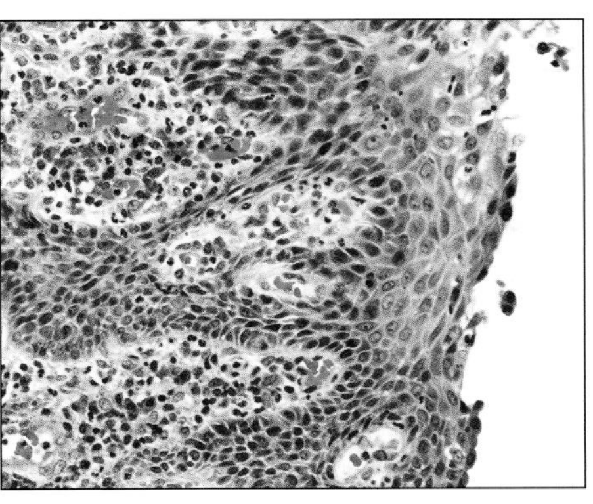

.7 A fissural cyst, with nspecific histologic ndings of stratified uamous lining d stromal chronic flammation. This is a sopalatine cyst.

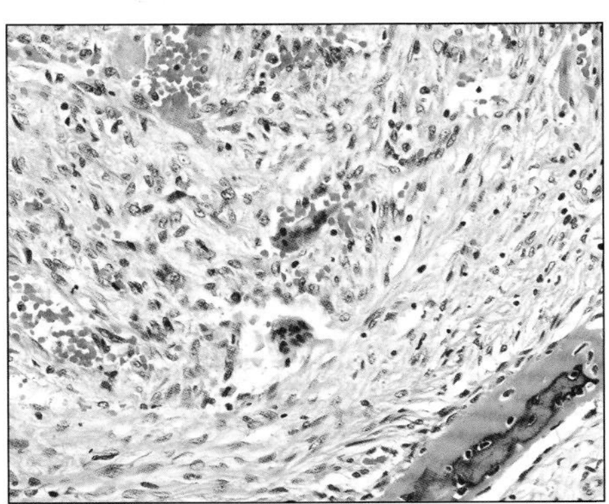

i12.8 A central giant cell granuloma with numerous giant cells in a cellular stroma. Note the fragment of bone, indicating intraosseous origin.

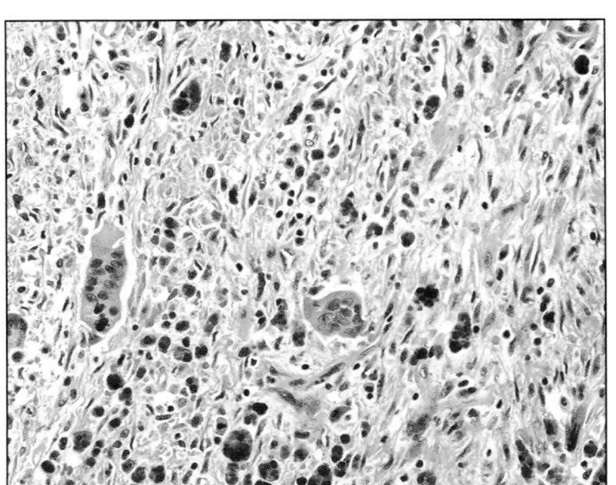

.9 A central giant cell anuloma with numerous emosiderin macrophages

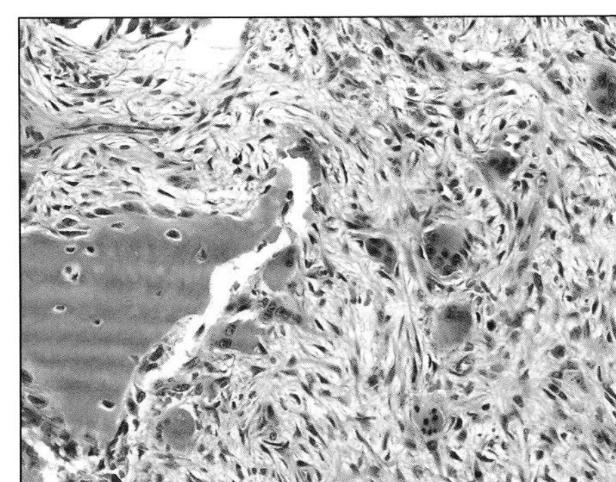

i12.10 A jaw lesion caused by primary hyperparathyroidism, simulating a central giant cell granuloma

ISBN 978-089189-5886

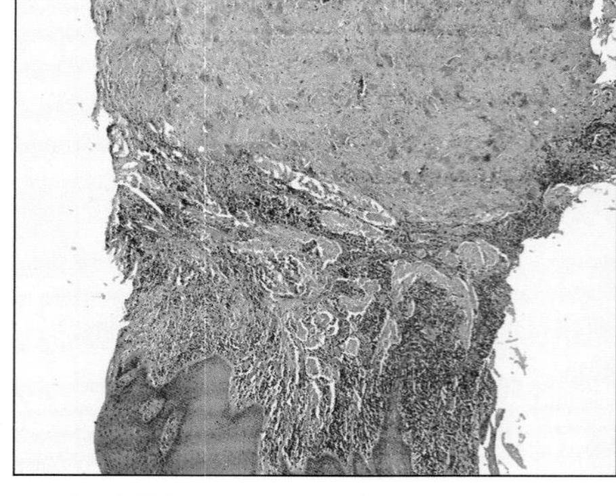

i12.11 A low-power view of a peripheral giant cell granulomas. The oral mucosa at the bottom of the photograph identifies the process as occurring in soft tissue and not in bone, as would be the case for a central giant cell granuloma.

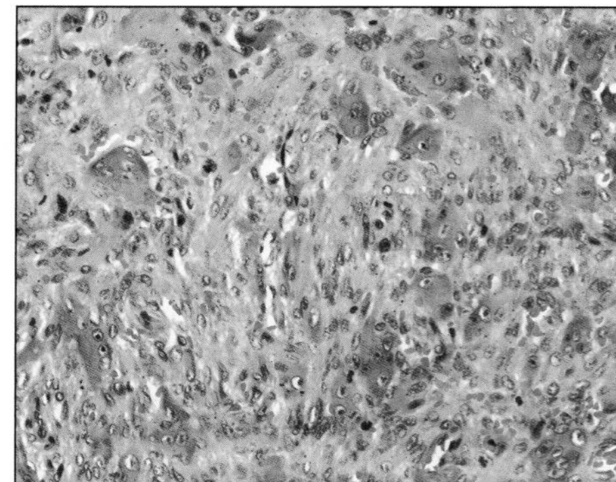

i12.12 A high-power view of the same case as in i12.11, illustrating that central and peripheral giant cell granulomas are essentially indistinguishable histologically.

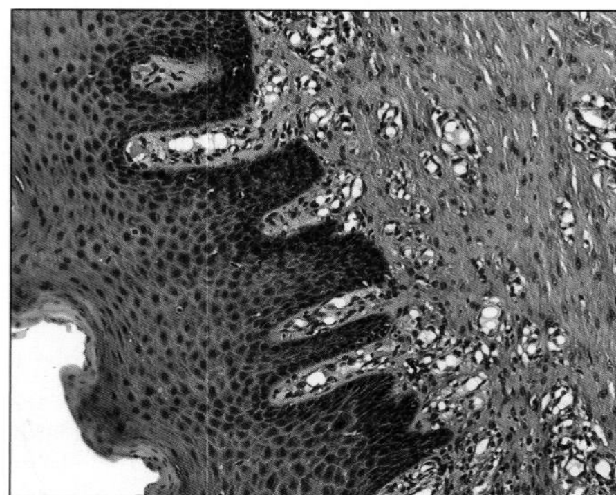

i12.13 A fibrosing epulis (epulis fissuratum) characterized by epithelial hyperplasia and a densely fibrotic stroma

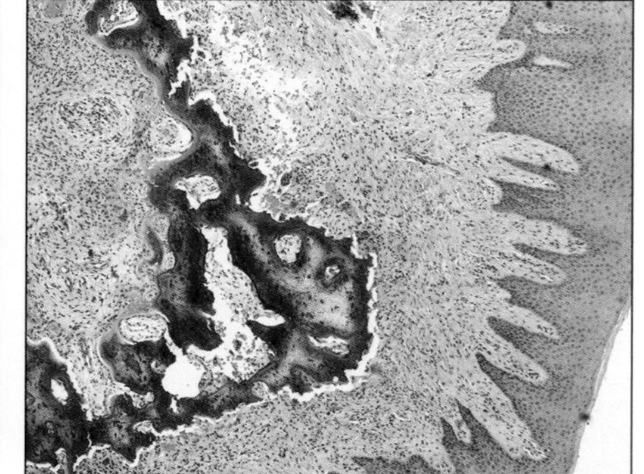

i12.14 A fibrosing epulis with metaplastic bone formation

Assoc. w/ ill-fitting dentures.

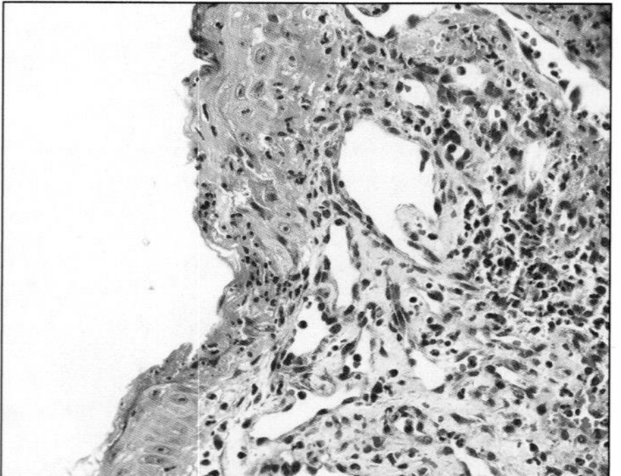

i12.15 A richly vascular epulis that is essentially a pyogenic granuloma

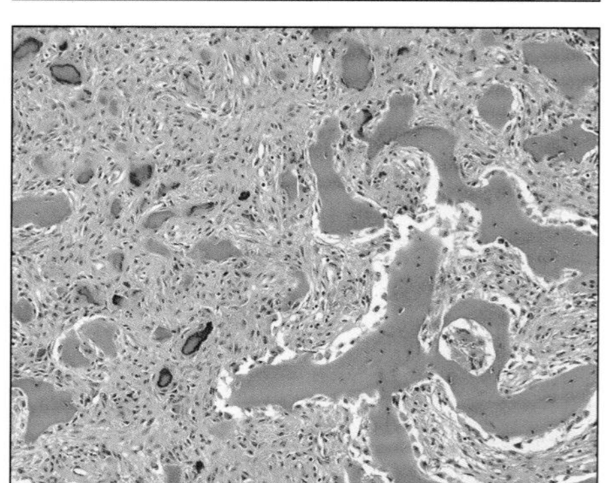

i12.16 A benign fibro-osseous lesion of the jaw, which could be fibrous dysplasia, ossifying fibroma, or any of the entities grouped together as osseous dysplasia

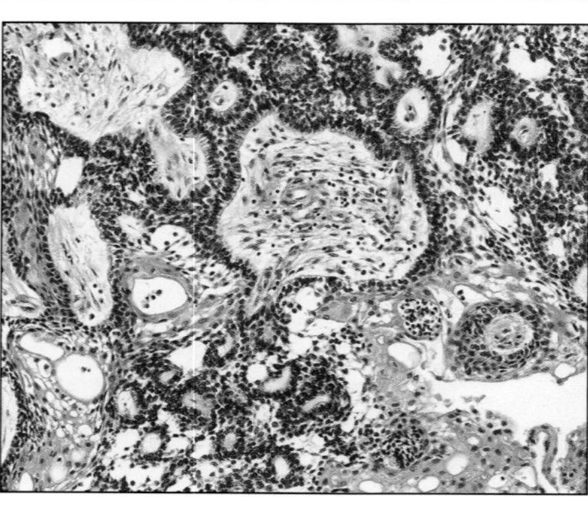

i12.17 An ameloblastoma in which basaloid cells surround less cellular areas

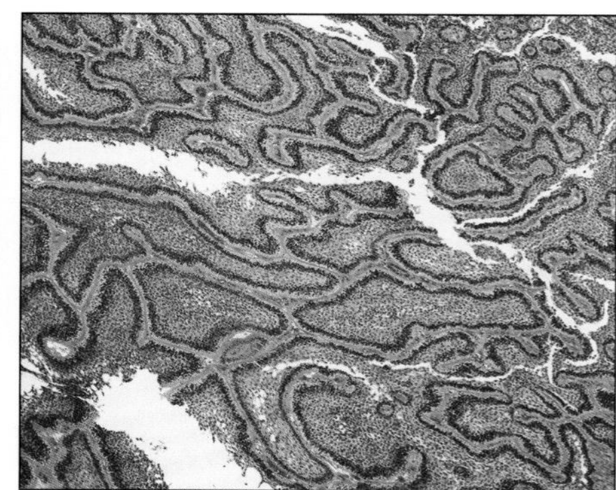

i12.18 An ameloblastoma with pronounced peripheral palisading, resembling basal cell carcinoma of the skin

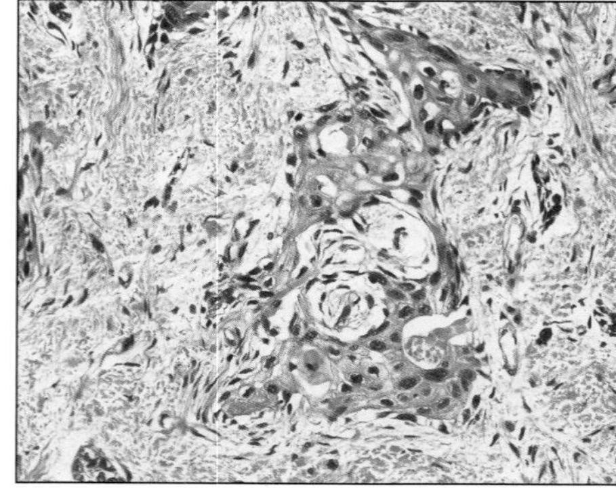

i12.19 A squamous form of ameloblastoma, an unusual form that does not have basaloid cells or a dimorphic population

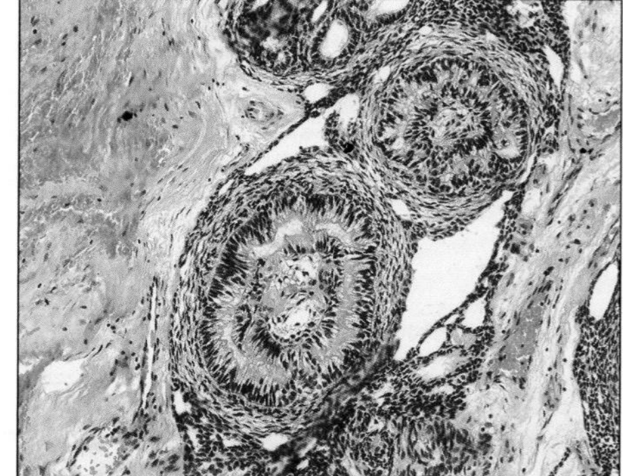

i12.20 An adenomatoid odontogenic tumor with concentric arrangements of uniform epithelial cells. The appearance here, in which a smaller ring of epithelial cells is inside a larger ring, with eosinophilic material between them, is commonly seen in this entity.

21 An odontogenic
xoma with a myxoid
trix within which there
few or no epithelial
ls. The matrix is
nctuated by occasional
od vessels.

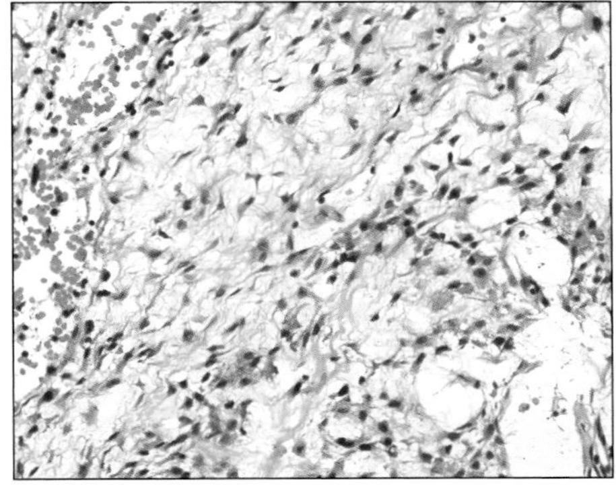

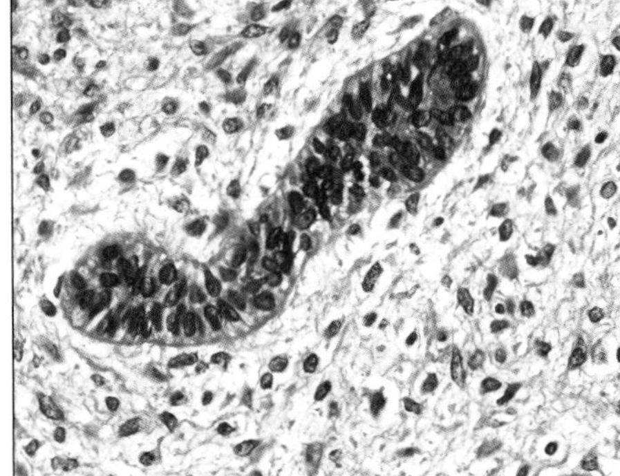

i12.22 An ameloblastic fibroma with a thin strand of epithelium in a fibromyxoid matrix

23 Another example of
ameloblastic fibroma
th islands of cells, on
periphery of which are
ithelial cells resembling
ose seen in i12.22 but in
center of which are
s cellular areas

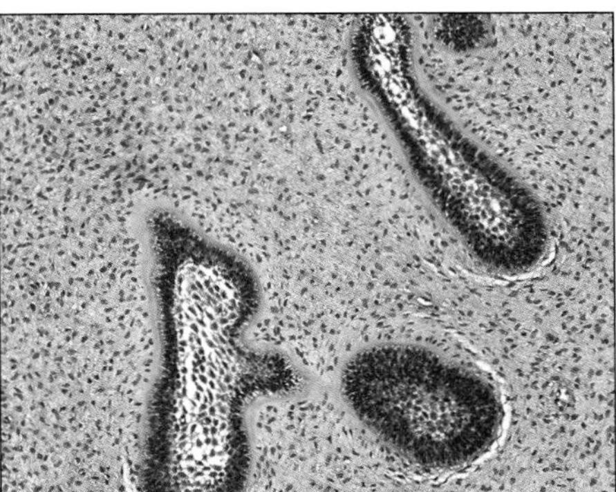

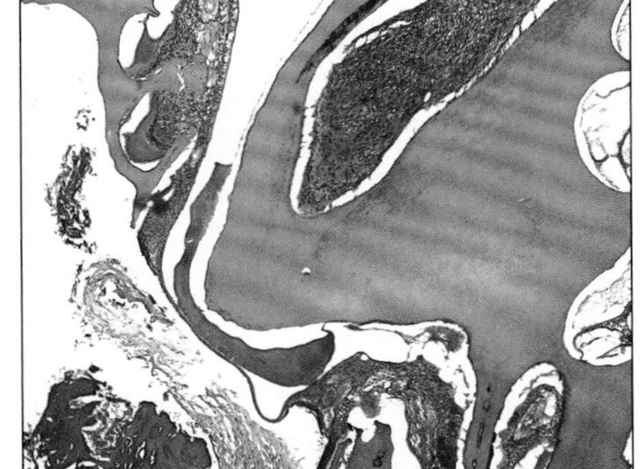

i12.24 A compound odontoma in which a small amount of dark pink enamel is noted in the left lower portion, adjacent to which is a large amount of pink-orange dentin. In the upper middle portion is a fibromyxoid stroma that resembles the dental papilla.

25 A compound
lontoma in which
amel is seen at the left,
ntin in the middle and
ntal papilla stroma at
e right

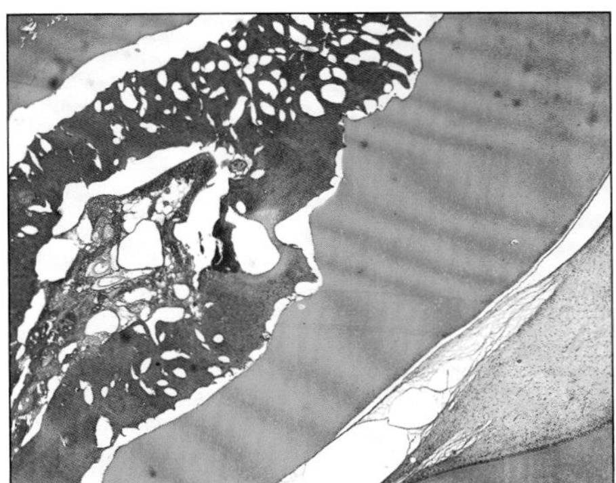

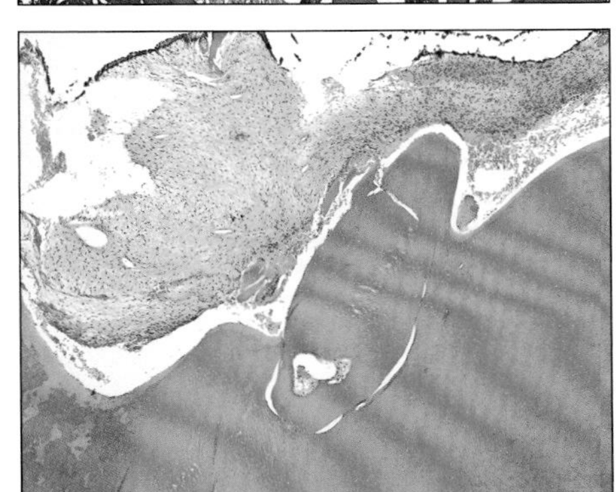

i12.26 A complex odontoma in which there is stroma in the upper portion while the lower portion is dentin. A thin layer of enamel can be seen overlying the dentin.

.27 A complex odontoma
th dentin in the left
wer portion and a
nall amount of enamel
sible in the fragment on
e right

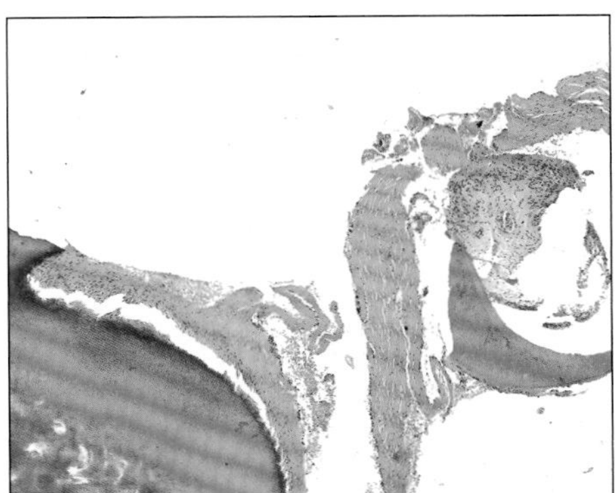

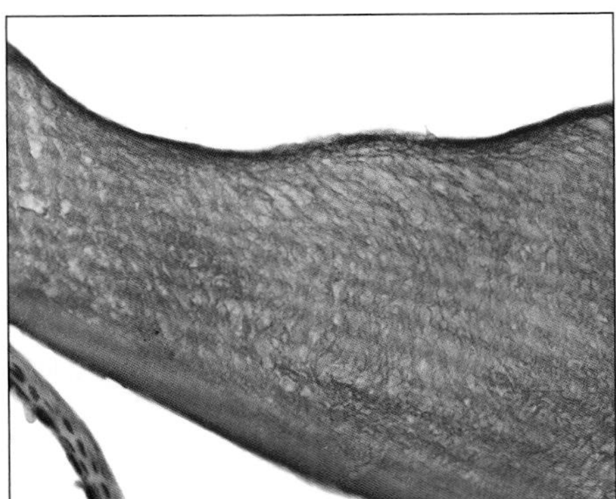

i12.28 A high-power view of enamel demonstrating the enamel rods that appear as very tiny channels

.29 The minute tubules
at are present within
entin

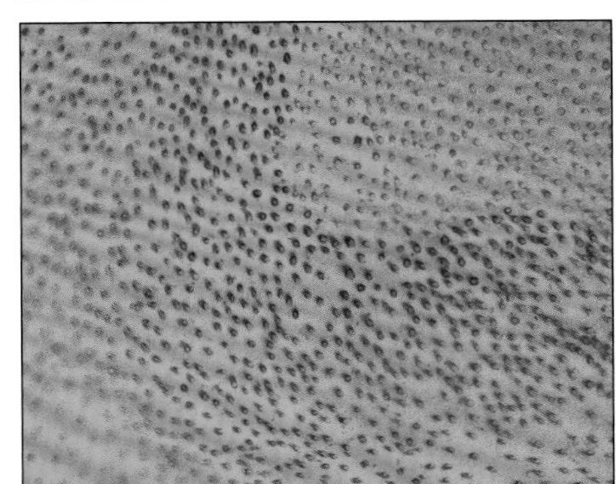

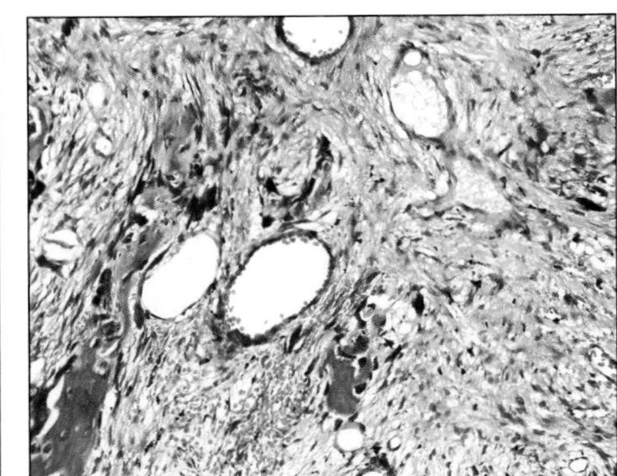

i12.30 A cementoblastoma demonstrating disorganized bone-like material in a stroma with giant cells

ISBN 978-089189-5886

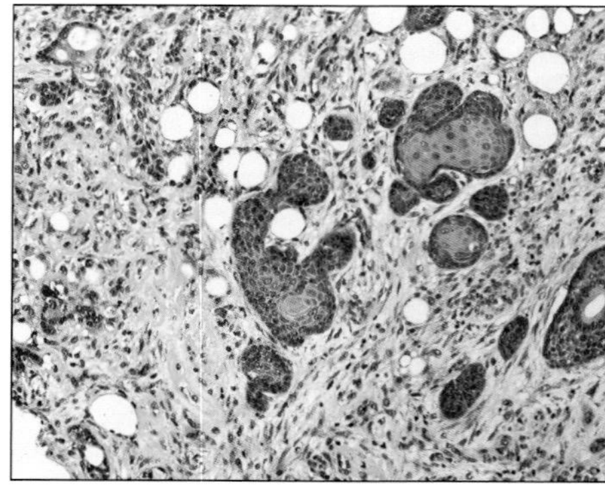

i12.31 Necrotizing sialometaplasia. The presence of squamous epithelium within the stroma may be alarming, but attention to the lobular architecture and the innocuous nuclei will prevent a misdiagnosis of squamous carcinoma.

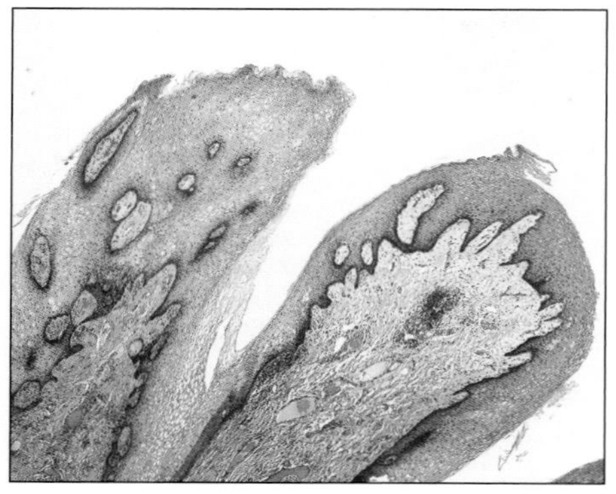

i12.32 Palatal papillomatosis secondary to ill-fitting dentures, demonstrating the hyperplastic epithelium and papillary architecture

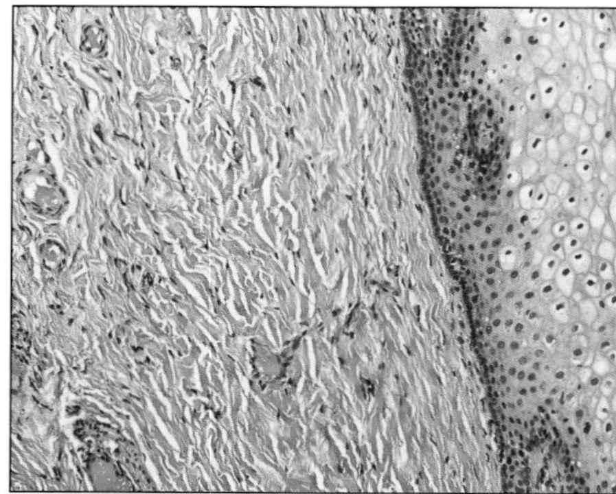

i12.33 A higher-power view of the same case as in i12.32, illustrating the fibrous stroma and the lack of significant epithelial atypia

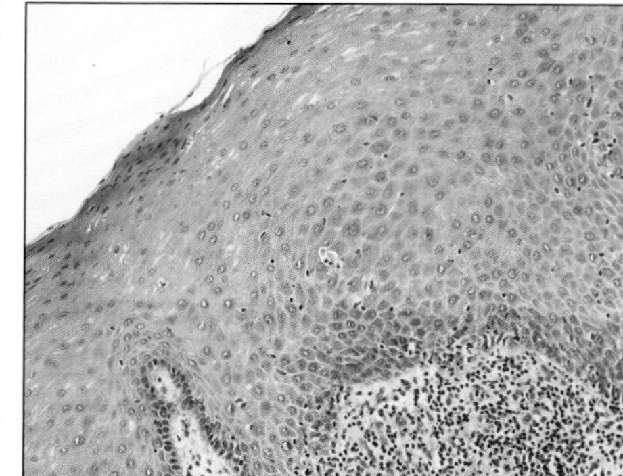

i12.34 A biopsy of a clinical leukoplakia, illustrating epithelial hyperplasia, hyperkeratosis, and parakeratosis. This case does not have intraepithelial neoplasia.

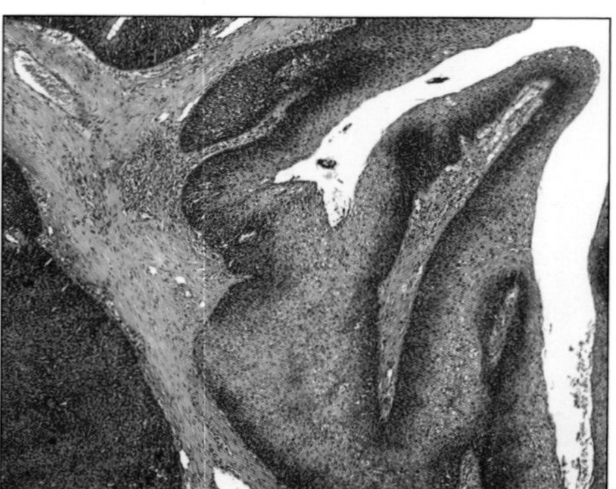

i12.35 A verrucous carcinoma in which there is verrucous epithelial hyperplasia on the surface

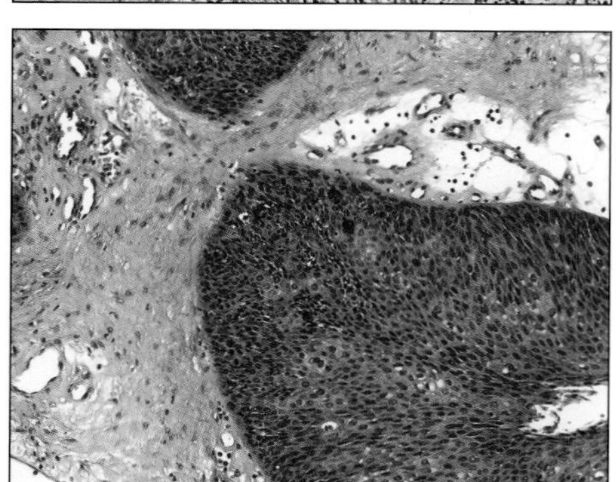

i12.36 The lower portion of the epithelium in a verrucous carcinoma, illustrating the markedly thickened, but well circumscribed rete pegs that push into the stroma without obvious invasion

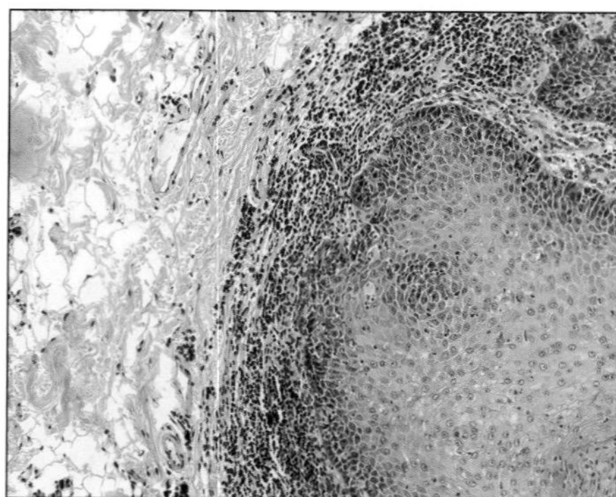

i12.37 Verrucous carcinoma with the lymphocytes and plasma cells that are typically found at the junction of the stroma and the lower portion of the epithelium

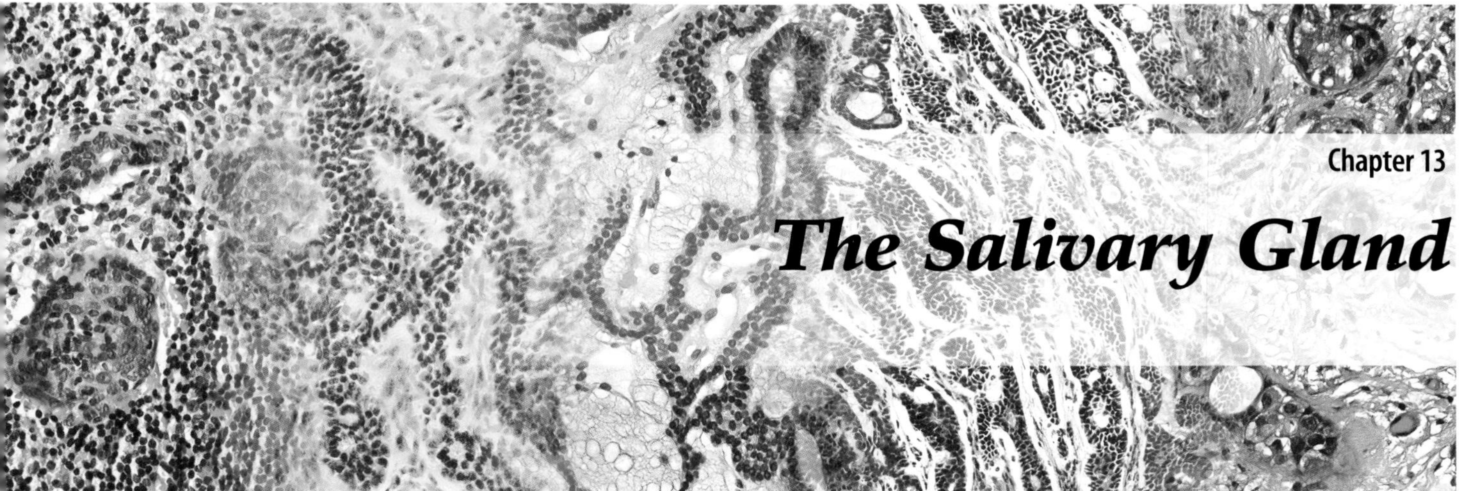

Chapter 13

The Salivary Gland

onneoplastic Processes

There is good agreement that cervical lymph nodes may ntain benign salivary gland inclusions [PMID15742261] or benign uamous inclusions. In contrast, it is conventional to regard yroid tissue within a lymph node as indicative of metastatic yroid carcinoma, provided that it is clear that the lymphoid sue forms a true lymph node.

The criteria for Sjögren syndrome are dry eyes, dry mouth, tensive lymphocytic infiltrate in a biopsy of the lacrimal gland of a salivary gland (biopsy of a minor labial salivary gland is mmon) i13.1, and serologic evidence of a systemic autoimmune sorder. The definitive diagnosis is a triad of the clinical, the opsy, and the laboratory. There should be at least 2 clusters of lymphocytes per 4 mm^2 in at least 4 lobules [PMID4589360]. The agnosis is never made in the presence of a lymphoma, graft vs st disease, Aids, or sarcoidosis.

Differentiating Sjögren syndrome from low-grade lymphoma salivary glands can be very difficult. The absence of clinical serologic evidence of Sjögren syndrome favors lymphoma, does the presence of lymphadenopathy unrelated to the livary glands. In unclear cases, it is wise to diagnose a mphoepithelial lesion, comment that the picture is consistent th either Sjögren syndrome or a lymphoma, and recommend nical correlation, serologic studies for autoimmune disease, d biopsy of enlarged lymph nodes, if any.

Salivary glands in Sjögren syndrome may contain imyoepithelial islands i13.2, though these are not neither ecific nor required for the diagnosis of Sjögren syndrome. espite the name, it is unclear if there are any true myoepithelial lls in these islands [PMID7598870].

An uncommon entity in the differential diagnosis of Sjögren sease is IgG4-related sclerosing sialadenitis. Sclerosing aladenitis is one of the autoimmune conditions that is sociated with elevated serum IgG4. This group of disorders discussed in Chapter 24, since autoimmune pancreatitis is the imary presentation. In IgG4-related sclerosing sialadenitis, ere is a lymphoplasmacytic infiltrate and fibrosis. There may a generalized adenopathy, with plasmacytic infiltration lymph nodes that simulates the plasma cell variant of astleman disease.

The term "Sicca syndrome" refers to dry eyes and dry mouth ly, without a demonstrable connective tissue disorder. The rm "Mikulicz disease" is rarely used now, but refers to a benign lymphoepithelial lesion which usually presents as a mass. Some, but not all, of these patients will have Sjögren syndrome. Given that the terminology is confusing under the best of circumstances, the term "Mikulicz disease" is best avoided.

Benign Salivary Neoplasms

A benign cystadenoma, often with oncocytic lining, is rarely found in the salivary glands, but most salivary cystic lesions are lymphoepithelial cysts. These are more likely developmental than neoplastic (a few are of branchial cleft origin, but most are epithelial inclusions), but are included here because they clinically present as a neoplasm and are an integral part of the differential diagnosis of cystic neoplasms.

Salivary glands, especially the parotid, may contain lymphoepithelial cysts. A minority of these are associated with HIV [PMID19550061, PMID19157503]. Unfortunately, there are no reliable histologic criteria upon which to distinguish these from the innocuous lymphoepithelial cysts that have no such association, though those cases associated with HIV often have multiple or bilateral cysts i13.3, whereas cases without this association are usually single. In either case, the lesion is composed of small cysts lined by stratified squamous epithelium i13.4, perhaps with focal areas of cuboidal or columnar lining, surrounded by a dense lymphoid population.

The Warthin tumor and oncocytoma are not discussed because they are rarely diagnostically difficult.

A few sebaceous glands may be found in the normal parotid. Rarely these will give rise to a neoplasm such as a sebaceous adenoma or sebaceous lymphadenoma i13.5a, i13.5b.

The mesenchymal component of a pleomorphic adenoma (mixed tumor) is often myxoid, may resemble cartilage i13.6, and may stain positively for glial fibrillary acidic protein and S100 [PMID2168672]. The epithelial portion contains both conventional epithelial cells and myoepithelial cells i13.7.

Malignancy may arise in an untreated pleomorphic adenoma, usually after 15-20 years [PMID18552001]. These cases of malignant transformation (carcinoma ex pleomorphic adenoma) are not to be confused with a carcinosarcoma or a so-called benign metastasizing pleomorphic adenoma. The diagnosis of carcinoma ex pleomorphic adenoma first requires the fundamental diagnosis of pleomorphic adenoma, either by the demonstration of a concomitant benign mixed tumor or by a

ISBN 978-089189-5886

secure history of a preexisting benign mixed tumor i13.8a, i13.8b. Proof of malignancy can come in the form of demonstrating metastases i13.8c, by the finding of widespread cytologically malignant cells (occasional bizarre cells in an otherwise bland tumor is not an indication of malignancy), by extensive necrosis, or by invasion of vascular spaces, perineural spaces, or the capsule. Malignancy can also be suspected if there are many mitotic figures, but there are no universally accepted numbers. Microcalcifications, an expansile nodule within the tumor, and sclerosis should arouse suspicion. An apparently infiltrating pattern of the tumor cells *within* the tumor is not helpful. Focal malignant change within an otherwise benign mixed tumor that does not invade the capsule or vessels is unlikely to behave clinically in a malignant fashion.

In contrast to carcinoma ex pleomorphic adenoma, the so-called metastasizing benign mixed tumor, which may represent multiple adenomas, has no histologic indication of malignancy and has a good prognosis.

Pleomorphic adenomas can be particularly troublesome on fine needle aspiration examination because adipocytes can be shredded as the tissue is pushed through a small-bore needle, resulting in a myxoid material that appears as the characteristic background material of this tumor type, but is actually incidental. This is especially possible on Wright-Giemsa or Diff-Quik stained smears, where both the adipose tissue and the myxoid material of a pleomorphic adenoma will stain metachromatically.

There are several neoplasms that are related to the pleomorphic adenoma. "Basal cell adenoma" is now the favored term for monomorphic adenoma, and is characterized by less conspicuous (though not absent) myoepithelial cells and a stroma that is more fibrous than myxoid. 4 growth patterns are recognized: trabecular, membranous, solid, and tubular. The most common pattern is the trabecular form i13.9. The membranous type consists of islands of cells, with smaller cells on the periphery and larger cells in the interior.

The basal cell adenocarcinoma may develop from the membranous pattern of basal cell adenoma and is distinguished from its benign counterpart by its lack of circumscription or encapsulation [PMID2326038].

The canalicular adenoma almost always arises in a minor salivary gland, usually on the upper lip or buccal mucosa, and is composed of a single layer of cuboidal to columnar cells, forming both trabeculae and glands i13.10 [PMID19639085].

The myoepithelioma is a rare benign neoplasm with a myxoid background, within which are scattered cells that stain for actin. These cells are usually spindled but may be epithelioid, plasmacytoid, clear cell, or oncocytic, and they may also stain for keratin, S100, or GFAP. The appearance of the cells and their staining characteristics may overlap with the pleomorphic adenoma, in which case the distinction between them rests on the greater cellularity and focal ductular differentiation in the latter, and on the actin positivity of all cells, even if of epithelioid appearance, and the less conspicuous gland formation, in the myoepithelioma i13.11.

Malignant Salivary Neoplasms

The malignant counterpart to the pleomorphic adenoma and the rare basal cell adenocarcinoma were discussed above. Adenoid cystic carcinomas are composed of basaloid cells, some of which have myoepithelial differentiation. They may have a variety of patterns, the most common of which is a cribriforming architecture in which duct structures enclose an amorphous eosinophilic material that is derived from the basement membrane i13.12. A tubular/ductule pattern occurs i13.13, as does a more aggressive solid pattern i13.14 that is only recognized by the focal presence of a more classic pattern or the immunohistochemical demonstration of actin or basement membrane material [PMID21353624]. This variety of patterns and its ability to occur in unexpected places outside of the salivary glands can make the adenoid cystic carcinoma diagnostically challenging, but generous sampling will usually disclose an area of classic cribriform morphology even in cases where another pattern predominates.

Because both the pleomorphic adenoma and the adenoid cystic carcinoma may have a variety of similar patterns, with a dimorphic epithelial-myoepithelial cell population and minimal pleomorphism, there may be cytologic and architectural overlap between the 2 neoplasms, particularly in cases where the adenoma lacks the characteristic myxoid background material or has a predominantly cribriform pattern that is more commonly seen in an adenoid cystic carcinoma. Generous sampling is the best pathway to a correct diagnosis, but in problematic situations, clusters of tumor cells with peripheral palisading or an appearance reminiscent of a cutaneous adnexal neoplasm suggest a pleomorphic adenoma, while duct structures with eosinophilic intraluminal material suggests an adenoid cystic carcinoma. Invasion of surrounding tissues, perineural invasion i13.15 within the tumor, or a clinical history of pain all point to an adenoid cystic carcinoma.

In problematic situations involving a cribriforming pattern, it may help to determine the nature of the material that is enclosed by the tumor cells. In an adenoid cystic carcinoma, but not in a pleomorphic adenoma, the material inside such clusters is derived from the basement membrane. If immunohistochemical stains for basement membrane components, such as collagen type 4 and laminin, are positive throughout the central material, an adenoid cystic carcinoma is suggested, while negative staining of the central material suggests a pleomorphic adenoma [PMID12539293, PMID12694353]. Adenoid cystic carcinomas with a solid pattern produce little basement membrane material but are unlikely to be confused with a pleomorphic adenoma. Some help might also be found in other immunohistochemical stains. For example, adenoid cystic carcinomas tend to stain for CD117 [PMID17539914] and elevated proliferation, as assessed by the immunohistochemical stain Ki-67, suggest malignancy [PMID10560511].

Many adenoid cystic carcinomas have a t(6;9)(q22-23;p23-24) that results in fusion of the *MYB* gene with the gene that encodes the transcription factor NFIB and causes overexpression of *MYB*. The translocation is detectable by FISH, and in most cases, immunohistochemistry will demonstrate the Myb protein in the nucleus, whereas the protein is rarely found in other salivary gland neoplasms [PMID21164292, PMID21572406].

An adenoid cystic carcinoma with a predominantly tubular/ ctule pattern may also resemble a canalicular adenoma or polymorphous low-grade adenocarcinoma. In these cases, s well to remember that both the canalicular adenoma and polymorphous low-grade adenocarcinoma have a strong edilection for minor salivary glands.

Epithelial-myoepithelial carcinoma is a rare low-grade alignant neoplasm with a multinodular pattern i13.16a and 2 ll types. Myoepithelial cells with clear cytoplasm predominate d may initially appear to be the only cell type. But closer udy will disclose, within clusters of myoepithelial cells, duct-rming cells with eosinophilic cytoplasm i13.16b. The epithelial-yoepithelial carcinoma behaves as a low-grade malignancy ith a high likelihood of local recurrence, but with a low elihood of distant metastasis.

Although acinar (or acinic) cell tumors often run a benign urse, they are now considered to be low-grade malignancies, d are called acinar (or acinic) cell carcinomas, because of their predictable behavior. Aggressive behavior is more likely if ere is necrosis or >2 mitotic figures per 10 high-power fields IID19309749]. The usual pattern is the formation of small glands .17, resulting in a microcytic architecture, often with nodules at are separated by fibrous tissue with chronic inflammation. ther patterns exist, including solid i13.18 and papillary-cystic. cinar cell carcinoma may rarely have relatively clear cytoplasm, it there will usually be some areas with more characteristic anular cytoplasm. Stromal desmoplasia is not usually seen.

There are 2 salivary gland tumors that have both squa-ous and glandular components—adenosquamous and ucoepidermoid carcinoma. Traditionally, mucoepidermoid rcinoma has lower grade nuclei than adenosquamous carci-oma i13.19. Extensive nuclear pleomorphism, large numbers mitoses, and necrosis suggest an adenosquamous carci-oma over a mucoepidermoid carcinoma [PMID6731349]. However, my experience, these differences may simply reflect the egree of differentiation of the tumor. The role of the patholo-ist in these situations is to identify a malignant neoplasm ith 2 components, and to assign a grade and stage.

Polymorphous low-grade adenocarcinoma (PLGA) occurs most exclusively in minor salivary glands. It has a number of ppearances, but all of them have relatively uniform nuclei. A olymorphous low-grade adenocarcinoma should be considered henever there is an adenocarcinoma in minor salivary glands ith low-grade nuclei and >1 architectural pattern. A low-ower pattern reminiscent of sclerosing adenosis of the breast is ommon i13.20. On closer study, PLGA may have glandular i13.21 r trabecular i13.22 pattern. Because of the nuclear uniformity, LGA is often mistaken for an adenoma. PLGA often invades essels or nerves, and often infiltrates the surrounding tissue, contrast to an adenoma.

PLGA may also simulate an adenoid cystic carcinoma or an acinar cell carcinoma. Again, realization that PLGA occurs in minor salivary glands and generous sampling will help in both of these differential diagnoses. PLGA lacks the myoepithelial differentiation of an adenoid cystic carcinoma, and the cells in an acinic cell carcinoma will have cytoplasm that is at least focally granular. Also, PLGA expresses bcl-2 [PMID9675591].

Salivary duct carcinoma has an appearance that is similar to intraductal carcinoma of the breast i13.23 but is an infiltrating carcinoma i13.24. These are high-grade neoplasms that metastasize distantly [PMID9059870]. Very rarely, there may be a true intraductal carcinoma in a salivary gland, and immunohistochemical stains for a myoepithelial layer or basement membrane may clarify the issue of invasion, as in the breast.

An occasional salivary gland adenocarcinoma cannot be classified and is designated adenocarcinoma, not otherwise specified (NOS). These may have a number of architectural patterns, but all are infiltrative and an appearance similar to invasive ductal carcinoma of the breast is typical i13.25a, i13.25b. Low-grade examples of adenocarcinoma, NOS may do well, but higher-grade examples are aggressive and tend to metastasize widely.

Core Points for the Salivary Glands

- Sjögren syndrome: autoimmune process.
  - Triad of dryness of the eyes and mouth, an extensive lymphocytic infiltrate in lacrimal or salivary glands, and serologic evidence of an autoimmune disorder.
  - Differential diagnosis includes the IgG4-related disorders.
- Lymphoepithelial cysts of the salivary glands: usually without significance
  - Often simple epithelial inclusion cysts
  - A minority may be of branchial cleft origin or associated with HIV.
- Common benign neoplasms of salivary glands:
  - Pleomorphic adenoma (mixed tumor)
  - Warthin tumor
  - Oncocytoma
  - Basal cell adenoma, and the related canalicular adenoma.
- Common malignant neoplasms:
  - Adenoid cystic carcinoma
  - Acinar (or acinic) cell tumor
  - Mucoepidermoid carcinoma.
- Less common malignancies:
  - Polymorphous low-grade adenocarcinoma
  - Almost exclusively in minor salivary glands
  - Salivary duct carcinoma
  - Adenocarcinoma, not otherwise specified.

ISBN 978-089189-5886

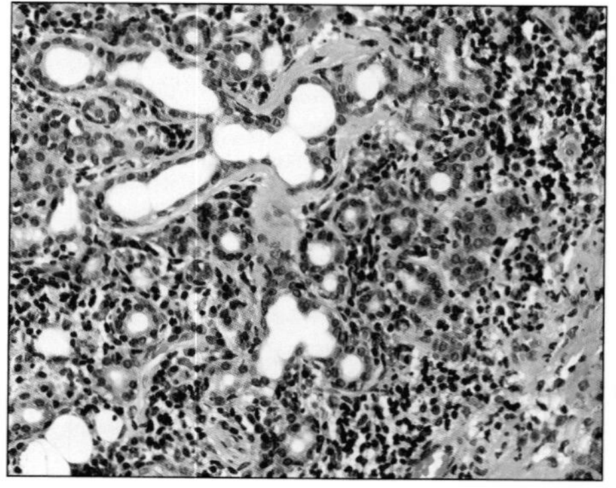

i13.1 A biopsy from a minor salivary gland in Sjögren syndrome, illustrating the extensive lymphocytic infiltrate

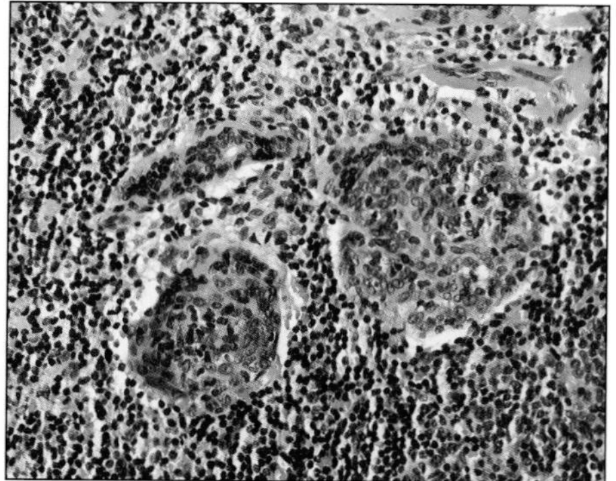

i13.2 A biopsy of a minor salivary gland in Sjögren syndrome illustrating the epimyoepithelial islands

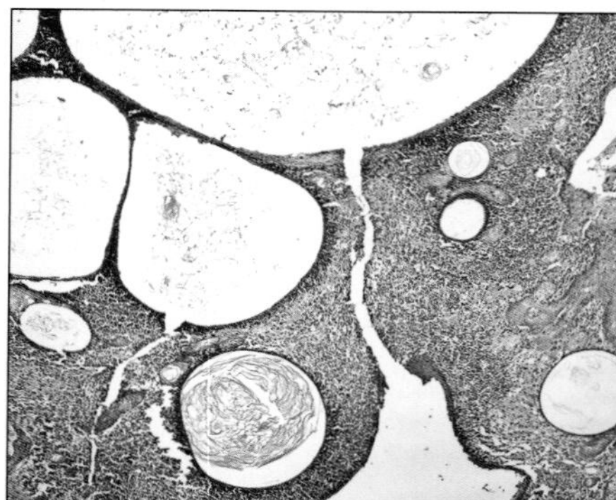

i13.3 A salivary gland with multiple lymphoepithelial cysts

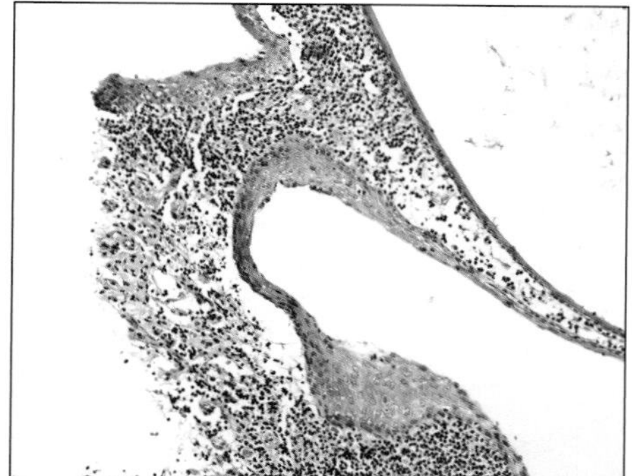

i13.4 A higher-power view of the same case as in i13.3, illustrating the benign stratified squamous epithelium lining the cysts

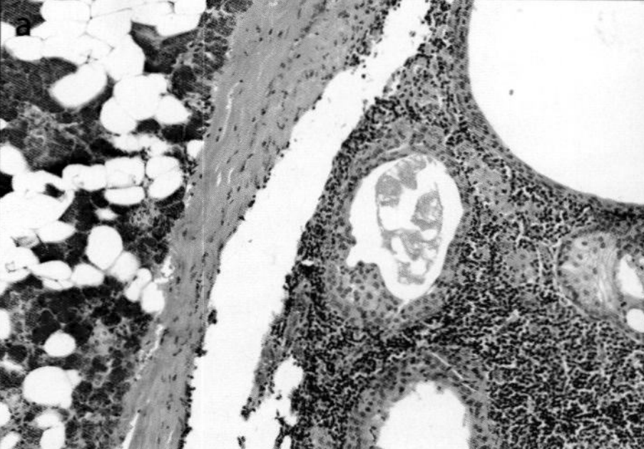

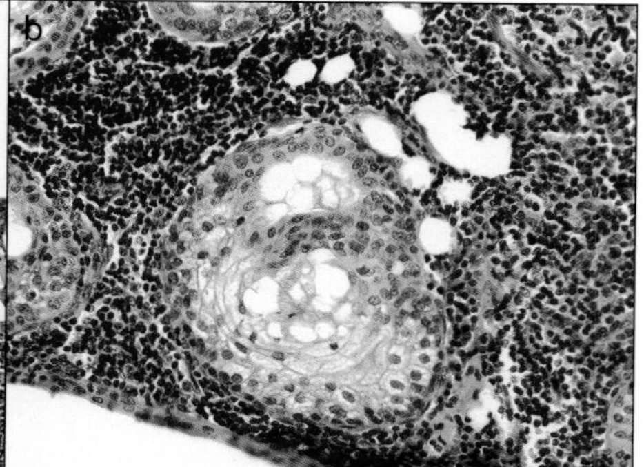

i13.5 **a** A low-power view of a sebaceous lymphadenoma of the parotid. Note the normal parotid tissue on the left. **b** A higher-power view of the same case as in i13.5a, illustrating sebaceous differentiation in the clusters of epithelial cells

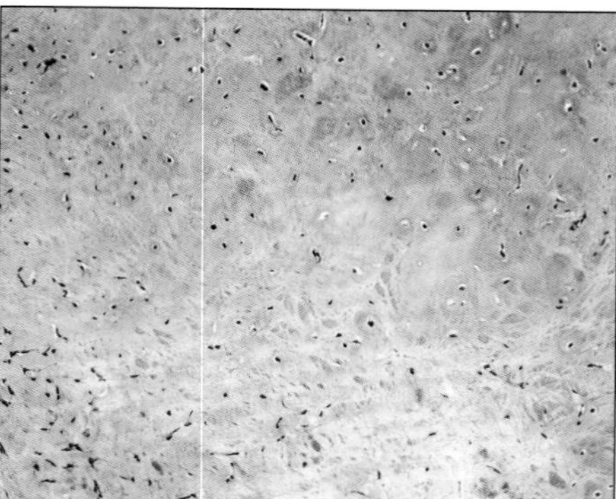

i13.6 The stroma of a pleomorphic adenoma often has a cartilaginous appearance

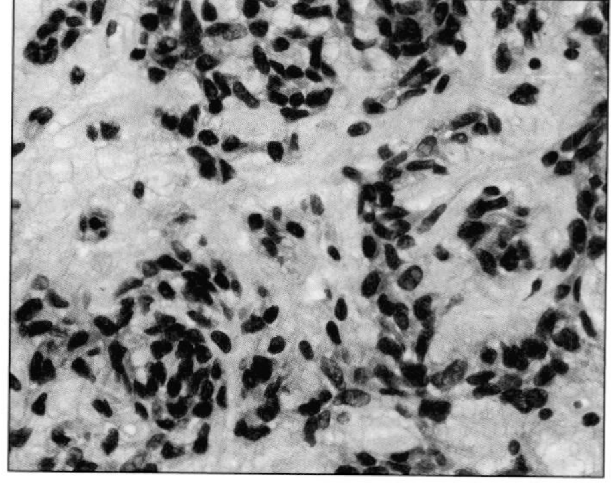

i13.7 The epithelial component of a pleomorphic adenoma consists of small, spindled cells that are of myoepithelial origin, as well as larger cells with ovoid to round nuclei

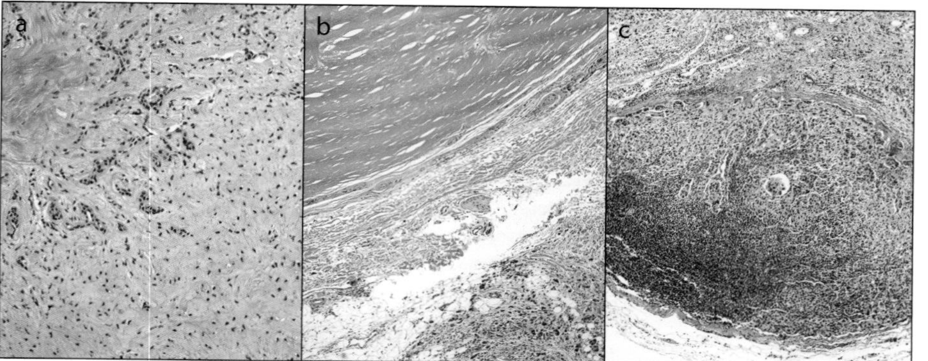

a Carcinoma ex pleomorphic adenoma. This image illustrates an ordinary, benign pleomorphic adenoma. **b** The same case as in i13.8a. In the upper right, the typical myxoid stroma has been largely replaced by a dense fibrous stroma, a consequence of the age of the lesion. In the lower left corner neoplastic cells have penetrated the capsule and acquired substantial nuclear atypia. **c** A higher-power view of the same case as in i13.8a, i13.8b. There is metastatic tumor to a lymph node as well as diffuse infiltration of neoplastic cells in the soft tissue above the lymph node.

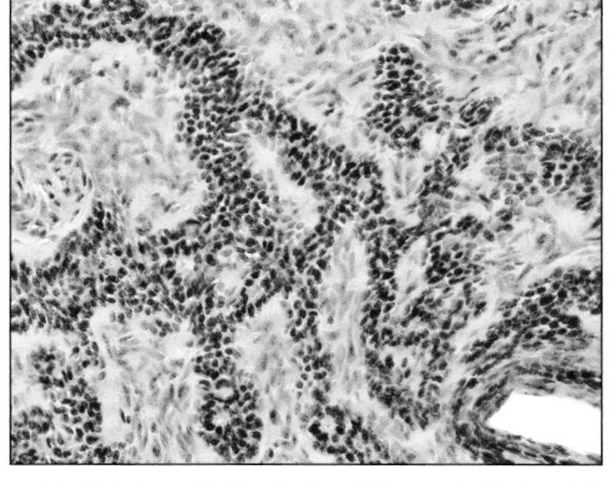

3 The trabecular form a basal cell adenoma. ote the relatively mono-orphic population of ba-oid cells with minimal oplasm and the cellular, rous stroma.

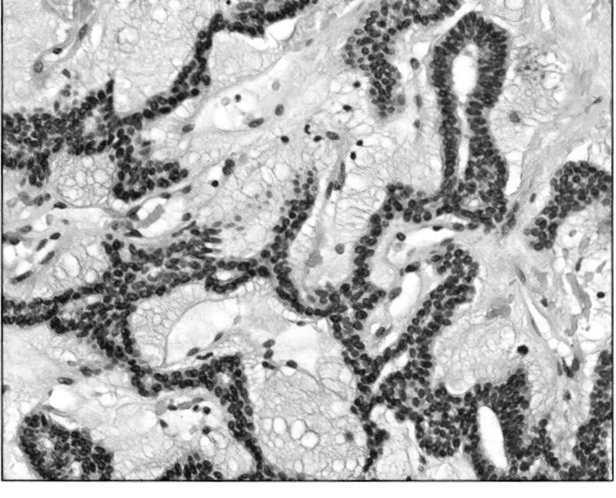

i13.9 A canalicular adenoma in which neoplastic cells form thin, often single-cell trabeculae, with occasional gland formation

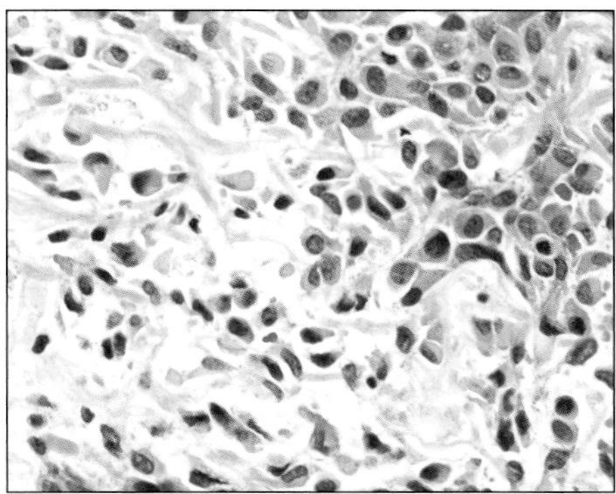

0 A myoepithelioma a minor salivary gland which the spindled, oepithelial component edominates over the unded epithelial cells t are prevalent in a mmon pleomorphic enoma

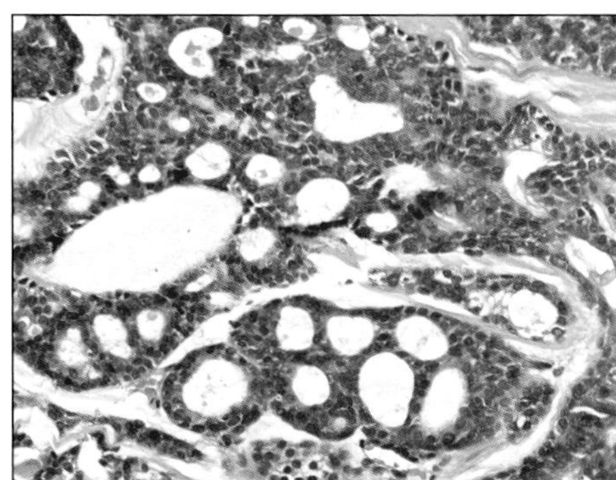

i13.11 The common cribriform pattern of an adenoid cystic carcinoma of the salivary glands

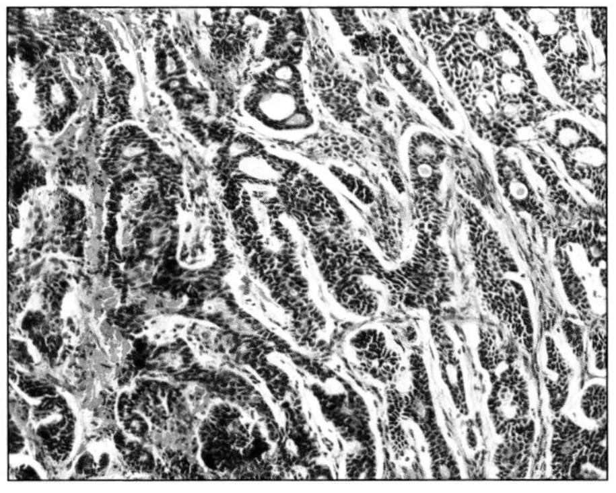

2 A tubular pattern of enoid cystic carcinoma. ote the focal cribriform ttern.

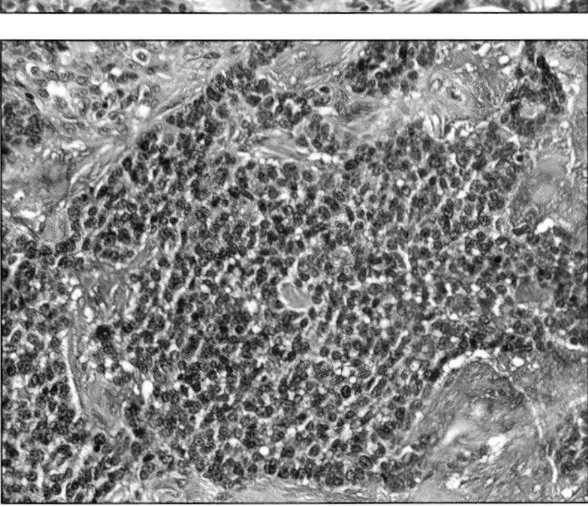

i13.13 A solid pattern of adenoid cystic carcinoma. Elsewhere in this case, a more classic cribriform arrangement was evident.

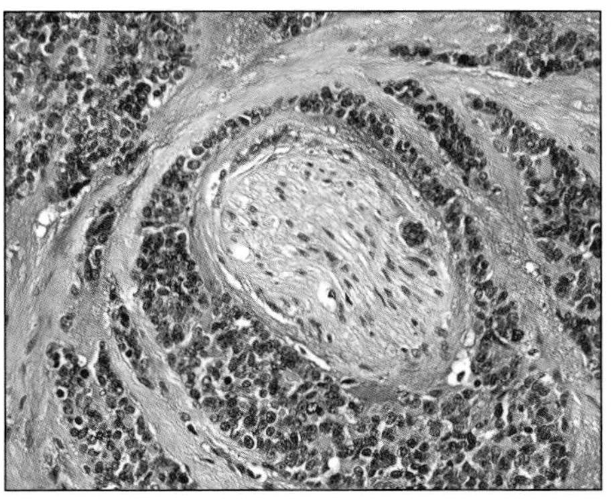

4 Perineural invan in an adenoid cystic rcinoma

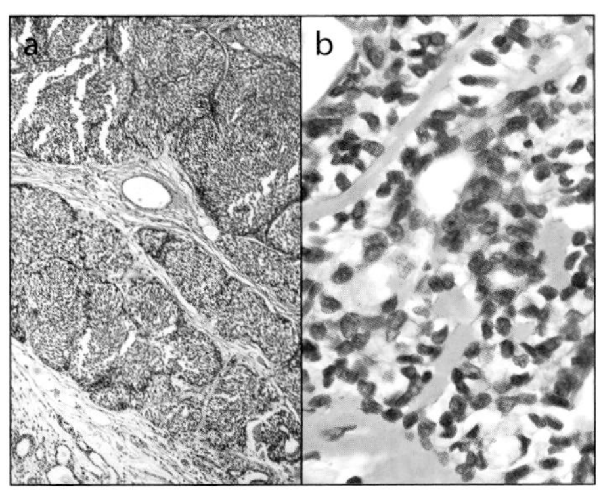

i13.15 **a** A low-power view of epithelial-myoepithelial carcinoma illustrating the multinodular growth pattern. Most cells have clear cytoplasm and a myoepithelial appearance. **b** A high-power view of the same case as in i13.16a, illustrating a second population of cells that form glands and have eosinophilic, rather than clear cytoplasm

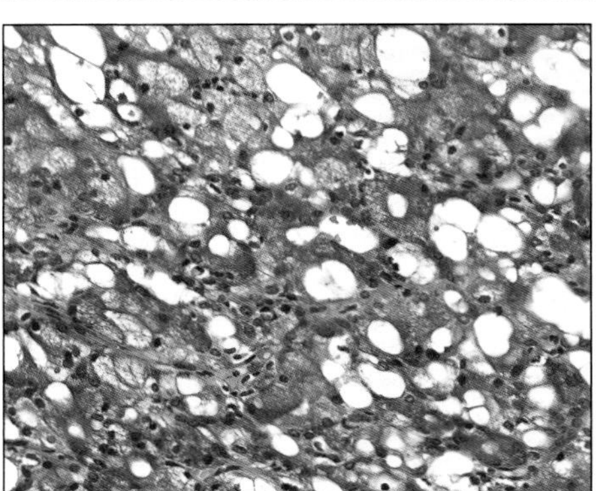

16 The most common pearance of the acinar l tumor is microcys-. consisting of small nds. Note the granular toplasm.

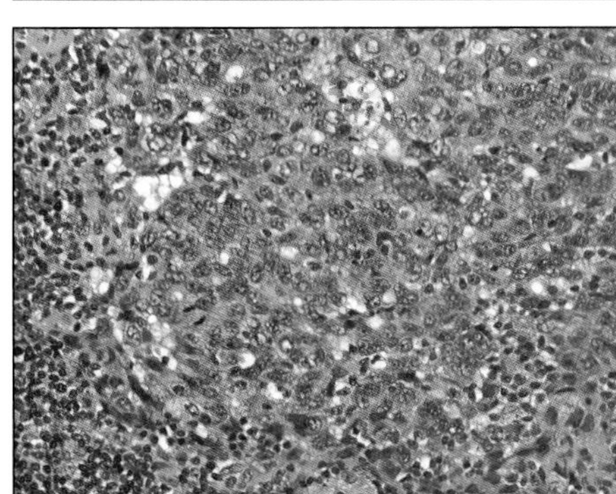

i13.17 A solid pattern of acinar cell tumor. Elsewhere, this case had more classic, microcystic areas.

ISBN 978-089189-5886

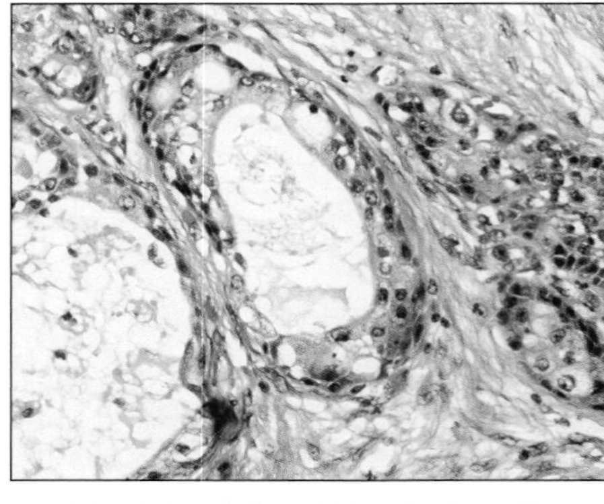

i13.18 Mucoepidermoid carcinoma. Note the overt squamous differentiation, especially on the right, while overt gland formation is evident on the left. The gland in the center is largely lined by squamous epithelium.

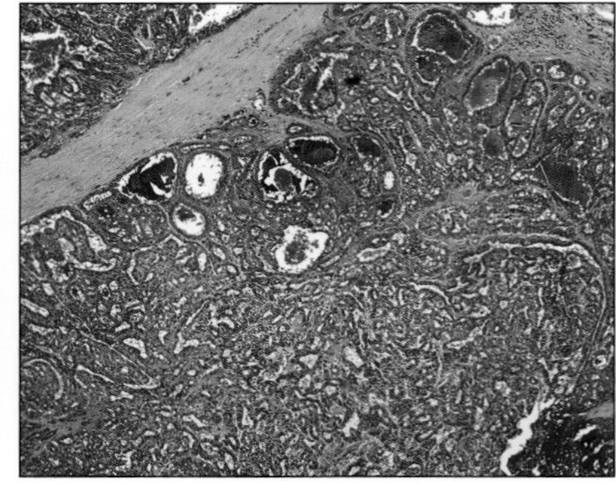

i13.19 A low-power view of a polymorphous low-grade adenocarcinoma (PLGA) resembling sclerosing adenosis of the breast

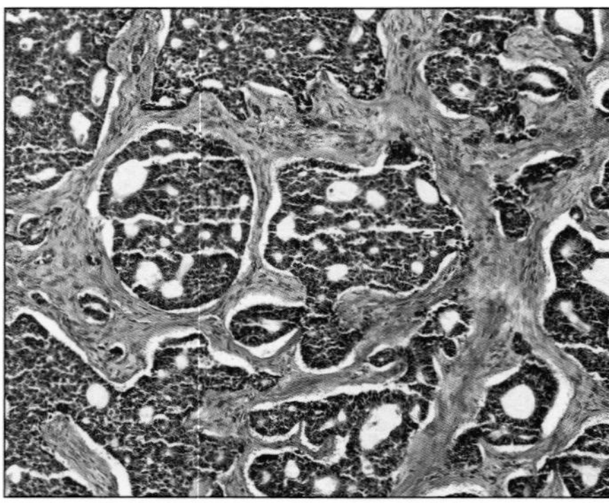

i13.20 PLGA with distinct gland formation

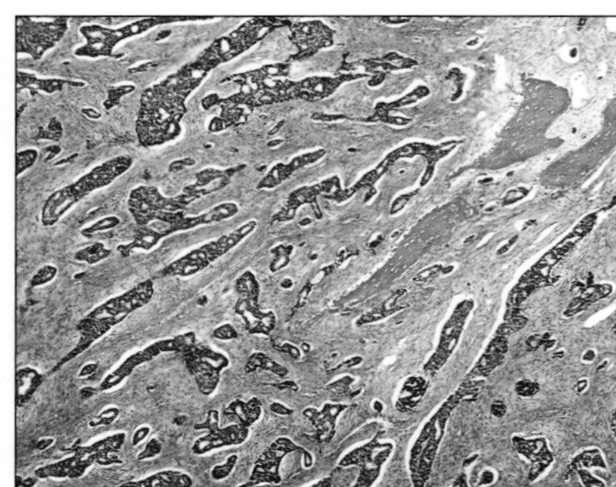

i13.21 Another example of PLGA with a trabecular growth pattern

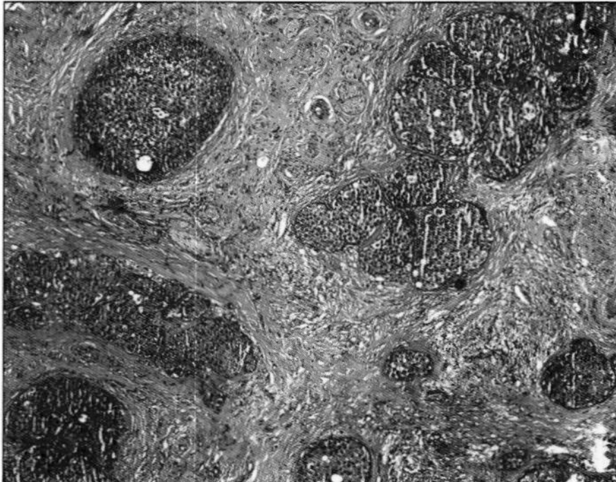

i13.22 Salivary duct carcinoma, which out of context is essentially indistinguishable from high-grade intraductal carcinoma of the breast

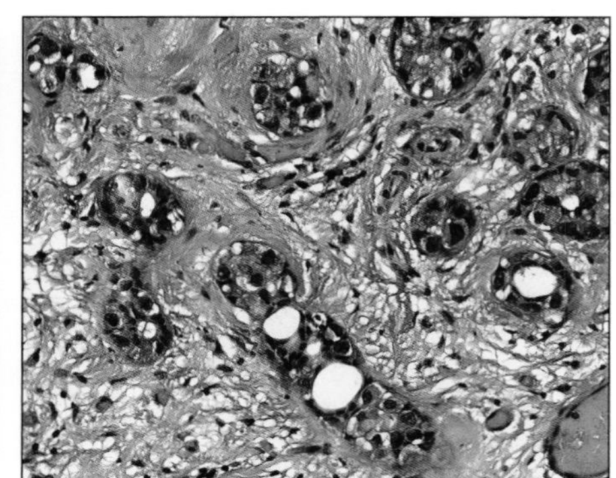

i13.23 Salivary duct carcinoma. The same case as in i13.23. The entire neoplasm is invasive, including the foci illustrated in i13.23, but this field illustrates the high-grade nuclei of salivary duct carcinoma as well as an area which is more immediately recognizable as infiltrating.

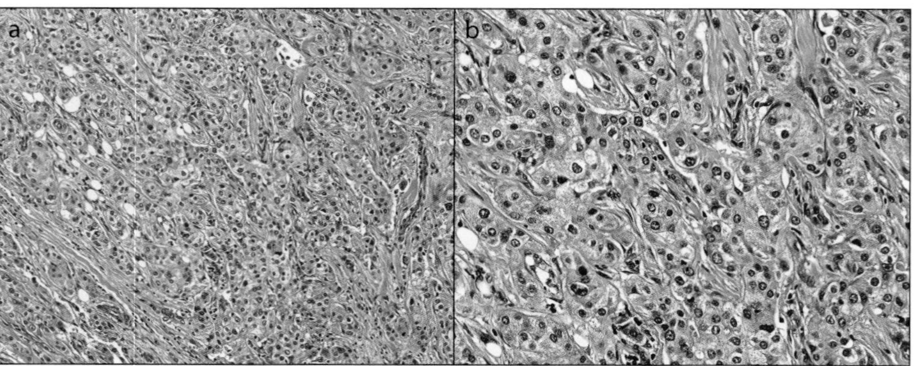

i13.24 **a** Salivary adenocarcinoma, not otherwise specified. This low-power view demonstrates a trabecular pattern that is reminiscent of invasive ductal carcinoma of the breast.

b A higher-power view of salivary adenocarcinoma, not otherwise specified, reinforcing the similarity to invasive ductal carcinoma of the breast

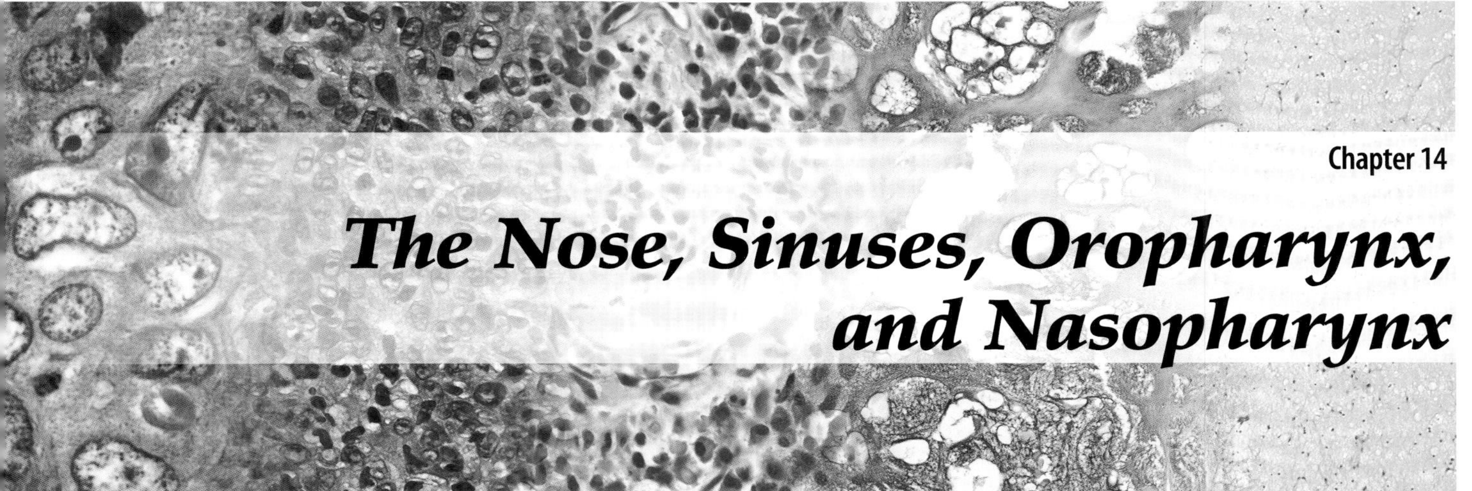

Chapter 14

The Nose, Sinuses, Oropharynx, and Nasopharynx

ıflammatory and Infectious Reactions

Most nasal polyps are not neoplasms, but simply clinical asses caused by nonspecific inflammation and edema i14.1. ı unusual cause of nasal polyps is allergic fungal sinusitis, hypersensitivity reaction to fungus (usually, but not always, *pergillus*) that is roughly a sinus counterpart to allergic bron- opulmonary aspergillosis. Both allergic fungal sinusitis and ergic bronchopulmonary aspergillosis are hypersensitivity actions in immunocompetent patients to noninvasive, other- ise innocuous fungal infection. There is increased mucin pro- ıction, and mucous plugs with eosinophils are characteristic. ıngi are *not* required for the diagnosis and may not be present a given mucus plug. The reason for this is that since the prob- m is a hypersensitivity reaction and not the actual fungus, the ganism may be present in small quantities and may be missed the sampling. In fact, the presence of a large amount of fun- ıs (fungus ball) in an immunocompetent patient suggests poor ainage more than a hyperimmune reaction. Chronic sinusitis the rule in allergic fungal sinusitis, often with nasal polyps.

In contrast to allergic fungal sinusitis, invasive fungal sinus- s is caused by fungi that play a direct pathogenic role, and e causative organism must be identified and treated. Most ses are caused by *Aspergillus* species, but some are caused by *ındida* or *Mucor* species. Fungi may be evident on H&E i14.2, ıt special stains (GMS or PAS) or culture are often needed identify them, and speciation can be very difficult without ılture. In particular, the distinction of *Aspergillus* from *Mucor* ecies on H&E is difficult. I generally recommend the GMS ain for fungi, as fungal organisms stained with this stain ually stand out more against the background than those ained by PAS. The antibody MUC5B stains almost all cases of *spergillus* and *Candida* while staining only a rare case of *Mucor* ecies. Moreover, the rare staining that is seen in *Mucor* spe- es is cytoplasmic, whereas it is in the cell wall of the hyphen the other fungi [PMID18439938]. In some cases, however, fungi nnot be speculated, or even detected, without molecular ethods or culture.

There are 2 unusual infectious processes that occur in the ose and sinuses. Rhinoscleroma is caused by *Klebsiella* species ıd has numerous foamy macrophages. Rhinosporidiosis is a ıronic granulomatous inflammation, with multiple polyps in e sinuses, caused by the protozoan *Rhinosporidium seeberi*, and endemic to only a few places, such as parts of India, Sri Lanka, and Brazil [PMID21814408].

Myospherulosis is a phenomenon that occurs in postopera- tive patients whose wounds have been packed with a petroleum product. It is caused by an interaction of the petroleum with erythrocytes, but may simulate a fungal infection, especially if there is a giant cell reaction i14.3.

Benign Neoplasms and Neoplasm-Like Conditions

Although there is some variation in the terminology of nasal papillomas, most use "Schneiderian papillomas" as a general term for all papillary lesions of the nose, sinuses, or nasophar- ynx. Major types of Schneiderian papillomas are fungiform (exophytic) and inverted. Fungiform papillomas are occasion- ally oncocytic i14.4. Although the inverted papilloma as a whole forms an exophytic mass, the individual collections of epithelial cells grow inward into the stroma i14.5.

The respiratory epithelial adenomatoid hamartoma (REAH) is a rare lesion of nasal cavity, nasal septum, sinuses, or naso- pharynx, derived from submucosal glands [PMID20237993], whose epithelial component may have goblet cells or may resemble a colonic adenomatous polyp, but are generally ciliated i14.6. The stroma may resemble a hemangiopericytoma i14.7 or an inflammatory myofibroblastic tumor, or it may be hyalinized. It may be confused with a low-grade sinonasal adenocarcinoma (discussed below) if it is found in the sinonasal area. In this situation, the cilia are a major distinguishing feature [PMID7639474].

A variety of vascular lesions occurs in the sinuses. The usual types of hemangioma occur in the sinuses, but perhaps the most enigmatic vascular lesion of the sinus area is the heman- giopericytoma. Hemangiopericytomas of the sinonasal area have the same appearance as those of other body sites i14.8 but usually have more myoid differentiation than the usual soft tissue hemangiopericytoma [PMID12766577] and therefore may be a different entity. For this reason, some call these tumors heman- giopericytoma-like to indicate that they may not be identical to their soft tissue counterparts. Sinonasal hemangiopericytomas usually behave in a benign manner with possible local recur- rence but not metastases, but as is the case for hemangiopericy- tomas in soft tissue, malignant forms occur and mitotic activity is the best guide to identifying these cases. As is the case for their counterparts in soft tissue, there is some feeling that even

ISBN 978-089189-5886

the benign examples, because of their potential for local recurrence, may be better regarded as low-grade malignancies.

The head and neck area is one of the more common sites for extranodal sinus histiocytosis with massive lymphadenopathy (SHML; also called Rosai-Dorfman disease), which often simulates a neoplasm. This condition is discussed in Chapter 2 **i2.65**, **i2.66** and should be excluded in all granulomatous/infectious diagnoses or in any situation where there are collections of macrophages or apparent Langerhans cells. SHML is associated with plasma cells and fibrosis. The principal cells stain for CD68, as do ordinary macrophages, and also stain for S100 and CD1a.

The angiofibroma occurs in the nasopharynx, primarily in young men and is characterized by a fibrous stroma with large numbers of vessels of varying caliber **i14.9**. Angiofibromas have testosterone receptors [PMID19626637]. Rarely, a pituitary adenoma will invade beyond the sella and present in the nasopharynx. Additional rare lesions in this site include craniopharyngioma, meningioma, plasmacytoma, and "glioma" (heterotopic glial tissue).

Malignant Sinonasal Neoplasms

The routine squamous cell carcinoma of the sinonasal area is omitted in this work, as it is rarely a diagnostic problem and is thoroughly discussed in other texts.

Sinonasal adenocarcinomas are relatively rare and are divided into intestinal and nonintestinal types, depending on the nature of the epithelium. Intestinal type adenocarcinomas of the sinonasal area tend to be associated with occupational exposure, particularly to wood dust [PMID11190758]. Intestinal-type sinonasal adenocarcinomas are generally of higher grade, and usually even the lower-grade examples of this tumor have moderate nuclear atypia, with an appearance similar to a colonic adenomatous polyp, often with small papillae, nuclei found throughout the epithelium (ie, pseudostratification), and a villous architecture. Intestinal metaplasia is common. Higher-grade forms of the intestinal type resemble a conventional colonic adenocarcinoma. Even lower-grade examples of intestinal type sinonasal adenocarcinomas are locally aggressive, with distant metastases in 13% of cases [PMID3953940].

The nonintestinal type of sinonasal adenocarcinoma is divided into low-grade and high-grade variants. The high-grade nonintestinal sinonasal adenocarcinoma is generally readily recognizable as malignant, but in contrast to both the high-grade nonintestinal form and the intestinal form, the low-grade nonintestinal type has uniform nuclei that are small and basally oriented, with little pseudostratification. The diagnosis of carcinoma cannot be made by nuclear appearance alone, and distinguishing a low-grade sinonasal adenocarcinoma of the nonintestinal type from an exuberant, florid benign polyp can be challenging. Particularly difficult is the distinction of a low-grade nonintestinal sinonasal adenocarcinoma from a REAH, since neither entity will have significant nuclear pleomorphism [PMID17198306]. Indeed, these 2 entities often are found together and may be associated [PMID19011560]. Lack of encapsulation and evidence of invasion, either radiographically or in the material available for histologic examination, favors a carcinoma, but encapsulation and invasion are likely to be difficult to assess on curetted material received by the pathologist, and a large benign polyp may erode adjacent bone from pressure effect, simulating invasion radiographically. A low-grade nonintestinal sinonasal adenocarcinoma has subtle pleomorphism and glandular crowding, with mild stratification and back-to-back gland formation [PMID7083137].

Fortunately, this is not as critical a distinction as might initially be imagined. Low-grade nonintestinal sinonasal adenocarcinomas are not aggressive and most will not recur after resection [PMID15714475]. Metastases are not to be expected and no deaths were noted in one long-term study [PMID19591973]. There is, in fact, a role for "watchful waiting" in the diagnosis of a problematic mass whose differential diagnosis resides between an exuberant polyp, REAH, and a low-grade sinonasal adenocarcinoma of the nonintestinal type. If the mass recurs after apparently complete surgical removal, it is likely a low-grade adenocarcinoma, in which case it can be effectively treated by additional surgery or radiation therapy, with reasonable assurance that the delay has caused no harm to the patient.

Sinonasal undifferentiated carcinoma (SNUC) is an aggressive neoplasm that is characterized by neoplastic cells with pleomorphic nuclei, often with small nucleoli, and a modest amount of cytoplasm [PMID19415944]. Mitoses are numerous. SNUC is distinct from the sinonasal adenocarcinomas of both the intestinal and nonintestinal types, and also differs from the undifferentiated *nasopharyngeal* carcinoma, discussed below, not only in the location, but also in its histologic appearance. It has smaller cells and smaller nucleoli than nasopharyngeal carcinoma. There is less syncytial growth, fewer lymphocytes, more necrosis, and no association with Epstein Barr virus (EBV). In contrast to undifferentiated nasopharyngeal carcinoma, SNUC usually lacks expression of cytokeratins 5/6 [PMID12459626].

The olfactory neuroblastoma (esthesioneuroblastoma) is a malignant neoplasm that arises from the olfactory epithelium of the upper portion of the nasal septum. Its cells may have a concentric arrangement, with or without rosettes, resembling the adrenal neuroblastoma **i14.10**. It may also have cytoplasmic fibers and may also resemble conventional neuroblastomas on electron microscopy. Adenocarcinoma should be excluded before the diagnosis of olfactory neuroblastoma is made, particularly if there are no fine cytoplasmic projections in the lumens. This may require immunohistochemical stains. Olfactory neuroblastomas may also have a solid growth pattern **i14.11**. The immunohistochemical profile of the olfactory neuroblastoma is very similar to that of the conventional neuroblastoma, and an additional feature is S100 positivity in the sustentacular cells that surround clusters of tumor cells [PMID19700942].

While extranodal natural killer (NK)-cell lymphomas are rare in any site, they are most commonly seen in the sinonasal area and the presence of any lymphoma in this site should prompt an exclusion of this entity, with immunohistochemical stains as described in Chapter 8. NK-cell lymphomas are discussed and illustrated fully in Chapter 8, but **i14.12** shows this entity associated with submucosal glands of a sinus.

In my experience, the only neoplasm of bone or cartilage that occurs with any frequency in the sinonasal area is the low-grade chondrosarcoma **i14.13**.

Ialignant Neoplasms of the Nasopharynx

Almost all carcinomas of the nasopharynx are squamous. ıe very rare adenocarcinomas in this region may simulate livary or thyroid papillary adenocarcinomas [PMID16844563]. ıe terminology for poorly differentiated carcinomas of the sopharyngeal region is somewhat confusing, as it is for neoısms of the sinonasal area, but these are forms of squamous ll carcinoma, rather than adenocarcinoma, as are encountered the sinonasal region. A few squamous cell carcinomas in the sopharynx will be overtly keratinizing. These should be diagısed as squamous cell carcinomas of the usual and common pe, but most nasopharyngeal carcinomas are nonkeratinizing.

The nonkeratinizing nasopharyngeal carcinomas are conlered to be differentiated if they exhibit the architectural aracteristics of squamous epithelium, such as stratification, tercellular bridges, or arrangement of cells in a "jigsaw" nfiguration, and undifferentiated if there are no squamous aracteristics at the H&E.

Nonkeratinizing nasopharyngeal carcinomas, particularly the undifferentiated type, have large nuclei with a markedly sicular chromatin pattern (with the chromatin disproportionıly on the periphery) and very prominent nucleoli. There is pically very little necrosis, often a partial syncytial growth ttern, and the neoplastic cells may be spindled. There are any lymphocytes, often causing confusion with lymphoma, ıd immunohistochemical stains are needed to identify the oplasm as a carcinoma. For this reason, these undifferentiıd carcinomas are sometimes called lymphoepithelioma. chitecturally, there are 2 forms in the undifferentiated nasoaryngeal carcinoma, one in which the neoplastic cells form hesive nests within a sea of lymphocytes level **i14.14a**, **i14.14b** ıd one in which the neoplastic cells are dispersed **i14.15a**, **i14.15b**. ıe latter type is particularly easy to confuse with lymphoma. cases where the nature of the neoplastic process (carcinoma lymphoma) is in doubt, it may be helpful not only to show at the atypical cells are epithelial, but also to show that the mphocytes are polyclonal. The undifferentiated nasophangeal carcinoma generally expresses cytokeratins 5 and 6 IID19077909] and is associated with EBV [PMID1847985]. EBV levels in asma predict risk of recurrence or metastasis of nasopharynal carcinoma [PMID21319149].

Ialignant Neoplasms of the Oropharynx

Like their nasopharyngeal counterparts, oropharyngeal uamous cell carcinomas may be keratinizing or nonkeratinizg. The former has a conventional appearance and is strongly sociated with smoking, but the nonkeratinizing oropharynal carcinoma, found primarily in the area of the palatine nsils and base of tongue, is associated with human papilloavirus (HPV) rather than smoking. Nonkeratinizing oropha ngeal squamous cell carcinomas may have an undifferentiıd morphology identical to the nasopharyngeal carcinoma **.16** [PMID20421782], but whereas nonkeratinizing *naso*pharyngeal rcinomas are associated with EBV, nonkeratinizing *oro*phangeal carcinomas are associated with HPV, especially type [PMID20551264]. HPV can be identified in 72% of nonkeratinizing opharyngeal carcinomas [PMID21777945]. Viral load testing for PV has been described in patients with nonkeratinizing oroıaryngeal carcinomas [PMID22240447].

These carcinomas are also associated with p16, a tumor suppressor protein that is overexpressed, but apparently misdirected, in many HPV-related processes [PMID16504868], as discussed in Chapter 46. Indeed, a positive immunohistochemical stain for p16 has greater sensitivity in the detection of HPV than in situ hybridization in head and neck squamous carcinomas [PMID21572401].

There are 2 potential consequences to the association of oropharyngeal carcinomas with HPV. First, despite a propensity for early metastasis to regional neck lymph nodes (often the presenting symptom), HPV-associated oropharyngeal nonkeratinizing squamous cell carcinomas are overall less aggressive than their keratinizing counterparts [PMID18270337]. For this reason, it is desirable to ascertain the HPV status of these carcinomas. Second, in dealing with metastatic squamous cell carcinoma of unknown primary in cervical lymph nodes, the finding of HPV suggests an oropharyngeal primary over a squamous carcinoma of the lung in cases where clinical and radiographic studies are not rewarding [PMID18300234].

Wegener and Its Differential Diagnosis

Midfacial necrotizing lesion (also called lethal midline granuloma) is a clinical designation that may have a number of pathologic correlates. The 3 most common of these are Wegener, angiocentric lymphoma, and idiopathic midline destructive disease.

A clue to the possibility of Wegener is an extensive and destructive neutrophilic infiltrate, often with eosinophils **i14.17**, associated with necrosis **i14.18**. Large numbers of lymphocytes and plasma cells are typical **i14.19**, and granulomas are often seen **i14.20**. Wegener usually, but not always, has necrotizing vasculitis of small- and medium-sized vessels **i14.21**, **i14.22**. Because there is an extensive inflammatory infiltrate, the affected vessels may be difficult to identify and staining for CD31 or CD34 may highlight damaged vessels.

Before the diagnosis of Wegener is made, neoplasia, infection, and intranasal drug abuse must be excluded. The diagnosis of Wegener should not be made until every effort to exclude an infectious etiology—including cultures—has been made. Once this is done, attention should then be turned to the 3 cardinal microscopic features of Wegener—granulomas, vasculitis, and necrosis—and to the presence or absence of involvement of the lungs and kidneys. If all 3 cardinal histologic features are present in the nasal midline, then involvement of the lung *or* kidney secures a diagnosis of Wegener. If only 2 histologic features are present in the nasal midline, then *both* the lung and kidney must be involved for a firm diagnosis. If only 1 of the 3 microscopic features is present, or if there are 2 microscopic features and only one other organ site, one can only be suspicious of systemic Wegener [PMID2337204], and a diagnosis of a limited form of Wegener is appropriate. One should be particularly suspicious of Wegener if the granulomas are destructive or are in vessel walls. Antineutrophilic cytoplasmic antibody (ANCA; discussed in more detail in Chapter 19) is an important supporting test for Wegener. Although neither cytoplasmic ANCA (c-ANCA) nor perinuclear ANCA (p-ANCA) is specific for Wegener, c-ANCA is more closely associated with Wegener than p-ANCA [PMID15804710].

Angiocentric lymphoma is a heterogeneous group, and this term is not specifically used in the WHO classification as a distinct entity. They are often of natural killer or natural killer/T-cell origin. As discussed in Chapter 8, true natural killer cell lymphomas are associated with EBV, occur disproportionately in Asian patients, and often in the nasal or nasopharyngeal area [PMID20614334]. The neoplastic cells may be large or small, often with nucleoli and clear cytoplasm. Widespread necrosis is almost always seen. In angiocentric T-cell lymphomas, blood vessel walls are invaded by neoplastic lymphocytes, but they not necrotic. There is often an accompanying polymorphous infiltrate [PMID11296995]. Although giant cells and true granulomas may occur in these lymphomas, they are unusual and their presence requires exclusion of Wegener or idiopathic midline destructive disease. In contrast to Asian patients, the rare angiocentric lymphomas of the nasal midline in Western patients are usually EBV-negative B-cell lymphomas.

Idiopathic midline destructive disease does not have true vasculitis, but may have secondary vasculitis. This diagnosis is achieved by the exclusion of infection, Wegener, lymphoma, and drug abuse [PMID7064915].

Core Points for the Nose, Sinus, and Pharynx

- Allergic fungal sinusitis: hypersensitivity reaction to fungus (usually *Aspergillus*).
  - o Essentially a sinus equivalent to bronchial allergic bronchopulmonary aspergillosis.
  - o Both occur in immunocompetent patients and are to be distinguished from true fungal infection.
- Hemangiopericytomas of the sinonasal area: same general appearance as those of other body sites but more myoid differentiation.
- Sinonasal adenocarcinomas: rare and occur in intestinal and nonintestinal forms.
  - o Must be differentiated from an exuberant nasal polyp and also from the respiratory epithelial adenomatoid hamartoma (REAH).
- Sinonasal undifferentiated carcinoma: aggressive, with pleomorphic nuclei.
- Nasopharyngeal squamous carcinomas of the nonkeratinizing and undifferentiated type: large nuclei, a vesicular chromatin pattern, and prominent nucleoli.
  - o Often accompanied by many lymphocytes (old term lymphoepithelioma)
  - o Often associated with Epstein Barr virus.
- Nonkeratinizing poorly differentiated squamous carcinomas of the oropharyngeal area: similar morphology to nasopharyngeal carcinomas.
  - o But often associated with human papillomavirus (HPV) rather than EBV.
  - o If associated with HPV, are overall less aggressive.
- Keratinizing oropharyngeal squamous carcinomas are generally not associated with HPV and tend to be more aggressive.
- Midfacial necrotizing lesion (lethal midline granuloma): clinical term
  - o Most common corresponding pathologic entities are Wegener granulomatosis, angiocentric lymphoma, and idiopathic midline destructive disease.
- Classic histologic triad of Wegener: granulomas, vasculitis, and necrosis
  - o Definitive diagnosis requires exclusion of neoplasia, infection, and drug abuse, and involvement of the lungs or kidneys.
  - o In difficult cases, the presence of antineutrophilic cytoplasmic antibody suggests Wegener.
- Angiocentric lymphoma: heterogeneous group, not a specific diagnosis.
  - o Often of the natural killer or NK/T immunophenotype.
- Idiopathic midline destructive disease: clinical diagnosis of mid facial necrotizing lesion, but no specific histologic diagnosis can be made.

.1 Nasal polyp
ıstrating pronounced
ıema of the stroma

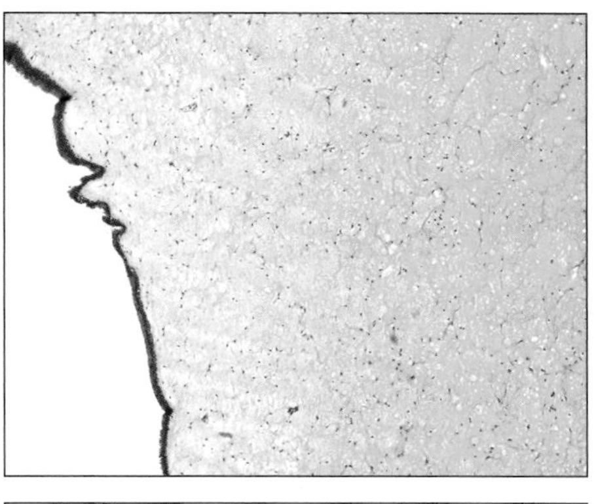

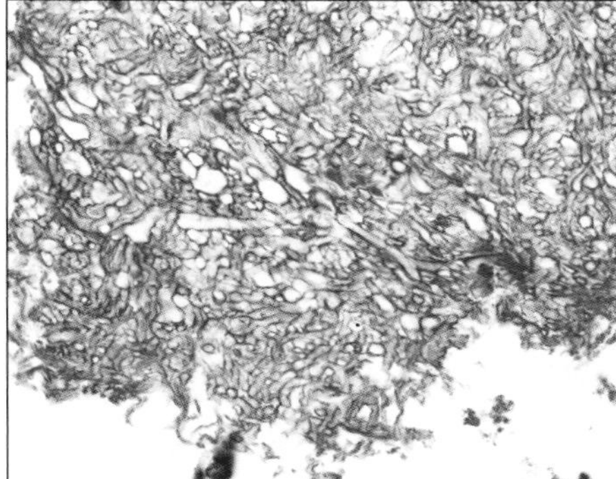

i14.2 Fungus infection of the sinus. This is *Mucor* mycosis.

.3 Myospherulosis, with
giant cell reaction to
e foreign petroleum
aterial

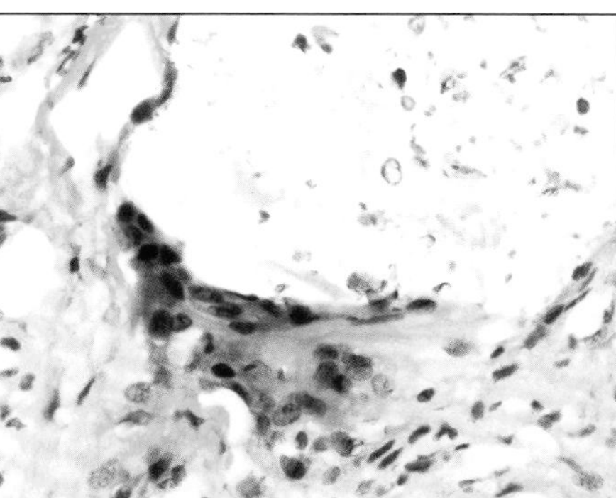

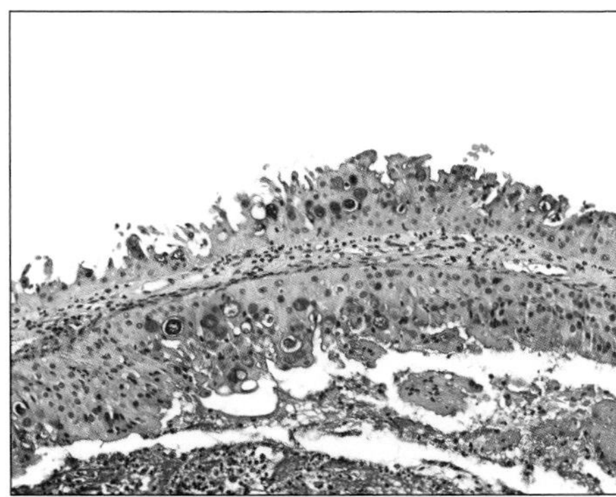

i14.4 Fungiform papilloma of the sinus of the oncocytic type

.5 Inverted papilloma of
e sinus. Note the overall
ophytic architecture
used by the entophytic
owth of nests of benign
uamous epithelium.

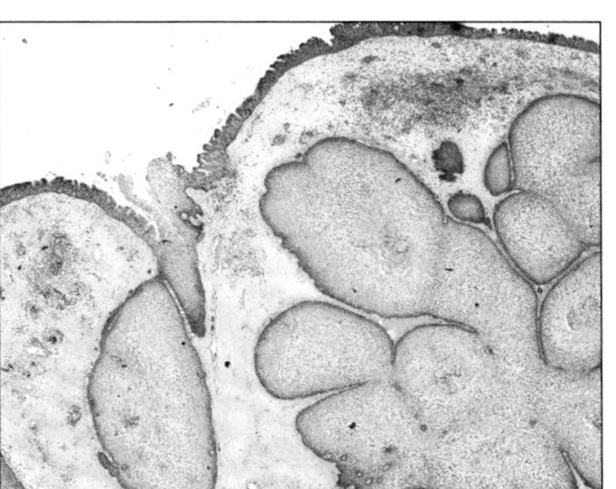

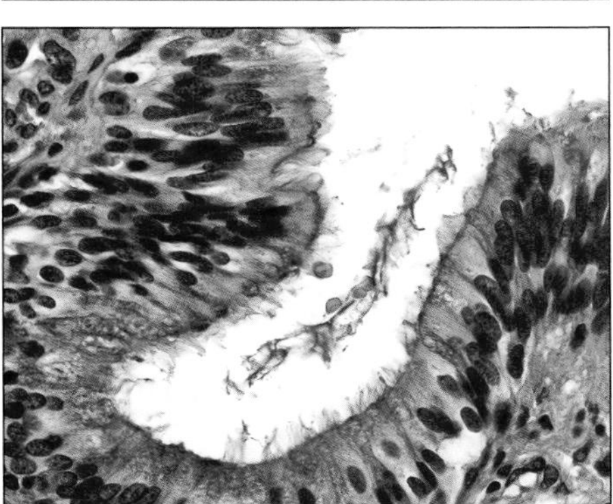

i14.6 The respiratory epithelial adenomatoid hamartoma (REAH). Note the goblet cells in the left lower portion while the left upper portion resembles a colonic adenomatous polyp. Note also that most of the cells are ciliated.

.7 Hemangiopericytoma-
ke stroma in a REAH

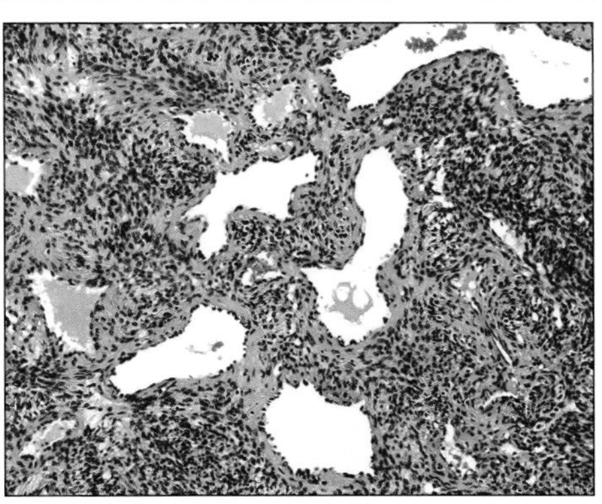

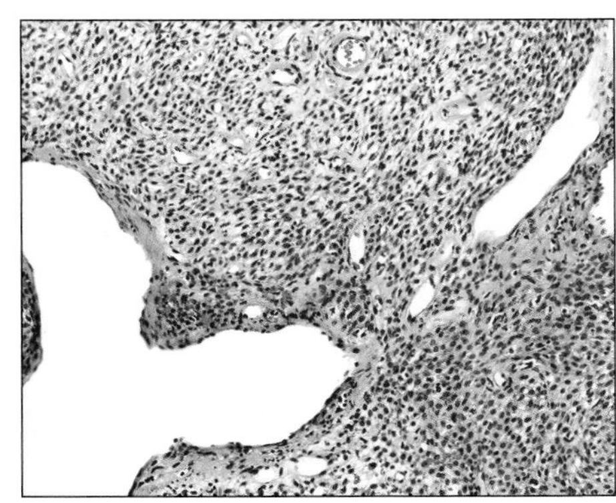

i14.8 Hemangiopericytoma of the sinonasal area. Unlike most hemangiopericytomas in soft tissue, this case was positive for actin immunohistochemical stain.

.9 An angiofibroma
 the nasopharynx in a
ung man, illustrating
ood vessels of differing
liber and a fibrous
roma

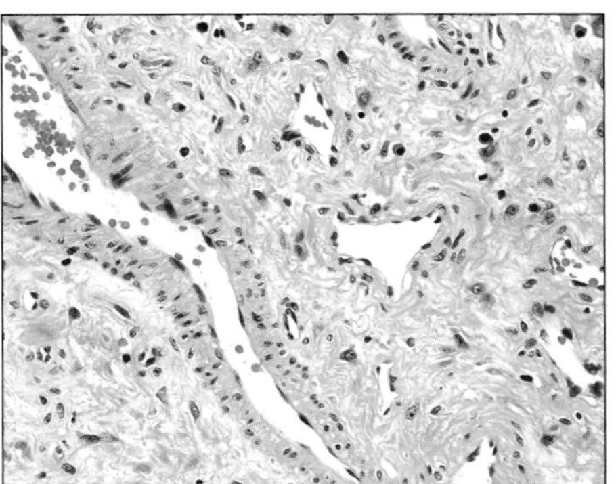

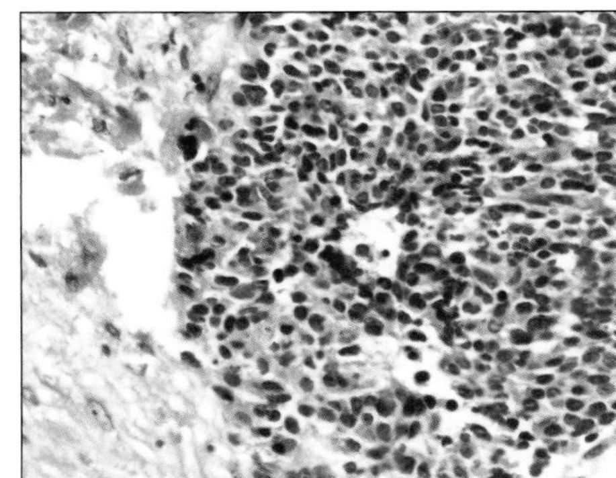

i14.10 An olfactory neuroblastoma with some neoplastic cells having a concentric arrangement. These attempts at rosette formation may simulate an adenocarcinoma.

ISBN 978-089189-5886

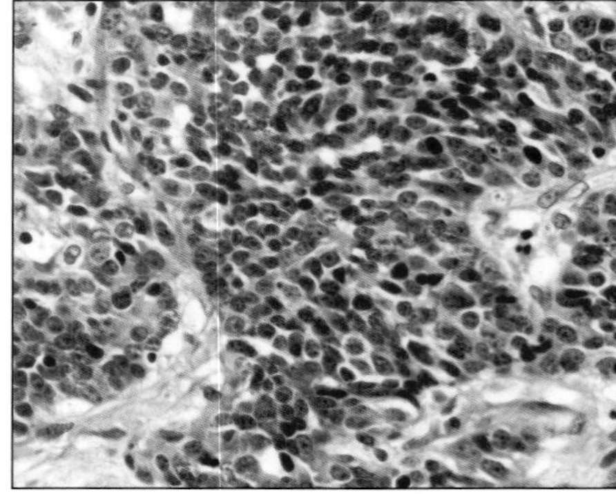

i14.11 Olfactory neuroblastoma with a solid growth pattern. This pattern may also be confused with adenocarcinoma.

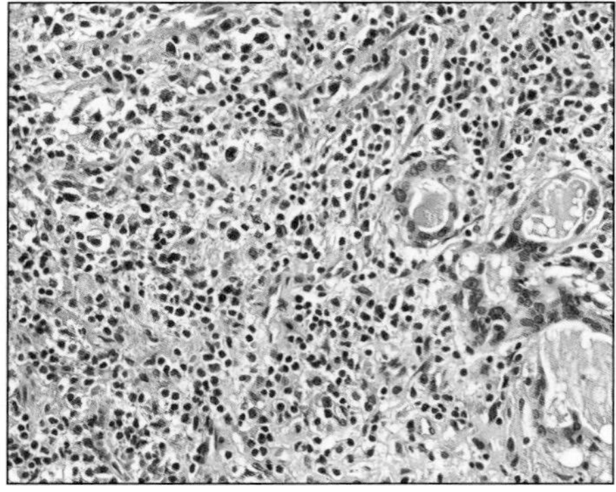

i14.12 Extranodal natural killer cell lymphoma of a sinus. Note the benign glands on the right side.

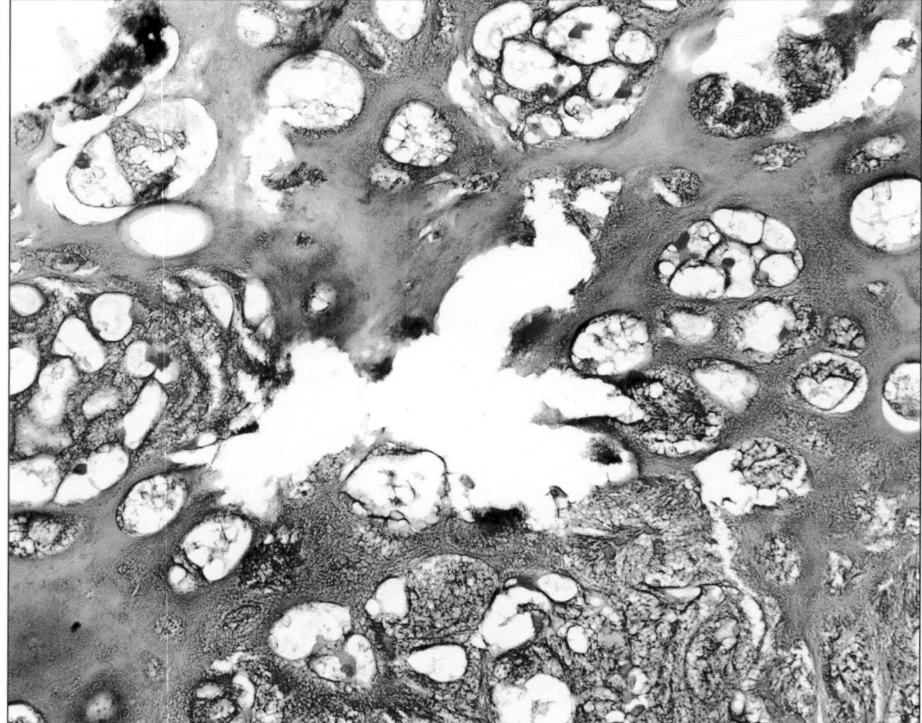

i14.13 Low-grade chondrosarcoma of the sinonasal area. As is always the case with bone or cartilaginous neoplasms, clinical and radiographic correlation is necessary for the correct diagnosis, but note the hypercellularity in the upper portions, with lacunae very close together.

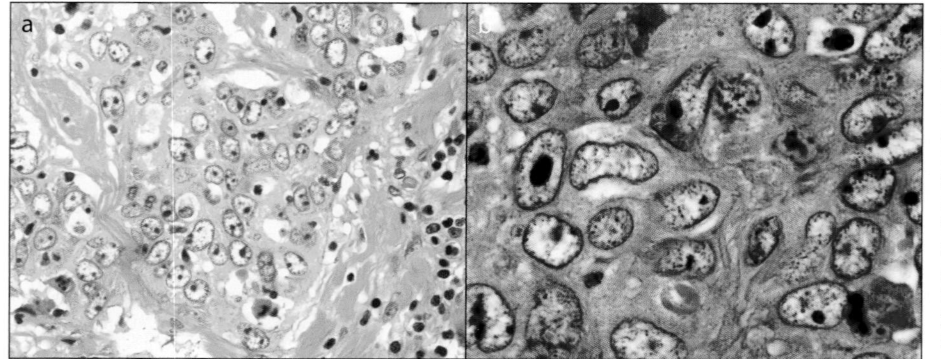

i14.14 **a** A nonkeratinizing, undifferentiated nasopharyngeal carcinoma in which the neoplastic cells form clusters. Note the lymphocytes on the right which accompany the clusters, but generally do not intermingle with the neoplastic cells therein.

b A high-power view of the same as case in i14.14a, illustrating the very large nucleoli and the vesicular chromatin pattern. Although this neoplasm is fundamentally undifferentiated, there is a very small amount of keratin in the lower middle portion, and from top to bottom along the center, the neoplastic cells fit together in a manner suggestive of squamous epithelium.

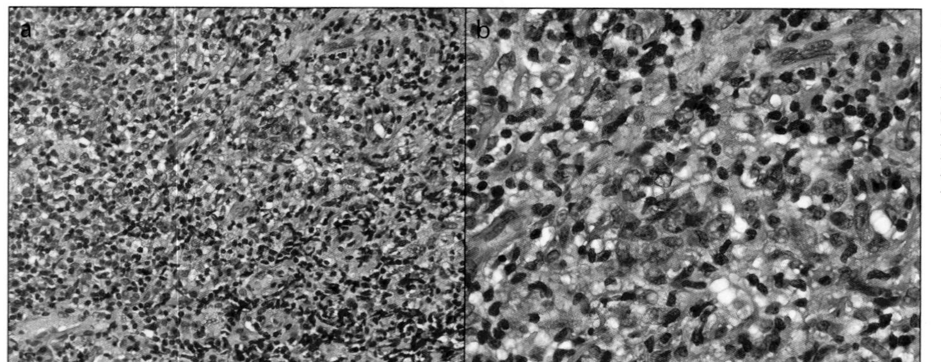

i14.15 **a** A nonkeratinizing undifferentiated nasopharyngeal carcinoma in which the neoplastic cells are dispersed among lymphocytes. The initial impression is lymphoma.

b A higher-power view of the same case as in i14.15a, in which the neoplastic cells are seen as larger cells with nucleoli scattered within the background benign lymphocytes.

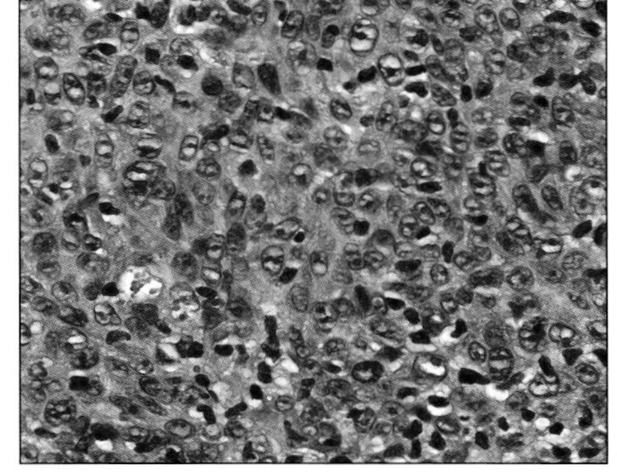

6 A nonkeratinizing differentiated cinoma of the or arynx (this case is m the tonsil). Note great similarity to nonkeratinizing differentiated sopharyngeal cinoma.

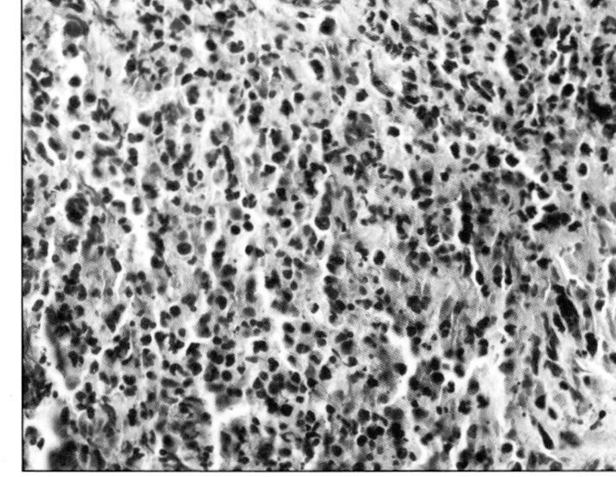

i14.17 The next 6 photomicrographs illustrate the many faces of Wegener granulomatosis. In this image, there are large numbers of neutrophils, mixed with eosinophils, and necrosis.

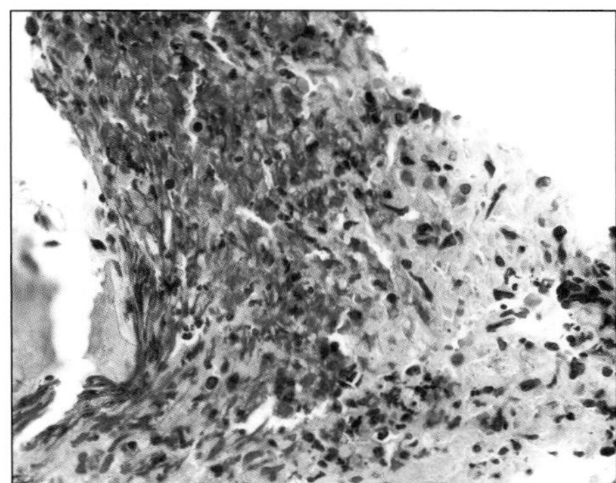

8 Another illustration necrosis in Wegener

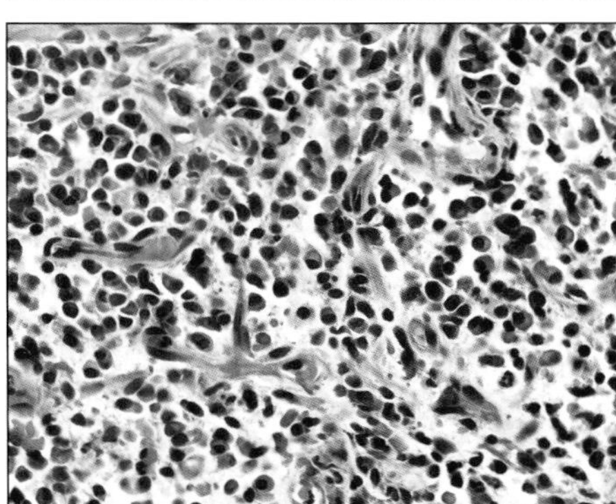

i14.19 Although acute inflammation and necrosis are common in Wegener, a lymphoplasmacytic infiltrate is typically seen in other areas.

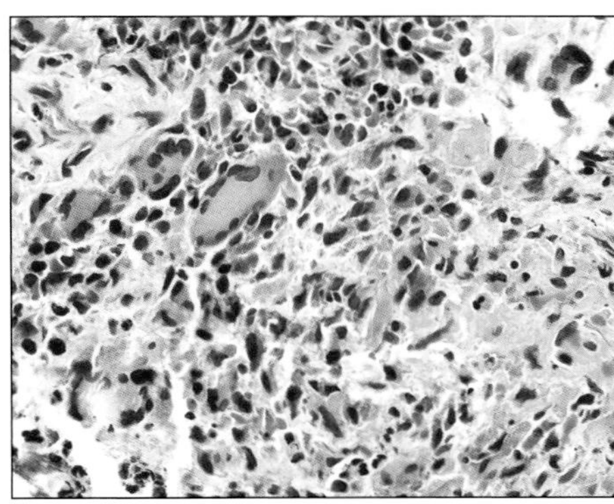

20 A granulomatous us in Wegener

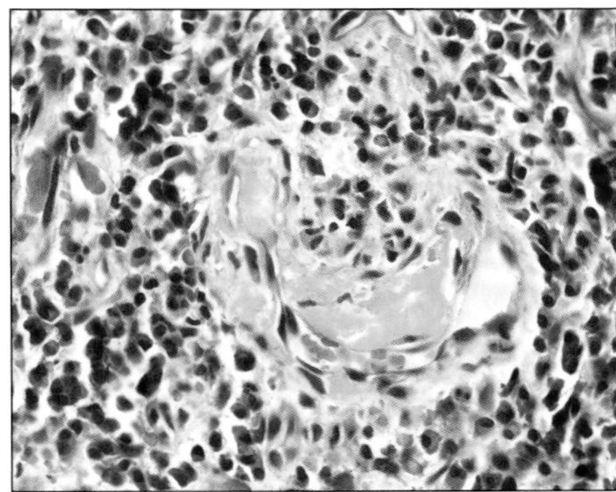

i14.21 Fibrinoid necrosis of the wall of a blood vessel, indicative of vasculitis, in Wegener granulomatosis. Fibrinoid necrosis resembles amyloid but is negative in a Congo red stain.

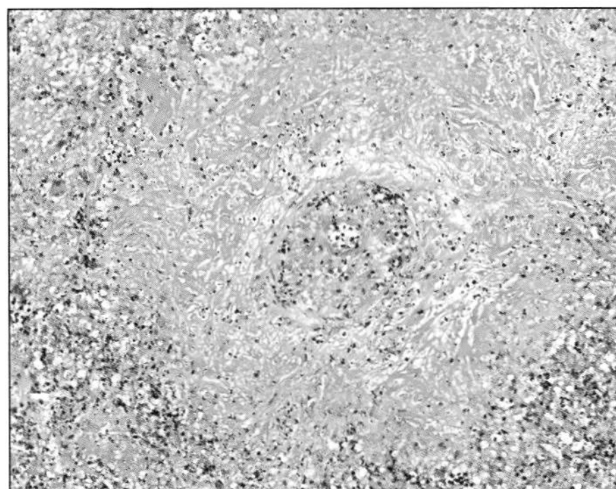

22 i14.17-i14.21 were from nasal septum, but this age is from Wegener nulomatosis of the ng, illustrating acute sculitis and geographic crosis.

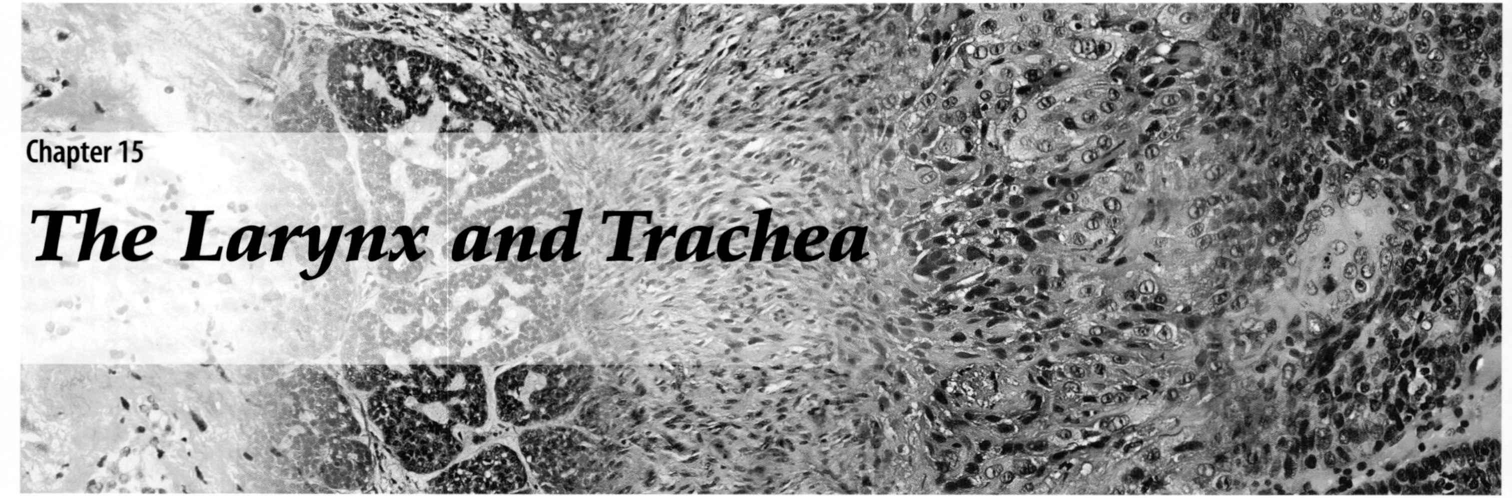

Chapter 15

The Larynx and Trachea

The false cords (more correctly called the upper vestibular folds) are above the true vocal cords. The space between the false vocal cords and the true vocal cords is the ventricle. The glottis refers only to the true cords and the commissure between them. The supraglottis extends from the tip of the epiglottis to the true cords. The subglottis (infraglottis) extends to the first tracheal cartilage. Normally, the epithelium of the larynx is of the pseudostratified, ciliated respiratory type, with the exception of the stratified squamous epithelium that is found on the true cords. However, squamous epithelium may be the rule throughout the larynx in smokers, and even in nonsmokers, occasional patches of squamous epithelium may be seen. By the time a lesion from the supraglottis or subglottis is biopsied, it is often lined by squamous epithelium. Except in situations of trauma or inflammation, the squamous epithelium is usually nonkeratinized.

Nonneoplastic Processes

The stroma in vocal cord polyps (also called laryngeal nodules) may be edematous i15.1, myxoid i15.2, collagenous/hyalinized i15.3, or a combination of these types. Trauma to the epithelium i15.4, with hyperkeratosis and parakeratosis i15.5 is common. Severely traumatized polyps may be ulcerated i15.6. There may be reactive atypia but there is no intraepithelial neoplasia (dysplasia). There may be fibrin deposition i15.7 and telangiectatic vessels. In a biopsy of an apparent polyp, if there is no stroma i15.5 it is wise to comment that a more significant process cannot be excluded.

In adults, squamous papillomas of the larynx may occasionally be multiple but are usually solitary and incidental. In contrast, laryngeal papillomas in children are almost always multiple and usually occur as a syndrome called juvenile-onset laryngeal papillomatosis i15.8, i15.9, which is associated with human papillomavirus (HPV) types 6 and 11. In children, these multiple lesions can be substantially obstructive, often requiring surgical removal or laser ablation [PMID10923940]. The differential diagnosis for these lesions in adults is a papillary squamous cell carcinoma.

Persistent, unexplained ulcers or areas of inflammation of the larynx or pharynx may occasionally be secondary to unsuspected esophageal reflux i15.10. The most vulnerable area is the subglottis [PMID20213655]. Often, such patients may not have a known history of gastroesophageal reflux and may not be aware of classic "heartburn" symptoms.

Epithelial hyperplasia of the larynx can be overdiagnosed as carcinoma. Exuberant hyperplasia, simulating carcinoma, may be associated with or caused by other entities, such as a stromal granular cell tumor.

Laryngeal Neoplasia and Intraepithelial Neoplasia

Common squamous cell carcinoma of the larynx and laryngeal intraepithelial neoplasia (dysplasia) are diagnosed by the same criteria as employed in other sites and are illustrated in i15.11 but not discussed here because they rarely pose diagnostic dilemmas and are well covered in a number of other texts. Here, we discuss only some unusual forms of squamous carcinoma.

The verrucous hyperplasia/verrucous carcinoma lesions, discussed in Chapter 12, are also encountered in the larynx i15.12 and can be diagnosed in the same manner. As was the case in the oral cavity, the pathologist can avoid the debate on the precise nature of the verrucous carcinoma because the imperatives are to identify any invasion and to assess the margins.

The papillary squamous carcinoma is a rare variant of invasive squamous carcinoma that has a papillary exophytic component i15.13 but invades into the stroma in the usual manner for a squamous carcinoma i15.14. Invasion may be difficult to prove in a biopsy of a papillary squamous carcinoma because the interface of the epithelium and stroma may not be well seen, but when a single papillary lesion is encountered in an older patient and there is significant atypia, a comment is in order that a papillary squamous carcinoma cannot be excluded.

The basaloid type of squamous carcinoma usually has an aggressive course. Basaloid tumors in this location are more likely to be variants of squamous carcinoma than true basal cell carcinoma. The initial appearance of a basaloid type of squamous carcinoma is that of a cutaneous basal cell carcinoma i15.15, but the nuclei are higher grade. Another clue to this diagnosis is the frequent (but not invariable) presence of areas of classic squamous cell carcinoma i15.16 or high-grade squamous dysplasia/carcinoma in situ i15.17. The basaloid type of squamous carcinoma may also resemble a high-grade neuroendocrine carcinoma (small cell carcinoma), and it is wise to exclude the latter entity before diagnosing a basaloid type of squamous carcinoma. If areas of a more typical invasive uamous carcinoma or of squamous carcinoma in situ are not en, immunohistochemical stains may be needed. Unlike a uroendocrine carcinoma, basaloid squamous carcinoma is gative for chromogranin and synaptophysin, and positive r low molecular weight cytokeratins 5/6 [PMID19077909]. High olecular weight keratin CK903 (also called 34βE-12) is more ely to stain basaloid squamous carcinoma. p63 is of less help, t will stain basaloid squamous carcinomas more diffusely d strongly than neuroendocrine carcinomas [PMID18284937].

The basaloid form of squamous carcinoma may also resemble enoid cystic carcinoma i15.18. Immunohistochemistry is useful this distinction, as S100 [PMID8393682] and p63 [PMID15529180] stain saloid squamous carcinomas more diffusely than adenoid stic carcinomas.

Laryngeal sarcomatoid carcinomas (carcinomas with rcomatous metaplasia) can be especially challenging because, is the case in other sites, the nonepithelial component can be rprisingly bland i15.19. Moreover, 1/4 to 1/2 will be negative for l epithelial markers [PMID2437812, PMID11812937, PMID2430474], increasing e already substantial temptation to designate the neoplasm a sarcoma. 63% of sarcomatoid carcinomas of the head and ck will be positive for p63 [PMID15976812], so this marker may lp separate sarcomatoid carcinomas from the very rare true rcomas of the larynx, but the best pathway to an accurate agnosis is generous sampling and awareness that sarcomatoid rcinoma is far more common than a sarcoma in an organ.

As in other sites, radiation therapy may cause significant ithelial atypia that simulates carcinoma, but there will not be infiltrative pattern, and there will usually be characteristic romal changes in radiation atypia. Acutely, radiation therapy uses necrosis i15.20. After a healing stage of acute and ronic inflammation i15.21, a chronic stage is reached and characterized by fibrosis i15.22, dilated vessels with mild dothelial atypia i15.23 and atypical, often bizarre, fibroblasts 5.24.

Core Points for the Larynx and Trachea

- Vocal cord polyps (laryngeal nodule): characteristic changes are in the stroma—edema, myxoid, and/or hyaline.
- Laryngeal papillomas: in adults, usually single and must be distinguished from papillary squamous carcinoma
    - In children, almost always multiple and usually indicate laryngeal papillomatosis, which is associated with HPV types 6 and 11.
- Persistent, otherwise unexplained laryngeal ulcers may be secondary to unsuspected esophageal reflux.
- Laryngeal squamous dysplasia and squamous carcinoma are diagnosed as in other sites
    - Pitfall: misinterpret reactive atypia in a polyp or hyperplasia overlying a stromal process.
- Verrucous lesions of the larynx: possible verrucous hyperplasia/carcinoma
    - Attention to focal invasion and margin status.
- Unusual variants of laryngeal squamous carcinoma: papillary and basaloid.
    - Papillary may have a deceptively bland exophytic surface but is invasive
    - Basaloid has an aggressive course.
- Sarcomatous processes, even if negative for epithelial markers, are more likely to be carcinomas with sarcomatous metaplasia than true sarcomas.

ISBN 978-089189-5886

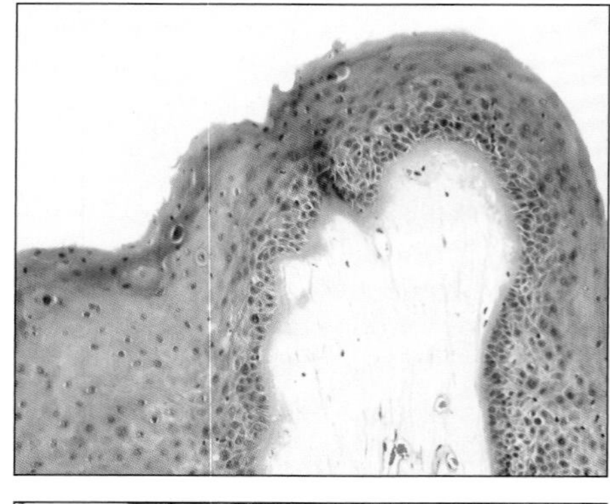

i15.1 A vocal cord polyp with an edematous stroma. Note the hyperkeratosis and parakeratosis, reflective of the trauma that is often seen in vocal cord polyps. This should not be interpreted as intraepithelial neoplasia.

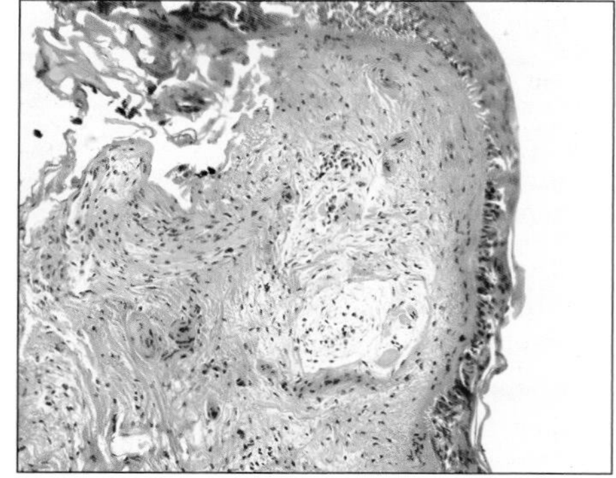

i15.2 A vocal cord polyp with a myxoid stroma

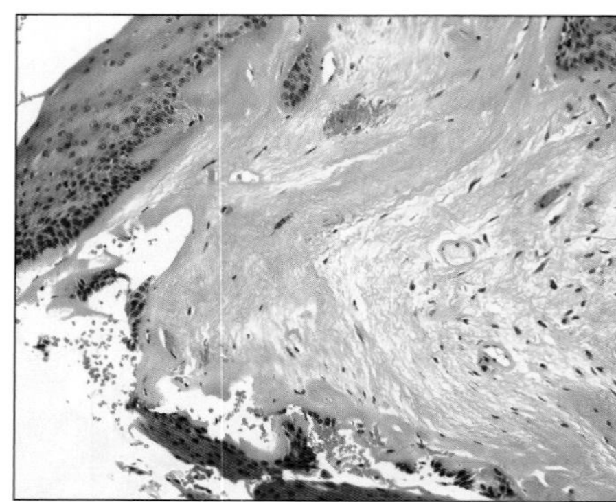

i15.3 A vocal cord polyp with a hyalinized stroma

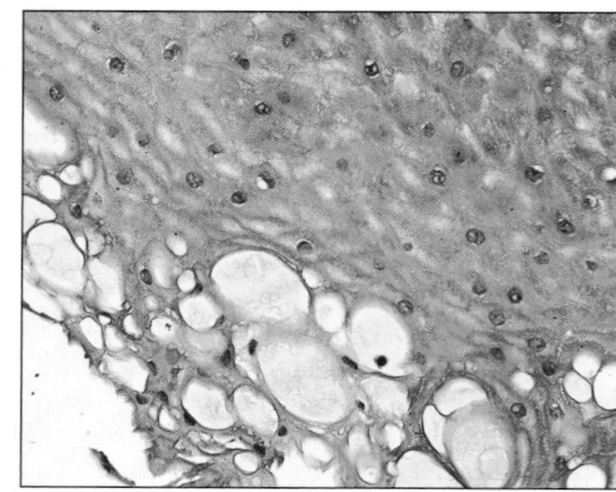

i15.4 A vocal cord polyp with trauma to the outer layers of the epithelium, as shown by ballooning change

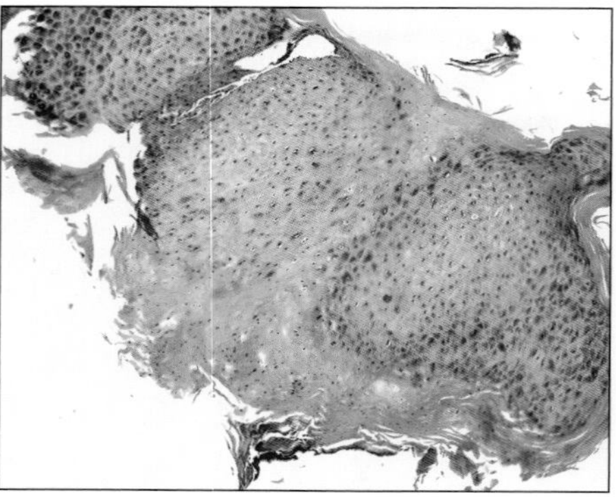

i15.5 A vocal cord polyp with severe hyperkeratosis and parakeratosis. While a carcinoma is exceedingly unlikely given the lack of significant epithelial atypia, it is wise to comment that no stroma is present.

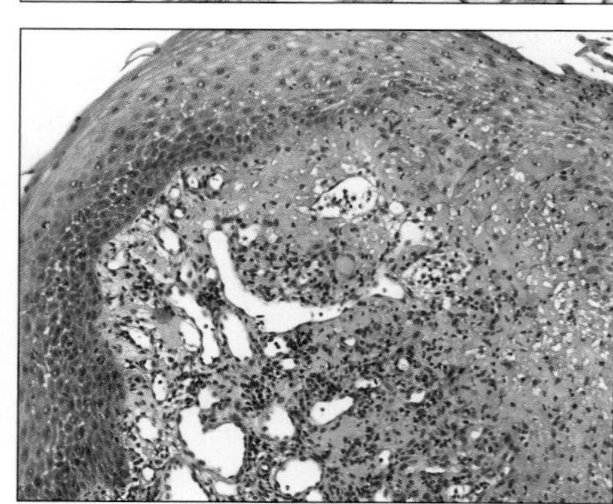

i15.6 A vocal cord polyp with ulceration and a granulation tissue response in the stroma

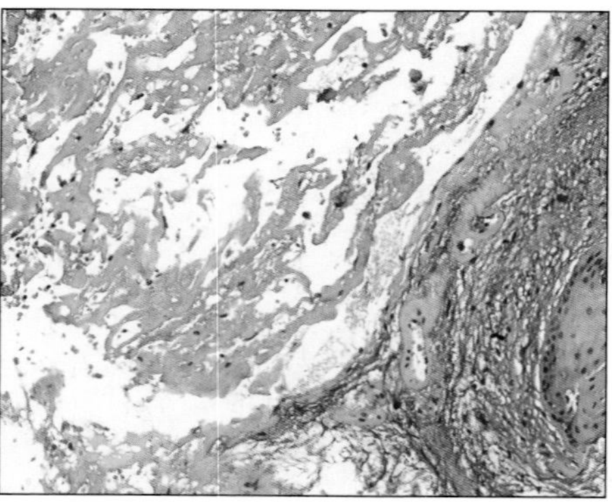

i15.7 A vocal cord polyp with fibrin deposition in the stroma, on the left. Note the myxoid change in the stroma just beneath the epithelium on the right.

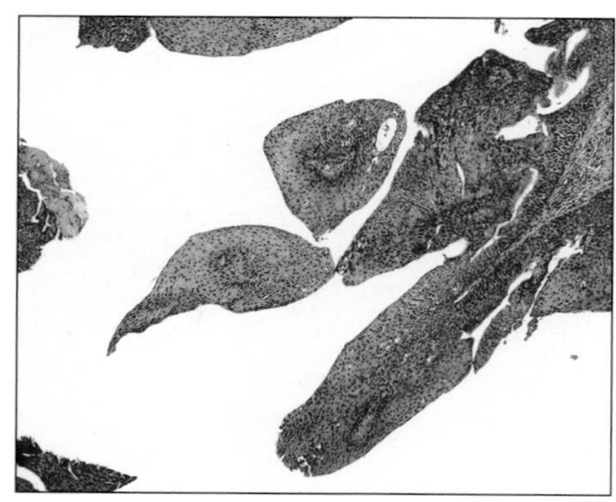

i15.8 Juvenile laryngeal papillomatosis

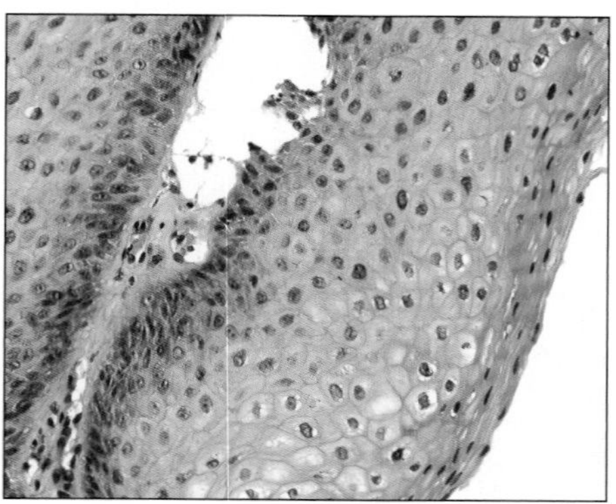

i15.9 A high power view of the same case as in i15.8, illustrating the mild epithelial atypia and small perinuclear haloes, as might be expected with infection by human papillomavirus (HPV). However, this atypia is unlikely to be significant because the HPV types are 6 and 11, which are low risk.

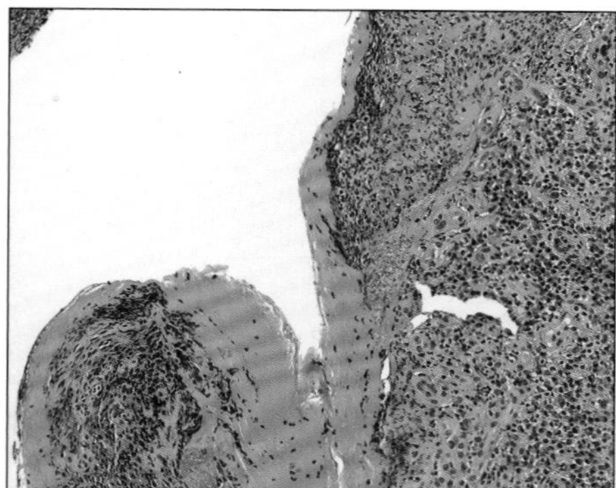

i15.10 Ulceration of the subglottis secondary to unsuspected gastroesophageal reflux

1 Carcinoma in situ
the larynx on the left
h a focus of invasive
amous cell carcinoma
the usual type on the
ver right

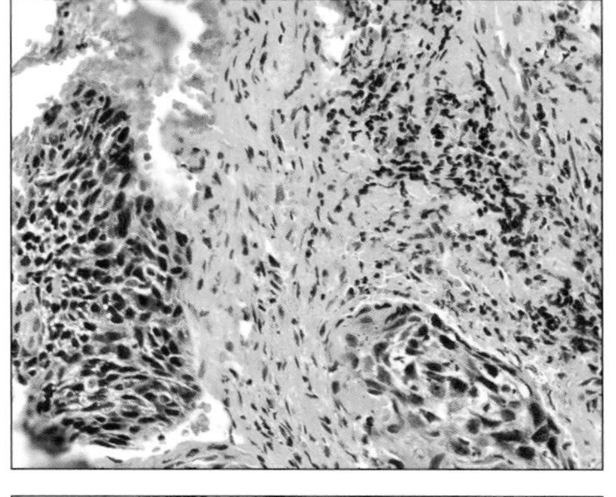

i15.12 A verrucous carcinoma of the larynx. Note the very broad rete pegs which push into the stroma, but the interface of the epithelium in the stroma remains smooth.

3 The exophytic
tion of a papillary
amous carcinoma
the larynx. The
pillae may or may not
monstrate carcinoma
situ.

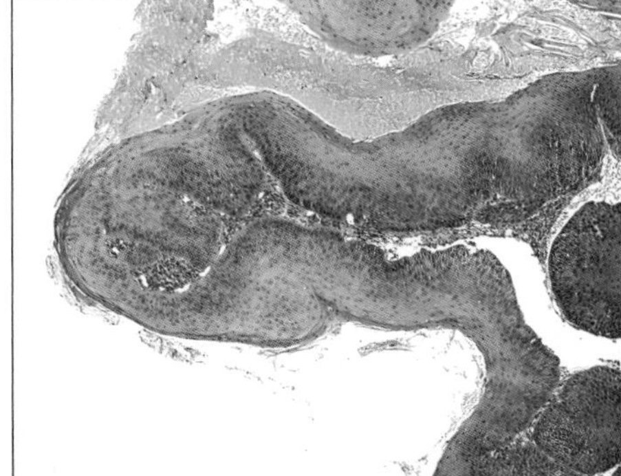

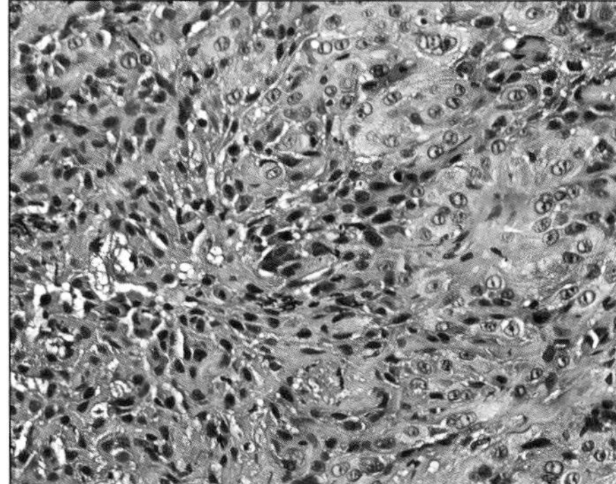

i15.14 The same case as in i15.13, illustrating invasive squamous carcinoma, with a relatively routine appearance, in the lower portion

15 A laryngeal
amous carcinoma
the basaloid type.
te the similarity to
utaneous basal cell
cinoma, but the nuclei
of higher grade.

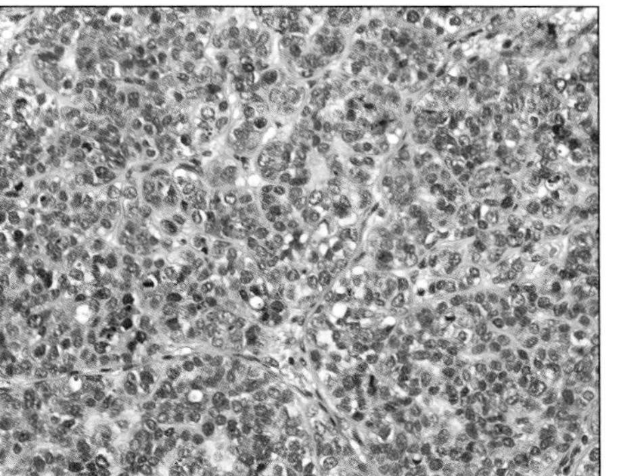

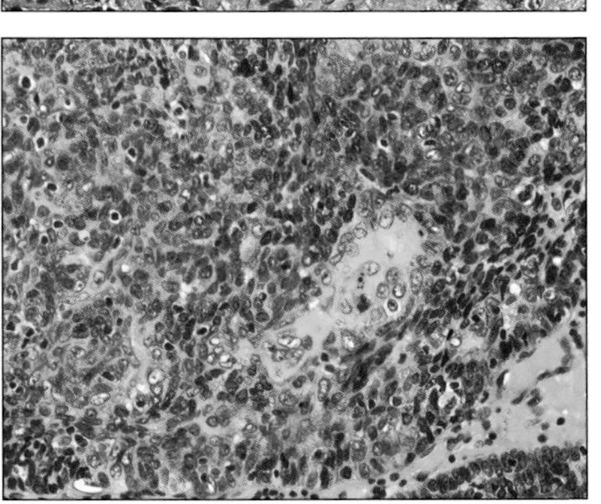

i15.16 A basaloid squamous carcinoma with a rare area of conventional keratinizing squamous carcinoma in the invasive portion

17 High-grade
uamous dysplasia/
cinoma in situ of
surface epithelium
erlying an invasive
saloid neoplasm
ntifies the invasive
mponent as squamous.

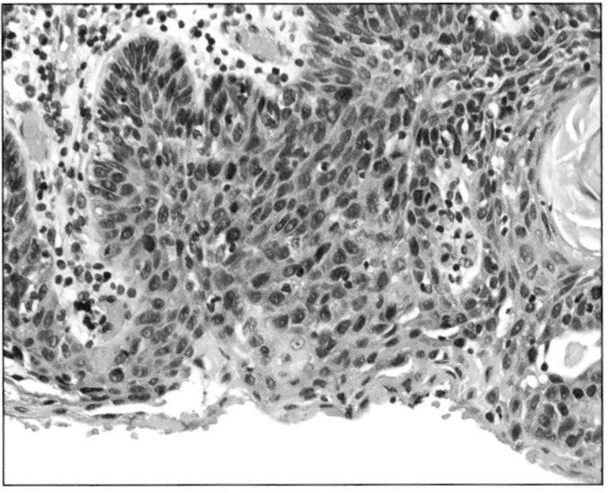

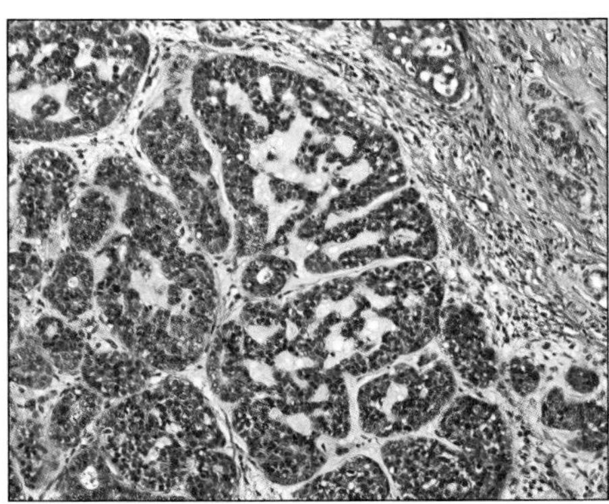

i15.18 A basaloid squamous carcinoma of the larynx resembling an adenoid cystic adenocarcinoma

19 A laryngeal
rcinoma with
rcomatous metaplasia
rcinosarcoma) with a
omal component that is
rprisingly bland and not
mediately recognizable
malignant. These cells
re keratin positive.

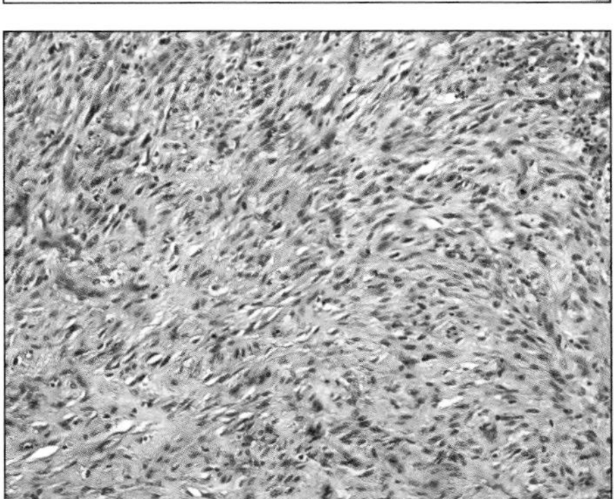

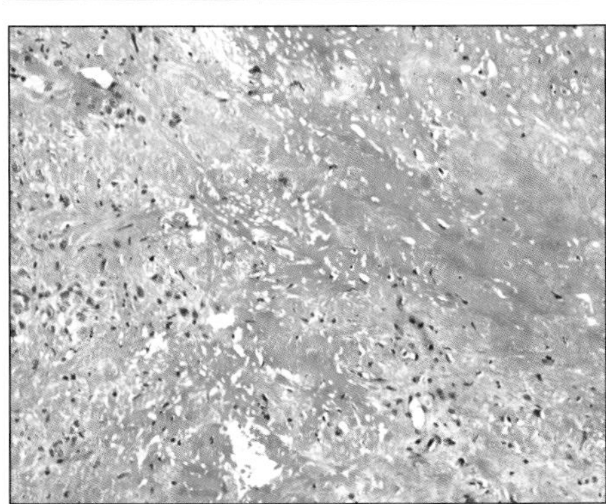

i15.20 Acute radiation injury manifest as necrosis

ISBN 978-089189-5886

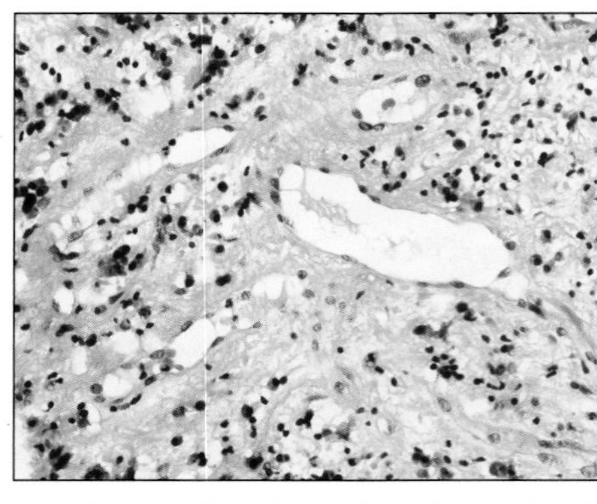

i15.21 The same specimen as in i15.20, illustrating a healing response consisting of acute and chronic inflammatory cells and new blood vessels

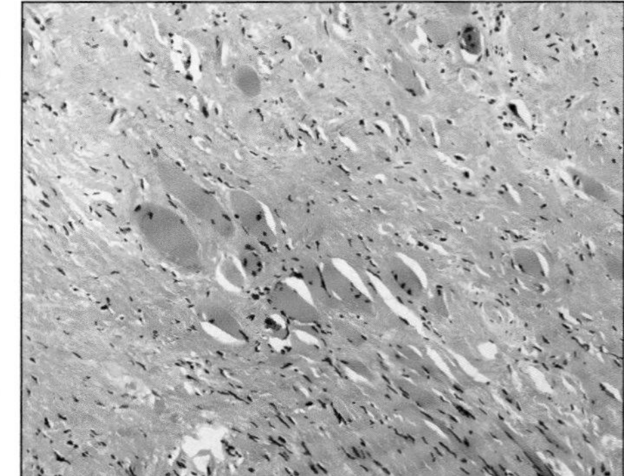

i15.22 The chronic stage of radiation change in which skeletal muscle is heavily infiltrated by fibrous tissue. The sequence of events from necrosis through a healing response to a fibrotic stage is classic healing and repair, as discussed in Chapter 7.

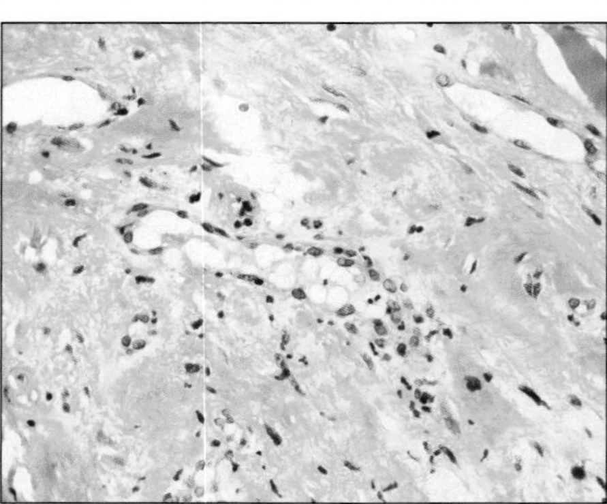

i15.23 Chronic radiation change may also be manifest as dilated capillaries, lined by slightly atypical endothelial cells, in a fibrous stroma without the inflammatory cells that were seen in the healing stage.

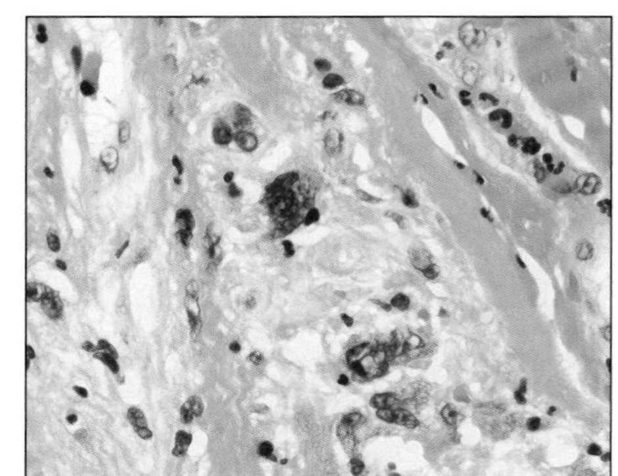

i15.24 Atypical, or even bizarre, fibroblasts are often seen in chronic radiation change

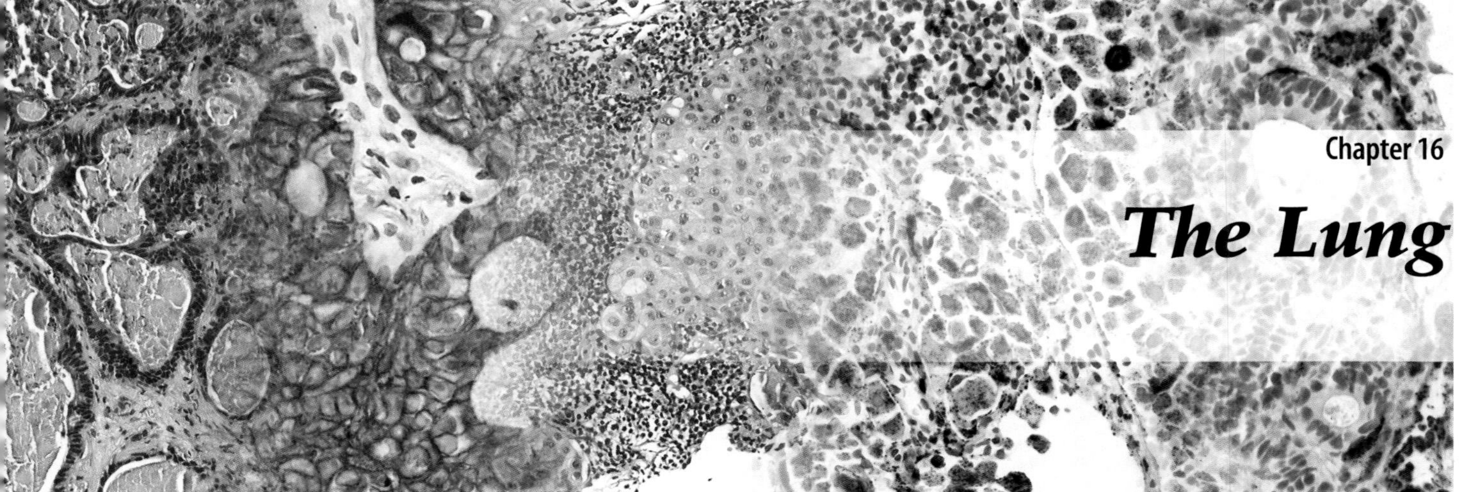

Chapter 16

The Lung

onneoplastic Lung Masses

A pulmonary hamartoma usually has a cartilaginous nponent i16.1, but rarely may not, in which case it often sembles a fibroadenoma i16.2.

Many congenital cystic processes in the lung may present a mass. These include adenomatoid malformation, connital lobar emphysema, bronchogenic cyst, congenital bronectasis, and pulmonary sequestration (a separation of lung sue from the bronchial tree).

Pulmonary hyalinizing granuloma is composed of dense, loidal-type collagen fibers, resembling sclerosing mediasitis, punctuated by small collections of lymphocytes i16.3. ectious agents have been found in some cases and should excluded, but the cause is usually unknown and may be toimmune. The diagnosis is made by exclusion and liberal npling, especially at its periphery, as a solitary fibrous nor may have a paucicellular, fibrotic central area that simtes a pulmonary hyalinizing granuloma. The prognosis good, but there is an association with lymphoproliferative sorders [PMID3799538].

enign Lung Masses

Lymphangiomyoma (lymphangioleiomyoma) usually volves the lung and mediastinum, and sometimes the retroritoneum. It is associated with tuberous sclerosis and often esents with a chylous effusion. Lesions consist of dilated nphatic vessels lined by large amounts of smooth muscle .4. Lymphangiomyomas are thought to be part of a group tumors called PEComas, which occur primarily in younger omen and are thought to arise from the perivascular epielioid cell [PMID19391667, PMID19604538]. Isolated masses respond ell to resection, but disseminated cases (lymphangiomyotosis or lymphangioleiomyomatosis) in the lung may lead progressive pulmonary dysfunction. Like other PEComas, nphangiomyomas are usually positive for HMB-45, actin, d desmin, and are often positive for CD1a [PMID18251780] and catenin [PMID21502434]. They are also positive for estrogen and ogesterone receptors, and respond to hormonal therapy ID11031360].

There may be some smooth muscle in a simple lymphanoma, and it may be problematic to distinguish a lymphangioyoma from a lymphangioma, particularly if there are multiple lesions (ie, lymphangiomyomatosis vs lymphangiomatosis). There is more muscle in a lymphangiomyoma, and it will form small masses rather than being restricted to lining vessels i16.5. In questionable cases, it is wise to favor a lymphangiomyoma (or lymphangiomyomatosis if there are multiple masses) in a young woman and favor a lymphangioma or lymphangiomatosis in a child or man.

The controversial entity "benign metastasizing leiomyoma" should also be excluded in these situations. Many patients with "benign metastasizing leiomyoma" have histories of hysterectomy for leiomyomas, suggesting to some that these are well differentiated metastatic leiomyosarcomas. Others, however, point out that many of these cases run a benign course, which would not be expected if they were metastatic malignancies. Another proposed explanation is the synchronous appearance of multiple leiomyomas that originate in situ [PMID7336571]. There is preliminary evidence that these tumors have a distinct cytogenetic profile that differs from that of the typical uterine myoma [PMID17460458]. Whatever may be the nature of this process, it does not express the HMB-45 that is seen in a lymphangiomyoma.

The sugar tumor is a benign tumor whose cells have clear cytoplasm i16.6. Like the lymphangiomyoma, the sugar tumor has similarities to PEComas and is sometimes grouped with them. The differential diagnosis for a benign sugar tumor includes glycogenated squamous cell carcinoma, primary adenocarcinoma, and metastatic clear cell carcinoma (eg, from the kidney or adrenal). In addition to the benign nuclear appearance and staining for HMB-45, sugar tumors may also stain for HMB-50, another melanosome-associated antigen, and for S-100. Sugar tumors are negative for epithelial antigens. Electron microscopy confirms premelanosomes [PMID11406665].

2 entities are difficult to classify as neoplastic or nonneoplastic: pulmonary meningothelial-like nodules (PMLNs; "tumorlets") and the so-called sclerosing hemangioma. Tumorlets are small collections of cells with small nuclei and minimal cytoplasm i16.7. They may cause brief concern for a neuroendocrine carcinoma, but they are minute incidental findings and are noninfiltrative, with uniform nuclei. They usually (but not always) stain negatively for synaptophysin and chromogranin, and are usually thought to be meningothelial rests rather than minute neuroendocrine neoplasms, as

was previously thought. However, DNA work has not proved that theory either, and some tumorlets do stain with neuroendocrine markers. Tumorlets may be a heterogeneous group, and some of them may be of neuroendocrine origin.

The sclerosing hemangioma remains an enigma. There are a variety of patterns in addition to the fibrous/angiomatous pattern from which the name is derived, such as papillary **i16.8** and solid, and a single tumor may have more than 1 pattern. The proliferation is demarcated from the surrounding tissue, without infiltration **i16.9**. Both the immunohistochemical [PMID2823596] and electron microscopic [PMID4342853, PMID225006] characteristics of the sclerosing hemangioma support an origin from pneumocytes, and these cases are increasingly being called pneumocytomas, though that term has also been criticized since it has not been proven that the cells are truly neoplastic. A minority may be true benign vascular neoplasms **i16.10**, and like the so-called "tumorlets," the sclerosing hemangioma may be a heterogeneous group of proliferations.

Pneumocytomas can resemble a bronchiolar carcinoma or a well differentiated invasive adenocarcinoma, so this entity—whatever name is used—should be excluded before either of those malignant diagnoses are made. Likewise, a bronchiolar carcinoma and a well differentiated adenocarcinoma should be excluded before the diagnosis of benign pneumocytoma is made. In the cases that are vascular, care should be taken to avoid the diagnosis of angiosarcoma. True angiosarcomas are rare in the lung, and as is the case for angiosarcomas in other sites, they are not well demarcated. As is always the case in any body site, beware of a well-demarcated "angiosarcoma." A final point regarding sclerosing hemangiomas is that if they have a fibrous/angiomatous pattern, Kaposi sarcoma should be excluded.

Other benign epithelial processes that can simulate malignant neoplasms are squamous metaplasia and transitional cell papilloma, both of which can simulate a well differentiated squamous cell carcinoma, and squamous cell papilloma with mucous cells, which can resemble a mucoepidermoid carcinoma.

Malignant Lung Neoplasms

Historically, lung carcinoma have been divided into small cell and non-small cell types, as the latter were amenable to potentially curable surgery in 10-15% of patients, whereas the former had invariably spread at least to mediastinal lymph nodes at the time of presentation and could therefore be treated only with chemotherapy and/or radiation therapy. For this reason, the time-honored first step in classifying a lung carcinoma is to correctly place it in the small cell or non-small cell category, which is not as simple as one might think. In 1 study, "9 pathologists with a special interest in pulmonary pathology" had only fair agreement in this most basic question [PMID20459535]. Once again, as we have seen in other situations, such as intraductal lesions of the breast [PMID1847606] and follicular lesions of the thyroid [PMID18854266, PMID15371949], the role of the "expert" appears exaggerated.

Non-Small Cell Lung Carcinomas (NSCLCs)

The 2004 WHO classification recognizes 3 principal types of non-small cell carcinoma (NSCLC)—squamous, adenocarcinoma, and large cell undifferentiated—though many non-small cell lung carcinomas have overlapping features [Travis ISBN978-9283224181].

Squamous cell carcinoma of the lung has the appearance of squamous carcinoma in other sites, and is diagnosed in the same way. It may be preceded by squamous dysplasia of the bronchi, which is also assessed in the same manner as elsewhere. If poorly differentiated, the squamous nature of the carcinoma is identified either by immunohistochemistry as discussed below or by finding focal areas that are better differentiated, with features such as intracellular or extracellular keratin, spinous intercellular connections, or clusters of cells that fit together like pieces of a jigsaw puzzle. Squamous carcinoma is often associated with hypercalcemia that is not caused by metastases. This is usually caused by a protein that resembles parathormone [PMID2885845], though prostaglandins have also been implicated.

Basaloid squamous carcinoma may occur in the lung and resemble the same tumor in the laryngeal or the genital area, with basaloid cells that have minimal cytoplasm. The squamous nature of these neoplasms can be discerned by identifying areas with squamous features **i16.11**, finding squamous carcinoma in situ, or by immunohistochemistry. The basaloid squamous carcinoma may also resemble a small cell carcinoma. Squamous carcinomas of any type, including basaloid, generally stain with p63 [PMID18284937], which is not expected in small cell carcinoma. Thyroid transcription factor 1 (TTF-1) is also helpful. Although originally described in thyroid tumors, TTF-1 is also expressed by 75% of primary lung adenocarcinomas [PMID17616654] and most small cell carcinomas [PMID11956814], but by few squamous cell carcinomas. Small cell carcinomas usually have neuroendocrine differentiation on immunohistochemical stains, especially synaptophysin [PMID2168288].

A detailed discussion of the types of pulmonary adenocarcinoma can be found in the WHO 2004 classification, but the major types are bronchiolar (or bronchoalveolar), acinar, papillary, solid, colloid (mucinous), signet ring, and mixed types. A pure bronchiolar carcinoma, by definition, must have no gland formation, no invasion of the parenchyma between alveolar walls, and a purely lepidic (along the septal walls) growth pattern. A pure bronchiolar carcinoma is rare, and much more commonly, a bronchiolar pattern is part of a mixed adenocarcinoma. The few cases of pure bronchiolar carcinoma are less aggressive [PMID17616987], and pure cases of bronchiolar carcinoma have been called adenocarcinoma in situ [PMID18834206].

There are 2 types of bronchiolar carcinoma, mucinous (also goblet cell or type I) and nonmucinous (or type II). The mucinous type has minimal nuclear atypia, with columnar cells that have abundant mucinous cytoplasm **i16.12**. The nonmucinous variant has less cytoplasm, more nuclear atypia, and often has "hobnail" nuclei (apical, appearing to protrude into the lumen) **i16.13**. The nonmucinous type of bronchiolar carcinoma seems to have differentiation toward Clara cells or type II pneumocytes. Either type may be focally papillary, but e diagnosis of bronchiolar carcinoma takes precedence over at of papillary carcinoma if there is no stromal invasion.

Distinguishing a bronchiolar carcinoma from reactive eumocytes can be notoriously difficult on biopsy material. e remarkable similarity of reactive pneumocytes and bron-iolar adenocarcinoma can not only cause the former to be erdiagnosed, but can also cause the latter to be missed. Few :falls in surgical pathology can wreak havoc in both direc-ns as can the distinction of reactive pneumocytes from onchiolar carcinoma.

Because reactive pneumocyte hyperplasia is usually a dif-se process, the presence of a discrete mass favors a bronchi-ar carcinoma, and one should be cautious in the diagnosis a bronchiolar carcinoma if there is not a defined mass that at least 1 cm. The presence of cilia favors a reactive process ID18708941].

Because the diagnosis of the mucinous form of bronchi-ar carcinoma is largely made by the abundant mucinous toplasm, the differential diagnosis between bronchiolar rcinoma and reactive atypia is particularly acute for the nmucinous form. In these situations, it is important to nsider the milieu. If the background is that of a fibroinflam-atory process, with abundant numbers of inflammatory lls and fibrosis, one should lean toward a reactive atypia less the evidence for neoplasia is compelling i16.14. There is other site in the body in which a fibroinflammatory back-ound calls more forcefully calls for a conservative interpre-tion. Particular caution is advised if the fibrosis forms small dules suggestive of bronchiolitis obliterans with organizing eumonia (BOOP; see following discussion on interstitial ng diseases).

Although reactive pneumocytes is the main differen-l diagnosis in bronchiolar carcinoma, a pneumocytoma d the so-called atypical adenomatous hyperplasia (AAH) ust also be excluded before the diagnosis is made. AAH controversial, but some feel that it is a distinct entity and precursor of adenocarcinoma [PMID11235908], and therefore portant to diagnose. If one subscribes to this viewpoint, d wishes to suggest AAH, its diagnosis requires a distinct, ell circumscribed, small (usually <0.5 cm) lesion, with gaps tween cells on microscopic study [PMID11829087]. To my mind, ven the nebulous nature of AAH and the inability of most aging studies to verify its central features—demarcation d small size—there is little to be gained by distinguishing tween reactive atypia and AAH. Even if the latter entity is stinct and premalignant, no therapy will be given upon its agnosis. The overarching issue is to separate reactive atypia d AAH on the one hand from bronchiolar carcinoma on e other.

In reactive atypia, the alveoli are lined by mildly atypical lls. There will be a few cells that, out of context, are indis-nguishable from those of bronchiolar carcinoma, but the erall atypia is less and there is often a gradation from early benign cells to cells that resemble malignancy or dis-ntinuity between the cells i16.15. Stratification is minimal .16. In bronchiolar carcinoma, there is a more uniform, con-ient population of clearly atypical cells, with increased cel-larity and crowding, resulting in confluence and crowding cells i16.17.

The features which point most convincingly to a bron-chiolar carcinoma are crowding of cells, with confluence, microtufting, focal stratification, generalized nuclear atypia, mitoses, and exfoliation of cells into the alveolar space [PMID17616987], and a clear demonstration of all, or at least most, of these findings is required for the definitive diagnosis of bronchiolar carcinoma.

In difficult cases, equivocation is often prudent and the better part of valor is to render a diagnosis along the lines of "atypical epithelium, cannot exclude a bronchiolar carci-noma." The term "atypical pneumocyte proliferation" has been suggested for these situations [PMID12951843]. One may then discuss the differential diagnosis of bronchiolar carcinoma and the difficulties of the particular case.

On resection material, it may be difficult to determine if there is a pure bronchiolar carcinoma or if there is focal inva-sion. Collapse or fibrosis of the wall may simulate invasion. Features favoring true invasion include irregularly shaped or small glands, a stromal response i16.18, i16.19, and high-grade nuclei. Many cases will have a bronchiolar pattern in some areas, but with focal invasion in other areas. It is wise to report these as adenocarcinomas with bronchiolar features so there will be no doubt about the invasive nature of the tumor. Some advocate giving the percentage of each type, though the clinical utility of this has not been established.

In 2011, a new classification of lung adenocarcinomas was proposed by the International Association for the Study of Lung Cancer, the American Thoracic Society, and the European Respiratory Society, in which adenocarcinomas are considered to be in situ, minimally invasive, or fully invasive [PMID22054879]. This proposed classification does not use the term bronchiolar carcinoma and places carcinomas of this type into the in situ category.

Poorly differentiated NSCLCs often have overlapping fea-tures of both squamous carcinoma and adenocarcinoma i16.20. While this is generally unlikely to make a clinical difference, an effort should be made to determine the precise histogen-esis, as there are unusual situations in which the exact type of tumor may have clinical implications. In these situations, staining for TTF-1 strongly suggests adenocarcinoma, while p63 and cytokeratins 5/6, which stain myoepithelial cells, are associated with squamous origin [PMID19170169, PMID21164283]. Staining with cytokeratin 7 or PE-10, an antibody to surfac-tant apoprotein A, suggests an adenocarcinoma [PMID16647951]. Napsin A, an enzyme involved in the synthesis of surfactant, is more sensitive and specific for lung adenocarcinoma than TTF-1 [PMID22288963], and in fact, a 2-antibody panel of napsin A and p63 accomplishes the distinction between adenocarci-noma and squamous carcinoma in almost all cases [PMID22288962].

Metastatic Carcinomas to the Lung

Many lung carcinomas are metastatic rather than primary. In these cases, the history of a previous carcinoma is often indispensable in the correct interpretation, and immunohisto-chemical stains may help. Foremost among these are cytoker-atins 7 and 20. All cells have 1 or more intermediate filaments that convey structural integrity to the cell. Intermediate fila-ments in nonepithelial cells include vimentin (found in cells of mesenchymal origin), the neurofilament proteins (found

ISBN 978-089189-5886

primarily in neural cells), glial fibrillary acidic protein (found primarily in glial cells), and desmin (found in muscle cells). In epithelial cells, this role is primarily filled by keratins, of which there are about 20 types, numbered 1-20. Epithelial cells from different tissues have different types of keratin, and these types are maintained in malignant transformation.

Differential Expression of Cytokeratins 7 and 20 Has Been Enormously Helpful in Elucidating the Primary Site of a Carcinoma

While cytoplasmic keratin expression is a hallmark of any epithelial cell, some types of keratin are expressed much more in certain epithelial cells than in others. The most clinically useful keratins in identifying a specific origin for an adenocarcinoma are cytokeratin 7 and cytokeratin 20 [PMID11937308].

In general, the following table of cytokeratin 7 and 20 positivities is useful:

7+, 20+	**Urothelial, pancreas, ovarian mucinous** A minority of the following tumors may be 7+, 20+: 10% of colon; 38% of gastric; 11% of lung adenocarcinomas; 7% of HCC; 12% of endometrial; 8% of prostatic; 16% of breast
7+, 20–	**Lung (adenocarcinoma), breast, serous and endometrioid ovarian, endometrium, mesothelioma, cholangiocarcinoma, squamous carcinoma of the cervix** A minority of the following tumors may be 7+, 20–: 11% of urothelial; 17% of gastric; 26% of pancreatic; 17% HCC; 8% of prostatic; 24% of renal; 18% of lung small cell carcinomas; 7% of ovarian mucinous
7–, 20+	**Colon** A minority of the following tumors may be 7–, 20+: 35% of gastric; 9% of pancreatic; 8% of lung squamous; 23% of prostate; 6% of renal; 3% of breast
7–, 20–	**HCC, renal, prostate, lung small cell carcinoma, lung squamous cell carcinoma** A minority of the following tumors may be 7–, 20-: 15% of colon; 10% of gastric; 17% of lung adenocarcinomas; 8% of endometrium; 31% of mesothelioma, 13% of cervical squamous carcinomas

A carcinoma in the lung that is not positive for cytokeratin 7 and negative for cytokeratin 20 should be suspicious for a metastatic tumor. In addition, as mentioned in the differentiation of primary lung adenocarcinoma from squamous carcinoma, most primary lung adenocarcinomas stain for 1 or more of the following: TTF-1, PE-10, and napsin A. Staining for napsin A is strongly suggestive of a primary lung adenocarcinoma [PMID21464700], though it may also be expressed by renal cell carcinomas [PMID22156835]. **i16.21-i16.23** illustrate how the adenocarcinoma in the lung is unlikely to be primary.

There are also immunohistochemical stains that point to a specific primary site other than lung. For example, if an intestinal metastasis is under consideration, nuclear staining for the transcription factor CDX2 is helpful, as this stains most adenocarcinomas of the lower gastrointestinal tract and would not be expected in primary pulmonary adenocarcinomas [PMID12548159, PMID12604886]. **i16.24a** shows how a positive CDX2 on the case shown in **i16.21**, **i16.22**, and **i16.23** identifies the adenocarcinoma in the lung as being of colonic origin, while **i16.24b** and **i16.24c** show how a positive napsin A identifies a metastatic adenocarcinoma in a lymph node as a lung primary.

Historically, the distinction of a primary lung carcinoma and a metastatic breast carcinoma has been very difficult because the cytokeratin 7 and 20 profiles are the same (CK7 positive, CK20 negative), and until recently, more specific stains have not been available. Positivity for estrogen receptor or progesterone receptor, or evidence of overexpression of *HER2* identifies the neoplasm as a metastasis from the breast, but many breast carcinomas will not demonstrate these findings. Mammaglobin and gross cystic disease fluid protein 15 (GCDFP-15) stain a minority of breast carcinomas, but staining is highly specific if present [PMID19217055]. If these markers are all negative, positivity for TTF-1, PE-10, or napsin A suggest a lung primary. **i16.24d** and **i16.24e** illustrate how a positive napsin A elucidates a breast adenocarcinoma as a metastasis from the lung.

Another difficult problem with lung adenocarcinomas is their distinction from mesotheliomas. Pleural-based masses may simulate parenchymal masses on radiographic studies, especially if the mass arises on the visceral pleura between 2 lobes of a lung. The immunohistochemical differences between adenocarcinoma and mesothelial cells are discussed more completely in Chapter 17, but positivity for TTF-1, PE-10, or napsin A suggests a pulmonary adenocarcinoma over a mesothelioma.

Mutations in Non-Small Carcinomas of the Lung

There are numerous mutations that have been described in NSCLC [PMID21277552], but at this writing, 4 are thought to have potential therapeutic benefit. The *ERB-B* family of genes codes for receptor tyrosine kinases, which are single transmembrane protein molecules that have an extracellular domain attached to an intracellular tyrosine kinase. The tyrosine kinase portion of the molecule initiates the intracellular response to the binding of a messenger molecule to the extracellular portion of the receptor. The 2 clinically most important *ERB-B* genes are the epidermal growth factor receptor gene (*EGFR*; sometimes called *ERB-B1* or *HER1*; on 7p12) and *HER2*, on chromosome 17.

ERB-B signaling pathways such as those used by the EGFR protein involve GTPases encoded by genes of the *RAS* gene family. The 3 principal members of the ras protein family are K-ras, H-ras, and N-ras, of which K-ras is the most important. In the normal situation, stimulation of the extracellular moiety of the EGFR protein leads to activation of the tyrosine kinase, which in turn leads to a series of reactions that stimulate K-ras.

Mutations or overexpression of *EGFR* or *HER2* are occasionally found in some malignancies. The most noted example is overexpression of *HER2* in some breast cancers, but a minority of lung or colon carcinomas may have a mutation in the *EGFR* gene that causes increased activity of the intracellular tyrosine kinase portion of the EGFR protein. Activating mutations in the EGFR tyrosine kinase domain are more likely in adenocarcinomas in nonsmoking women and are particularly common in nonmucinous bronchiolar carcinomas in Asian women [PMID20855837]. 90% of these mutations are either deletions in exon 19 or a missense mutation that results in L858R (arginine for leucine substitution at amino acid 858) in the tyrosine kinase domain [PMID20156777].

Gefitinib (Iressa) and erlotinib (Tarceva), inhibitors of the tracellular tyrosine kinase moiety of the EGFR protein, are little clinical benefit in most cases of NSCLCs, but are bencial in the minority of patients with a mutation in *EGFR*, d their use in these patients can result in better outcomes an conventional chemotherapy [PMID20573926]. Consequently, tivating mutations in the tyrosine kinase portion of the GFR protein are favorable because they enhance therapeutic sponse to either antibodies that block the extracellular main of EGFR protein, or to inhibitors of the intracellar tyrosine kinase moiety of the receptor [PMID19644023], and is necessary to identify this subset of NSCLC patients. nfortunately, many patients who initially respond to tyrone kinase inhibitors will subsequently become resistant. any of these cases result from a group of tumor cells that ve a second mutation that results in T790M (ie, codon mber 790 codes for methionine instead of threonine), in the GFR protein, and which become dominant after exposure to rosine kinase inhibitors [PMID17699786]. Initially, immunohistoemistry for the EGFR protein was not clinically useful, but ow, antibodies specific for the proteins resulting from the 2 ost common mutations, while not as sensitive as molecular sting, can identify most positive patients and obviate e need for molecular testing if there is a positive result MID20093391]. PCR examination for these mutations, combined ith FISH studies that look for gene amplification, are approiate in cases that are negative by immunohistochemistry.

A separate minority of NSCLCs may have an activating utation in the "downstream" K-ras protein, and these mutaons have very different clinical consequences. Activating utations in K-ras uncouple it from EGFR and confer tonomy to it, sharply diminishing response to chemotheraeutic agents [PMID19855375]. Mutations in *EGFR* and *K-RAS* genes not occur together, and since mutations in *K-RAS* are more mmon (tending to occur in older patients and in smokers) d will not respond to tyrosine kinase inhibitors, a mutation this gene may be searched for first, unless the patient is unger or has no smoking history [PMID19855375]. *K-RAS* mutaon analysis is usually done by direct sequencing, but newer d shorter methods, such as allele-specific PCR and meltrve analysis, are coming to the fore [PMID21745016].

An uncommon mutation in NSCLCs is an inversion on romosome 2p that results in a fusion gene formed from rts of anaplastic lymphoma kinase (*ALK*) and the echiderm microtubule-associated protein-like 4 (*EML4*) gene, und in up to 7% of patients [PMID17625570] i16.25. The ALK proin is a kinase, and a kinase inhibitor is beneficial in these ses [PMID20979469]. Simple increases in the copy number of *ALK* e more common i16.26, but appear to lack clinical signifince [PMID21107285].

Non-small lung tumors that are positive for the nucleotide cision repair enzyme ERCC1 are resistant to platinumsed chemotherapeutic agents, while those that are negative e prognostically worse without any adjuvant chemotherapy it will respond more to platinum-based chemotherapy MID20944091].

Neuroendocrine Carcinomas of the Lung, Including Small Cell Carcinoma

The 2004 WHO classification of lung malignancies recognizes 4 neoplasms with neuroendocrine features: typical carcinoid, atypical carcinoid, small cell carcinoma, and large cell neuroendocrine carcinoma [Travis ISBN978-9283224181].

To avoid confusion, it is desirable to report both the older and newer terminology in neuroendocrine carcinomas. A carcinoid tumor is a grade 1 neuroendocrine carcinoma, an atypical carcinoid is a grade 2, and a small cell carcinoma is a grade 3 neuroendocrine carcinoma. Grade 1 neuroendocrine carcinomas are characterized by nuclear uniformity, minimal mitotic activity, and no necrosis i16.27. A trabecular growth pattern is common i16.28 and rosettes are often found i16.29. Occasionally, the cells are spindled i16.30.

Grade 2 neuroendocrine carcinomas still have relatively uniform nuclei i16.31, but there is extensive necrosis i16.32 or >2 mitotic figures per 10 high-power fields [PMID20462655]. If the nuclei are pleomorphic or if the mitotic count is >20 per 10 high-power fields, the neoplasm is a small cell carcinoma.

Small cell carcinomas are often not observed in their pristine state because of poor preservation, necrosis, or crush artifact. Where well seen, the cells of small cell carcinoma have pleomorphic nuclei with relatively fine chromatin and minimal cytoplasm i16.33. Only with poor preservation is nuclear detail lost or a coarse chromatin texture seen i16.34. Mitoses and necrosis are common i16.35. Because of the minimal cytoplasm and delicate nuclei, crush artifact and linear streaking of chromatin are common i16.36.

A major problem in biopsy material is that small cell carcinomas can be indistinguishable from lower-grade neuroendocrine carcinomas or clusters of lymphocytes in the presence of crush artifact. An assiduous search for well-preserved cells is the best assurance of an appropriate diagnosis. A malignant diagnosis should not be rendered on or because of crushed cells or linear streaks of chromatin. Other cell types, especially lymphocytes, can display this feature. Just as reactive pneumocyte atypia in a fibroinflammatory background is the pitfall for adenocarcinoma in the lung, so crush artifact without viable, identifiable tumor cells is the primary cause of an inappropriate diagnosis of small cell carcinoma. If more viable areas do not permit a distinction on H&E study, immunohistochemical stains may help but must be used cautiously because they are not reliable when performed on damaged cells and care must be taken to ensure that the stains are interpreted in viable cells. If there are an insufficient number of viable cells, it is wise to equivocate.

As mentioned, differentiating a small cell carcinoma from a poorly differentiated NSCLC is a greater problem than one might initially believe [PMID20459535]. The cells of small cell carcinoma are not necessarily small and may overlap in size with those of NSCLCs. A more reliable feature than cell size in this important distinction is the indistinctness of the nucleoli in small cell carcinomas, but this is not foolproof and immunohistochemistry may be required.

Small cell carcinomas are of neuroendocrine origin but are often negative for chromogranin. They are usually at least focally positive for synaptophysin and TTF-1. In addition, N-CAM (CD56) and MAP-2 are markers associated with neuroendocrine differentiation in lung tumors [PMID12605092]. CD117 stains most small cell carcinomas, as well as some large cell neuroendocrine carcinomas [PMID18091382]. Neuron-specific enolase (NSE) is also a neuroendocrine marker, but is too nonspecific for effective use (indeed, it is called by a variety of derisive names, such as "nonspecific enolase" and "now stains everything"). In my experience, the most helpful stains in the identification of a neuroendocrine neoplasm are chromogranin, synaptophysin, and CD56 **i16.37a**, **i16.37b**, **i16.37c**, **i16.37d**. These 3 markers performed on well-preserved cells will identify almost all neuroendocrine carcinomas and exclude both poorly differentiated non-small carcinomas and clusters of lymphocytes. A good argument can be made that TTF-1 is as good or better than chromogranin, but it must be remembered that TTF-1 also stains most pulmonary adenocarcinomas.

If the differential diagnosis is between a small cell carcinoma and a poorly differentiated adenocarcinoma, TTF-1 is unlikely to help, as both of these neoplasms are often positive. In addition to neuroendocrine markers, helpful immunohistochemical stains include cytokeratin 7, PE-10, and napsin A. While most pulmonary adenocarcinomas stain strongly with cytokeratin 7, most small cell carcinomas stain weakly or not at all [PMID20398190, PMID10987260]. Only about half of lung adenocarcinomas stain with PE-10, but positive staining essentially excludes a small cell carcinoma [PMID11956814], as does staining with napsin A. **i16.38-i16.41** illustrate the use of immunohistochemical stains to identify a poorly differentiated carcinoma as an adenocarcinoma rather than a small cell or squamous carcinoma.

If the concern is to distinguish between a small cell carcinoma and a poorly differentiated squamous cell carcinoma, in addition to neuroendocrine stains **i16.38a**, **i16.38b**, helpful immunohistochemical stains include TTF-1, high molecular weight keratin, and p63, as small cell carcinomas are usually positive for TTF-1 and negative for HMW keratin and p63, while poorly differentiated squamous carcinomas are usually the reverse: negative for TTF-1, and positive for p63 and HMW keratin [PMID15309021]. Cytokeratin 5/6 staining suggests squamous carcinoma over either small cell carcinoma or adenocarcinoma [PMID18091384], but once neuroendocrine differentiation has been excluded, p63 and napsin A are most helpful in suggesting either a squamous or adenocarcinoma, respectively [PMID22288962]. **i16.42**, **i16.43**, **i16.44**, and **i16.45** illustrate the use of immunohistochemical stains to identify a poorly differentiated carcinoma as squamous rather than a small cell or adenocarcinoma.

Rarely, overlapping morphologic features between a small cell carcinoma and an NSCLC will be confirmed by immunohistochemical stains **i16.46**, **i16.47**, **i16.48**.

Once neuroendocrine markers establish the diagnosis of a neuroendocrine carcinoma, Ki-67 is helpful in classifying neuroendocrine neoplasms and preventing an overdiagnosis of small cell carcinoma. Ki-67 will generally stain no more than 2% of cells in a grade 1 neuroendocrine carcinoma, from 2-20% in a grade 2 carcinoma, and at least 25% of cells in a small cell carcinoma. Ki-67 staining in excess of 60% is commonly seen in small cell carcinomas **i16.49** [PMID21043816, PMID15644774].

Immunohistochemical staining for the phosphorylated form of the histone H3 (PHH3) may also be helpful. This histone undergoes phosphorylation in mitosis, concomitant with chromatin condensation [PMID2401299]. Because PHH3 is found only in the actual mitosis phase, as opposed to Ki-67, which is found in any cell that is committed to mitosis, the threshold numbers for classification of neuroendocrine lung tumors will be smaller with staining for this antigen than with Ki-67 [PMID21757598].

A small cell carcinoma may resemble a lymphoma, particularly if there is crush artifact, in which case the presence of necrosis, nuclear molding, and nuclear pleomorphism point to a small cell carcinoma. A small cell lymphoma will have more uniform nuclei, but immunohistochemical stains are essential. One might assume that the immunohistochemical differentiation of any carcinoma from a lymphoma would begin with keratin, and indeed, small cell carcinomas typically have focal or weak keratin staining **i16.50**, while lymphomas do not. However, keratin staining can be inconsistent in small cell carcinomas, and they are usually negative for high molecular weight keratin [PMID15309021], so a better immunohistochemical panel for this situation is synaptophysin, CD56, TTF-1, and CD45. This panel includes 3 stains that are likely to be positive in small cell carcinomas, while the CD45 addresses possible lymphoid lineage. Negativity for CD79 and CD3, encompassing almost every stage of B and T lymphocytes, respectively, provides additional assurance that the neoplasm is not lymphoid.

Large cell undifferentiated carcinoma is diagnosed when there is an NSCLC that does not demonstrate any of the features of squamous or adenocarcinoma by either H&E morphology or immunohistochemistry. This category may contract now that many poorly differentiated squamous carcinomas and adenocarcinomas can be identified by immunohistochemistry. Some cases of large cell undifferentiated carcinoma have neuroendocrine features by immunohistochemistry, but the therapeutic implications of the diagnosis of large cell neuroendocrine neoplasms are unclear at this time. Some feel these should be treated as small cell carcinomas because the neuroendocrine differentiation is the most significant feature, while others feel that the neuroendocrine features are less important in large cell undifferentiated carcinomas. The pathologist need not weigh in on this controversy but should either perform and document neuroendocrine stains, as well as p63 and napsin A, on any NSCLC that is not a straightforward squamous or adenocarcinoma, or indicate a willingness to do so if desired.

are Malignant Lung Neoplasms

The 2004 WHO classification recognizes 5 subtypes of rcomatoid carcinoma: pleomorphic, spindle cell, giant cell, rcinosarcoma, and pulmonary blastoma. The first 3 types e poorly differentiated NSCLC whose principal histologic atures follow from their names. The carcinosarcoma is a orly differentiated NSCLC with sarcomatous metaplasia.

Pulmonary blastoma is a type of carcinoma with sarco-atous metaplasia. It occurs in young to middle-aged adults. ie biphasic variant is often characterized by tubules that e lined by tall columnar cells, looking somewhat like the ands of an adenomatous colonic polyp or an endometrioid rcinoma, in a stroma of immature mesenchymal cells .51. There may be squamous metaplasia adjacent to the ands. The spindle stroma is neoplastic but usually stains for mentin only, and not for epithelial markers.

The pleuropulmonary blastoma occurs in children younger an 10 and has a somewhat similar appearance to the mes-chymal component of a pulmonary blastoma i16.52. The ithelial component is likely entrapped rather than a com-nent of the neoplasm. The pleuropulmonary blastoma ay have cystic areas and heterologous areas that are of esenchymal derivation, especially cartilage or muscle. It is garded by some as a type of blastoma, and by others as a fferent entity. A pleuropulmonary blastoma should be con-lered when addressing cystic masses in young children that ve a mesenchymal stroma without an epithelial component.

Salivary-type neoplasms may rarely occur in the lung. ie most common of these rare tumors are the adenoid stic carcinoma and the mucoepidermoid carcinoma, which e diagnosed as in salivary glands. Pulmonary lymphoid oliferations are diagnosed as in other sites. Mesenchymal oplasms, including those of muscle, nerve sheath, fibro-stiocytic, and vascular origin, may occur in the lung, and e diagnosed as discussed in Chapter 2, *once a metaplastic rcinoma is excluded.*

The only mesenchymal tumor that merits special atten-on is the epithelioid hemangioendothelioma, a low-grade igiosarcoma that is found occasionally in the lung, liver, spleen, and that may be multinodular or bilateral. The oplastic endothelial cells in an epithelioid hemangioendo-elioma have an epithelial appearance, and the neoplasm is kely to have zonation, with fibrosis centrally and more cellu-rity peripherally i16.53. Immunohistochemical stains (CD31 id CD34) may be needed to appreciate the vascular nature the cells. The stroma may predominate, especially in the nter, and, in conjunction with the epithelioid appearance the cells, can make an erroneous diagnosis of sclerosing rcinoma easy. A complete immunohistochemical panel, cluding vascular markers and epithelial membrane antigen, essential, as a minority of epithelioid hemangioendothe-omas may have some keratin positivity [PMID19492891].

An epithelioid hemangioendothelioma can simulate an flammatory myofibroblastic tumor. Inflammatory myofi-oblastic tumors may have areas of variable cellularity but ill not have a distinct increase in cellularity towards the periphery. The neoplastic cells are negative for CD31 and CD34, and they are likely to stain for actin and ALK.

An epithelioid hemangioendothelioma may also resemble a solitary fibrous tumor, as both will have areas of greater cellularity and prominent vascularity. Immunohistochemical stains may again be required, employing both vascular markers and antigens typical of solitary fibrous tumor, such as CD99 and bcl-2.

Lymphomatoid granulomatosis is a rare, angiocentric, necrotizing lymphoproliferative disorder that is primarily found in the lung. The old use of the term "lymphomatoid granulomatosis" likely encompassed several distinct entities, including angiocentric T-cell lymphomas, T-cell rich B-cell lymphomas, and Wegener granulomatosis. The entity is currently defined as a neoplastic proliferations of Epstein Barr virus-infected B cells with a large number of accompanying, nonneoplastic T cells [PMID8037289], and is characterized by large, atypical B lymphocytes admixed with smaller T lymphocytes, infiltrating the walls of blood vessels and bronchi [PMID19732432]. Vascular invasion i16.54 and necrosis are common, but granulomas are not necessarily seen. In addition to the lungs, lymphomatoid granulomatosis can affect the upper respiratory tract, the skin, and the central nervous system.

Unusual Inflammatory Lung Conditions

Pulmonary Wegener is diagnosed as discussed in Chapter 14 for the sinonasal area. Some believe there is a bronchocentric form of Wegener that is restricted to the lungs, but it is unclear if this is a true subtype of Wegener, or simply cases in which involvement of other organs has not yet been found.

Churg-Strauss syndrome and microscopic polyangiitis should be excluded before a diagnosis of pulmonary Wegener is made. Churg-Strauss syndrome (allergic angiitis and granulomatosis) is a systemic vasculitis with eosinophilia, manifest in the lung as a necrotizing vasculitis with eosinophils, and often with granulomas. In contrast to Wegener, skin, nerves, and heart are commonly affected in Churg-Strauss, whereas the sinonasal area and the kidneys rarely are. ANCA is usually positive. Microscopic polyangiitis is a small vessel vasculitis that involves the kidney and the lung, and it should always be excluded in any case in which vasculitis is found in either of those locations.

Bronchocentric granulomatosis is caused by an abnormal response to *Aspergillus* and is characterized by mucous and acute inflammatory cells in a bronchial lumen, surrounded by giant cells [PMID1092235].

Pneumocystis carinii, originally thought to be a protozoan and now known to be a fungus [PMID16444423], can be exceptionally subtle, especially if it is not known that the patient is immunocompromised. A clue to the diagnosis is that this organism may cause the alveoli to fill with an amorphous foamy to lightly eosinophilic material i16.55.

"Bronchopulmonary dysplasia" is a clinical term and a clinical diagnosis, based on persistence of lung problems from the neonatal period, usually requiring continued assistance with ventilation. There are variable morphologic manifestations, including continued hyaline membrane formation, fibrosis, large alveoli (indicating poor septation), vessels with changes of hypertension, etc. All of these changes are less severe now than formerly because of the advent of artificial surfactant and the reduced use of oxygen in the neonatal period.

Interstitial Lung Disease

Only a cursory treatment of interstitial lung diseases will be offered here. For a more comprehensive discussion, the reader is referred to the time-honored text edited by Katzenstein [Katzenstein ISBN978-0721600413].

Liebow began the relevant and useful classification of idiopathic interstitial lung disease [Liebow ISBN978-0808904304]. Since this pioneering work, the classification of interstitial lung disease has undergone several modifications. BOOP was well described in 1985 [PMID3965933] and diffuse alveolar damage (DAD) was well characterized in 1990 [PMID2134041].

In 1998, Katzenstein and Myers did not include BOOP in the category of interstitial pneumonitis since it is primarily intraluminal rather than interstitial, and also eliminated lymphoid interstitial pneumonia (LIP) since it had been shown to be a lymphoproliferative disorder (associated with immunocompromised patients). They also added the entities AIP (AIP) and nonspecific interstitial pneumonia (NSIP) [PMID9563754].

In 2002, the American Thoracic Society and the European Respiratory Society re-introduced LIP because by then immunohistochemistry and molecular studies permitted the identification of both neoplastic and nonneoplastic forms. The 2002 classification recognized 6 other types of idiopathic interstitial lung disease: idiopathic pulmonary fibrosis (IPF), NSIP, cryptogenic organizing pneumonia, AIP, respiratory bronchiolitis-associated interstitial pneumonia, and diffuse interstitial pneumonitis (DIP). They continued to omit BOOP [PMID11790668].

Transbronchial and transcutaneous biopsies are important in the initial workup of a possible interstitial process because they can exclude a neoplasm or an obvious infectious process. Once this is done, however, and an interstitial pneumonitis appears likely, an open biopsy is often required for a precise diagnosis.

In assessing any interstitial process in the lung, both the geographical extent (focal or diffuse) and the relative ages of lesions (ie, the presence or absence of temporal uniformity) in the involved areas should be considered. Often, valuable information can be obtained from a wedge biopsy without even using a microscope [PMID18384206], though I have found that inverting a microscope eyepiece and taking advantage of the ensuing 10-15× magnification is valuable.

Those conditions that *primarily* thicken the septae and do not have significant acute pneumocyte damage are called chronic fibrosing interstitial pneumonias. These include usual interstitial pneumonia (UIP) and NSIP.

UIP is the prototype pulmonary fibrosing condition. It is idiopathic, although there is some association with autoimmune disorders and immune complexes have been demonstrated in some cases. Changes are neither diffuse nor uniform. There is an uneven pattern of involvement, and a wedge biopsy shows some areas of nearly normal lung alternating with areas of varying degrees of fibrosis. Moreover, in the abnormal areas, changes are seen at all stages, ranging from interstitial inflammation with reactive pneumocytes to early, fibroblastic fibrosis **i16.56** to well developed fibrosis **i16.57** [PMID16304242]. However, by definition, hyaline membranes are not seen unless there is a superimposed acute event.

Although the histologic findings of UIP can be seen in asbestosis and autoimmune disorders, UIP is usually idiopathic and is associated with the clinical syndrome of IPF. UIP/IPF can usually be reliably diagnosed by CT, in conjunction with clinical symptoms, though lung biopsy is nearly always performed for a definitive diagnosis and treatment plan. The clinical course of UIP is invariably progressive, but there is substantial variation in the velocity of progression. Right heart failure and cor pulmonale often result and the process will eventuate in honeycomb lung [PMID18366757].

One of the entities in the differential diagnosis of UIP is simple atelectasis. In UIP, while the fibrosis is often most severe just under the pleura, it will invariably extend, in a vaguely linear manner, into the remainder of the lung. In contrast, in atelectasis, the fibrosis is only subpleural and is sharply demarcated from the remainder of the lung.

The other group of chronic, fibrosing interstitial pneumonitis is NSIP. Like UIP, NSIP has patchy involvement, but in contrast to UIP, of those areas that are involved, there is temporal uniformity. In contrast to UIP, response to steroids is often good and some patients will recover completely [PMID8291652].

While UIP and NSIP are manifest as *chronic* lung injury, DAD and AIP (Hamman-Rich syndrome) are the primary forms of severe *acute* lung injury. DAD is the morphologic counterpart to adult respiratory distress syndrome (ARDS). It is the pattern of acute injury resulting from any number of etiologies, such as shock, chemicals, oxygen toxicity, drugs, some infections, etc [PMID788524]. In DAD, there is initially edema, hemorrhage, and fibrin deposition, followed by hyaline membrane formation **i16.58**. Hyaline membranes are amorphous eosinophilic material lining alveoli in cases of acute injury such as DAD and AIP. Intuitively, it is easy to assume that hyaline membranes are composed only of material from necrotic pneumocytes, but their precise composition and mechanism of formation remain unclear. Immunohistochemical studies suggest that alveolar epithelium may be only a minor constituent and that there may also be components from damaged endothelial cells. It may also be that the composition may differ in different types of interstitial lung disease or different etiologies [PMID17187083]. In DAD and AIP, there may be reactive pneumocyte hyperplasia and atypia, with squamous metaplasia around foci of fibrosis. In DAD, the changes are usually geographically diffuse and temporally uniform. The prognosis is usually poor.

AIP has a sudden onset, usually in young adults. By definition, the cause is unknown. The histologic changes are diffuse, temporally uniform, and resemble those of well developed DAD. AIP is essentially an acute, idiopathic form of DAD, and it is sometimes called idiopathic ARDS. Although there is a high mortality, some patients do recover fully.

DAD and AIP may lead to interstitial fibrosis, but in con-ast to UIP and NSIP, the fibrosis follows from injury to veolar cells and subsequent incorporation of hyaline mem-ane material into septal fibrosis. If a fibrosing condition is condary to DAD or AIP, the patient likely has a history of vere acute pulmonary dysfunction consistent with ARDS, well as evidence of continued acute injury.

Desquamative interstitial pneumonitis (DIP) is strongly nked to cigarettes, has many intraalveolar macrophages 5.59, and also has mild interstitial fibrosis. The nature of the lls in the alveolar spaces was long a matter of controversy, it their identity as macrophages, not desquamated alveolar lls, has now been secured [PMID6990759]. Changes in DIP are dif-ise and temporally uniform. An occasional macrophage may multinucleated, but large numbers of multinucleated cells, articularly if they have phagocytized other inflammatory lls, requires the exclusion of a pneumoconiosis. Langerhans ll histiocytosis should also be excluded. Interstitial changes DIP are minor. There is usually a good response to steroids.

Respiratory bronchiolitis is one of a number of forms of nall airway disease. Respiratory bronchiolitis is related to IP and is characterized by macrophages in the distal air-ays. It is also strongly linked to smoking and responds will steroids [PMID3565934].

Cellular bronchiolitis is another form of small airway dis-ise in which there is chronic inflammation around small rways. If lymphoid follicles are formed, the process is called llicular bronchiolitis. Constrictive bronchiolitis obliterans is concentric fibrosis of small airways.

BOOP is a condition that is a final pathway for a variety conditions that primarily affect small airways [PMID3965933]. here is young, cellular fibrosis, often with a myxoid com-onent, in and around bronchioles. The bronchioles are nevenly affected and the interstitium is relatively spared. iagnostic clues to BOOP are a paucity of bronchioles and e presence of small, rounded, well demarcated nodules of oung, cellular fibrous tissue i16.60, the result of obliteration bronchi. The prognosis is usually favorable with steroid eatment.

Another condition that preferentially affects small airways smokers is Langerhans cell histiocytosis (formerly called osinophilic granuloma or histiocytosis X). There is disagree-ent over whether Langerhans cell histiocytosis of the lung a neoplasm or a reactive process, but there is evidence of a onal proliferation [PMID8008029]. It is strongly associated with garette smoking. There may be intraalveolar macrophages, it the primary finding is a peribronchial distribution of ixed inflammation, including eosinophils and Langerhans lls i16.61. CD1a and S-100 may be needed to highlight the tter cells. Langerhans cells will also stain with CD68, but is does not differentiate them from ordinary macrophages. he inflamed areas may have a stellate shape, and in older sions, the inflammation may diminish, leaving stellate ars. In older cases, where the Langerhans cells may no nger be demonstrable, the low-power appearance of small, eribronchial stellate scars suggests this diagnosis. Many atients recover spontaneously, and the prognosis is usually ood, particularly if the patient stops smoking or if steroids re instituted [PMID8372949]. The difficult part of diagnosing a Langerhans proliferation is to think of it. Langerhans cells resemble ordinary macrophages, and the number of Langerhans cells diminishes in older lesions. Eosinophils may not be prominent. If the diagnosis is confirmed, a minority of cases will have Langerhans proliferations in other sites.

Other conditions associated with eosinophils include chronic eosinophilic pneumonia and allergic bronchopul-monary aspergillosis. Chronic eosinophilic pneumonia is associated with drugs, with fungus (usually *Aspergillus*), and often with a history of asthma. There may be intraalveolar col-lections of eosinophils mixed with lymphocytes, plasma cells, and macrophages. The vasculitis and necrosis that are seen in Churg-Strauss, another condition associated with eosinophils, are absent [PMID5773637].

Allergic bronchopulmonary aspergillosis is characterized by hypersensitivity to *Aspergillus*. These are not immuno-compromised patients who are besieged by the organism. The problem is a hypersensitivity reaction. Allergic broncho-pulmonary aspergillosis is often associated with asthma and peripheral eosinophilia [PMID19723372], and if chronic, may result in a histologic appearance that is similar to chronic eosino-philic pneumonia.

The right middle lobe is prone to atelectasis. This occa-sionally predisposes the area to poor clearance, followed by pneumonia, eventually resulting in broncheictasis (bronchi-ectasis is rarely a primary finding and is usually secondary to obstruction or inflammation). This is called middle lobe syn-drome. There will be focal fibrosis and chronic inflammation along airways. This is a chronic process, and the diagnosis is not made in the presence of acute pneumonia. The same pro-cess may occur in the lingula to a lesser extent.

Asbestosis demonstrates a nonspecific interstitial fibrosis that is indistinguishable from that seen in UIP. Indeed, asbes-tosis is a cause of UIP, and the only way to make the diagnosis of asbestosis on H&E examination is to find the asbestos. These particles are usually coated with iron, so an iron stain may help. Such iron-coated particles are called ferruginous bodies, but other types of materials, if coated with iron, are also called ferruginous bodies. Electron microprobe analysis (in which the sample is bombarded with a beam of electrons, after which the elements are identified by the wavelengths emitted) provides definitive confirmation and subtyping of the asbestos fibers [PMID507508]. Recently, work has been done in the molecular mechanism of injury in asbestosis [PMID11811924].

Lymphoid interstitial pneumonitis (LIP) is seen in immu-nocompromised patients (especially those with AIDS), in autoimmune disorders, and in certain drug reactions, and is characterized by an intense lymphoid infiltrate primarily in the interstitium i16.62. LIP is a heterogeneous group of lym-phoid proliferations, some of which are neoplastic and some of which are not. The nonneoplastic varieties differ from a low-grade lymphoma in the absence of a distinct mass, the absence of significant destruction or displacement of lung tissue, the mature and innocuous appearance of the indi-vidual cells, and the presence of germinal centers. However, immunophenotyping of the cells, with demonstration of polyclonality, is necessary in most cases to identify the pro-cess as nonneoplastic [PMID7544761, PMID7638448]. Hypersensitivity pneumonitis (extrinsic allergic alveolitis) is an occupational

ISBN 978-089189-5886

pneumonia that resolves with cessation of the offending agent. Many cases are caused by *Actinomycetes*, though reactions to other organisms, such as *Aspergillus* species, are well documented. Changes are initially patchy, but may become diffuse. There is interstitial lymphoplasmacytic inflammation with only minimal fibrosis i16.63 unless exposure has been long-term, in which case slight fibrosis may be evident. Vaguely defined granulomas may be seen, but eosinophils are rare, despite their common association with hypersensitivity and allergic reactions. There is general temporal uniformity. In acute cases, the inflammation, though interstitial, is often near bronchioles, and a bronchiolar component may occasionally be seen. Small peribronchial granulomas, macrophages in airspaces, and BOOP-like areas may be seen, and if so, the combination suggests the diagnosis of hypersensitivity pneumonitis. Any patchy inflammation without significant fibrosis, in the right clinical setting, suggests this diagnosis [PMID3389449]. The differential diagnosis includes sarcoidosis, BOOP, and LIP. BOOP usually has fewer granuloma-like areas and less lymphoplasmacytic inflammation. While chronic exposure can lead to mild interstitial fibrosis, identification of and removal of the inciting agent generally leads to remission and an excellent prognosis.

A more recent addition to the list of interstitial lung disorders is the IgG4-related autoimmune disorders. As discussed in Chapter 24, these are a group of disorders that are characterized by fibrosis and a lymphoplasmacytic infiltrate, with most of the plasma cells expressing IgG4. The lung findings are as seen in other sites and there may also be an endothelialitis [PMID19623032].

Core Points for the Lung

- Congenital lesions of the lung: hamartoma and numerous cystic processes.
- Lymphangiomyoma and the so-called "sugar tumor": PEComas, thought to arise from the perivascular epithelioid cell.
  - This family of tumors is positive for HMB- 45.
- Sclerosing hemangioma: heterogeneous group
  - Most are now thought to be proliferations of alveolar lining cells (pneumocytomas) rather than proliferations of endothelial cells.
- Neuroendocrine carcinomas: carcinoid, atypical carcinoid, and small cell carcinoma
  - Generally positive for synaptophysin and CD56.
  - May also express chromogranin, and small cell carcinoma tends to be positive for TTF-1.
  - A high mitotic rate as identified by Ki-67 favors a small cell carcinoma over a lower grade neuroendocrine neoplasm.
- Lymphomas or benign lymphoid nodules may also have crush artifact and appear to be small cell carcinoma.
  - IHC may be necessary
  - But both H&E interpretation and IHC should be performed on viable cells that have not been crushed.
- Small cell vs non-small cell lung carcinoma remains important.
- Small cell carcinoma vs poorly differentiated adenocarcinoma: negativity for neuroendocrine markers and positivity for cytokeratin 7, PE-10, or napsin A suggests an adenocarcinoma.
- Small cell carcinoma vs poorly differentiated squamous cell carcinoma: high molecular weight keratin and p63 staining suggests squamous origin.
- Significance of neuroendocrine differentiation in the so-called large cell undifferentiated carcinoma is unclear.
  - Any non-small cell lung carcinoma that is not clearly a squamous carcinoma or an adenocarcinoma can be investigated for neuroendocrine differentiation.
- Non-small cell lung carcinomas often have features of both squamous carcinoma and adenocarcinoma.
  - p63 expression favors squamous origin while TTF-1, PE-10, or napsin A expression favors an adenocarcinoma.
- Bronchiolar carcinoma: Not invasive into the parenchyma.
  - Mucinous and nonmucinous types.
  - Principal differential diagnosis is reactive pneumocytes.
  - A radiographically defined mass favors a bronchiolar carcinoma while the presence of cilia or a fibroinflammatory background favors a reactive process.
  - Cellular crowding with stratification and tufting favors a neoplastic process, as does mitotic activity and exfoliation of cells into the alveolar space.
- 4 mutations which have potential relevance in some cases of non-small cell lung carcinoma:
  - Epidermal growth factor receptor gene
  - *K-RAS* gene
  - A fusion product of the *ALK* and *EML4* genes
  - A mutation in the nucleotide excision repair enzyme ERCC1.
- The primary site of metastatic neoplasms requires a clinical history and immunohistochemical characterization.
  - Most useful immunohistochemical stains are cytokeratins 7 and 20.
- Also important to differentiate a pulmonary adenocarcinoma from a mesothelioma, as discussed in Chapter 17.
- Clues to a possible pulmonary Wegener: necrosis, tissue destruction, severe acute inflammation, vasculitis, and granulomas.
  - Must exclude neoplasia and infection
  - Concomitant involvement of the sinonasal area or the kidney is typically seen in pulmonary Wegener.

Transbronchial and transcutaneous biopsies are important in the diagnosis of interstitial lung disease as a first step by excluding a neoplasm or an infectious process.

- o But once interstitial pneumonitis appears probable, an open biopsy is often required.
- o Geographical extent and the presence or absence of temporal uniformity are important observations.

Usual interstitial pneumonitis (UIP): primary, idiopathic, fibrosing condition that corresponds to the clinical syndrome of idiopathic pulmonary fibrosis.

- o Abnormal areas are unevenly distributed throughout the lung.
- o Lesions of different ages.

Asbestosis: histologic appearance indistinguishable from UIP

- o Can only be diagnosed by the identification of asbestos.

- Diffuse alveolar damage: morphologic counterpart to adult respiratory distress syndrome
  - o Results from acute pneumocyte injury from many causes.
- Bronchiolitis obliterans with organizing pneumonia (BOOP): may be a final pathway for a number of conditions that damage small airways.
  - o Often evident as small, rounded nodules of cellular fibrous tissue and a paucity of bronchioles.
  - o Unlike many other interstitial lung disorders, BOOP often responds to steroid treatment.
- Allergic bronchopulmonary aspergillosis: a hypersensitivity reaction to aspergillus. Hypersensitivity pneumonitis: may occur as a reaction to a number of agents.
  - o Histologic changes are multifocal and temporally uniform.
  - o There may be minimal fibrosis.

ISBN 978-089189-5886

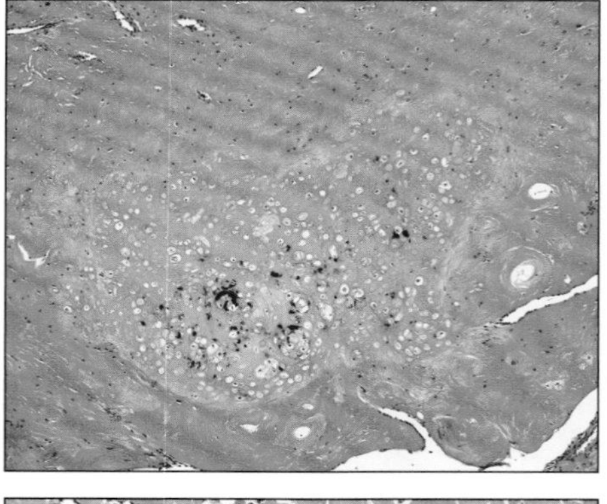

i16.1 A cartilaginous hamartoma of the lung. Focal calcification is common.

i16.2 A pulmonary hamartoma without cartilage. Note the similarity to a fibroadenoma of the breast.

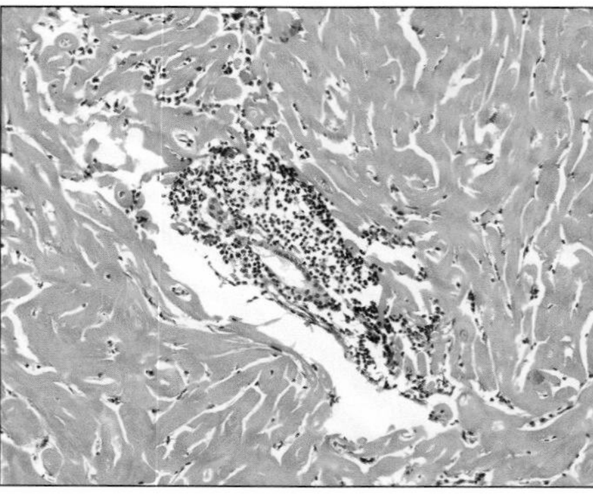

i16.3 Pulmonary hyalinizing granuloma, illustrating the very dense collagenous fibrosis

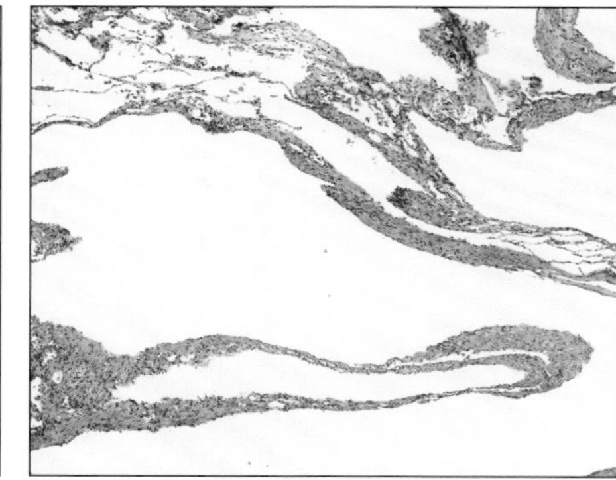

i16.4 Lymphangiomyoma consisting of dilated lymphatic channels that are lined by much larger amounts of smooth muscle than are typically seen in lymphatic vessels

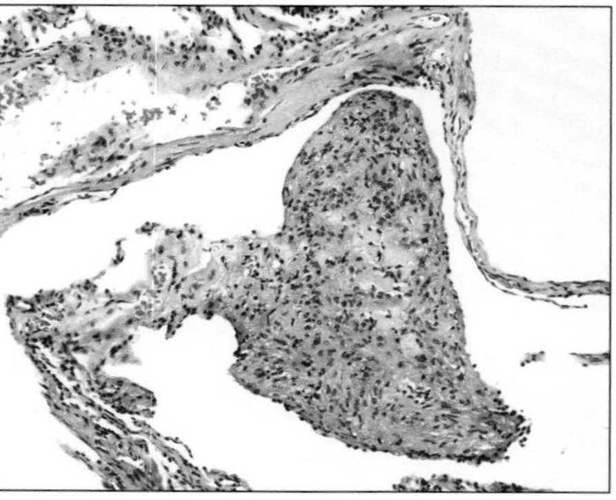

i16.5 A high-power view of a lymphangiomyoma illustrating that the smooth muscle in the wall may form small masses

i16.6 The so-called "sugar tumor," a benign neoplasm with clear cytoplasm

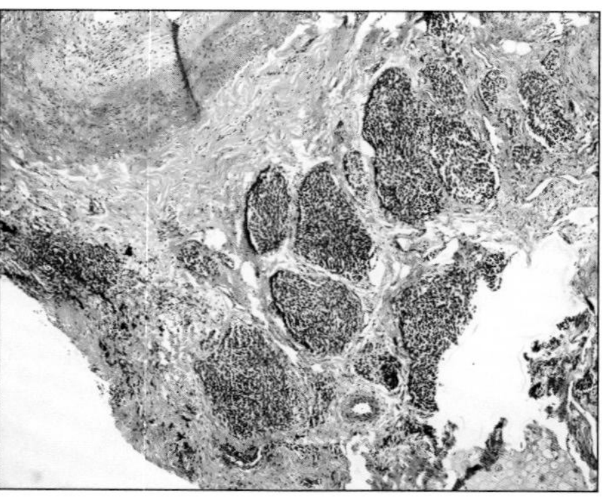

i16.7 So-called "tumorlets," small clusters of cells that are incidental findings but may resemble a small neuroendocrine carcinoma

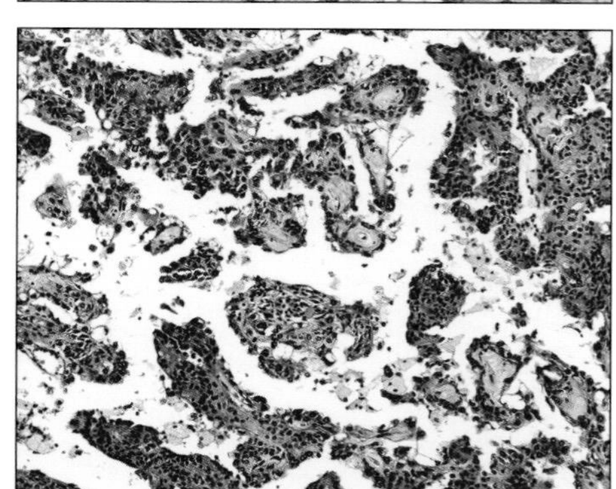

i16.8 A so-called sclerosing hemangioma, with a papillary architecture, likely derived from pneumocytes

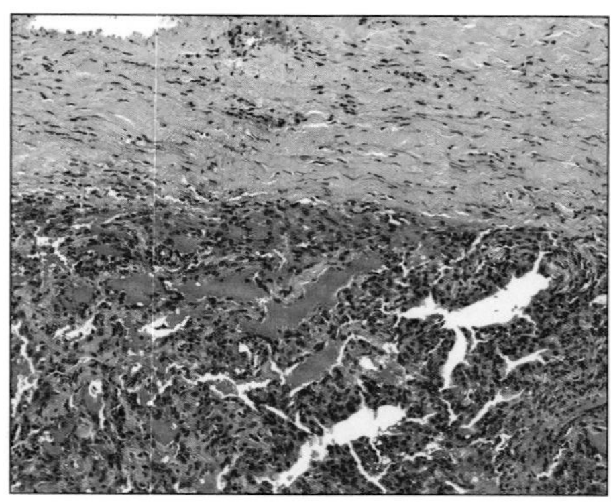

i16.9 All members of the sclerosing hemangioma family, whatever their histogenesis, are well circumscribed and generally encapsulated.

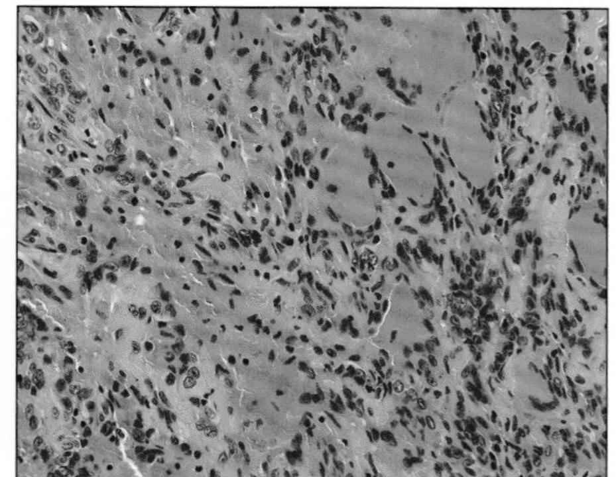

i16.10 A sclerosing hemangioma that, unlike most examples in this group, may truly be a benign vascular neoplasm

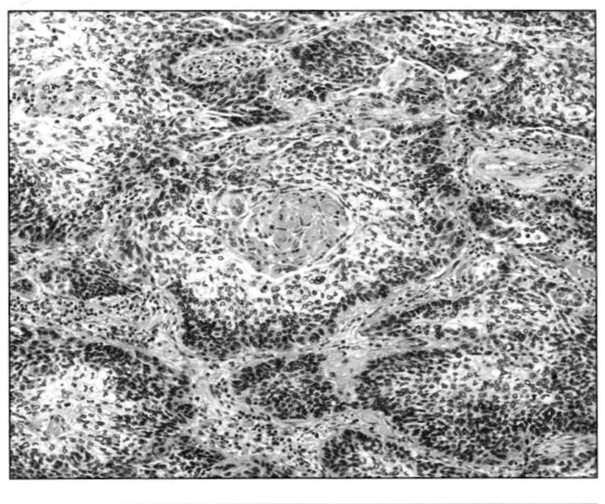

1 A basaloid type of
uamous carcinoma
th a small focus of
nventional, keratinizing
uamous carcinoma in
e center

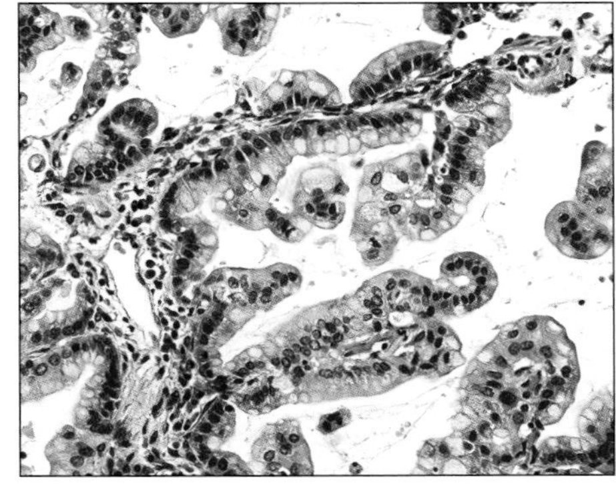

i16.12 A mucinous form of bronchiolar carcinoma. Note the small, uniform, basally oriented nuclei. The clue to this form of bronchiolar carcinoma is the abundant mucinous cytoplasm. Note also the micropapillary architecture.

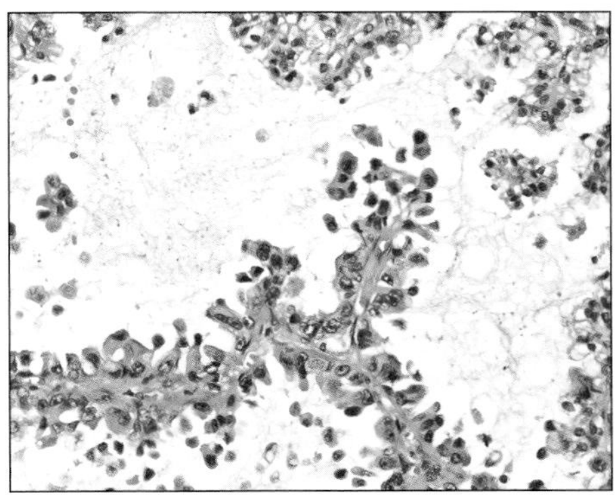

13 The nonmucinous
riant of bronchiolar
rcinoma. This form
s less cytoplasm and
ore nuclear atypia
an the mucinous form.
ote the apical nuclei,
th focal stratification,
d microtufts that are
und in the lumen. Note
so the micropapillary
chitecture.

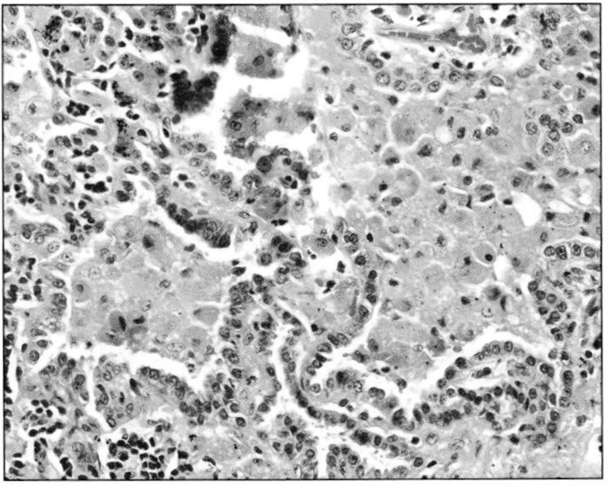

i16.14 Reactive pneumocyte atypia. Note inflammatory cells on the left, suggesting a benign process. These cells cannot be of the mucinous form of bronchiolar carcinoma because they lack the abundant mucinous cytoplasm, but they also lack the nuclear crowding and stratification that would be expected in a nonmucinous bronchiolar carcinoma (compare to i16.13).

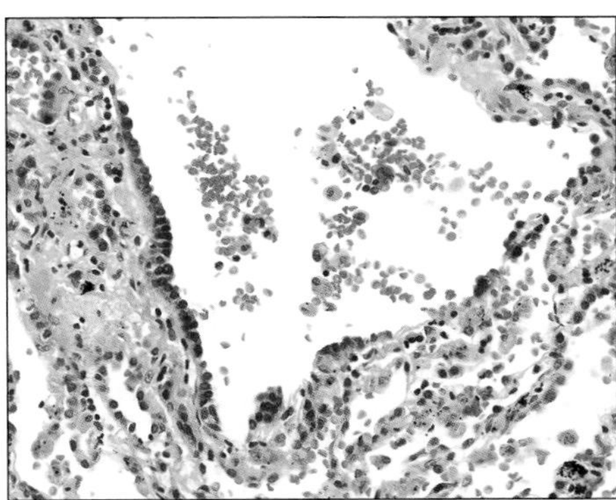

15 Another example of
nign pneumocyte atypia.
ote that the problematic
lls are restricted to the
t side rather than lining
e entire dilated alveolus,
would be expected in
onchiolar carcinoma.
ote also the discontinuity
the right side, with
ypical pneumocytes
terspersed with
eumocytes that have
t, inconspicuous nuclei.

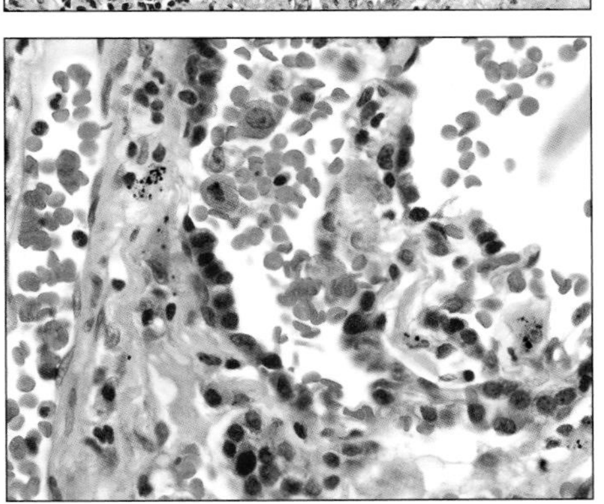

i16.16 A higher-power view of the same case as in i16.15. Again, in contrast to i16.13, the atypical area lacks significant nuclear crowding and stratification.

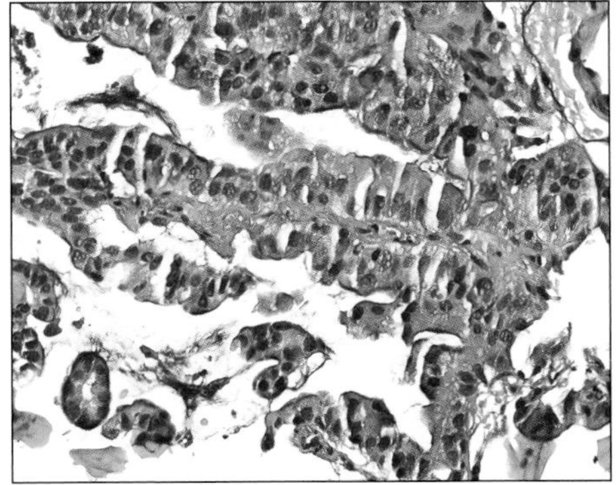

.17 Another example of
onchiolar carcinoma
ustrating uniform
uclear enlargement with
ratification and nuclear
owding, resulting in
icrotuft formation,
atures not generally seen
reactive atypia

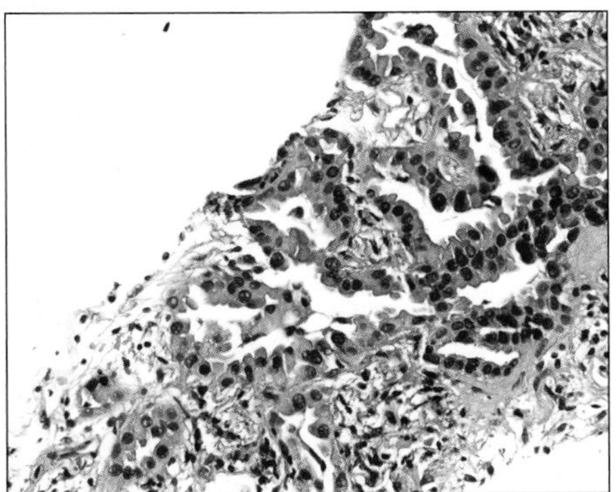

i16.18 An adenocarcinoma of the lung that is both bronchiolar and invasive. A noninvasive bronchiolar carcinoma is seen at top, but at bottom, there are smaller glands that are separated by a fibroblastic stroma rather than by alveolar septae.

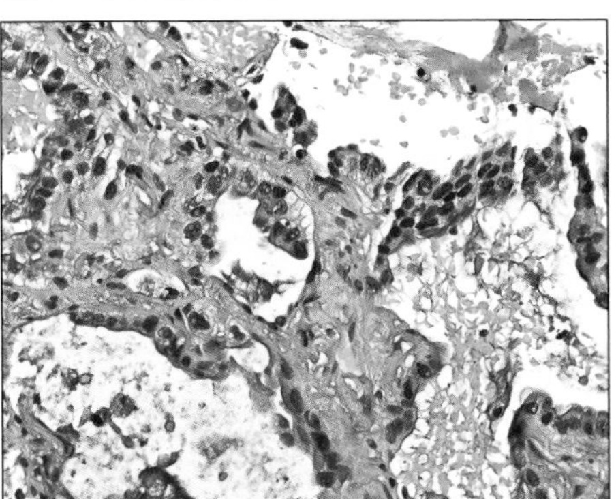

.19 Another
lenocarcinoma of
e lung that is both
onchiolar and invasive.
n the right there is a
onchiolar carcinoma
ithout invasion, but
ft of center, the fibrotic
roma indicates a reaction
invasion.

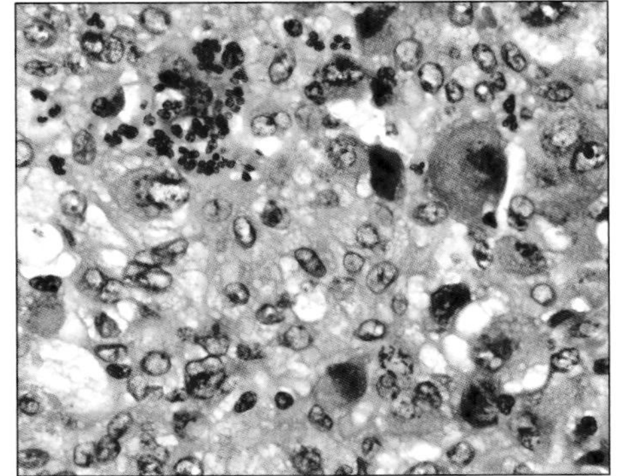

i16.20 A poorly differentiated non-small cell carcinoma with features of both squamous and adenocarcinoma. A large tumor cell to the right of center has coarse chromatin and possible cytoplasmic keratinization. Another tumor cell below center also has coarse nuclear chromatin and probable cytoplasmic keratinization. On the other hand, many other tumor cells have a vesicular chromatin pattern and appear to form glands.

ISBN 978-089189-5886

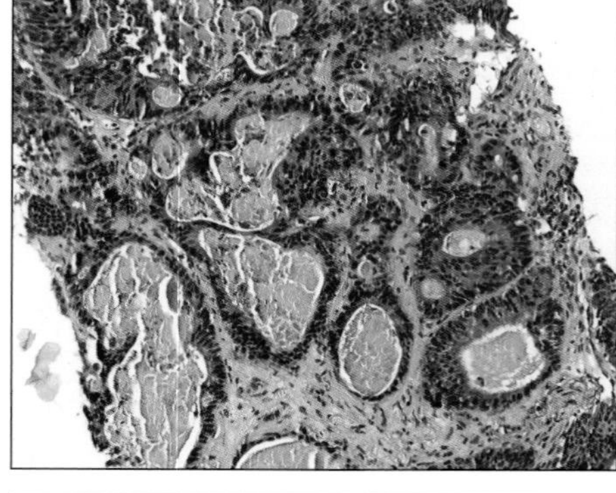

i16.21 Metastatic colon cancer to the lung. The tall columnar cells in the lower right and the necrosis in the upper left may suggest colonic origin, but immunohistochemical stains are necessary.

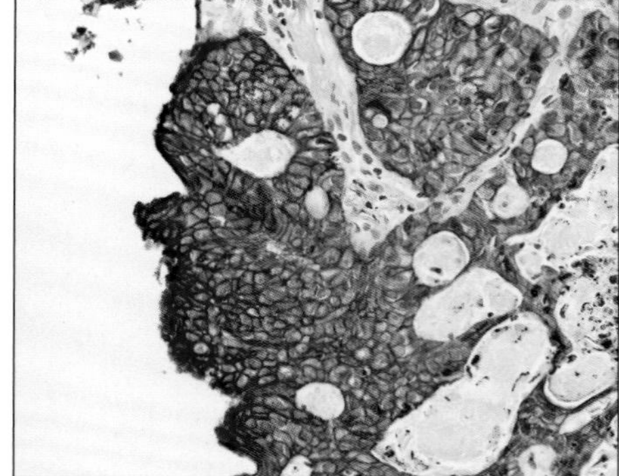

i16.22 The same case as in i16.21, demonstrating positive staining for cytokeratin 20, which is unusual in a primary adenocarcinoma of the lung.

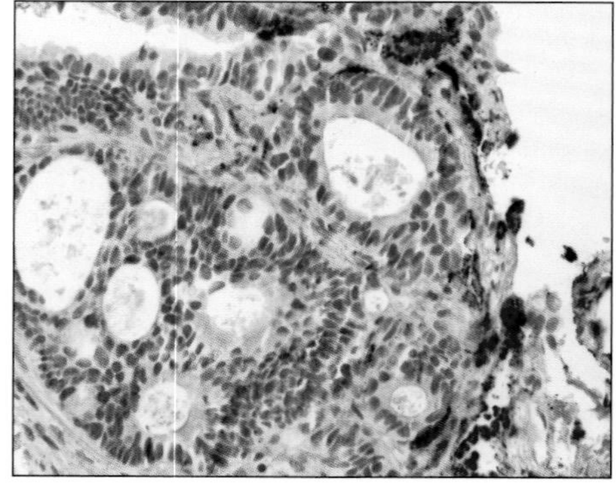

i16.23 The same case as in i16.21, demonstrating negative staining for napsin A, another indication of probable metastatic origin. Note the normal staining of the benign pneumocytes on the right, furnishing an excellent internal control.

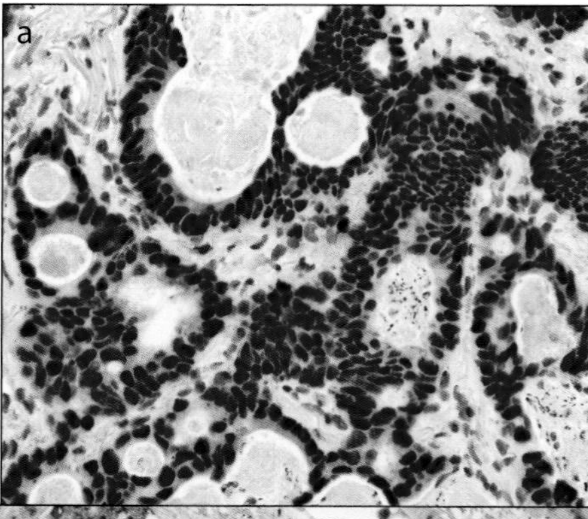

i16.24 **a** The same case as in i16.21, demonstrating positive staining for CDX2, confirming lower gastrointestinal tract origin

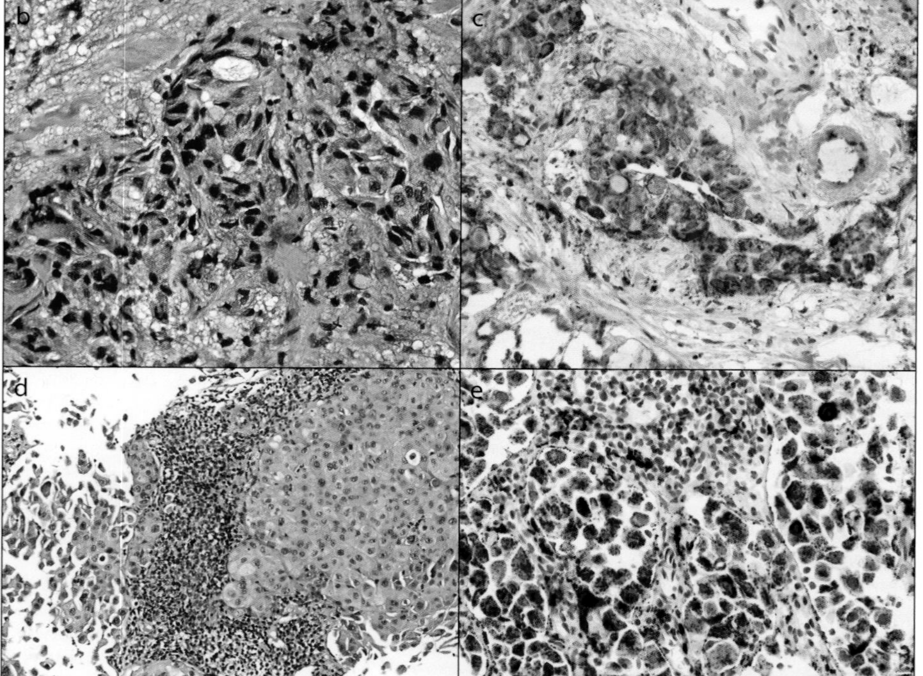

b Metastatic adenocarcinoma to a lymph node

c The same case as in i16.24b, illustrating positivity for napsin A. This suggests a lung primary, a diagnosis that was confirmed by numerous additional immunohistochemical studies.

d A poorly differentiated adenocarcinoma in the breast. With the large number of lymphocytes, medullary carcinoma of the breast is a possibility, as is a metastatic hepatocellular carcinoma. The neoplasm was positive for cytokeratin 7 and negative for cytokeratin 20, suggesting that a metastatic hepatocellular carcinoma was unlikely, but not helpful in the distinction of a primary breast carcinoma from a pulmonary metastasis.

e The same case as in i16.24d. This positive napsin A identifies this carcinoma as a metastasis from the lung. Because no one immunohistochemical stain secures a definitive diagnosis, the napsin A was part of a large panel. In addition to napsin A, the neoplasm was positive for TTF-1. It was negative for mammaglobin, gross cystic disease fluid protein-15, ER, PR, and Heppar1.

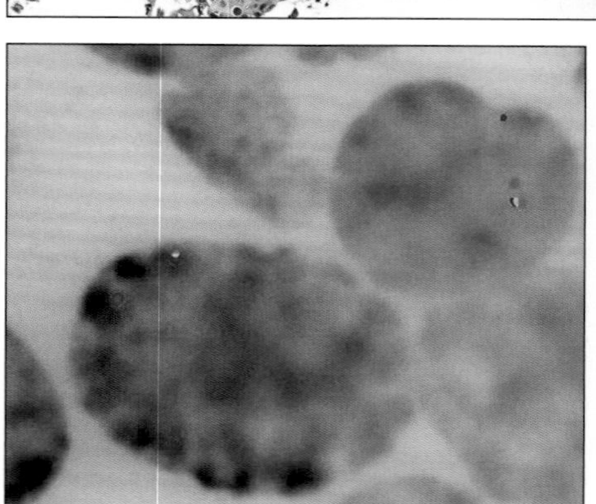

i16.25 A break apart FISH study for the *ALK/EML* translocation in non-small cell lung cancer. 2 probes of different colors are used that hybridize to areas immediately adjacent to the breakpoint. Both probes hybridize to the gene of interest. Each cell has one area in which the colors remain adjacent, and one in which they are separated, indicating that this patient has a translocation on 1 of the 2 chromosomes.

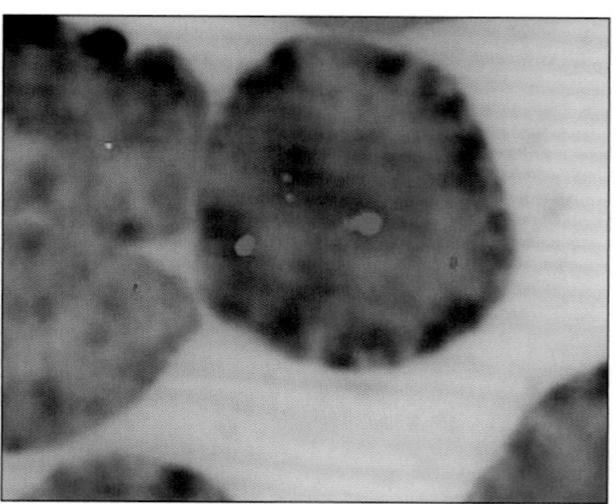

i16.26 FISH study for the *ALK/EML* translocation in non-small cell lung cancer. This cell in a break apart FISH study has 5 signals. 2 of these are small separated red and green signals, indicating a translocation, but also has 3 additional green signals for which there is no red counterpart anywhere. This indicates amplification without translocation of the portion of the *ALK* gene that this probe hybridized to.

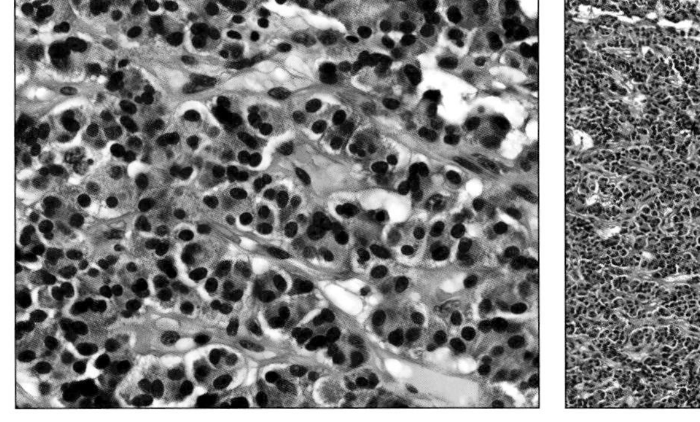

27 A grade 1 neuroen-
crine carcinoma (carci-
id tumor) demonstrat-
; small, uniform nuclei,
noderate amount of
sinophilic cytoplasm,
mitotic activity, and no
crosis

i16.28 A trabecular growth pattern is common in grade 1 neuroendocrine carcinomas

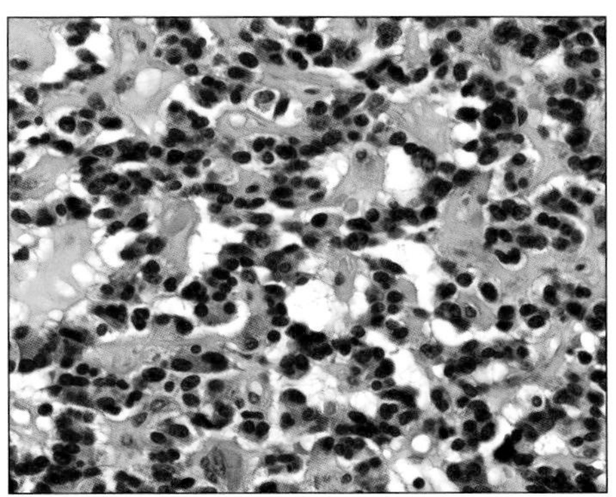

29 Rosette formation in
ide 1 neuroendocrine
cinoma

i16.30 A spindle cell grade 1 neuroendocrine carcinoma

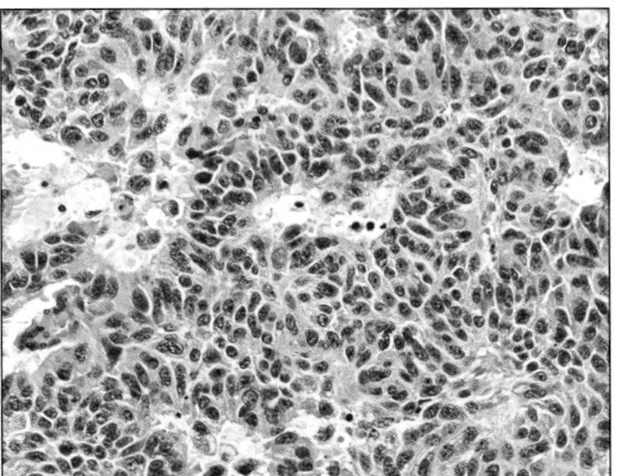

31 A grade 2
uroendocrine carcinoma
ypical carcinoid). The
oplasm has relatively
iform nuclei and cell-
-cell, is very difficult
distinguish from a
ide 1 neuroendocrine
cinoma.

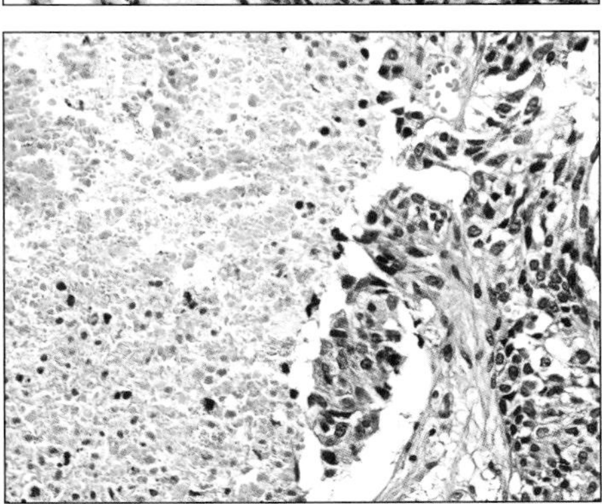

i16.32 Necrosis in a grade 2 neuroendocrine carcinoma

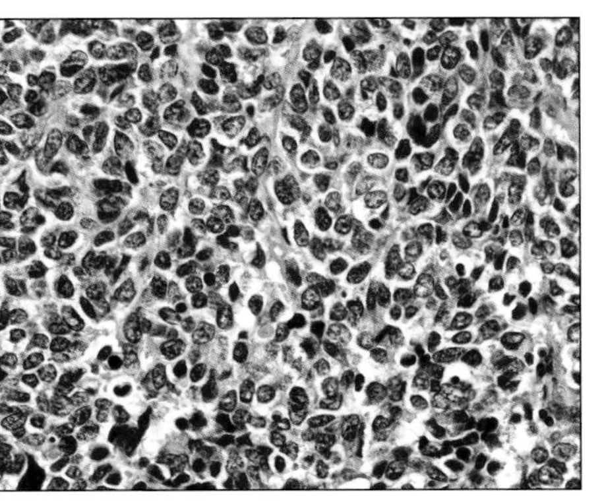

33 Well preserved cells
a small cell carcinoma.
ote the relatively fine
romatin, indistinct
cleoli, and minimal
toplasm.

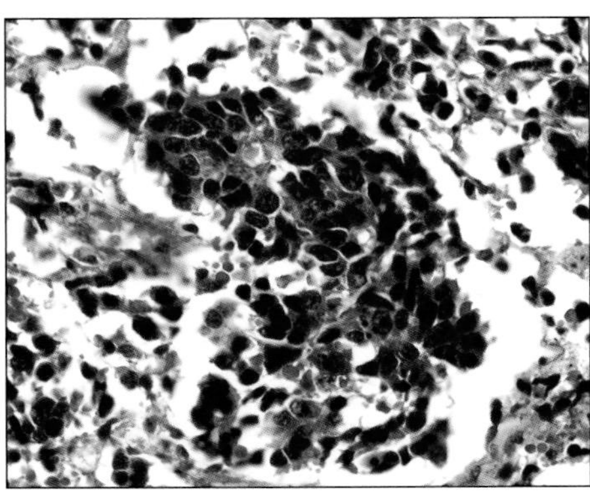

i16.34 Small cell carcinoma in a less well preserved state, causing the chromatin to appear coarse

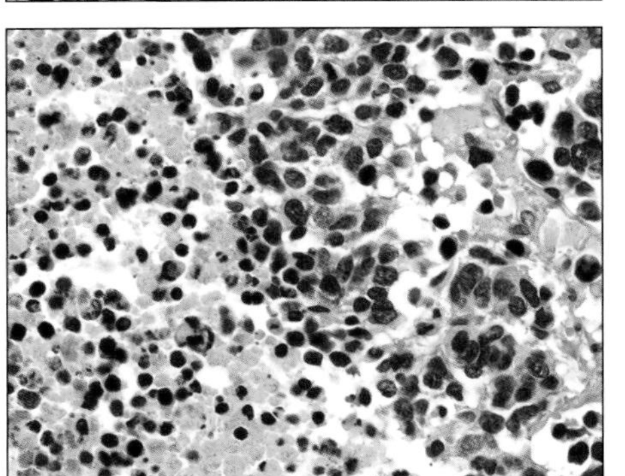

35 Necrosis in a small
ll carcinoma. Note
e well preserved cells
the right, and the
ryorrhectic cells on the
t.

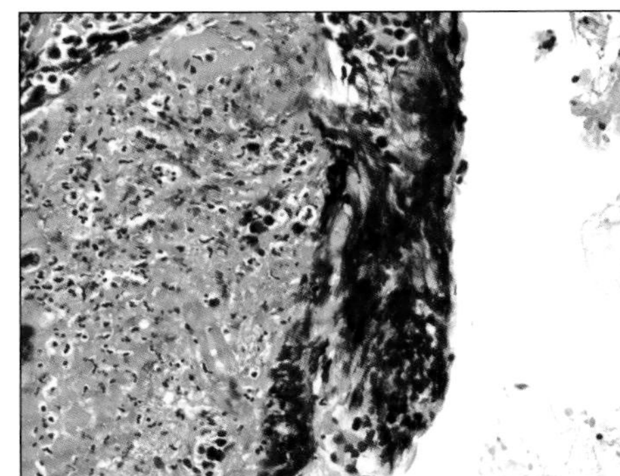

i16.36 Crush artifact and chromatin streaking in small cell carcinoma

ISBN 978-089189-5886

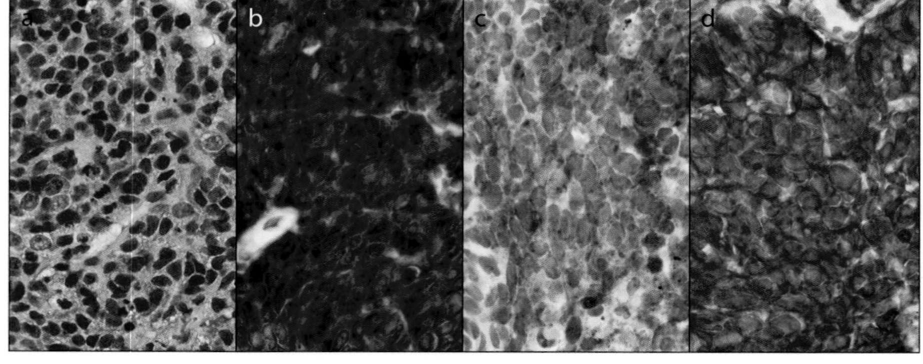

i16.37 a-d Small cell carcinoma. **a** is an H&E. Note the mixture of well-preserved cells with fine chromatin (primarily on the left) and less well-preserved cells with coarse or smudged chromatin. In **b** (synaptophysin), note the intense cytoplasmic positivity. In **c** (chromogranin), note the much less intense cytoplasmic staining (some small cell carcinomas are negative for chromogranin). In **d** (CD56), note the cell membrane staining (CD56 is neural cell adhesion molecule).

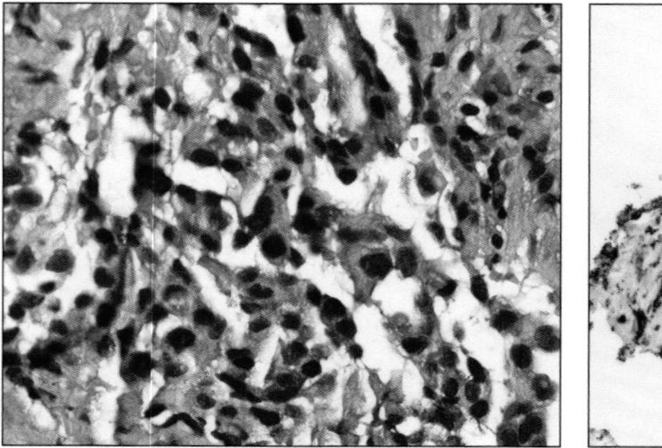

i16.38 A poorly differentiated malignant neoplasm in the lung without obvious gland formation or keratinization

i16.39 The same case as in i16.38 with a positive stain for napsin A

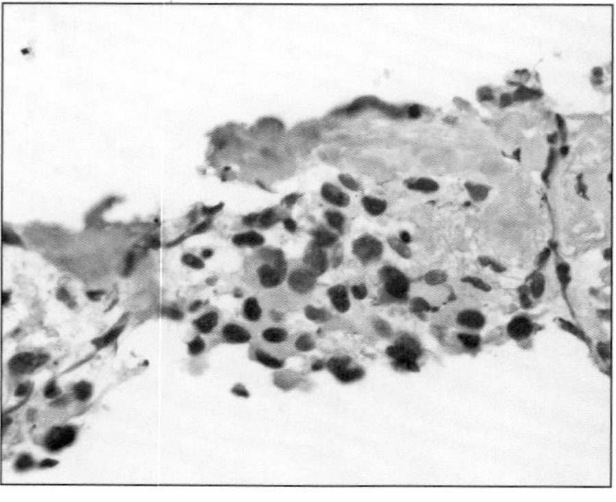

i16.40 The same case as in i16.38 with a negative synaptophysin stain, essentially excluding neuroendocrine origin

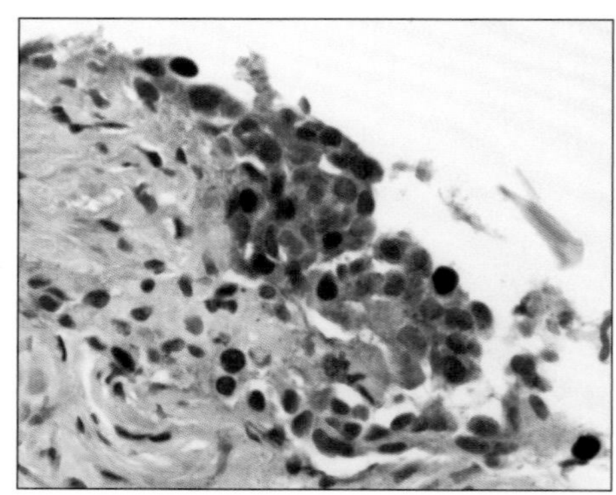

i16.41 The same case as in i16.38, demonstrating cytoplasmic positivity for p63. However, since p63 is a nuclear stain, this is actually a negative stain and is a point against a squamous cell carcinoma. The immunohistochemical panel identifies the tumor in i16.38 as a poorly differentiated adenocarcinoma.

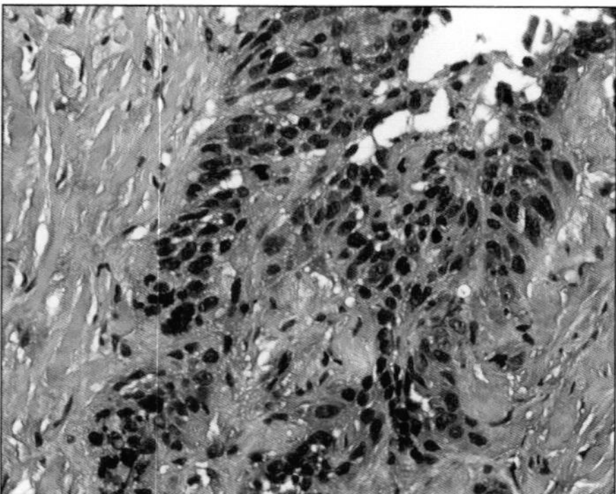

i16.42 Another poorly differentiated carcinoma of the lung without obvious keratinization or gland formation

i16.43 A negative CD56 stain on the same case as in i16.42, essentially excluding a neuroendocrine origin

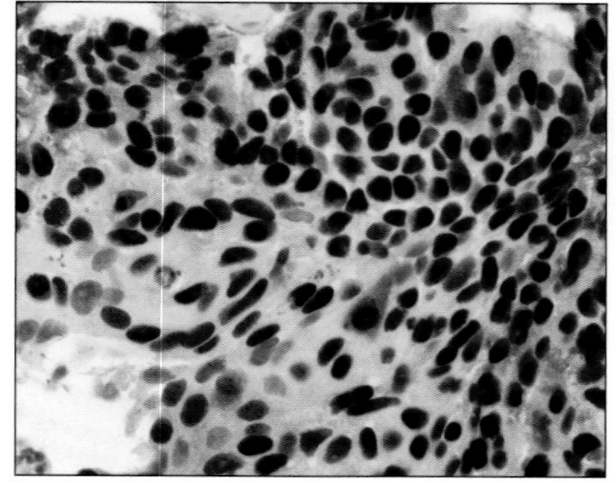

i16.44 A positive p63 stain on the same case as in i16.40, indicating squamous origin

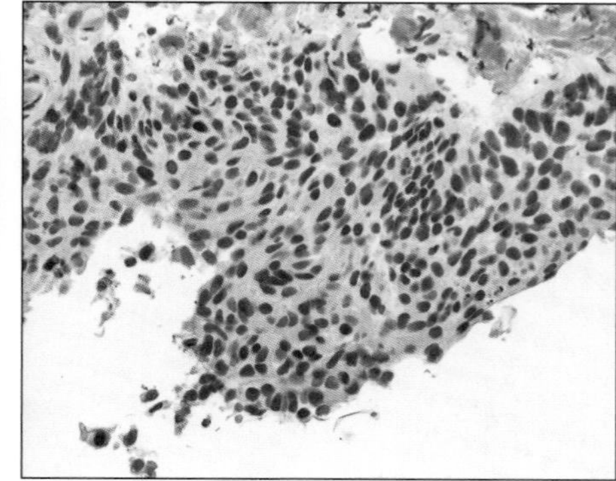

i16.45 A negative napsin A stain on the same case as in i16.42. The immunohistochemical stains performed on the poorly differentiated carcinoma of i16.42 identify it as a poorly differentiated squamous carcinoma rather than a small cell or an adenocarcinoma.

6 Another poorly erentiated carcinoma he lung with no cific features. On E, this could be a all cell carcinoma, oorly differentiated amous carcinoma, or adenocarcinoma.

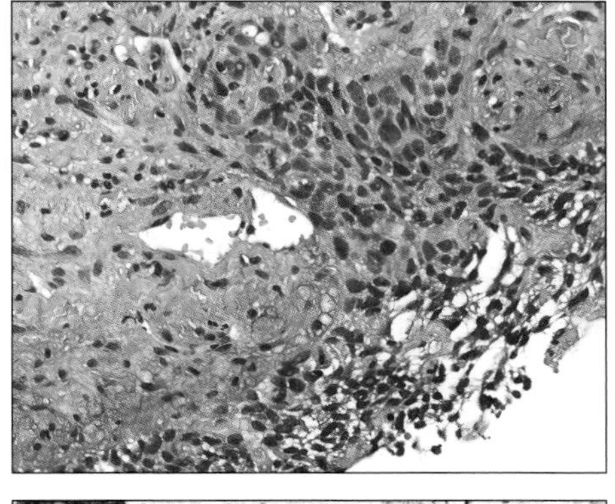

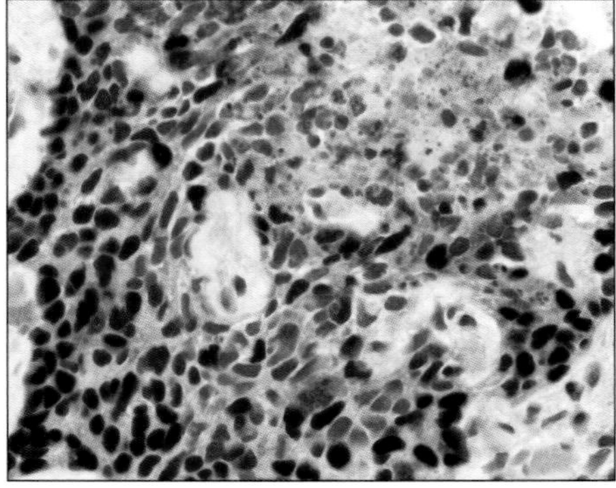

i16.47 A p63 stain on the same case as in i16.46. Note that some of the neoplastic cells are clearly positive, with obvious staining in the nucleus, while other cells appear negative.

8 A CD56 stain on same case as in 46 demonstrating itivity. This unusual e has overlapping tures between a poorly erentiated squamous carcinoma and a small carcinoma.

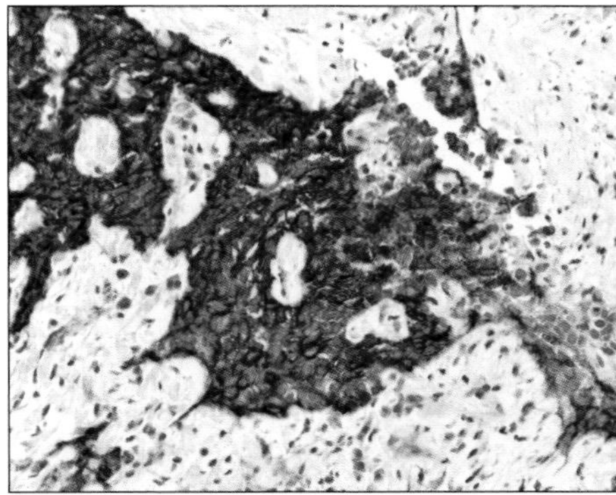

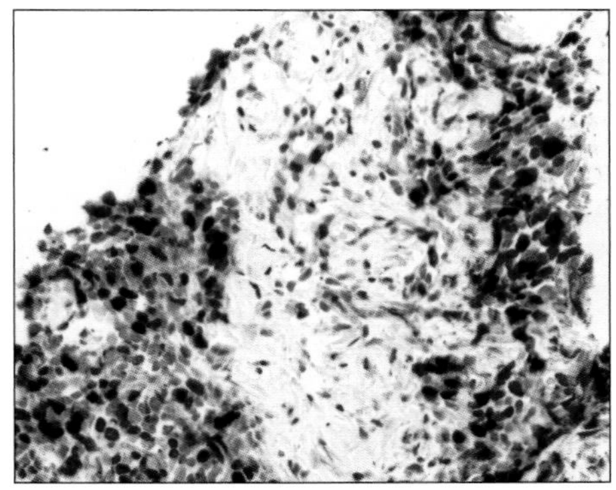

i16.49 Ki-67 immunohistochemical stain of a small cell carcinoma. The majority of the neoplastic cells are positive, far exceeding what would be expected in a grade 1 or grade 2 neuroendocrine carcinoma.

0 Small cell carcinoma ung metastatic to the r, stained with AE1/ 3. The positivity is very ak compared to the mal bile duct (upper nt). By itself, this weak in would be insufficient secure a diagnosis of all cell carcinoma over mphoma. While small carcinoma is an epi-lial neoplasm, keratin ining is not a good way dentify it.

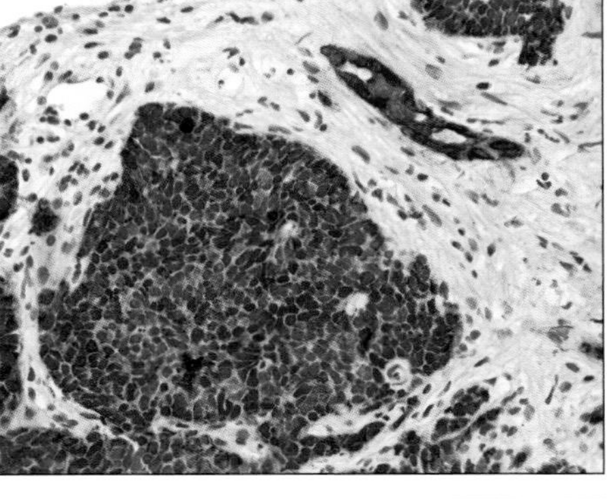

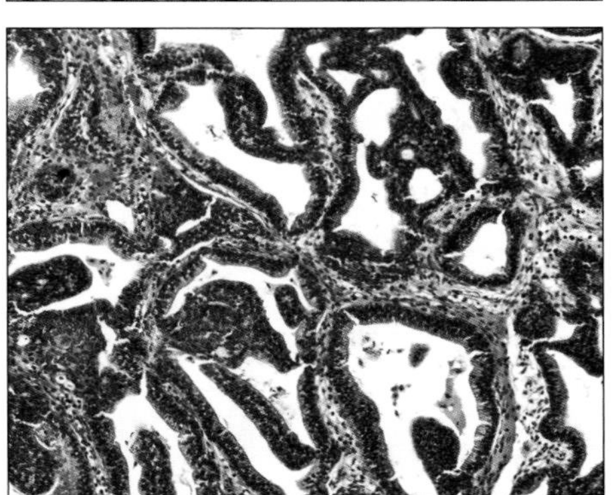

i16.51 A pulmonary blastoma with a characteristic biphasic appearance. The epithelial component consists of tubules resembling a colonic adenomatous polyp. The stroma consists of immature mesenchymal cells.

2 A pleuropulmonary stoma consisting nost completely of mature mesenchyme, h a minor epithelial nponent that has likely en trapped

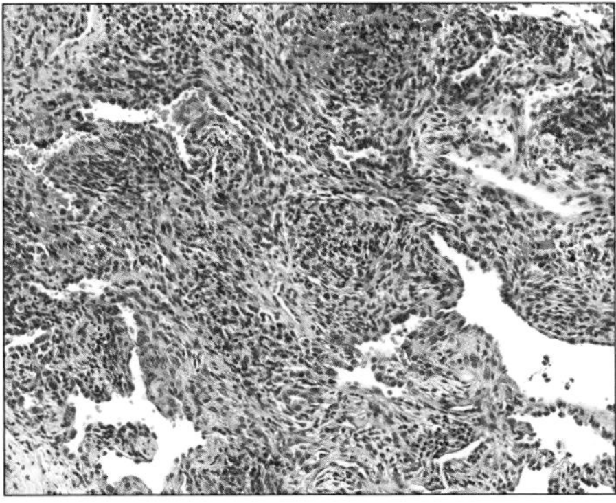

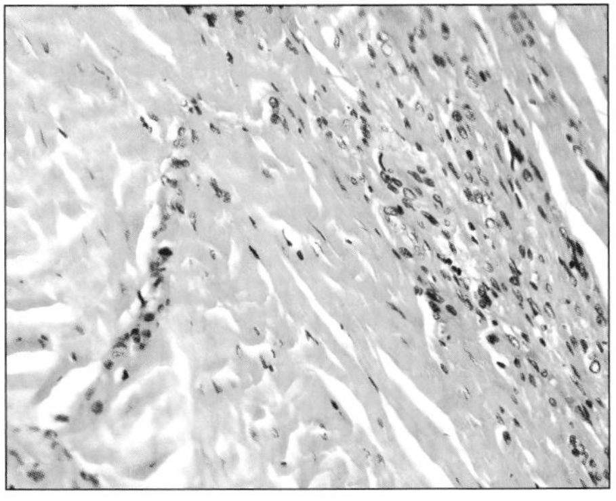

i16.53 An epithelioid hemangioendothelioma. Note the collagenous area on the left, with minimal cellularity and the much larger number of blood vessels and much greater endothelial cellularity on the right.

4 Lymphomatoid nulomatosis with scular invasion by nphocytes, many of ich are not neoplastic

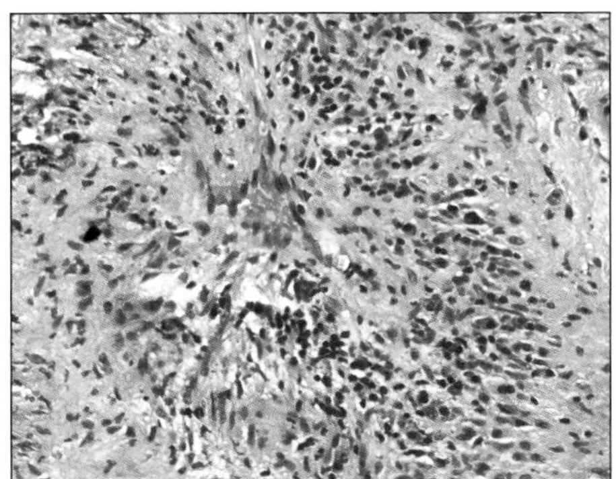

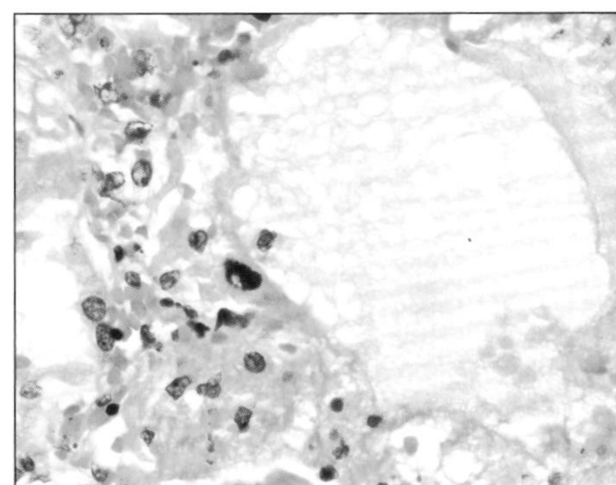

i16.55 *Pneumocystis carinii*. This was confirmed by a GMS stain, but on H&E, note the frothy intraalveolar material. This patient also had CMV, as seen by the inclusion body to the left of center.

ISBN 978-089189-5886

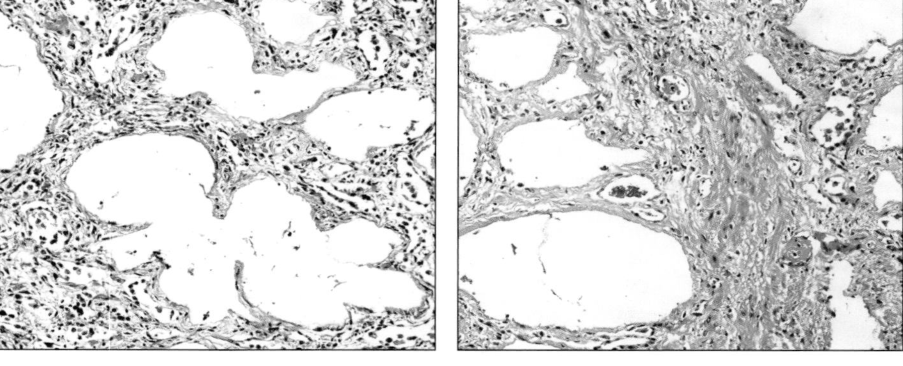

i16.56 UIP. This focus has not yet reached end stage and still has inflammatory cells and fibroblastic cellularity.

i16.57 Another focus in the same biopsy as i16.56, demonstrating a later stage of the process, with less cellularity and denser fibrous tissue

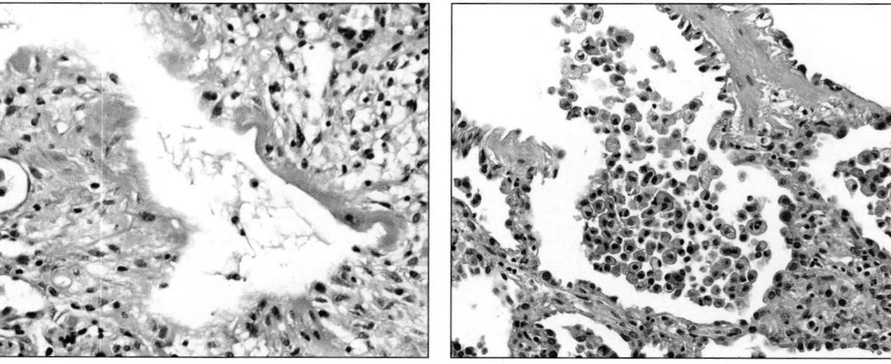

i16.58 Diffuse alveolar damage with hyaline membrane formation

i16.59 Desquamative interstitial pneumonitis with many intraalveolar macrophages

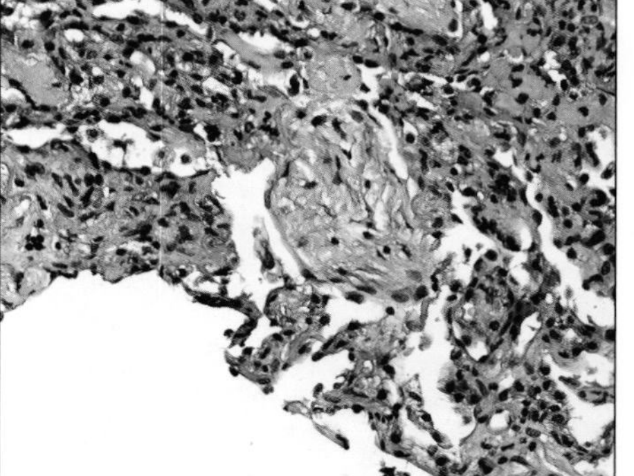

i16.60 Bronchiolitis obliterans with organizing pneumonia. Note the small rounded nodules of cellular fibrosis.

i16.61 Langerhans cell histiocytosis. While a few eosinophils are seen in the upper left, the diagnostic cell type is the Langerhans cell, a member of the histiocyte family that is important in immunity.

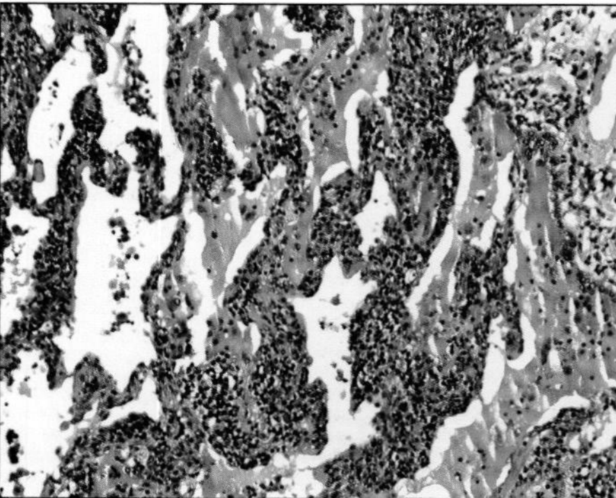

i16.62 Lymphoid interstitial pneumonitis, with abundant lymphocytes filling and distending the interalveolar septae

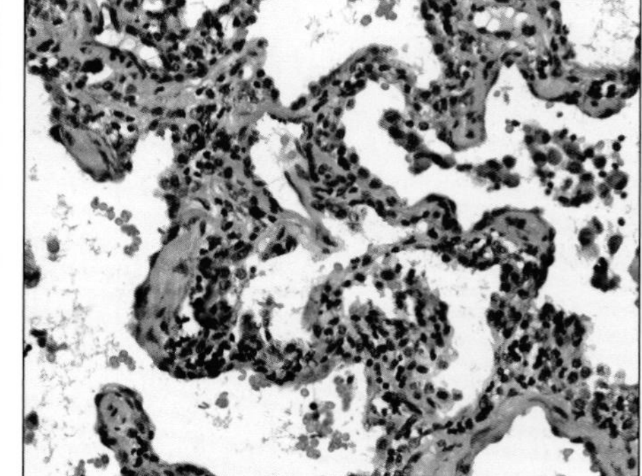

i16.63 Hypersensitivity pneumonitis, with a modest lymphoplasmacytic infiltrate in the interalveolar septae. Note the small amount of septal fibrosis at the left, which neither precludes the diagnosis nor portends an aggressive course.

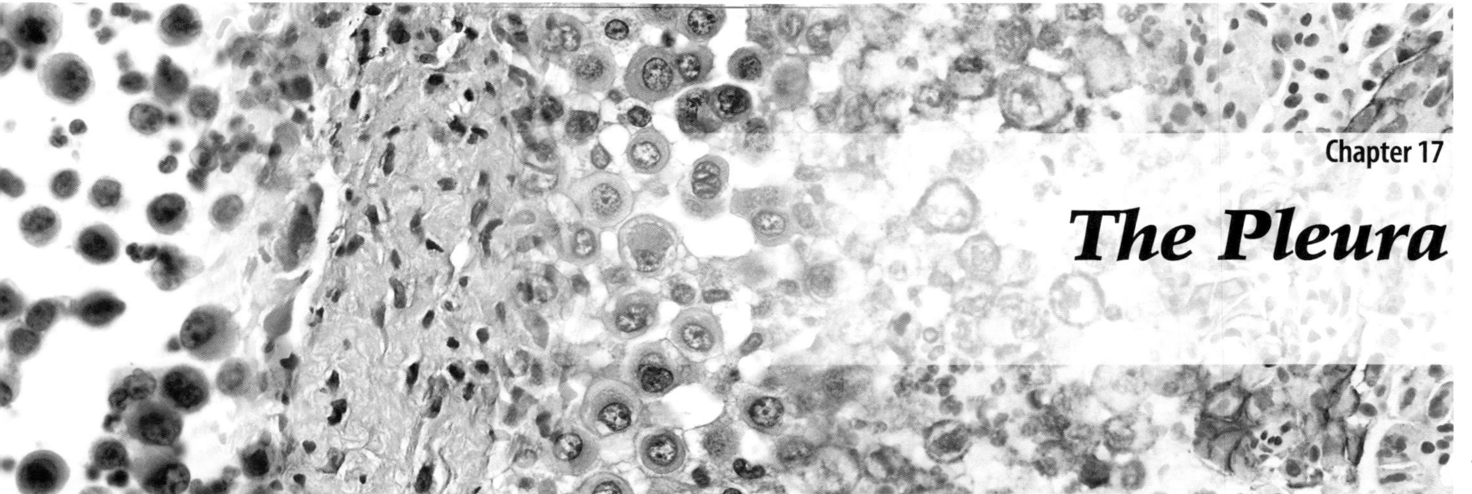

:esothelial Cells vs Metastatic Carcinoma

Distinguishing a mesothelial proliferation from metastatic enocarcinoma in effusions is often exceptionally difficult and :en requires immunohistochemical stains. For this reason, a raffin-processed cell block is preferred, as this is more amenble to immunohistochemical stains.

In recent years, there have been dozens of publications con:rning immunohistochemical stains that preferentially highht either mesothelial cells or adenocarcinoma. Different studies ve arrived at slightly different percentages of cells that stain for articular antibody, but there is agreement that B72.3, Ber-EP4, OC-31, and CD15 stain adenocarcinomas with much greater quency than mesothelial cells and do so in a membranous patn. CEA and Bg-8 preferentially stain the cytoplasm of adenorcinomas. TTF-1 stains the nuclei of adenocarcinomas of lung d thyroid origin. From the other direction, there is agreement at WT-1 preferentially stains the nuclei of mesothelial cells, retinin stains both the nuclei and the cytoplasm of mesothelial ls, and thrombomodulin stains mesothelial cells in a memanous pattern. These results have been confirmed by multiple idies (eg, PMID16554731) and can be accepted with reasonable rtainty i17.1-i17.6.

Because no single stain is perfect, a panel should be employed, d antigens that are associated preferentially with both mesoelial cells and carcinoma should be used. For example, a mprehensive panel of 12 antibodies is certainly effective in disguishing between mesothelioma and pulmonary adenocarcima [PMID16554731], but in these days of cost containment, a smaller of antibodies, selected so that some will highlight epithelial lls while others highlight mesothelial cells, should be sufficient reliably distinguish between the 2 processes. Smaller panels at retain excellent sensitivity and specificity include calretinin, T1, and thrombomodulin to stain mesothelial cells and CEA highlight adenocarcinoma [PMID17316414], as well as calretinin to in mesothelial cells and Bg-8 and CD15 to stain epithelial cells IID19152187].

These panels will require constant updating as new marks are demonstrated. For example, the lymphatic endothelial arker D2-40 has been shown to have high sensitivity (96%) and gh specificity for mesothelium, staining both benign and alignant mesothelial cells in a membranous pattern. D2-40 also ins a number of tumors, including many seminomas, adrenal rtical tumors, schwannomas, and cutaneous adnexal tumors IID19098468]. At this writing, the only adenocarcinoma that is liketo be in the differential diagnosis of a problematic proliferation cells in a pleural or peritoneal specimen and that is routinely stained by D2-40 is ovarian serous carcinoma (65% of which will also stain in a membranous pattern) [PMID15389250].

Once immunohistochemical stains disclose an adenocarcinoma, additional stains may help to identify the primary site. Foremost among the second round of stains, should an adenocarcinoma be present, are cytokeratins 7 and 20 [PMID11937308]. Additional markers include estrogen receptor, progesterone receptor, CGDFP-15, mammaglobin (positivity of any of which suggests a breast primary) [PMID19217055], TTF-1, PE-10, and napsin A (staining for which points to a lung carcinoma) [PMID11668468]. CDX2 staining with negative mesothelial markers supports a lower gastrointestinal adenocarcinoma.

Occasionally, a squamous carcinoma may simulate a mesothelioma in an effusion and immunohistochemical stains are needed. While a history of squamous carcinoma of the lung with a positive effusion and negative mesothelial markers generally secures a diagnosis of metastatic squamous carcinoma, p63 is effective in identifying squamous cell carcinomas in effusions, staining 80% of squamous carcinomas, and few mesothelial proliferations or adenocarcinomas [PMID18064689]. Cytokeratins 5/6 also generally show a preference for squamous cells over adenocarcinoma or mesothelial cells [PMID18064689], suggesting that p63 is currently the best marker of squamous cells. P63 is a transcription factor that is found in the basal layer of multilayered epithelia and is thought to maintain the proliferative potential of this layer, thus permitting multilayering [PMID21151771]. This is why it is useful in identifying squamous as opposed to glandular epithelium, and in demonstrating a myoepithelial or basal layer underlying glandular epithelium in tissues such as breast and prostate.

Malignant Mesotheliomas and Their Mimics

Most malignant mesotheliomas occur in the pleura. There are 3 types of malignant mesotheliomas: epithelial i17.7, i17.8, sarcomatous (also called fibrous or spindle cell) i17.9, and mixed. If a sarcomatous mesothelioma is paucicellular and densely fibrotic, it may be called a desmoplastic mesothelioma. There are a number of types of epithelial mesothelioma, the most common of which, called the tubulo-papillary form i17.10, resembles an adenocarcinoma and is distinguished therefrom by the immunohistochemical stains discussed above.

In any biopsy of a pleural or peritoneal lesion for which a mesothelioma is a consideration, the first requirement is to ensure the mesothelial nature of the cells and to exclude a metastatic carcinoma, as the epithelial variant of malignant mesothelioma can be indistinguishable from carcinoma on

H&E. Immunohistochemical stains as described above can be employed if needed, as the principles in distinguishing a mesothelial proliferation from metastatic carcinoma are the same in effusions, biopsies, and resection material **i17.11**, **i17.12**, **i17.13**.

Once it is clear that the cells are of mesothelial origin, attention can be directed to the benign vs malignant nature of the mesothelial cells. In any mesothelial lesion—pleural or peritoneal—invasion must be proven to diagnose malignancy **i17.14**, **i17.15**. Once metastatic carcinoma is excluded by immunohistochemical stains, it is the presence of invasion more than the appearance of the nuclei that histologically confirms a malignant mesothelial process on biopsy material [PMID16253023]. Atypical cells whose mesothelial nature is confirmed by immunohistochemical staining are not sufficient for the diagnosis of any form of mesothelioma because there is substantial overlap in appearance between reactive mesothelial cells and those from mesothelioma.

If invasion cannot be proven in a pleural biopsy whose problematic cells have been shown to be of mesothelial origin, it is wise to indicate that clinical correlation is needed to exclude a malignancy because the biopsy may not have captured an invasive focus. If the mesothelial nature of a clinically worrisome mass is confirmed, but invasion cannot be proven, a presumptive diagnosis of mesothelioma can be rendered on the basis of clinical and radiographic findings (eg, large or multifocal) in conjunction with the morphology and immunohistochemical characterization of the cells in the biopsy.

While the demonstration of invasion is indispensable in the diagnosis of a malignant mesothelial proliferation, some assistance may be forthcoming from both immunohistochemistry and DNA studies. There are several forms of mesothelial hyperplasia that are uncommonly encountered as small nodules. The antibody GLUT-1 is reported to stain malignant mesotheliomas and lung carcinomas, but not benign mesothelial cells [PMID17192790], and IMP3 has been reported to stain only malignant mesothelial proliferations [PMID21566519]. The demonstration of aneuploidy (a chromosome number that is not a multiple of 23), an increased number of nucleolar organizing regions, and the demonstration of a 9p21 deletion by FISH are suggestions that the mesothelial cells are malignant [PMID18306350], but at this writing, the value of both immunohistochemistry and DNA studies await confirmation, and either histologic invasion or compelling clinical/radiographic findings must be present for a firm diagnosis of mesothelioma.

A pleural plaque is a localized, simple collagenous proliferation with scattered fibroblasts and entrapped mesothelial cells **i17.16**. Its benign nature is usually evident both radiographically and histologically. A much greater diagnostic pitfall is that desmoplastic mesothelioma—a malignant neoplasm—can greatly resemble the nonneoplastic entity fibrinous pleuritis. In differentiating these 2 entities, it is particularly imperative to remember that invasion must be demonstrated before a malignant diagnosis is rendered. Fibrinous pleuritis may have substantial nuclear atypia **i17.17** and may appear to invade the adjacent tissue, but keratin or calretinin staining will show that the actual mesothelial cells—the putative malignant cells—fail to invade, and that the "invasion" is actually caused by a fibroinflammatory exudate **i17.18**.

Solitary Fibrous Tumors

Most cases of what were called benign, solitary fibrous mesothelioma are now called solitary fibrous tumor (SFT; also called localized fibrous tumor) [PMID12118790], though SFT may occur in other locations and may rarely be malignant. The term "solitary fibrous tumor" is preferred over "solitary fibrous mesothelioma" because SFTs are thought to arise from submesothelioblasts rather than from mesothelial cells and are not associated with asbestos exposure [PMID9447390].

SFTs often have alternating hypocellular and hypercellular areas **i17.19** and a hemangiopericytoma-like vascular pattern (ie, thin-walled, dilated vessels that often branch) **i17.20**. Like hemangiopericytomas, most SFTs are positive for bcl-2 [PMID9669348], and often positive for CD99 [PMID19929175] and CD34 [PMID17669989]. This similarity in H&E appearance and immunohistochemical profile suggests that there is a relationship between SFT and hemangiopericytoma or that they may be the same entity [PMID19444101].

The H&E appearance of most SFTs is distinct from an epithelial mesothelioma, but they must be differentiated from the sarcomatous form of mesothelioma and from the unusual entity hyaline pleural plaque, which consists of dense collagen and occurs predominantly in the lower pleura in men, especially those with a history of asbestos exposure [PMID10434462].

Core Points for the Pleura

- IHC can distinguish a mesothelial proliferation from a metastatic adenocarcinoma.
  - o If such stains indicate an adenocarcinoma, additional stains may identify the primary tumor.
- IHC is less effective in distinguishing a mesothelial proliferation from a metastatic squamous carcinoma.
  - o p63 and cytokeratins 5/6 suggest a squamous carcinoma
  - o But the main value of immunohistochemistry in these cases is to exclude mesothelial origin.
- Once the mesothelial nature of a proliferation has been confirmed, IHC does not distinguish benign from malignant processes.
  - o Demonstration of invasion required for histologic diagnosis of malignant mesothelioma, though persuasive radiographic evidence of a malignant neoplasm provides reasonable certainty.
- 3 types of malignant mesothelioma:
  - o Epithelial
  - o Sarcomatous (also called fibrous or spindle cell)
  - o Mixed
- Fibrinous pleuritis: may resemble desmoplastic mesothelioma, especially if entrapped mesothelial cells within the exudate simulate invasion.
  - o IHC may demonstrate that the mesothelial cells are dispersed in fibroinflammatory tissue adjacent to the pleura rather than invading into it.
- Solitary fibrous tumor (SFT): most cases once regarded as localized, benign fibrous mesothelioma are now recognized as SFT.
  - o Must be distinguished from the sarcomatous form of mesothelioma.
  - o Localized nature of the SFT.
  - o SFT and the hemangiopericytoma share many morphologic and immunohistochemical characteristics and are the same entity, or at least related.

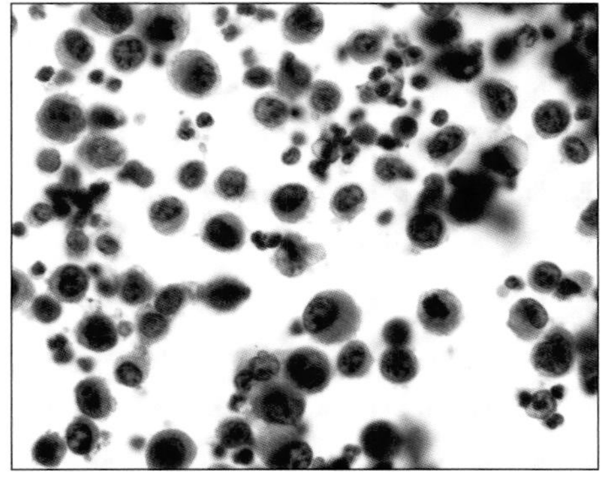
A cytology ·paration of a malignant ·ural effusion. Although ·re is significant nuclear ·pia, the neutrophils ·ggest that confirmation ·malignancy is prudent.

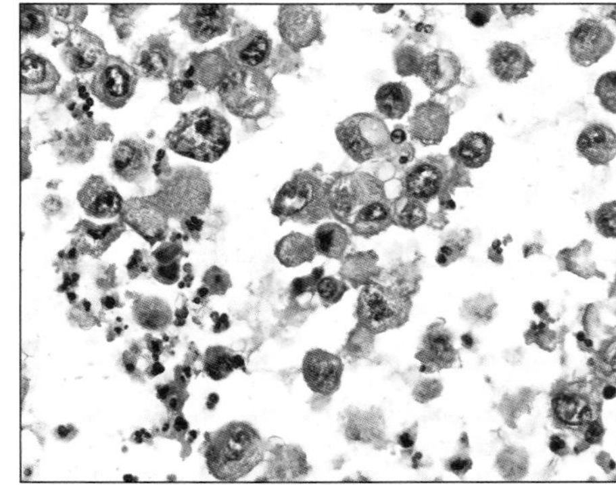
i17.2 A cell block prepared from the same case as in i17.1. Again, the significant atypia makes malignancy very likely, but acute inflammation is still apparent, suggesting that a reactive atypia may not be completely excluded.

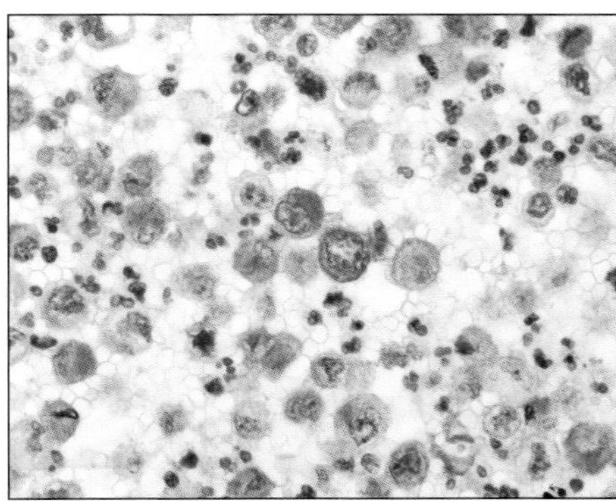
CEA stain ·formed on the cell ·ck, demonstrating ·oplasmic staining ·some of the ·ls, confirming ·enocarcinoma

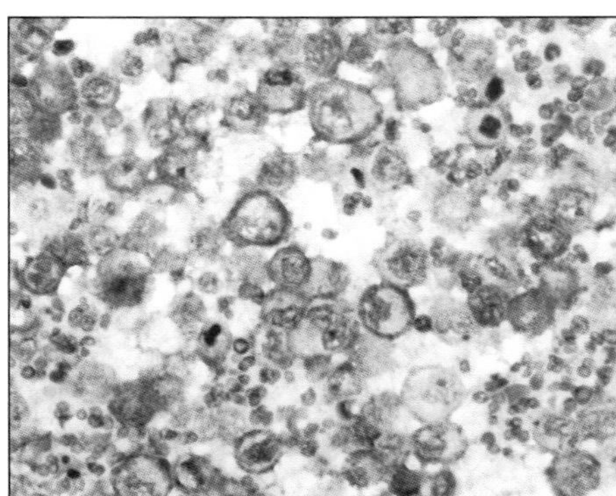
i17.4 Ber-EP4 stain of the same case as in i17.1, demonstrating cell membrane positivity of the adenocarcinoma cells

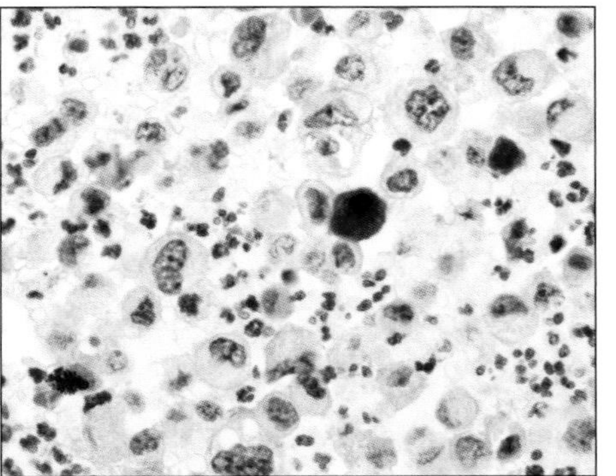
Calretinin stain on ·same case as in i17.1, ·monstrating only a rare ·nign mesothelial cell

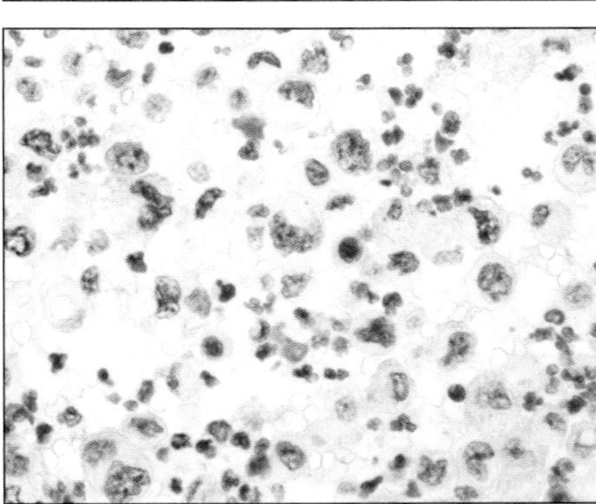
i17.6 WT-1 stain, demonstrating only a rare benign mesothelial nucleus

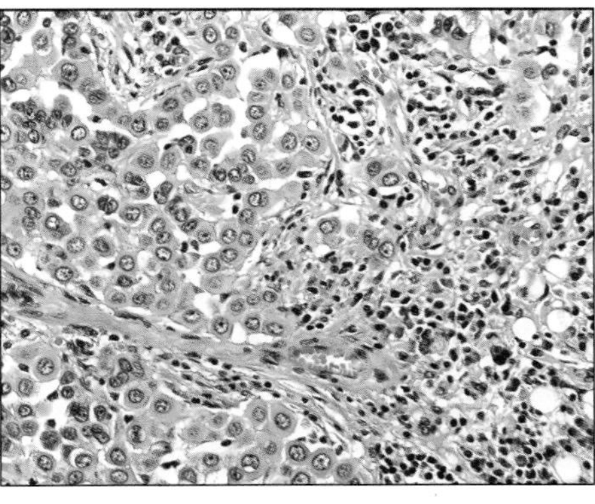
An epithelial ·lignant mesothelioma ·the diffuse type, ·ading into the pleura

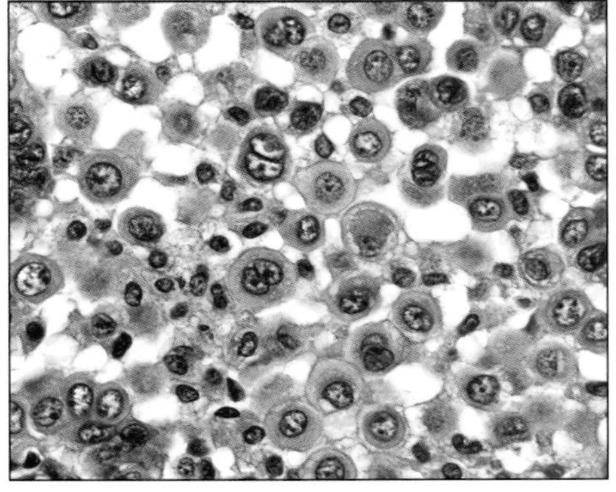
i17.8 A higher-power view of i17.7, showing that some mesothelial characteristics are still recognizable. Note occasional binucleated cells, demarcation of endoplasm and ectoplasm in the central cell (endoplasm is the darker perinuclear cytoplasm and the ectoplasm is a lighter peripheral cytoplasm), and the "windows," very small spaces between adjacent mesothelial cells.

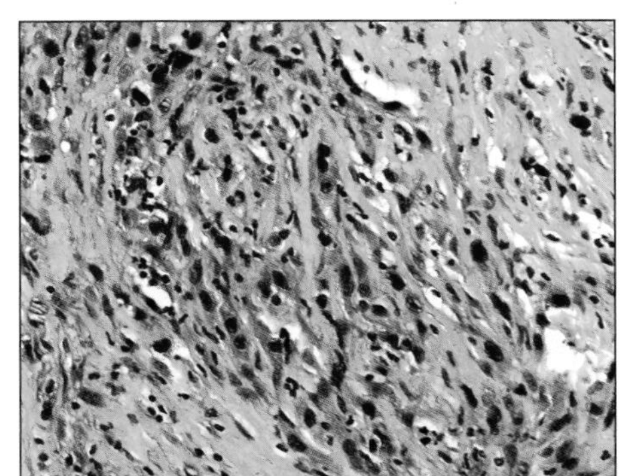
A sarcomatous ·lignant mesothelioma

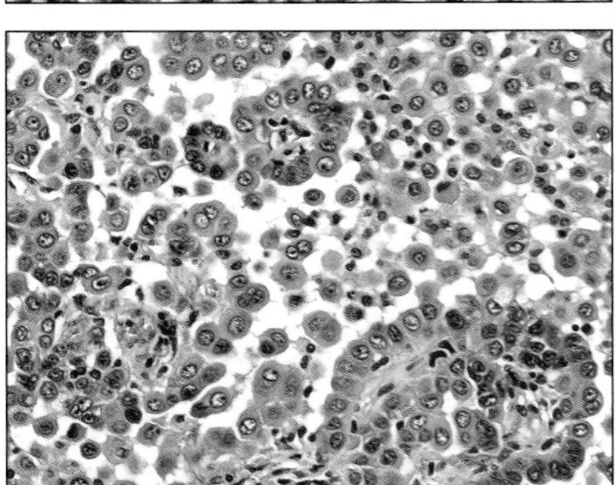
i17.10 A tubulo-papillary form of epithelial mesothelioma

ISBN 978-089189-5886

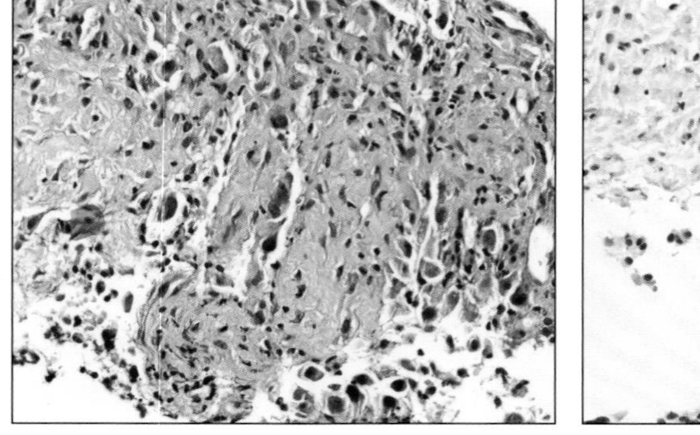

i17.11 A malignant neoplasm invading into the pleura, requiring immunohistochemical characterization to distinguish between a malignant mesothelioma and a metastatic adenocarcinoma

i17.12 The same case as i17.11, illustrating a negative calretinin stain

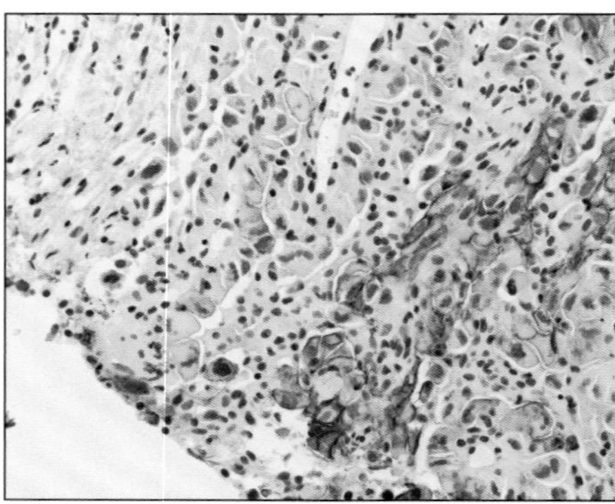

i17.13 The same case as in i17.11, illustrating a positive stain for MOC-31 in a membranous pattern. The negative calretinin and the positive MOC-31 identify the neoplasm as an adenocarcinoma.

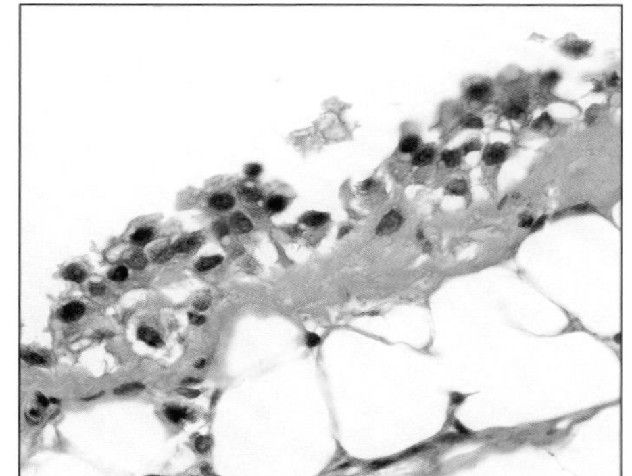

i17.14 Mesothelial cells with nuclear atypia and stratification, but a firm diagnosis of malignant mesothelioma cannot be made because there is no invasion.

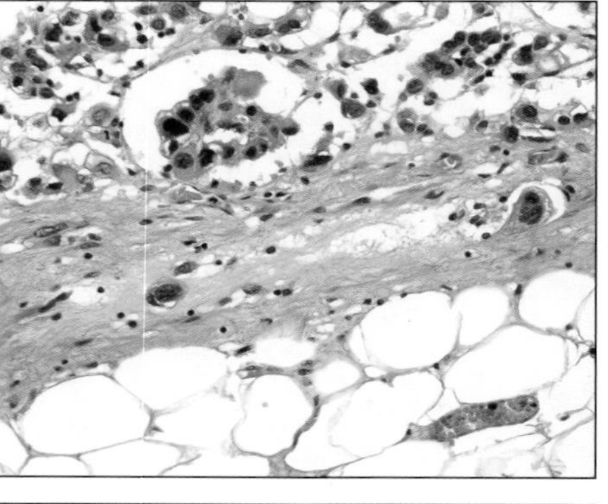

i17.15 While the atypical and very hyperplastic mesothelial cells in the upper portion of the photograph strongly suggest malignancy, a malignant diagnosis is secured only by a very small number of cells invading into the central fibrous portion.

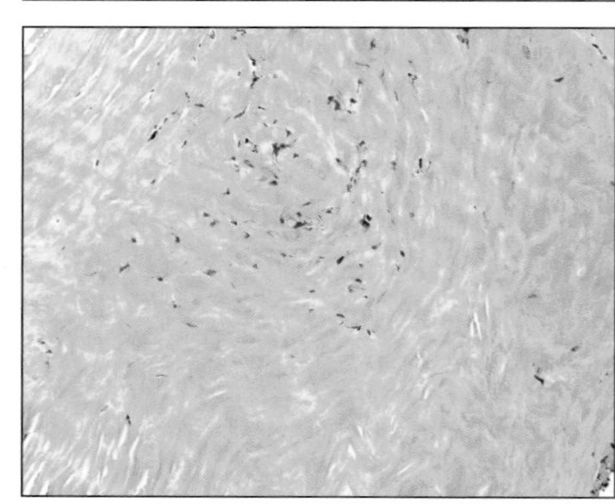

i17.16 A pleural plaque, with collagenous stroma and low cellularity

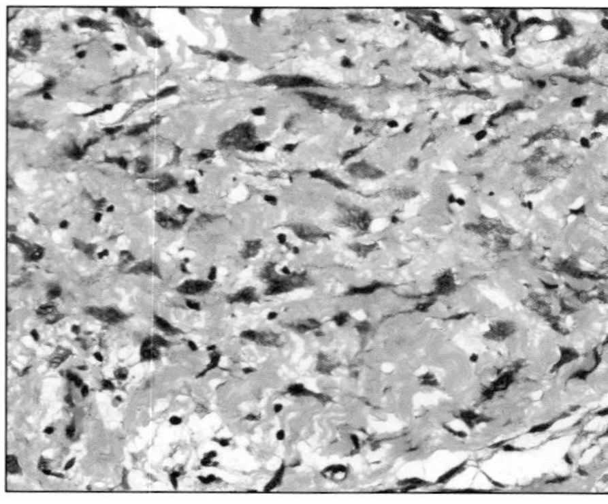

i17.17 Atypical cells in the stroma of a pleural biopsy, suggesting a malignant process

i17.18 The same case as in i17.17, demonstrating that this is fibrinous pleuritis. The atypical cells in i17.17 are actually reactive fibroblasts.

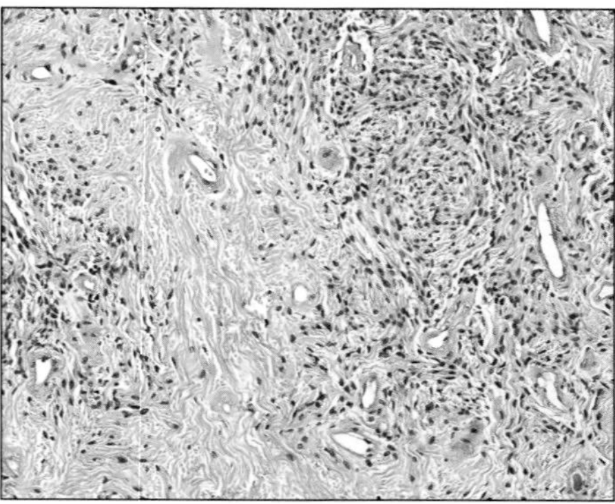

i17.19 A solitary fibrous tumor demonstrating areas of low cellularity intermingled with hypercellular areas

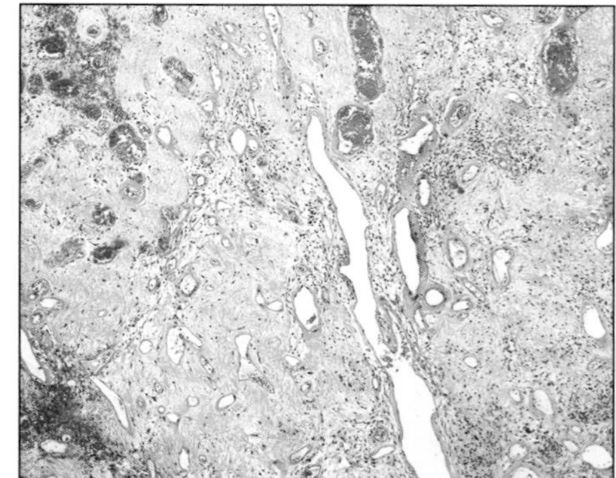

i17.20 A solitary fibrous tumor with a hemangiopericytoma-like vascular pattern (thin-walled, dilated vessels). The morphologic and immunohistochemical similarities between the solitary fibrous tumor and hemangiopericytoma suggest they are related or identical entities.

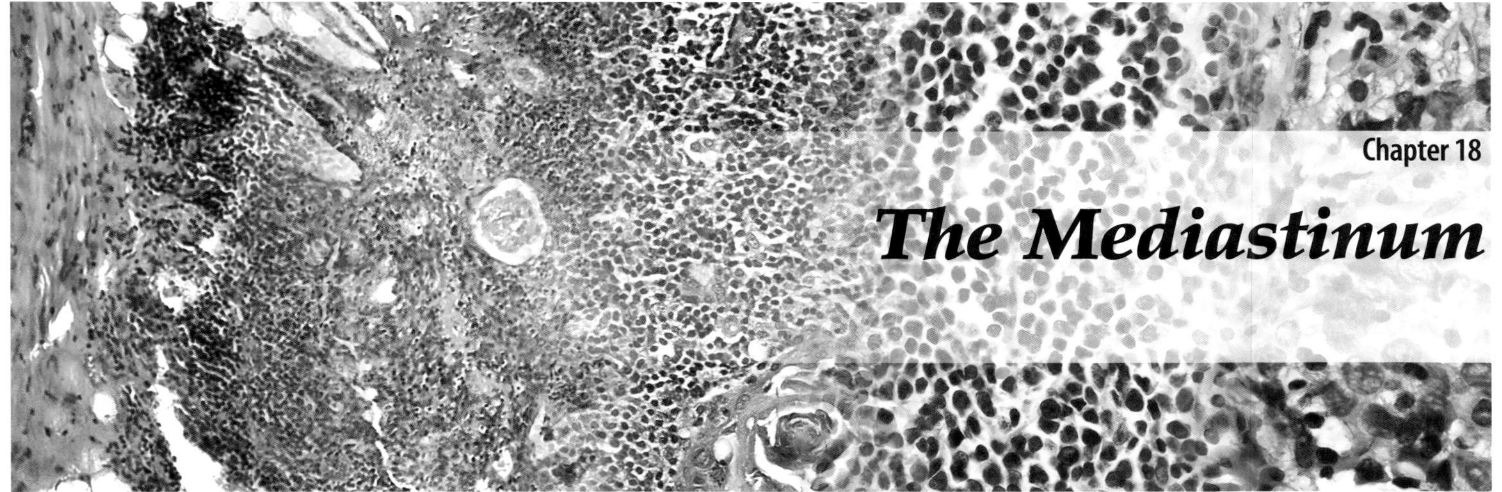

Nonneoplastic Anterior Mediastinal Lesions

Many mass lesions of the mediastinum are nonneoplastic cysts. These cystic masses are primarily bronchogenic, thymic, lymphangiomas, and mesothelial lined (coelomic) [PMID20207297]. Lymphangiomas and mesothelial-lined cysts are rarely a diagnostic challenge. Intrapulmonary bronchogenic cysts communicate with the airways, and therefore are exposed to pathogens. Because they may lack normal clearance mechanisms, they often become infected. In contrast, mediastinal bronchogenic cysts do not communicate with airways, and are therefore not exposed to pathogens and are usually asymptomatic.

Other than these cysts, most anterior mediastinal processes, cystic or neoplastic, involve the thymus. The normal thymus consists of lobules that are separated by thin bands of fibrous tissue. Each lobule has a light staining medulla surrounded by a darker staining cortex. Hassall corpuscles are small concentric arrangements of keratinizing squamous cells in the medulla i18.1. Both the cortex and the medulla consist primarily of T cells, but there are a few B cells in the medulla.

Thymic cysts are lined by squamous, cuboidal, or columnar epithelium, with or without cilia. It is prudent to exclude a bronchogenic cyst if cilia are seen. Thymic cysts may be unilocular i18.2 or, more commonly, multilocular i18.3. Unilocular cysts are usually congenital, while multilocular are usually acquired. The epithelium of thymic cysts may be lost in some areas, and cholesterol clefts, hemorrhage, necrosis, and granulation tissue may all be found in the lumen i18.4.

While the innocuous nuclei in thymic cysts should prevent an overdiagnosis of squamous carcinoma, they can easily be confused with a cystic thymoma. This is especially true of the proliferating subtype of multilocular cyst, in which there is hyperplasia of the squamous lining of the cysts [PMID1709608]. A significant amount of epithelium between cysts, not connected to any cyst lining, suggests a thymoma.

Although the major neoplasm that is potentially missed in a cystic mass is a thymoma, lymphomas and germ cell tumors may also "hide" in what appears to be a thymic cyst. Missing a neoplasm in a cystic mass of the thymus is especially problematic on fine needle aspiration or core biopsy. In these specimens, the presence of a cyst should always elicit a comment that a neoplasm cannot be excluded in this material.

Major noncystic, nonneoplastic anterior mediastinal masses include thymic hyperplasia, benign lymphadenopathy, and sclerosing mediastinitis. In children, thymic germinal centers are common, and weight is the key indicator of thymic hyperplasia. In adults, thymic germinal centers are rare, and many regard their presence, not weight, as the key indicator of thymic hyperplasia. The defining feature of the thymus in most patients with myasthenia gravis is follicular lymphoid hyperplasia i18.5 or a thymoma, not a simple increase in weight. 2/3 of patients with myasthenia gravis will have follicular hyperplasia of the thymic lymphoid tissue, and many of the remainder will have a thymoma [PMID3677008]. In any case, the terminology used should indicate whether the hyperplasia is secondary to an increase in thymic tissue or to follicular hyperplasia of lymphoid tissue.

Lymphoid processes are addressed as in other sites and as discussed in Chapter 8. The only comment here is that while Castleman disease may indeed involve the anterior mediastinal lymph nodes and clinically appear to be a thymic process i18.6, care must be taken not to misinterpret Hassall corpuscles as the atrophic germinal centers of the hyaline vascular type.

Sclerosing mediastinitis usually occurs in the anterior mediastinum and has minimal cellularity i18.7, except in the rare cases in which it is diagnosed early, when there are still numerous fibroblasts and inflammatory cells. Sclerosing mediastinitis is associated with *Histoplasma* in about 1/2 of cases. Some of the remaining 1/2 are part of the IgG4 related autoimmune sclerosing disorders [PMID16426926]. Sclerosing mediastinitis may calcify, in which case it may be called a calcifying fibrous pseudotumor. The caveat in these situations is not to miss a paucicellular, desmoplastic carcinoma, desmoplastic mesothelioma, or a nodular sclerosing Hodgkin disease.

Epithelial Neoplasms of the Anterior Mediastinum

The mediastinum is home to many neoplastic processes, many of which contain several types of "passenger" cells in addition to the neoplastic cells. For this reason, immunohistochemical characterization is usually indispensable in correctly evaluating neoplasms in this location.

Thymomas, by definition, have bland epithelial cells. If the epithelial cells are overtly malignant, the correct diagnosis is thymic carcinoma, not thymoma. Rare Hassall corpuscles may be seen in thymomas, but the normal thymic corticomedullary architecture is usually vague or absent in thymomas, owing in part to the atrophy of the gland in adults and in part to the effacement of whatever amount of normal thymic architecture remains.

The traditional classification of thymomas is lymphocyte predominant (or lymphoepithelial), if they are >66% lymphocytes **i18.8**, epithelial predominant if they are >66% epithelial cells **i18.9**, mixed if neither the epithelial nor lymphoid population exceeds 66%, and spindle cell **i18.10**.

While the squamous cells may be readily identifiable in a lymphocyte predominant thymoma, they may also be subtly dispersed in a sea of lymphocytes, and the nonneoplastic lymphocytes may so perfectly resemble a lymphoproliferative disorder that the correct diagnosis is impossible without immunohistochemical identification of the epithelial component **i18.11**. Another benefit of immunohistochemical stains in these situations is to prove polyclonality of the lymphocytes. Encapsulation **i18.12** favors a thymoma over a lymphoma. Many thymomas have anastomosing bands of collagen within them, demarcating them into lobules, and this finding also favors a thymoma if lymphocytes are abundant **i18.13**.

An odd finding in many thymomas is that of perivascular spaces, in which cysts form adjacent to or around capillaries. These initially appear to be dilated capillaries, and the capillary may indeed be somewhat dilated, but closer study shows that the space primarily surrounds the vessel **i18.14**.

Cystic thymomas are distinguished from nonneoplastic thymic cysts by the amount of thymic epithelium. Thymic cysts usually have little epithelium outside of the lining of the cysts **i18.3, i18.15a, i18.15b**. Even in the proliferating subtype of the multilocular cyst, the epithelium is generally associated with cysts. In contrast, in cystic thymomas, most of the epithelium is not associated with cysts **i18.16**. A keratin stain is helpful in differentiating cystic thymoma from thymic cyst because it highlights the amount and location of the epithelium. A thick capsule and angular anastomosing bands of collagen within the tumor favor a thymoma over a thymic cyst, just as they favor a thymoma over a lymphoid process. The presence of recognizable normal cortical-medullary architecture favors a nonneoplastic cyst, but absence of normal architecture is not helpful since the normal architecture is likely to be attenuated from atrophy and a thymic cyst may disrupt whatever normal structure remains. Fortunately, given that thymomas are indolent if not invasive, the distinction of a thymic cyst from a cystic thymoma is not generally critical if the mass is noninvasive.

The 2004 WHO classification [Travis ISBN978-9283224181] focuses on the morphology of the tumor cells rather than the number of lymphocytes. While the WHO recognizes many subtypes of thymoma, type A thymomas generally have spindle cells, type B have round cells, and type C thymic neoplasms are frank squamous cell carcinomas.

For any type of thymoma (as opposed to overt thymic carcinoma), the important issue is whether or not the neoplasm is clinically invasive. Therefore, many now simply classify these tumors as thymoma if they are well circumscribed and noninfiltrative, and invasive (or atypical) thymoma if they are not **i18.17**. Stage is much more important than histologic type. Specifically, once the diagnosis of thymoma is made, and overt thymic carcinoma is excluded, the key question is not the ratio of epithelial cells to lymphocytes or the shape of the cell, but the presence or absence or infiltration into adjacent tissues [PMID18514131]. At this writing, this single feature supersedes morphology, immunohistochemistry, and DNA characteristics in the prognosis of thymomas that are not overtly cytologically malignant.

There are many types of thymic carcinoma, but major varieties include classic squamous **i18.18**, basaloid squamous **i18.19**, spindle cell squamous, adenosquamous/mucoepidermoid, and lymphoepithelioma-like. The rare lymphoepithelioma-like thymic carcinoma has large nuclei, a vesicular chromatin pattern and prominent nucleoli, with background lymphocytes **i18.20a**, **i18.20b**, resembling undifferentiated nasopharyngeal carcinomas. The unusual varieties may be accompanied by a focus of more conventional squamous carcinoma, but if they are not, immunohistochemical stains may be needed, particularly to distinguish the basaloid variety of squamous carcinoma from a neuroendocrine neoplasm. In addition to possible foci of conventional squamous carcinoma and immunohistochemistry, thymomas, even atypical ones, are at least partially encapsulated, while thymic carcinomas are not. Lymphoepithelioma-like thymic carcinomas are not encapsulated, and have more nuclear pleomorphism and larger nucleoli.

If there is difficulty distinguishing between a thymoma and a thymic carcinoma, or a carcinoma of another type, immunohistochemistry may assist, as thymic carcinomas are reported to express CD5 [PMID9620029, PMID9930146] CD70 [PMID10800994], and bcl-2 [PMID12877732] more than either thymomas or carcinomas of other organs.

Nonepithelial Neoplasms of the Anterior Mediastinum

The nonepithelial anterior mediastinal neoplasms, except the thymolipoma, are discussed elsewhere in this work, and they have also been reviewed [PMID19054157], so they will not be discussed in detail here. The most common nonepithelial anterior mediastinal neoplasms are the lymphomas. Hodgkin disease is the most common mediastinal malignancy and may occur either in the thymus or in mediastinal lymph nodes. When Hodgkin disease is present in the thymus, it must be distinguished from a thymoma. Because most thymomas have nodules of tumor in a fibrous stroma, nodular sclerosing Hodgkin is a particular potential mimic of a thymoma **i18.21**. One should be suspicious of Hodgkin disease in a thymic mass if there are eosinophils, but the identification of Reed-Sternberg cells or variants **i18.22**, followed by immunohistochemical verification, is imperative for the diagnosis.

Except for Hodgkin disease, the most common nonepithelial malignancy in the anterior mediastinum is a specific type of diffuse large cell non-Hodgkin lymphoma called the primary mediastinal large B-cell lymphoma, which occurs mostly in young to middle-aged women and often demonstrates substantial fibrosis **i18.23** [PMID3953939]. They may have cells that resemble Reed-Sternberg cells, and the similarity to Hodgkin disease can be striking i18.24. Indeed, they have immunophenotypic and molecular characteristics that are intermediate between a Hodgkin and a non-Hodgkin lymphoma and which are discussed in Chapter 8.

The primary mediastinal large B-cell lymphoma can also resemble a carcinoma, and because the neoplastic cells are large and are often associated with smaller lymphocytes, this entity can also resemble a seminoma. Mediastinal tumors that might be a diffuse large cell lymphoma should therefore receive broad immunohistochemical characterization, including CD15, CD30, CD45, a B marker, a T marker, keratin, and placental alkaline phosphatase (for germ cell tumors). Of particular importance is that 70% of primary mediastinal large B-cell lymphomas may stain with CD30 [Swerdlow ISBN978-9283224310]. Hence, the importance of a complete immunohistochemical characterization, as a false diagnosis of Hodgkin disease or anaplastic lymphoma is avoided by recognizing that the neoplastic cells are negative for CD15 and positive for CD45, CD20, and CD79.

A third lymphoma encountered in the anterior mediastinum is the lymphoblastic lymphoma, characterized on H&E by a monomorphic population of small lymphocytes with fine chromatin i18.25, i18.26. This entity is discussed in Chapter 8, but the caveat here is to be careful not to overdiagnose a lymphoblastic lymphoma because of the large number of immature T cells that are found in the normal thymus. Full immunohistochemical characterization is necessary, but a TdT stain will not help, as it will be positive in both normal and neoplastic lymphocytes. In difficult cases, it may be necessary to perform T-cell receptor gene rearrangement studies.

One can also encounter an inflammatory myofibroblastic tumor (formerly called inflammatory pseudotumor) in the mediastinum. This may resemble sclerosing mediastinitis, but circumscription and plasma cells favor an inflammatory myofibroblastic tumor. Extensive fibrosis, paucicellularity, and infiltration favor sclerosing mediastinitis. Immunohistochemical stains may be of benefit in the identification of an inflammatory myofibroblastic tumor, as discussed in Chapter 2.

Other anterior mediastinal tumors include carcinoid tumor (the spindle cell variety of which may resemble the spindle cell thymoma), paraganglioma, parathyroid tumors arising from ectopic parathyroid tissue, germ cell tumors i18.27, and mesotheliomas, all of which are diagnosed as in other sites. The thymolipoma is a lipoma with a small amount of admixed benign thymic and lymphoid tissue i18.28. Thymolipomas can be quite large, but are circumscribed [PMID8539231].

Middle and Posterior Mediastinal Lesions

Neoplasms of the middle mediastinum are rare, as the heart almost completely occupies this area. A useful mnemonic regarding the posterior mediastinum is that most neoplasms in this location are neural in nature. Nerve sheath tumors, such as schwannomas i18.29 and neurofibromas, are commonly seen in the posterior mediastinum, as are ganglioneuromas. The latter tumor has, in addition to the large ganglion cells, a background that resembles a neurofibroma i18.30. In addition to the larger cells, a ganglioneuroma also differs from a neurofibroma in that it is encapsulated.

The only other process to occur with any frequency in the posterior mediastinum is the enteric cyst, which often has a squamous or gastrointestinal lining surrounded by a double muscle layer, as is seen in the gastrointestinal tract [PMID4741443].

Core Points for the Mediastinum

- Thymic cysts: single of multiloculated, 1-2 cell layer lining, with epithelium associated with the cyst.
  - o Bronchogenic cyst: lining may be ciliated.
- Thymomas: encapsulated squamous neoplasms without compelling nuclear atypia.
  - o Some classifications of thymomas have employed the number of lymphocytes or the shape of the cells
  - o But the presence or absence of infiltration is the most important feature.
  - o Those thymomas that infiltrate are atypical thymomas, but even they are at least partially encapsulated.
- The lymphocyte-predominant thymoma must be distinguished from a lymphoma.
  - o H&E and immunohistochemical findings suggest epithelial origin
  - o May also help to show that the lymphocytes are polyclonal and nonneoplastic.
- Thymic carcinoma: a form of squamous carcinoma
  - o Significant nuclear atypia, infiltration, and lack of a capsule.
- Most common non-epithelial neoplasms of the anterior mediastinum:
  - o Hodgkin disease
  - o Primary mediastinal large B-cell lymphoma
  - o Lymphoblastic lymphoma.
- The middle mediastinum is the home of the heart and rarely of concern in surgical pathology.
- Most neoplasms of the posterior mediastinum are neural in nature, such as nerve sheath tumors and ganglioneuromas.

ISBN 978-089189-5886

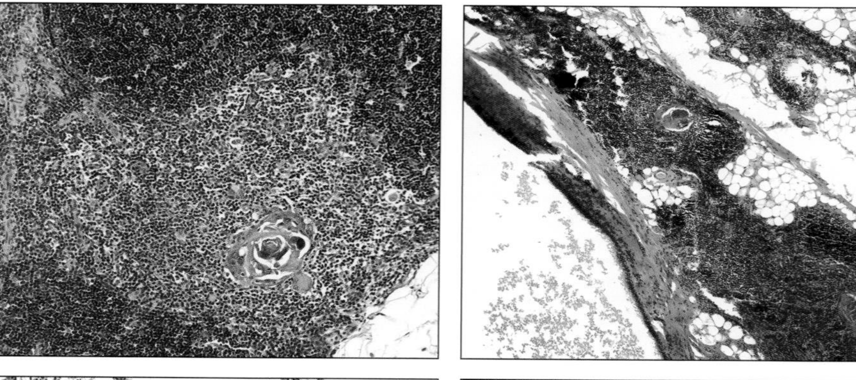

i18.1 Normal thymus. The lighter-staining medulla is surrounded by the darker cortex. A Hassall corpuscle is present in the medulla.

i18.2 A unilocular thymic cyst

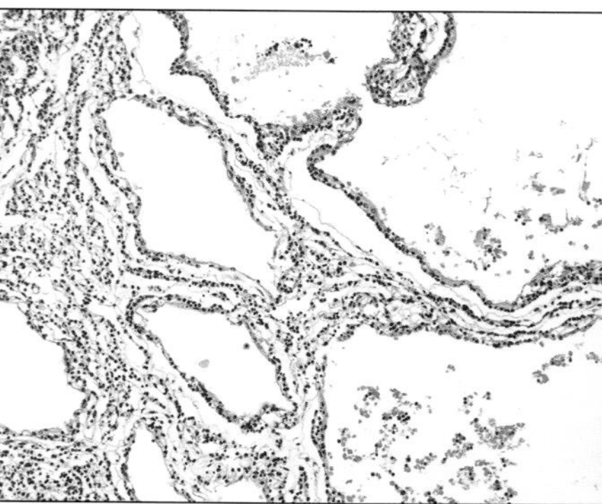

i18.3 A multilocular thymic cyst. Note the absence of epithelium except for the lining of the cysts.

i18.4 A thymic cyst in which the epithelial lining has been lost and replaced with cholesterol clefts

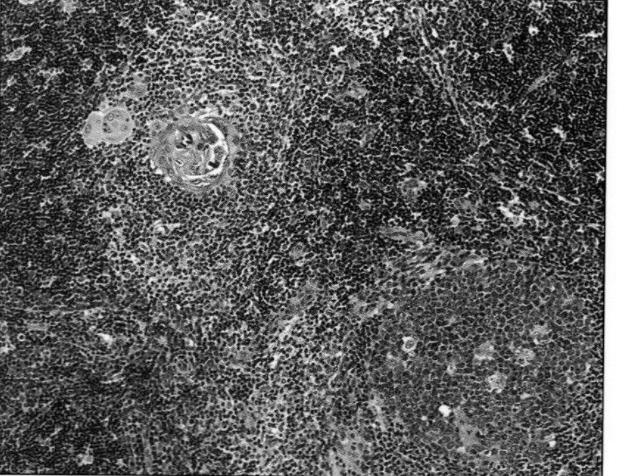

i18.5 Follicular lymphoid hyperplasia in the thymus. Note the germinal center in the lower right, which is unusual in an adult. This patient had myasthenia gravis.

i18.6 Castleman disease involving anterior mediastinal lymph nodes. Note the characteristic small artery entering an atrophic germinal center.

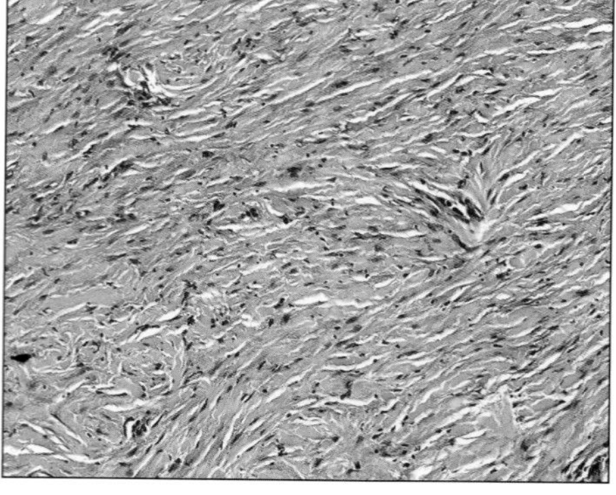

i18.7 Sclerosing mediastinitis, with characteristic dense collagenous fibrosis

i18.8 A lymphocyte predominant thymoma. The slightly larger cells, with less condensed chromatin, are the squamous neoplastic cells.

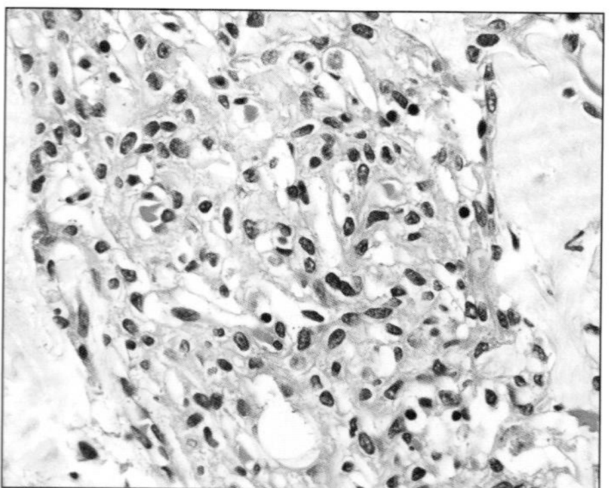

i18.9 An epithelial predominant thymoma

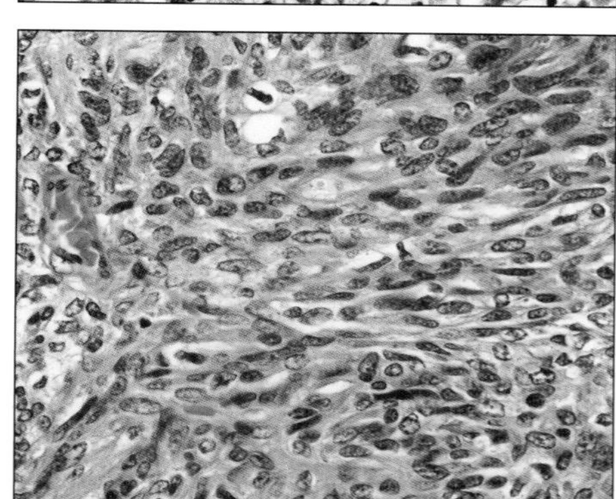

i18.10 A spindle cell thymoma

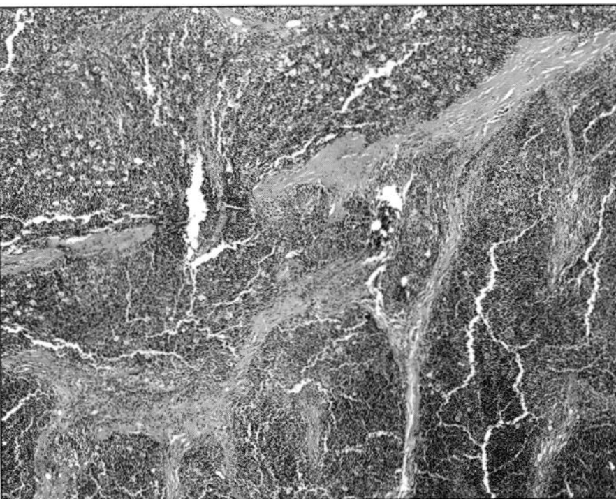

i18.11 A lymphocyte predominant thymoma with an inconspicuous epithelial component. The larger cells in this photograph are the keratin positive, neoplastic squamous cells. The lymphocytes are non-neoplastic.

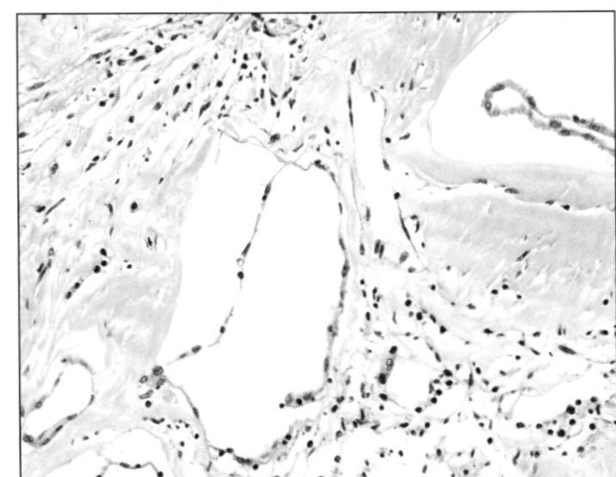

i18.12 The same case as in i18.11, demonstrating encapsulation

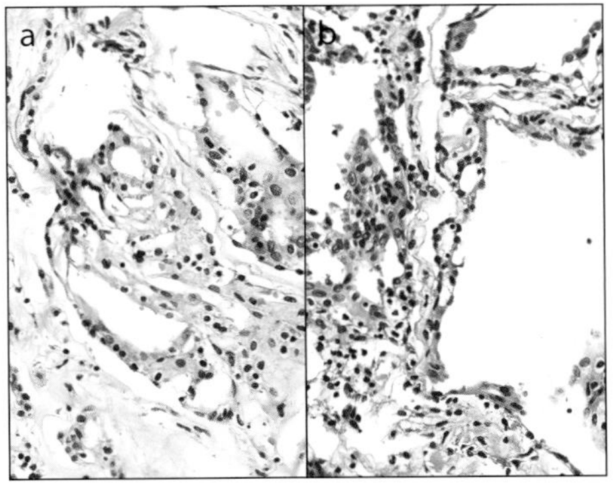

i18.13 The same case as in i18.11, demonstrating anastomosing bands of collagen, forming lobules, which would be unusual in a lymphoma

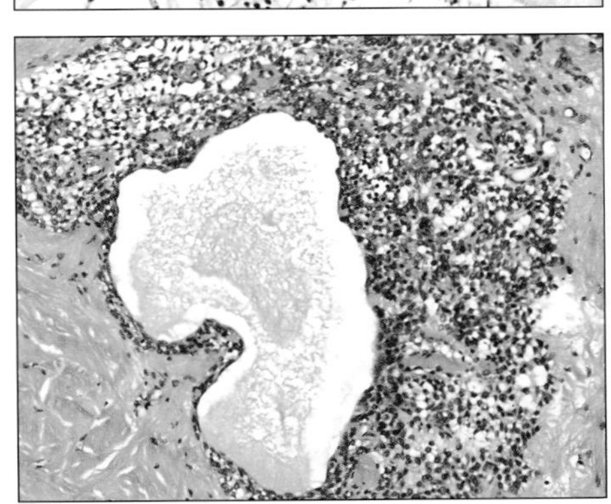

i18.14 The perivascular clear spaces that are characteristic of thymomas

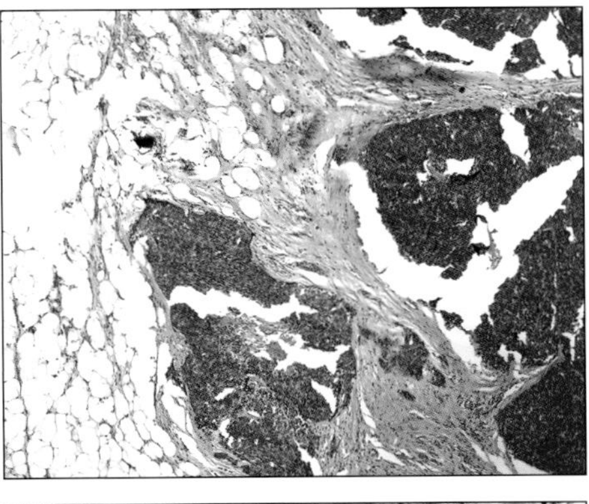

i18.15 **a** A multiloculated thymic cyst with increased epithelium, but the epithelium still lines the cysts. **b** A multiloculated thymic cyst simulating a thymoma, but the epithelium is contained within the cysts.

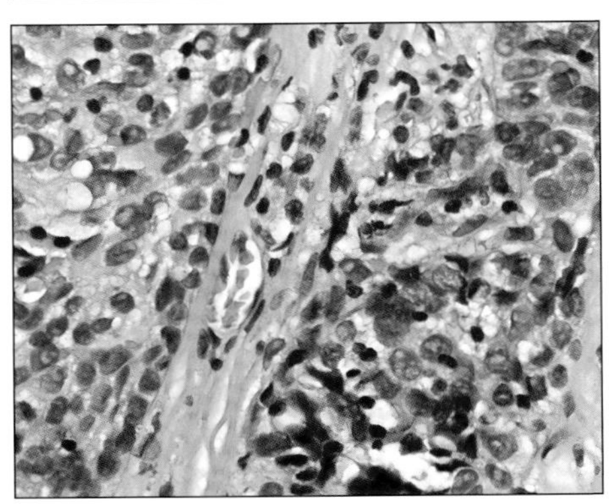

i18.16 A cystic thymoma, with appreciable epithelium that is not associated with the cyst

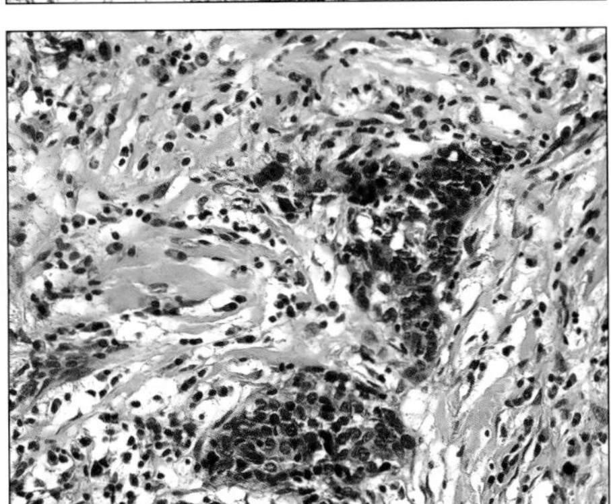

i18.17 Invasion of the capsule by an invasive thymoma

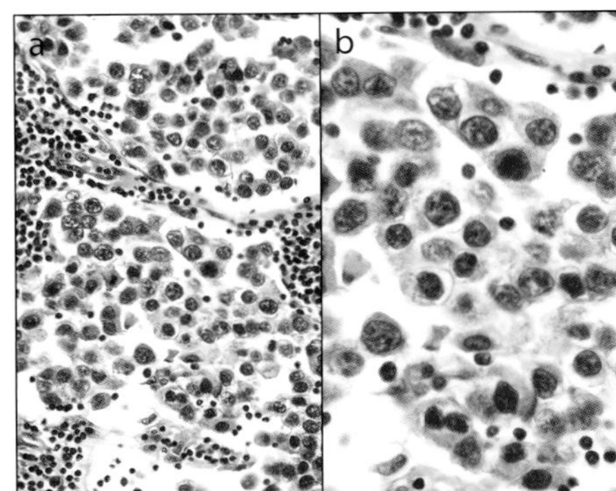

i18.18 Thymic carcinoma of a classic or usual type

i18.19 Thymic carcinoma of the basaloid type

i18.20 **a** Thymic carcinoma of the lymphoepithelioma-like type **b** A higher-power view of the same case as in i18.20a, illustrating the vesicular chromatin pattern and prominent nucleoli. Note the striking similarity to the undifferentiated nasopharyngeal carcinoma.

ISBN 978-089189-5886

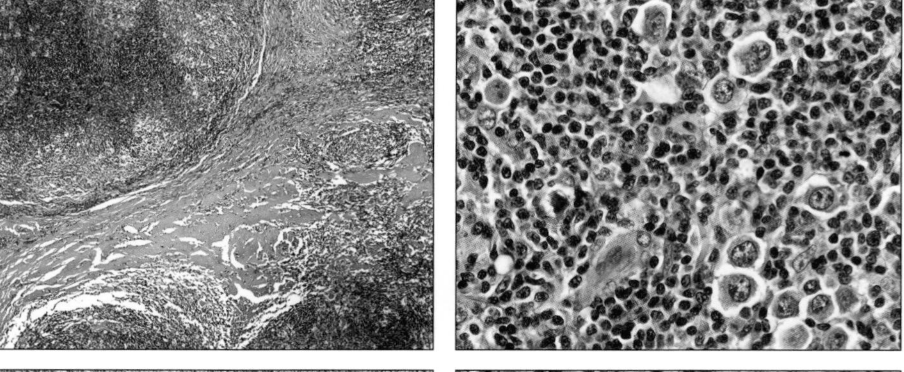

i18.21 Nodular sclerosing Hodgkin disease of the anterior mediastinum. The fibrosis and the formation of the lobules cause this neoplasm to resemble a thymoma.

i18.22 A higher-power view of the same case as in i18.21, illustrating Reed-Sternberg variants

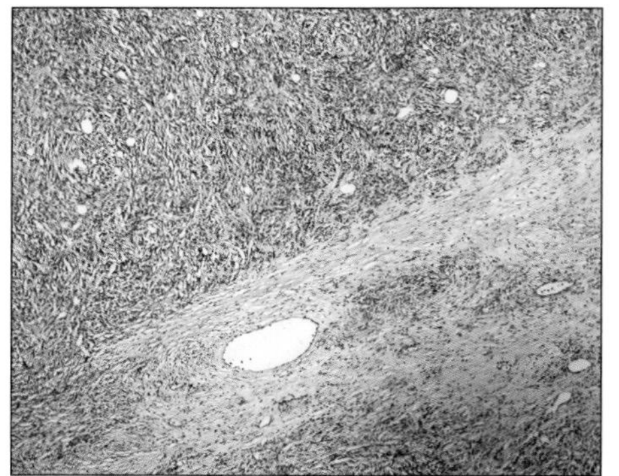

i18.23 Primary mediastinal large B-cell lymphoma. At low power, note the similarity to a thymoma or to nodular sclerosing Hodgkin disease.

i18.24 A higher-power view of the same case as in i18.23. Note the similarity of the neoplastic cells, particularly the large one in the center, to Reed-Sternberg variants in Hodgkin disease, underscoring the need for immunohistochemical characterization of anterior mediastinal processes.

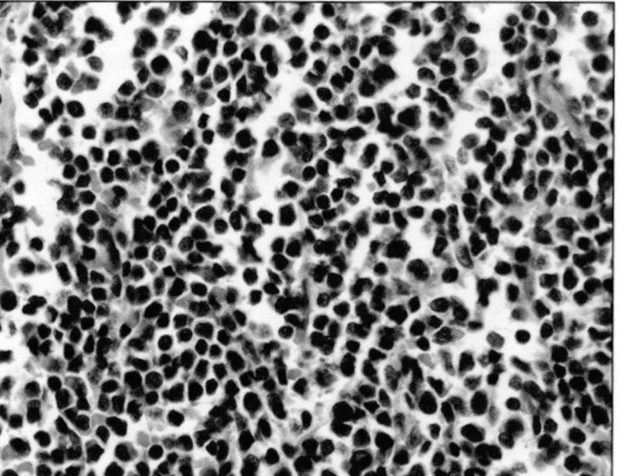

i18.25 Lymphoblastic lymphoma of the anterior mediastinum. Note the monomorphic population of small lymphocytes with no normal thymic or lymph node architecture.

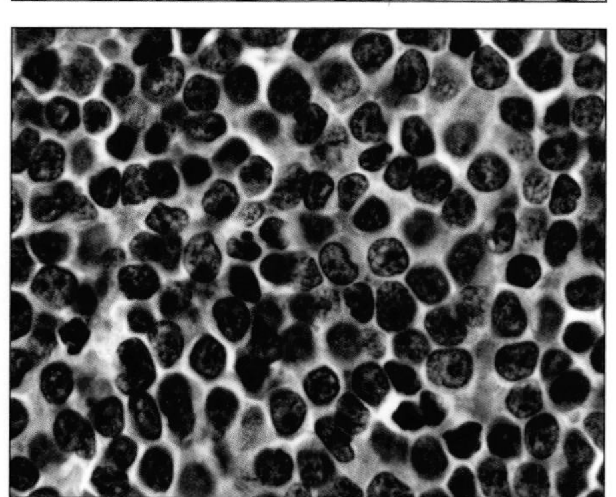

i18.26 A higher-power view of the same case as in i18.25, illustrating the fine chromatin that is characteristic of lymphoblastic lymphoma

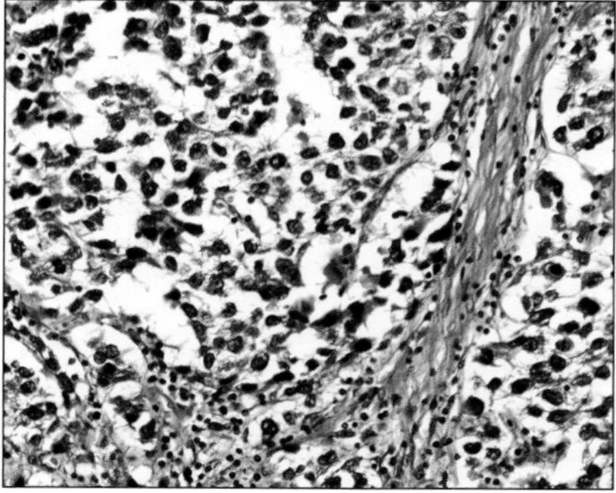

i18.27 A seminoma of the anterior mediastinum, with an appearance identical to that in the gonads, with neoplastic cells separated by septae containing lymphocytes

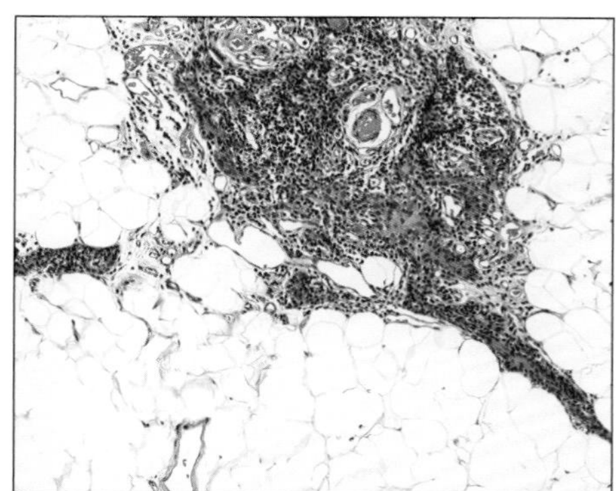

i18.28 A thymolipoma with a small amount of residual thymus tissue. Note the few benign squamous cells at the lower portion of the thymic tissue, in the center.

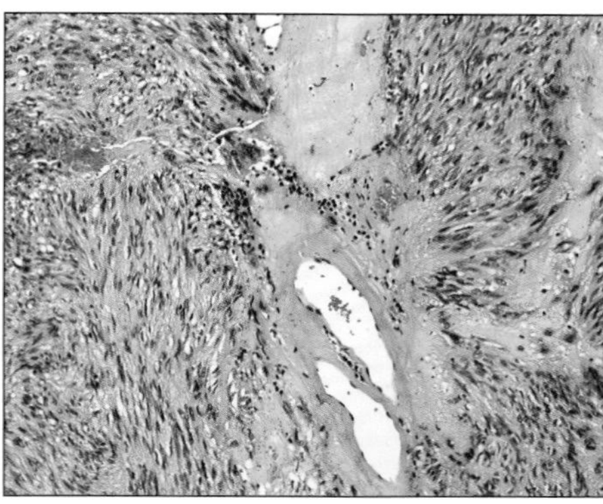

i18.29 A schwannoma of the posterior mediastinum, with the thickened hyalinized vascular walls that are often seen in schwannomas

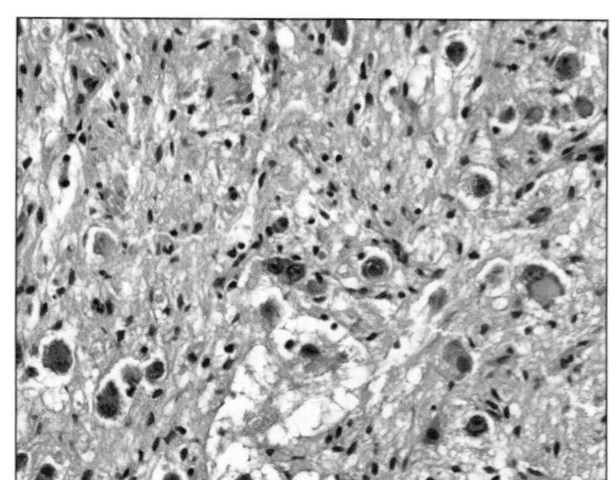

i18.30 A ganglioneuroma of the posterior mediastinum. Note the large ganglion cells, with nucleoli, in a background that resembles a neurofibroma.

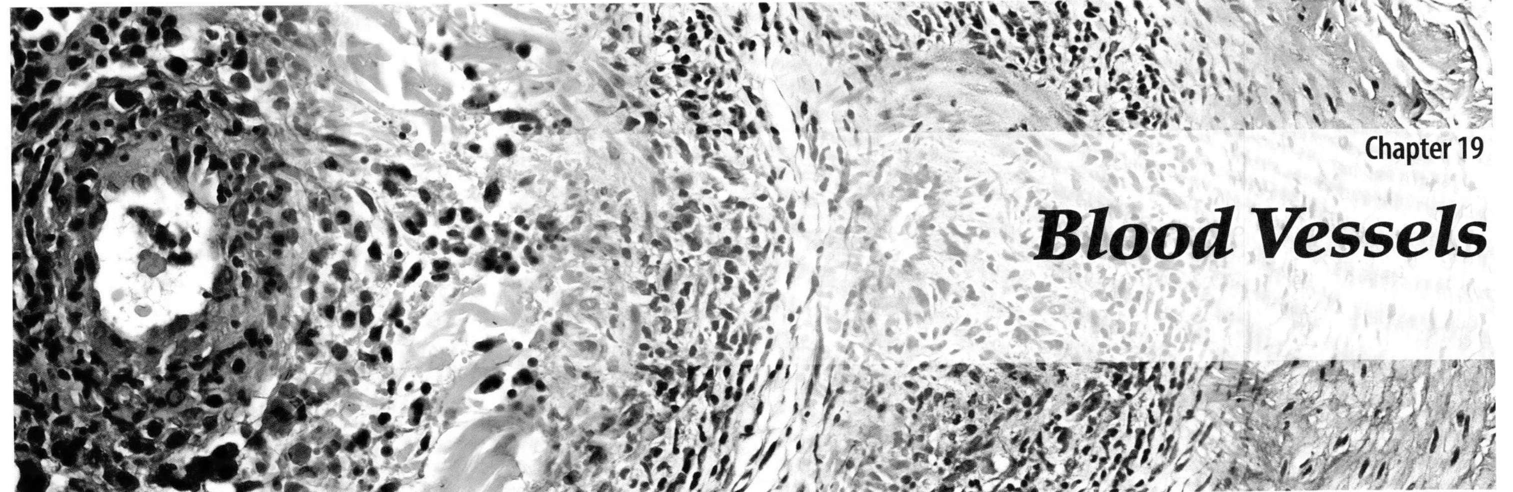

Chapter 19

Blood Vessels

No attempt is made here to discuss the pathology of the heart because, with rare exceptions (transplant specimens and endocardial samples to assess rejection), cardiac tissue is not part of the practice of surgical pathology. Here, we will consider only the group of disorders called vasculitis, with a brief closing comment on a fascinating hypothesis on the pathogenesis of atherosclerosis.

Vasculitis is a primary inflammation of blood vessels that leads to necrosis of the wall of the vessel, thrombi, and occlusion of the vascular lumen, followed by ischemia and necrosis of the surrounding tissue. Because most types of vasculitis have a predilection for vessels of a particular size, a primary vasculitis tends to affect vessels of only 1 caliber (ie, only small vessels, or only medium-sized vessels). While the acute inflammation may spread to surrounding areas because the vasculitis compromises blood flow and leads to necrosis, it remains at least as intense in and around the vessels as in other areas. There is an association between vasculitis and autoimmune disorders, so the finding of either of these should elicit the exclusion of the other.

The 2 difficulties in the diagnosis of primary vasculitis are to differentiate it from secondary inflammation of blood vessels and to appreciate that there is a more chronic stage that lacks the classic features. Like any other anatomic structure, blood vessels may be secondarily involved in severe inflammatory processes. Clues that a putative acute vasculitis is secondary include a generalized inflammatory background that involves other structures as much as it does blood vessels, the involvement of vessels of different calibers, failure of the inflammatory cells to achieve a transmural distribution within the vascular wall, less swollen endothelial cells, lack of necrosis of the vessel wall, and lack of fibrin microthrombi **i19.1a**, **i19.1b**. Characteristics of primary vasculitis include inflammation in the vessel wall that is greater than in the surrounding areas, necrosis of the wall, thrombi, endothelial damage, and karyorrhectic neutrophilic debris [PMID20055902]. Extravasated erythrocytes, secondary to loss of vascular integrity, are supportive, but not diagnostic.

As primary (ie, etiologic) vasculitis evolves, its morphology changes. In the acute stage, primary vasculitis has transmural acute inflammatory cells (usually neutrophils, though eosinophils predominate in some types and are diagnostically important), necrosis of the vessel wall, swollen endothelial cells, and fibrin microthrombi.

With time, the inflammation in the vessel wall becomes less acute, and lymphocytes replace acute inflammatory cells. Necrosis and fibrin microthrombi are less conspicuous. It may be difficult to appreciate that inflammation of the vessels was the inciting event. It is debatable whether or not there is a true primary "lymphocytic" vasculitis (ie, with lymphocytes in the vascular wall), but it is important to consider a chronic phase of what had been an acute vasculitis when encountering a "lymphocytic" vasculitis.

Once the diagnosis of a primary vasculitis is established, the next task is to assess the caliber of the involved vessels. Large vessel vasculitis is seen in temporal and Takayasu arteritis. Medium-sized vessels are affected in periarteritis (or polyarteritis) nodosa, Kawasaki disease, and granulomatous angiitis of the central nervous system. While most cases of vasculitis of large and medium caliber are idiopathic and probably autoimmune, a minority of cases are directly linked to medications or viruses [PMID19007534].

Small vessel vasculitis is seen in Wegener, Churg-Strauss, microscopic polyangiitis, cutaneous leukocytoclastic vasculitis, Henoch-Schönlein purpura, rheumatoid vasculitis, most cases of drug-induced vasculitis, and cryoglobulinemic vasculitis. Leukocytoclastic vasculitis is associated with immune complexes. Henoch-Schönlein purpura is a form of leukocytoclastic vasculitis with deposits of IgA [PMID16581560]. Microscopic polyangiitis is a necrotizing glomerulonephritis, often with lung involvement causing pulmonary hemorrhage. It is a more common cause of pulmonary-renal syndrome than Goodpasture syndrome.

Kawasaki disease (also called mucocutaneous lymph node syndrome) is a leading cause of vasculitis in young children. It affects many organs, but especially the heart, and often causes aneurysms [PMID22018429]. But in adults, the primary vasculitis conditions that are commonly encountered are temporal arteritis, periarteritis (or polyarteritis) nodosa, leukocytoclastic vasculitis, and Wegener.

Temporal arteritis (also called giant cell arteritis or cranial arteritis) affects larger vessels, especially the temporal artery, and is likely to cause significant visual disturbances. While the term "temporal arteritis" has been discouraged because other forms of vasculitis may affect this vessel, I prefer the term because giant cells are often not present, especially if the patient has been treated with steroids prior to the biopsy, or if the biopsy is obtained an appreciable time after onset. Indeed, it is more likely that a biopsy of a temporal artery affected by

ISBN 978-089189-5886

this entity will *not* have giant cells than it is that the vessel is affected by another type of vasculitis, since temporal arteritis and Takayasu arteritis are the only common vasculitides that affect larger vessels. I do not recommend the term "cranial arteritis" because any of the vasculitides may involve the cranium. While any vasculitis can be associated with an autoimmune disorder, temporal arteritis is associated with polymyalgia rheumatica in up to 50% of cases [PMID1807817].

The normal temporal artery in older patients virtually always has intimal hyperplasia **i19.2**, and this finding alone is never sufficient for the diagnosis. The normal temporal artery in older patients may also show focal fragmentation of the internal elastic membrane, but the structure of the wall is intact [PMID1807817]. Likewise, calcification confined to the media is much more likely to be medial calcific sclerosis (Monckeberg medial stenosis) than any stage of temporal arteritis.

Giant cells and granulomas may be present *in the active, untreated stage* of temporal arteritis **i19.3**, **i19.4**, **i19.5** [PMID1807817], but with progression or treatment, the inflammation lessens, and the histologic picture becomes one of nonspecific chronic inflammation in the wall **i19.6**, perhaps with partial replacement of the muscular layer by fibrous tissue, and a focal disruption of the internal elastic membrane **i19.7a**, **i19.7b**. Because giant cells are unlikely to be found in the chronic stage, the term "temporal arteritis" is preferable to "giant cell arteritis."

A diagnosis of healed arteritis is appropriate if there is a thrombus **i19.8** or obvious scarring in the wall that significantly disrupts the media, not just the elastic membrane. Another indication of long-standing temporal arteritis is capillaries in the media (vasa vasorum), which are not usually seen in the temporal artery [PMID1807817]. As in any body site, neovascularity is an indication of subacute or chronic inflammation. While an elastic stain to assess the internal elastic membrane and a trichrome stain to assess collagen deposition may be helpful, they are rarely necessary in my experience.

Because temporal arteritis is a discontinuous process—meaning that one segment is affected while an adjacent portion is not—a comment might be added in negative biopsies that the results of the biopsy should not preclude treatment if the clinical impression is compelling. Indeed, almost 1/2 of patients with sufficient signs and symptoms of temporal arteritis to warrant treatment for vasculitis will have negative biopsies, either because the biopsy fortuitously missed an involved area, because treatment has mitigated the histologic features, or because the patient has another type of vasculitis affecting other vessels, clinically simulating temporal arteritis [PMID1807817].

Rheumatologists and surgeons may feel comfortable that the biopsy is long enough to avoid a false negative, but this is not always true, and they are less likely to appreciate that treatment, and chronicity can make the histologic changes subtle. In most biopsies of the temporal artery there will be surrounding soft tissue that has small vessels and nerve fibers. Inflammation of either of these **i19.9** likely indicates temporal arteritis that is not evident in the main specimen because of the skipping nature of the arteritis [PMID11407699] or a different kind of vasculitis affecting smaller vessels that may have clinically simulated temporal arteritis.

While temporal arteritis is often confined to the temporal artery, these patients are at risk for the development of extracranial arteritis, and this should be suspected if there are signs of ischemia in other sites [PMID19560390].

Periarteritis nodosa involves medium-sized vessels in any organ or body site. Unlike temporal arteritis, a biopsy is rarely performed to diagnose periarteritis nodosa. Rather, it is occasionally encountered as an unsuspected finding in surgical specimens **i19.10a**, **i19.10b**. Once it is diagnosed, however, the clinician must be made aware that many patients will have systemic symptoms, and that a workup for autoimmune disorders and systemic vasculitis is appropriate. Angiograms of liver, kidney, or mesentery may assist in the diagnosis of periarteritis nodosa, as it predisposes to aneurysms in these locations. Some cases of periarteritis nodosa patients have anti-MPO [PMID7933581].

The most common small vessel vasculitis conditions are Wegener and leukocytoclastic vasculitis. Wegener is discussed in Chapter 14. Leukocytoclastic vasculitis is usually seen in the skin and is the most common group of primary cutaneous vasculitis (cutaneous vasculitis involves small vessels because the skin generally lacks larger blood vessels). Leukocytoclastic vasculitis is usually associated with immune complexes [PMID16581560] and can be caused by infection, autoimmune processes, drug reactions, hypersensitivity reactions, and malignancy. It can be localized (eg, the cutaneous disorders granuloma faciale and erythema elevatum diutinum) or generalized.

As is the case for other vasculitis conditions, leukocytoclastic vasculitis has different histologic features at different stages in its evolution, and the picture that is seen in most textbooks is only valid for a classic, fully developed case. In its classical appearance, neutrophils are seen in the vascular wall and the endothelial cells, damaged by the inflammation, are enlarged **i19.11**. There may be fibrinoid necrosis of the wall **i19.12**. Fibrin microthrombi may form on the damaged endothelium. Interstitial neutrophils may be prominent **i19.13**.

However, the late stages of leukocytoclastic vasculitis may not have this appearance. In later stages, there may be a mixed infiltrate in the wall with lymphocytes predominating, and frank necrosis may not be obvious **i19.14**. Older lesions of leukocytoclastic vasculitis may resemble a "lymphocytic" vasculitis, and an older manifestation of leukocytoclastic vasculitis should be excluded when there is a "lymphocytic" vasculitis. Indeed, it is debatable if there is a true pure lymphocytic vasculitis, and such an appearance should prompt the exclusion of other conditions that result in lymphocytes within vascular walls, such as chronic vasculitis or a lymphoproliferative disorder.

Small vessel vasculitides are more likely to be associated with antineutrophilic cytoplasmic antibody (ANCA) than those affecting larger vessels, and in fact, the presence or absence of ANCA is a basis for the sub-classification of small vessel vasculitides. ANCA is actually a collection of proteins and is initially screened by immunofluorescence (IFA). IFA is a technically difficult procedure that requires a fluorescent microscope and is dependent on the precise preparation and fixation of the target and on the experience of the interpreter. Samples that are positive by IFA are then assessed by enzyme immunoassay (EIA; originally and still occasionally called enzyme-linked immunosorbent assay [ELISA]) for specific proteins, but there are at least 6 antigens that can generate a positive IFA, some of which cannot be identified by EIA, so a failure to identify a specific antigen by EIA does not invalidate the IFA test, and the IFA test remains essential until all antigens have been characterized and can be assayed by EIA [PMID19922728]. For example, many patients with inflammatory bowel disease have a positive IFA for which no specific antigen can be identified on EIA testing [PMID11370121].

The 2 most common specific antigens in ANCA are myeloperoxidase (MPO) and proteinase 3 (PR3) [PMID19815703]. There is a partial association between the location of the fluorescent signal in the IFA screening test and the final antigen that is identified.
in the IFA screening test and the final antigen that is identified.
Cytoplasmic ANCA (c-ANCA) is a more diffuse, coarse, and granular staining than p-ANCA **i19.15**. It is likely to be PR3 on EIA. Anti-PR3 is associated with Wegener granulomatosis [PMID20614334], and >90% of Wegener patients will have anti-PR3, while only 10% will have anti-MPO [PMID15804710]. Anti-MPO is strongly associated with Churg-Strauss, microscopic polyangiitis, polyangiitis overlap syndrome, and crescentic (or rapidly progressive) glomerulonephritis, a renal-limited form of microscopic polyangiitis.

Because there is imperfect correspondence between c-ANCA and PR3 and between p-ANCA and MPO, and not every positive IFA has an identified antigen by EIA, I recommend specifying the specific antigen that is found on EIA, if possible, or indicating that the patient has a positive ANCA of unknown specificity, in addition to indicating that there is a positive c-ANCA or p-ANCA. Even if this more detailed information has no immediate clinical application, it may be beneficial at some point in the future.

Those vasculitides that typically have a positive ANCA include Wegener, Churg-Strauss, microscopic polyangiitis, and some cases that are drug induced [PMID19560390, PMID20878509], while cryoglobulinemic vasculitis and those that are associated with immune complexes, such as leukocytoclastic vasculitis and Henoch-Schönlein purpura, tend to be ANCA-negative [PMID20617753].

In addition to the vasculitides, ANCA may be seen in several forms of autoimmune liver disease, especially autoimmune chronic hepatitis and primary sclerosing cholangitis [PMID18626795], up to 75% of inflammatory bowel disease patients, especially active ulcerative colitis (but also 20% of Crohn disease) [PMID19858012], as well as some autoimmune disorders, especially lupus and rheumatoid arthritis. However, at this time, the role of ANCA is essentially limited to the vasculitides, and only to their diagnosis. There is no consensus on the advisability of using ANCA to monitor severity of vasculitis or response to treatment.

We close our consideration of disorders of blood vessels with a hypothesis concerning atherosclerosis, which is now considered by many to be a response of the arterial wall to injury of the endothelium—in effect, to be a manifestation of vasculitis and the healing process. In this hypothesis, the sequence of steps is as follows [PMID22204378]:

1. Endothelial injury, with increased permeability
2. Deposition of cholesterol from LDL beneath the endothelium
3. Endothelial cells produce cytokines that attract monocytes
4. Migration of monocytes into the subendothelial space, and their activation, possibly by LDL
5. Smooth muscle cells or stem cells migrate into subendothelial space from the media, in response to chemotactic factors
6. Secretion of immune-stimulating cytokines and growth factors by the cells within the plaque
7. Smooth muscle and fibrous proliferation in subendothelial space
8. Sequelae, such as thrombi, ulceration, hemorrhage

If this view is correct, our understanding of atherosclerotic vascular disease changes from a simple mechanical obstruction to an immune system-mediated process. Paradoxically, the normal functioning of the immune system may actually be the primary culprit.

Core Points for Blood Vessels

- Primary vasculitis: must be distinguished from secondary involvement in an inflammatory milieu.
- Characteristics of primary vasculitis
  - Inflammation that is more intense in the walls of blood vessels
  - Necrosis of the wall
  - Thrombi
  - Restriction of vascular inflammation to vessels only one caliber
- Vasculitis may also have a chronic phase in which the classic features are not present.
- Many cases of primary vasculitis are idiopathic
  - But there is an association between vasculitis and autoimmune disorders
  - Some cases are linked to drugs or infection.
- Most types of vasculitis preferentially affect vessels of a particular size
  - Large vessel vasculitis: temporal and Takayasu.
  - Medium sized vessels: periarteritis (or polyarteritis) nodosa, Kawasaki disease, and granulomatous angiitis of the central nervous system affect.
  - Small vessels: Wegener, Churg-Strauss, microscopic polyangiitis, cutaneous leukocytoclastic vasculitis, Henoch-Schönlein purpura, rheumatoid vasculitis, most cases of drug-induced vasculitis, and cryoglobulinemic vasculitis.
- Leukocytoclastic vasculitis and Henoch-Schönlein purpura are associated with immune complexes.
- Small vessel vasculitides are often associated with antineutrophilic cytoplasmic antibody (ANCA) and can be subdivided by the presence or absence of ANCA.
  - Wegener, Churg-Strauss, microscopic polyangiitis are typically ANCA positive.
- Most commonly encountered primary vasculitis conditions:
  - Leukocytoclastic vasculitis
  - Wegener
  - Temporal arteritis
  - Periarteritis nodosa
- Patients with temporal arteritis have usually been treated with steroids before biopsy, so classic findings may be muted.
  - Any acute or chronic inflammation in the wall, or disruption of the normal architecture, suggests arteritis if the clinical context is appropriate.
- Even if the biopsy is generous, the discontinuous nature of temporal arteritis is always a consideration.
  - A negative biopsy should not preclude treatment.

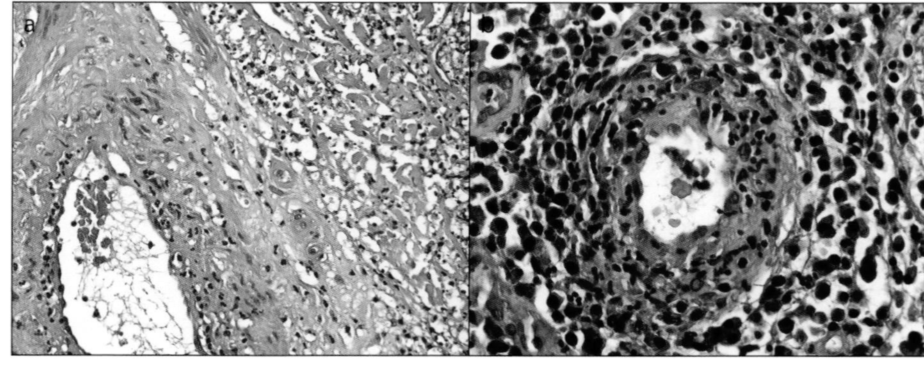

i19.1 **a** Secondary vasculitis. Note that the wall of the blood vessel is less inflamed than the surrounding tissue and that the vascular wall is undamaged.

b Secondary vasculitis. There are large numbers of neutrophils in the vascular wall, but it is undamaged. The adjacent plasma cells were part of the granulation tissue in which this vessel lay. These neutrophils are simply passing through the vessel wall to their destinations in the tissues.

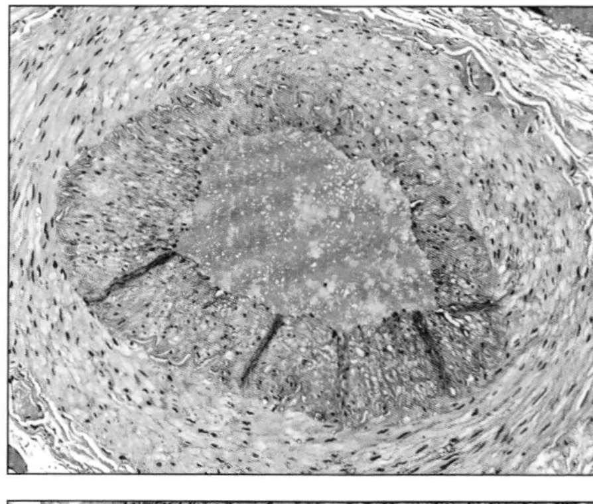

i19.2 Intimal hyperplasia in a temporal artery biopsy

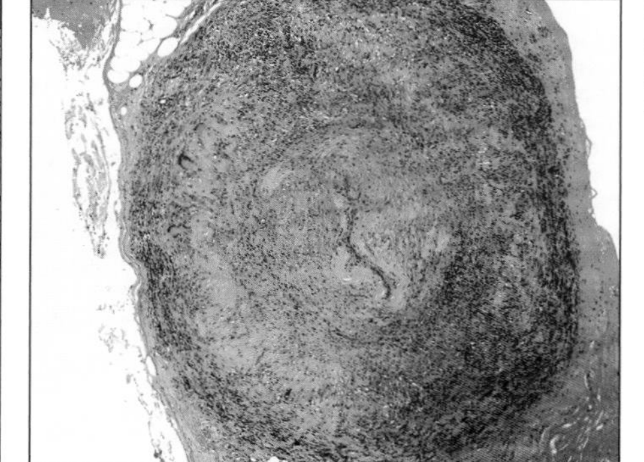

i19.3 Active temporal arteritis, with giant cells and severe chronic inflammation

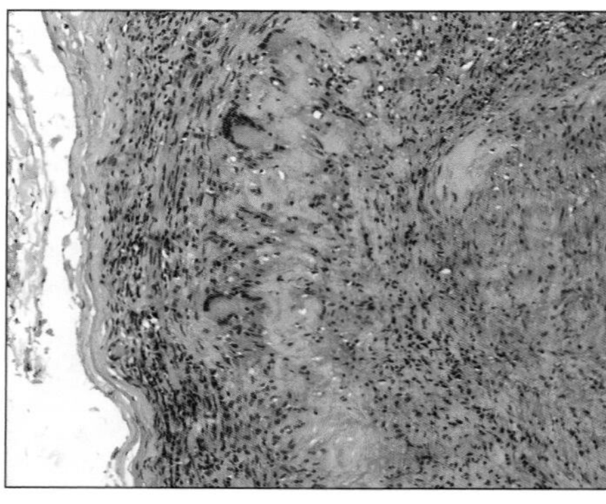

i19.4 A higher-power view of the same case as in i19.3

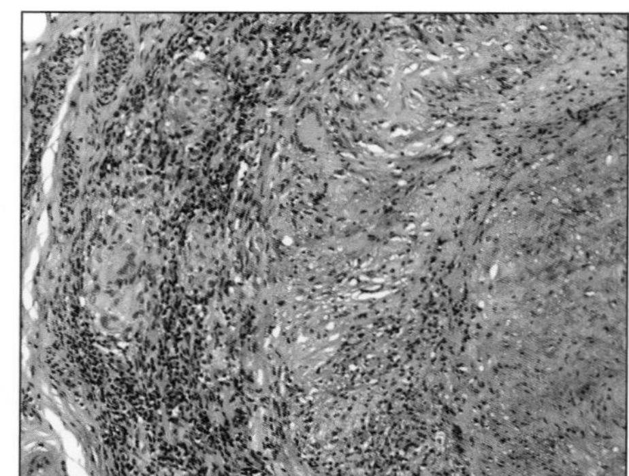

i19.5 Active temporal arteritis with granulomas

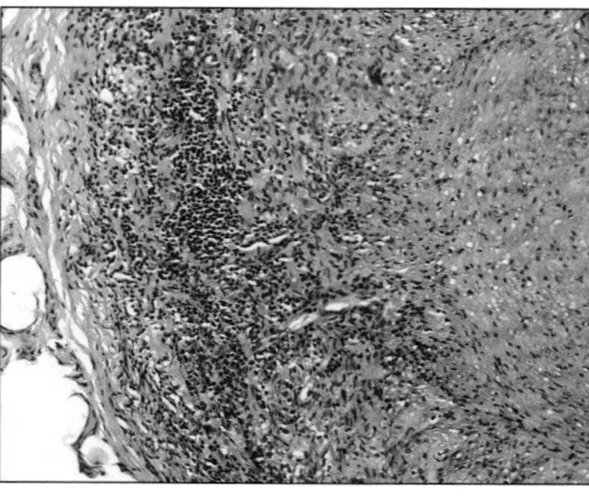

i19.6 Temporal arteritis with nonspecific chronic inflammation in the wall

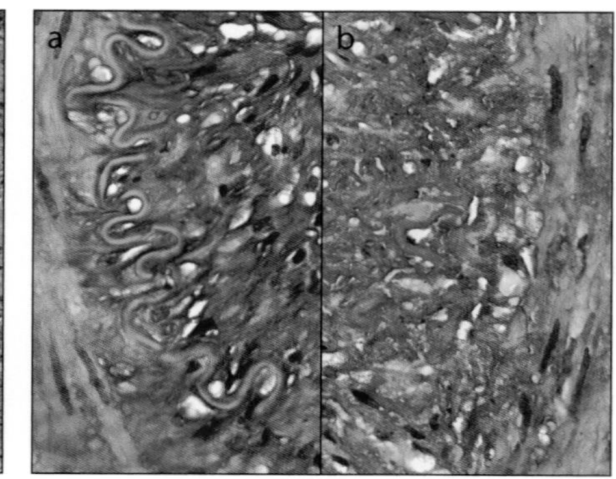

i19.7 **a** The internal elastic membrane can be seen reasonably well on H&E. It is an intact, continuous wavy line to the right of center in this normal temporal artery biopsy. **b** The internal elastic membrane is focally identified as disrupted, discontinuous slightly amphophilic fragments just to the left of center.

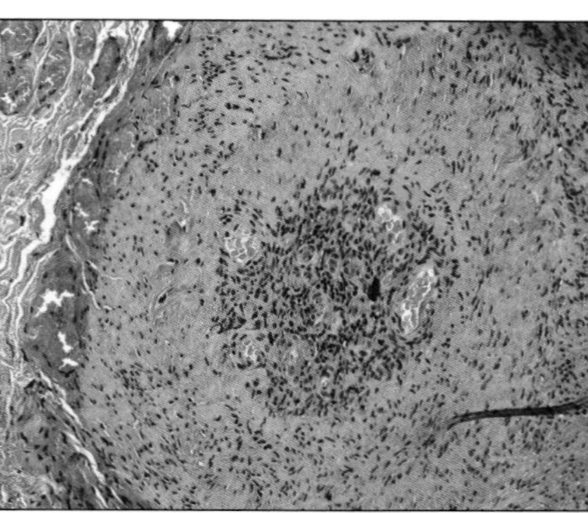

i19.8 A thrombus, with recanalization, in chronic temporal arteritis

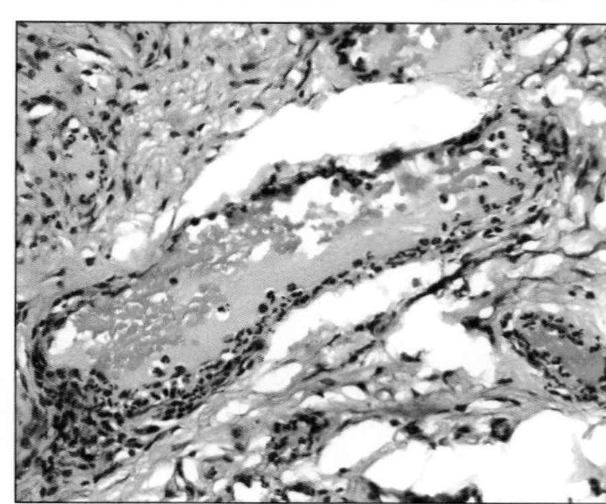

i19.9 Acute inflammation of the small blood vessels surrounding the temporal artery

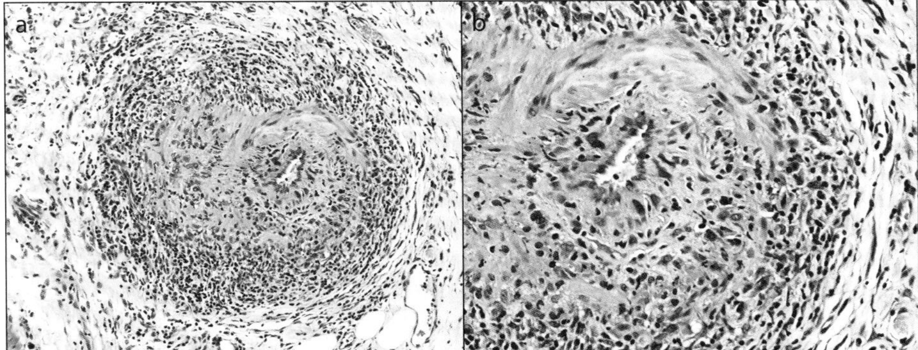

i19.10 **a** Periarteritis nodosa found incidentally in a cholecystectomy

b A higher-power view of the same blood vessel as in i19.10a

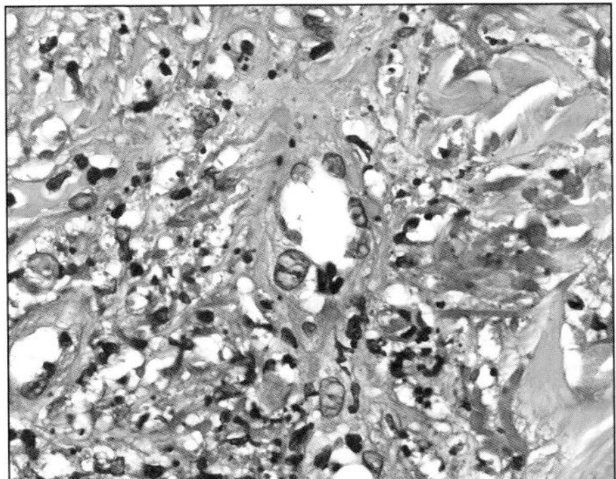

i19.11 Active leukocytoclastic vasculitis. Neutrophils have so extensively infiltrated the walls of small blood vessels that they are difficult to discern. Note the markedly enlarged endothelial cells in the center.

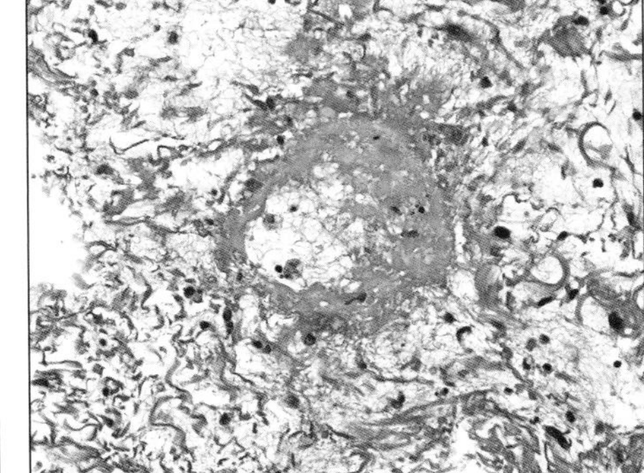

i19.12 Fibrinoid necrosis of the wall of a small blood vessel in leukocytoclastic vasculitis

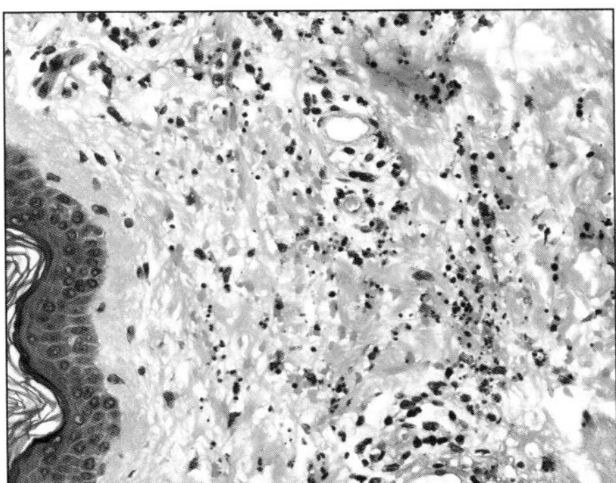

i19.13 Prominent interstitial neutrophils in leukocytoclastic vasculitis

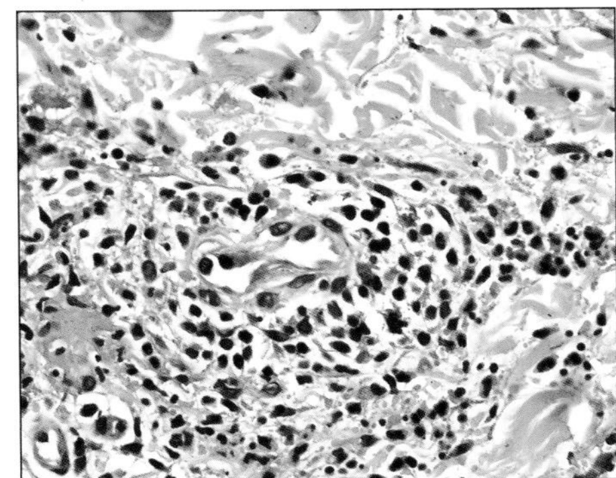

i19.14 Chronic leukocytoclastic vasculitis in which neutrophils have substantially replaced neutrophils in the vascular wall

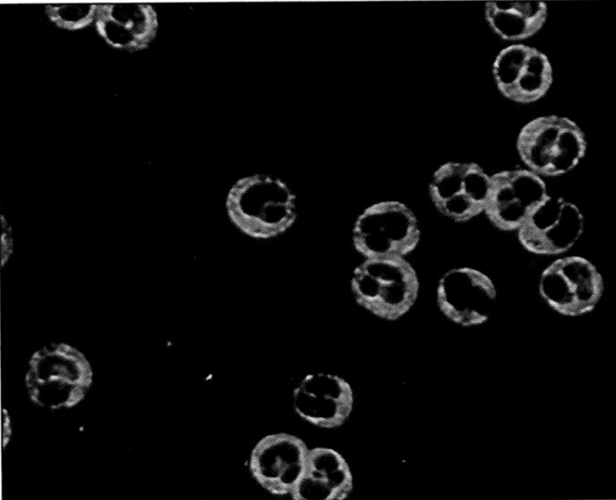

i19.15 Positive antineutrophilic cytoplasmic antibody (ANCA). The trilobed nucleus is negative and dark, while the cytoplasm fluoresces green. This diffuse, coarse staining of the cytoplasm is characteristic of c-ANCA. This positive initial fluorescent screening test was later more specifically identified as proteinase 3 and the patient was shown to have Wegener granulomatosis.

ISBN 978-089189-5886

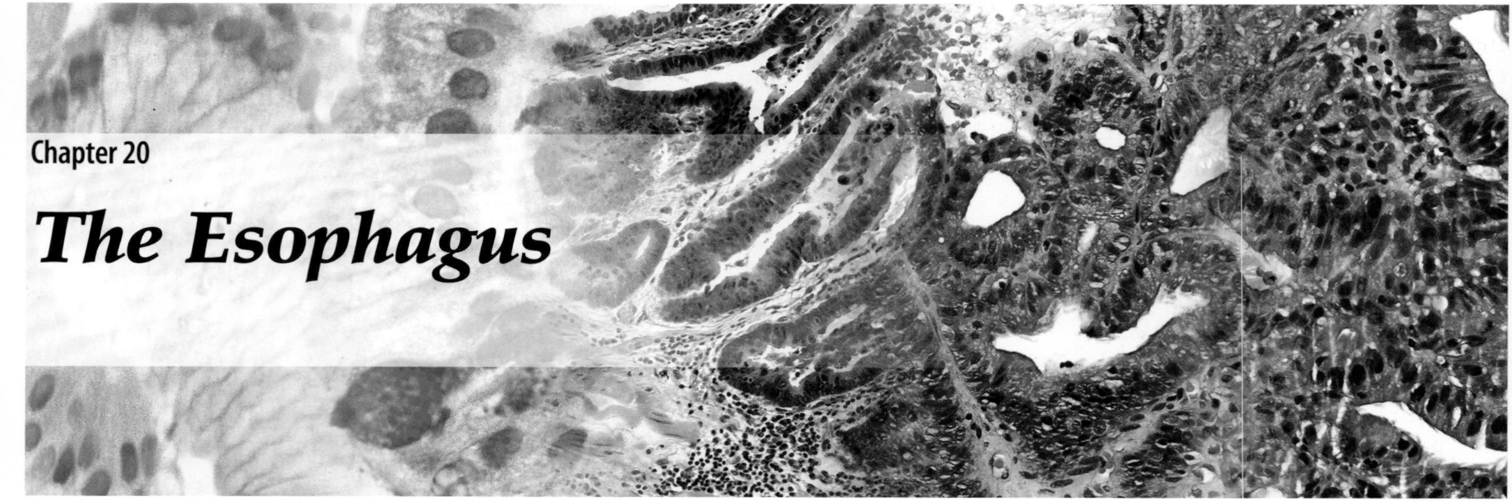

Chapter 20

The Esophagus

The only terms pertaining to normal esophageal anatomy that commonly concern pathologists are "rings" and "webs." Esophageal webs are folds of mucosa and rings are circumferential folds. Rings in the lower esophagus are called Schatzki rings. These terms refer to endoscopic findings, without histologic correlates, but they are often used by gastroenterologists.

Gastroesophageal Reflux Disease (GERD) and Barrett Esophagus

In adults, glandular epithelium in the esophagus indicates early gastroesophageal reflux disease (GERD). The presence of acid on the basal layer of squamous epithelium in the esophagus leads to a defensive glandular metaplasia, as this type of epithelium is better able to withstand acidic pH than squamous epithelium. The first recognizable precursor to reflux is a multilayered epithelium that appears squamous in the lower portions and glandular in the upper portion i20.1 [PMID11342767]. Eosinophilic inflammation follows. Eosinophils are a reasonably reliable indicator of early GERD in most cases but are not specific. Indeed, there is an idiopathic eosinophilic esophagitis (EE), discussed below, that is quite distinct from GERD. Barrett esophagus occurs when intestinal metaplasia forms in preexisting nonspecific glandular metaplasia.

Although in theory, there are other types of specialized intestinal epithelium, such as Paneth cells or neuroendocrine cells, the only form of intestinal metaplasia that is considered in the diagnosis of Barrett esophagus is the goblet cell because this is the only this cell type significantly predisposes to the development of adenocarcinoma [PMID10907312]. Simple gastric mucosa, without goblet cells, above the gastroesophageal junction (GEJ) does not increase the risk of adenocarcinoma and is not considered Barrett esophagus.

The goblet cell is an intestinal cell type in which there is a single, large cytoplasmic vacuole, filled with acidic mucopolysaccharides (as opposed to the neutral mucopolysaccharides of common glandular cells), that pushes the nucleus to the basal portion of the cell and pushes the cytoplasmic boundaries outward, so that the lateral borders of the cell are curved, as in a goblet, breaking the strict "picket fence" appearance of a row of columnar cells. The cytoplasm is slightly amphophilic rather than strictly eosinophilic as in normal glandular cells i20.2. "Pseudogoblet" cells share some features with true goblet cells in that the cytoplasm appears demarcated into a vacuole, but they lack acidic mucopolysaccharides and therefore have eosinophilic rather than amphophilic cytoplasm on H&E examination i20.3.

The old definition of Barrett esophagus was the presence of glandular epithelium, with or without intestinal metaplasia, 2 cm or more above the GEJ, the theory being that glandular epithelium may be found in normal patients up to 2 cm above the apparent junction. The current definition of Barrett esophagus is glandular epithelium, *with the presence of intestinal metaplasia*, in the esophagus near the GEJ [PMID18341497]. This definition of Barrett esophagus is superior to the older definition for 2 reasons. First, the GEJ is not always distinct, and even experienced endoscopists may have difficulty precisely localizing the junction, especially if there is a hiatal hernia. One may not know where to measure from. The second and more important reason for the new definition of Barrett esophagus is that the presence of intestinal metaplasia specifically, not simply glandular epithelium, predisposes to adenocarcinoma. The wisdom of the new definition is illustrated by short segment Barrett, which is defined as glandular epithelium with intestinal metaplasia that extends for <2 cm above the GEJ. Since this is shorter than the distance that nonmetaplastic glandular epithelium may be found above the normal GEJ, in the older definition, short segment Barrett would never be recognized because it would always fall within the spectrum of normality, and such patients, who are at increased risk of adenocarcinoma, would not be recognized and properly monitored.

The normal esophagus may contain a few glands in the submucosa. These are generally small glands with a distinct lobular distribution i20.4a. Some of the cells in these glands may resemble goblet cells and may have acidic mucopolysaccharides i20.4b. However, the presence of these submucosal glands does not require any followup or surveillance because there has been no metaplasia (ie, there has been no change in the type of epithelium). If the biopsy has been fragmented, the submucosal location of these glands may no longer be evident, but clues to recognizing normal submucosal glands include small, tightly cohesive clusters of small glands that do not intermingle with the squamous epithelium. It is wise to insist on the presence of goblet cells *in the surface epithelium*, so as to be sure that there has been a true change in the type of epithelium.

We now come to the first of 3 controversies: what constitutes intestinal metaplasia? Definitive, well-formed goblet cells can usually be reliably identified on H&E. An alcian blue stain performed at pH 2.5 stains acidic mucopolysaccharides and may highlight goblet cells because normal glandular cells have only neutral mucopolysaccharides and therefore will not stain with alcian blue, while the acidic mucopolysaccharides in goblet cells cause them to stain strongly and diffusely with alcian blue i20.5. Immunohistochemical stains may also assist in identifying goblet cells. Hep (also called HepPar 1) [PMID12826887], CDX2, villin [PMID18343784], and MUC2 [PMID21602660] all stain goblet cells in Barrett esophagus, but not normal gastric epithelium. The first 3 of these usually do not stain nongoblet epithelium, but in patients with goblet cells, MUC2 usually also stains nongoblet epithelium that is adjacent or very close to goblet cells, suggesting that its expression may be an early indicator of metaplasia.

However, a question arises regarding the use of special stains in identifying goblet cells. Some feel that they are sufficiently well seen on H&E that no special stains are necessary, and that such stains may inappropriately highlight "pseudogoblet" cells, causing a false diagnosis of Barrett, although in my experience, alcian blue does not cause false positive staining of "pseudogoblet" cells. Certainly, if an alcian blue stain is employed, care must be taken to avoid interpreting normal esophageal submucosal glands, which will be alcian blue positive [PMID16995451], as intestinal metaplasia. Fortunately, in many of these situations, the diagnosis of Barrett esophagus has been established by a previous biopsy in which there were definitive goblet cells on the surface, eliminating any need to perform special stains.

A second area of controversy concerns glandular cells whose cytoplasmic mucin is partially demarcated into an amphophilic vacuole on H&E or for which an alcian blue stain discloses dispersed staining for acidic mucopolysaccharides, seen as wisps of blue cytoplasm i20.6a, i20.6b. While such cells are clearly not goblet cells, they are also clearly different from glandular cells that have only neutral mucopolysaccharides. Should such cells be regarded as having early or partial intestinal metaplasia, with the beginnings of a transformation to the acidic mucopolysaccharides that characterize goblet cells, or are they a variant of normal that has no significance? Most favor the latter position, which is well articulated in the excellent text by Odze and Goldblum [Odze ISBN978-1416040590], and regard such cells as pseudogoblet cells.

I am in full sympathy with this viewpoint, but the molecular pathology of very early intestinal metaplasia has not been well characterized, so we do not know when the patient becomes at increased risk for adenocarcinoma (ie, we do not know where the "tipping point" is). Perhaps we will learn that immunohistochemical staining or molecular techniques identify cells that have made an irreversible commitment to intestinal metaplasia, but until the sequence leading to intestinal metaplasia is elucidated at the molecular level and it is clearly established that dispersed acidic mucopolysaccharides are not associated with any increased risk of adenocarcinoma, I recommend a comment to the effect of, "No definitive intestinal metaplasia seen, but cannot rule out early or partial intestinal metaplasia." This does not label the patient with a diagnosis of Barrett, but it leaves the door open until we have more data. It seems unlikely that such a comment will significantly increase the number of endoscopies the patient will undergo in the forthcoming years, and even if it does, the inconvenience of an upper endoscopy is minimal, and until we know more, I recommend that we take full advantage of *the only tool we have* to detect early esophageal adenocarcinoma. The esophageal biopsy, followed by the identification of a different form of mucopolysaccharide, is the esophageal equivalent of the Pap smear. Let us make full use of it.

The third controversy concerns the significance of goblet cells in biopsies from the GEJ in the absence of an endoscopic appearance of Barrett. Approximately 20% of endoscopically normal patients may have intestinal metaplasia of the gastric cardia. Moreover, as discussed at the beginning of Chapter 21, the mucosal zones of the stomach are not sharply demarcated, and mucosa of the fundic/body type is often found in the cardia. Indeed, some have questioned if there even is a true cardiac-type mucosa in the stomach [PMID10716154]. In any event, biopsies of the GEJ may have parietal cells or intestinal metaplasia of gastric origin i20.7.

Historically, many have felt that intestinal metaplasia anywhere around the GEJ predisposes to adenocarcinoma and mandates closer followup, and that it does not matter whether the metaplasia is in the esophagus or the gastric cardia. Others, however, have countered that intestinal metaplasia of the gastric cardia may be related to *H pylori*, with no significant predisposition to adenocarcinoma [PMID10729733]. According to this view, while goblet cells in the stomach represent a true metaplasia, there is no need for increased surveillance because there is no increased risk of carcinoma. While this issue has not been completely settled, it is likely that the definitive diagnosis of Barrett esophagus requires the presence of intestinal metaplasia on the surface epithelium in fragments that are not of gastric origin. At this time, a comment to the effect of "gastric-type epithelium with intestinal metaplasia of uncertain significance" might be made.

Goblet cells may be rare in Barrett esophagus in children [PMID2252419] (probably because the process is not sufficiently developed), so some feel that the old definition of Barrett, which is simply the presence of glandular mucosa >2 cm above the GEJ, should be used in children. To my mind, we should use the same definition in children and adults, but comment in children that even without goblet cells, we may have the first stage of what will become Barrett. Indeed, in any biopsy that shows glandular mucosa without intestinal metaplasia, a comment might be made that metaplasia, and thus definitive Barrett esophagus, is not excluded because not every biopsy necessarily captures a metaplastic focus, and that some degree of surveillance may be indicated.

A final comment regarding Barrett esophagus is that much more widespread use of upper gastrointestinal screening will be needed to maximize the effectiveness of the advances in this area. Screening colonoscopies beginning at age 50 are now well accepted, and to my mind, upper gastrointestinal screening at the time of colonoscopy, while the patient is already sedated and in the endoscopy suite, seems the most efficient method of screening for esophageal carcinoma and its precursors.

Dysplasia in Barrett Esophagus

Although conceptualized after squamous dysplasia, the concept of glandular dysplasia is now well established in many sites. The sequence of reflux→Barrett→dysplasia→adenocarcinoma is well enough established that patients with Barrett esophagus undergo periodic surveillance with biopsies to monitor for dysplasia. In taking biopsies for dysplasia, more tissue is better. Especially when high-grade dysplasia has been documented or is suspected, jumbo forceps are recommended, and endoscopic mucosal resection, which uses saline injection to lift up the mucosa prior to biopsy, is preferable [PMID16330950].

The Common Colonic Adenomatous Polyp Is the Guide for Low-Grade Glandular Dysplasia throughout the Gastrointestinal Tract

The principal differential diagnosis for glandular dysplasia in Barrett esophagus is reactive atypia. As is the case anywhere, caution is needed in diagnosing a carcinoma-directed dysplasia if there is severe concomitant acute inflammation. A reactive process is generally favored over dysplasia if there is only slight nuclear enlargement i20.8a, i20.8b or if there is severe acute inflammation. In cases where the distinction between reactive atypia and low-grade dysplasia cannot be made with certainty, a diagnosis of "indefinite for dysplasia" is recommended.

In "indefinite for dysplasia" in Barrett esophagus, there is glandular crowding i20.9a, and nuclei are enlarged i20.9b but still relatively uniform, with indistinct nucleoli. Nuclear stratification is generally limited and does not involve the entire epithelial thickness. There is still a moderate amount of mucin in the cytoplasm [PMID12692197, PMID11936261]. These cases are subject to interobserver variation even among excellent pathologists. One person's "indefinite for dysplasia" is another person's reactive atypia and a third person's low-grade dysplasia.

Low-grade dysplasia is characterized by slight glandular crowding, with nuclear enlargement and hyperchromasia. Stratification is not pronounced, however, and cytoplasm is readily apparent in the apical portion of the cell. Chromatin is relatively coarse in most cells and nucleoli are small i20.10a, i20.10b, i20.10c [PMID12692197, PMID11936261]. Roughly, low-grade glandular dysplasia of the esophagus resembles a routine colonic adenomatous polyp, and we will return to this analogy when we consider glandular dysplasia in other contexts throughout the gastrointestinal tract.

Historically, most have felt that the surface should be affected in any dysplasia, with some degree of nuclear atypia and stratification i20.11a, i20.11b, and it has been recommended that the diagnosis of dysplasia be questioned, or that a diagnosis of "indefinite for dysplasia" rather than definitive dysplasia be rendered if the surface epithelium is uninvolved i20.12a, i20.12b, i20.12c. However, a study of apparent esophageal glandular dysplasia that was confined to the lower epithelium, without surface involvement, not only showed that these patients had a significantly higher incidence of associated adenocarcinoma but also had aneuploid DNA or a loss of heterozygosity in chromosomes 9p or 17p, findings which have been observed in esophageal adenocarcinoma [PMID16625087].

There has been variable experience regarding the percentage of patients with low-grade glandular dysplasia who will progress to a more significant process. One study concluded that about 2/3 of patients with low-grade dysplasia will regress, and the actual incidence of progression to high-grade dysplasia or adenocarcinoma is 0.6% per year [PMID16630761], while another found a higher incidence of progression if the diagnosis of low-grade dysplasia was agreed upon by 2 or more pathologists [PMID20461069].

In high-grade dysplasia, there are significant abnormalities both architecturally and in nuclear appearance. Architecturally, the glands are crowded, often back-to-back without intervening stroma i20.13a, with branching and infolding, or with a cribriform arrangement. There is full thickness nuclear stratification and sharply diminished cytoplasm i20.13b. The nuclei are enlarged, hyperchromatic, and variable, often with a vesicular chromatin pattern (ie, the chromatin is on the periphery of the nucleus, and the nuclear center is clear), prominent nucleoli, and significantly increased mitoses i20.13c [PMID11936261, PMID19864239]. As low-grade glandular dysplasia in Barrett esophagus roughly resembles a colonic adenomatous polyp, so high-grade dysplasia roughly resembles a colonic adenomatous polyp with high-grade dysplasia. For all practical purposes, a diagnosis of high-grade dysplasia is tantamount to a diagnosis of adenocarcinoma in situ.

There is appreciable interobserver variation in the diagnosis of both low-grade and high-grade glandular dysplasia in Barrett esophagus, even among so-called "specialists." In one study, there was only fair agreement at best in the diagnosis of low-grade dysplasia among "gastrointestinal pathologists" [PMID11151865]. One might expect better agreement among "experts" in the diagnosis of high-grade dysplasia and carcinoma in esophageal biopsies, but there was poor agreement even among "gastrointestinal pathologists who see a high volume of Barrett cases" [PMID18671819]. In dysplasia in Barrett esophagus, we see once more, as we have in intraductal lesions of the breast, in follicular lesions of the thyroid, and in small cell vs non-small cell carcinomas of the lung, that all "experts" cannot possibly be better than a good general pathologist if they cannot agree among themselves.

Immunohistochemical staining for α-methylacyl-coenzyme A racemase (AMACR; commercially available as P504S) may be helpful in detecting high-grade dysplasia, as it stains essentially no normal Barrett epithelium, no cases of reactive atypia, few cases of low-grade dysplasia, but 64% of cases of high-grade dysplasia and 75% of esophageal adenocarcinomas [PMID16996568]. In cases where the diagnosis of dysplasia is secure and the question is the degree, p53 expression shifts the odds to a high-grade process [PMID16835318], but the diagnosis of any degree of dysplasia is still largely a matter of good H&E interpretation.

Although the sequence of reflux→Barrett→low-grade dysplasia→high-grade dysplasia→adenocarcinoma is well established, only a minority of patients with dysplasia—even high-grade dysplasia—will develop carcinoma [PMID11375943], and only about 5% of resection specimens removed for high-grade glandular dysplasia of the esophagus will have invasive adenocarcinoma [PMID19864239]. Because only a minority of patients with high-grade dysplasia will have invasive carcinoma if a resection is performed, and given the technical difficulty and morbidity of a resection, attention has focused on nonsurgical means of treating high-grade dysplasia. Many nonsurgical ablation methods have been tried, including radiofrequency, cryoablation, and photodynamic therapy.

Photodynamic therapy has shown great promise in preventing high-grade dysplasia from progressing to invasive adenocarcinoma. In this technique, a photosensitizing agent called porfimer sodium (Photofrin) is injected intravenously. Photofrin is a mixture of porphyrin units formed by ester linkages and is absorbed more by high-grade dysplastic and cancer cells than by normal cells. After 1 to 3 days, little of the agent remains in normal cells, but enough persists in dysplastic or early cancer cells that the application of laser light at 630 nm produces a series of reactions eventuating in superoxide (O_2–) and hydroxyl radicals. These destroy the cell both directly and indirectly by compromising its blood supply and activating the immune system [PMID21180605]. Radiofrequency ablation for Barrett esophagus without dysplasia is being investigated, but at this writing, only high-grade dysplasia is uniformly acted upon [PMID21180605].

Inflammatory Conditions in the Esophagus Unrelated to Barrett

Eosinophils are associated with early reflux, and occasional eosinophils suggest early reflux even in the absence of glandular epithelium. However, large numbers of this cell type may suggest a diagnosis of EE rather than GERD. EE is a distinct entity that is often accompanied by atopy, and allergies to food, medications, or environmental agents. There may be a mild peripheral eosinophilia [PMID21836470].

EE is best known of primary eosinophilic gastrointestinal disorders (EGIDs). Other entities in the EGID group are very rare, but almost certainly exist. For example, the number of well-documented cases of eosinophilic colitis does not exceed 100 at this writing, but enough cases have been recognized to identify it as an EGID [PMID21922029].

EE is usually treated with anti-inflammatory agents, often steroids, rather than with proton pump inhibitors, as is the case for reflux. The question therefore arises as to the distinction of eosinophilia secondary to reflux from that caused by EE. EE is usually found in the proximal or mid esophagus, without glandular epithelium. The presence of eosinophils in the distal esophagus or in association with glandular epithelium on a biopsy suggests that reflux should be excluded. If eosinophils do not sharply outnumber neutrophils, the diagnosis of EE is unlikely. Additionally helpful is that EE often has a characteristic endoscopic appearance.

There have been publications on the number of eosinophils necessary for the diagnosis of EE, most of which have concluded that the diagnosis of EE should be particularly suspected if there are large numbers of eosinophils (>15/HPF) or if there are eosinophilic microabscesses [PMID18061097]. Epithelial edema i20.14a and degranulation of the eosinophils i20.14b are possibly associated with EE. All this said, however, in the lower esophagus, there is great overlap in the histologic features, including the number of eosinophils, between EE and GERD [PMID19642735]. In one study, 70% of patients with large numbers of eosinophils in biopsies of the lower esophagus had GERD, not EE [PMID18289205]. In children, overlap between the histologic findings of EE and reflux has been observed, and the distinction can be especially challenging [PMID19209168].

pH and manometric data may be needed to exclude reflux and secure a diagnosis of EE if the biopsy is from the distal esophagus or if it contains glandular epithelium. Alternatively, the gastroenterologist might keep an open mind and consider changing the therapy if treatment directed at one entity does not appear effective. The exclusion of reflux and the willingness of the gastroenterologist to change therapy are more important than a specific number of eosinophils. Biopsies from the proximal esophagus with large numbers of eosinophils are more likely to be EE unless there is a long column of Barrett continuously extending from the gastroesophageal junction.

Lymphocytes are commonly seen in the lamina propria throughout the gastrointestinal tract, but not within the epithelium. A unique form of chronic inflammation, seen in many areas of the gastrointestinal tract, is manifest as lymphocytes that are within the epithelium (although they are not actually within the epithelial cells). Lymphocytic esophagitis is characterized by large numbers of intraepithelial lymphocytes, but its nature has not yet been clarified [PMID19700939]. Intraepithelial lymphocytes are much more important in the colon.

Esophageal biopsies with severe neutrophilic acute inflammation or which have detached clusters of neutrophils should be studied for *Candida*. Even large numbers of organisms can be surprisingly subtle in an exudate i20.15a and a special stain (GMS or PAS) might be beneficial i20.15b. Esophageal biopsies that have acute neutrophilic inflammation and are negative for *Candida*, consideration should be given to pill esophagitis. Many older or debilitated patients have difficulty swallowing the many large pills that are prescribed and these cause an acute inflammatory reaction as they become wedged in the esophagus i20.16.

Carcinomas of the Esophagus

Common squamous and adenocarcinomas of the esophagus are not discussed, since they are rarely a diagnostic challenge and are well covered elsewhere, but there is a basaloid variant of squamous carcinoma of the esophagus, as is the case for the head and neck area, the lung, and the genital region i20.17a. Basaloid tumors in any of these locations are more likely to be variants of squamous carcinoma than true basal cell carcinoma or a neuroendocrine neoplasm. As is the case for other body sites, areas of classic squamous cell carcinoma or squamous carcinoma in situ establish the diagnosis, but these areas may not always be present. Positivity for p63, cytokeratin 5/6, and high molecular weight keratin, as discussed in Chapters 15 and 16, suggests this diagnosis. Even without overt squamous differentiation, neoplastic cells with more eosinophilic cytoplasm than their counterparts may suggest the need for these stains i20.17b.

ISBN 978-089189-5886

Core Points for the Esophagus

- Reflux leads to glandular metaplasia in the lower portion of the esophagus.
  - The addition of intestinal metaplasia in the form of goblet cells completes the transformation to Barrett esophagus
  - Predisposition to esophageal adenocarcinoma.
- Problematic situations in the diagnosis of Barrett:
  - Submucosal glands in the normal esophagus
  - Intestinal metaplasia in the proximal stomach
  - Hiatal hernia
  - Incomplete intestinal metaplasia
  - Intestinal metaplasia in children.
- These difficulties notwithstanding, the understanding of the sequence of reflux → Barrett → dysplasia → adenocarcinoma, and the development of effective surveillance, is a success story.
- Low-grade glandular dysplasia in Barrett esophagus is characterized by glandular crowding and nuclear enlargement
  - But the nuclei remain relatively uniform and have indistinct nucleoli.
  - Nuclear stratification is generally limited to the lower half of the epithelium.
  - Overall appearance is similar to that of a common colonic adenomatous polyp.
  - Principal differential mimic of low-grade glandular dysplasia is reactive atypia.
- High-grade glandular dysplasia in Barrett esophagus is characterized by abnormalities in both architecture and nuclei.
  - Glands are crowded, often without intervening stroma.
  - Epithelium often folds out from the gland or into its lumen, or there may be a cribriform arrangement within the lumen.
  - Nuclei are not only enlarged and hyperchromatic, but also more variable than in low-grade dysplasia,
  - Vesicular chromatin pattern and prominent nucleoli.
  - Full thickness nuclear stratification and sharply increased mitoses.
  - Overall appearance is similar to a colonic adenomatous polyp with high-grade dysplasia.
- Eosinophilic esophagitis (EE): usually distinct clinical and endoscopic findings.
  - Histologic distinction from Barrett esophagus can be difficult because eosinophils are found in reflux.
  - Origin from the proximal esophagus and the absence of glandular epithelium suggest eosinophilic esophagitis.
  - In difficult situations, pH and manometric data may be needed, and empiric treatment may be needed.
- Squamous dysplasia and carcinoma of the esophagus are diagnosed as in other body sites.
- Basaloid squamous carcinoma may have little indication of squamous origin
  - Search for areas of classic squamous cell carcinoma or squamous carcinoma in situ.
  - If none, IHC needed to establish the squamous nature of the neoplasm.

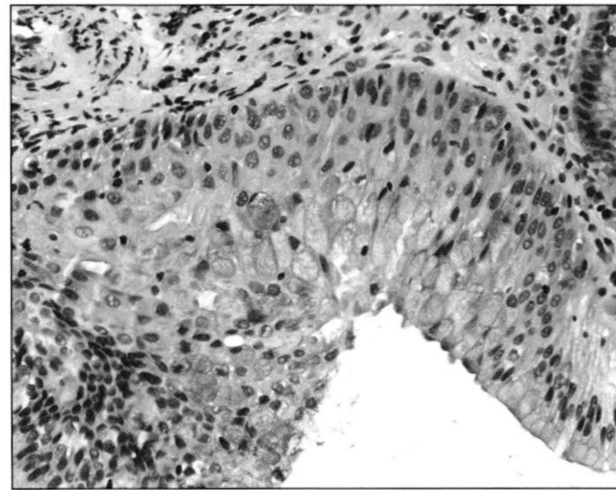

i20.1 Barrett esophagus demonstrating the transition from stratified squamous epithelium, evident on the upper portion of the photograph, to glandular epithelium, evident in the lower portion. Intestinal metaplasia has already begun even though the squamous epithelium has not yet been completely replaced.

i20.2 A goblet cell demonstrating a single cytoplasmic vacuole, filled with amphophilic acidic mucopolysaccharide material, with rounded cytoplasmic borders

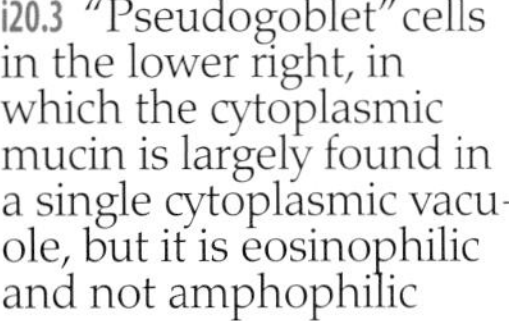

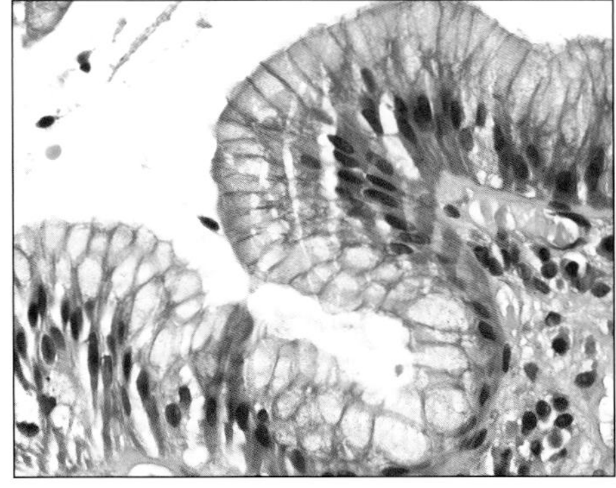

i20.3 "Pseudogoblet" cells in the lower right, in which the cytoplasmic mucin is largely found in a single cytoplasmic vacuole, but it is eosinophilic and not amphophilic

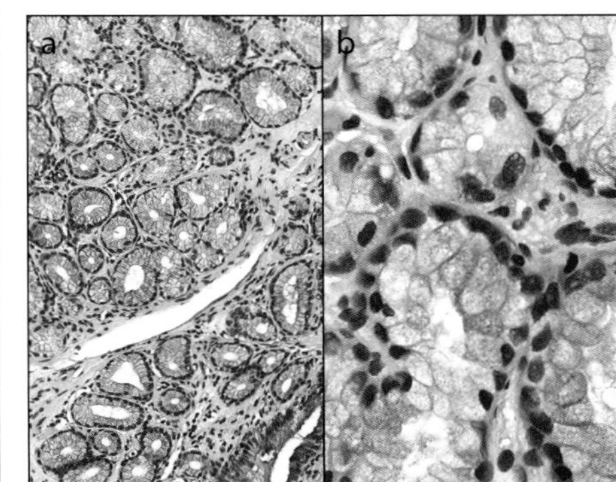

i20.4 **a** The submucosal glands that are often found in the normal esophagus. Note the small glands and cohesive lobular pattern. **b** The cells in normal esophageal submucosal glands may have some amphophilic acidic mucopolysaccharide material.

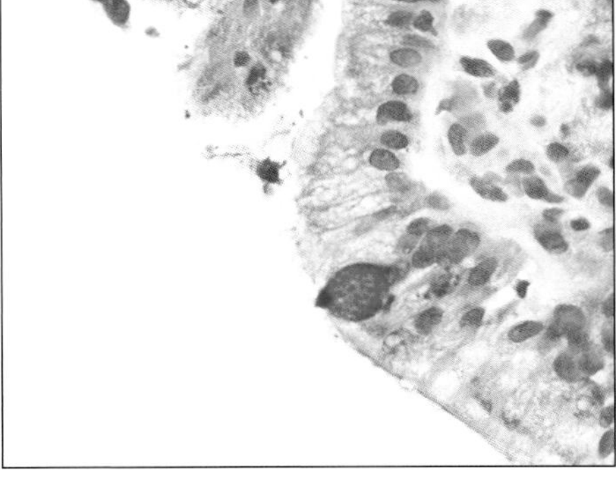

i20.5 An alcian blue stain highlighting a rare goblet cell

alcian blue
pH 2.5
acidic
mucopolysaccharide
normal gland
alcian blue
negative

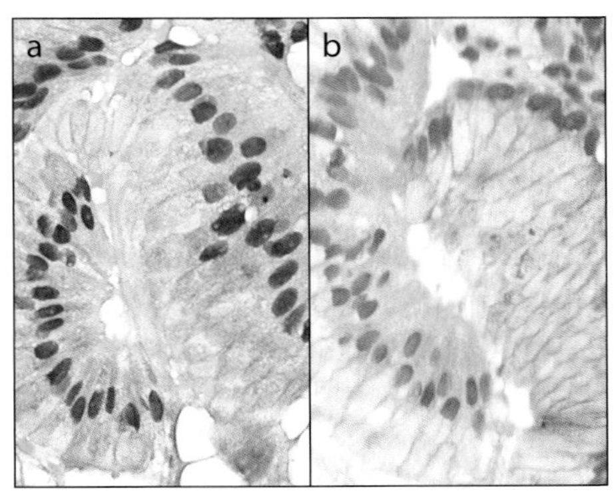

i20.6 **a** A biopsy of the gastroesophageal junction in which some glandular cells on the surface have slightly amphophilic cytoplasm, but no distinct goblet cells **b** The same case as in i20.6a, stained with alcian blue. This stain confirms the presence of acidic mucopolysaccharides, but goblet cells are not seen.

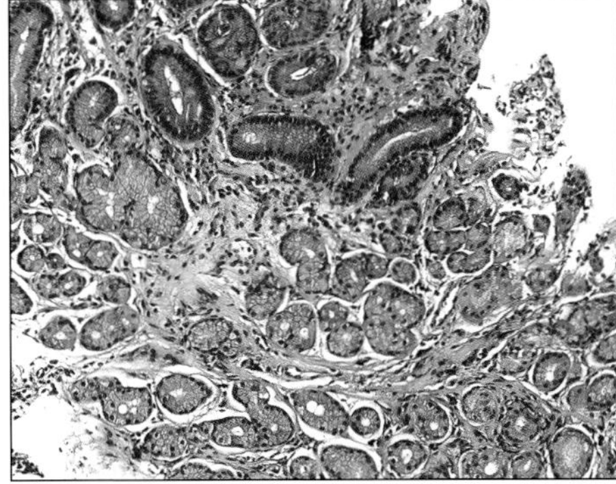

i20.7 A biopsy of the GE junction demonstrating gastric-type mucosa of the fundic/body type (as indicated by the parietal cells in the lower portion of the photograph) and intestinal metaplasia in the upper portion

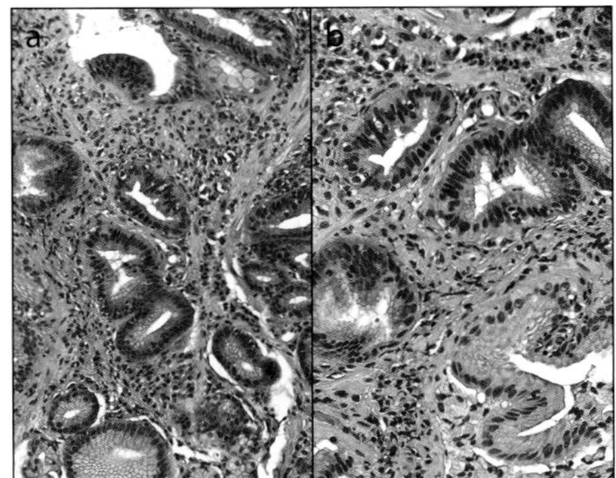

i20.8 **a** Mild glandular atypia in Barrett esophagus **b** A higher-power view of the same case as in i20.8a. The nuclei of the glands in the central and upper portion are larger than those in normal gland in the lower right, but the enlargement is minimal and there are no other features to suggest dysplasia.

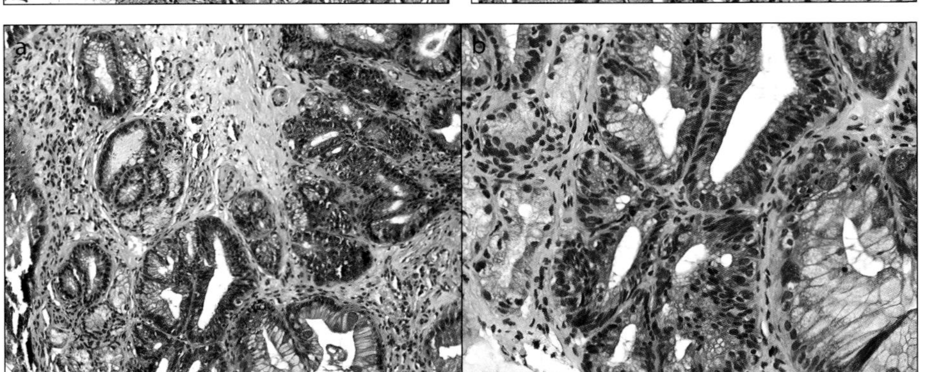

i20.9 **a** Barrett esophagus with glandular atypia that is indefinite for dysplasia. There is mild glandular crowding and slight nuclear enlargement.

b The same case as in i20.9a, highlighting the slight glandular crowding and mild nuclear enlargement

ISBN 978-089189-5886

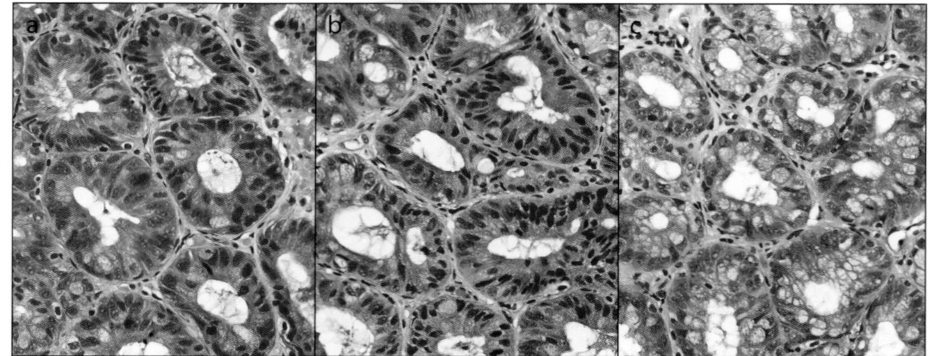

i20.10 **a** Low-grade glandular dysplasia in Barrett esophagus. Note the resemblance to a colonic adenomatous polyp and also note the nuclear stratification on the surface. **b-c** Low-grade glandular dysplasia in Barrett esophagus. The glands are crowded, but not markedly so. The nuclei are generally confined to the lower half of the cell with a good amount of cytoplasm and in some cases, retention of goblet cells. Although an occasional nucleus has a vesicular chromatin pattern with a small nucleolus, most maintain a coarse chromatin pattern with indistinct nucleoli, as would be seen in an ordinary colonic adenomatous polyp.

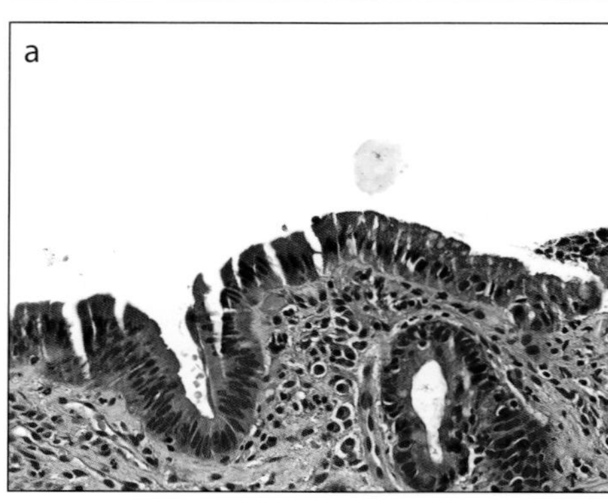

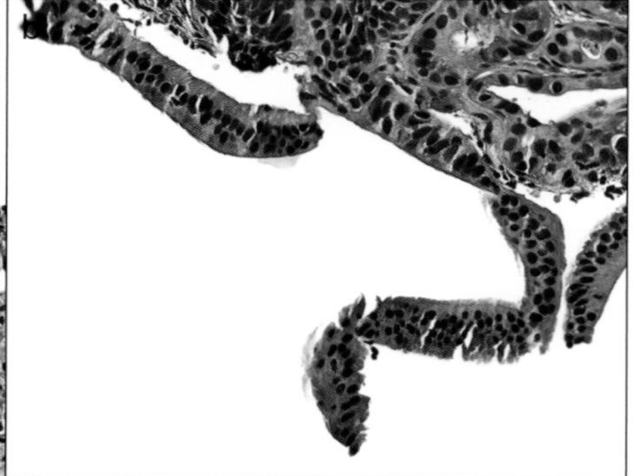

i20.11 **a** Barrett esophagus, in which there is slight stratification of the nuclei on the surface on the left side, as opposed to the normal surface on the right side, in which there is only a single, small, round basal nucleus **b** Another example of Barrett esophagus in which the surface epithelium demonstrates nuclear enlargement and stratification. Surface involvement is neither necessary nor specific for the diagnosis of dysplasia, but its presence does suggest a diagnosis of either indefinite for dysplasia or low-grade dysplasia over reactive atypia.

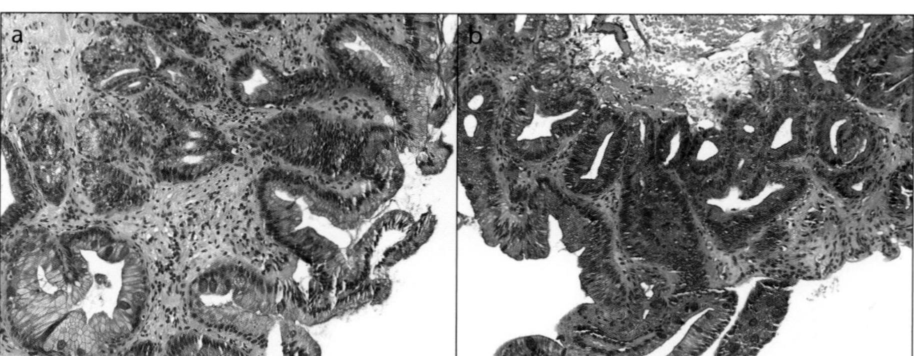

i20.12 **a, b** Barrett esophagus with slight glandular atypia but an uninvolved surface epithelium. This does not exclude dysplasia, but it suggests that a definitive diagnosis of dysplasia is unlikely. In i20.12b, the normal surface epithelium is seen at lower left.

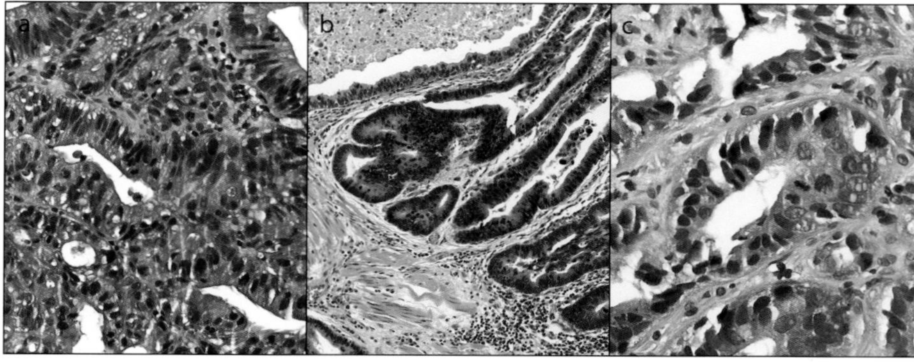

i20.13 **a** High-grade glandular dysplasia in Barrett esophagus illustrating marked glandular crowding, often to the exclusion of intervening stroma. **b** A resection specimen demonstrating high-grade glandular dysplasia in Barrett esophagus. Note the full thickness nuclear stratification and the sharply diminished cytoplasm in the glandular cells. **c** Another biopsy example of high-grade glandular dysplasia in Barrett esophagus illustrating the vesicular chromatin pattern and prominent nucleoli that are typically found in high-grade dysplasia. Note the nuclear stratification, the minimal amount of cytoplasm, and the mitotic figure just to the right of center.

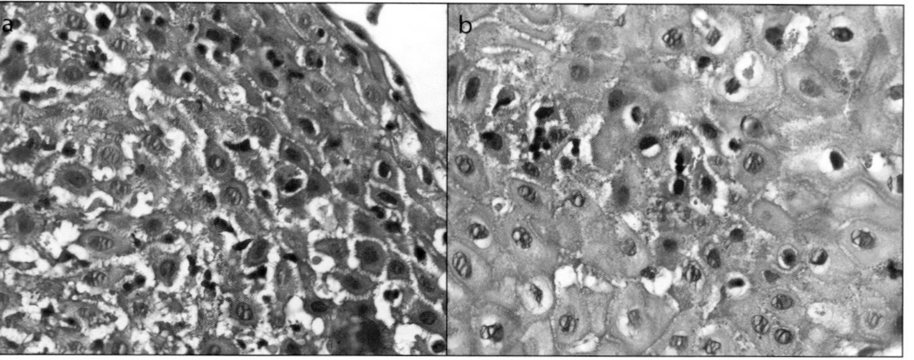

i20.14 **a** Eosinophilic esophagitis with marked epithelial edema, as indicated by the spaces between the cells. Because of the tight intercellular connections caused by desmosomes, squamous epithelial cells often remain connected even in the presence of extensive edema. **b** Eosinophilic esophagitis with loss of cell membrane integrity of the eosinophils, resulting in extracellular granules

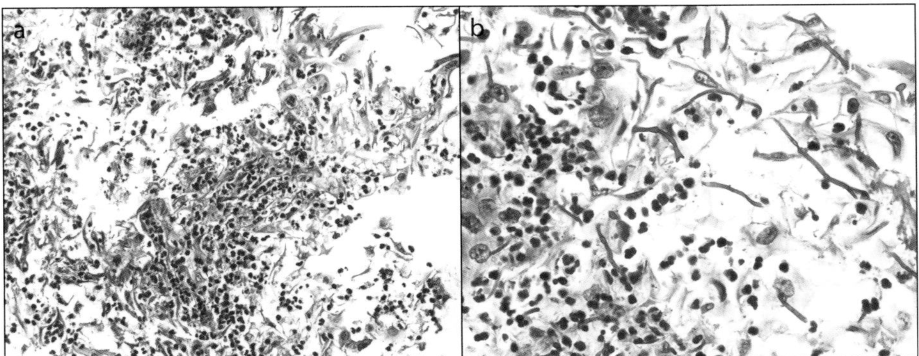

i20.15 **a** A collection of neutrophils and debris in an esophageal biopsy

b The same field as in i20.15a, stained with PAS, demonstrating numerous *Candida* organisms

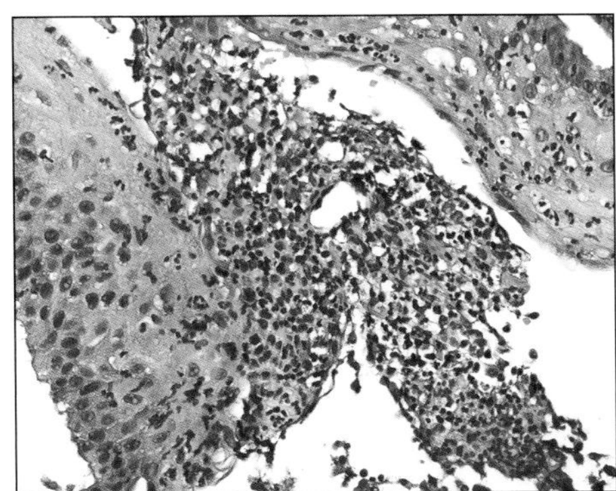

i20.16 Pill esophagitis in an esophageal biopsy from an older patient. The biopsy did not demonstrate glandular epithelium, significant numbers of eosinophils, or *Candida*.

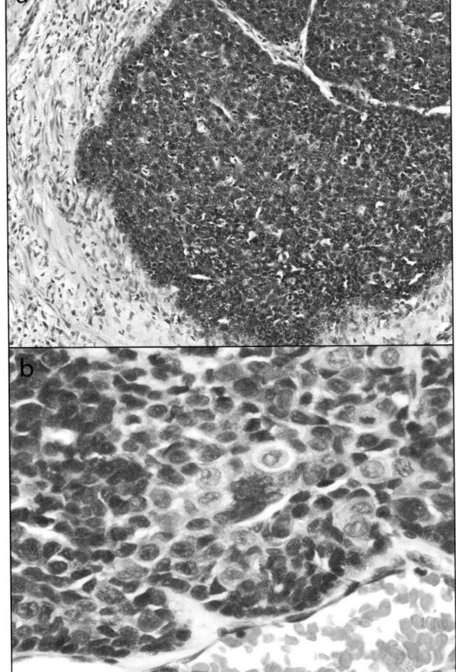

i20.17 **a** The basaloid variant of invasive squamous carcinoma of the esophagus

b The same case as in i20.17a, illustrating a small focus in which the neoplastic cells have a sufficient amount of eosinophilic cytoplasm to raise suspicion for squamous carcinoma

ISBN 978-089189-5886

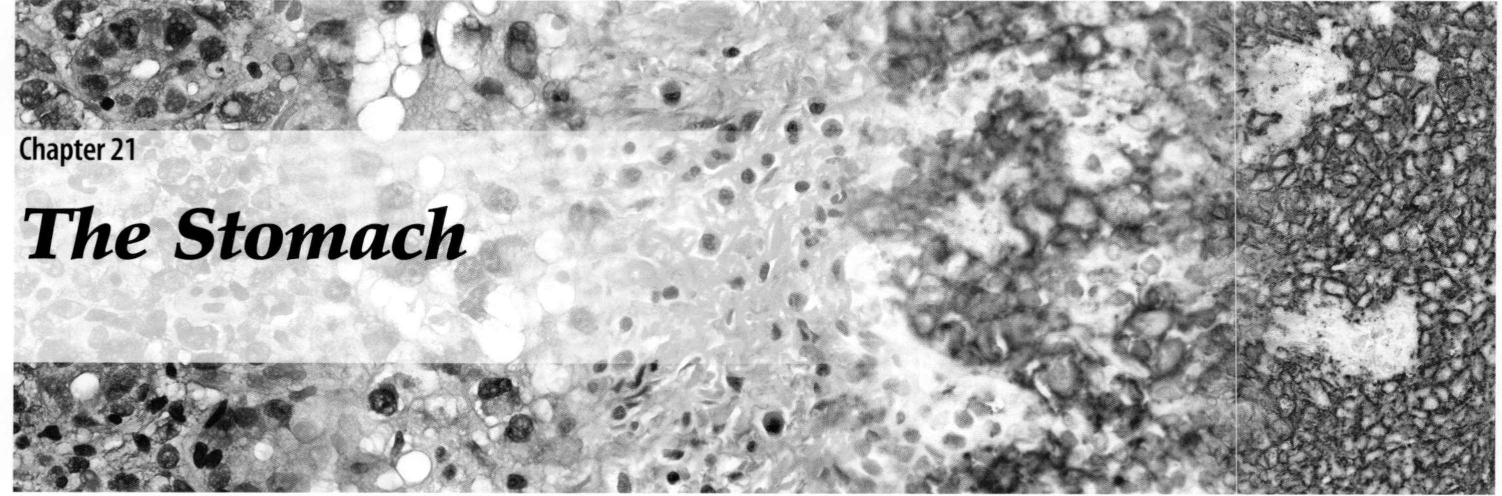

Chapter 21

The Stomach

Normal Histology of the Stomach

Nowhere in surgical pathology is the terminology of the normal specimen more confusing than in the stomach. Paradoxically, the word "pit" refers to the superficial part of the epithelium. Adding to the confusion is the fact that this superficial region can also be called "the crypts," another word normally associated with depth or lower regions. The origin of these 2 terms for the superficial portion of the epithelium is that this portion consists of invaginations of the surface epithelium, and early microscopists were more impressed with these invaginations than by the overall superficial location of the region. Perhaps the least confusing term for the superficial portion of the epithelium is "the foveola" (ie, a small fovea, which is Latin for "pit"). The deeper portion of the epithelium contains the glands, which empty into the foveola i21.1.

The most proximal portion of the stomach is the cardiac region. The fundus and body are the central portions. The most distal portion, the pylorus, is essentially a continuation of the antrum. The mucosa of the fundus and body is thicker than the mucosa of either the proximal or distal portion and contains more parietal and chief cells. In the fundus and body, the glands are 3-4 times the thickness of the foveolar i21.2. In contrast, the mucosa of the pylorus, antrum, and cardia does not generally contain parietal or chief cells and is thinner i21.3. In these locations, the glands have about the same thickness as the foveola. There are therefore essentially only 2 types of mucosa in the stomach. The pyloric-antral mucosa in the distal region and the cardiac mucosa on the one hand, and the thicker mucosa of the fundus and body on the other. However, these zones are poorly demarcated and there is very imperfect correspondence between the anatomic zone and the type of epithelium that is encountered histologically. Parietal cells, the hallmark of the mucosa of the fundus and body, may occasionally be seen in other zones [Owen ISBN978-0781762410] and are commonly seen in biopsies from the gastroesophageal junction adjacent to squamous epithelium i21.4, clearly indicating origin in the cardiac region. In fact, the very existence of a cardiac portion of the stomach has been challenged [PMID10716154].

Gastritis

Numerous classifications of gastritis have been offered, the 2 most commonly used of which are those of Whitehead [PMID5015372] and the more recent updated Sydney system [PMID8827022]. In the frankly rather complicated Sydney system, gastritis is divided into acute or chronic, and the latter is further divided into nonatrophic forms (often *H pylori*), atrophic forms (eg, autoimmune and multifocal atrophic gastritis), and forms with specific features (granulomatous, lymphocytic, and eosinophilic gastritis).

Acute gastritis is evident as neutrophils within the epithelium i21.5. While the Whitehead system for chronic gastritis is perhaps slightly outdated in regard to *Helicobacter* gastritis, it is otherwise excellent, still very much applicable, and simpler than other systems. The Whitehead system is based on the type of mucosa, the grade and activity of the inflammation, and the presence or absence of intestinal metaplasia. The 2 major categories of the Whitehead system are chronic superficial gastritis and chronic atrophic gastritis. In chronic superficial gastritis, inflammation is confined to the foveola. The normal lamina propria of the stomach contains minimal numbers of lymphocytes, and any significant number of such cells permits a diagnosis of chronic gastritis i21.6, though it may not be possible to distinguish between chronic superficial gastritis and chronic atrophic gastritis on a mucosal biopsy.

Severe and prolonged full thickness mucosal inflammation may result in chronic atrophic gastritis i21.7. Whereas the normal antrum has 3-4 glands in the wall, a reduction to 1 or 2 glands is suggestive of atrophy. In severe atrophy, there is almost complete loss of glands, often with intestinal metaplasia (ie, goblet cells, as described in Barrett esophagus). The degree of inflammation may be diminished in severe gastric atrophy, as the inflammatory process apparently "burns itself out."

Lymphocytic gastritis is a special type of chronic gastritis that tends to spare the glands and affect the overlying foveola. *Helicobacter* infection must be excluded before this diagnosis is made. The cells in lymphocytic gastritis are mostly T cells, suggesting that this process is likely a T-cell response to an antigen [PMID19700939].

Helicobacter *Gastritis*

Helicobacter pylori is a gram-negative bacillus whose etiologic role in the pathogenesis of gastric ulcer and adenocarcinoma led to the Nobel Prize for Barry Warren and Robin Marshall in 2005 [PMID6145023]. Although *H pylori* may be associated with acute gastritis, this stage may not be biopsied. Many cases of chronic gastritis are caused by *H pylori* and chronic gastritis of the follicular type (ie, with lymphoid follicles) **i21.8** is very often associated with *H pylori* [PMID12162525].

There are many strains of *H pylori*, and excellent progress has been made in the characterization of the molecular mechanism of *Helicobacter* infections [PMID19712163]. Some gram-negative bacteria can make exotoxins, as do gram-positive bacteria, but they can also be pathogenic by 2 other mechanisms. First, they can release endotoxin, part of the lipopolysaccharide from the cell wall, upon death and cell lysis. Endotoxin plays a major role in many cases of septic shock. Second, gram-negative bacteria can release proteins that may act as toxins or function in shielding the bacteria from the host immune system, but unlike exotoxins, they act locally, on the external surface of the bacterial cell oe on the surface of the host cell, or are injected into the host cell's cytoplasm. Gram-negative bacteria need a more complicated secretion system than their gram-positive counterparts because they have a double-layered cell wall and because their secretions, instead of diffusing away like exotoxins, may also cross the plasma membrane of the eukaryotic host. Gram-negative bacteria have evolved 6 major systems of conveying their proteins from their cytoplasm to the exterior [PMID20419401, PMID19605938].

Some strains of *H pylori* secrete a locally-acting toxin of this type, encoded by cytotoxin-associated gene A (*CAGA*). The cagA protein enters epithelial cells, causing them to release cytokines that attract neutrophils [PMID21088410]. The recruitment of neutrophils raises the pH of the local environment. The beneficial effect for the host is that excessive acidity facilitates reflux and contributes to esophageal adenocarcinoma, so *H pylori*, by raising the pH, can reduce reflux. On the other hand, the damage to the gastric epithelial cell not only promotes ulceration, but also gastric adenocarcinoma. Progress is being made in understanding the mechanism of gastric carcinogenesis [PMID19111390].

H pylori eradication has helped greatly in reducing ulceration and adenocarcinoma of the stomach, but potentially leaves us with an increased incidence of reflux and esophageal adenocarcinoma. The effect of *H pylori* on gastric mucosa is augmented if the bacteria also produce a toxin encoded by the vacuolating cytotoxin gene. This toxin, vacA, creates vacuoles in the epithelial cell. All *H pylori* make vacA, but only some strains make the m1 and s1 types, which are more toxic [PMID20512250]. A strain that makes both cagA and one of the toxic types of vacA predisposes to gastric ulceration and carcinoma.

H pylori can be seen in H&E stained biopsies as small curved rods on the luminal surface or in pits, although the eosinophilic organism can be difficult to distinguish from the surrounding mucus **i21.9a**, **i21.9b**. Special stains for *H pylori* are usually not necessary in routine cases for which there is no clinical concern or history, and in which there is no significant mucosal inflammation [PMID16538056], but it is particularly important to exclude *H pylori* when there is an ulcer, a history of an ulcer, a high clinical suspicion, severe acute mucosal inflammation, or a previously documented infection for which therapeutic efficacy is being assessed. In situations of special concern, a negative H&E examination cannot be depended on, and an additional measure is helpful. The historical gold standard for the identification of *H pylori* is culture, though this is technically difficult and cannot be done on formalin-fixed biopsies. A simple toluidine blue or Diff-Quik provides somewhat greater contrast between the organism and the surrounding mucus and may suffice **i21.10a**, **i21.10b**, but fragments of mucus simulate the organism, and the bacteria may not have the classic curved shape after treatment. Therefore, if there is significant clinical concern and the H&E examination is negative, immunohistochemistry is recommended because of its high sensitivity and specificity **i21.11** [PMID18834216].

A rapid urease test is available for gastric biopsy specimens, which has excellent specificity but poor sensitivity [PMID12700494]. There is a stool test for the antigen which has been reported to have 75% sensitivity (comparable to histopathology) and 82% specificity [PMID20455396]. There is a breath test for the urease produced by the organism, and the absence of antibodies to *H pylori* is helpful in excluding infection, though their presence simply indicates past exposure, and does not address the question of current infection [PMID17382278].

Nonneoplastic and Polypoid Conditions of the Stomach

Gastric xanthoma (also called xanthelasma) is a condition of unknown cause characterized by collections of macrophages in the lamina propria **i21.12** [PMID19915233]. The stomach is the only gastrointestinal organ in which macrophages may commonly be found in the normal state.

Gastric antral vascular ectasia (GAVE) occurs in the antrum and is endoscopically manifest as the so-called watermelon stomach. GAVE is similar to the vascular ectasia (formerly called angiodysplasia) of the right colon. Histologically, there are dilated capillaries under the surface, perhaps with fibrin microthrombi, but the diagnosis is made endoscopically.

The most common cause of enlarged mucosal folds without a distinct mass is a normal variant or a reactive change. Other causes include Menetrier disease, Zollinger-Ellison syndrome, and hypertrophic hypersecretory gastropathy. Menetrier disease is characterized by foveolar hyperplasia, often with glandular atrophy, reduced acid secretion, increased protein secretion, and hypoalbuminemia. Zollinger-Ellison syndrome has glandular rather than foveolar hyperplasia and increased parietal cells. Acid production is sharply increased, but protein secretion is not. Hypertrophic hypersecretory gastropathy has features of both Menetrier disease and Zollinger-Ellison syndrome.

Polypoid change secondary to mucosal prolapse, which is common in the left side of the colon, is rare in the stomach because of its much greater size, but may occur if there has been an anastomosis to the small bowel.

Hyperplastic polyps are primarily caused by foveolar hyperplasia **i21.13**, resulting in elongated and distorted pits, though occasional chief and parietal cells can be seen. Fundic gland polyps are primarily hyperplasias of the glands under the pits. Because of the location of these polyps in the fundus

ISBN 978-089189-5886

and body, where chief and parietal cells are numerous, and because the hyperplasia occurs in the deeper portion of the mucosa, where these cells are found, chief and parietal cells are much more numerous in fundic gland polyps than in hyperplastic polyps. Dilatation of glands is a typical feature of fundic gland polyps i21.14. Long-term use of proton pump inhibitors for reflux increases the incidence of fundic gland polyps [PMID19830554].

Adenomatous polyps are rare in the stomach but are occasionally encountered, and when they are, their appearance and significance (ie, low-grade dysplasia) are that of a typical colonic adenomatous polyp i21.15. A familial polyposis syndrome should be excluded when a gastric adenomatous polyp is encountered.

The inflammatory fibroid polyp occurs in the gastrointestinal tract, usually in the stomach. It consists of loose connective tissue in the submucosa i21.16a, i21.16b, with variable numbers of inflammatory cells, often admixed with areas of collagen i21.16c and areas of greater cellularity i21.16d. There may be numerous small blood vessels, many of which are surrounded by a hypocellular zone with concentric fibrosis. Eosinophils or plasma cells may be prominent in the more cellular or fibrotic areas. The inflammatory fibroid polyp may be of myofibroblastic origin. If a gastrointestinal polyp resembles nodular fasciitis or an inflammatory myofibroblastic tumor, an inflammatory fibroid polyp should be considered. Also, if a mass appears to be a benign stromal tumor, but has many eosinophils or plasma cells, an inflammatory fibroid polyp should be excluded.

Gastric Lymphoid Proliferations

Gastric lymphomas are diagnosed as in other sites and as discussed in Chapter 8, so only 2 entities, the marginal zone lymphoma and the diffuse large B-cell lymphoma, are discussed here. The most common low-grade gastric lymphoma is a mucosa-associated lymphoma that is usually of the marginal zone type i21.17a-e. As is the case for marginal zone lymphomas anywhere, those in the stomach may have a monocytoid, plasmacytoid, or small lymphocytic appearance.

Because *H pylori* is often associated with an intense lymphoid response and it can be impossible to distinguish a reactive lymphoid hyperplasia in response to *H pylori* from a low-grade lymphoma of the extranodal marginal zone type on H&E sections, it is wise to exclude this organism before the diagnosis of low-grade lymphoma is made. Indeed, most gastric marginal zone lymphomas arise in a setting of chronic infection with *H pylori* [PMID21970484], reflecting the fact that this type of lymphoma anywhere is associated with long-term stimulation by microbial or autoimmune antigens [PMID16397126].

Those lymphoid proliferations that have a t(11;18)(q21:q21), resulting in an *AP12/MALT1* fusion, are likely to be marginal zone lymphomas, but some of these lymphomas lack this translocation, so its absence does not ensure a benign lymphoid process [PMID15577674]. While the presence of this translocation suggests neoplasia over a reactive lymphoid infiltrate, the diagnosis of a low-grade lymphoma in the stomach should be made if and only if a thorough search for *H pylori* is negative and the process has failed to respond to antibiotics directed against the bacterium.

Other than adenocarcinoma, the most common malignancy in the stomach is the diffuse large B-cell lymphoma, which can simulate a poorly differentiated adenocarcinoma nearly perfectly on H&E i21.18a, i21.18b. It is prudent to perform immunohistochemical stains before rendering a diagnosis of either type of neoplasm i21.18c, i21.18d.

Gastric Dysplasia

Gastric dysplasia in flat mucosa is not as well characterized as glandular dysplasia in the esophagus and colon, and even greater interobserver variation is to be expected, but in general, the criteria are similar to those employed in assessing glandular epithelium in Barrett esophagus [PMID9023391]. Reactive atypia is characterized by prominent nucleoli, but a large amount of cytoplasm, so that the nucleus to cytoplasmic ratio is unchanged. The chromatin is open, with minimal clumping i21.19. As is the case in other sites, if the nucleolus is subtracted in the mind's eye, there will be little of concern, and as in other sites, an acutely inflamed background suggests reactive atypia.

Cases that are indefinite for dysplasia have slight glandular crowding and mild nuclear enlargement with chromatin clumping, without less prominent nucleoli, and with slightly diminished cytoplasm i21.20. They have basal nuclei without stratification, and a normal surface epithelium. In short, they have a reactive appearance, but without nucleoli or significant inflammation.

Low-grade gastric dysplasia is characterized by glandular crowding with nuclear enlargement and hyperchromasia, elongated nuclei with clumped chromatin, generally indistinct nucleoli, some diminution of cytoplasmic mucin, and slight stratification i21.21 [PMID9023391, PMID17996792]. As is the case for esophageal low-grade glandular dysplasia, the appearance is reminiscent of a typical colonic adenomatous polyp.

High-grade dysplasia is essentially synonymous with adenocarcinoma in situ, and attempts to distinguish between them are likely futile. Gastric high-grade dysplasia/adenocarcinoma in situ is similar to that in Barrett esophagus (illustrated in Chapter 20, i20.13a-c) and is characterized by severe glandular crowding with significant nuclear enlargement and hyperchromasia, sharply reduced cytoplasm, and full-thickness nuclear stratification. Mitoses are clearly increased, and some will be apical, adjacent to the lumen. Some nuclei will be vesicular, with peripheralized chromatin, and nucleoli will often be prominent [PMID9023391, PMID17996792]. It is generally reasonable to regard any glandular epithelium in the gastrointestinal tract that resembles a typical colonic adenomatous polyp as low-grade dysplasia and any such epithelium that resembles a colonic adenomatous polyp with high-grade dysplasia as demonstrating high-grade dysplasia.

Gastric Adenocarcinoma

Only 3 points are made about gastric adenocarcinoma because it is well covered in other works. First, although old, the Lauren classification of gastric carcinomas [PMID14320675] remains clinically useful. It simply divides them into intestinal (also called tubular, meaning that glands are formed), diffuse (without glands, with or without signet ring cells), and mixed. The incidence of the intestinal type varies among populations, but the incidence of the diffuse type does not. It may be that loss of the cell adhesion molecule E-cadherin is a basic defect in diffuse gastric carcinoma, as it seems to be in lobular carcinoma of the breast [PMID11345240, PMID17545690].

Second, paradoxically, the highest-grade gastric carcinoma, the diffuse type, may be the most difficult to detect in biopsy material. A few signet ring cells in the lamina propria are easily overlooked or mistaken for macrophages i21.22a, i21.22b. In contrast to macrophages, the cells of a signet ring adenocarcinoma often have a single vacuole. Moreover, this vacuole often pushes the nucleus to the periphery of the cell and indents it, causing it to depart from a round contour i21.23a, i21.23b (compare to i21.23c. Occasionally, the mucin in a signet ring cell is condensed into a distinct eosinophilic droplet i21.24. One should therefore be wary of nuclei that are eccentrically located in the cell or are not round. An eccentric, indented or ovoid nucleus is often a better indicator of malignancy than nuclear size, especially if it is adjacent to a distinct cytoplasmic vacuole. If there is any question as to the nature of a cell, a simple keratin immunohistochemical stain will identify the epithelial nature of the cell and resolve the matter, as dispersed vacuolated cells in the stroma that are keratin positive are almost certainly carcinoma i21.25a, i21.25b.

Third, as discussed and illustrated above i21.18a-d, immunohistochemical stains are often required to distinguish between a diffuse adenocarcinoma and a diffuse large-cell lymphoma. Reactive epithelial atypia and intimate intermingling of lymphoma cells and residual glands may make the distinction impossible without immunohistochemical stains i21.26.

Some cases of gastric adenocarcinoma overexpress Her2 and may benefit from Trastuzumab (Herceptin) therapy, as is the case for breast carcinomas [PMID20728210], though data are very preliminary at this writing.

Gastric Stromal Tumors

Gastrointestinal stromal tumors (GISTs), as the name implies, are unique to the gastrointestinal tract and often occur in the stomach. Most GISTs that are not of muscle or nerve sheath origin appear to originate from the interstitial cells of Cajal, which are pacemaker cells between axons and muscle cells that permit peristalsis. Cajal cells are named after the great Spanish neuroscientist Santiago Ramón y Cajal (1852-1934). They are positive for CD117 (c-kit) [PMID15613856, PMID17090188], a receptor tyrosine kinase (ie, a transmembrane protein with an intracellular tyrosine kinase) that binds extracellular ligand, then phosphorylates other proteins to initiate the intracellular response [PMID20533592]. CD117 is a proto-oncogene, meaning that it is normal protein that can become an oncogene through a gain of function mutation. CD117 may be found in many types of tumors and at this writing, gain of function mutations of CD117 have been etiologically implicated in 5 types of tumors: GISTs, mastocytosis, chronic myelogenous leukemia, a subset of acute myelogenous leukemia, and seminoma. The drug imatinib (Gleevec), in addition to targeting the tyrosine kinase that results from the *BCR/ABL* translocation in chronic myelogenous leukemia, can also inhibit the tyrosine kinase moiety of CD117, and may be beneficial in some cases [PMID19343301].

Up to 95% GISTs that are not of nerve sheath or muscle origin express CD117, and of the minority that do not, about 1/3 have a gain of function mutation in a structurally similar protein called platelet-derived growth factor receptor α (PDGFRA) [PMID18648736]. A number of activating mutations, often point mutations, are found in the genes that code for CD117 or PDGFRA in GISTs. While many of these aberrant forms of CD117 or PDGFRA are inhibited by imatinib, some mutations are associated with imatinib insensitivity [PMID12522257]. These forms may cause a poor response initially or a relapse as a resistant clone is selected for during imatinib therapy. Sunitinib can be employed as a second-line agent in these cases. Rather than simply finding these proteins by immunohistochemistry, it is likely to become important to genotype CD117 or PDGFRA [PMID20947481].

DOG1, a chloride channel protein, is also strongly associated with GISTs, and has a high sensitivity and specificity. DOG1 is especially useful in gastric GISTs, those of epithelioid morphology, and those that have a mutation in PDGFRA [PMID20418677]. Less than 3% of GISTs are negative for both CD117 and DOG1 by immunohistochemistry [PMID19606013].

Most GISTs are spindle cell neoplasms i21.27. The differential diagnosis of a spindle cell GIST includes neoplasms of muscle and nerve sheath, spindle cell carcinoma, fibromatosis, inflammatory myofibroblastic tumor, melanoma, mesothelioma, and angiosarcoma. Immunohistochemistry is usually needed for a secure diagnosis, focusing on the demonstration of CD117 and DOG1, and verifying negativity for actin, S-100, keratin, melan A, calretinin, and CD31. GISTs may rarely express keratin [PMID20502319], and fibromatosis may rarely have focal positivity for CD117 [PMID21970485], but a panel will reveal the correct diagnosis. A rare stromal neoplasm is epithelioid and may simulate a signet ring adenocarcinoma, yet another pitfall involving this entity i21.28a-d.

While some still use the term "gastrointestinal autonomic nerve tumor" (GANT), it appears to be synonymous with GIST [PMID11474281], and to my mind, the term "GANT" should not be routinely used, as it does not have a universal meaning. I recommend the term "GIST" for any stromal tumor that expresses CD117, followed by a comment on any other positive immunohistochemical stains, because it is readily understood by clinicians and opens the door to tyrosine kinase inhibitor therapy. The important points are as follows:

1. Any gastrointestinal stromal tumor should be immunohistochemically stained for epithelial and mesothelial markers to exclude a carcinoma with sarcomatous metaplasia and a mesothelioma. If an apparent GIST or an unusual gastrointestinal tumor stains for keratin alone or only for keratin and vimentin, and is negative for other markers (CD117, DOG1, CD34, actin, desmin, S100, calretinin), it is probably a carcinoma with sarcomatous metaplasia.
2. Once a carcinoma with sarcomatous metaplasia and mesothelioma are excluded, the tumor should be stained for nerve sheath and muscle markers, positivity for either of which suggests a more specific diagnosis. However, even if such differentiation is found, positivity for CD117 mandates a diagnosis of GIST because the therapeutic implications of CD117 positivity are critical. While

ISBN 978-089189-5886

muscle or nerve sheath differentiation is important to note, and may suggest origin from a cell type that is not the interstitial cell of Cajal, CD117 status must still be ascertained because of the therapeutic implications.

3. Tumors that are negative for CD117, with or without evidence of muscle or nerve sheath differentiation, may be candidates for molecular study of PDGFRA. Again, the possible opportunity to employ imatinib must not be missed if a tumor is CD117 negative or appears to be a muscle or nerve sheath tumor. Staining for epidermal growth factor receptor may also be indicated, as expression of this protein has been found in 96% of GISTs [PMID17643098]. Although this has no therapeutic implications at this writing, documentation of EGFR overexpression may permit improved therapy at some time in the future, as more therapeutic agents targeting tyrosine kinases are developed.
4. A statement should be made on its malignant potential. The behavior of gastric stromal tumors is very difficult to predict, but the study of Miettinen et al [PMID15613856] showed that the best predictions were based on a combination of size and mitotic activity. Gastric stromal tumors are likely benign if they are smaller than 6.0 cm *and* have only rare mitoses. They are of uncertain malignant potential if they are between 6.0 and 10.0 cm *or* have 2-4 mitoses per 50 high-power fields. They should be considered clearly malignant if they are >10.0 cm *or* have >5 mitoses per 50 high-power fields. In addition to these criteria, nuclear uniformity and stromal hyalinization favor a benign course, while mucosal invasion and a myxoid stroma suggest the possibility of a more aggressive course [PMID12023574].

Core Points for the Stomach

- There are several classifications of gastritis, but the most important aspect is that it may be caused by *Helicobacter pylori*.
- *H pylori* can often be seen on H&E or detected by a rapid urease test.
  - o Toluidine blue or Diff-Quik can slightly increase sensitivity.
  - o Best test, though usually not necessary, is immunohistochemistry.
- Gastric extranodal marginal zone lymphoma: can be impossible on routine H&E sections to distinguish from lymphoid hyperplasia response to *H pylori*.
  - o Reactive lymphoid proliferations lack a t(11;18)(q21:q21) that is often present in gastric lymphomas
  - o Unresponsiveness to antibiotics is often a better indication of a lymphoid neoplasm because marginal zone lymphomas may also lack t(11;18)(q21:q21).
- Diffuse large B-cell lymphoma requires IHC to exclude a poorly differentiated adenocarcinoma.
- Gastric polyps: many are fundic gland polyps, with chief and parietal cells.
  - o Hyperplastic and adenomatous are also found.
  - o Inflammatory fibroid polyp occurs primarily in the stomach.
- Gastric dysplasia: criteria similar to those in Barrett esophagus or colonic polyps, but not as well established.
- Gastric adenocarcinoma: 2 types, those that form glands (intestinal type) and those that do not (diffuse type).
- Loss of the cell adhesion molecule E-cadherin may be the underlying problem in diffuse gastric carcinoma, as it is in lobular carcinoma of the breast,
  - o These 2 malignancies may occur together in mutations of *CDH1*, the gene that codes for E-cadherin.
  - o Diagnosis of diffuse gastric carcinoma can be difficult because the neoplastic cells resemble macrophages or a large cell lymphoma.
  - o A keratin stain can be helpful.
- Gastric stromal tumors: exclude a metaplastic carcinoma and origin from nerve sheath or muscle
  - o Neoplasm is likely derived from interstitial cells of Cajal, and to be positive for CD117 (c-kit), or in rare cases, for PDGFRA.
  - o Testing for CD117 and PDGFR important, even if evidence of muscle or nerve origin, because neoplasm may respond to imatinib.
  - o These proteins have often undergone a gain of function mutation that may not be detectable by immunohistochemistry, so genotyping may become increasingly important.
  - o Prognostication is difficult, but size and mitotic activity important.

i21.1 Normal gastric mucosa. The foveola is on the lower right while the pits are on the upper left.

i21.2 Normal gastric mucosa of the fundus/ body type, with numerous parietal cells

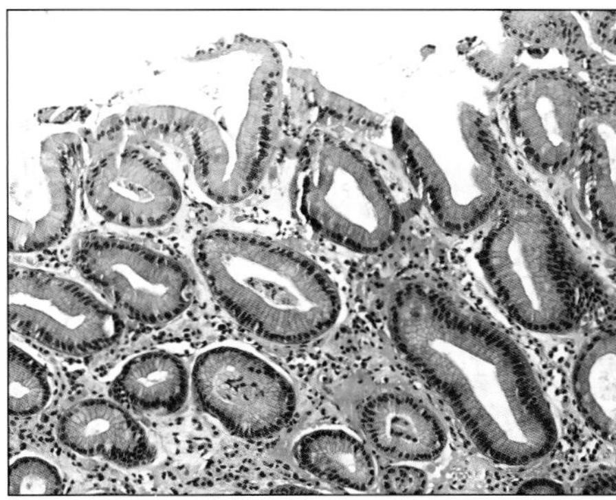

i21.3 Gastric mucosa of the antral type, without parietal cells

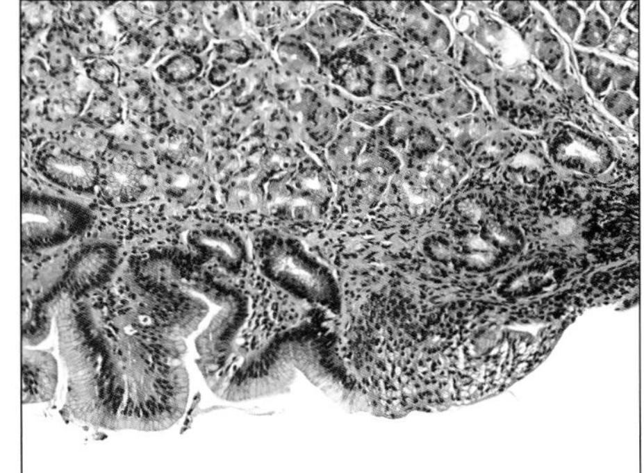

i21.4 A biopsy from the gastroesophageal junction (note the very small amount of squamous epithelium in the lower center) with numerous parietal cells, illustrating that many patients simply do not have a "cardiac" form of gastric mucosa

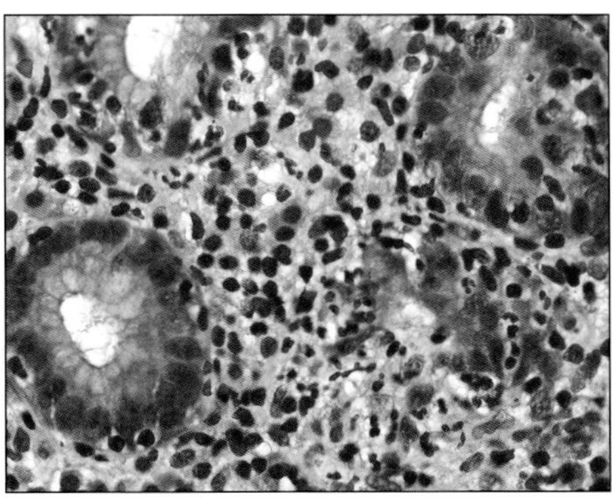

i21.5 Acute gastritis. The gland in the lower right has been severely damaged by neutrophils, which have also infiltrated other glands.

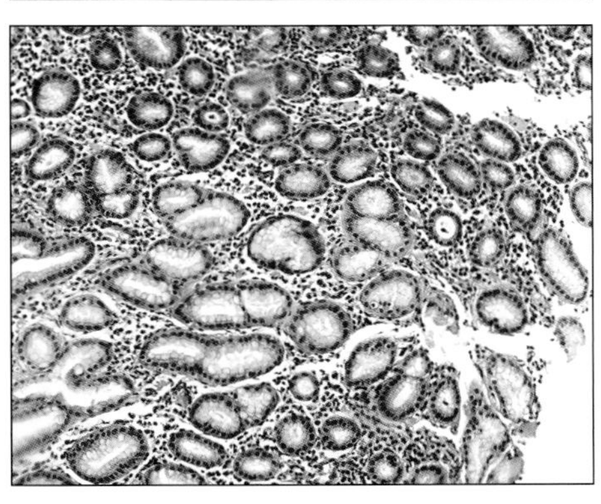

i21.6 Chronic gastritis, evident as an increased number of lymphocytes and plasma cells in the lamina propria

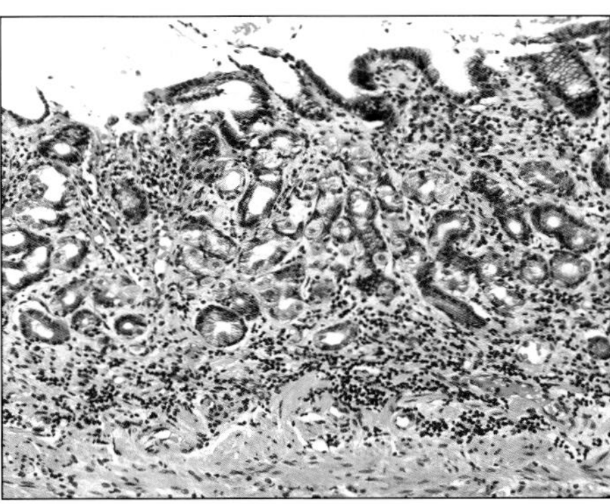

i21.7 Chronic atrophic gastritis, in which the mucosa is thin and contains abundant lymphocytes in the lamina propria

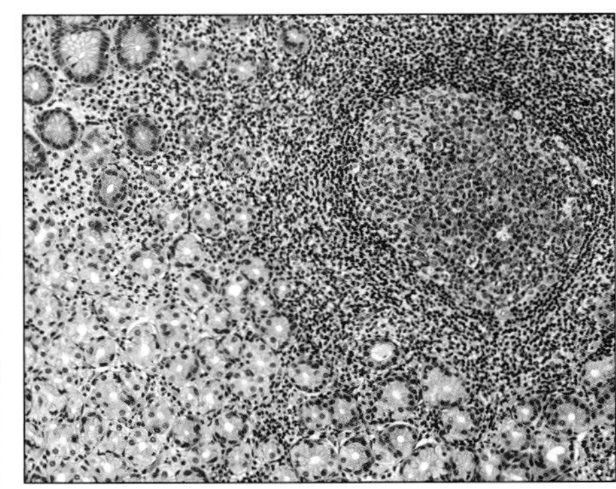

i21.8 Follicular gastritis. Note the germinal center in the lymphoid follicle. This type of chronic gastritis is often associated with *H pylori*, as was this case.

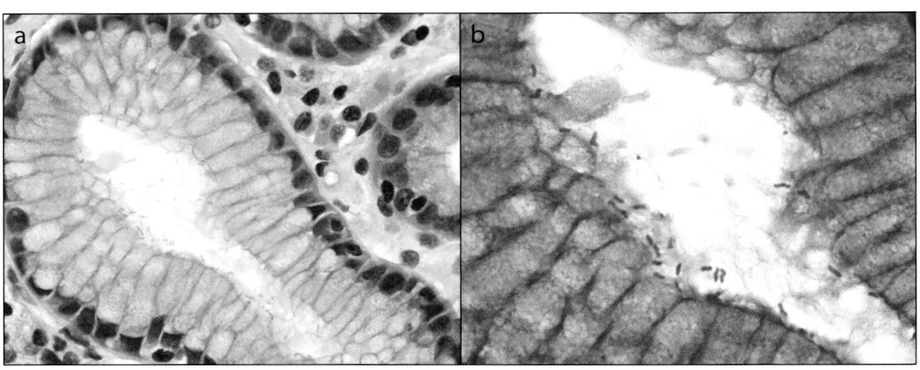

i21.9 **a, b** *H pylori* seen on H&E. Note the curved shape of the bacillus.

ISBN 978-089189-5886

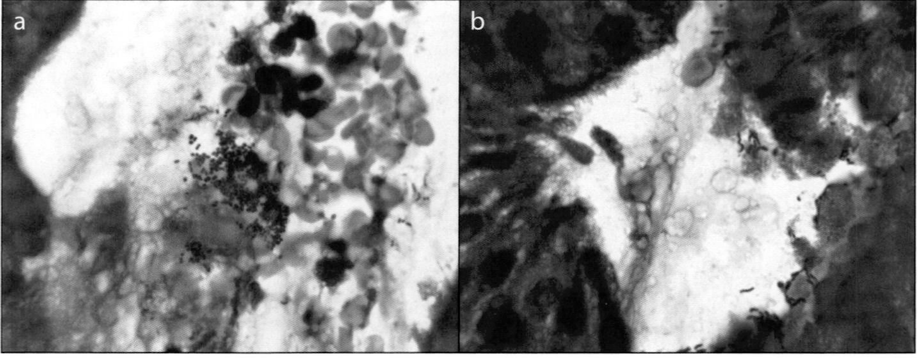

i21.10 **a** A Diff-Quik stain for *H pylori*. A few *H pylori* organisms are seen on the right, but in the center there are bacteria of a different type, illustrating that *H pylori* is not the only species of bacteria that may be found in gastric biopsies.

b A Diff-Quik stain demonstrating *H pylori*. Note that most organisms hug the apical portion of epithelial cells so as to be immersed in protective mucin. As is the case in H&E stain, the organism stains the same color in Diff-Quik as the cytoplasm of the epithelial cells, making the contrast only marginally better than with H&E.

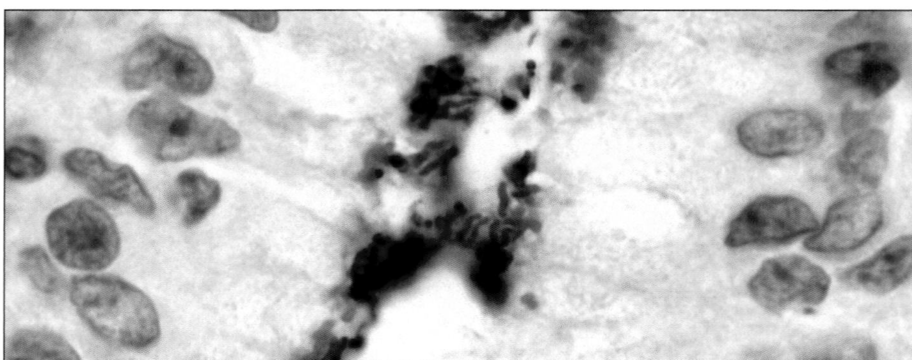

i21.11 An immunohistochemical stain for *H pylori*. Note again the curved nature of the bacillus, its propensity to be found immediately adjacent to the apical surface of the epithelial cell, and the superior contrast provided by the immunohistochemical stain since the organism is a completely different color from the counterstained epithelial cells.

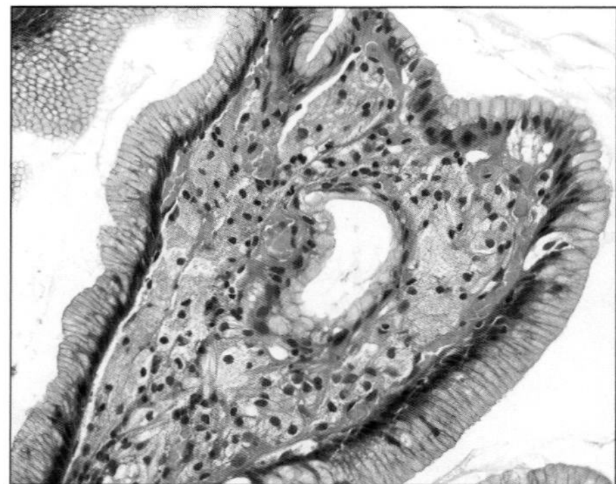

i21.12 Gastric xanthoma (xanthelasma), characterized by collections of macrophages in the lamina propria

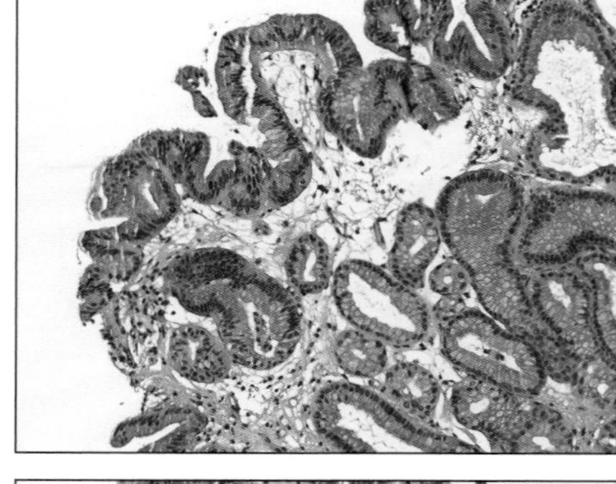

i21.13 A hyperplastic polyp of the stomach, characterized by hyperplasia of the foveola

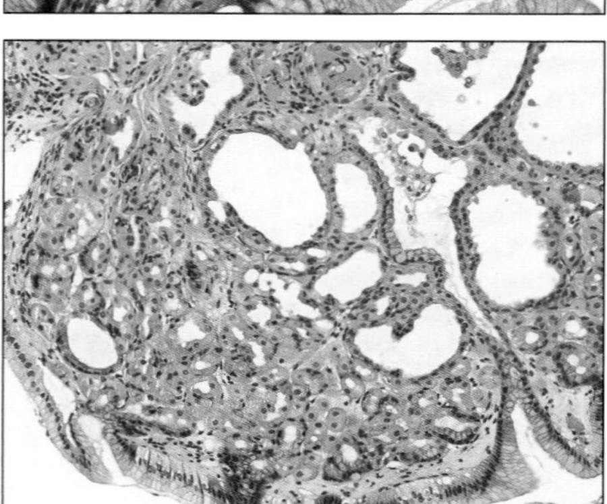

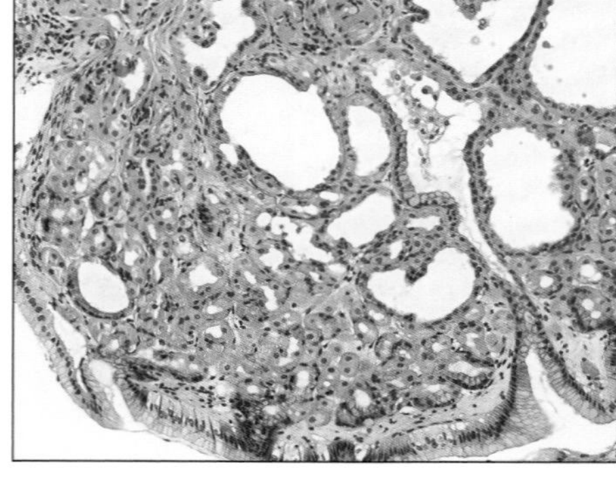

i21.14 A fundic gland polyp, characterized by the presence of numerous parietal cells and dilated glands

i21.15 An adenomatous polyp of the stomach, with an appearance essentially identical to its colonic counterpart

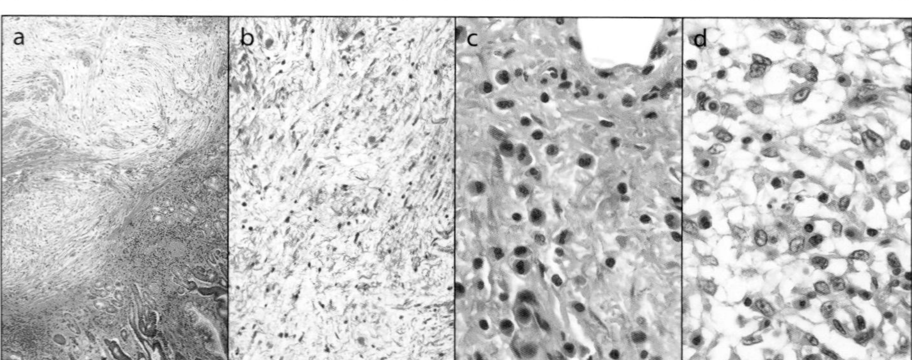

i21.16 **a** An inflammatory fibroid polyp. Note the myxoid change in the submucosa.
b A higher-power view of the same case as in i21.16a, illustrating the "tissue culture" appearance that resembles nodular fasciitis (compare to i3.2)
c A more collagenous area of an inflammatory fibroid polyp. Note the numerous eosinophils and occasional plasma cells.

d A cellular area in a gastric inflammatory fibroid polyp. The numerous eosinophils and mononuclear cells have a myofibroblastic appearance. These cells resemble myofibroblasts in an inflammatory myofibroblastic tumor i3.7. This resemblance, and the occasional staining of inflammatory fibroid polyps for muscle antigen, has suggested that this polyp may be of myofibroblastic origin.

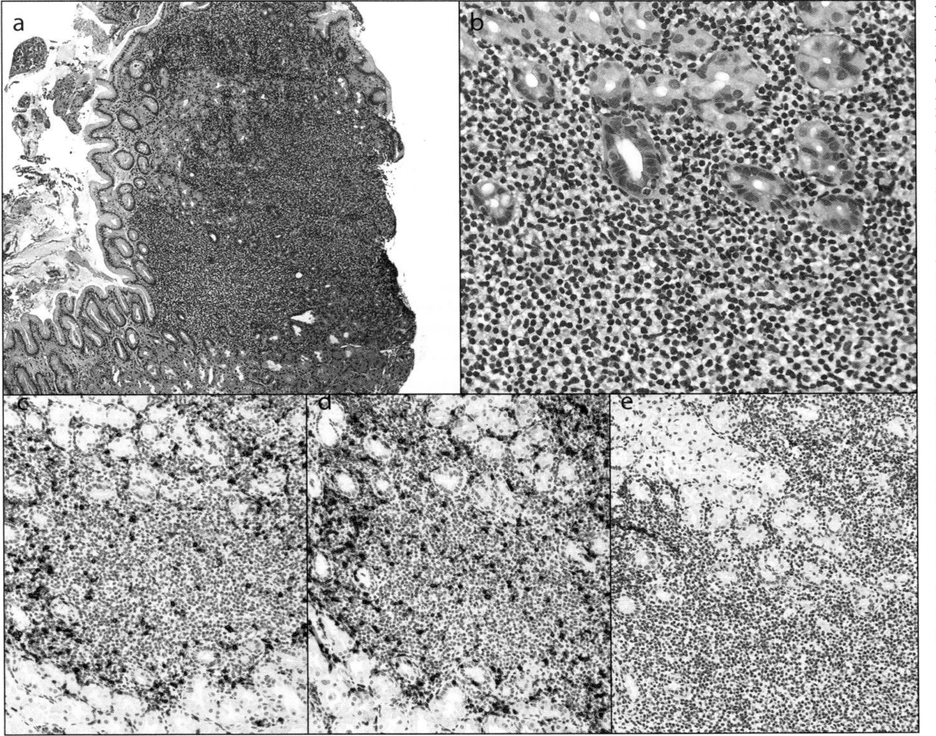

i21.17 **a** A gastric marginal zone lymphoma. Note the apparent mass effect. **b** A higher-power view of the same case as in i21.17a. Note that the lymphoid infiltrate has damaged some glands, causing them to drop out, a finding not expected in chronic gastritis or follicular gastritis. Note also the clear cytoplasm of the lymphocytes, indicating that this marginal zone lymphoma is of the so called "monocytoid" type. **c, d** A CD5 stain of the same case as in i21.17a. It appears that many of the neoplastic lymphocytes are positive for CD5, suggesting a possible mantle-cell lymphoma. However, CD5 also stains T cells, and when this stain is compared to the CD3 stain in i21.17d, it is seen in almost all of the CD5 positive cells are T cells and that the neoplastic cells are actually CD5 negative. Only if a lymphoproliferative disorder can be shown to be of B lineage and to express CD5 without expressing CD3 can it be concluded that it is a CD5 positive process. **e** The same case as in i21.17a with negative CD10 stain, identifying this process as negative for both CD5 and CD10. While a lymphoplasmacytic lymphoma may also be negative for both CD5 and CD10, this double negativity in a gastric lymphoid infiltrate with a "monocytoid" morphology strongly suggests the diagnosis of marginal zone lymphoma.

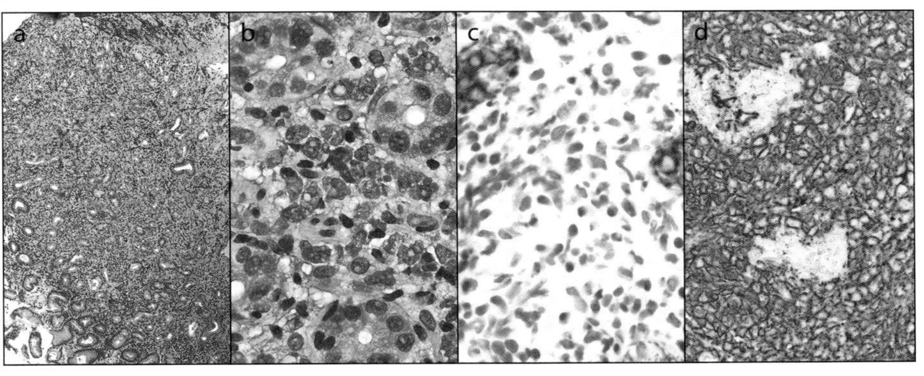

i21.18 **a** Another process that diffusely infiltrates the gastric mucosa **b** A higher-power view of the same case as in i21.18a, illustrating that the neoplastic cells are of much higher grade than a typical marginal zone lymphoma **c** The same case as in i21.18a with a negative keratin stain and an excellent internal control in the form of 2 benign gastric glands developed by the process **d** A CD20 stain of the same case as in i21.18a, indicating that this is a diffuse large B-cell lymphoma

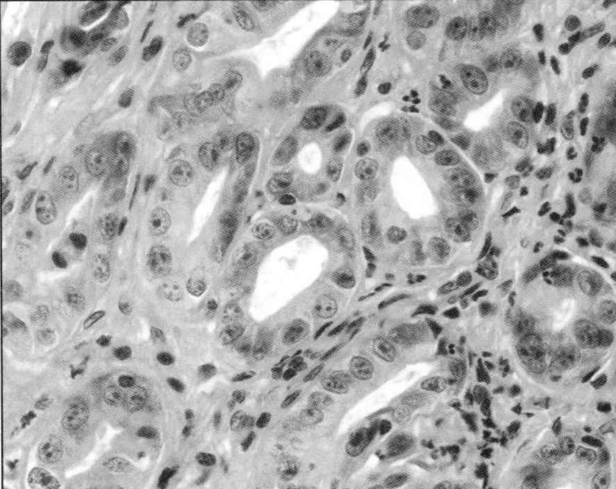

i21.19 Reactive atypia in a gastric biopsy. The nuclei are enlarged, but are not hyperchromatic or pleomorphic. Rather, they are uniform and accompanied by an increased amount of cytoplasm. These cells lack disturbing features other than the nucleoli. The acute inflammatory cells on the right support a conservative interpretation of this atypia.

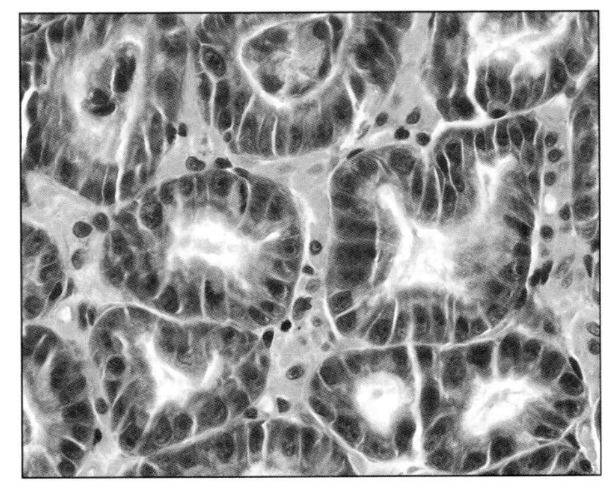

i21.20 A gastric biopsy with glandular atypia that is indefinite for dysplasia. The nuclei have more clumped chromatin and generally less conspicuous nucleoli than in a clearly reactive atypia. There is also an increase in the nucleus to cytoplasmic ratio. However, the nuclei remain relatively uniform and are basally oriented.

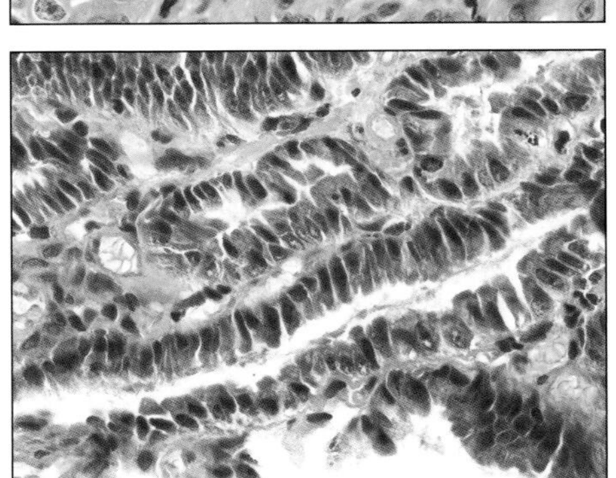

i21.21 A biopsy of flat gastric mucosa with low-grade dysplasia. The appearance is that of an adenomatous polyp, had this been a polypoid process.

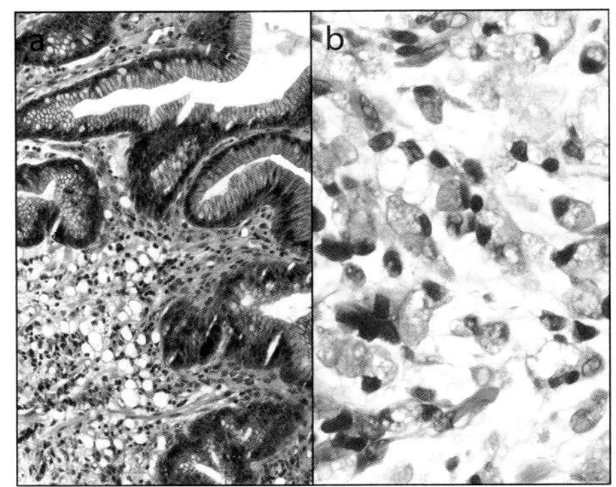

i21.22 **a** A gastric biopsy in which the lamina propria is sharply expanded, and many stromal cells have clear cytoplasm. At low power, malignancy is not obvious; many acute inflammatory cells in the lower center suggest a benign inflammatory process with numerous macrophages. **b** The same case as in i21.22a at higher power, illustrating that some of the stromal cells are in fact signet ring adenocarcinoma cells

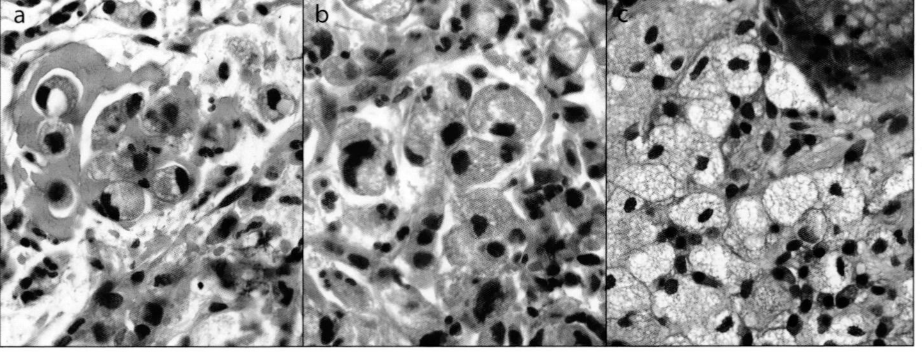

i21.23 a, b High-power views of signet ring adenocarcinoma. Although the neoplastic cells are small, the nuclei are somewhat enlarged and quite hyperchromatic. They are eccentrically located and often indented. **c** For comparison, a high-power view of gastric xanthoma. The nuclei in these macrophages are slightly smaller than in the signet ring adenocarcinoma cells and are generally centrally located since they lack the single cytoplasmic mucin vacuole that pushes the nucleus to the periphery.

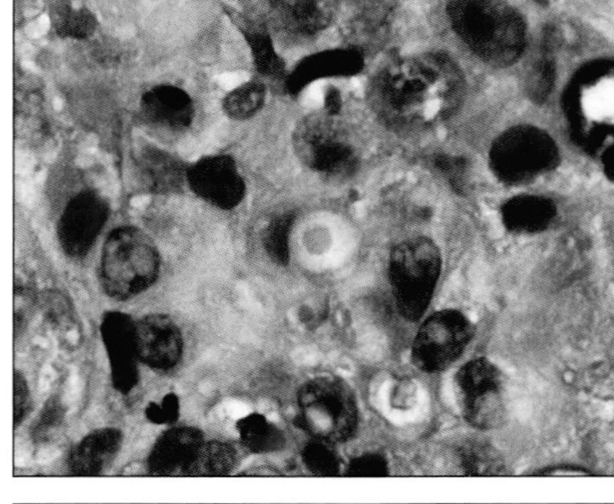

i21.24 A signet ring adenocarcinoma cell in which mucin has condensed within the cytoplasmic vacuole. Cells of this nature are sometimes called "owl's eye cells."

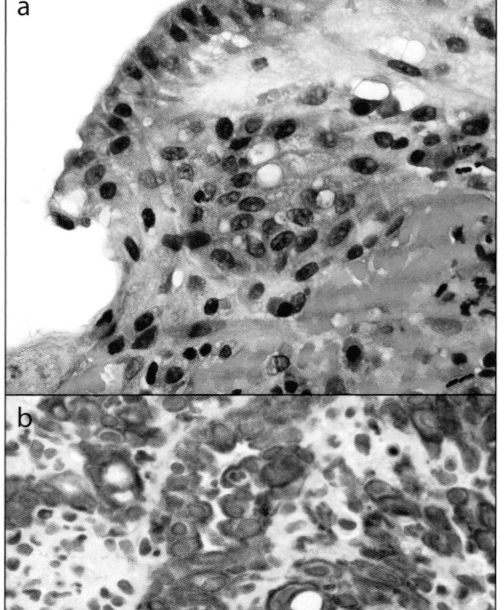

i21.25 a A gastric biopsy in which the stroma contains a few vacuolated cells whose nuclei are generally not alarming and which do not demonstrate an obvious infiltrative pattern. Note also the acute and chronic inflammatory cells in the lower right central portion of the photograph, suggesting a possible reactive process. **b** The same case as in i21.25a, stained for keratin. While 2 benign glands stain just to the left of center, the cells in the right half of the photograph are signet ring adenocarcinoma cells.

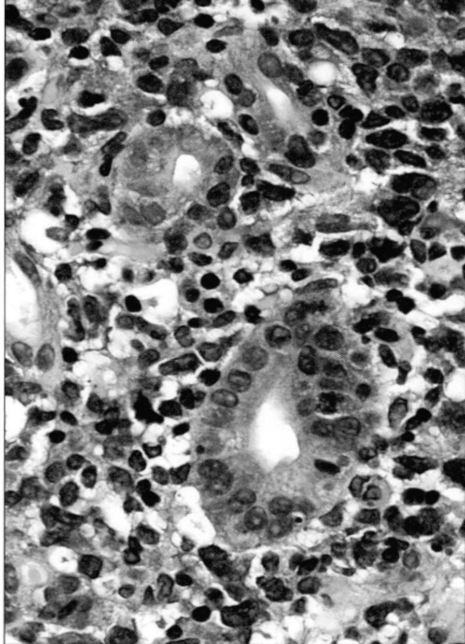

i21.26 A diffuse large B-cell lymphoma of the stomach, confirmed by immunohistochemistry, in which there is appreciable reactive atypia of the residual glandular epithelium and intermingling with the lymphoma cells, making it difficult to discern that there are actually 2 populations of cells.

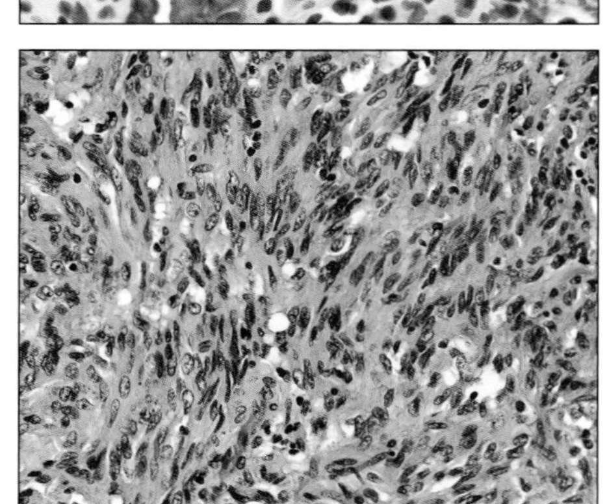

i21.27 A CD117 positive gastrointestinal stromal tumor of the stomach with a spindled appearance

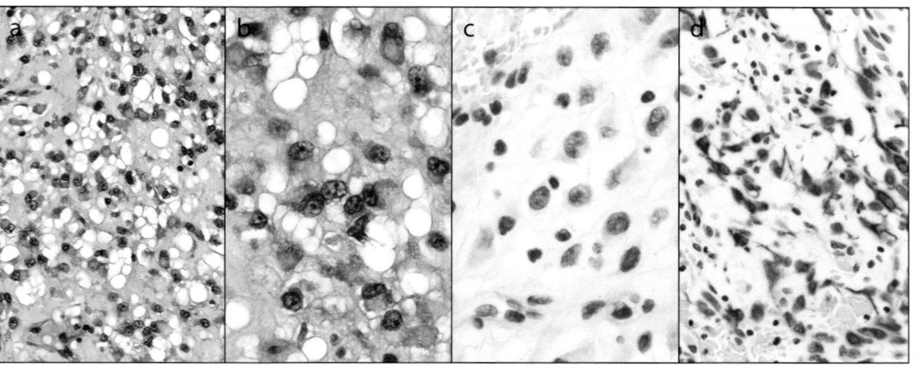

i21.28 a A gastric tumor with numerous vacuolated cells suggesting a signet ring adenocarcinoma **b** The same case as in i21.27a at higher power, highlighting the nuclear atypia and the vacuolated cells, further suggesting the possibility of a signet ring adenocarcinoma **c** The same case as in i21.27a, with a negative keratin stain **d** The same case as in i21.27a. This case was negative for CD117, but this positive desmin stain identifies the neoplasm as being an epithelioid smooth muscle tumor. Because desmin is one of the intermediate filaments, it is a cytoplasmic stain.

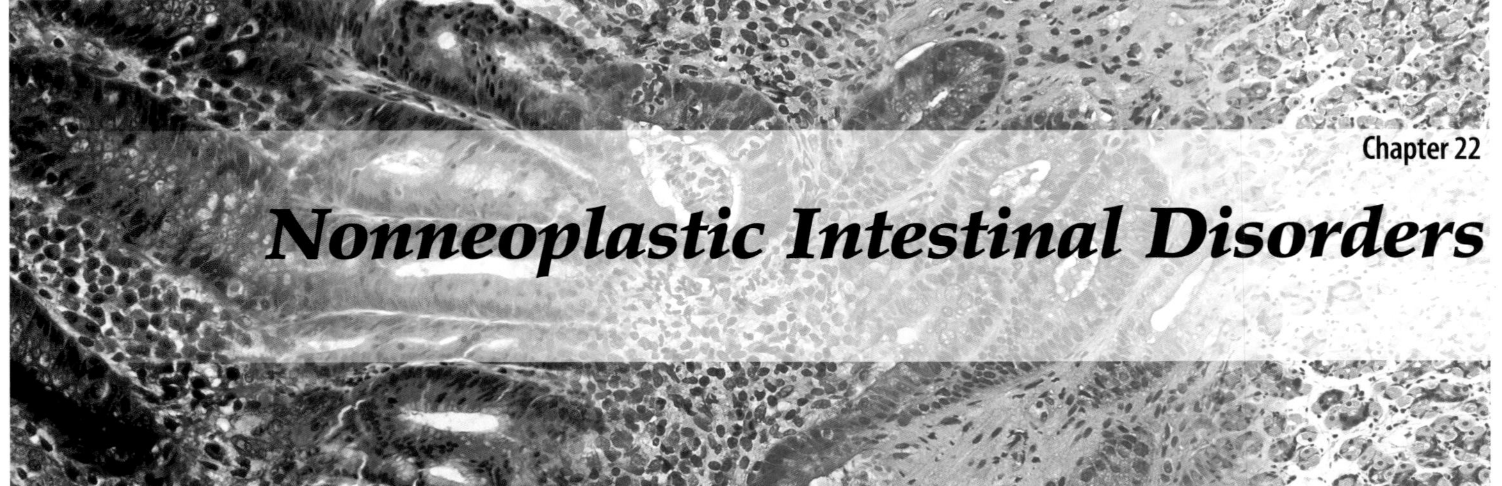

In addition to its role in digestion and absorption, the gastrointestinal tract has other vital roles. Indeed, before we begin the discussion of the intestinal tract, we need to ponder a little-remembered fact—the bowel, and especially the colon, is the only organ that is actually an ecosystem. Gastric acid holds bacterial numbers to low levels in most of the small bowel, but beginning in the distal small bowel and increasing dramatically in the colon, huge numbers of commensal bacteria (there are 10 times as many bacteria in the gastrointestinal tract as there are cells in the human body) form an ecosystem that serves to keep the pathogenic bacteria at bay. In fact, the colon is 2 ecosystems because in addition to the enormous number of bacteria in the lumen, there is a biofilm on the mucosal surface. A biofilm is a collection of microorganisms, usually bacteria, that are adherent to a surface. In a biofilm, the organisms often secrete extracellular molecules that facilitate the adherence of the organisms to the surface or to each other [PMID22189663]. Derangements of this delicate ecological balance are certainly a factor in many bacterial infections, especially after the use of antibiotics. Changes in the ratios of gut bacterial species have been implicated in inflammatory bowel disease [PMID16819463].

Even apart from its many commensal bacteria, the gastrointestinal system is an integral part of the immune system. The enormous numbers of lymphocytes and plasma cells in the gut are critical in reacting to the innumerable foreign antigens that have gained entry through that pathway. Lymphoid follicles, although concentrated in the ileum, are dispersed throughout the gut and serve a function similar to lymph nodes. Overlying these lymphoid follicles are flattened surface cells termed "M" (for membranous or microfold; also called follicle-associated epithelial cells) cells. Whereas other epithelial cells of the intestines are effective in excluding antigen penetration, M cells do the opposite—they facilitate entry of antigens and microorganisms and their transport to the subjacent lymphoid tissue through the process of transcytosis [PMID11193574].

The gastrointestinal tract is also an important endocrine organ. It may be that the aggregate of all endocrine cells in the gut exceeds that of any other endocrine organ. The function of these enteroendocrine cells is unclear, but over 30 different hormones are made in the gut, and it seems clear that the future will bring great knowledge about the role of these cells in both normal function and pathologic conditions [PMID21518048]. The immune and endocrine functions of the bowel have caused it to be called "the forgotten organ."

Gluten-Sensitive Enteropathy (Celiac Disease)

Celiac disease has a strong genetic predisposition and is strongly associated with HLA-DQ2, though only a minority of patients with this genotype will develop celiac disease. The disease is caused by the inappropriate production of peptides that bind to HLA class 2 (especially HLA-DQ2) molecules. These peptides result from the deamidation (glutamine to glutamic acid) of the peptides of α-gliadin, a constituent of gluten, by the enzyme transglutaminase. After the action of transglutaminase, the modified gliadin can then bind to HLA class 2 molecules and initiate an immune response that activates T cells, which then damage epithelial cells and release γ interferon. The transglutaminase also crosslinks a glutamine residue from the gliadin to a lysine residue of the enzyme itself, resulting in an epitope that is recognized by the immune system. This is thought to be the mechanism of formation of the antitransglutaminase antibodies that are characteristic of celiac disease [PMID19634568].

The diagnosis of celiac disease is more challenging than many realize because both the clinical presentation and endoscopic appearance of celiac disease may be quite variable. Many patients do not have the classic endoscopic appearance of cracked earth mucosa, and half do not have diarrhea. Some patients may have only anemia or arthritis, and a minority may have neurologic symptoms, depression, or fatigue [PMID16968605]. 15-25% of celiac disease patients have dermatitis herpetiformis [PMID17075969]. With a greater appreciation of the variety of symptoms and improved serologic testing, it is now understood that about 1% of all people have celiac disease, a prevalence that approaches *100 times* what had been previously believed [PMID19902715].

The histologic hallmarks of the duodenum are well developed villi and Brunner glands i22.1. Brunner glands are submucosal mucous glands i22.2a, though they may extend into the mucosa i22.2b or form hyperplastic nodules i22.3. Glands in the intestinal tract are also called crypts and in the small bowel are seen as the depressions between villi The normal ratio of villus to gland length should be between 3:1 and 5:1 i22.1. Villi may be shorter over Brunner glands or lymphoid aggregates i22.3. This ratio is sharply diminished in well developed celiac disease as villi become atrophic to absent i22.4a, i22.4b. Historically, even an occasional normal villus was accepted as essentially normal architecture and likely exclusive of celiac disease. Now, with better understanding of the many clinical manifestations of the disease and improved serological testing, more subtle histologic features are recognized, and the histology can be graded by the Marsh system [PMID1727768], in which stage 1 has an increase in intraepithelial lymphocytes with generally intact villous architecture i22.5a, i22.5b. The lymphocytes are usually disproportionately in the surface epithelium and are predominantly CD3+ T lymphocytes. Marsh stage 2 still maintains recognizable villi, but they are shorter, with an increase in gland length i22.6. Stage 3 has obvious villous flattening, while stage 4 has atrophy and loss of villi, resulting in an appearance that is essentially indistinguishable from colonic mucosa. In practice, Marsh stage 1 or 2 is rarely seen in a biopsy. Marsh stage 1 is more commonly seen in relatives of patients with celiac disease or patients who have related conditions (dermatitis herpetiformis, etc) than in actual celiac disease. I recommend caution in the diagnosis of Marsh stage 1 celiac disease unless there is a positive antitransglutaminase, a family history, or concomitant dermatitis herpetiformis. In North America, villous atrophy is still the usual histology of celiac disease at any stage, and severe villous atrophy almost always means celiac disease. The histologic appearance of the villi will improve after a gluten-free diet, but this improvement lags behind the clinical improvement and is often incomplete, with partial villous atrophy remaining.

Although some degree of histologic abnormality is found throughout the small bowel in all celiac disease patients, changes vary regionally and are generally more severe proximally [PMID20372112]. About 10% of patients have pronounced villous atrophy only in the duodenal bulb (the most proximal portion of the duodenum) [PMID21606978]. These findings underscore that a biopsy to diagnose celiac disease or to assess efficacy of therapy should generally include the duodenal bulb, despite the long-standing and legitimate concern that Brunner gland hyperplasia or ectopic gastric mucosa may render bulb biopsies difficult to interpret.

Antitransglutaminase IgA antibodies have a sensitivity of nearly 100% and a specificity of 98% in well developed cases, making them superior to antiendomysial or antigliadin IgG or IgA antibodies [PMID16185576]. The sensitivity and specificity at earlier stages is likely to be somewhat lower, and there may or may not be a role for the antigliadin antibody test in the early stages, but IgA antitransglutaminase is the test of choice. The incidence of serum IgA deficiency in celiac patients is 2-3%, much higher than in the general population [PMID18217518]. For this reason, a serum total IgA level should accompany testing for IgA antitransglutaminase, to ensure that a negative result is not secondary to general IgA deficiency. Testing for IgG antitransglutaminase is recommended in patients who are IgA deficient. Rare patients can only be properly assessed after a gluten-free dietary trial.

With dietary compliance, elevated antibody levels will fall and the histologic appearance will return towards normal, though histologic improvement lags behind serological improvement, may take a few months, and may not be complete i22.7a, i22.7b.

With the excellent sensitivity of blood tests, one might question the need for a biopsy if patients with symptoms and a positive blood test show clear improvement upon institution of a gluten-free diet, but a biopsy continues to be a mainstay in diagnosis, in large part because it provides a baseline against which to measure the effectiveness of therapy.

Collagenous sprue, in which the subepithelial collagen layer of the duodenum is markedly thickened, reminiscent of collagenous colitis, is a rare complication of celiac disease, though not all agree that collagenous sprue derives from celiac disease. Lymphoma, especially enteropathy-associated T-cell lymphoma (discussed subsequently), is a rare complication of celiac disease.

Partial villous atrophy in a duodenal biopsy is usually indicative of celiac disease that has responded to a gluten free diet, but may also be seen in tropical sprue (an enigmatic entity that responds to B12, folate, and antibiotics), dermatitis herpetiformis, infections, stasis syndromes, and autoimmune enteropathy.

Unusual Small Bowel Conditions

Microvillous inclusion disease (MID; originally called familial enteropathy) is an autosomal recessive condition causing intractable diarrhea and steatorrhea in infants. In MID, brush border components necessary for absorption are abnormally located in the interior of the cytoplasm. Historically, this diagnosis required electron microscopy, but cytoplasmic staining (as opposed to apical staining) with CD10, CEA, alkaline phosphatase, and PAS, in conjunction with complete villous atrophy, is also considered diagnostic [PMID12131157].

Abetalipoproteinemia is characterized by lack of apoprotein B, normally found in the cytoplasm and required to make chylomicrons from fatty acids. Without the ability to make chylomicrons, the intestinal cell cannot export the fat it has absorbed and quickly becomes saturated. Eventually, the cell is distended with fat and no further absorption of fats can occur, leading to steatorrhea. In abetalipoproteinemia, fat can be detected in vacuolated cells with a fat stain, but the biopsy should be performed at least 6 hours after a meal, and the diagnosis must be confirmed by low levels of apoprotein B and low serum chylomicrons [PMID18611256].

Giardia is about the size of an epithelial nucleus. In profile, it is sickle shaped i22.8. A trichrome stain is recommended if giardiasis is suspected, but ova and parasite examination is likely to be more rewarding than a small bowel biopsy. Even better is a stool antigen test, which offers excellent sensitivity and specificity, and is simpler and faster than a morphologic search for the organism or its ova [PMID1864930].

Inflammatory Bowel Disease

Ulcerative colitis (UC) and Crohn disease (CD) are the 2 manifestations of inflammatory bowel disease (IBD). Both are idiopathic. While a mucosal variant of CD has been described, and UC may occasionally involve the submucosa to a limited extent, for all practical purposes, UC is a mucosal disease while CD is transmural. In resection material, restriction of the changes to the mucosa makes CD highly unlikely and extensive submucosal involvement makes UC highly unlikely.

UC must involve the rectum to some extent. It is not required that the entire colon be involved, but whatever portion is involved must be continuous with an involved rectum, with no "skip" areas. A definite diagnosis of UC requires all of the following features: diffuse disease, involving the rectum, limited to the large intestine, with no skip lesions, no deep fissural ulcers, no sinus tract, and no transmural lymphoid aggregates or granulomas. Ulcerative proctitis is a limited form of UC with an identical histologic appearance.

In mucosal biopsies, active ulcerative colitis has severe mucosal inflammation, often with crypt abscesses, which are collections of neutrophils, occasionally with eosinophils, in the lumens of glands i22.9, frequently with partial destruction of the glandular wall i22.10. While the terms "gland" and "crypt" are synonymous n the intestinal tract, the term "gland abscess" is not used. Although crypt abscesses are not specific for UC, and may occur in CD or other forms of colitis that are not IBD (especially infectious colitis), their presence in large numbers requires exclusion of UC, especially if there is also architectural distortion.

A hallmark of IBD, whether active or quiescent, is that the architecture is disturbed. This is particularly true for UC, while CD may have more subtle or focal architectural abnormalities. Even in acute presentations of UC in patients who have no known history of that disorder, mucosal biopsies in adults usually show some evidence of chronicity in the form of architectural distortion. Mild architectural distortion may occasionally be seen in some cases of severe infectious colitis, such as that caused by salmonella, *Shigella*, or *E coli* O157, but the presence of well developed architectural abnormalities suggests IBD unless there is strong evidence of another process, and one should question the diagnosis of IBD in an adult if biopsies show no architectural distortion.

There are 4 principal manifestations of architectural distortion. First, the luminal border is irregular rather than smooth i22.11a (compared to i22.11b. Second, the number of glands is decreased i22.12a, i22.12b. Third, remaining glands are short and may not reach the muscularis mucosa i22.13. Fourth, glands may be branched i22.14 [Goldman ISBN978-0683180077]. Architecture should not be assessed near a lymphoid aggregate, as this may cause minor focal architectural distortion in normal patients.

An increased number of lymphocytes and plasma cells in the lamina propria is also characteristic of IBD. In the normal biopsy, the number of lymphocytes and plasma cells decreases in the lower portion of the lamina propria, near the muscularis mucosa i22.15, while in IBD, this reduction is diminished, so that chronic inflammatory cells in the lamina propria are increased and more evenly distributed i22.16. In practice, however, it is difficult to appreciate a significant increase in chronic inflammatory cells in the lamina propria. Moreover, increased stromal chronic inflammation is a nonspecific finding. In assessing architectural distortion in mucosal biopsies, and the chronicity that it implies, it is wise to focus on the epithelium.

A definite diagnosis of CD requires evidence of a transmural process, such as submucosal and subserosal fibrosis, dilated lymphatics, hypertrophic nerves, and lymphoid aggregates in the bowel wall i22.17. In colonoscopy, where only the mucosa can be visualized, longitudinal ulcers parallel to the length of the bowel (fissuring ulcers, aphthous ulcers (punctate and deep) i22.18, and endoscopic evidence of intervening normal mucosa are characteristic of CD. While granulomas are associated with CD i22.19, they are seen in less than half of mucosal biopsies and are not specific for CD.

The uniformity that characterizes UC at the gross and endoscopic level generally continues at the microscopic level. Mucosal biopsies in UC tend to have a more uniform distribution of inflammation than those from CD, with all biopsies affected and with relatively even distribution of inflammation within individual biopsies. Focal active colitis, which refers to a patchy distribution of acute inflammation within a biopsy i22.20, is more suggestive of CD [PMID9720510, PMID9191008].

Foci of IBD that are severely inflamed may have a polypoid appearance, in which case the polyp is said to be an inflammatory pseudopolyp i22.21. The polypoid appearance of an inflammatory pseudopolyp arises from a combination of inflammation, edema, and often a granulation tissue response.

Quiescent cases of IBD will have little or no acute inflammation, but will generally have some form of architectural distortion, as described above.

Current bowel preparations may cause mild acute inflammation in the surface epithelium, but this will not be a major finding, the glands are not affected, and most importantly, preparation will not distort the architecture. There need be no fear that changes from the preparation will cause a false diagnosis of IBD.

By definition, the rectum must be involved in UC, and in adult patients, a *completely normal* rectum, both endoscopically and histologically upon examination of multiple rectal biopsies, excludes this diagnosis. However, mild architectural distortion in a rectal biopsy, even without acute inflammation, keeps UC in the differential diagnosis. Biopsies from children with IBD generally have features that are similar to those in adult IBD patients, except that architectural distortion may not yet be well developed. For this reason, while a completely normal set of rectal biopsies excludes UC in adults, the rectum may be normal in children with UC.

By definition, UC is restricted to the colon and cannot involve the ileum except for backwash ileitis, a term used to describe those patients who have UC, not CD, but who also have involvement of the terminal ileum (an older term for this is "cecal kick"). The diagnosis of backwash ileitis requires an otherwise secure diagnosis of UC, and the cecum must be at least moderately involved. There must be continuity from the cecal involvement to the involved areas of the terminal ileum, and the degree of inflammation in the cecum must equal or exceed that of the terminal ileum. By these criteria, about 6% of chronic UC patients—usually with more severe disease—will be found to have backwash ileitis. Ileal biopsies of backwash ileitis are histologically indistinguishable from UC. The cause of backwash ileitis is unknown, but its presence does not contraindicate an ileal pouch if the diagnosis of UC is secure and CD is excluded [PMID16880149]. In practice, backwash ileitis rarely causes a misdiagnosis of CD. A clearly inflamed terminal ileum without concomitant and equal cecal involvement excludes backwash ileitis and therefore excludes UC.

Occasionally, even serial sets of mucosal biopsies may not permit a definitive distinction between UC and CD. In these cases, the important point is to secure a diagnosis of IBD and exclude a carcinoma-directed dysplasia. The passage of time will usually clarify the situation before the distinction between UC and CD becomes critical, if it ever does. In the meantime, a general diagnosis of IBD or indeterminate colitis can be made.

The term "indeterminate colitis" arose when surgical pathologists examined colectomy specimens, usually from patients with fulminant colitis, that had overlapping features of CD and UC. Because radiographic studies and capsule endoscopy are now diagnostic modalities, a colectomy is no longer required for the diagnosis of indeterminate colitis. As long as etiologies other than IBD are excluded, the term can be appropriately used in any situation where the evidence from all sources shows overlap of diagnostic criteria for UC and CD [PMID15990620]. Even in patients who have had resections for IBD, indeterminate colitis, or overlapping features of UC and CD, it occurs in approximately 5-10% of cases, usually fulminant.

Serologic testing to differentiate between UC and CD has been disappointing. At this writing, serological tests are not helpful, either in establishing the diagnosis of IBD or in distinguishing CD from UC. About half of UC patients have perinuclear antineutrophilic cytoplasmic antibody (p-ANCA) and about half of CD patients have antibodies to *Saccharomyces cerevisiae* (ASCA). In addition to this low sensitivity, neither test is specific [PMID19902862]. Consequently, neither of these tests should be done until it is clear that the patient has IBD (ie, neither is a screening test), all other attempts to differentiate between UC and CD have failed, and therapeutic decisions require the maximal probability of differentiation between UC and CD. Therapy in indeterminate colitis is difficult, particularly regarding possible colectomy, as an ileal pouch may fail if the patient actually has an unusual form of CD.

Although the molecular basis of IBD is not understood, progress is being made in CD. About 30% of these patients have a loss of function mutation in the gene *IBD1*, which encodes for NOD2 (also called CARD15), an intracellular receptor in monocytes for certain bacterial peptides, the stimulation of which increases the activity of the transcription factor NFκB, which in turn induces proinflammatory cytokines [PMID11385577]. Thus, at least comes cases of CD may be a result of a defective response to gut bacteria.

A major pitfall in the histologic diagnosis of IBD is to overinterpret nonspecific focal acute colitis. Most patients with focal acute colitis without architectural distortion or specific features will not have any form of inflammatory bowel disease. In some of these patients, the inflammation is secondary to medications (especially NSAIDS) or infection, but in many, the cause is unknown [PMID22092396].

A major clinical mimic of inflammatory bowel disease is irritable bowel syndrome (IBS). Endoscopically, there is a clear distinction between *active* inflammatory bowel disease and IBS, as the mucosa in the latter condition is not significantly inflamed, but endoscopically distinguishing *quiescent* IBD from IBS is much more difficult. Biopsies are helpful, because those from IBS patients are either normal or have only mild nonspecific acute inflammation, and do not have the architectural distortion seen in quiescent cases of IBD.

Dysplasia in Ulcerative Colitis

Because of the greatly increased incidence of colonic carcinoma in UC, surveillance colonoscopies have been instituted in these patients. For this surveillance to be effective, the pathologist must recognize the early stages of adenocarcinoma. Active UC leads to severe reparative changes that can simulate dysplasia. As is the case in the esophagus and stomach **i20.8**, **i21.19**, reparative nuclei tend to be more uniform in size and shape than dysplastic nuclei, with an open chromatin pattern **i22.22**. Although they often have prominent nucleoli, if the nucleolus is subtracted out in the mind's eye, a relatively innocent nucleus results. It is generally customary not to diagnose dysplasia in IBD in areas of active inflammation.

The histologic criteria for dysplasia in UC have been extensively described (eg, PMID18942763, PMID19770847, PMID20524866), but a useful rule of the thumb is that in general, low-grade dysplasia in UC resembles that in Barrett esophagus **i20.10** and resembles an ordinary adenomatous polyp, with mildly variable, ovoid nuclei that have coarse chromatin, indistinct nucleoli, and minimal stratification **i22.23a**, **i22.23b**. Because distinction between reparative atypia and low-grade dysplasia is difficult, an indefinite category is recognized **i22.24**.

High-grade dysplasia in UC resembles its counterpart in Barrett esophagus **i20.13** and resembles an adenomatous polyp with high-grade dysplasia, with glandular crowding, epithelial cells with rounded nuclei that have a vesicular chromatin pattern (ie, with the chromatin primarily on the periphery of the nucleus) and prominent nucleoli, full thickness stratification, and increased mitoses **i22.25**.

The manifestation of dysplasia as a mass lesion (DALM; dysplasia associated with a lesion or mass) **i22.26** is particularly problematic [PMID19770847, PMID10406230]. In patients with UC, it is impossible to determine with certainty if a mass with adenomatous change is an incidental adenomatous polyp or an area of low-grade dysplasia resulting from the UC. There is preliminary evidence that β-catenin and p53 staining may help distinguish between a sporadic adenomatous polyp and a DALM in UC, with the positivity for the former suggesting an incidental polyp, and positivity for the latter suggesting a DALM [PMID19897978], but this is a developing area. Likewise, there are suggestions of cytogenetic differences between common polyps and DALM [PMID10746669], but this finding also awaits maturity.

Until there is clarification, such lesions should be regarded as DALM unless the patient is in an age group where an ordinary adenomatous polyp might be expected *and* the lesion is in an area that is not thought to be significantly involved by UC (ie, there is little acute inflammation or architectural distortion in the adjacent mucosa).

Some feel that any DALM—even those with only low-grade dysplasia—is an indication for colectomy unless *all* of the following are met: the patient is older, a negative base or stalk can be found, the patient can be followed, and there is no dysplasia in the adjacent mucosa. There is a general consensus that DALM, even with high-grade dysplasia, can be very closely followed without colectomy if the dysplasia is completely excised, there is no dysplasia of the surrounding flat mucosa, and there is increased surveillance and frequent biopsies [PMID15168373, PMID15224277, PMID10579970].

Management of low-grade dysplasia in flat mucosa is controversial [PMID16292084] but can often be addressed by very close surveillance and frequent biopsies of the surrounding area. On the other hand, any DALM with any incompletely excised dysplasia, or any high-grade dysplasia in flat mucosa warrants colectomy [PMID16292084].

Diversion Colitis and Pouchitis

There are 2 confusing terms that arise from surgical therapy. "Diversion colitis" (also called disuse colitis or defunctionalized bowel) refers to changes that take place in the unused portion of colon in patients who have had colostomies or ileostomies. The histologic changes in diversion colitis may perfectly mimic those in IBD i22.27a, i22.27b, but there may be follicular lymphoid hyperplasia with muscular hypertrophy and fibrous hyperplasia of the submucosa i22.27c [PMID12352238]. Diversion colitis is thought to be secondary to loss of some unknown trophic factor conveyed by short chain fatty acids in the stool, since administration of these fatty acids is beneficial [PMID2909876].

"Pouchitis" refers to the presence of bloody diarrhea in patients who have an ileal pouch after colectomy for UC. Pouchitis has a number of causes, one of which is CD that was thought to be UC (2-7% of cases). Some cases are secondary to bacterial overgrowth and may respond to antibiotics. Other cases of pouchitis are not caused by either of these processes and remain idiopathic. Biopsies of the pouch may look remarkably normal for the patient's symptoms i22.28a, and even when the biopsy is abnormal, the usual picture is one of nonspecific inflammation or indeterminate IBD i22.28b, i22.28c rather than classic UC or CD [PMID18237865, PMID2182398]. Because it is difficult to tell if the pouchitis patient has CD, bacterial overgrowth, or one of the other causes of pouchitis, many clinicians will try antibiotics regardless of the biopsy results.

Collagenous Colitis and Lymphocytic Colitis

Historically, the term "microscopic colitis" referred to any colitis in which the mucosa appeared normal endoscopically, but for which microscopic study demonstrated abnormalities. This included any number of situations, including subtle or quiescent forms of IBD, collagenous colitis, or lymphocytic colitis. While the term "microscopic colitis" is still used, many believe it is now preferable to use the term "collagenous colitis" or "lymphocytic colitis," not only because they are more specific, but also because "microscopic colitis" may be construed as a mild form of IBD that is only identifiable microscopically.

The gastrointestinal tract has occasional lymphocytes within the epithelium. These intraepithelial lymphocytes are a heterogeneous group, and can be of several immunophenotypes. Many are of the CD8 cytotoxic type, expressing α and β chains in their T-cell receptors, while others are of the γ-δ type [PMID9530144]. The function of these intraepithelial lymphocytes is not known, but it is clear that they are a normal finding to an extent, but that excessive numbers are associated with and probably cause a watery diarrhea.

By definition, patients with lymphocytic colitis must have diarrhea. Moreover, the diarrhea must be watery and not bloody. Bloody diarrhea suggests IBD, a severe infectious colitis, or ischemia. The criteria for lymphocytic colitis are >20 intraepithelial lymphocytes per 100 epithelial cells (ie, >1 per 5 epithelial cells) i22.29a, usually associated with an increased lymphoplasmacytic infiltrate in the lamina propria i22.29b and sometimes with occasional eosinophils i22.29c or surface injury, in conjunction with an appropriate clinical picture [PMID2912870]. The surface epithelium is usually more affected than that of the glands i22.29d. The intraepithelial lymphocytes in lymphocytic colitis are predominantly CD8 positive, α-β receptor T lymphocytes [PMID8677934], but as is the case for celiac disease, the immunophenotype of the intraepithelial lymphocytes is of limited diagnostic value. The proximal colon may be more affected than the distal colon, but changes may be patchy and some areas may fall within normal limits even in well defined cases, so biopsies from multiple regions are necessary to establish the diagnosis. Occasionally, there is an increased number of intraepithelial lymphocytes, but not enough for a secure diagnosis i22.29e, in which case one can comment that early lymphocytic colitis cannot be excluded or the gastroenterologist may offer a therapeutic trial directed at lymphocytic colitis. There is an approximate correlation between the severity of lymphocytic infiltrate and the severity of symptoms. In some, but not all, cases of lymphocytic colitis, there is also thickening of the subepithelial collagen layer, and the diagnosis of lymphocytic/collagenous colitis may be appropriate.

While most cases of lymphocytic colitis are idiopathic, there is an association with some drugs, including NSAIDS, lansoprazole (Prevacid), and ranitidine (Zantac), and there is also an association with autoimmune disorders, including celiac disease, type I diabetes, Hashimoto thyroiditis, linear IgA disease, psoriasis, and autoimmune hepatitis [PMID19700939].

Brainerd diarrhea is histologically identical to lymphocytic colitis, but its epidemiological characteristics suggest a point source of an infectious agent [PMID8764747]. The diagnosis requires an epidemic setting. Brainerd diarrhea causes severe chronic watery diarrhea, but it is eventually self-limited.

Like lymphocytic colitis, collagenous colitis causes watery diarrhea and shows a predilection for middle aged to older women. It is diagnosed by an increased thickness of the subepithelial collagen layer, which is normally so thin as to be nearly invisible i22.30a. The diagnosis is ideally made in well-oriented sections i22.30b, but can be suggested in sections that are slightly tangential i22.30c. Beyond this fundamental feature, there is a wide spectrum of inflammatory changes that may or may not be seen in collagenous colitis. It may have an increased numbers of intraepithelial lymphocytes, in which case the diagnosis of lymphocytic/collagenous colitis may be appropriate i22.30d. It may also have occasional eosinophils and surface injury i22.30e. Indeed, 30% of collagenous or lymphocytic patients may have significant acute inflammation (including crypt abscesses), and about 5% may have architectural distortion [PMID12409717]. On the other hand, many cases of collagenous colitis do not have significant acute or chronic inflammatory changes in the lamina propria or in the epithelium.

ISBN 978-089189-5886

In difficult cases, the thickness and nature of the subepithelial collagen layer is best evaluated with a trichrome stain. PAS stain will not assist in the diagnosis because the material that is deposited does not contain glycoproteins. When studied with a trichrome stain, the collagen layer may have several appearances. Sometimes, there is only a thickened collagen layer **i22.30f**, in which case 10 µm has been recommended as a minimum thickness for the diagnosis. But in other cases, the collagen may be fragmented or frayed, with an indistinct lower border that merges imperceptibly into the lamina propria **i22.30g**. Erythrocytes or capillaries may be trapped within it **i22.30h** [PMID10562895].

The changes of collagenous colitis are often patchy, and as is the case for lymphocytic colitis, multiple biopsies are needed and the characteristic changes should be seen in more than 1 fragment. The transverse colon is most commonly affected in collagenous colitis and the descending colon is affected in 80-95% of cases, but the rectum is often spared [PMID10638608]. The terminal ileum may be affected. The severity of symptoms does not correlate with the thickness of the collagen layer in collagenous colitis. Like lymphocytic colitis, collagenous colitis is associated with celiac disease [PMID18701946].

Ischemic Colitis

Ischemia is usually a mucosal abnormality, but can be transmural if prolonged and severe. The most affected areas of the colon are the splenic flexure and rectosigmoid. Acute ischemia is characterized by superficial ulceration and necrosis, often with hemorrhage **i22.31a**, but this stage because is rarely biopsied. Subacute ischemia, the first stage that is likely to be biopsied, demonstrates damage to glands in addition to active inflammation and may resemble inflammatory bowel disease on a mucosal biopsy **i22.31b** [PMID794801, PMID6759364]. Chronic ischemia has a classic, nearly pathognomonic appearance of atrophic glands in a fibrotic, hyalinized lamina propria **i22.31c**, **i22.31d** [PMID9199649]. In chronic ischemia, the architecture is distorted, but not in the same way as in IBD.

Older patients indeed get inflammatory bowel disease, but ischemic colitis should be excluded in older patients before a diagnosis of IBD is made. Hemosiderin macrophages suggest ischemia, but a diligent search may uncover focal areas of the atrophic glands and dense, hyalinized stroma that secure a diagnosis of chronic ischemia, or areas in which the architectural distortion of IBD is evident. The presence of a concomitant heart or lung comorbidity increases the odds that an apparent case of inflammatory bowel disease is actually ischemia.

It has been my consistent experience, as well as that of others, that the pathologist can only very rarely identify the etiology of ischemia. Mesenteric thrombi are likely to either escape the pathologist's detection or be in a portion of a mesenteric vessel that was not removed. Volvulus and intussusception are likely to be rectified by the surgeon as the specimen is removed. Vasculitis (usually periarteritis nodosa) is a cause of ischemia and can be identified by the pathologist, but is only rarely the culprit.

Mucosal Prolapse Syndromes and Conditions Resulting from Mucosal Injury

Mucosal prolapse is a name given to a variety of conditions that can cause a fold of mucosa to prolapse into the lumen, exposing it to mechanical traction and compression. Nomenclature is somewhat confusing because the same process has historically been given different names in different sites. These conditions include prolapsing mucosal folds in diverticular disease, the so-called solitary rectal ulcer syndrome, inflammatory cloacogenic polyp, and localized colitis cystica profunda. All of these conditions can cause ulceration and inflammation that can endoscopically simulate a focus of IBD. The histologic appearance may also simulate IBD **i22.32a**, though there is often a fibromuscular hyperplasia of the lamina propria **i22.32b**. There may also be glandular atrophy, simulating chronic ischemia **i22.32c** [PMID17204024, PMID19861563]. Indeed, chronic mucosal prolapse appears to cause compression of blood vessels, resulting in ischemia [PMID12456946].

The mucosal prolapse syndromes involve the colon from the sigmoid to the ano-rectal junction. Mucosal prolapse in the sigmoid is usually secondary to diverticular disease (the term "diverticular disease" is preferred to the older terms "diverticulosis" and "diverticulitis"). Mucosal prolapse from diverticular disease is a leading cause of a false diagnosis of IBD in mucosal biopsies from the sigmoid colon.

Solitary rectal ulcer syndrome is a double misnomer. Only about half of these patients have ulcers, and 20% have >1 lesion. The characteristic fibromuscular hyperplasia is often best seen adjacent to the ulcerated areas. The cause is likely pressure or traction from inspissated stool.

The inflammatory cloacogenic polyp is a mucosal prolapse syndrome that occurs at the junction of the colonic and squamous mucosa and may clinically simulates hemorrhoids. It is lined primarily by colonic epithelium but may have some squamous epithelium. It is distinguished from the solitary rectal ulcer by its location at the ano-rectal junction, its clinical similarity to hemorrhoids, and the occasional presence of squamous epithelium.

Perhaps the most confusing of the mucosal prolapse syndromes is localized colitis cystica profunda. Localized colitis cystica profunda typically occurs in the rectum when mucosal damage from an inflammatory process allows the mucosa to grow inward into the stroma, resulting in ectopic glands and mucous cysts **i22.32d**. Localized colitis cystica profunda may be a form of solitary rectal ulcer [PMID1483723], and its appearance is similar to that of the solitary rectal ulcer except for the additional presence of displaced glands and mucinous cysts. Mucosal prolapse may be the inciting event that damages the mucosa and allows the ingrowth of glands into the stroma.

Localized colitis cystica profunda is not to be confused with generalized colitis cystica profunda, which is not a mucosal prolapse syndrome. Generalized colitis cystica profunda is associated with generalized colitis of any etiology, especially IBD or radiation therapy [PMID19388808]. The basic process and appearance is the same as for localized colitis cystica profunda—mucosal injury furnishes an avenue for glands to gain entry into the lamina propria, resulting in mucinous cysts lined by displaced epithelium—but a much larger area is involved.

Generalized colitis cystica profunda, in turn, is not to be confused with pneumatosis cystoides intestinalis, which is the presence of intestinal gas in the stroma. In pneumatosis cystoides intestinalis, air rather than epithelium or pools of mucin is trapped in the intestinal wall. A key feature that distinguishes pneumatosis cystoides intestinalis from either form of colitis cystica profunda is that the spaces are not lined by epithelium i22.33a.

Pneumatosis cystoides intestinalis occurs in a fulminant and benign form. The fulminant form occurs mostly in infants with necrotizing enterocolitis, indicating severe and widespread mucosal damage. The benign form occurs primarily in adults, usually in the colon (pneumatosis coli). It is more localized, is associated with increased luminal pressure or cracks in the mucosa, and may occur as a response to mucosal injury from colitis, usually IBD. Pneumatosis cystoides intestinalis is often asymptomatic in adults. The collections of gas in the stroma may elevate areas of the mucosa, resulting in what may appear to be multiple polyps endoscopically. There is an inflammatory response, often with giant cells i22.33b. Occasionally, collections of giant cells are more prevalent than the cysts i22.33c. Clusters of giant cells in the stroma without other explanation should raise suspicion for pneumatosis cystoides intestinalis.

Displaced Epithelium vs Invasive Adenocarcinoma

A mucosal prolapse syndrome or a previous biopsy may cause benign epithelium to be pushed from the surface into the stroma, simulating invasive adenocarcinoma. A particularly difficult situation arises when an adenomatous polyp has either been subjected to traction or compression by the fecal stream (this occurs primarily on the left side), or has been biopsied i22.34a [PMID17372755, PMID4810096, PMID11557782]. In these situations, displaced epithelium will have changes of dysplasia, heightening concern.

The following findings suggest benign, displaced epithelium rather than invasion:

1. The overlying epithelium may be adenomatous, but there is no carcinoma in situ i22.34b.
2. The nuclei in the problematic focus either appear unremarkable or no worse than the nuclei of the overlying adenomatous epithelium i22.34c.
3. There is no stromal desmoplasia.
4. There may be lamina propria around the questionable epithelium because it has been carried with the epithelium into the stroma i22.34d. Lamina propria is not generally seen in invasive carcinoma.
5. There may be hemosiderin deposited in the displaced focus, as displaced epithelium, either from traction or a biopsy, tends to cause bleeding i22.34e, i22.34f.
6. There may be physical continuity between benign surface epithelium and the problematic focus in the stroma.
7. A subtle layer of muscularis mucosa may envelop the problematic focus i22.34g, i22.34h.

If there is mucin, displaced epithelium will tend to be on the periphery of the pools of mucin i22.34i, whereas it is intermingled with the mucin in a mucinous carcinoma.

In contrast, superficial invasion i22.35a is associated with one of more of the following findings:

1. There is high-grade dysplasia/carcinoma in situ overlying the problematic stromal focus i22.35b.
2. The problematic epithelium resembles that of an adenomatous polyp with high-grade dysplasia (rounded nuclei, vesicular chromatin, nucleoli, glandular crowding, stratification, mitoses), rather than a routine adenomatous polyp i22.35c.
3. There are no hemosiderin macrophages or lamina propria in the problematic focus i22.35d.
4. Continuity between carcinoma in situ on the surface and a collection of epithelium in the stroma is especially worrisome for invasion, but at the same time, the inability to establish continuity between a focus of atypia on the surface and a stromal focus after serial levels also suggest invasion. In any situation of displaced epithelium vs invasive carcinoma, a large number of levels are often illuminating. In the case depicted in i22.35a, for example, extensive serial levels never showed continuity between the surface and stromal clusters.

Infectious Colitis

It is now understood that differentiating an infectious colitis from active inflammatory bowel disease cannot be done on the basis of the location of the neutrophils, as had been thought. Rather, the pivotal criterion for an infectious etiology is the absence of architectural distortion. With only rare exceptions, infectious colitis is an acute process that does not disturb the fundamental architecture of the mucosa i22.36 [Odze ISBN978-1416040590]. By contrast, IBD is a chronic process, even if it presents acutely, and there is almost always some degree of architectural distortion even in the initial biopsies or in quiescent cases.

There are no specific histologic features that can identify the organism in infectious colitis. *Clostridium difficile* causes severe necrosis of the surface epithelium and the upper portions of glands, resulting in the classic "mushroom-shaped' exudate on the surface that might be a histologic clue on biopsy examination i22.37, but this is nonspecific, and it is generally not possible for the pathologist to determine which organism is responsible in cases of infectious colitis.

Hemorrhagic colitis syndrome is an emerging public health concern and is usually caused by strains of *E coli* that make a toxin similar to the Shiga toxin (Stx) that is produced by *Shigella dysenteriae*. *E coli* makes 2 toxins that are very similar in structure to Shiga toxin, Shiga-like toxin 1 and Shiga-like toxin 2 (Stx-1 and Stx-2, also called SLT-1 and SLT-2, or verotoxin). Stx-2 is much more toxic that Stx-1. The Shiga and Shiga-like toxins have 6 subunits, 1 A component and 5 B components and are members of a group of toxins called AB5 toxins (the toxins produced by *Vibrio cholerae* and *Bordetella pertussis*, while slightly different from the Shiga and Shiga-like toxins, are also AB5 toxins). The 5 B subunits form a pentamer that binds to a component of the cell membrane called globotriaosylceramide

(Gb3). After binding, the A subunit enters the cell and is then cleaved into 2 smaller subunits, one of which, A1, binds to the ribosome and disrupts protein synthesis by cleaving an adenine base from ribosomal RNA [PMID20023663, PMID11595626].

In addition to inhibiting protein synthesis, the Shiga and Shiga-like toxins may also induce apoptosis by a pathway unconnected to the inhibition of protein synthesis. Apoptosis is particularly important in the gastrointestinal symptoms, since intestinal cells lack the Gb3 receptor for Stx-1 and Stx-2 [PMID10801274]. Apoptosis, rather than inhibition of protein synthesis, also appears to be the major mechanism of renal injury [PMID19124603].

The Stx toxins exert an especially potent effect on vascular endothelium, neurons, and renal epithelium, accounting for the symptoms of thrombotic thrombocytopenic purpura/hemolytic uremic syndrome that often accompany hemorrhagic colitis syndrome.

E coli O157:h7 (the O refers to an antigen in the lipopolysaccharide of the outer membrane that all gram-negative bacteria possess) is the major cause of hemorrhagic colitis syndrome and has emerged as a public health menace because of its association with epidemics. In 2010, another *E coli* strain, O145, was also found to produce Stx-1 and Stx-2, with similar symptoms. Unlike most infectious processes, *E coli* O157:h7 may cause mild architectural distortion i22.38.

While *Clostridium difficile* is the main culprit in antibiotic-associated colitis, *Klebsiella oxytoca* is also associated with antibiotics and may cause similar symptoms to *C difficile*. It should be excluded whenever *C difficile* is a clinical concern, but that organism cannot be identified [PMID17151365].

Amebiasis is easy to miss in biopsies, as the organisms very closely resemble macrophages. Amebiasis is characterized by severe acute inflammation, often with ulceration and crypt abscesses. Although the architecture is generally intact, the degree of acute inflammation may simulate active inflammatory bowel disease. Any collection of apparent macrophages in colon biopsies performed for diarrhea requires the exclusion of amoebae. In problematic cases, immunohistochemical stains may be needed, but at the H&E level, *Entamoeba histolytica* has prominent nucleoli i22.39 and often phagocytized erythrocytes. In such cases, a reliable travel history must be obtained from the gastroenterologist and passed on to the pathologist.

"Typhlitis" is an obsolete term that referred either to a neutropenic enterocolitis that occurs in immunocompromised patients secondary to bacterial infection or to a hemorrhagic necrosis, commonly of the cecum and ascending colon, of probable ischemic origin. The term is best avoided and replaced by a description of the findings and the probable etiology.

In assessing a biopsy for diarrhea, special attention should be given to the very minute zone from the immediate luminal border to the subepithelial collagen layer i22.30a. In this area will be pathogens that are adherent to the external surface of the cell membrane, pathogens in the cytoplasm of the surface epithelium, any inflammatory cells in the surface epithelium, and the thickened collagen layer of collagenous colitis. Other than the identification of architectural distortion and significant acute inflammation, there is no assessment in a mucosal biopsy that is more important than this tiny region.

Unusual opportunistic organisms like *Isospora* and *Enterocytozoon bieneusi* appear as intracytoplasmic inclusions of surface enterocytes, but electron microscopy may be required for the diagnosis [PMID8739472]. A clue to unusual cytoplasmic pathogens is that the tip of the enterocyte nucleus will often be indented or indistinct.

Mycobacterium avium intracellulare (MAI) is characterized by macrophages in the lamina propria [PMID10989639], illustrating the need to study macrophages in the lamina propria of immunocompromised patients. The differential diagnosis for MAI is Whipples disease and xanthoma/xanthelasma. Except in the stomach, where xanthoma/xanthelasma is relatively common, large numbers of macrophages in the lamina propria merit respect if the patient is immunocompromised.

The Appendix

Little will be said here of acute appendicitis because it is rarely a diagnostic challenge. The appendix remains of unknown function, and acute appendicitis remains of unknown etiology. Because a number of extrinsic processes may secondarily involve the wall of the appendix, mucosal acute inflammation must be found for the diagnosis of acute appendicitis, and the only time the diagnosis is difficult is when there is inflammation of the wall, but not of the mucosa, in which case it may be necessary to submit more of the gross specimen. There are occasional cases in which the pathologist cannot secure a diagnosis of acute appendicitis with complete certainty, and the surgeon must exclude other causes based on clinical judgment and operative findings. While some have cautioned that luminal neutrophils do not prove mucosal inflammation because they may flow into the appendix from another site, in my experience luminal neutrophils secure a diagnosis of primary acute appendicitis.

A different histologic picture occurs in the so-called interval appendectomy. Surgeons may occasionally postpone an appendectomy, in which case the pathologist will not see an acute appendicitis, but rather a more subtle chronic inflammation, often with macrophages and lymphocytes, rather than neutrophils, in the wall i22.40a, and chronic inflammatory cells in the surrounding adipose tissue i22.40b. The clinical history of an earlier presentation and clinical diagnosis of acute appendicitis may be needed in these cases. If the appendix was ruptured in the initial presentation, pools of mucin may be seen in the appendectomy and must be carefully studied to exclude a mucinous carcinoma of the appendix. A paucity of epithelial cells in the mucin, their benign appearance, and the absence of in situ or invasive carcinoma anywhere else in the specimen suggest a benign process i22.40c, i22.40d.

A peculiar occurrence in appendectomy specimens is that lymphocytes may fill and distend capillaries, causing a resemblance to a lymphoid nodule [PMID20002767]. It has also been my experience that a "nodule" of intravascular lymphocytes can simulate a carcinoid tumor i22.41.

Rarely, the entity of granulomatous appendicitis will be encountered. Although at one time thought to be an appendiceal manifestation of CD, granulomatous appendicitis is now believed to be a separate entity, but 5-10% of these patients will develop CD [PMID15807470], suggesting that granulomatous appendicitis may be a collection of disorders. Granulomatous appendicitis is typically distinguished from CD by the large number of granulomas. Some cases of CD do not have any granulomas, and very few cases will have the large numbers typically seen in granulomatous appendicitis. Nevertheless, the report should indicate the inability to exclude CD of the appendix and such patients should be monitored for possible CD.

Unusual Conditions in the Bowel

The incidence of radiation proctitis is thankfully decreasing now, with more precisely target external radiation, and with brachytherapy, but is still relatively commonly encountered. Acute radiation proctitis histologically presents as nonspecific acute inflammation and ulceration i22.42a. Chronic radiation proctitis demonstrates damage to glands and fibrosis of the stroma i22.42b, often with dilated capillaries i22.42c, common findings in chronic radiation change in any site.

Although Meckel diverticulum may have variant locations, most are on the antimesenteric border, and are 10-30 cm proximal to the ileocecal valve. 2/3 have ectopic gastric mucosa i33.43 [PMID18322689]. The principal differential diagnosis for Meckel diverticulum is an enteric duplication cyst.

The mucosa of enteric duplication cyst (sometimes simply called a duplication cyst) in the colon or small bowel may not precisely match that of the adjacent bowel, and they may also have ectopic gastric mucosa [PMID12469471]. Proof that the cyst does not communicate with the adjacent bowel suggests an enteric duplication cyst over a Meckel diverticulum. A more complex wall, with muscularis propria or nerves, also favors an enteric duplication cyst, as Meckel are simple diverticula.

Graft vs host disease (GVH) occurs in the setting of bone marrow transplant, when the recipient's immune system has been iatrogenically destroyed and the donor's marrow may then have free rein to attack patient tissues. Donor T lymphocytes attack recipient proteins, primarily those of the HLA system [PMID19282026]. Major manifestations are in the skin, liver, and gastrointestinal tract. GVH in the colon is graded on a scale of 1-4. Grade 1 GVH is characterized by single cell necrosis, grade 2 by crypt abscesses, grade 3 by extensive loss of epithelium i22.44, and grade 4 by total or nearly total loss of epithelium [Sale ISBN978-0893522209].

Vascular ectasia of the colon (formerly called angiodysplasia) occurs in the right colon and is a leading cause of lower gastrointestinal hemorrhage. Theories of its pathogenesis include compression of veins in the wall, with consequent backing up of blood and dilatation of vessels, and a degeneration of the vascular wall [PMID18711303]. It is immensely difficult to make the diagnosis from a gross and microscopic examination of a resection specimen. The principal role of the pathologist is to exclude other etiologies, after which the correct diagnosis is made by clinical correlation and exclusion. If there is time during the acute bleeding episode, radiographic studies may help localize the bleeding to the right colon.

Ceroidosis (brown bowel syndrome) is a brown discoloration of the bowel wall that occurs in longstanding malabsorption. Ceroidosis results from the deposition of lipofuscin-like material in the external muscle layer and in the muscularis mucosa, and can occur anywhere in the GI tract. Vitamin E deficiency may be the ultimate cause, as absence of its antioxidant properties is thought to be responsible for the accumulation of pigment [PMID423605].

Fibrosing colonopathy affects the terminal ileum and right colon and is seen in patients who have received enzyme supplements for pancreatic deficiency, such as those who have cystic fibrosis or have undergone partial pancreatic resection [PMID15455984]. The mechanism for this association is unclear. The major differential diagnosis for fibrosing colonopathy is progressive systemic sclerosis (scleroderma).

Hirschsprung disease, an absence of ganglion cells in the colonic wall, occurs in both a syndromic form (ie, associated with other abnormalities) and a nonsyndromic form. In 80% of cases, the absence of ganglion cells occurs only in the rectosigmoid area (the so-called short form), while in the remaining 20% of cases (the so-called long form), aganglionosis may extend throughout the colon and even involve the distal ileum [PMID20610192]. The long form is associated with mutations in the *RET* gene [PMID18280283], and in assessing biopsies for Hirschsprung disease, H&E examination can be supplemented with immunohistochemical staining for the Ret protein. Ganglion cells are positive for Ret protein in a paranuclear position, and such staining is slightly more sensitive in the identification of ganglion cells than H&E [PMID16753599].

Core Points for Nonneoplastic Intestinal Disorders

- Celiac disease: clinical presentation and endoscopic appearance may be variable.
  - Antitransglutaminase IgA is the best serological test, but a normal result must be accompanied by a demonstration of normal serum total IgA.
- Ulcerative colitis (UC): almost completely mucosal, must affect the rectum, cannot affect the terminal ileum without also affecting the cecum, and has no skip areas.
- Crohn disease (CD): transmural, though this cannot be appreciated in a mucosal biopsy, and may or may not affect the rectum or the terminal ileum.
- IBD mucosal biopsy usually has some architectural distortion, such as irregularity of the luminal border, reduction in the number of glands, shortening of the remaining glands, and branching of glands.
  - Architectural distortion may be the only indication of IBD in quiescent times, and the only means of distinguishing it from irritable bowel syndrome, a clinical mimic.
- Low-grade dysplasia in UC: resembles an ordinary adenomatous polyp.
- High-grade dysplasia: resembles an adenomatous polyp with severe dysplasia.
  - Diagnosis of dysplasia should be made with caution in the presence of significant acute inflammation.
- Low-grade dysplasia in flat mucosa and dysplasia-associated lesion or mass (DALM) with negative margins can often be managed conservatively
- Colectomy is often performed for high-grade dysplasia in flat mucosa or a DALM with any dysplasia at a resection margin.

- Diversion colitis/defunctionalized bowel: idiopathic inflammatory condition occurring in a portion of colon that is no longer functional.
  - May perfectly resemble IBD histologically.
- Pouchitis: is a series of conditions causing bloody diarrhea in patients who have an ileal pouch after colectomy for UC.
  - Some cases are Crohn disease that was thought to be ulcerative colitis
  - Other cases respond to antibiotics
  - Many cases are idiopathic
- Lymphocytic colitis and collagenous colitis: watery diarrhea
  - Disproportionately affect middle aged and older women.
  - Overlapping features and occasional acute inflammation, but lymphocytic colitis is characterized by large numbers of intraepithelial lymphocytes
  - Collagenous colitis has thickening or fraying of the subepithelial collagen layer, or entrapment of cells within it.
- Mucosal prolapse syndromes: left colon, mimic IBD or ischemia.
- Pitfall: a false-positive diagnosis of carcinoma from mucosal prolapse
  - Clues: innocuous nuclei, the absence of carcinoma in the overlying epithelium, absence of stromal desmoplasia, lamina propria surrounding the problematic cells, and the presence of hemosiderin.
- Infectious colitis is best distinguished from IBD by the absence of architectural distortion.
- Ischemic colitis: acute stage has superficial necrosis.
  - Subacute stage resembles IBD.
  - Chronic ischemia: atrophic glands and a fibrotic, hyalinized stroma.

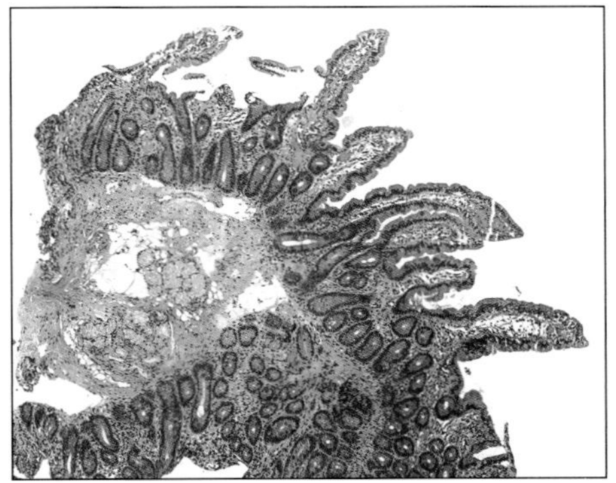

i22.1 Normal duodenal mucosa with well developed villi. Brunner glands are readily noted in the submucosa.

i22.2 **a, b** Normal duodenal mucosa with Brunner glands in the submucosa and extending into the mucosa

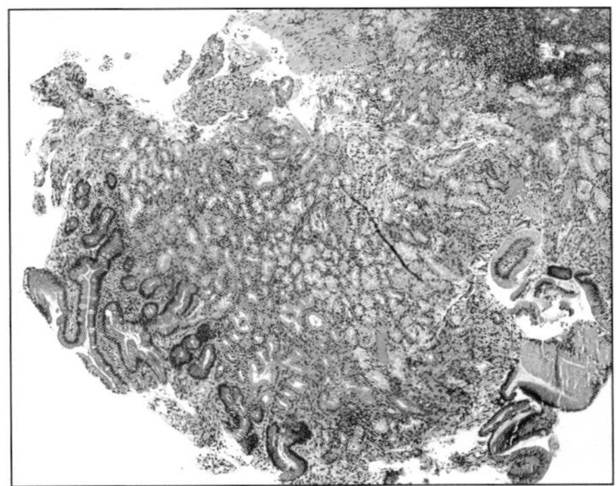

i22.3 Brunner gland hyperplasia. Note the diminished villi over the hyperplastic nodule, a normal finding.

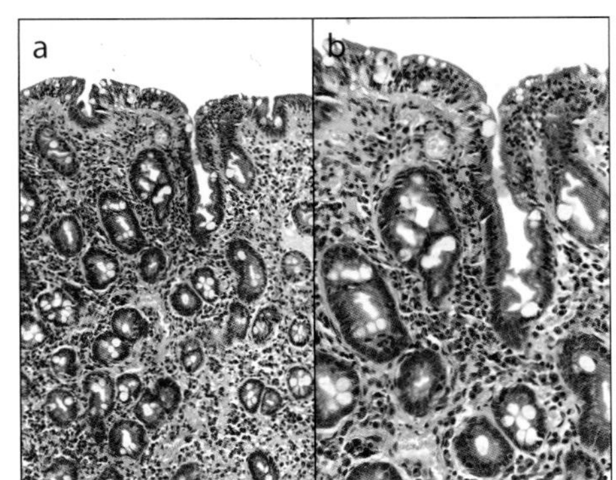

i22.4 **a** Well developed celiac disease with essentially absent villi, causing resemblance to colonic mucosa.
b A higher-power view of the same case as in i22.4a, illustrating the numerous intraepithelial lymphocytes

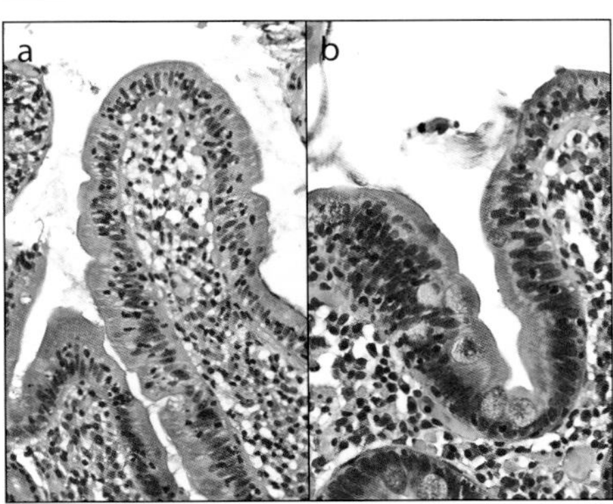

i22.5 **a, b** Marsh stage 1 celiac disease with preserved villi but with numerous intraepithelial lymphocytes

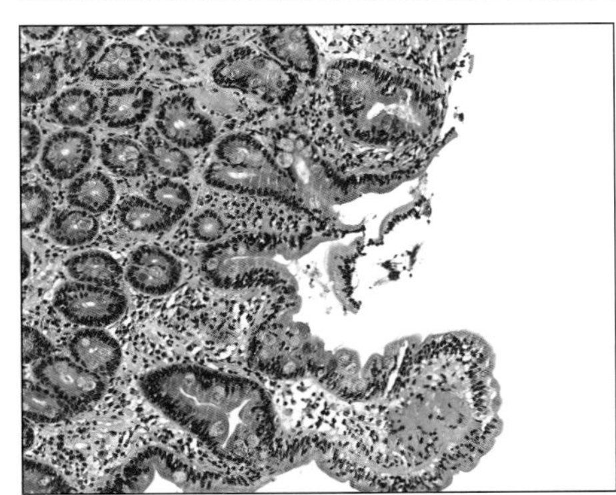

i22.6 Marsh stage 2 celiac disease with attenuated, but still readily apparent villi and intraepithelial lymphocytes

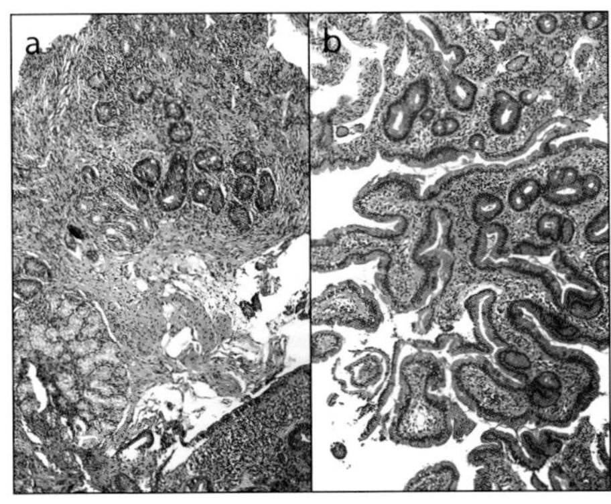

i22.7 **a** Well developed celiac disease prior to the institution of a gluten-free diet
b The same patient 6 months later after compliance with a gluten-free diet

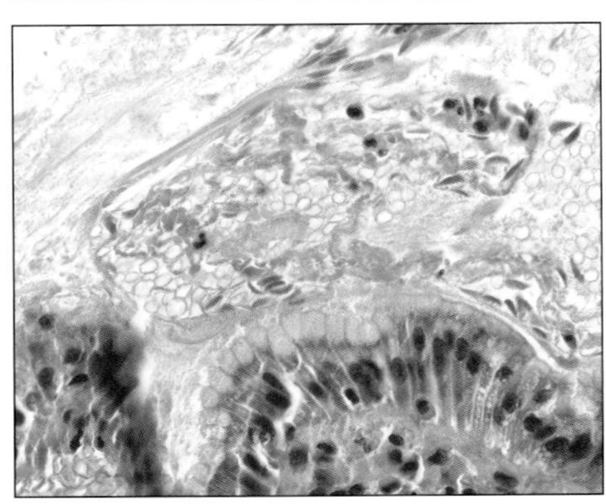

i22.8 *Giardia*, evident as minute basophilic sickle-structures, primarily adjacent to the apical border of the cytoplasm

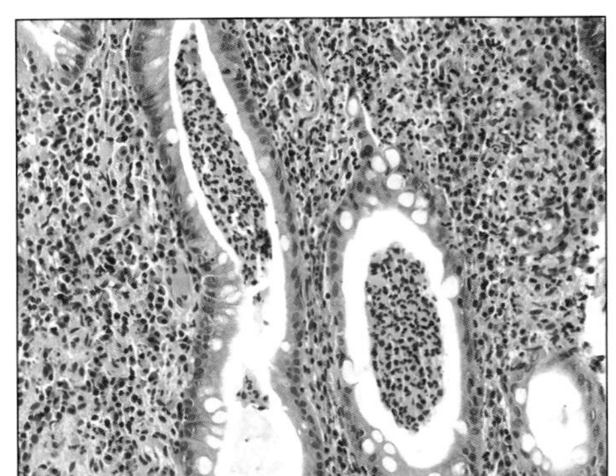

i22.9 Crypt abscesses in active ulcerative colitis

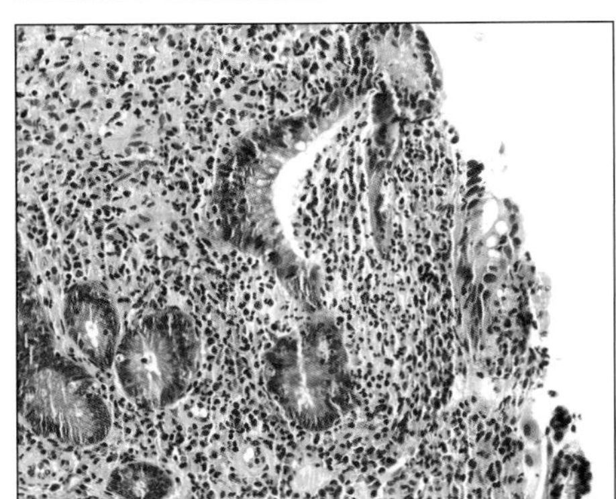

i22.10 A crypt abscess with destruction of the glandular wall

ISBN 978-089189-5886

i22.11-i22.16 illustrate architectural distortion in inflammatory bowel disease.

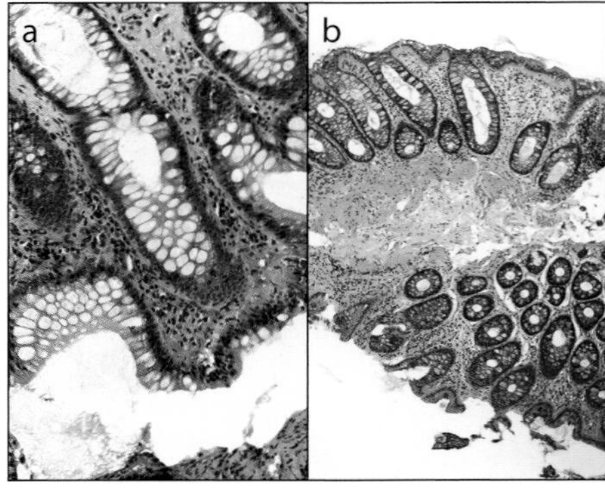

i22.11 **a** illustrates an irregular luminal border. Compare to **b**, which illustrates a normal, regular luminal border in the upper portion of the photograph. The lower portion of i22.11b is also normal, but is tangentially sectioned.

i22.12 **a, b** Dropout of glands in inflammatory bowel disease. Note the paucity of acute inflammation in these examples of quiescent ulcerative colitis.

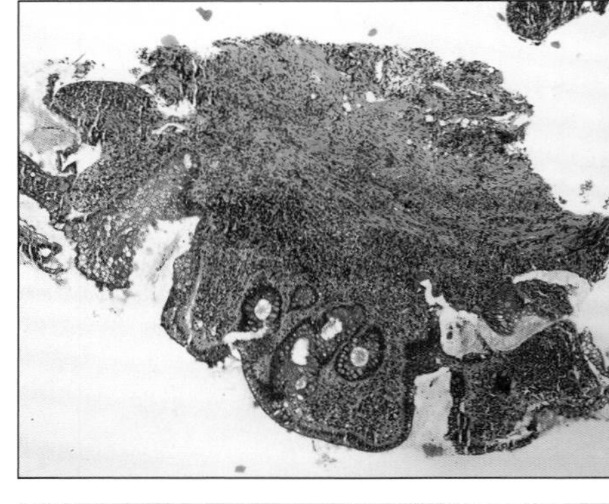

i22.13 Quiescent inflammatory bowel disease in which the glands fail to reach the muscularis mucosa

i22.14 Quiescent inflammatory bowel disease in which the glands are irregularly shaped

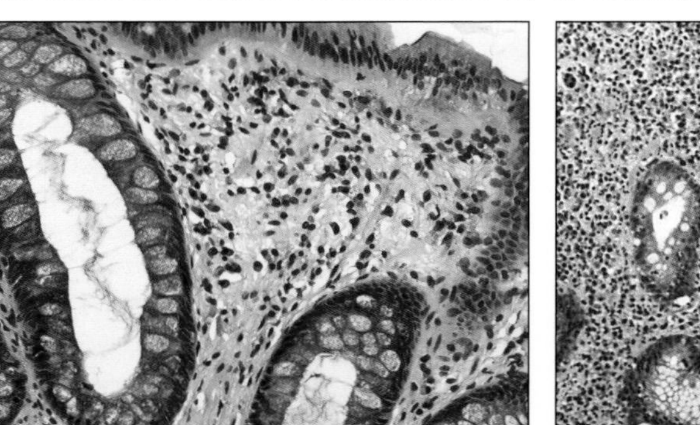

i22.15 A normal biopsy in which the chronic inflammatory cells in the lamina propria decrease moving from the apical surface to the muscularis mucosa

i22.16 Quiescent inflammatory bowel disease in which the lamina propria contains an increased number of chronic inflammatory cells and there is no tapering towards the muscularis mucosa

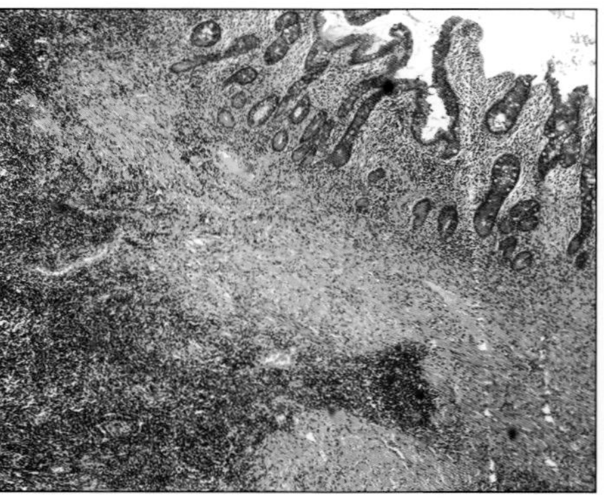

i22.17 Crohn disease with fibrosis and a lymphoid aggregate in the submucosa

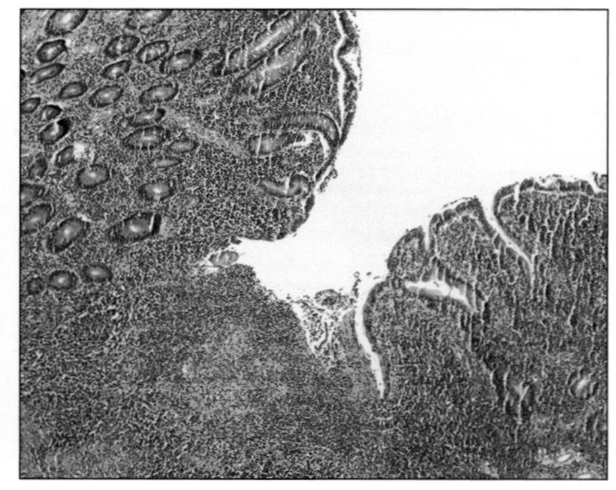

i22.18 An aphthous ulcer in Crohn disease

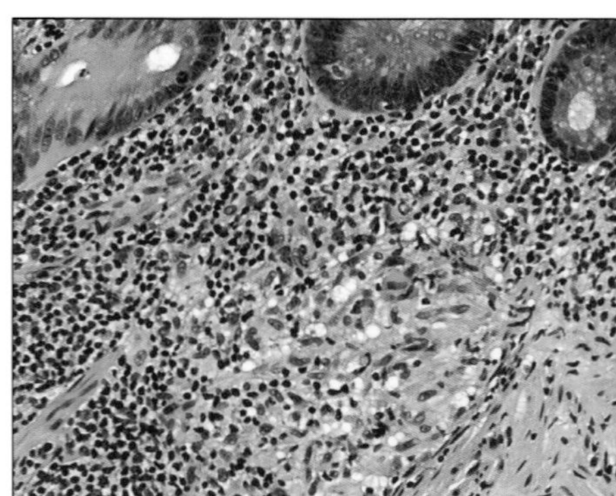

i22.19 A granuloma in Crohn disease

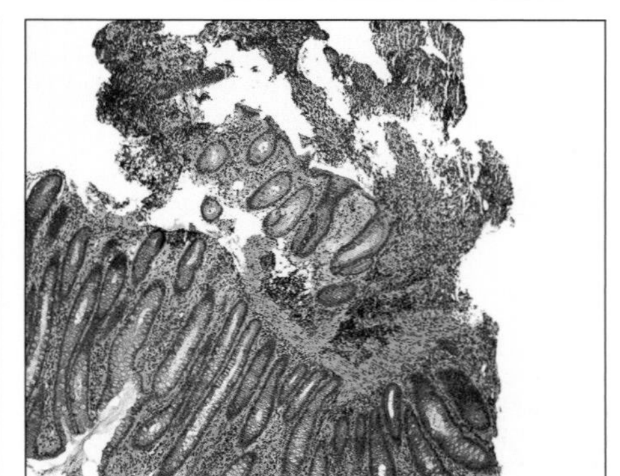

i22.20 A mucosal biopsy of Crohn disease in which the acute inflammation is very focal. While not diagnostic of Crohn disease, punctate acute inflammation is more suggestive of Crohn disease than ulcerative colitis.

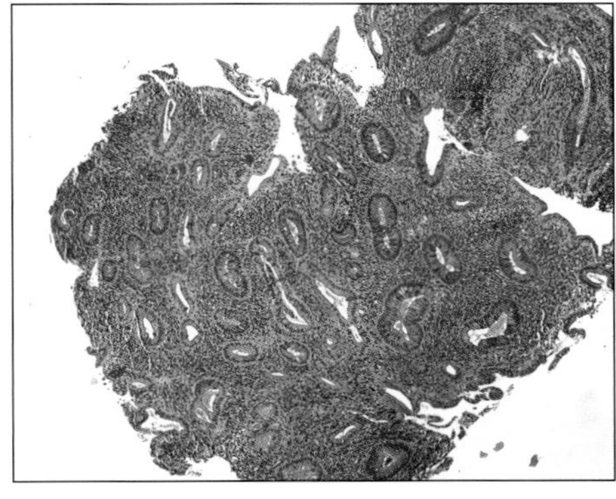

i22.21 An inflammatory pseudopolyp in ulcerative colitis. There is no dysplasia in this polyp.

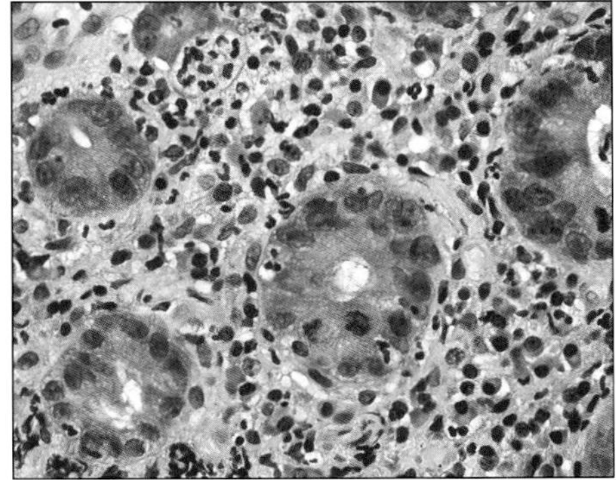

i22.22 Reactive atypia in active ulcerative colitis. Note the relative nuclear uniformity, the abundant amount of cytoplasm, and the open chromatin pattern. Also note the active acute inflammation.

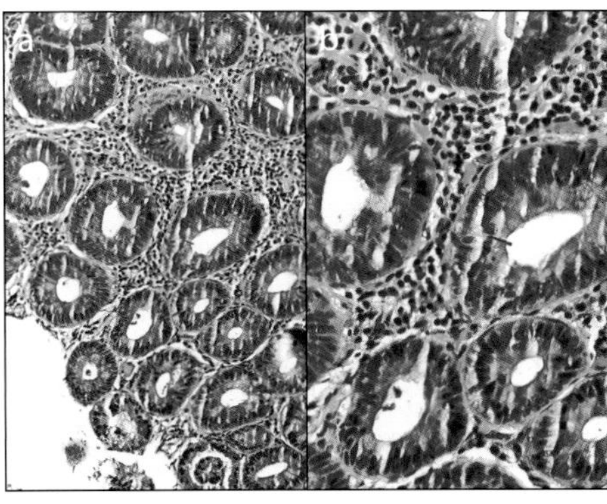

i22.23 **a** Low-grade dysplasia in ulcerative colitis. Note the resemblance to a colonic adenomatous polyp with relatively coarse chromatin, indistinct nucleoli, and minimal stratification.
b A higher-power image of the same case as in i22.23a

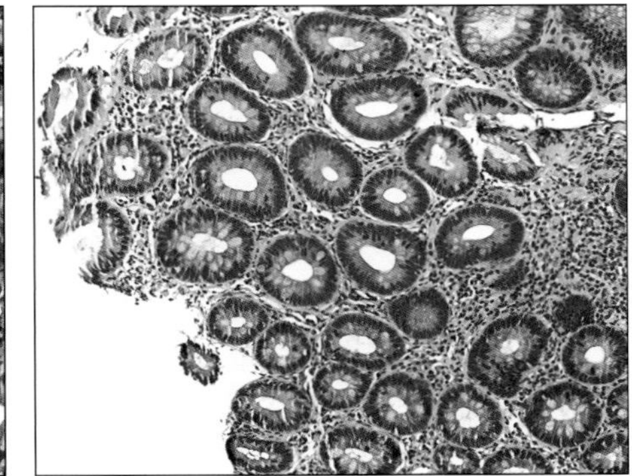

i22.24 Ulcerative colitis with atypia that is indefinite for dysplasia. If this were a routine colonic polyp, one would struggle with whether or not there was true adenomatous change.

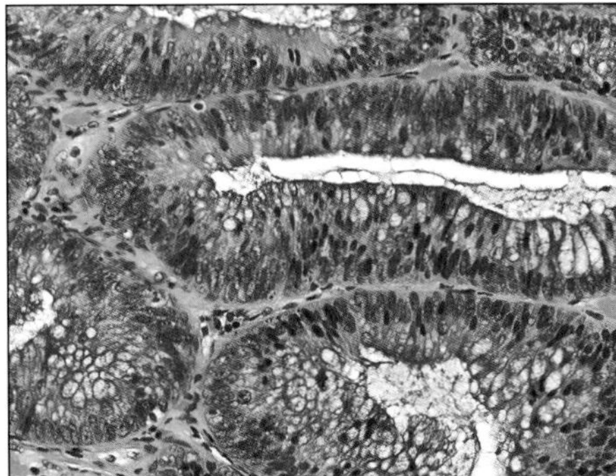

i22.25 High-grade dysplasia in ulcerative colitis. Note the more open chromatin pattern, with occasional nucleoli, relative to low-grade dysplasia. Also note the full-thickness stratification.

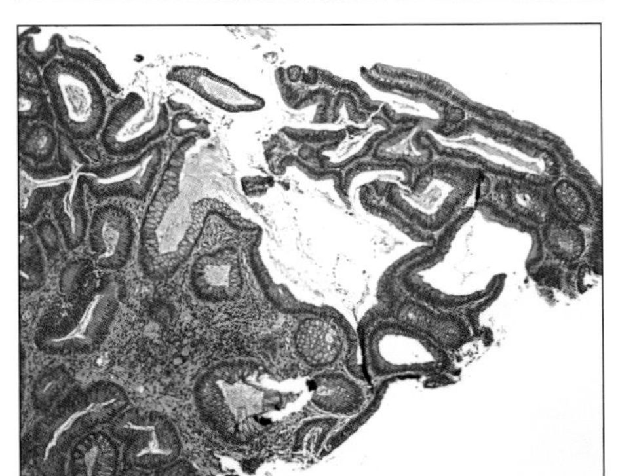

i22.26 A dysplasia-associated lesion or mass (DALM) in a patient with ulcerative colitis. This polyp demonstrates low-grade dysplasia, unlike the simple inflammatory pseudopolyp illustrated in i22.21.

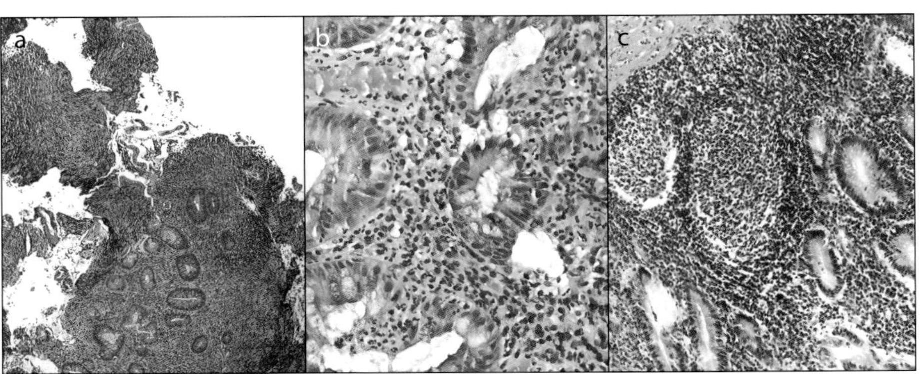

i22.27 Diversion colitis.
a simulates active ulcerative colitis perfectly.
b is a high-power view of diversion colitis, again simulating ulcerative colitis perfectly, with crypt abscesses.
c illustrates the lymphoid follicles that are occasionally seen in diversion colitis.

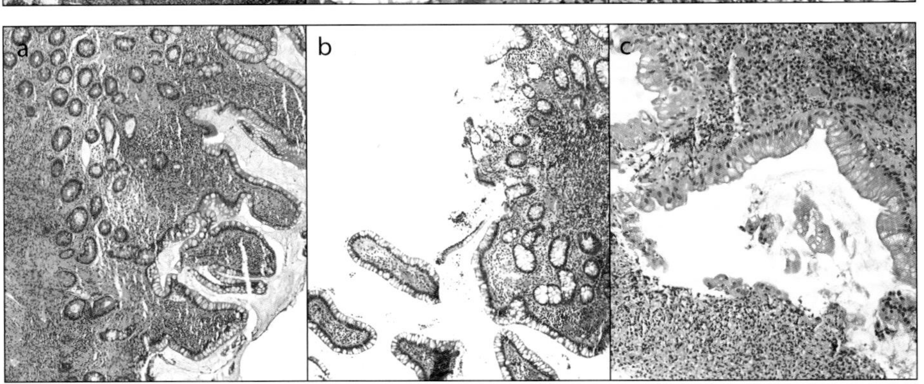

i22.28 Pouchitis.
a illustrates relatively unremarkable small bowel mucosa, even in a patient with significant symptoms.
b illustrates mild inflammation with attenuation of the villous architecture, again in a patient with significant symptoms.
c illustrates severe acute inflammation with ulceration, but in a nonspecific pattern.

ISBN 978-089189-5886

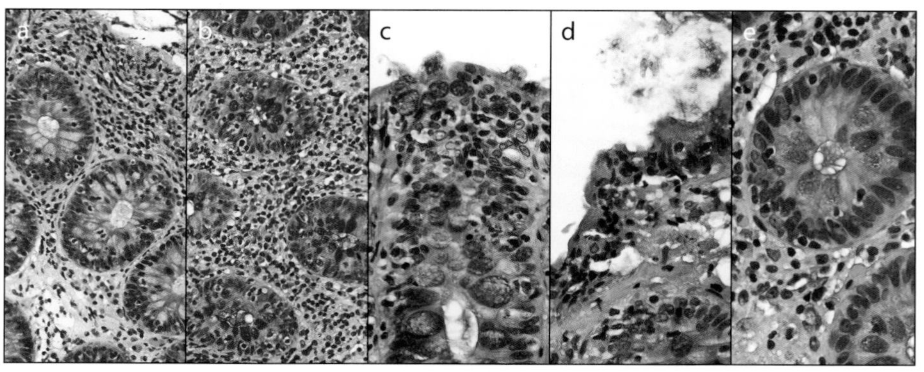

i22.29 Lymphocytic colitis. **a** illustrates numerous intraepithelial lymphocytes. **b** illustrates both numerous intraepithelial lymphocytes and the increased number of lymphocytes in the lamina propria that is characteristically seen in this entity. **c** illustrates the eosinophils that are often focally present. **d** illustrates the predilection of the lymphocytes for the surface epithelium in many cases. **e** A biopsy from a middle-aged woman with watery diarrhea. Lymphocytic colitis is suspected but this set of biopsies did not conclusively establish that diagnosis.

i22.30 **a** The normal subepithelial collagen layer in the colon, barely visible as a very thin pink line between the basal cell membrane of the surface epithelium and the erythrocytes **b** Collagenous colitis on H&E in well-oriented sections **c** Even in this tangential section, it is clear that the collagen layer surrounding the gland in the lower right is significantly thicker than normal. **d** In this biopsy there is both thickening of the subepithelial collagen layer and increased intraepithelial lymphocytes, illustrating that collagenous colitis and lymphocytic colitis are often related and occur together. **e** Like lymphocytic colitis, collagenous colitis may have occasional eosinophils. **f** Collagenous colitis as illuminated by a trichrome stain, highlighting a markedly thickened subepithelial collagen layer **g** Collagenous colitis in which the subepithelial collagen layer is frayed with a lower border that is less distinct than the upper border. Note the entrapped erythrocytes and capillaries. **h** A higher-power view of entrapment of capillaries by the collagen layer in collagenous colitis

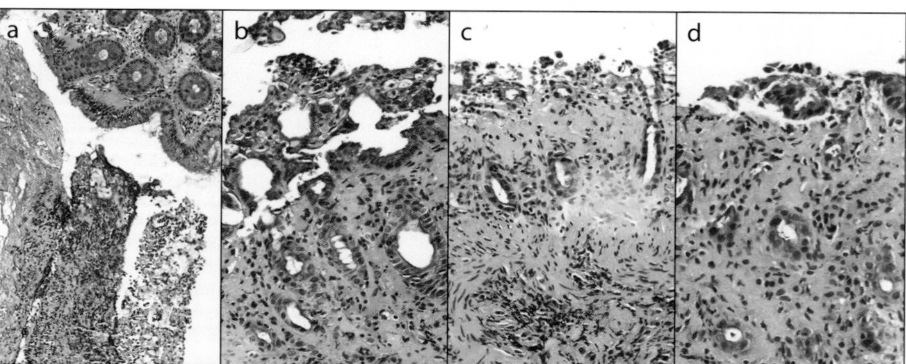

i22.31 **a** Acute ischemic colitis, illustrating a nonspecific ulceration **b** The more usual histologic picture of ischemic colitis with acute inflammation on the right but chronicity apparent on the left with atrophic glands and a fibrotic stroma **c, d** Another illustration of the atrophic glands and fibrotic stroma that is characteristic of chronic ischemic colitis

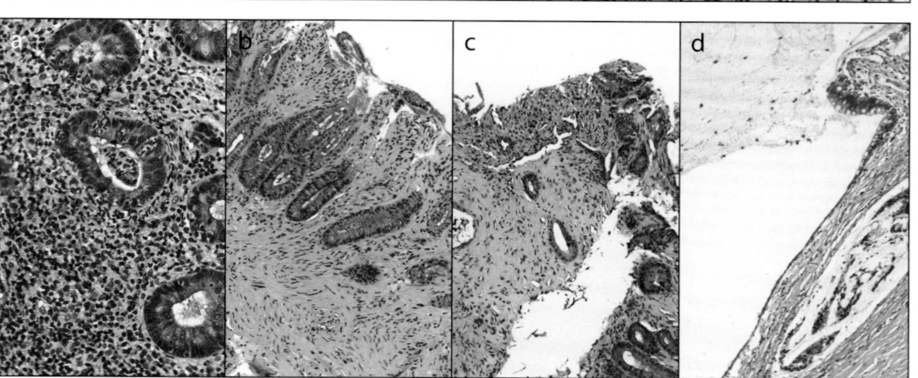
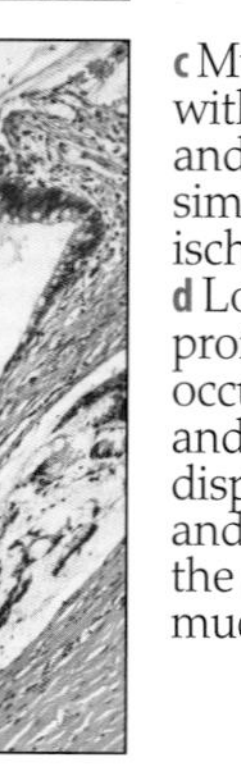

i22.32 **a** Mucosal prolapse simulating ulcerative proctitis, with acute inflammation and crypt abscesses **b** Mucosal prolapse with fibromuscular hyperplasia of the lamina propria **c** Mucosal prolapse with stromal fibrosis and glandular atrophy, simulating chronic ischemia **d** Localized colitis cystic profunda. This case occurred in the rectum and demonstrates displaced epithelium and cyst formation in the stroma, likely due to mucosal injury.

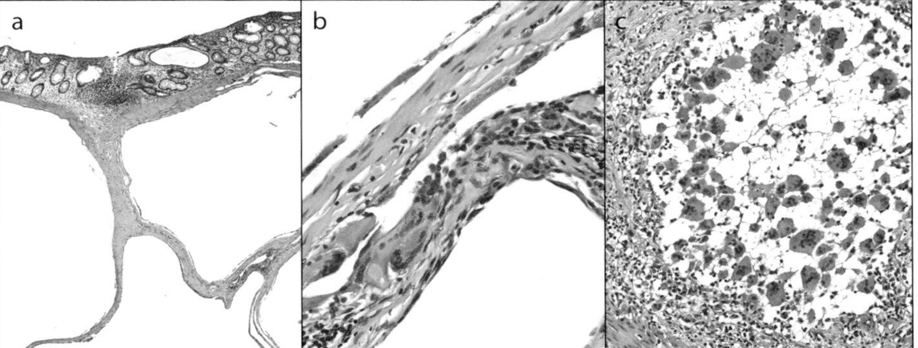

i22.33 **a** Pneumatosis cystoides intestinalis in which the stroma contains cystic spaces that are not lined by epithelium **b** The same case as in i22.33a, illustrating the lack of epithelial lining of the cyst and the presence of giant cells **c** Another case of pneumatosis cystoides intestinalis in which giant cells are prevalent

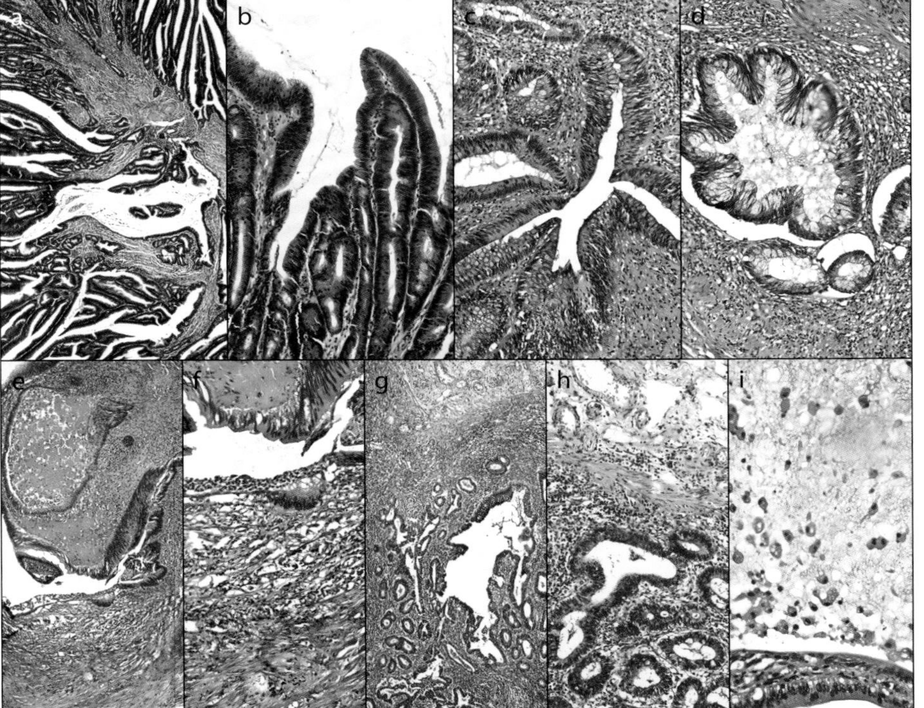

i22.34 **a** An adenomatous polyp that has been biopsied and which has adenomatous epithelium displaced into the stroma **b** The same case as in i22.34a in which the surface epithelium demonstrates adenomatous change but not carcinoma **c** Atypical epithelium in the stroma, initially worrisome for invasive carcinoma, but lacking sufficient atypia for that diagnosis **d** A problematic focus of atypical epithelium in the stroma, but it is surrounded by lamina propria. **e, f** Displaced epithelium in the stroma, associated with hemosiderin macrophages, a consequence of the previous biopsy **g** A focus of atypical epithelium that appears to penetrate deeply into the stroma, relative to the surface epithelium visible at the bottom of the photograph **h** A higher-power view of the same case as in i22.34g, illustrating that the problematic focus is surrounded by muscularis mucosa **i** A mucinous deposit associated with displaced epithelium, causing concern for a mucinous carcinoma in the stroma, but the epithelium is on the periphery of the mucin rather than intermingled with it.

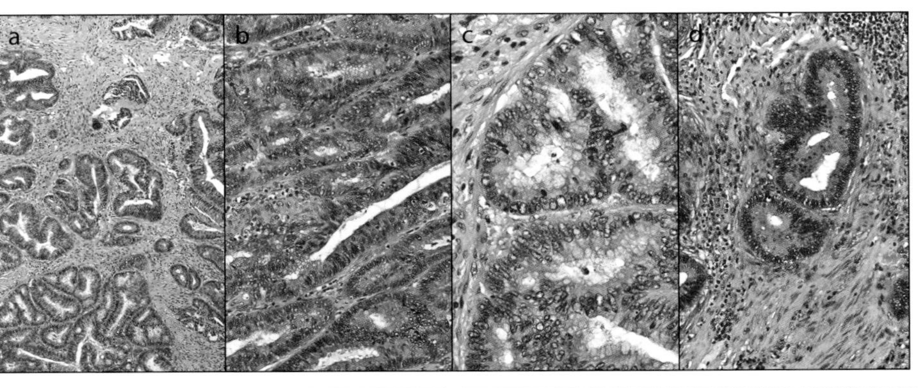

i22.35 **a** A superficially invasive colonic adenocarcinoma **b** The surface epithelium of the case that is illustrated in i22.35a, illustrating adenocarcinoma in situ, not just adenomatous change, increasing the likelihood that the problematic focus depicted in i22.35a is invasive **c** A higher-power view of the problematic focus in the stroma in the case illustrated in i22.35a, illustrating that this epithelium is more atypical than would be expected in adenomatous epithelium. Compare with the displaced epithelium in the stroma in i22.34c. **d** Another view of a superficially invasive carcinoma, demonstrating the lack of lamina propria

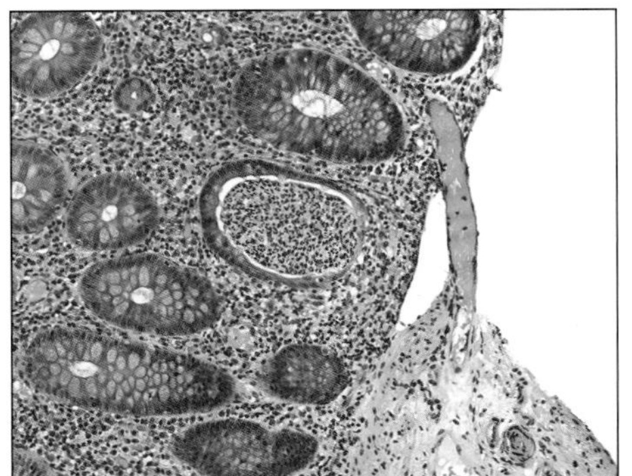

i22.36 Acute infectious colitis. Note the crypt abscess but the retention of the normal architecture, with no damaged epithelial structures and none of the features of architectural distortion associated with inflammatory bowel disease, depicted in i22.11-i22.16. This patient had a positive culture for *Salmonella*.

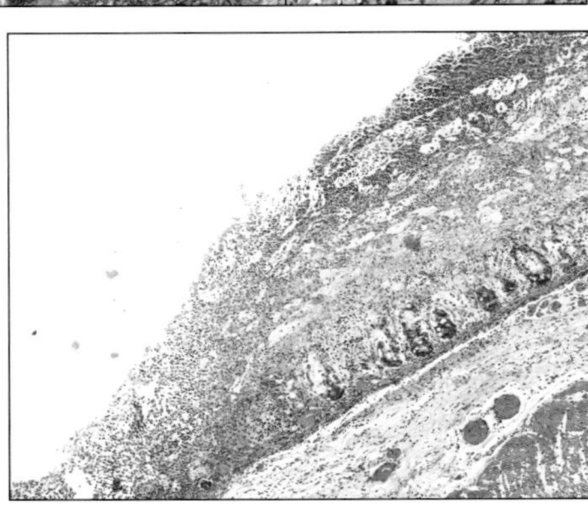

i22.37 A mucosal biopsy from a patient with *Clostridium difficile*, illustrating the "mushroom-shaped" exudate on the surface

ISBN 978-089189-5886

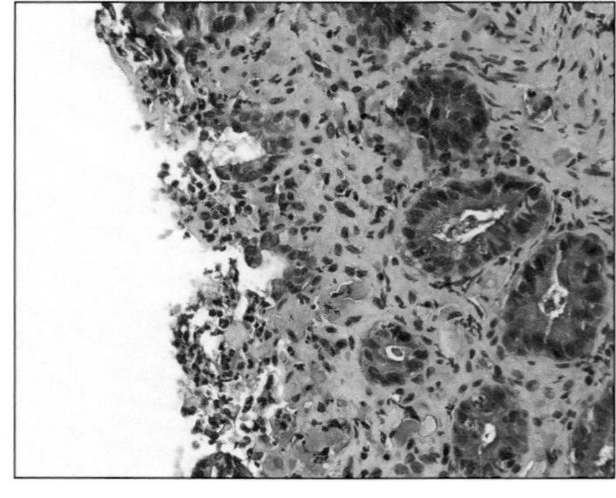

i22.38 A mucosal biopsy from a patient subsequently found to have *E coli* O157:h7. Note the acute inflammation on the surface, but also the slight glandular atrophy and mild stromal fibrosis, features that are not usually seen in an infectious colitis.

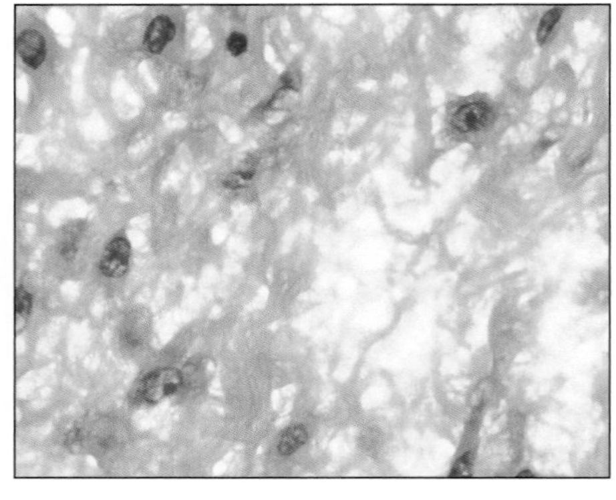

i22.39 Amebiasis in a biopsy of a mucosal ulcer. The organisms resemble histiocytes and immunohistochemistry is often required for a diagnosis from a mucosal biopsy, but the prominent nucleoli suggests the possibility of amebiasis.

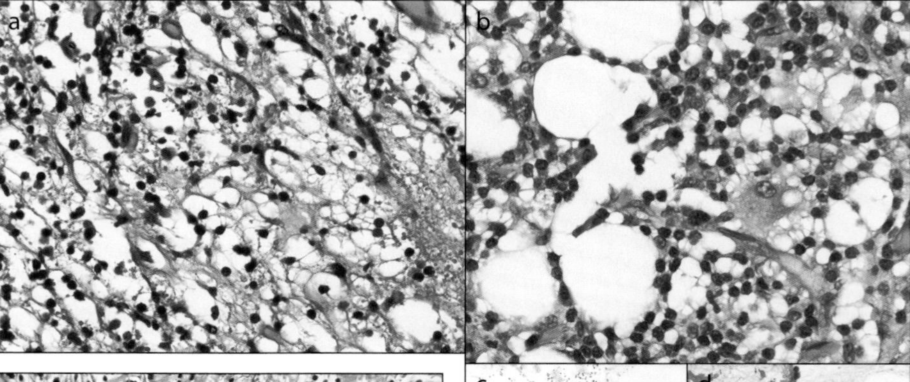

i22.40 **a** An interval appendectomy in which macrophages and lymphocytes, rather than neutrophils, predominant throughout the wall

b An interval appendectomy in which chronic inflammatory cells are found in the periappendiceal adipose tissue

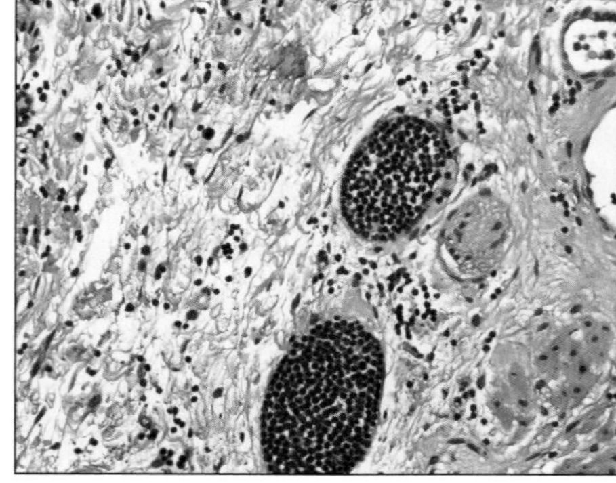

i22.41 An appendectomy specimen in which lymphocytes fill and distend a capillary, simulating a cluster of low-grade neuroendocrine carcinoma (carcinoid tumor). Immunohistochemical stains disclosed the lymphoid nature of these cells and were negative for all neuroendocrine markers.

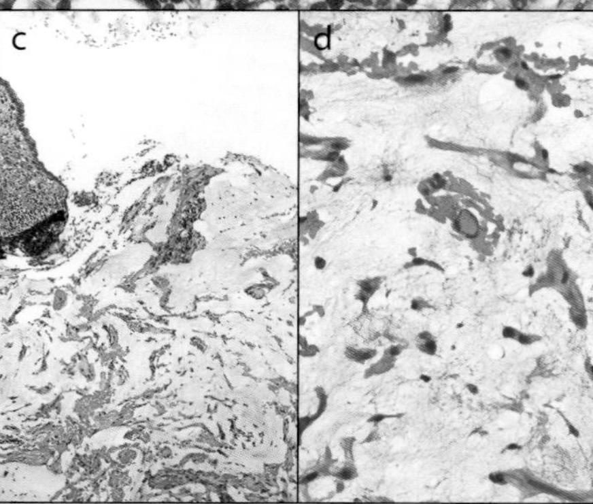

c An interval appendectomy in which a pool of mucin (a consequence of previous rupture) simulates a mucinous carcinoma
d The same case as in i22.41c, illustrating the absence of epithelial cells in the pool of mucin. The capillaries indicate a reparative response.

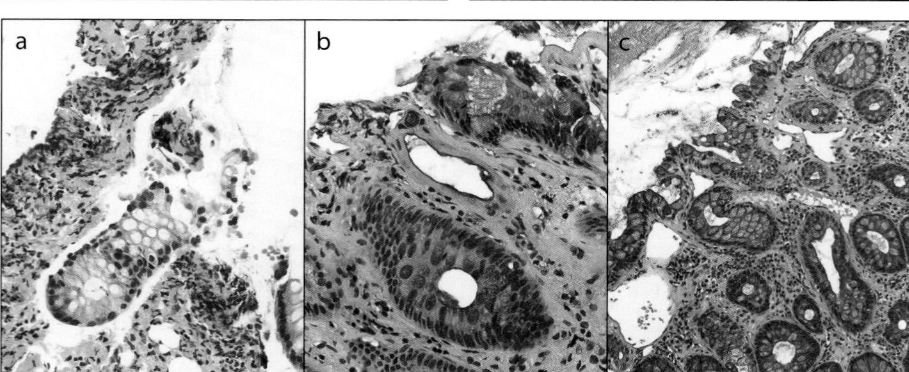

i22.42 **a** Acute radiation proctitis, with nonspecific ulceration
b Chronic radiation proctitis with stromal fibrosis and damage to the gland in the center

c Chronic radiation proctitis with dilated capillaries

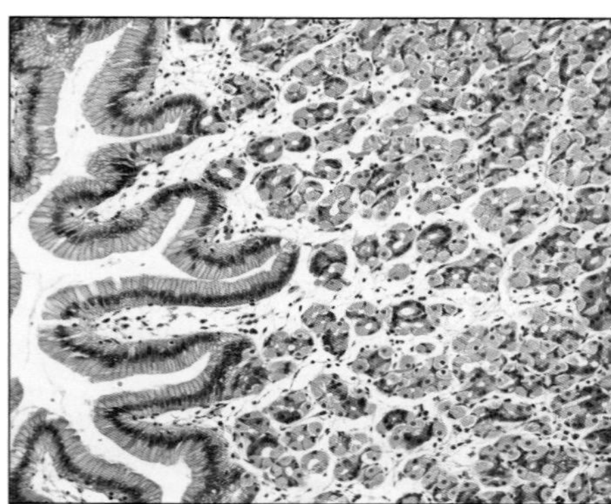

i22.43 Meckel diverticulum, with ectopic gastric mucosa. Note the parietal cells.

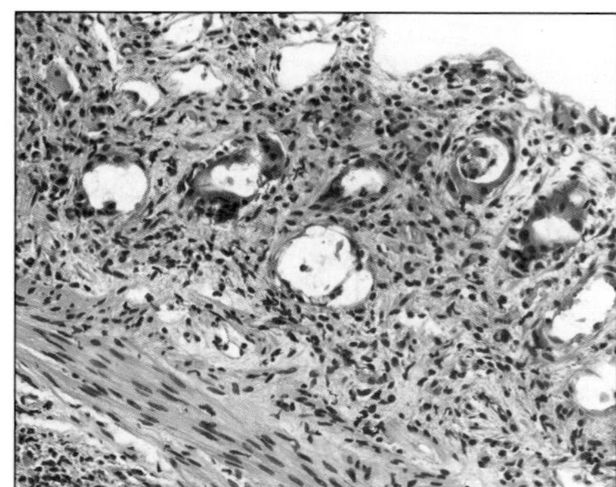

i22.44 Graft vs host disease in a colonic mucosal biopsy from a patient who has received bone marrow transplant. Note the extensive damage to and loss of glands.

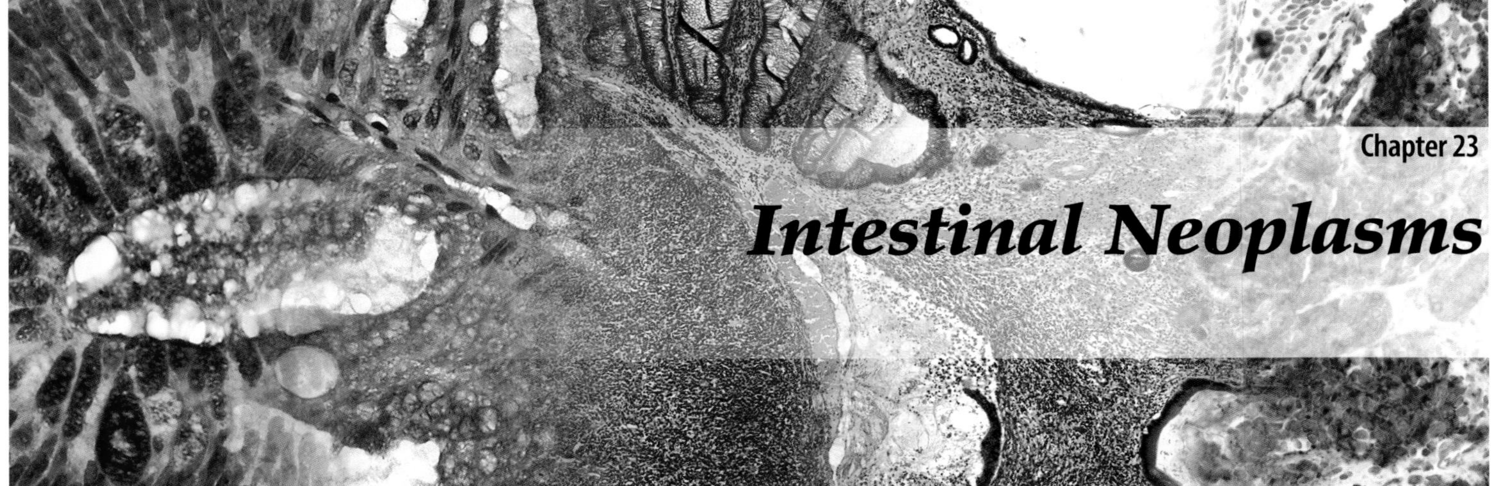

Chapter 23 Intestinal Neoplasms

There are 3 common nonneoplastic conditions of the proximal small bowel that can endoscopically simulate neoplasia: Brunner gland hyperplasia i22.3, heterotopic gastric mucosa i23.1, and heterotopic pancreas i23.2. Heterotopic gastric mucosa occurs in the proximal small bowel. Heterotopic pancreas may occur in the stomach or proximal small bowel. The distribution of acinar and islet elements is irregular in heterotopic pancreas, and normal pancreatic architecture may not be apparent.

In the small bowel, gastrointestinal stromal tumors (GISTs), lymphomas, neuroendocrine tumors, serosal mesotheliomas, and metastatic tumors are all more common than primary adenocarcinomas, and all of these should be excluded before a diagnosis of primary small bowel adenocarcinoma is made.

Intestinal Stromal Neoplasms

Because the H&E morphology, the immunohistochemical characteristics, and the molecular biology of intestinal GISTs are the same as those in the stomach [PMID17090188], they are diagnosed in the same way and with the same differential diagnosis as their gastric counterparts. However, the criteria for malignancy are different, and GISTs in the intestinal tract are more likely to be malignant than those in the stomach [PMID12094372]. Duodenal GISTs, for example, are usually malignant if they are very cellular, have 2 or more mitoses per 50 high-power fields (HPF), or are >4.5 cm in size, whereas these findings would be of far less concern in the stomach. In the jejunum, ileum, and colon, definitive criteria for malignancy have been elusive. A benign course can rarely be guaranteed in these locations, and the pathologist is better advised to offer an educated estimate about possible metastatic potential based on size, mitotic activity, and location. If a GIST in the intestinal tract is >5 cm *or* has >1 mitoses per 10 HPF, it is likely malignant i23.3a, i23.3b [PMID12094370, PMID12094372].

As is the case for gastric GISTs, the differential diagnosis of intestinal GISTs includes muscle and nerve sheath neoplasms, spindle cell carcinoma, inflammatory myofibroblastic tumor, mesothelioma, melanoma, and angiosarcoma. In addition, 2 other entities are encountered in the mesentery and enter the differential diagnosis for intestinal GISTs. These are mesenteric fibromatosis and sclerosing mesenteritis.

Although mesenteric fibromatosis and sclerosing mesenteritis occur in the mesentery rather than the wall of the gastrointestinal tract, they may clinically, grossly, and microscopically simulate an intestinal GIST. As is the case with fibromatoses in general (see i3.8a, i3.8b, i3.9, i3.10), mesenteric fibromatosis consists of uniform spindled cells in a stroma that may be focally myxoid or collagenous, but is not inflamed i23.3c-e. Mesenteric fibromatosis is unencapsulated and may sometimes infiltrate into the wall of the bowel, closely simulating a GIST [PMID16418255].

Sclerosing mesenteritis is an inflammatory condition of unknown etiology, but possibly associated with abdominal trauma or surgery, that eventuates in fibrosis through the normal reparative process. It has several appearances depending on when it is examined. Early lesions have a myxoid stroma with fat necrosis i23.3f. Neutrophils are rare, but scattered eosinophils may be seen in some cases [PMID20351487]. Chronic inflammation, perhaps with germinal centers and lipid-laden macrophages, follows i23.3g. The necrotic fat may be separated into lobules by septae. Sclerosis, perhaps with calcification, is seen in old lesions i23.3h. Fat necrosis and inflammation, consequences of the healing process, separate sclerosing mesenteritis from mesenteric fibromatosis. While sclerosing mesenteritis may initially simulate a GIST, it is not infiltrative and will not involve the bowel wall [PMID16418255].

The distinction of mesenteric fibromatosis from sclerosing mesenteritis can be important, but it is much more important to separate these entities from a GIST. GISTs are usually positive for CD117 and DOG1. Also, GISTs rarely express β-catenin. Sclerosing mesenteritis may express this protein, but not in the nucleus. Nuclear staining for β-catenin strongly suggests mesenteric fibromatosis over either GIST or sclerosing mesenteritis [PMID12360044].

Intestinal Lymphoid Proliferations

Proliferations of mucosa-associated lymphoid tissue may be reactive or neoplastic and can be immunohistochemically characterized, if necessary, in the same way as lymphoid proliferations elsewhere. Reactive lymphoid hyperplasia is particularly common in the terminal ileum. Low-grade lymphoid neoplasms of the intestines are often called MALTomas, but this term is not helpful clinically, and a specific immunophenotype is needed.

Immunoproliferative small-intestinal disease (also called Mediterranean lymphoma or α chain disease) is a lymphoma characterized by diarrhea, malabsorption, weight loss, and abdominal pain, and is usually found in the second or third decade. On biopsy, there is a diffuse plasma cell infiltrate mixed with small lymphocytes that immunohistochemically stain as marginal zone cells. Both the plasma cells and the small lymphocytes express monoclonal α chains without a light chain. Antibiotics may cause regression, and for this reason, this diagnosis should not be made without an antibiotic trial, as is the case for apparent extranodal marginal zone lymphomas of the stomach. Those cases that are truly neoplastic generally stain as marginal zone lymphomas [Nakemura ISBN 978-9283224327, PMID3683173].

Enteropathy-associated T-cell lymphoma (EATCL) is a T-cell lymphoma, often of the small intestine, that is associated with ulceration and malabsorption **i23.4a**, **i23.4b**. A disproportionate number of patients with EATCL have a history of celiac disease [Müller-Hermelink ISBN 978-9283224327]. EATCL should be excluded in situations where there is malabsorption or ulceration in the presence of a lymphoid infiltrate or large numbers of apparent macrophages, as the neoplastic lymphocytes in EATCL may resemble macrophages. Some cases of EATCL have gains of 9q [PMID12414511].

Mantle cell lymphomas are also common in the gastrointestinal tract, where they are often polypoid. Most small lymphoid polyps are benign **i23.5**, but mantle cell lymphomas are also common in the gastrointestinal tract are often polypoid. Many cases of polyposis of the bowel secondary to lymphoma are mantle cell lymphomas **i23.6a**, **i23.6b**.

Colonic Polyps and Adenocarcinoma

Little will be said about the interpretation and reporting of common colonic carcinoma, as this topic is well covered in other works.

Juvenile polyps are hamartomas of the lamina propria and have cystically dilated glands separated by expanded lamina propria, often with appreciable acute inflammation **i23.7**. They are most commonly seen in children but are sometimes seen in adults. Because of the concomitant acute inflammation, juvenile polyps were formerly called inflammatory polyps, but the latter term is no longer used because it is ambiguous and may connote a polyp of a different type, especially an inflammatory pseudopolyp secondary to inflammatory bowel disease, and might mislead the clinician into believing there is another pathologic process. A juvenile polyp may be a sporadic finding, but juvenile polyposis is an autosomal dominant syndrome.

Peutz-Jeghers polyps are hamartomas of smooth muscle. While the epithelial component may predominate, the core of smooth muscle results in a characteristic low-power arborizing appearance that is more orderly than a juvenile polyp **i23.8**. Sporadic Peutz-Jeghers polyps occur, but these are less common than sporadic juvenile polyps, and most patients with a Peutz-Jeghers polyp will have Peutz-Jeghers syndrome, which is autosomal dominant and occasionally associated with malignancies, especially of the breast and gastrointestinal tract [PMID20581245, PMID20051941].

The hyperplastic polyp is the simplest of all colonic polyps and it characterized by epithelial hyperplasia that has a "sawtooth" appearance on the surface **i23.9a**. In the interior, the hyperplasia results in glands with infoldings **i23.9b**. Nuclei remain small and basal **i23.9c**. There is no increase in malignant potential in the hyperplastic polyp.

The serrated adenoma has a low-power appearance similar to that of a hyperplastic polyp, with "sawtooth" epithelial hyperplasia and retention of ample cytoplasm **i23.10a**. But whereas the nuclei of a hyperplastic polyp are small and basal, those of the serrated adenoma are enlarged, round to ovoid, with a somewhat vesicular (peripheralized) chromatin pattern and occasional nucleoli **i23.10b**. The serrated adenoma may also have focal nuclear stratification **i23.10c** and mitoses, some of which may be close to the luminal surface. Some have defined a serrated adenoma architecturally, on the basis of the location of the serrations relative to the surface or lower layers of the epithelium. However, to my mind, it is a postulate in pathology that malignant potential is derived more from the appearance of the nucleus than from cellularity or architecture—a lesson first taught by Dr Papanicolaou—and I recommend that the diagnosis of serrated adenoma be based on nuclear morphology.

The biologic potential of the serrated adenoma appears to be that of an adenomatous polyp, and it may be helpful to state in parentheses that the serrated adenoma is essentially a type of adenomatous polyp [PMID16191506, PMID20551824].

In general, the nuclei of adenomatous polyps are enlarged and elongated, with coarse chromatin and small nucleoli **i23.11a**, **i23.11b**. They are larger than the nuclei of hyperplastic polyps, though a hyperplastic polyp may artifactually appear to be adenomatous if the section is thick **i23.12a**, **i23.12b**. Typical adenomatous polyps have only mild stratification of nuclei, largely limited to the lower half of the epithelial thickness **i23.11b**.

The terms "adenoma" and "adenomatous polyp" are interchangeable. Some adenomatous polyps have a villous architecture **i23.13**, and these may be called villous adenomas if entirely composed of a villous pattern or tubulovillous adenomas if partially of such a pattern. In this nomenclature, the term "tubular adenoma" refers to an adenomatous polyp without a villous component. However, because all of these types of adenomatous polyps have the same malignant potential and the only architectural features that are important to note are glandular crowding, irregular shapes, and nuclear stratification (as discussed in the following section on dysplasia in adenomatous polyps), these subclassifications of adenomatous polyps serve little point and potentially confuse the clinician, who simply needs to know the degree of dysplasia, and if possible, the completeness of removal.

i23.13a-c compare the nuclei of hyperplastic polyps, serrated adenomas, and adenomatous polyps. While there are exceptions among individual cells in any given polyp, and sweeping statements are to be avoided, in general, the nuclei of hyperplastic polyps are smaller than the other types **i23.14a**. The nuclei of serrated adenomas and adenomatous polyps are of roughly equal size, but in most cells, the nuclei of the former type are rounder and have a more open chromatin pattern **i23.14b**, while those of an adenomatous polyp are more spindled, with coarser chromatin and less prominent nucleoli **i23.14c**.

There are situations in which it is difficult to definitively classify a polyp. Indeed, some polyps are a mixture of 2 or even all 3 types **i23.14d**. In situations where it is difficult to distinguish between types of colonic polyps, I recommend leaning toward the "higher" diagnosis (eg, serrated adenoma or adenomatous polyp instead of hyperplastic polyp or adenomatous polyp instead of mixed hyperplastic-adenomatous polyp) so as to ensure adequate surveillance.

Mucosal prolapse may act alone and cause a polyp that endoscopically simulates one of the more conventional polyps i23.15a, or it may be superimposed on an existing polyp of a routine type i23.15b. Less common colonic polyps include those caused by leiomyomas of the muscularis mucosa i23.16, lymphoid follicles i23.5, and ganglioneuromas i23.17a-c.

Dysplasia in Adenomatous Polyps

Few areas are more controversial than the matter of dysplasia in colonic adenomatous polyps. The first concept to realize is that by definition, *all* adenomatous polyps have low-grade adenocarcinoma-directed dysplasia. For this reason, specific mention of low-grade dysplasia in a typical adenomatous polyp is unnecessary and is likely to confuse the clinician into believing that the polyp has a greater biologic potential than it actually has. The lowest degree of dysplasia that should be specifically mentioned is intermediate-grade dysplasia, but the WHO classification recognizes only the categories of low-grade dysplasia (ie, no "added" dysplasia) and high-grade dysplasia [Hamilton ISBN 978-9283224327]. Any mention of dysplasia should include a comment that ordinary adenomatous polyps have low-grade dysplasia, so the clinician can see how many "steps" above an ordinary adenomatous polyp this particular polyp is.

Assessment of dysplasia in polyps must work hand-in-glove with increased colon cancer screening. If the pathologist can identify those polyps that have a higher degree of dysplasia, the complete removal of those polyps and more frequent surveillance of those patients augment the effectiveness of colon cancer screening. The 3 criteria that are most consistently useful in identifying adenomatous polyps that have increased dysplasia are irregularly shaped or crowded glands, nuclear stratification, and severe nuclear atypia [Hamilton ISBN 978-9283224327, PMID11554160, PMID7959660]. "Irregularly shaped or crowded glands" refers to glands that have irregular contours or a cribriform appearance, or abut each other without intervening stroma i23.18a, i23.18b. Nuclear stratification refers to nuclei that are found in the upper half of the epithelium i23.18c. Severe nuclear atypia refers to a nuclear appearance that is indistinguishable from that of an invasive carcinoma. Specifically, the nucleus of an adenomatous polyp with high-grade dysplasia is large and round, rather that the elongated nucleus of the usual adenomatous polyp, and often has vesicular chromatin and a prominent nucleolus i23.18d. Large numbers of mitoses, especially in the upper portion of the epithelium, may also be considered, though this tends to reflect the degree of stratification. Villous architecture is no longer generally regarded as independently significant.

Although these 3 broad criteria are generally agreed upon, there is wide interobserver variation in how they are applied. Some will diagnose high-grade dysplasia if only 1 of the above findings is present, and others will diagnose intermediate-grade dysplasia if 1 or 2 criteria are present. To my mind, it is prudent to accept 1 of the above findings as still within the spectrum of a routine adenomatous polyp (ie, low-grade dysplasia), while 2 or more suggest high-grade dysplasia, which is essentially synonymous with adenocarcinoma in situ (AIS). In borderline situations, it might be reasonable to make a "lower" diagnosis if there is a well defined negative stalk or base, and a "higher" diagnosis if the lesion is incompletely removed.

There is no consensus on the term "intramucosal carcinoma." Some do not use the term since the distinction of AIS from intramucosal invasion is unlikely to be clinically significant because the mucosa lacks lymphatic vessels except for rare lymphatic channels in the muscularis mucosa [PMID12926829], and therefore, there is no chance of metastases in intramucosal carcinoma. Others believe that intramucosal invasion is a recognizable step between AIS and submucosal invasion. Among the latter group, some believe that the diagnosis of invasion into the mucosa requires the same criteria as are used to identify invasion anywhere, including a desmoplastic stroma i23.19a. Others believe intramucosal invasion can be inferred from extensive, confluent areas of AIS in the mucosa, even without a stromal reaction i23.19b, i23.19c. The important point is to verify that there has not been invasion into the submucosa, because invasion into the submucosa introduces the possibility for metastases. The muscularis mucosa can be difficult to identify in polyps, making it potentially problematic to determine if an adenocarcinoma is invasive only into the mucosa or also into the submucosa. In questionable cases, a trichrome stain or an immunohistochemical stain for actin may highlight the muscularis mucosa.

The management of situations in which carcinoma in a polyp invades into the submucosa is not completely settled. Many feel it is permissible to manage these cases by polypectomy alone if the carcinoma is not poorly differentiated, there is no vascular invasion, and there is a stalk or base that can be shown to be negative [PMID1395979]. Not everyone is comfortable with this approach, however, and there is a risk of nodal metastases in these situations, ranging from 2-25% in differing studies [PMID7305483]. The precise risk of management by polypectomy alone is difficult to assess, probably because of disagreement regarding whether or not the stalk is invaded, and if so, whether or not its base is truly negative, and how thoroughly lymph node dissection is performed after resection.

Although there are a number of syndromes that involve colonic neoplasms, there are 2 major colon carcinoma syndromes, one with polyposis (familial adenomatous polyposis) and one without polyposis (hereditary nonpolyposis colon cancer syndrome; also called Lynch syndrome). Gardner syndrome is familial adenomatous polyposis with extraintestinal manifestations. Both of these syndromes are inherited in an autosomal dominant manner.

Colorectal Cancer Screening

At this writing, traditional colonoscopy is far and away the best method of early detection. The colonoscopic detection of flat premalignant lesions is challenging, but newer endoscopic methods using dyes (so-called chromoendoscopy) or magnification are promising. Colonography (the "virtual" colonoscopy by CT scan) requires the same preparation as the traditional procedure—universally acknowledged as the most trying part of the test—and is therefore only slightly less inconvenient to the patient. Colonography also introduces the dilemma of what to do if a polyp is found. Must it be removed? The literature is settling on the matter at this writing, but there is support for a protocol of recommending colonoscopy and removal of polyps

>1 cm and not pursuing polyps that are <0.5 cm, with a gray zone in between [PMID20501711, PMID20451813, PMID20451812].

Stool testing for occult blood is a very poor surrogate for colonoscopy and simply serves to identify a group of patients who need further testing. When testing for occult blood is indicated, a fecal immunochemical test is recommended over the traditional hemoccult cards because it uses a monoclonal antibody that is specific for human hemoglobin and therefore avoids interference from dietary hemoglobin [PMID16998938].

Testing of plasma for methylated DNA sequences that are associated with malignancies is another promising avenue of screening. Since methylation of a promoter site diminishes the transcription of a gene (this is a form of epigenetic regulation of the genome, discussed in Chapter 47), hypermethylation of promoters of tumor suppressor genes can silence them and thereby lead to neoplasia. The detection of methylated DNA for the gene septin 9 (SEPT9) in plasma may be helpful in screening for colon cancer [PMID19406918]. For reasons that are not yet clear, hypermethylation of genes that do not serve a known tumor suppressor function may also be associated with neoplasia. The vimentin gene, which codes for an intermediate filament structural protein and is not a known tumor suppressor, is hypermethylated in many colon carcinomas, and the identification of this in stool specimens is a promising means of early colon cancer detection [PMID18759824].

The Colectomy Specimen

In addition to an assessment of tumor differentiation in general, I recommend that the pathologist comment on the degree of differentiation of the tumor at the advancing front in colon carcinomas, as this may be less differentiated than the bulk of the tumor **i23.20a**, **i23.20b**. Reduced differentiation or buds of tumor cells branching from a larger cluster at the advancing front correlate with increased lymph node metastases in T1 (submucosally invasive) colon carcinomas [PMID20473277].

As is the case for so many other tumors, attempts to identify important prognostic variables other than tumor grade and stage have met with mixed results at best. Supposedly independent prognostic variables in colon carcinoma that may portend an aggressive course include microacinar architecture, neuroendocrine differentiation (if confirmed by immunohistochemical stains), tufting of tumor cells, and CD10 expression. A Crohn-like lymphoid or granulomatous reaction has been suggested as a favorable finding. As is the case for other sites, firmly established independent prognostic variables are elusive and even when successfully identified, add only indirectly to patient care.

An area of controversy is the number of lymph nodes that the pathologist should recover in the gross examination of a colon cancer resection. Some have opined that if no positive nodes are found, anything less than 12 lymph nodes constitutes a suboptimal examination and is a potential false negative. The difficulty with such broad, sweeping statements is that there is variability in the number of pericolic nodes among patients, fewer nodes will be expected in shorter resections, the number of nodes varies from place to place in the colon, and nodes are rendered less conspicuous by neoadjuvant chemotherapy. Moreover, in 2007, Wong et al found that a higher number of total lymph nodes recovered does not increase the detection of positive nodes and does not impact survival [PMID18000198]. Kukreja et al found similar results 2 years later [PMID19620539] and offered a particularly important conclusion that the designation of "Centers of Excellence," with probable financial implications for the laboratory or hospital, should not be based on lymph node recovery.

It has been my consistent experience that there are cases that simply do not have 12 pericolic lymph nodes. To my mind, if a thorough initial examination does not recover 12 nodes, the specimen should be reexamined after additional fixation in an attempt to increase the number, and the report should indicate that a second gross examination was performed. However, if 2 examinations do not recover any positive lymph nodes and the total is <12, the clinician needs to understand that neither he nor his patient has in any way been shortchanged. The best scholarship is not to demand an absolute standard in all cases without considering the many causes of variability, but rather to set a goal, make every effort to meet it, and accept and explain deviations on a case by case basis where necessary.

There is interest in sentinel lymph node examination in colon carcinomas. Some preliminary data suggest that sentinel node examination is often a reasonable substitute for a full lymph node dissection, especially in colon (as opposed to rectal) carcinomas [PMID19261431]. An additional benefit of sentinel lymph node examination is that it potentially obviates much of the controversy concerning the number of nodes recovered. However, not all of the early experience has been promising. Bertagnolli et al found a 54% false negative rate [PMID15383790].

Ano-rectal carcinomas are occasionally treated by neoadjuvant chemotherapy or radiation therapy before surgery. In these cases, the pathologist may be called upon to assess the effect of the neoadjuvant therapy after resection. A 5-tiered system has been proposed [PMID21771024], but in most cases, an evaluation of viable tumor cells and fibrosis suffices **i23.21a-c**.

Intestinal Carcinomas with Neuroendocrine Differentiation

Most intestinal neoplasms with neuroendocrine differentiation are pure, low-grade neuroendocrine carcinomas (carcinoid tumors) in the appendix **i23.22** or terminal ileum **i23.23**. The rectum is also a relatively common site. Low-grade neuroendocrine carcinomas are usually indolent, especially in the appendix, though those in the terminal ileum may be aggressive **i23.24a**, **i23.24b**.

The World Health Organization currently lists 3 categories of tumors with features of both a neuroendocrine tumor and an adenocarcinoma [Klimstra ISBN 978-9283224327]. The first of these is a carcinoid with a tubular pattern, in which a lumen is enclosed by a single layer of cells with the same uniform appearance as those forming low-grade neuroendocrine carcinomas in a trabecular pattern **i23.25**. This neoplasm is probably a pure carcinoid (ie, low-grade neuroendocrine carcinoma) that can resemble an adenocarcinoma because the neuroendocrine rosettes resemble glands. It is relatively indolent, especially if it occurs in the appendix.

The second neoplasm with morphologic features of both a neuroendocrine carcinoma, and a conventional adenocarcinoma is one in which individual cells have features of both a neuroendocrine tumor and an adenocarcinoma. This is often manifested as the so-called goblet cell carcinoid, because individual cells may have both neuroendocrine features and a distinct cytoplasmic vacuole i23.26a, i23.26b. Although not as aggressive as a conventional adenocarcinoma, goblet cell carcinoids have metastatic potential and warrant a hemicolectomy [PMID20524865].

The third tumor in this category is the mixed neuroendocrine carcinoma-adenocarcinoma, which consists of separate areas of each tumor type i23.27a-c. Because of its pure adenocarcinoma component, it is more aggressive than a goblet cell carcinoid and will behave as a conventional adenocarcinoma. This category includes neoplasms that initially appear to be goblet cell carcinoids, but that are actually a mixture of a conventional carcinoid and a mucinous signet ring adenocarcinoma i23.28a-c.

Neoplasms with features of both a neuroendocrine tumor and an adenocarcinoma may overlap, both morphologically and immunohistochemically. The unqualified term "adenocarcinoid" is confusing, and is used by some as synonymous with goblet cell carcinoid and by others as a mixed neuroendocrine carcinoma-adenocarcinoma. I recommend avoiding this term, or at least descriptively qualifying it if used.

Very rarely, there will be a high-grade neuroendocrine carcinoma (small cell carcinoma) that is primary in the gastrointestinal tract i23.29a-d.

Unusual Intestinal Neoplasms

The medullary carcinoma is a form of undifferentiated colonic carcinoma. It resembles a breast medullary carcinoma, with highly pleomorphic nuclei and occasionally prominent nucleoli. There is very little gland formation, if any i23.30. Cytoplasmic mucin is inconspicuous and usually cannot be demonstrated. Lymphocytes may be adjacent to or within the tumor. The medullary carcinoma should be excluded in any colorectal carcinoma that has minimal gland formation or a neuroendocrine appearance but is negative for neuroendocrine markers. Medullary colonic carcinomas tend to arise from defective DNA repair and have both microsatellite instability and a deficiency of the mismatch repair protein MLH1. In addition, they differ from conventional colon carcinomas in that they are usually positive for calretinin, a marker that is used to stain mesothelial cells and is negative for CDX2 [PMID18992917]. Despite the alarming nuclear appearance and the minimal gland formation, the colonic medullary carcinoma has a better prognosis than conventional colon carcinomas.

The appendix may be the site of an ordinary colonic adenocarcinoma, of the full range of neuroendocrine tumors described above, or of mucinous tumors that are difficult to evaluate. Although simple mucoceles do exist, most mucinous distention of the appendix is caused by a neoplasm, and certainly, any such distention or any pools of mucin found in an appendix should prompt the submission of the entire specimen. Appendiceal mucinous neoplasms may be adenomas, mucinous tumors of uncertain malignant potential (UMP), or fully malignant mucinous adenocarcinomas i23.31a, i23.31b.

Appendiceal mucinous neoplasms are the most common cause of pseudomyxoma peritonei, even in the presence of a mucinous ovarian neoplasm [PMID17511804]. Any peritoneal mucinous deposit should be closely examined for epithelial cells, using immunohistochemical stains if necessary, but even if none are found, it is wise to examine the appendix.

Molecular Pathology in Colorectal Cancer

Many colon carcinomas have some chromosomal abnormality. Among the numerous chromosomal abnormalities that have been reported are losses of 8p or 18q [PMID20709793]. However, most colon cancers arise through 1 of 2 mechanisms related to individual genes, not to chromosomal abnormalities. 80% of colon cancers and the vast majority of sporadic cases are thought to arise from accumulated abnormalities of tumor suppressor genes, such as *P53*, *APC*, *K-RAS*, and *SMAD4*. This pathway to neoplasia has been well described by Vogelstein (eg, [PMID15286780]). A minority of colon cancers arise as part of a syndrome, the 2 most common of which are familial adenomatous polyposis (FAP; also called adenomatous polyposis coli [APC]) and hereditary nonpolyposis colon cancer syndrome, both of which are discussed in Chapter 46.

While there has long been anecdotal feeling that rectal adenocarcinomas may have a different behavior from those arising elsewhere in the colon, recent work in the molecular biology of adenocarcinomas from the rectum and colon has shown that this is not the case, and that rectal adenocarcinomas are not different from general colonic adenocarcinomas [PMID22810696].

Increased understanding of the molecular biology of colorectal carcinoma is beginning to find clinical application. The *ERB-B* family of genes encodes transmembrane proteins that contain an intracellular tyrosine kinase that is important in initiating the intracellular response to extracellular growth factors. The epidermal growth factor receptor gene (*EGFR*) and *HER2* are members of this family. Just as some cases of breast cancer overexpress *HER2* and are candidates for treatment with trastuzumab (Herceptin), some cases of colon cancer overexpress the EGFR protein. If overexpression is found (immunohistochemistry is usually used to identify these cases), cetuximab (Erbitux) or panitumumab (Vectibix), monoclonal antibodies that bind to the extracellular domain of the EGFR protein and diminish its signaling capacity, may be beneficial [PMID20524863]. These drugs have a roughly comparable effect on the EGFR protein to that of Herceptin on the Her2 protein.

As is the case for lung cancer, the Ras protein family, of which K-ras is the most important, receives input from the EGFR protein. The normal, wild-type form of the *K-RAS* gene is found in 50-70% of colorectal cancer patients. In these patients, the signaling pathway distal to EGFR is normal, and blockade of the receptor may be helpful. However, 30-50% of colorectal carcinoma patients have a gain of function mutation in *K-RAS*, usually from a mutation in codons 12 or 13 [PMID19644023]. These patients do not benefit from EGFR blockade, presumably because the mutant K-ras protein is autonomous and does not require activation by the EGFR pathway. For this reason, before therapy with cetuximab or panitumumab is instituted to blockade EGFR, colon cancers are often tested for a mutation in *K-RAS* [PMID19117687]. In addition to *K-RAS*, mutations in the genes *BRAF* or *PIK3CA* may result in proteins that function independently of the EGFR protein and therefore negate the benefit of EGFR blockade [PMID19738166]. It is worthwhile to retest a colorectal carcinoma for these mutations if a metastasis occurs because the genotype of a metastasis may differ from the primary [PMID21704278].

Gefitinib (Iressa) and erlotinib (Tarceva) are inhibitors of the intracellular tyrosine kinase moiety of EGFR. At this writing, they are used in some cases of advanced non-small cell

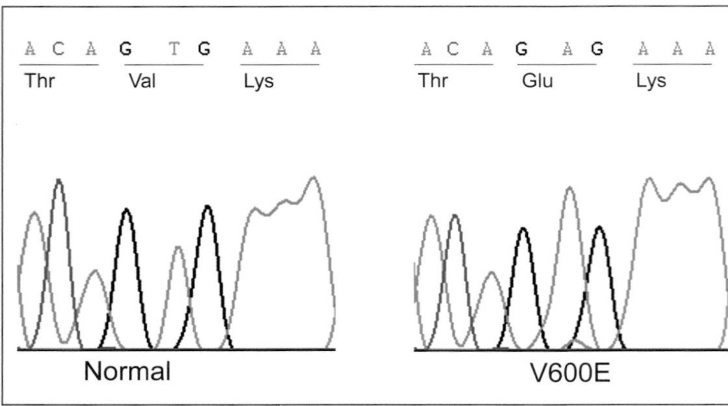

f23.1 A V600E (glutamate instead of valine at amino acid position 600) mutation in the *BRAF* gene in a sporadic colorectal carcinoma. The relevant codon is in the center and is a GTG on the left (coding for valine) but a mutated GAG (coding for glutamate) on the right.

carcinoma of the lung and are in phase II trials for colorectal carcinomas [PMID20524863]. They, or similar drugs, may find their way into use in some cases of colon cancer, but since they still target part of the EGFR molecule, there presumably will still be the problem of mutations conferring autonomy to downstream genes.

The V600E mutation in the *BRAF* gene found in some cases of thyroid cancer, is also found in some cases of sporadic colorectal carcinomas that have microsatellite instablity (discussed in Chapter 46) [PMID20489114] f23.1. Attention is being focused on this subgroup because there is an inhibitor of the Braf enzyme (vemurafenib).

The Anal Canal

"Anal canal intraepithelial neoplasia" (ACIN or AIN) is accepted terminology for squamous dysplasias in this location, reflecting the movement toward the terminology "intraepithelial neoplasia" instead of "dysplasia" in all sites. AIN is graded on a scale of 1-3, using the same criteria as are used in the cervix i23.32a-c. Anal canal squamous carcinomas are strongly associated with human papillomavirus, especially types 16 and 18 [PMID11231953, PMID11231961]. Interestingly, as is the case for high-grade cervical intraepithelial neoplasia, 90% of cases of AIN 2 or 3 are positive for the protein P16INK4a (usually just called p16, discussed in Chapter 46). Many cases of AIN also demonstrate staining for the proliferation marker Ki-67 in cells above the basal layer [PMID16819320].

The anal canal is one of the sites in which the verrucous carcinoma may be found i23.33. The diagnosis of verrucous carcinoma is made here as in other locations, but as in other sites, the precise terminology is less important than identifying invasion and assessing resection margins.

The terms "transitional" and "cloacogenic" are not used now, and these carcinomas are best thought of as squamous carcinomas of the basaloid type, as are encountered in other sites i23.34. Invasive carcinomas of the anal canal should simply be called squamous carcinomas, with a comment on whether it is of the common or basaloid type.

Core Points for Intestinal Neoplasms

- Intestinal GISTs: morphologic, immunohistochemical, and molecular characteristics parallel those in the stomach.
- Intestinal lymphomas: evaluated as in other sites.
- Mantle cell lymphomas of the gastrointestinal tract often present as polyps, but most lymphoid polyps are benign.
- Immunoproliferative small-intestinal disease (Mediterranean lymphoma): a low-grade lymphoma, with plasma cells
  - Often accompanied by diarrhea and malabsorption
  - Predominantly affecting patients in the second or third decade
- Enteropathy-associated T-cell lymphoma (EATCL): a high-grade lymphoma associated with ulceration and malabsorption
- Juvenile polyps: hamartomas of the lamina propria
  - Characterized by dilated glands and acute inflammation
- Peutz-Jeghers polyps: hamartomas of smooth muscle
- Hyperplastic polyp: "sawtooth" epithelial hyperplasia, with nuclei that are small and basal
- Serrated adenoma: serrations of a hyperplastic polyp, but nuclei are enlarged and round, with vesicular chromatin and occasional nucleoli.
  - Nuclear stratification and mitoses are common. The individual nuclei of a serrated adenoma are larger than those of a hyperplastic polyp, and rounder, with more vesicular chromatin, than those of an adenomatous polyp.
- Adenomatous polyps: nuclei are elongated, with coarse chromatin and small nucleoli, and differ from those of either the hyperplastic polyp or the serrated adenoma.
  - Low-grade dysplasia by definition.
- Adenomatous polyps with high-grade dysplasia: irregularly shaped or crowded glands, nuclear stratification, and severe nuclear atypia.
- Most cases in which carcinoma in a polyp invades into the submucosa can be managed by polypectomy if:
  - The carcinoma is not poorly differentiated
  - There is no vascular invasion
  - There is a negative stalk or base
- Most colon cancers are sporadic and arise from abnormalities of tumor suppressor genes, such as *K-RAS* and *P53*.
- Some colon cancers overexpress epidermal growth factor receptor (EGFR)
  - Blockade of its extracellular portion or inhibition of its intracellular tyrosine kinase portion may be beneficial.
- But 30-50% of colorectal carcinoma patients have a gain of function mutation in the *K-RAS* gene
  - The K-ras protein is decoupled from EGFR and the tumor is refractory to either extracellular blockade of EGFR or inhibition of its intracellular tyrosine kinase.

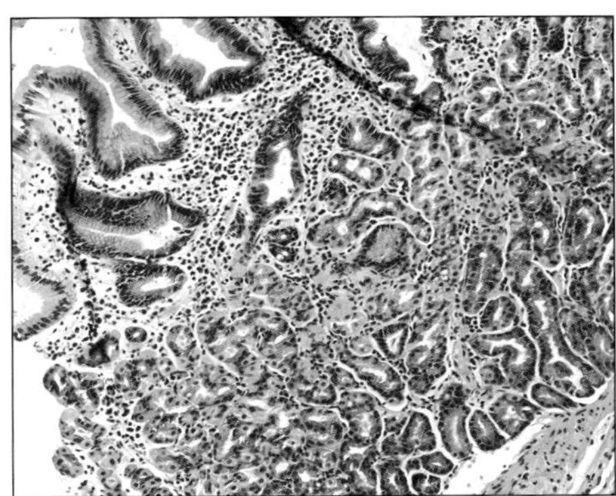

i23.1 Heterotopic gastric mucosa in the duodenum

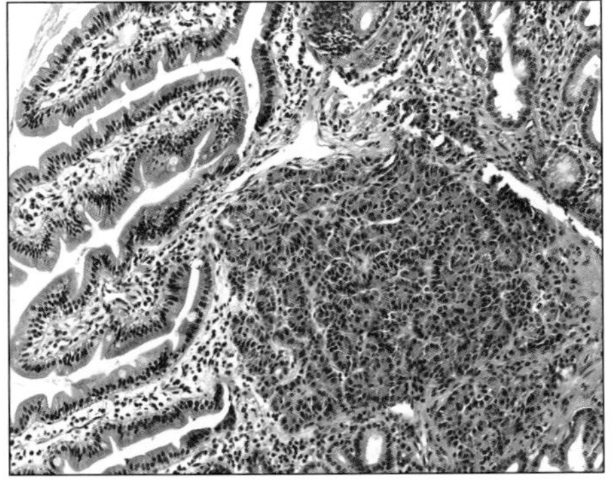

i23.2 Heterotopic pancreatic tissue in the duodenum

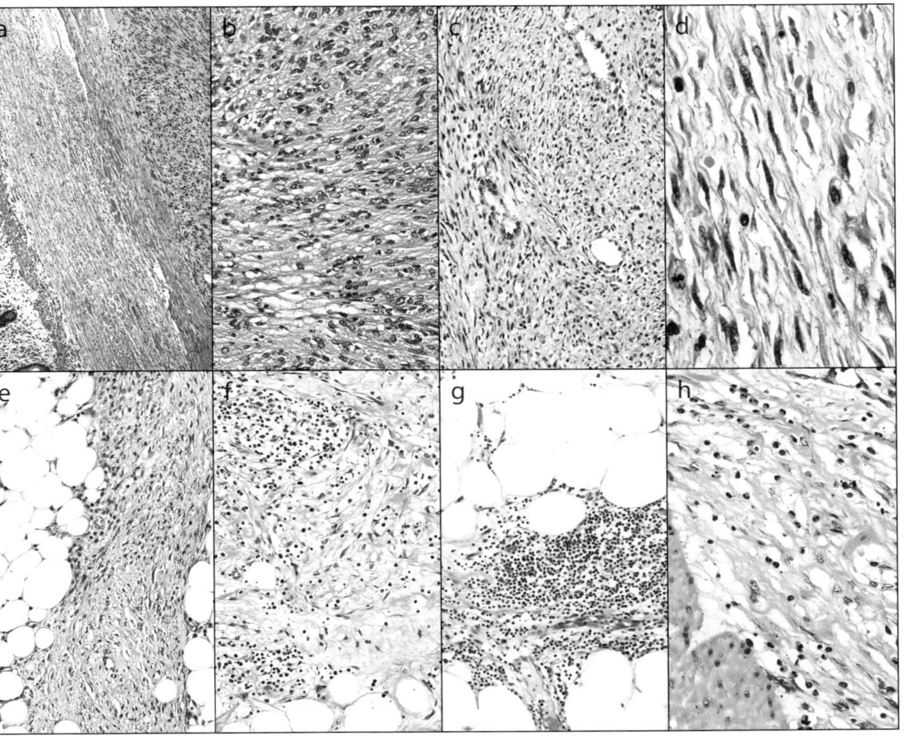

i23.3 a A gastrointestinal stromal tumor of the colon **b** A higher-power view of the same case as in i23.3a. This neoplasm was positive for CD117 and was of uncertain malignant potential. **c** Mesenteric fibromatosis. As is the case for fibromatosis in other sites, there is a uniform proliferation of fibroblasts in a stroma that varies from myxoid to collagenous. **d** A high-power view of the same case as in i23.3c, illustrating the nuclear uniformity **e** Mesenteric fibromatosis infiltrating lobules of fat in the mesentery. This process may also infiltrate the bowel wall, simulating a GIST. **f** Sclerosing mesenteritis. Fat necrosis, which is typically seen in the early stages of this entity. **g** A later stage of sclerosing mesenteritis in which chronic inflammation is present. Lipid-laden macrophages are also commonly seen at this stage, and there may be overt lymphoid follicles. **h** Long-standing sclerosing mesenteritis with collagenous fibrosis. Note that the process extends to the muscularis propria on the left, but, unlike mesenteric fibromatosis, will not infiltrate it.

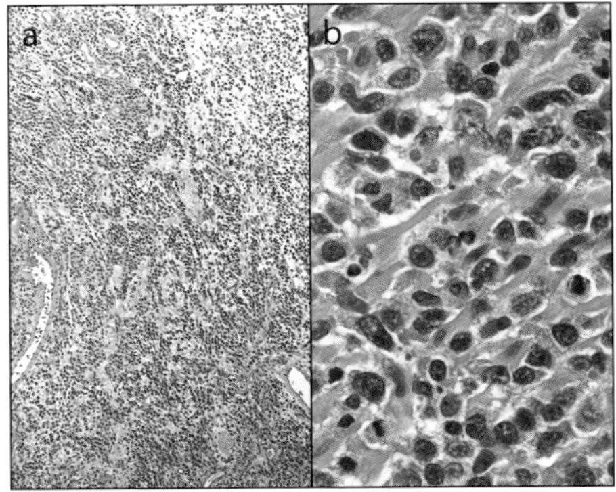

i23.4 a Enteropathy-associated T-cell lymphoma of the small intestine **b** Enteropathy-associated T-cell lymphoma. A higher-power view of the same case as in i23.4a.

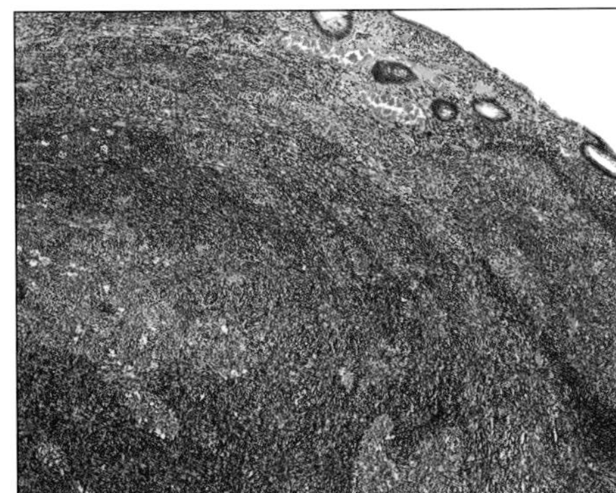

i23.5 Lymphoid hyperplasia of the colon, resulting in an endoscopically evident polyp

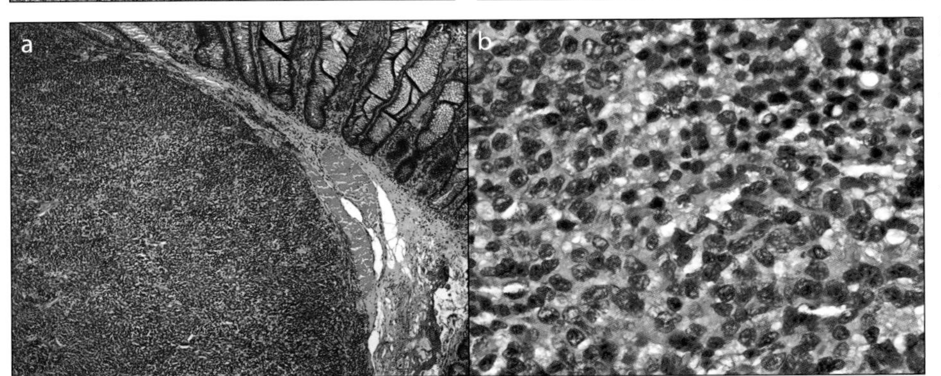

i23.6 a Mantle zone lymphoma of the colon, resulting in an endoscopically evident polyp **b** A higher-power view of the same case as in i23.6a, illustrating the uniform population of small lymphocytes that is characteristic of mantle cell lymphoma. These cells were positive for bcl-1.

ISBN 978-089189-5886

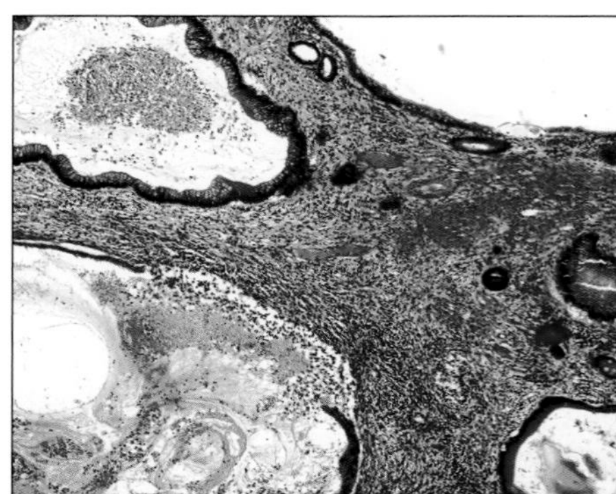

i23.7 A juvenile polyp of the colon, with sharply expanded lamina propria and acute inflammation

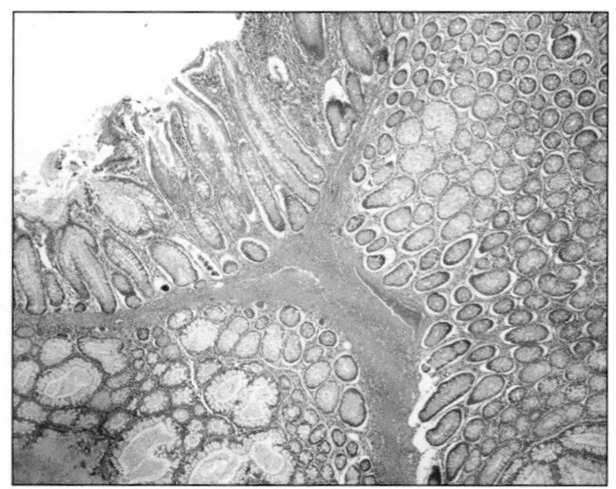

i23.8 A Peutz-Jeghers polyp. Although the bulk of the polyp is composed of epithelium, the fundamental process is hyperplasia of the smooth muscle from the muscularis mucosa, resulting in an arborizing appearance.

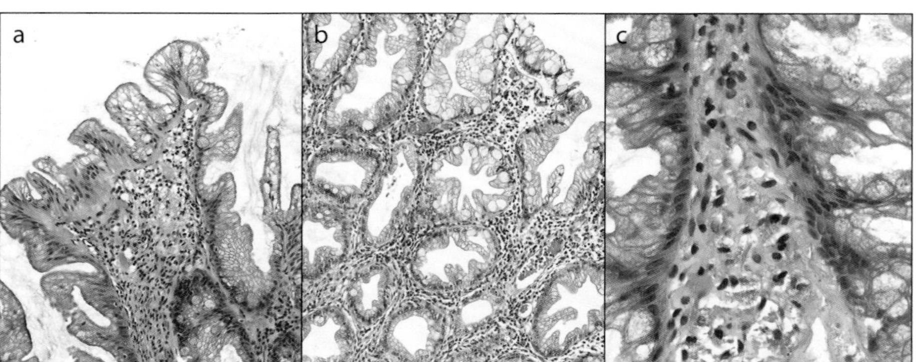

i23.9 **a** A hyperplastic colonic polyp with "saw tooth" hyperplasia of the surface epithelium **b** The interior of a colonic hyperplastic polyp, where the epithelial hyperplasia has resulted in infolding **c** The nuclei of a hyperplastic polyp are small, uniform, and basal, with minimal nucleoli

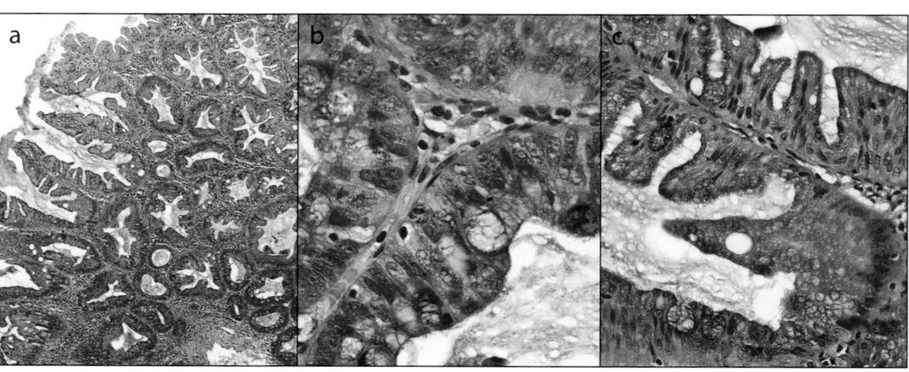

i23.10 **a** A serrated adenoma. The low-power appearance is virtually identical to that of a hyperplastic polyp. **b** The same case as in i23.10a, illustrating the nuclei of a serrated adenoma, which are significantly larger than those of a hyperplastic polyp. Note the generally open chromatin pattern, with small nucleoli. **c** A serrated adenoma with nuclear stratification

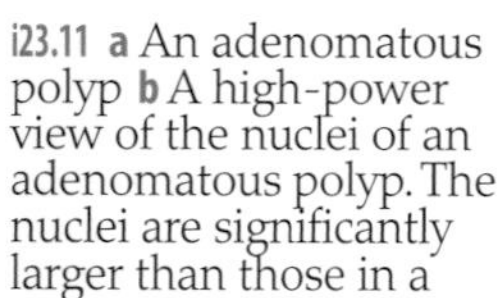

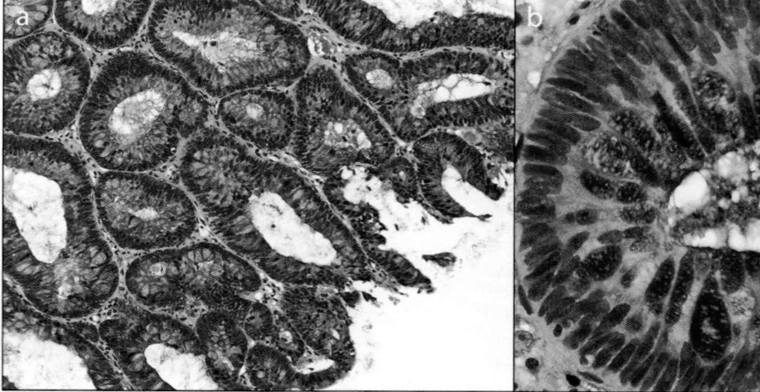

i23.11 **a** An adenomatous polyp **b** A high-power view of the nuclei of an adenomatous polyp. The nuclei are significantly larger than those in a hyperplastic polyp, but they are more spindled, with coarser chromatin and less distinct nucleoli than the nuclei of a serrated adenoma.

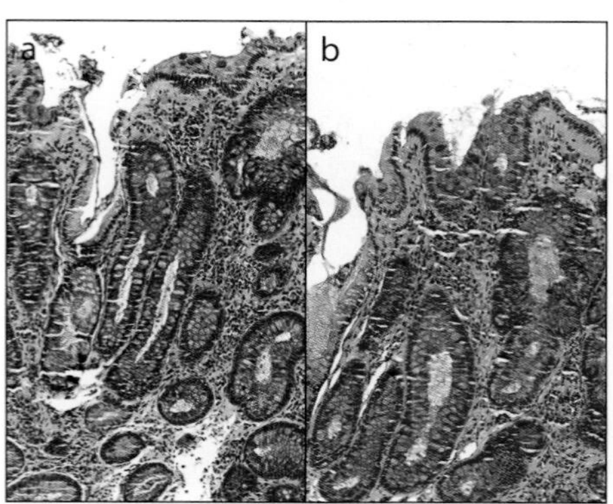

i23.12 **a** A colonic polyp that appears adenomatous in a thick section but **b** hyperplastic in the thinner section

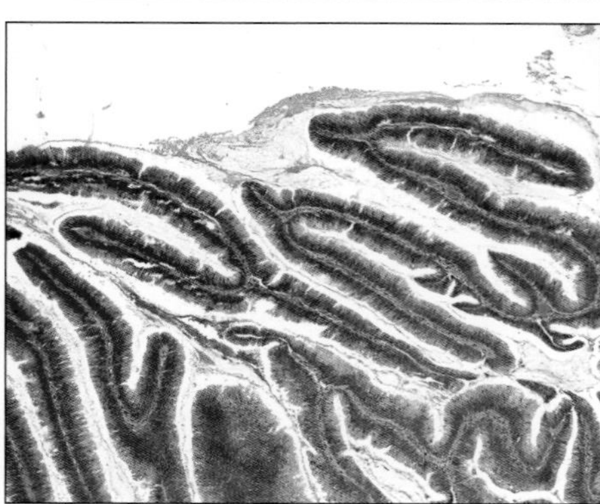

i23.13 An adenomatous polyp with a villous architecture (villous adenoma)

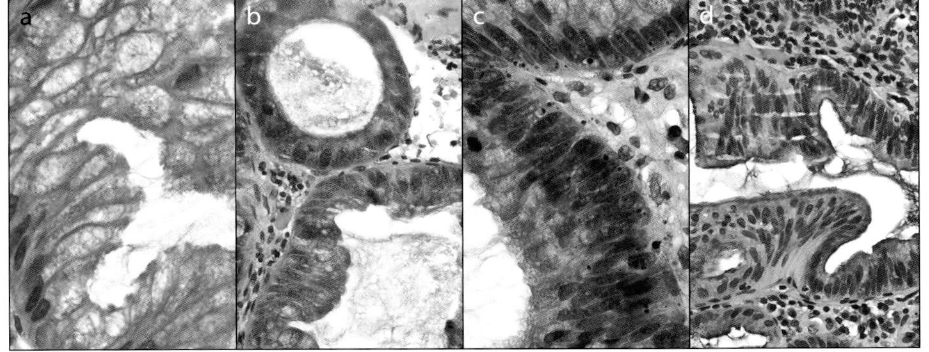

i23.14 Side-by-side comparisons of the nuclei in **a** a hyperplastic polyp, **b** a serrated adenoma, and **c** an adenomatous polyp.

d shows a polyp in which a gland has an abrupt transition between an area of adenomatous change and an area of serration and nuclear stratification. In the lower right corner of the photograph, still in the polyp, there is a gland with the small nuclei characteristic of a hyperplastic polyp.

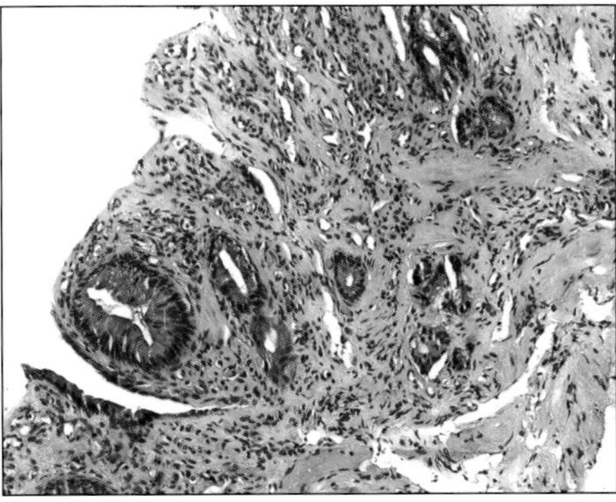

i23.15 Mucosal prolapse that resulted in an endoscopically evident polyp. Mucosal prolapse superimposed on a hyperplastic polyp in the sigmoid. Note the stromal fibrosis in the left-center.

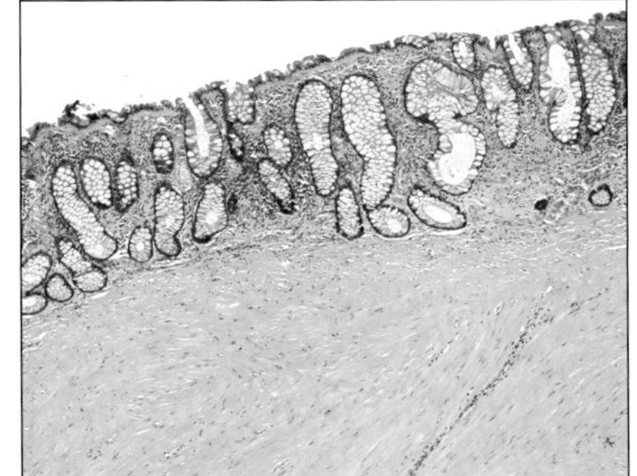

i23.16 A leiomyoma of the muscularis mucosa

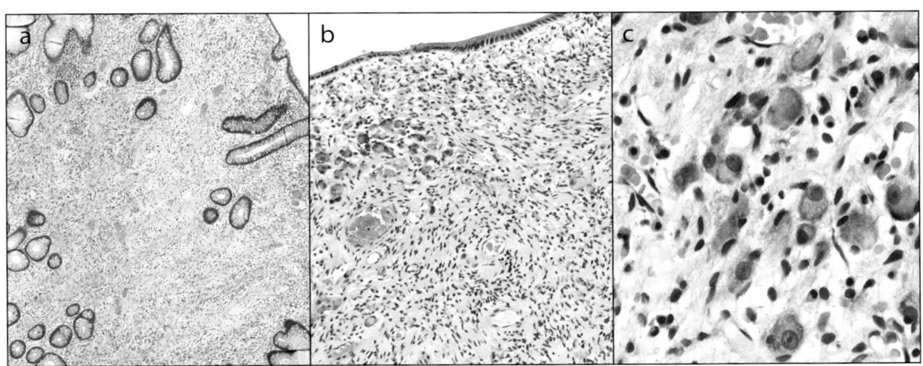

i23.17 A ganglioneuroma of the colon, presenting as a polyp. **a** is a low-power view illustrating the schwannoma-like stroma that pushes aside the glands.
b illustrates the stroma and the ganglioneuroma cells.

c illustrates the characteristic prominent nucleoli and abundant amphophilic cytoplasm of ganglioneuroma cells.

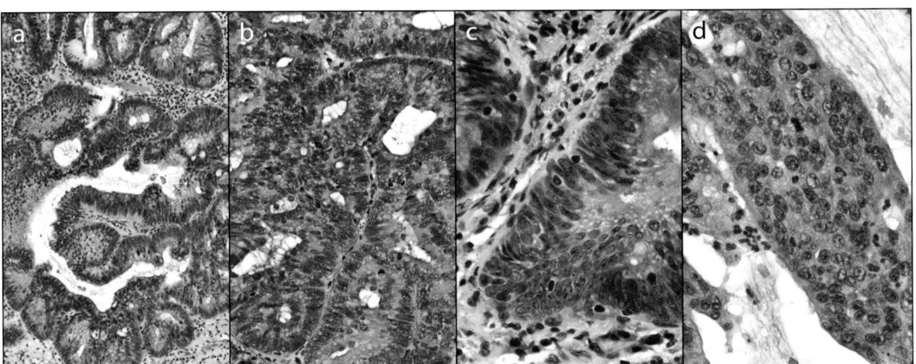

i23.18 The 4 images of i23.18 illustrate the features of an adenomatous polyp with high-grade dysplasia.
a-b Glandular crowding in an adenomatous polyp

c Nuclear stratification in an adenomatous polyp
d An adenomatous polyp with rounded nuclei, open chromatin, and nucleoli, nuclear features that are not usually seen in an adenomatous polyp

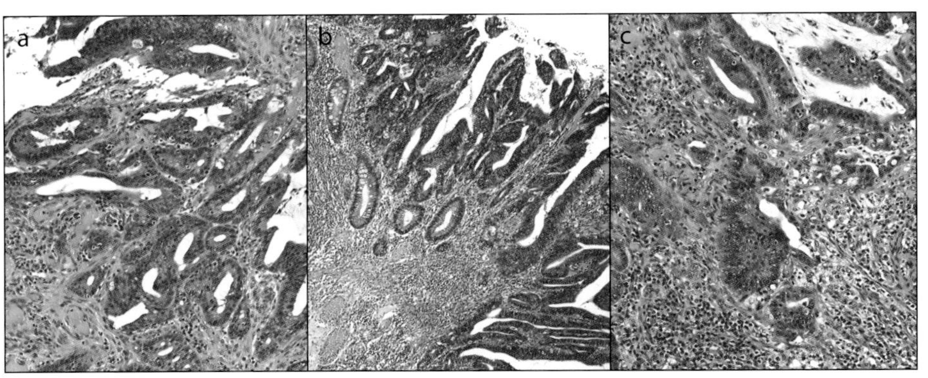

i23.19 Intramucosal adenocarcinoma. A small amount of muscularis mucosa can be seen in the upper right. The remainder of the photograph is mucosa but the normal lamina propria has been displaced with a fibrotic stroma, an indication of invasion.

b, c Other examples of intramucosal adenocarcinoma inferred by the glandular crowding rather than by stromal desmoplasia. The muscularis mucosa is to the upper left in **b** and to the lower right in **c**.

ISBN 978-089189-5886

i23.20 **a** The superficial portion of a colonic adenocarcinoma. This portion of the tumor, just below the muscularis mucosa, is a routine, gland-forming, moderately differentiated adenocarcinoma.

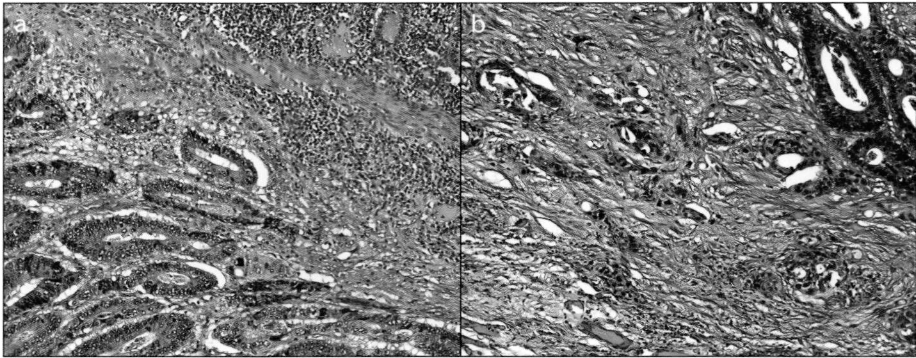

b The same case as in i23.20a, illustrating the deepest portion of the tumor, which is less well differentiated

i23.21 **a, b** A rectal adenocarcinoma which was treated with neoadjuvant chemotherapy and radiation therapy prior to resection. There is appreciable necrosis and elimination of the surface component, but residual viable tumor remains in the stroma.

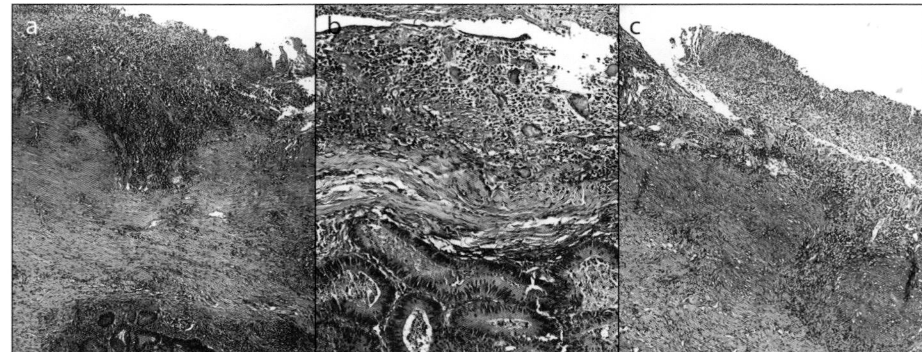

c Another case of rectal adenocarcinoma treated with neoadjuvant therapy, with complete response. There was no residual tumor in the resection specimen.

i23.22 A low-grade neuroendocrine carcinoma (carcinoid tumor) in the appendix

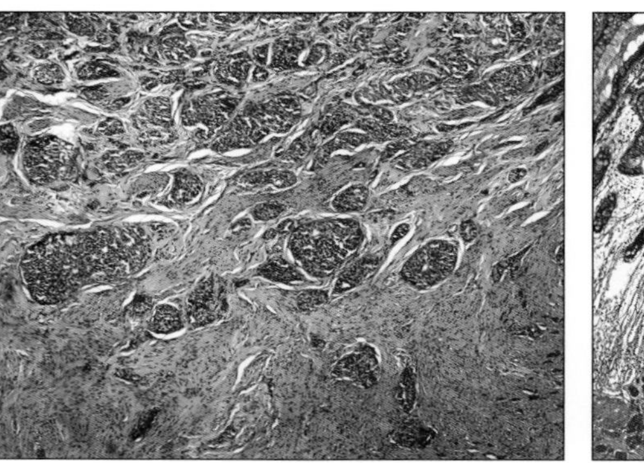

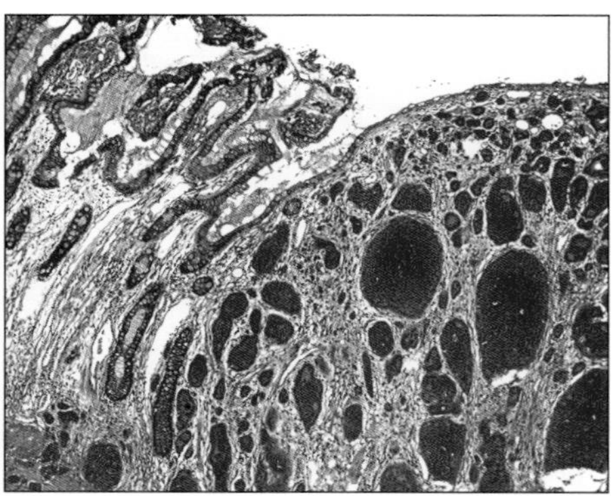

i23.23 A low-grade neuroendocrine carcinoma of the terminal ileum

i23.24 **a** A low-grade neuroendocrine carcinoma of the terminal ileum metastatic to a lymph node **b** A higher-power view of the same case as in i23.24a. Note the extensive lymphatic invasion adjacent to the lymph node and also note that despite the aggressive behavior the neoplasm continues to have low-grade nuclei.

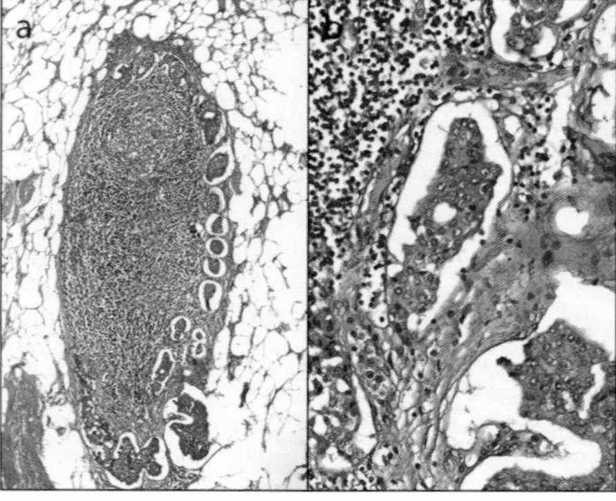

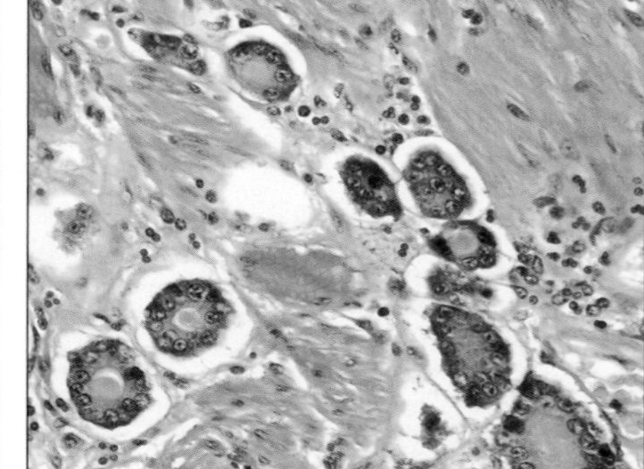

i23.25 A low-grade neuroendocrine carcinoma with a tubular pattern in which concentric arrangements simulate the glands of an adenocarcinoma. This case, from the tip of the appendix, was positive for neuroendocrine markers and negative for cytoplasmic mucin.

i23.26 **a, b** A neuroendocrine carcinoma with cytoplasmic vacuolization (so called goblet cell carcinoid).

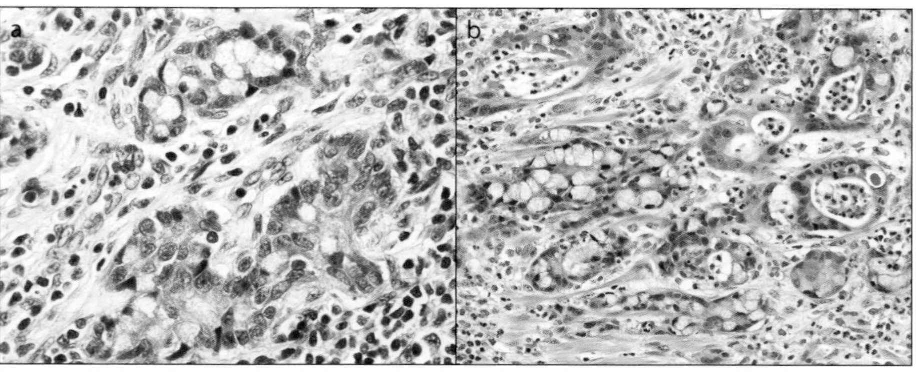

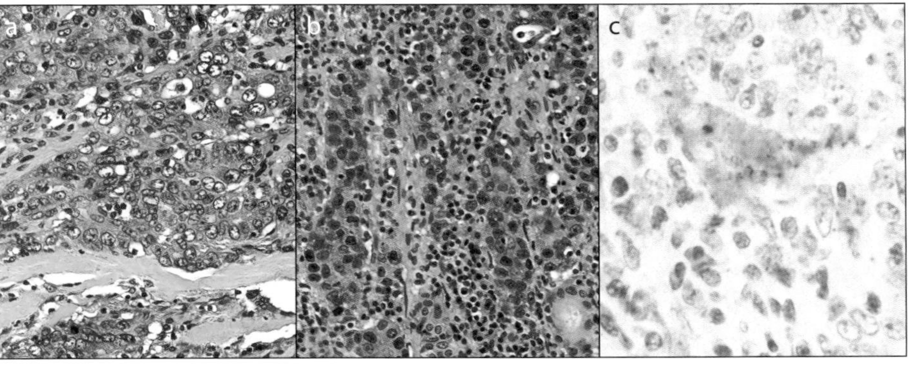

i23.27 A mixed neuroendocrine carcinoma-adenocarcinoma. **a** illustrates a high-grade adenocarcinoma with subtle gland formation in the upper right. **b** illustrates a routine low-grade neuroendocrine carcinoma, with a trabecular growth pattern, immediately adjacent to the focus in i23.27a. **c** is a focally positive synaptophysin stain in the adenocarcinoma component.

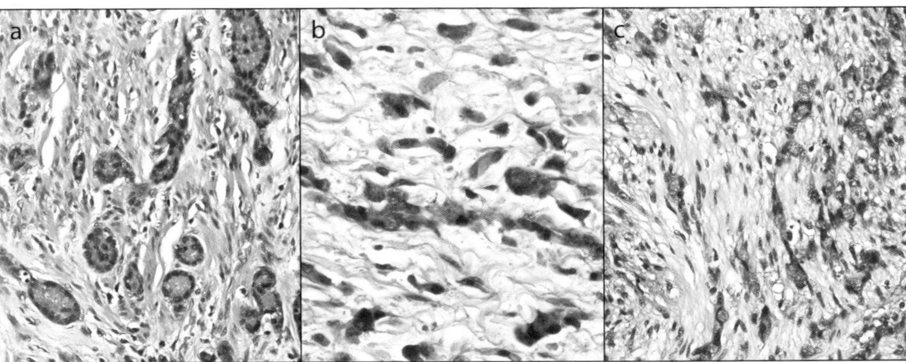

i23.28 Another example of a mixed neuroendocrine carcinoma-adenocarcinoma in which the adenocarcinoma component (seen in **b** and **c**) initially appears to be a goblet cell carcinoid. However, in addition to the distinctly mucinous nature of the cytoplasm, unusual in a lower-grade goblet cell carcinoid, **c** illustrates perineural invasion, identifying the neoplasm as an aggressive signet ring adenocarcinoma accompanied by a low-grade neuroendocrine component.

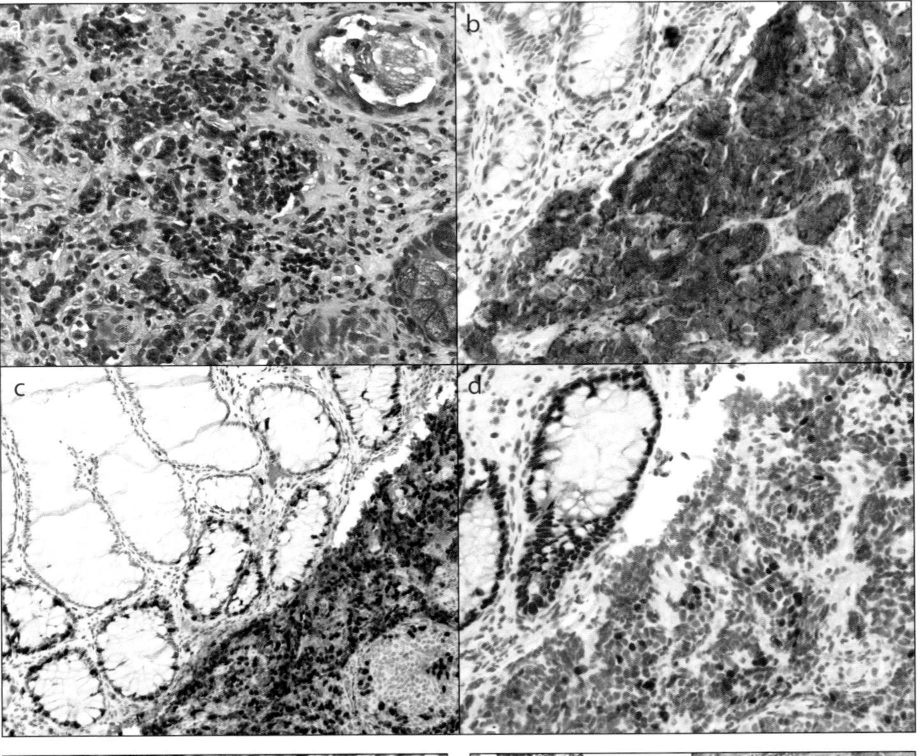

i23.29 **a-c** A primary high-grade neuroendocrine carcinoma (small cell carcinoma) of the colon. In a note the paucity of cytoplasm and the hyperchromasia of the nuclei. **b** is a positive synaptophysin immunohistochemical stain, confirming the neuroendocrine nature of the process. **c** is Ki-67 immunohistochemical stain to assess proliferation. Almost all of the neoplastic cells are positive, with a nuclear staining pattern. The rounded cluster that is negative in the lower right corner is a lymphoid nodule. This very high proliferation rate identifies the carcinoma as being high grade, and is not seen in a grade 1 or grade 2 neuroendocrine carcinoma. An interesting feature of this stain is that the basal layer of the benign colonic epithelium, running diagonally from the lower left to the upper right is almost uniformly positive, indicating a high rate of proliferation, while the remainder of the colonic epithelium, in the upper left portion of the photograph, moving towards the lumen, is negative. The basal layers of gastrointestinal mucosa, the skin, and the myeloid line in the bone marrow have the fastest turnover rates of any tissue. **d** is a CDX2 stain, the positivity of which suggests a colonic origin. Pulmonary small cell carcinomas are generally negative for CDX2. This patient did not have a pulmonary mass.

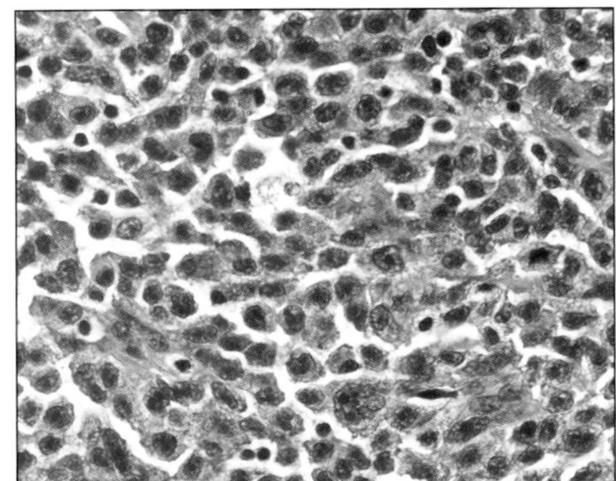

i23.30 A colonic medullary carcinoma with high-grade nuclei, prominent nucleoli, and no gland formation.

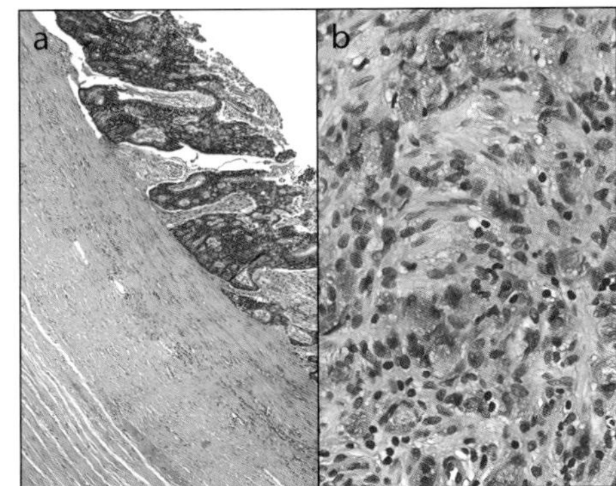

i23.31 A mucinous adenocarcinoma of the appendix. **a** illustrates an in situ component while **b** illustrates a poorly differentiated, signet ring invasive component.

ISBN 978-089189-5886

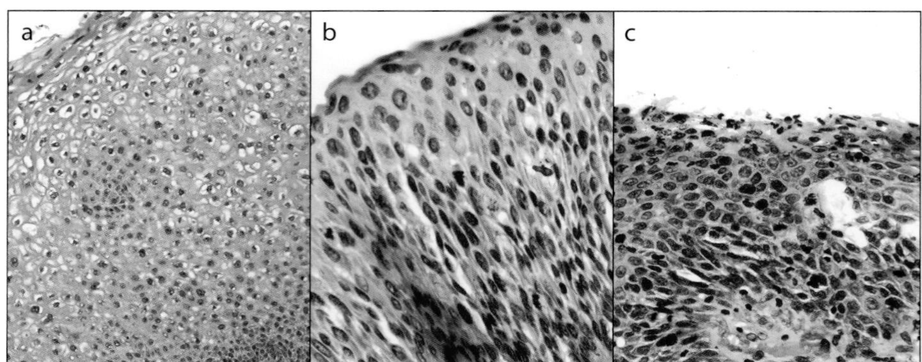

i23.32 Anal intraepithelial neoplasia.
a illustrates AIN1. Note the resemblance to CIN1 of the cervix, with diminished maturation and mild nuclear enlargement. The prominent perinuclear halos reflect the association of AIN with human papillomavirus, as is the case for CIN.
b illustrates AIN2. Note the sharp reduction in maturation, the mitotic figure in the center, well above the basal layer, and the dyskeratotic cells near the surface.
c illustrates AIN3/ squamous carcinoma in situ. Note the almost complete absence of maturation and the mitotic figures.

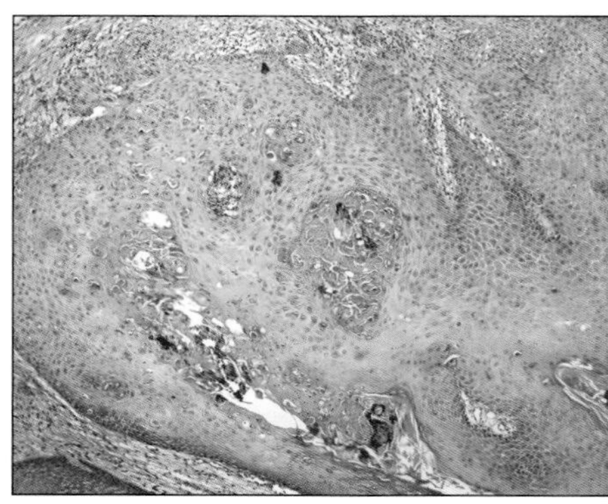

i23.33 A verrucous carcinoma of the anal canal. As is typical of this entity there is a large bulbous protrusion into the stroma, but the interface of the epithelium and the stroma remains smooth and there is no stromal reaction.

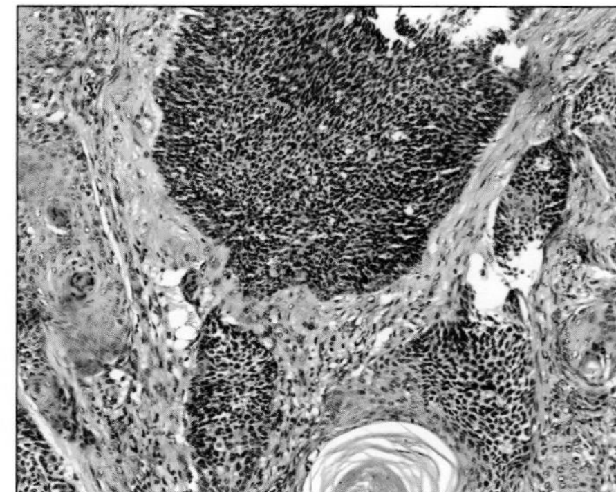

i23.34 A squamous cell carcinoma, primarily of the basaloid type, of the anal canal (formerly called transitional cell or cloacogenic carcinoma of the anus)

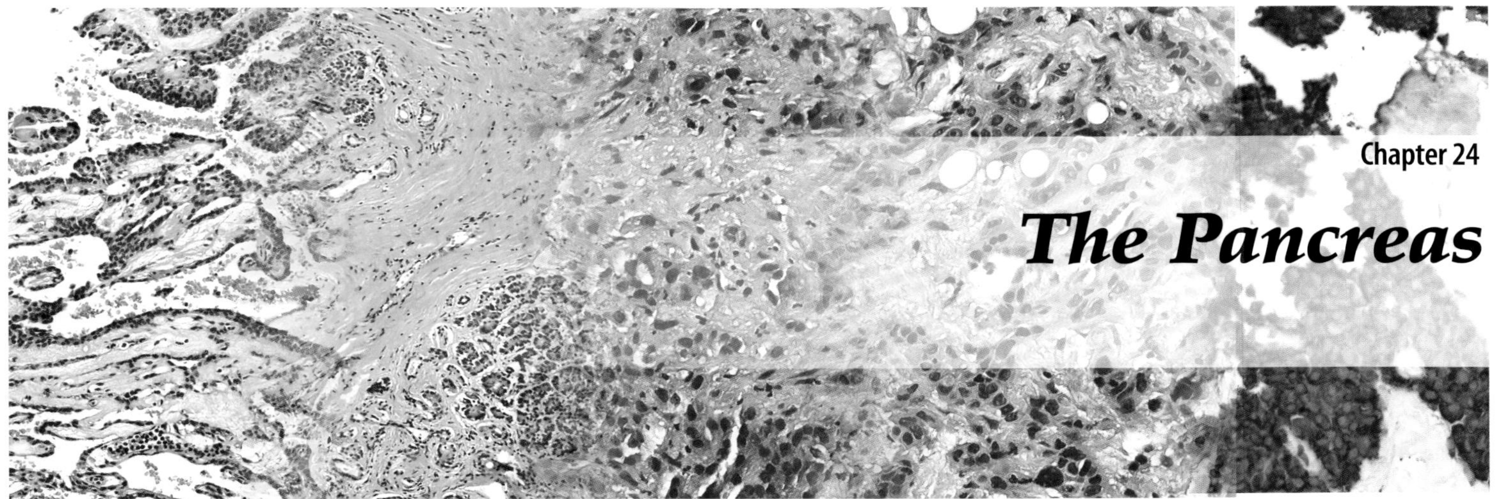

Chapter 24

The Pancreas

Developmental Anomalies

There are 3 developmental anomalies of the pancreas that are potentially encountered in common practice. Annular pancreas, in which the pancreas wraps around the duodenum, has potential clinical importance because it can cause obstruction. Pancreas divisum occurs when the major ducts of the dorsal and ventricle components fail to fuse, in which case part of the pancreas is drained by the duct of Santorini into a minor papilla, while the duct of Wirsung drains into the papilla of Vater. Heterotopic pancreas is usually an incidental finding of a small nodule in the stomach or duodenum.

Nonneoplastic Conditions of the Pancreas

No comments will be made about the principal nonneoplastic condition of the pancreas, type I diabetes, because the surgical pathologist has no contribution to make to the diagnosis and treatment of this disorder. Likewise, pancreatic pseudocysts and acute pancreatitis are commonly encountered in clinical medicine, but are not generally part of the purview of the surgical pathologist.

Chronic pancreatitis is important to the surgical pathologist for 2 reasons. First, biopsies of chronic pancreatitis may simulate adenocarcinoma. With time, the lymphoid infiltrate may give way to sclerosis. In most areas, the lobular pattern remains evident i24.1a, i24.1b, but especially on needle biopsy material, the normal architecture may be distorted and benign glands may appear infiltrative i24.2. Second, a subgroup of patients with chronic pancreatitis has autoimmune pancreatitis, which is one of the IgG4 fibroinflammatory conditions.

Since autoimmune pancreatitis was proposed in 1995 [PMID7628283], it has not only been well characterized but has also become the prototype of the IgG4-related fibroinflammatory conditions. The IgG4-related autoimmune disorders are autoimmune fibroinflammatory conditions that affect many body sites, either singly or in combination. Among the many other possible sites are lymph nodes (simulating the plasma cell type of Castleman disease), the mediastinum (accounting for many of the cases of sclerosing mediastinitis that are not associated with infection), the liver and biliary tract (sclerosing cholangitis), salivary glands (autoimmune sialadenitis), the retroperitoneum (retroperitoneal fibrosis), thyroid (Riedel thyroiditis), orbital region (fibrotic orbital pseudotumor), kidneys (autoimmune tubulointerstitial nephritis), lung (autoimmune interstitial pneumonitis), and prostate. There are numerous reports of IgG4-related fibroinflammatory processes in additional sites, and the full extent and nature of this process has not yet been elucidated. While most cases of IgG4 autoimmune disorders involve the pancreas, some do not [PMID16426926].

Because of the association with IgG4, the term "IgG4-related systemic sclerosing diseases" has been proposed for this group of disorders [PMID19817887]. In these conditions, serum IgG4 is elevated and there may be autoantibodies or anemia. The primary histologic finding is fibrosis with a lymphoplasmacytic infiltrate. Biopsies of autoimmune pancreatitis, for example, demonstrate chronic fibrosing pancreatitis that may be difficult to distinguish from chronic pancreatitis unrelated to an IgG4 fibroinflammatory process except for the presence of large numbers of lymphocytes and plasma cells, and possibly also phlebitis [PMID18609677]. Occasional eosinophils may be seen.

An IgG4-related sclerosing disorder should be excluded when a fibroinflammatory process is found in one of the above sites, and can be suspected if >1 body site is affected. While the presence of plasma cells in tissue sections has very poor sensitivity for an autoimmune etiology, plasma cells that express IgG4 in the tissue are suggestive of an autoimmune process, and for that reason, an immunohistochemical stain for IgG4 and a serum IgG4 level may be helpful. The IgG4-related sclerosing disorders often respond well to systemic steroid therapy, and immunosuppressants may also be used [PMID18609677].

The IgG4-related sclerosing disorders are not to be confused with fibromatosis, which may also affect many sites. In the fibromatoses, the fibrosis is more cellular, less collagenous, and less associated with inflammatory cells, and is not associated with the ancillary findings of elevated serum IgG4 or the presence of IgG4-secreting plasma cells in the tissues. The distinction is most important in the retroperitoneum, where both types of processes—retroperitoneal fibrosis and retroperitoneal fibromatosis—occur with some frequency [PMID18609677].

Autoimmune pancreatitis often presents as a mass, simulating carcinoma. In cases where autoimmune pancreatitis is difficult to differentiate from adenocarcinoma, the immunohistochemical demonstration of IgG4 in plasma cells, elevated serum IgG4 levels, and the demonstration of other areas of involvement in addition to the pancreas favor a benign process. In addition, the antibody AIP1-7 is reported to stain 95% of cases of autoimmune pancreatitis, but only 5% of pancreatic adenocarcinomas [PMID19940298].

Pancreatic Neoplasia

As is the case for many body sites, morphologic changes that are precursors to adenocarcinoma have been identified. Pancreatic intraepithelial neoplasia (PanIN) is increasingly recognized as an identifiable precursor to adenocarcinoma, though at this writing, the pathology community is still gaining experience in the reproducible use of this concept [PMID11342768].

Pancreatic adenocarcinoma of the common type is virtually always lethal and rarely operable. It shares with lung carcinoma the tragic properties of being undetectable until it is too late and frequently occurring in middle-aged people, significantly shortening life. There are a number of variants of pancreatic adenocarcinoma, including microglandular, adenosquamous, mucinous, and anaplastic.

The great difficulty for the pathologist in the diagnosis of pancreatic ductal adenocarcinoma is to distinguish it from reactive atypia and fibrosis secondary to chronic pancreatitis. Unlike other body sites, the pathologist cannot simply suggest a resection in a problematic lesion in the pancreas, since a resection is associated with high morbidity and indeed is rarely indicated even in cases of proven malignancy. The pathologist must successfully address the issue on biopsy material.

Duct structures that invade into the perineural space or into vascular structures are diagnostic of carcinoma, as are duct structures that are found in extra-pancreatic adipose tissue. However, one is rarely "fortunate" enough to encounter these findings, even in a carcinoma. More likely indicators of malignancy include generalized nuclear enlargement and hyperchromasia (occasional atypical nuclei can be seen in pancreatitis), large numbers of mitotic figures, ducts that are haphazardly distributed, without a normal acinar/lobular architecture, ducts with an irregular contour, and partial or incomplete duct formation i24.3a-d [PMID19260744]. Both adenocarcinoma and chronic pancreatitis will have stromal fibrosis, but the fibrosis in a malignancy tends to surround small clusters of cells.

A Ki-67 immunohistochemical stain for cells committed to division is helpful, as are the immunohistochemical demonstration of p53 and MUC1 [PMID19260744]. The antibody KOC reportedly stains pancreatic carcinomas and high-grade PanIN significantly more than benign or inflamed pancreas [PMID15644775]. Strong staining for IMP3 suggests an adenocarcinoma, while benign pancreatic tissue is generally negative or weakly positive [PMID21566520]. An immunohistochemical stain for CA19-9 (carbohydrate antigen 19-9) on a biopsy will be positive in benign or malignant pancreatic tissue, but the serum level of this marker is much higher in pancreatic adenocarcinoma than in benign pancreatic disease [PMID20007080]. MicroRNAs (discussed in Chapter 44) appear very promising at this writing in differentiating pancreatic carcinoma from reactive atypia [PMID19636633].

Cystic tumors of the pancreas are designated as serous or mucinous. Serous adenomas have abundant small cysts i24.4, accounting for their alternative name of microcystic adenoma. These cysts are lined by benign cuboidal cells with clear cytoplasm because of a high glycogen content.

Mucinous cystic neoplasms almost always occur in women [PMID21769313]. Unless a mucinous neoplasm is clearly malignant, most would say that it should be called uncertain malignant potential, because generous sampling may disclose more cellular areas i24.5a-c, and even simple mucinous neoplasms can be clinically troublesome [PMID19260748]. The terms "borderline" and "low malignant potential" are also acceptable in pancreatic mucinous neoplasms. However, others feel that mucinous tumors that appear to be completely benign adenomas in all areas i24.6 can be safely diagnosed as such [PMID10674612]. We will need more experience with bland mucinous tumors of the pancreas and probably a greater understanding of them at the molecular level before we can finally put to rest the uncertainty regarding pancreatic mucinous cystic neoplasms.

Further confusing the diagnosis of pancreatic mucinous neoplasms is the entity intraductal papillary mucinous neoplasm, a cellular intraductal proliferation with copious mucin production. Despite the name, some of these neoplasms have foci of invasion. Even when noninvasive, local resection is not always curative, presumably because of multifocal disease [PMID12404225].

The solid-pseudopapillary tumor (formerly called solid and papillary tumor) has a predilection for young women but may occur in all ages and in both genders. It has a much more favorable prognosis than adenocarcinoma, and surgery is often curative [PMID19845185]. In the solid-pseudopapillary tumor, fibrovascular cores may be readily apparent i24.7a, subtle i24.7b, or altogether absent in the more solid areas i24.7c. There is relative nuclear uniformity and solid areas may resemble a neuroendocrine tumor in biopsy material i24.7c and may have focal expression of synaptophysin [PMID11023097]. The solid-pseudopapillary tumor should be excluded before a diagnosis of a neuroendocrine neoplasm is made, and vice versa. In addition, the solid areas of a solid-pseudopapillary tumor may resemble an acinar cell tumor. Helpful features are that the solid-pseudopapillary tumor often has myxoid change in the cores i24.7d, i24.7e and small clusters of macrophages [PMID3812876]. Indeed, the prominence of myxoid change in the cores is why the term "pseudopapillary" is used, in contrast to the well developed fibrovascular cores of true papillations. CD10 [PMID11023097] and progesterone receptors [PMID17001154] may be expressed.

As is the case in the salivary glands, pancreatic acinar (or acinic) cell tumors are now considered low-grade adenocarcinomas of unpredictable behavior. As is also the case in the salivary gland, there are a variety of patterns, including acinar i24.8a, microacinar, and solid i24.8b. Nucleoli are variable, and may be prominent i24.8c, but the important diagnostic features in acinar carcinoma are relatively low-grade nuclear pleomorphism and granular cytoplasm i24.8d.

The important mimics of an acinar cell tumor are a neuroendocrine tumor, the solid-pseudopapillary tumor, and a microglandular or solid variant of common pancreatic adenocarcinoma. The latter will have more nuclear pleomorphism and less granular cytoplasm, but it is wise to employ immunohistochemical stains to exclude these neoplasms before diagnosing acinar cell carcinoma in the pancreas. Acinar cell carcinomas may have mild focal staining for neuroendocrine markers, but not the diffuse staining that indicates a neuroendocrine tumor. Also, immunohistochemical staining for trypsin and chymotrypsin will identify the neoplasm as an acinar cell carcinoma and not a neuroendocrine neoplasm. CD10 and progesterone receptor suggest a solid-pseudopapillary tumor. If these stains are all negative, the odds favor a pancreatic adenocarcinoma of the usual, more aggressive type that is demonstrating a microglandular or solid pattern.

In the pancreas, the terms "endocrine tumor," "islet cell tumor," and "neuroendocrine tumor" are often used interchangeably. Pancreatic neuroendocrine tumors are a diverse group genetically, biochemically, and clinically [PMID19411317]. Pancreatic neuroendocrine tumors usually have the appearance of a low-grade neuroendocrine neoplasm (ie, carcinoid tumor; i24.9a, but may have a variable appearance and may rarely have appreciable nuclear pleomorphism. For this reason, an islet cell tumor should be excluded in any unusual appearing pancreatic neoplasm that does not seem to "fit" into an established category. The most important immunohistochemical stains are synaptophysin to establish neuroendocrine differentiation and Ki-67 to establish a low grade i24.9b-d.

Islet cell tumor can be broadly grouped into 2 classes—those that are hormonally/biochemically functional and those that are not. The former group often comes to attention because of the products of the tumor, while the latter group is usually not detected until there are local effects or metastases. The product, if any, cannot be discerned at all from H&E examination. Surgery is the mainstay of treatment in this type of tumor [PMID19281699].

As is the case for endocrine neoplasms elsewhere, behavior is highly unpredictable and there are no absolute histologic indicators of malignancy in pancreatic endocrine tumors. To some extent, behavior correlates with the product, if any, made by the neoplasm (eg, gastrinomas are more likely to be malignant than insulinomas). Histologic findings that are may be associated with a malignant course in islet cell tumors include invasion of adjacent tissue, vascular or perineural invasion, extensive and generalized nuclear pleomorphism, high mitotic index (2/10 HPF), and necrosis [PMID8982376], but there remains a considerable amount of uncertainty i24.9e. Some feel that CK19 positivity confers a more aggressive course to a pancreatic endocrine neoplasm and makes it effectively malignant [PMID15316313]. A multiple endocrine neoplasia (MEN) syndrome should be clinically excluded when a pancreatic endocrine neoplasm is found.

Core Points for the Pancreas

- Chronic pancreatitis: a mimic of adenocarcinoma on biopsy material
  - May also indicate an IgG4 fibroinflammatory condition.
- Morphologic indicators of malignancy: generalized nuclear enlargement and hyperchromasia, brisk mitotic activity, loss of normal acinar/ductal architecture, irregularly shaped or partially formed ducts, and fibrosis surrounding small groups of atypical cells that do not form ducts.
- Pancreatic cystic tumors: serous or mucinous.
  - Serous adenomas have small cysts and contain glycogen.
  - Some mucinous neoplasms are clearly malignant
  - Some believe that the remainder should be designated as uncertain malignant potential, while other feel that a mucinous adenoma may occasionally be comfortably diagnosed.
- Solid-pseudopapillary tumor: predilection for young to middle-aged women
  - Generally not aggressive
  - Its papillary nature may be indistinct, but the stroma and the cores of the papillae are often myxoid and nuclei are low grade.
- Pancreatic acinar (or acinic) cell tumors: now considered low-grade adenocarcinomas of unpredictable behavior.
  - Several growth patterns, but common features are generally uniform nuclei, even in cases with prominent nucleoli, and granular cytoplasm.
  - A neuroendocrine tumor, a solid-pseudopapillary tumor, and a microglandular or solid form of adenocarcinoma must be excluded.
- Pancreatic neuroendocrine tumors (also called endocrine tumor or islet cell tumor): genetically and biochemically diverse.
  - They may secrete any of a number of hormones, and many secrete none at all.
  - Generally have the appearance of a carcinoid tumor.

ISBN 978-089189-5886

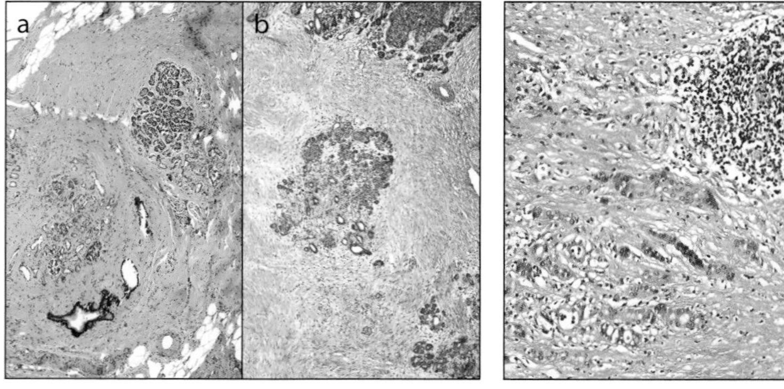

i24.1 **a-b** Chronic fibrosing pancreatitis. Note the retention of the lobular pattern.

i24.2 Another example of chronic fibrosing pancreatitis in which the epithelial cells below the lymphoid nodule, though benign, appear to have an infiltrative pattern. This area could be treacherous on a needle biopsy.

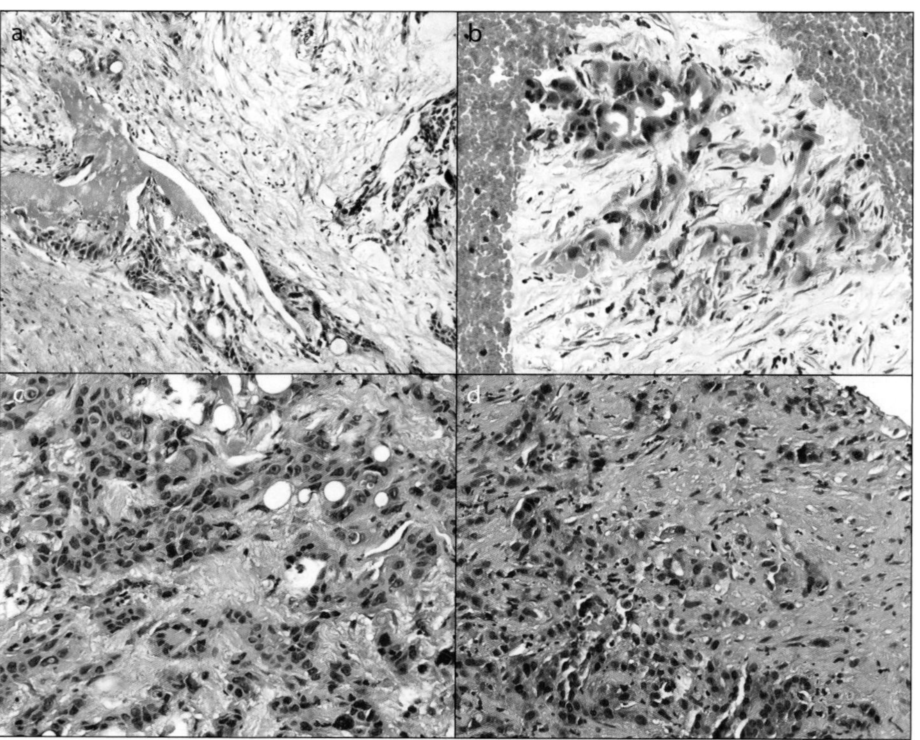

i24.3 These 4 images demonstrate invasive ductal adenocarcinoma of the pancreas. In all 4 images, note the generalized nuclear atypia, with enlargement and hyperchromasia, the incomplete gland formation, and the infiltrative pattern. There is also stromal desmoplasia, best illustrated in **d**, but this is a suboptimal criterion in the pancreas because dense fibrosis is often seen in chronic pancreatitis.

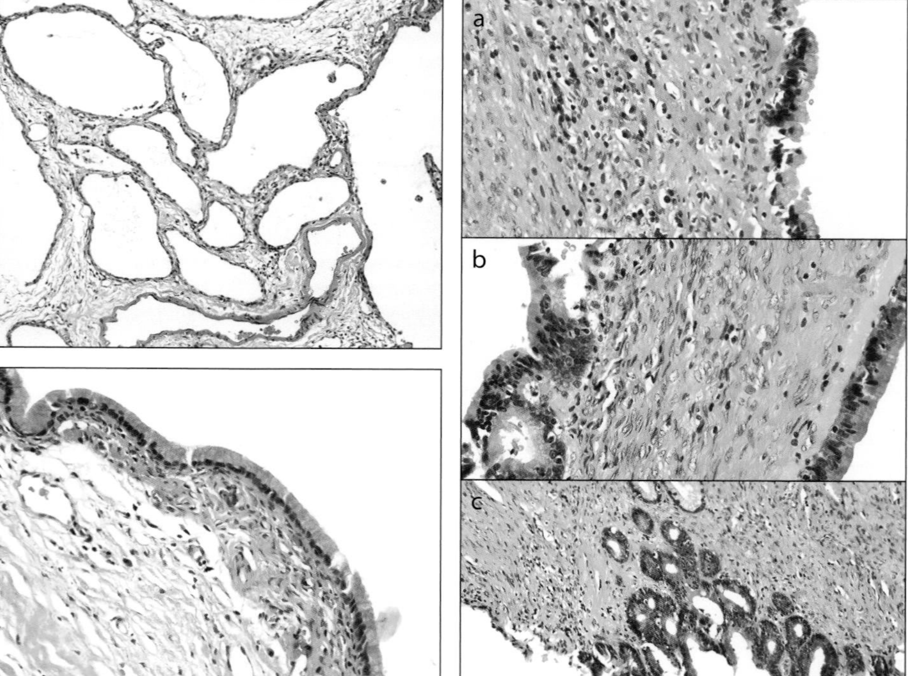

i24.4 A serous cystadenoma of the pancreas. The small cysts that are seen here account for the alternative name of microcystic adenoma.

i24.5 A mucinous cystic neoplasm. All 3 images come from the same case. Although **a** suggests a mucinous cystadenoma, **b** demonstrates dysplastic mucinous lining on the left and **c** demonstrates microinvasive mucinous carcinoma.

i24.6 Another mucinous cystic neoplasm in which the entire lining was a single, simple layer as seen here. While there is no universal agreement, many feel that a neoplasm of this nature can be diagnosed as a mucinous cystadenoma.

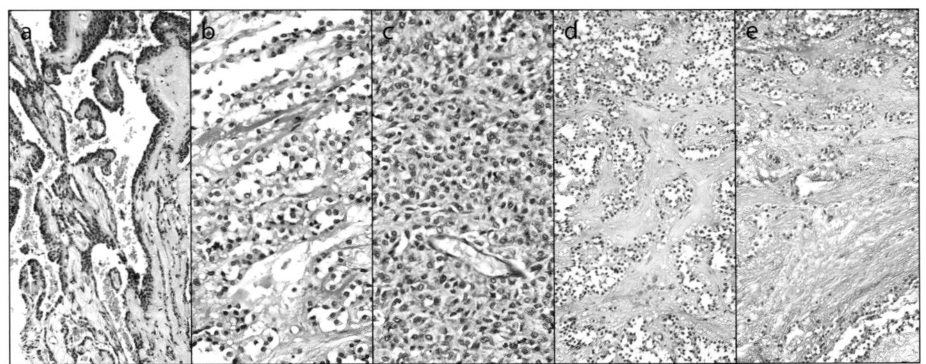

i24.7 A solid-pseudopapillary tumor of the pancreas. **a** demonstrates well defined papillations. In **b** the papillations are much more subtle. **c** demonstrates the solid component of a solid-pseudopapillary tumor, with no papillations at all. Note the continued nuclear uniformity, even in solid areas. Note also the resemblance to solid variants of a neuroendocrine neoplasm or an acinar cell tumor, and if a solid-pseudopapillary tumor consists predominantly of solid areas, immunohistochemical stains may be necessary. **d** illustrates the myxoid nature of most of the papillations, accounting for the term "pseudopapillary." **e** demonstrates a myxoid change that is often seen in the stroma apart from any papillary areas.

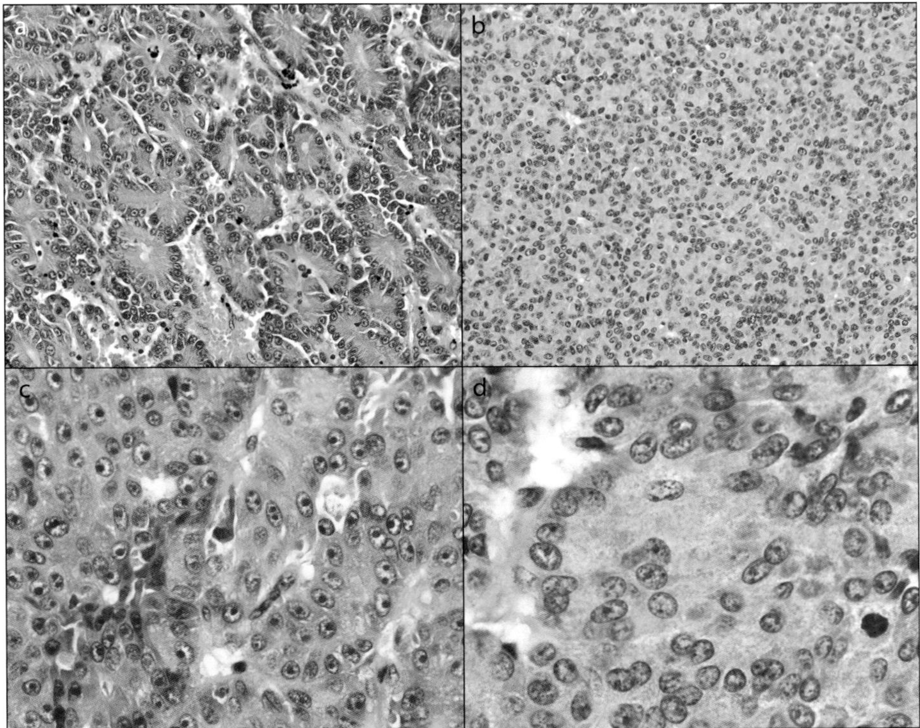

i24.8 **a-b** An acinar (or acinic) cell tumor of the pancreas. **a** illustrates the acinar pattern of this tumor and is distinguished from a high-grade adenocarcinoma by the relative nuclear uniformity. **b** illustrates a solid pattern. This pattern may resemble the solid areas in a solid-pseudopapillary tumor or a neuroendocrine neoplasm. **c** An acinar cell tumor with prominent nucleoli. Although the nucleoli are alarming, note the continued nuclear uniformity, in contrast to a ductal adenocarcinoma. **d** An illustration of the granular cytoplasm in an acinar cell tumor

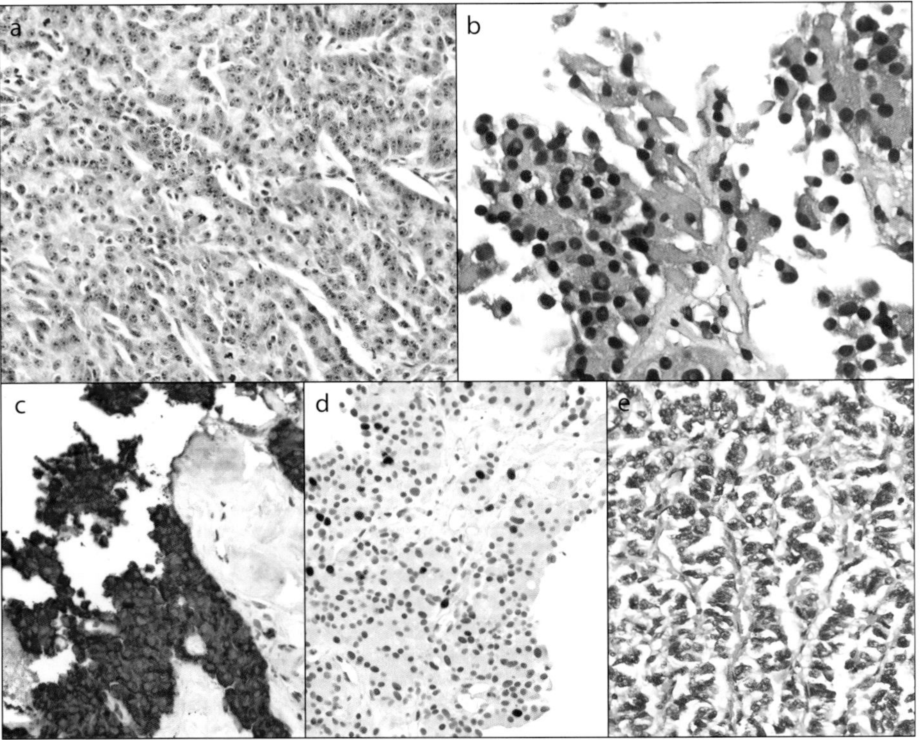

i24.9 A pancreatic neuroendocrine tumor (islet cell tumor). **a** illustrates the similarity to a low-grade neuroendocrine carcinoma (carcinoid tumor) that might be seen in a variety of sites. **b** illustrates a low-grade neuroendocrine tumor of the pancreas on needle biopsy. **c** is the same case as in i24.9b, with a synaptophysin stain, establishing neuroendocrine origin. **d** is the same case as in i24.9b, with a Ki-67 stain demonstrating minimal proliferation, identifying the process as a low-grade neuroendocrine tumor. **e** illustrates a low-grade pancreatic neuroendocrine tumor, but this neoplasm metastasized and was clinically aggressive, illustrating that there is poor correlation between the nuclear appearance and biologic potential.

ISBN 978-089189-5886

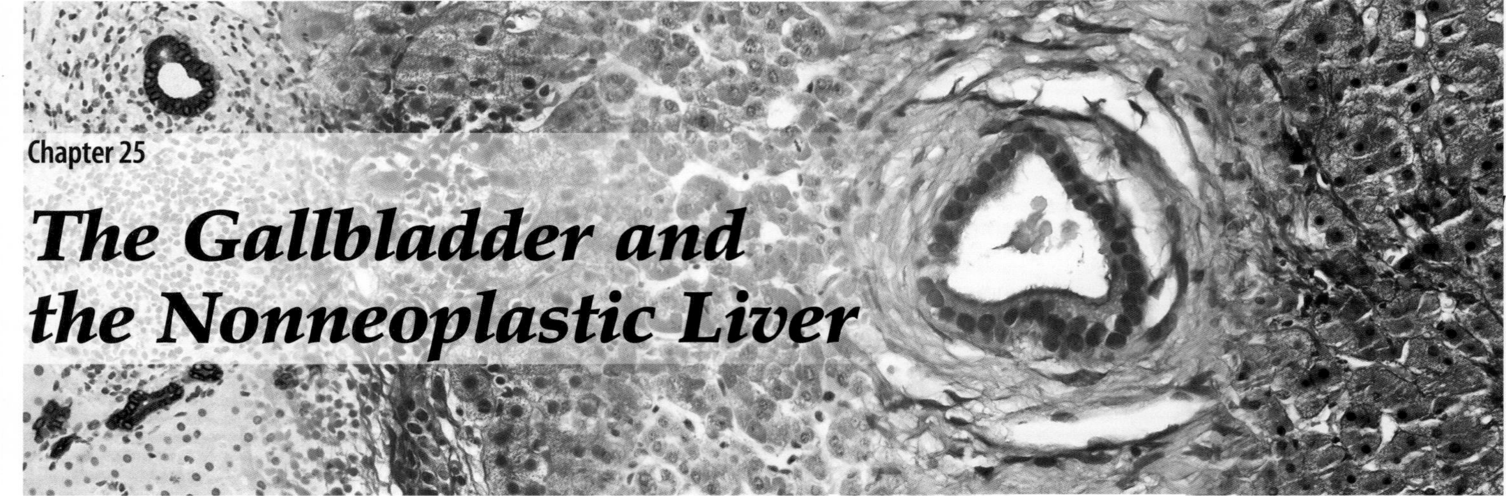

The Gallbladder and the Nonneoplastic Liver

The Gallbladder

Rokitansky-Aschoff sinuses are invaginations of the surface epithelium and communicate with the lumen. Ducts of Luschka are subserosal, smaller, and do not communicate with the lumen. They may represent Rokitansky-Aschoff sinuses that have been separated from the lumen i25.1. The so-called adenomyoma of the gallbladder is simply a complex mixture of Rokitansky-Aschoff sinuses and a hyperplastic stroma i25.2.

Gallstones result from a combination of stasis, followed by supersaturation, and nucleation [PMID18992590]. They are composed of cholesterol, calcium bilirubinate, or calcium carbonate, usually in some combination. Only 10% are composed of only 1 type of material. 90% of cases of acute cholecystitis are associated with demonstrable stones, and in all probability, the remaining cases are associated with stones that have been passed and are no longer evident.

The pathologist should not "stretch" for a diagnosis of chronic cholecystitis in an otherwise normal gallbladder for 2 reasons. First, occasional chronic inflammatory cells are typically found in the lamina propria in the gallbladder, as they are generally throughout the gastrointestinal tract, likely related to immune function, such as secretory IgA. Second, there is no need to "save" the surgeon from criticism for a supposedly unnecessary operation because preoperative radiographic procedures will have documented biliary dysfunction. However, if the number of lymphocytes is obviously increased, the diagnosis of chronic cholecystitis is reasonable and potentially important. There are also unusual forms of chronic cholecystitis that merit mention, including follicular i25.3, eosinophilic, and xanthogranulomatous types. In any form of chronic cholecystitis, there is little correlation between the severity of the inflammation and severity of the symptoms.

Nothing will be said here about neoplasms of the gallbladder because they are rarely a diagnostic challenge. Adenocarcinoma of the gallbladder is usually unresectable at diagnosis, but rare cures may be obtained if the malignancy is an incidental finding in a gallbladder removed for the usual reasons i25.4.

Normal Hepatic Histology

More than in any other organ, the normal histology of the liver can be confusing. The situation is compounded by the presence of 2 competing nomenclatures. In the older lobular view of hepatic architecture, the basic unit is called a lobule, the center of which is the central vein. Blood enters the periphery of the lobule through branches of the portal vein and hepatic artery, percolates through the sinusoids between the rows of hepatocytes, and leaves the lobule via the central vein i25.5. In this nomenclature, the term "lobule" usually refers to the hepatocytes themselves, as opposed to the structures of the portal area.

The newer acinar conception attempts to more accurately reflect the functional unit of the liver and the direction of blood flow. In the acinar nomenclature, the basic unit of function is called the acinus, the center of which is the portal area, not the central vein. The acinus is divided into 3 zones based on the direction of blood flow. Zone 1 is the periportal area, zone 2 is the sinusoidal region, and zone 3 is the area around the central vein. The acinar nomenclature is preferred by many academicians, but to my mind, does not offer any advantages to the practicing pathologist. Moreover, the lobular terminology is more familiar and less confusing to most clinicians.

The blood becomes less oxygenated as it moves through the sinusoids and toward the central vein. Consequently, in low flow states, such as cardiac failure, the greatest histologic changes are to be expected near the central vein. On the other hand, as the blood moves toward the central vein, hepatocytes metabolize any toxic exogenous agents, such as drugs, that are in the blood, occasionally causing those that are closest to the portal areas to be more damaged than those near the central vein because they have taken a more "direct hit" from toxic agents.

The bile flows in a direction that is opposite to that of the blood. Bile is made by hepatocytes and then secreted into the bile canaliculi that are between 2 hepatocytes. Bile canaliculi have no lining except the cell membranes of the adjacent hepatocytes. Bile canaliculi coalesce into the canals of Hering, which are lined by both bile duct epithelium and hepatocytes, and are usually not seen in histologic examination. The canals of Hering, in turn, coalesce into bile ductules (also called cholangioles). Bile ductules are lined exclusively by biliary epithelium and are also generally inconspicuous, though they may be increased in number and visible in conditions that are associated with obstruction. If bile ductules are seen, they have an indistinct lumen that if seen at all, does not exceed approximately 20 µm in diameter. They are usually seen in the periphery of the portal area, and they are accompanied by venules, not arterioles. Bile ductules merge into bile ducts (more properly called interlobular bile ducts), which are the commonly seen and familiar biliary structures in the portal areas, and which are accompanied by an arteriole. The commonly seen biliary structure in liver biopsies is the bile *duct*, not the bile *ductule* [Sternberg ISBN0-88167-621-7].

Approach to the Liver Biopsy

More than in any other organ, the productive interpretation of liver biopsies requires the integration of ancillary information, including a clinical history, the results of serological testing for hepatitis B and C viruses, and the results of testing for an autoimmune process. There are 3 screening tests that are used to exclude an autoimmune liver disease. These are antinuclear antibody (ANA), antimitochondrial antibody (AMA), and antismooth muscle antibody (ASMA). These tests are usually performed by immunofluorescence. Enzyme immunoassay (EIA) tests are technically easier and more reproducible among different observers, provided that the specific antigen is known, and attempts are underway to replace immunofluorescence testing with EIA testing whenever possible. The antismooth muscle antibody, for example, is often replaced now with an EIA test for filamentous actin (F-actin). This EIA test has greater sensitivity and equivalent specificity to antismooth muscle immunofluorescence testing [PMID17227520].

In addition to the routine H&E stained slides, a panel consisting of iron stain, PAS stain with diastase, and trichrome stain to assess fibrous tissue are often performed. Hepatic iron stores are quite subtle on H&E examination, and the identification of such stores is crucial in excluding liver pathology secondary to iron overload syndromes. The trichrome stain highlights connective tissue, and usually confirms H&E findings in that regard, though it occasionally reveals fine collagen fibers in the lobule that might escape detection on H&E. The PAS stain is primarily to identify the rare patient who has accumulation of α-1-antitrypsin, and in most cases is the least important of the special stains.

Duct Obstruction and Atresia

Large duct obstruction can be secondary to a variety of conditions, such as stones, tumor, primary sclerosing cholangitis, atresia of the extrahepatic ducts, etc. A similar histologic picture is seen in each case, with acute inflammation, cholestasis, extravasation of bile secondary to rupture of bile ducts, proliferation of bile ductules, and edema i25.6. With chronicity, there is a partial replacement of neutrophils by lymphocytes, less edema, and eventual fibrosis, with loss of some bile ducts. The parenchyma is relatively spared in large duct obstruction.

Intrahepatic biliary atresia occurs in a syndromic form called Alagille syndrome [PMID803282] and in a nonsyndromic form. These 2 forms have histologic features that are different from extrahepatic atresia or obstruction, but similar to each other. In both forms of intrahepatic biliary atresia, there is cholestasis with loss of interlobular bile ducts i25.7, often with a modest proliferation of ductules. The diagnosis is made by assessing the degree of loss of interlobular bile ducts. Normally, about 70% of portal areas have at least 1 bile duct, and most portal areas have 1 or 2 bile ducts on average. An average of <1/2 duct per portal area (ie, <1 bile duct per 2 portal areas) is consistent with this diagnosis, but only true interlobular ducts, not ductules, should be counted. Although not every arteriole will always have an accompanying duct, the presence of many arterioles that are not accompanied by a bile duct raises suspicion of ductulopenia.

Iron Overload Syndrome and Hereditary Hemochromatosis

Increased amounts of iron i25.8 can be seen in the liver in a variety of conditions, such as hereditary hemochromatosis, ethanol consumption, and multiple transfusions. Without additional information, such as ethanol and transfusion history and genetic evaluation for hereditary hemochromatosis, morphologic examination cannot establish the etiology. Therefore, the anatomic diagnosis to be made when large amounts of iron are seen in the liver is *iron overload syndrome*. i25.9a, i25.9b illustrate hereditary hemochromatosis.

Older terminology distinguished between hemosiderosis and hemochromatosis, but "hemosiderosis" is an old term that is likely to cause confusion and its use is discouraged. The term "hemochromatosis," on the other hand, has a specific meaning and refers to an iron overload syndrome caused by a genetic defect in iron metabolism. The underlying abnormality in hereditary hemochromatosis is increased absorption of dietary iron. This results in accumulation of iron stores since there is minimal ability to excrete excess iron. In patients of Caucasian descent, hemochromatosis usually refers to hereditary hemochromatosis type 1, now known to be caused by a defect in the *HFE* gene.

The product of the *HFE* gene is a protein, similar in structure to an HLA class 1 molecule, that binds to the transferrin receptor and inhibits transferrin from binding to its receptor [PMID11729128]. While the details of the action of transferrin and its modulation by the HFE protein are quite complicated, the HFE protein reduces the uptake of iron from transferrin by the cell [PMID10085150]. Abnormalities in the HFE protein are less able to bind to the transferrin receptor and therefore less able to reduce iron uptake [PMID10087990]. *HFE* mutations therefore facilitate the unloading of iron from transferrin into the cell.

There are 2 well described abnormalities of the *HFE* gene—a change from cysteine to tyrosine at position 282 (abbreviated C282Y, Y being the single letter abbreviation for tyrosine) and a change from histidine to aspartic acid at position 63 (H63D, D being the single letter abbreviation for aspartic acid) [PMID20542038]. There are occasional cases stemming from mutations of *HFE* at other foci. C282Y is the most common form of hereditary hemochromatosis. Type 1 hereditary hemochromatosis is autosomal recessive, but there is incomplete correspondence between the relevant liver function tests (transferrin saturation and ferritin level) and the severity of symptoms. A common method of detecting abnormalities of the *HFE* gene is polymerase chain reaction of the

HFE gene, followed by digestion and gel electrophoresis, after which the position of bands on the gel in a genetic variation will differ from that of the normal gene **i25.10**.

The hepatic iron *concentration* is the tissue iron concentration in micromoles per gram of dry liver weight. Because iron accumulation in the liver increases with age, it is important to compare the patient's hepatic iron stores with age-matched controls. The hepatic iron *index* is the iron concentration divided by the patient's age. Hepatic iron index is used primarily to follow patients once the diagnosis of hereditary hemochromatosis has been made, but may rarely have utility in the diagnosis of hemochromatosis because genetic testing does not cover all possible abnormalities of the *HFE* gene. An iron index of 1.9 or greater is usually more consistent with homozygous hereditary hemochromatosis than other etiologies [PMID2373481], but even in these rare situations, it is essential to exclude other possible causes. If untreated, hereditary hemochromatosis will cause fibrosis and eventually, cirrhosis. Treatment of type 1 hereditary hemochromatosis by chelation has been disappointing and the mainstay of treatment is phlebotomy [PMID18061062].

Type 1 hemochromatosis (ie, abnormalities of the *HFE* gene) is the most common type, but is largely restricted to patients of Caucasian descent. There are numerous other types of genetic iron-overload syndromes that are not related to the *HFE* gene [PMID17729390]. These are rare overall, but account for the majority of cases in non-Caucasian patients.

To understand these other types of hemochromatosis, we need to briefly review iron metabolism [PMID16450011]. The major sources of iron are dietary and erythrocyte breakdown. Ferroportin is a protein found on the surface of several types of cells, such as hepatocytes, cells of the gastrointestinal mucosa, and macrophages of the mononuclear phagocytic system (formerly called reticuloendothelial system, consisting of macrophages in the spleen and the Kupffer cells in the liver, which break down erythrocytes). These cells are the ones that are likely to contain iron through 1 of the 2 sources, and therefore, the cell types that can release iron to transferrin. Release of iron from these cells is made possible by ferroportin, located on the surface of these cells. Ferroportin moves iron from the cytoplasm to the extracellular surface, where it can be accessed and removed by transferrin and taken to the liver. Hepcidin is a hormone made by the liver that binds to and inactivates ferroportin. It is believed that hepatocytes release hepcidin when either transferrin becomes saturated or there is an excess of iron in hepatocytes. Elevated levels of hepcidin lead to increased intracellular iron in nonhepatocytes and decreased amounts of hepcidin lead to decreased intracellular iron stores in nonhepatocytes [PMID15514116]. Hemojuvelin is a modulator of hepcidin.

Juvenile hemochromatosis (also called type 2) is distinct from and more serious than the type 1 form. It exhibits extensive fibrosis early on, often with cholestasis and giant cell formation. Juvenile hemochromatosis is caused by abnormalities in either the *HEPCIDIN* (also called *HAMP*) gene or the *HEMOJUVELIN* (*HJV*; originally called *HFE2*) gene. Mutations in the *HEPCIDIN* gene cause type 2B hemochromatosis, while mutations in *HEMOJUVELIN* cause type 2A hemochromatosis. There is some evidence in rare cases of an interaction between the *HFE* and *HEPCIDIN* genes as a cause of the disease (digenic inheritance) [PMID12915468].

An abnormality in the gene for transferrin receptor 2 is a rare cause in adults (type 3 hemochromatosis) [PMID10802645]. Type 4 hemochromatosis is secondary to mutations in the protein ferroportin. Abnormalities in ceruloplasmin may also cause iron overload. Though associated with copper metabolism, plasma ceruloplasmin also transforms ferrous iron (Fe^{++}), which crosses the cell membrane, into ferric iron (Fe^{+++}), which is the only form of iron that transferrin can transport. Diminished ceruloplasmin increases intracellular iron by impairing the oxidation of ferrous to ferric iron, thus impeding its movement across the cell membrane and its access to transferring [PMID17541408].

Wilson Disease

Copper is absorbed in the GI tract and stored in intestinal cells. To reduce toxicity, it is complexed in the intestinal cell with a protein called with metallothionein [PMID19482593]. An enzyme called copper-transporting ATPase 1 (ATP7A), on the cell membrane of intestinal cells, permits the copper to be transported to the liver, bound to albumin. Mutations of *ATP7A* gene result in the accumulation of copper in intestinal cells, resulting in a total copper deficiency called Menkes disease, a severe X-linked disorder.

Once in the hepatocyte, some of the copper is bound to metallothionein, as it was in the intestinal cell, and stored. Hepatic copper is excreted into bile canaliculi or into the blood. If transferred to blood, copper binds to apoceruloplasmin to form ceruloplasmin, which is an α2-globulin that binds 6 copper atoms and supplies copper to peripheral organs.

Excretion of copper into either bile canaliculi or into the blood requires a membrane-associated copper transport protein called ATP7B (also called Wilson disease protein). Mutations in the *ATP7B* gene, which encodes the ATP7B protein, cause Wilson disease [PMID18568852]. The *ATP7B* gene is on chromosome 13q14.3, consists of 21 exons, and has over 200 described mutations. The defective ATP7B protein cannot facilitate either blood or biliary copper excretion. There is a reduction in the conversion of apoceruloplasmin into ceruloplasmin, explaining the low levels of this protein in these patients, and there is also a buildup of copper in hepatocytes. Wilson disease is inherited in an autosomal recessive manner, with a disease frequency between 1 in 5,000 and 1 in 30,000 and a carrier frequency of approximately 1 in 90.

Initially in Wilson disease, delivery of copper to other organs is diminished, but eventually, excess copper damages the hepatocytes (the mitochondria are especially vulnerable), causing free copper (not complexed to ceruloplasmin) to be spilled into the blood. The systemic delivery of free copper following hepatocyte damage results in deposits in the proximal renal tubules (leading to Fanconi syndrome) and to deposits in the periphery of Descemet membrane of the cornea (causing the characteristic golden-brown Kayser-Fleischer rings) [PMID18568852].

Wilson disease is characterized by low ceruloplasmin and initially by low total serum copper levels, but there are important qualifications on both of these criteria. Ceruloplasmin is an acute phase reactant and may be in the normal range as part of a general acute reaction. At the time of presentation, serum copper is likely to be increased because of the spillage of free copper into the blood from damaged hepatocytes. Indeed, copper often spills from the blood into the urine and a 24-hour urinary copper excretion is a helpful test [PMID18568852]. Normal 24-hour urinary copper excretion is between 20 and 50 μg per day, but in Wilson disease, excretion may be >100 μg per day. If additional testing is needed, a liver biopsy can be performed, and a measurement of hepatic copper content can be estimated by mass spectroscopy or atomic absorption spectroscopy. The degree of hepatic copper elevation can be estimated from quantitative studies performed on a paraffin block [PMID7942601] Radioactive copper uptake will be also sharply diminished because of hepatocyte damage.

The basic histologic findings at all stages are nonspecific, including fatty change, a portal lymphocytic infiltrate, and cytoplasmic invagination into nuclei, resulting in nuclear clearing that is often called nuclear glycogenation i25.11a, i25.11b. These are all features that are commonly seen in other entities. There is a special stain for copper that may help i25.11c, but it is rarely used since the diagnosis is more readily established by clinical findings and molecular testing. Chronic hepatitis, with fibrosis and cirrhosis, may eventually result.

Because of the nonspecific histologic findings, the diagnosis of Wilson disease cannot be made from a liver biopsy. The clinical features are more diagnostic (the classic diagnostic triad is low ceruloplasmin, Kayser-Fleischer rings, and neurologic symptoms pertaining to the extrapyramidal system), but since 1/3 of patients will lack 1 of more of these features, genetic testing is emerging as the gold standard for the diagnosis of Wilson disease. Treatment is by chelation of copper, usually by D-penicillamine, but trientine and ammonium tetrathiomolybdate are newer potential agents [PMID18568852].

α-1-Antitrypsin (α1AT) Deficiency

α-1-antitrypsin (α1AT) is a protein that is made in the liver and secreted into the blood, where it finds its way into a variety of tissues. α1AT is a member of the serine protease inhibitor family and is coded for by the *A1AT* gene on 14q31-32.3. Its function is to check the activity of several proteolytic enzymes.

α1AT deficiency is an autosomal recessive disorder that affects about 1 in 3000 people, with a carrier frequency of about 3%. The normal *A1AT* genotype is MM. Abnormal genotypes result in α1AT molecules that cannot be adequately excreted from the liver. This results not only in liver problems from the accumulation of the protein within hepatocytes, but also in emphysema because decreased serum levels of α1AT result in diminished restraint of trypsin-like enzymes, such as elastase, in the lung.

In addition to the normal M allele, there are numerous others, the most common being the Z and S alleles. While MZ heterozygotes and SS homozygotes may have symptoms, most severe cases of liver disease are caused by the ZZ genotype [PMID19961268]. The ZZ form of α-1-antitrypsin is likely functional, but it does not move properly through the endoplasmic reticulum and through the secretory pathway, probably because of aggregation. Biochemists use the term "novel property" to describe a protein whose intrinsic function (ie, enzymatic or structural) is essentially normal, but which has some other property (in this case, aggregation) that prevents the fulfillment of its complete in vivo role.

While α-1-antitrypsin deficiency may cause neonatal hepatitis, with a severe histologic appearance, the major histologic manifestation in adults is eosinophilic cytoplasmic globules because of aggregation of the protein [PMID7518264]. These are subtle on H&E examination i25.12a and require confirmation with special stains. PAS stain with diastase digestion to remove glycogen (PAS-D) is a good first line stain to highlight the accumulated α1AT i25.12b, i25.12c, but if this stain is suggestive of the accumulation of α1AT, confirmation of the identity of the globules should be secured with immunohistochemical staining for the protein unless the patient is known to have α1AT deficiency because diastase digestion of glycogen may be incomplete and the residual glycogen may simulate α1AT globules and because other PAS-positive, diastase-resistant proteins may be present.

The definitive identification of these globules by PAS and immunohistochemical staining can be followed by the genetic confirmation of an abnormal allele and documentation of diminished serum levels of the protein. Treatment for α1AT deficiency is intravenous administration of the normal enzyme [PMID20650978].

Acute Hepatitis

Acute hepatitis of any etiology primarily affects the lobule (or parenchyma; the actual hepatocytes as opposed to the portal areas). There may be acute inflammatory cells, but the major findings are ballooning of hepatocytes, disruption of the normal trabecular/sinusoidal architecture i25.13a, and necrosis of individual hepatocytes (Councilman bodies) i25.13b. In hepatitis of any etiology, with chronicity, the process in the lobule largely resolves, and the changes are found primarily in and around portal areas, though as subsequently discussed, some changes in the lobule are likely to remain in chronic hepatitis secondary to ethanol. Because acute hepatitis is rarely biopsied, and even in ethanol, the changes of chronic hepatitis are primarily in the portal area, the pathologist can generally expect a medical liver biopsy to show changes predominantly in the portal areas.

Viral Hepatitis

Although other hepatitis viruses, such as hepatitis E, are major causes of liver disease in developing countries, in North American and Europe viral hepatitis generally refers to hepatitis B or C. Hepatitis A is a cause of a self-limited hepatitis that only very rarely becomes chronic. Hepatitis B is a DNA virus, while hepatitis C is a single-stranded RNA virus that has never been isolated in culture. Hepatitis D (δ) is a virus that can only infect patients who are already infected by hepatitis B.

In chronic viral hepatitis, the portal areas have an increased number of lymphocytes (occasional plasma cells and eosinophils may also be seen) and may also be expanded by fibrous tissue. As long as the changes are confined to the portal areas i25.14a, i25.14b, there is a mild chronic hepatitis that is likely to resolve, or at least to be clinically inconsequential (this was formerly called chronic persistent hepatitis). However, if *either* the chronic inflammatory cells or the fibrous tissue extend into the adjacent hepatocytes at the junction of the portal area and the lobule (the limiting plate), then interface hepatitis is present and there is a potentially significant chronicity **i25.15a**, **i25.15b**. Interface hepatitis was formerly called piecemeal necrosis because some of the hepatocytes at the limiting plate may become necrotic as they intermingle with chronic inflammatory cells or fibrous tissue that migrate from the portal area, and liver biopsies demonstrating this finding were formerly said to have chronic active hepatitis. A trichrome stain affords an optimal assessment of possible interface hepatitis by defining the boundary between the portal area and the limiting plate, so that any lymphocytes that have crossed it can be more readily identified, and by highlighting any fine collagen fibers that may extend into the limiting plate **i25.16a**, **i25.16b**.

The histologic changes in chronic hepatitis B and C are very similar, and in both viruses, the inflammatory process triggers a fibrosis that may eventuate in cirrhosis. Hepatitis B may cause a homogeneous cytoplasm in hepatocytes, classically referred to as "ground glass" [PMID19399798], while hepatitis C may cause slight fatty change and mild lymphocytic infiltration of bile ducts (Poulson phenomenon), but only serological tests can definitively identify the responsible virus. Even δ hepatitis has no specific histologic features.

Numerous classification systems has been proposed to assess the various processes at work in liver biopsies for viral hepatitis [PMID7503362, PMID7847283, PMID17486049]. Assuming that the acute stage is not biopsied, the fundamental diagnosis is *chronic hepatitis*, followed by a description of etiology, findings, and extent. The Knodell system, also called hepatic activity index (HAI), was among the first. It combines 4 assessments into 1 score. 3 of these assessments pertain to inflammation in 3 different regions—portal, periportal, and lobular—while the assessment is of fibrosis. The result is a single composite score [PMID7308988]. This was a well-conceived system, but the combining of necrosis/inflammation with fibrotic activity was questioned, as these represent very different stages of the process, with potentially different clinical implications.

The Ishak modification of the Knodell system [PMID7560864] removed the combined inflammatory/fibrosis score, and scores the 2 processes separately. It also established a fourth category for confluent necrosis, graded 0-6. The Ishak system provides rich detail regarding the status of the necroinflammatory component, but it is difficult to employ in a manner that is reproducible from one observer to another. The Scheuer system simplified the Knodell process, and reported inflammation and fibrosis separately [PMID7751577, PMID1808228]. In the Scheuer system, inflammation is assessed on a scale of 0-4 and reported as a *grade* according to the following criteria:

- Grade 0 is normal
- Grade 1 is portal inflammation without interface hepatitis
- Grade 2 is mild interface hepatitis
- Grade 3 is moderate interface hepatitis
- Grade 4 is severe interface hepatitis or bridging necrosis

Fibrosis is then separately assessed and reported as a *stage* as follows:

- Stage 0 is normal
- Stage 1 is expanded portal tracts without significant extension into the limiting plate
- Stage 2 is extension into the limiting plate without bridging fibrosis
- Stage 3 is bridging fibrosis
- Stage 4 is cirrhosis

A useful mnemonic for both Scheuer grading and staging is that in both cases, a grade or stage 2 refers to a process that has moved out of the portal area and into the limiting plate. **i25.17**, **i25.18**, and **i25.19** illustrate the Scheuer system in the classification of cases of hepatitis C. Hepatitis B is rarely encountered or biopsied now because of vaccination, but these images also illustrate the histologic changes encountered in that virus.

To my mind, the Scheuer system remains the most useful for the reporting of chronic viral hepatitis because of its ease of use, reproducibility, ease of clinician understanding, and excellent correlation with the clinical situation. As subsequently discussed, it has been proposed that stages 3 and 4 be conflated into a category of "advanced stage."

In hepatitis of any cause, there has been debate as to whether the degree of activity (ie, interface hepatitis) or the extent of fibrosis is more important in therapeutic decisions. While it is wise to comment on both processes, in biopsies of hepatitis C at least, it appears that the stage of fibrosis is a more important clinical indicator than the degree of inflammation because inflammatory activity waxes and wanes while fibrosis progresses essentially linearly. Moreover, some cases of chronic viral hepatitis have superimposed acute changes from another process, such as ethanol consumption or medications **i25.20**, and fibrosis is less affected by these changes [PMID21970487].

Several studies of biopsies taken to assess hepatitis have found differences in grade and stage in different areas of the liver [PMID12385448, PMID11774953], but this has not been a universal finding [PMID11866299], and it is not established that any such differences outweigh the added risk and expense of simultaneously performing 2 biopsies [PMID21970487]. In an effort to avoid sampling error, and perhaps to obviate the need for a biopsy altogether, various surrogate serum testing panels have been proposed and are generally used in conjunction with an algorithm that takes into account the age and gender of the patient. The pluses and minuses of these serum tests relative to biopsy have been examined [PMID19207962]. While some have suggested that serum testing can theoretically avoid sampling error in a biopsy, thus permitting a more accurate assessment of changes over time, it has not yet been shown to replace the biopsy, and at this writing, the biopsy remains a time-honored and reliable means of assessing both the severity and progression in hepatitis.

If possible, liver biopsies should be compared to previous biopsies and a comment made on any progression. However, because of the possibility of sampling error, clinical data must be factored into a judgment as to whether or not there is progression.

Detection of hepatitis B infection by serology is generally done by finding the surface antigen, or by finding antibodies to the core, surface, or E antigen. The important qualifications are that the surface antigen fades away with time and its absence does not guarantee a negative status. Likewise, the presence of antibodies only to surface antigen is seen most commonly in patients who have been vaccinated.

For hepatitis C, most laboratories employ an EIA test as an initial screen. A negative test effectively excludes hepatitis C, but false positives occur, and even in cases that are true positives, the test does not fractionate IgM and IgG, and therefore cannot distinguish past from current infection. Therefore, patients with a positive EIA should not be reported as positive for hepatitis C, but rather should be tested by PCR for viral RNA, the presence of which confirms active infection. Some believe that patients who are EIA positive, viral RNA negative should have a second PCR test performed after a couple of months to ensure that the EIA result was either a false positive or that the infection has been cleared. Because about 20% of patients will clear hepatitis C without treatment, a positive EIA followed by a 2 negative RNA quantitations does not necessarily mean the EIA was a false positive, but it does mean that there is no active infection and that treatment is not needed.

The RIBA (recombinant immunoblot assay) is another test for antibodies to the hepatitis C virus, using recombinant proteins as the antigens and performed in a manner similar to a Western blot. Some feel that patients with a positive EIA and a negative PCR should be tested by RIBA. Such patients who are RIBA negative can then be assumed to have had a false-positive EIA, while those who are RIBA positive can be assumed to have had a true-positive EIA, but to have cleared the virus. However, since neither group will be treated, it is unclear if RIBA testing of PCR-negative patients is necessary, though the second group presumably has lifelong immunity and need not be tested again. Many laboratories are dispensing with RIBA and going directly to PCR confirmation and viral load testing after a positive EIA.

While there is no good therapy for hepatitis B, much progress has been made in the treatment of hepatitis C. Therapy for hepatitis C is indicated when there is interface hepatitis (Scheuer grade or stage 2), and is usually a combination of pegylated (conjugated to polyethylene glycol) α interferon and ribavirin (a synthetic nucleoside analogue). In 2011, the FDA approved both boceprevir (Victrelis) and telaprevir (Incivek), in combination with peginterferon and ribavirin, for genotype 1. Boceprevir is the first HCV protease inhibitor to be approved.

Before therapy for hepatitis C is instituted, the specific genotype is determined by sequencing a portion of the viral genome. There are 6 major genotypes of hepatitis C, and many subtypes. Depending on where one draws the line between a genotype and a subtype, the number of genotypes could be as high as 11. These genotypes respond differently to treatment. For example, genotype 1 requires a longer treatment time than genotypes 2 and 3 [PMID21473834].

Viral load (quantitation) is also determined before initiation of therapy. Several methods can be used, but quantitative polymerase chain reaction, as discussed in Chapter 45, is becoming standard. The viral load forms a baseline against which the effectiveness of therapy can be monitored. Viral load testing by different methodologies cannot be readily compared, and even within the same technique, any change in viral load that is <3-fold is unlikely to be clinically significant.

Autoimmune Liver Disease

The International Autoimmune Hepatitis Group first proposed criteria for the diagnosis of autoimmune liver disease in 1993. The group issued revised criteria in 1999 [PMID10580593] and again in 2008 [PMID18537184]. There are a variety of forms of autoimmune liver disease, some affecting the lobule (ie, hepatocytes) and others primarily centered on the bile ducts [PMID11068543]. The 2 primary manifestations of autoimmune liver disease in the biliary tree are primary sclerosing cholangitis and primary biliary cirrhosis.

Primary Sclerosing Cholangitis

Sclerosing cholangitis can occur as part of the IgG4-related autoimmune sclerosing disorders, but *primary* sclerosing cholangitis (PSC) is an autoimmune process that appears separate and unrelated to the IgG4 group of disorders [PMID20821235]. PSC usually primarily involves the extrahepatic biliary ducts, but patients often have concomitant involvement of the intrahepatic bile ducts. Patients with involvement of the large, extrahepatic ducts usually have characteristic radiologic findings upon imaging of the extrahepatic biliary tree by ERCP. The minority of patients with exclusively small duct PSC has a somewhat better prognosis than large duct PSC, though these patients may go on to develop large duct PSC [PMID19166657]. PSC is associated with p-ANCA (antimyeloperoxidase) in about 80% of cases, and is also associated with inflammatory bowel disease [PMID17486048].

The histologic changes in PSC can be subtle and the clinical and laboratory data are important in the diagnosis. Liver biopsy in cases of extrahepatic PSC may show the changes of large duct obstruction (cholestasis, portal edema, extravasated bile, neutrophils, proliferation of ductules, etc), as described above and illustrated in i25.6, but these are often not seen, making the diagnosis of extrahepatic PSC difficult without imaging studies of the extrahepatic ducts. i25.21a illustrates the acute inflammation that is seen in some cases of extrahepatic PSC. i25.21b shows the proliferation of cholangioles that may be seen in the small duct form, accompanying ductulopenia, but this feature is not necessarily present, and even if it is, there may confusion with primary biliary cirrhosis (PBC).

Some bile ducts in PSC will appear normal, but others may be surrounded by concentric, "onionskin" periductal fibrosis i25.21c, i25.21d, which if present, is an important histologic clue to the diagnosis. The portal fibrosis in PSC may encroach upon the limiting plate i25.21e and eventuate in cirrhosis i25.21f. 10-30% of patients with primary sclerosing cholangitis will develop cholangiocarcinoma.

Primary Biliary Cirrhosis

Primary biliary cirrhosis (PBC) in an autoimmune disorder found predominantly in middle aged women and characterized by AMA. The specific target of the AMA is the E2 subunit of pyruvate dehydrogenase, an enzyme complex involved in oxidative phosphorylation and found in the mitochondria [PMID19603170].

Liver function tests demonstrate increases in the canalicular enzymes alkaline phosphatase and GGT more than in the transaminases AST and ALT, but this is nonspecific and serves primarily to identify a group of patients for whom AMA testing is indicated.

The early changes are lymphocytic infiltration into portal areas and bile ducts i25.22a. Unless the bile ducts are clearly damaged, which is unusual in the early stages, or unless there are granulomas surrounding them i25.22b, i25.22c, but only 1/2 of cases of PBC have granulomas), the early stages—before there is ductulopenia—are histologically nonspecific and can resemble chronic hepatitis. Spillover into the adjacent parenchyma (interface hepatitis) often follows, but in the early stages, it may not be obvious that the bile ducts are the target and a chronic hepatitis may be suspected. In the early stages, a clue to the diagnosis of PBC, in the absence of granulomas, is a propensity of the lymphocytes to center on or near the bile ducts, an infiltration of biliary epithelium by lymphocytes, or a disruption of the basement membrane surrounding the bile duct.

Following this nonspecific early stage, there is damage to biliary epithelium, loss of ducts, disorganized proliferation of biliary epithelium i25.22d, i25.22e, and proliferation of ductules (cholangioles) [PMID19603170]. Once bile ducts are clearly the target of lymphocytic attack or become reduced in number i25.22f, the diagnosis becomes more apparent. About 70% of portal areas have a demonstrable bile duct, usually close to an artery, and the average portal area has 1 or 2 interlobular bile ducts. If this number is reduced to <0.5 bile ducts per portal area, there is a significant loss of ducts, and a duct-centered process such as PBC or PSC should be favored over a chronic hepatitis (but cholangioles must not be counted, as these are not reduced in number and may even be increased). The later stages are clearly centered on the bile ducts, but even then, unless there are granulomas, the process can resemble a small duct PSC. The clinical information (age and gender of patient, presence or absence of IBD, results of imaging studies of the extrahepatic bile ducts, and presence or absence of AMA) is indispensable in making the correct diagnosis.

In problematic cases, such as suspected PBC with negative AMA, immunohistochemical stains may highlight biliary epithelium, without staining hepatocytes, thereby elucidating the location and degree of organization of biliary epithelium. Cytokeratins 7 and 19 will do this [PMID20459548], but in my experience, the intermediate molecular weight keratin AE-1 nicely stains bile duct epithelium, but not hepatocytes [PMID8863666], and is ideal for demonstrating disorganized biliary epithelium that is intermingled with large numbers of lymphocytes and difficult to appreciate on H&E examination i25.22g.

The Scheuer system for viral hepatitis has been successfully adapted for primary biliary cirrhosis, since both processes are centered on portal areas, though the status of the biliary epithelium is perhaps more important than the Scheuer grade for inflammation. Grading and staging are essentially the same as for its use in viral hepatitis i25.22h-j. For both viral hepatitis and primary biliary cirrhosis, the Scheuer system conveys all the needed information and is much easier to reproducibly employ than more complicated systems.

Treatment of PBC is with ursodeoxycholic acid (UDCA), and prognosis has improved sharply in the last 2 decades [PMID19603170], but if unchecked or treated too late, PBC continues to cirrhosis, in which case transplant is the only current therapeutic option.

5-10% of cases of PBC by both serum enzyme levels and histologic findings are negative for AMA (a positive antinuclear antibody, often with a speckled pattern, or a positive anti-smooth muscle antibody is almost always found in these cases; an autoimmune process directed at biliary epithelium without any positive serological test is very rare). These cases have been designated autoimmune cholangitis, but the traditional term "AMA-negative PBC" seems completely appropriate since these unusual cases are indistinguishable from classic AMA-positive cases in every other way [PMID18251980]. Almost 1/2 of AMA-negative cases of PBC will be positive for unusual specific nuclear antigens [PMID21188646, PMID21185272].

Autoimmune Hepatitis

Autoimmune hepatitis (AIH) is a chronic autoimmune process directed against the hepatocytes in the lobule rather than against biliary epithelium. AIH has no specific histologic features. Its appearance varies with the stage of its evolution, the presence or absence of a concomitant autoimmune process involving the biliary epithelium, such as PBC or PSC, and the effects of treatment. In pure form, AIH generally has the appearance of chronic hepatitis, with interface hepatitis and sparing of centrilobular hepatocytes, in accord with the general principle that chronic inflammatory conditions in the liver affect the portal area and limiting plate i25.23a-c. Plasma cells are vaguely suggestive of AIH, but are far from sensitive or specific, and clinical and laboratory correlation, and serologic and histologic exclusion of a biliary component, are needed for the diagnosis [PMID21055683]. A true acute form of AIH exists, but is rare. Most cases of acute AIH are actually acute exacerbations of chronic AIH [PMID21595804].

Type 1 AIH accounts for 80% of cases. Many of these occur in younger women. Type 1 AIH is associated with antismooth muscle antibody and/or ANA (the ANA is usually a homogeneous pattern).

Type 2 AIH is associated with antiliver and kidney microsomal antibody (LKM antibody; the word "microsome" refers to an in vitro preparation of the endoplasmic reticulum). LKM antibodies are directed against components of cytochrome p450 and antiliver cytosol type 1, a peptide found in hepatocyte cytoplasm [PMID18528935]. Most patients with type II AIH are children.

Type 3 AIH has antibodies to antigens that were previously called soluble liver proteins (SLA) or liver-pancreas (LP) antigen. Because SLA and the LP antigen have been shown to be identical, they are often referred to as SLA/LP antigen [PMID18528935]. SLA/LP antigen cannot be detected by immunofluorescence [PMID2880112], and therefore may be missed on routine screen. Type 3 AIH may also have antismooth muscle. In contrast to types 1 and 2, these patients usually do not have systemic manifestations of autoimmune disease. The histologic appearance of all of these types of AIH is nonspecific except for possible occasional plasma cells.

Overlap syndrome has clinical and histologic features of both AIH and PBC i25.24a, i25.24b, or more rarely, AIH and PSC [PMID19072425]. It may have a positive AMA and ANA, usually with a homogenous pattern.

Alcoholic and Nonalcoholic Fatty Liver Disease (NAFLD)

By definition, viral and autoimmune etiologies have been excluded in the categories of alcoholic and nonalcoholic fatty liver disease (NAFLD), and alcohol consumption is excluded in NAFLD. The former exclusion—viral and autoimmune processes—is generally relatively easy, not only because of the availability of good serologic testing, but also because unlike viral and autoimmune processes, alcoholic and NAFLD tend to cause steatosis in the lobule i25.25a, cytoplasmic invagination into hepatocyte nuclei i25.25b, and if the process progresses to fibrosis, there is usually a deposition of fine collagen in the lobule as well as or in lieu of portal expansion i25.25c, i25.25d, though all of these findings are seen in viral and autoimmune processes.

The second exclusion—alcoholic from nonalcoholic fatty liver disease—is much more difficult. Alcoholic liver disease classically causes macrovesicular fat and micronodular cirrhosis, but these historical observations are of little practical use. Likewise, alcohol may have a slightly greater propensity to cause Mallory bodies (also called Mallory-Denk bodies), which are cytoplasmic collections of keratin filaments (specifically, cytokeratins 8 and 18 that have been attached to the protein ubiquitin) [PMID18805482], and neutrophilic infiltration than NAFLD i25.26, but for all practical purposes, alcoholic liver disease cannot be distinguished histologically from nonviral, nonautoimmune, nonalcoholic fatty liver disease. Moreover, it is often difficult to get a reliable history on the use of alcohol and there is no good blood test at this time to determine if a patient is drinking. The opinion that an AST level that is disproportionately elevated relative to ALT suggests ethanol is fraught with difficulty because there are both mitochondrial and cytosolic forms of both AST and ALT [PMID2302779, PMID7602770] and AST is found in many other tissues (muscle, heart, erythrocytes, kidney, brain).

Both GGT and alkaline phosphatase are canalicular enzymes that are elevated in obstructive conditions, as opposed to the transaminases AST and ALT, which reflect hepatocyte injury, but ethanol often directly results in elevated GGT apart from obstruction [PMID17045579]. Carbohydrate-deficient transferrin (CDT), and mean corpuscular volume of erythrocytes (MCV) are also helpful [PMID17045579, PMID17579567]. A serum level of GGT that is disproportionately elevated relative to alkaline phosphatase, CDT, and increased MCV are the best tests to suggest ethanol, but even in combination, are not perfect. Great caution is needed in drawing conclusions regarding an alcohol etiology from serum testing. *Indeed, the distinction cannot be made on a biopsy.*

NAFLD encompasses both nonalcoholic steatosis (ie, simple fatty change) and nonalcoholic steatohepatitis (NASH; fatty change with inflammation), and eventually cirrhosis in a minority of cases. NAFLD is now believed to be a hepatic manifestation of metabolic syndrome. The prevalence of NAFLD is difficult to determine because some cases are caused by surreptitious ethanol consumption but is probably is at least 10% in developed countries and is growing because of the epidemic of obesity.

2 polymorphisms in apolipoprotein C3, C482T and T455C, are associated with NAFLD [PMID20335584]. Apolipoprotein C3 inhibits hepatic lipase, and because these polymorphisms increase the concentration of apolipoprotein C3, lipase activity is decreased, resulting in increased amounts of triglycerides in the hepatocytes.

The Scheuer system is usually reserved for portal area-centered processes, such as chronic viral hepatitis and autoimmune processes, and another system, usually a modification of the Knodell or Ishak systems, is used in NAFLD. The most recent assessment system for NAFLD is the Clinical Network Scoring System by Kleiner, Brunt, and their coworkers [PMID15915461]. The following 3 categories are initially assessed in the Kleiner and Brunt system: steatosis (0-3), lobular inflammation (0-3), and hepatocyte ballooning (0-2). Steatosis involving <5% of the parenchyma is considered a variant of normal and is scored as a zero. 5-33% steatosis receives a score of 1, 33-66% a score of 2, and anything >66% receives a score of 3. A single focus of lobular inflammation per 200× field is scored as a 1, 2-4 such foci is scored as a 2, and >4 foci is scored as a 3. Occasional ballooned hepatocytes are scored as 1, while numerous foci of ballooning are a 2. Mallory bodies are often seen in any form of steatotic liver disease, and are not specifically scored.

NAFLD activity score (NAS) is the sum of the above 3 and is scored (0-8). NAS is really an assessment of steatohepatitis vs simple steatosis. NAS of 0-2 is likely not NASH, but is better regarded as simple steatosis without significant inflammation. A NAS of 3-4 is borderline for NASH, and a NAS of higher than 5 is considered diagnostic of NASH. i25.27a-c illustrate a Kleiner and Brunt activity score of 4/8, 2 for steatosis, 1 for lobular inflammation, and 1 for ballooning change.

Once the diagnosis of NASH is made as above, the Kleiner and Brunt system then separately assesses fibrosis on a scale of 0-4. The fibrosis in nonalcoholic liver disease, like the inflammation, tends to be more lobular-centered than portal-centered, and to surround individual hepatocytes or small groups of hepatocytes in the parenchyma, forming a delicate mesh. For this reason, the fibrosis in NAFLD is also scored differently from the Scheuer system, and is scored 0-4. Any process whose fibrosis is restricted to the lobule, even if moderate, is scored as a 1. Likewise, those rare cases in which the fibrosis is restricted to portal or periportal areas also receive a score of 1. A score of 2 is given for processes that demonstrate both lobular and portal or periportal fibrosis. Bridging fibrosis is a 3 and cirrhosis is a 4. i25.27d illustrates a fibrosis score of 1/4 in the same case as in i25.27a-c.

After the diagnosis of NASH is established in a case of NAFLD, and fibrosis is assessed, a global NASH score is issued. The global NASH score is the sum of NAS and fibrosis, and can range from 0-12. In the case illustrated in i25.27a-d, the fibrosis is minimal, 1/4, and the global score is 5/12. The fibrosis score can also identify a process as more serious than the NAS would suggest. i25.28a-d illustrate a case with a similar NAS of 4/8, but with cirrhosis. The advantages of this system is that it is specific to steatotic processes that remain primarily centered in the lobule, rather than processes, such as chronic viral and AIH, that become centered in the portal area.

Although the Kleiner and Brunt system provides for independent assessments of inflammation and fibrosis, in my opinion, borderline activity scores should be considered NASH if there is any fibrosis. For example, a NAS of 3/8 is a low activity score, equivocal between simple steatosis and steatohepatitis, but if there is also a fibrosis score of 1/4, the inflammation, mild though it is, must have had some consequence. In borderline situations, a persistent (longer than 6 months) elevation of transaminases should tip the scales to a mild steatohepatitis. Serum levels of cytokeratin 18 fragments may differentiate simple steatosis from true steatohepatitis. Values of CK-18 fragments above 395 U/L point to steatohepatitis with a sensitivity of 85.7% and specificity of 99.9%. A cutoff value of 380.2 U/L resulted in a sensitivity of 90.5% and specificity of 94.4% [PMID17352011].

Nonalcoholic steatosis and steatohepatitis are real entities, to be sure, but a leading cause of apparent nonalcoholic liver disease is unacknowledged ethanol consumption. Therefore, although the scoring system of Kleiner and Brunt was developed for nonalcoholic liver disease, it would seem to be applicable to alcoholic liver disease as well, since the 2 processes cannot be differentiated histologically. To my mind, once viruses and autoimmune processes are excluded by appropriate serological testing, and a histologic appearance of steatosis/steatohepatitis that is centered in the lobule is encountered, it is prudent to employ the Kleiner and Brunt scoring system even if the apparent etiology is ethanol.

Cirrhosis

Cirrhosis is a final outcome many processes that cause chronic liver disease, but in common practice, cirrhosis is most frequently encountered in viral and autoimmune processes, and in ethanol use. Cirrhotic nodules are considered regenerative. Historically, it was considered important in cases of cirrhosis to indicate if the cirrhosis was micronodular (nodules that were 0.3 cm or less) or macronodular (nodules >0.3 cm in diameter). The idea behind this was that there was an association between the size of the nodules and the likely etiology (eg, ethanol tends to cause micronodular cirrhosis). Today, however, it is understood that the size of cirrhotic nodules is of very limited value in determining the etiology. Complete testing and a thorough history are much more informative. Moreover, with time, cirrhotic micronodules tend to coalesce into macronodules.

It is useful to comment on the activity of any cirrhosis. Active cirrhosis has continued interface hepatitis, while an inactive cirrhosis has a sharp demarcation between the septae and the parenchyma. The number of lymphocytes in the septae is not prognostically or therapeutically useful, but the degree of ongoing interface hepatitis may be.

Advances in the treatment of hepatic disorders leading to cirrhosis have led to exciting new ideas on diagnosis and reporting, and to 2 new conceptions regarding cirrhosis. First, until recently, cirrhosis was considered to be fundamentally distinct from bridging fibrosis, representing a significant further progression. Second, cirrhosis has historically been considered to be irreversible. A liver biopsy that demonstrated cirrhosis was considered inherently different from one that demonstrated bridging fibrosis in both its severity and its irreversibility.

Regarding the first new conception, it has been recommended that the term "advanced stage" replace either bridging fibrosis or cirrhosis, reflecting newer thinking that the "breakpoint" is no longer between bridging fibrosis and cirrhosis, but rather between no or minimal fibrosis and bridging fibrosis [PMID22180471].

Regarding the second new conception, it is now clear that therapy can not only arrest the inciting agent, but can actually lead to a reduction in fibrous tissue, perhaps even partially reversing cirrhosis. Tentative criteria have been established for the determination and assessment of regression of cirrhosis [PMID11079009], but in practice, at this time, regression is best verified by comparison of a biopsy to a previous biopsy. Admittedly, this raises the issue of sampling error, but until histologic criteria are firmly established, it is our best approach.

The future will undoubtedly bring better a understanding of the molecular mechanisms of liver disease, and of the mechanism and recognition of regression of cirrhosis, but the important points at this time are that the report should recognize the essential similarity between bridging fibrosis and cirrhosis and should indicate not just the degree of fibrosis, but also the etiology, activity, and risk factors for worsening fibrosis or the development of carcinoma. For example, instead of indicating "chronic hepatitis C with bridging fibrosis, no definitive cirrhosis," the report might say "chronic hepatitis C, advanced stage, with activity, and with hepatocyte dysplasia." If there is evidence of regression, this should also be mentioned (eg, "chronic hepatitis C, advanced stage, but with features of regression").

For clarity, I recommend reporting both the "old' and "new" systems. For example:

> Liver biopsy: Chronic hepatitis C with bridging fibrosis, no definitive cirrhosis (chronic hepatitis C, advanced stage, with activity, by criteria proposed by the International Liver Pathology Study Group)

Drug-Induced Hepatitis

Although there are no specific histologic features of a drug-induced hepatitis, eosinophils, granulomas, fatty change, and cholestasis are characteristic, and exogenous agents should be excluded when any of these histologic findings are present.

Although fatty change is often seen in drug-induced hepatitis, the Kleiner and Brunt system is not recommended because the overall histologic findings in drug-induced hepatitis are rather dissimilar from fatty liver disease. The Roenigk scale [PMID5548272] is sometimes used to assess liver morphology in patients on methotrexate, which is used for psoriasis and some autoimmune disorders, especially rheumatoid arthritis. Roenigk scale 1 is mild steatosis **i25.29**, 2 is moderate steatosis without fibrosis, 3a is mild fibrosis, 3b is bridging fibrosis, and Roenigk scale 4 is cirrhosis. In this system, methotrexate can be continued with caution in 3a, but should be stopped in stage 3b.

Unusual Forms of Hepatitis

The diagnosis of nonspecific idiopathic neonatal hepatitis is made less often now, as the etiology of cholestatic syndromes of the neonatal period can now be determined in most cases.

Nevertheless, about 20% of cases remain idiopathic. Viruses are suspected in many of these cases, but a viral etiology can be shown in only about 20% of cases. Neonatal hepatitis has no specific histologic features, but lobular disarray, cholestasis, giant cells, and extramedullary hematopoiesis are commonly seen **i25.30a**, **i25.30b** [PMID20871223].

Primary recurrent pyogenic cholangitis (Oriental cholangiohepatitis) is now called hepatolithiasis, as most cases can be shown to result from the intrahepatic formation of stones [PMID17127192]. Hepatolithiasis resembles primary sclerosing cholangitis, with a bile duct-centered inflammatory process with fibrosis and ductule proliferation, but usually has more acute inflammation.

Graft vs Host Disease and Transplantation Pathology of the Liver

With the success of both bone marrow and solid organ transplantation, the pathologist is increasingly called upon to evaluate organs that are either attacked by allographic T lymphocytes in bone marrow recipient (graft vs host disease [GVHD]) or by the patient's own immune system in solid organ transplantation (rejection). Both GVHD and rejection have different stages and manifestations, occasionally with overlapping histologic features. Clinical correlation is essential, as the biopsy is never the only means by which GVHD or rejection is diagnosed. The most fundamental clinical question is "Did the patient receive a liver or a bone marrow transplant?" The answer to that question tells the pathologist whether to be on guard for the histologic signs of GVHD or organ rejection. The second question is the time since the transplant, and the third consideration is the clinical situation.

Acute GVHD occurs in bone marrow transplants and results when donor T lymphocytes react to proteins on host cells, primarily those of the HLA system. The clinical manifestations of acute GVHD occur primarily in the skin, gastrointestinal tract, and liver. In acute GVHD of the liver, there is damage to biliary epithelium (edema, vacuolization, and necrosis), with T-lymphocyte infiltration of the portal tracts and occasionally of the venous endothelium (endothelialitis) [PMID19282026]. Although the inflammation of the endothelium is inconstant, it is essentially diagnostic if found. Early GVHD can be difficult to diagnose because hepatocyte damage secondary to vascular compromise may be the predominant histologic feature, but bile duct damage or endothelialitis is required for the diagnosis. Any hepatocyte damage in a patient who has received a bone marrow transplant should elicit a search for the diagnostic features of acute GVHD.

Chronic GVHD affects primarily the skin, liver, eyes, and mouth. The etiology of chronic GVHD is less well understood than acute GVHD, and the variety of agents that are available for acute GVHD are not yet available for chronic GVHD, which is usually treated with a combination of cyclosporine and prednisone [PMID16426941]. In chronic GVHD of the liver, there is cholestasis and elevated transaminases, resulting in a clinical picture that resembles acute viral hepatitis. Histologic findings also resemble acute hepatitis [PMID11093733], but with the additional finding of damage to biliary epithelium that may rarely progress to the near absence of bile ducts [PMID15765790], making chronic GVHD a rare cause of the so-called vanishing bile duct syndrome (along with PSC, PBC, and some cases of chronic rejection of transplanted livers). Hepatocytes may be damaged, but this is less likely than in acute GVHD, and such damage is only in conjunction with damage to bile ducts.

In liver transplantation, hyperacute rejection (thankfully rare) is primarily humoral and is manifest as an immediately obvious (often intraoperative) compromise of the organ. There is a necrotizing arteritis with neutrophils and necrosis. Likewise, acute humoral rejection also primarily involves the vasculature.

On the other hand, acute cellular rejection is characterized by a mixed portal infiltrate, including T lymphocytes and usually also eosinophils, attacking the bile duct epithelium and the venous endothelium [PMID16892531]. By definition, there is no overt bile duct loss, and acute cellular rejection somewhat resembles acute GVHD. Arteritis and necrosis may occur in severe cases, but if they do, the changes are less severe and occur later than in hyperacute rejection. The hepatocytes are not directly attacked, but may be secondarily affected by ischemia. Mild (grade 1) acute cellular rejection involves <50% of portal areas. Moderate or grade 2 involves >50% of portal areas. Severe cellular rejection has spillover of inflammation into the parenchyma or damage to hepatocytes.

Chronic rejection has a vascular form, characterized by intimal and subintimal fibrosis and deposition of macrophages, eventuating in luminal compromise and ischemic damage to hepatocytes, and a biliary form in which there is injury to and loss of bile ducts [PMID16892531]. These 2 forms of rejection may occur simultaneously, but the vascular changes are more prominent in vessels of larger caliber than are typically sampled in a core biopsy, leaving the pathologist with histologic abnormalities that predominantly involve the biliary epithelium. Chronic biliary rejection can be a cause of vanishing bile duct syndrome. The biliary manifestation of chronic rejection can be difficult to distinguish from severe acute cellular rejection if there is no vascular component, especially in the early stages of chronic rejection, since the bile ducts are the target in both processes [PMID16892531]. This is problematic because acute cellular rejection, even if severe, is potentially reversible, while chronic rejection is likely irreversible. Intimal macrophages or fibrosis suggest chronicity, and there is usually less inflammation in chronic rejection than in acute rejection. Mild, or grade 1, chronic biliary rejection has only bile duct loss, whereas grades 2 and 3 have superimposed cholestasis, fibrosis, or hepatocyte damage.

ISBN 978-089189-5886

Core Points for the Gallbladder and the Nonneoplastic Liver

- Acute large duct obstruction or extrahepatic atresia: cholestasis, rupture of bile ducts with extravasation of bile, proliferation of bile ductules, and acute inflammation.
- Intrahepatic atresia: decreased bile ducts and increased ductules.
- Hereditary hemochromatosis: one of the iron overload syndromes.
  - o Type 1 from mutations in the *HFE* gene, usually either C282Y or H63D.
  - o Other types may be more common in non-Caucasian patients.
- Wilson disease: abnormal forms of copper transport protein ATP7B from mutations in the *ATP7B* gene.
  - o Acute stage: fatty change, a portal lymphocytic infiltrate, and nuclear glycogenation
  - o Chronic stage: fibrosis and cirrhosis
- Alpha-1-antitrypsin (A1AT): regulates other enzymes.
  - o Normal genotype for the *A1AT* gene is MM.
  - o Abnormal alleles—notably the Z and S alleles—result in impaired secretion of A1AT from the liver.
  - o Symptoms from hepatic compromise secondary to intrahepatic accumulation of the protein and from emphysema secondary to unimpeded activity of enzymes such as elastase in the lung.
  - o PAS stain is a screening test on hepatic biopsy
  - o Definitive diagnosis requires IHC for A1AT, followed by demonstration of diminished serum levels of A1AT and confirmation of a mutation in the gene.
- Diagnosis of either hepatitis B or C requires clinical and serologic information.
  - o Acute viral hepatitis: rarely biopsied, affects lobule.
  - o Chronic viral hepatitis: affects portal areas and limiting plate.
  - o Mild or early chronic viral hepatitis: either inflammatory cells or fibrous tissue encroaches on the limiting plate.
  - o Determination of viral load at diagnosis monitors the effectiveness of therapy, especially for hepatitis C.
- Autoimmune hepatitis: directed against hepatocytes.
  - o 3 types, all primarily affect hepatocytes at the limiting plate
  - o Biopsy looks like chronic hepatitis.
- Sclerosing cholangitis: primary or secondary.
  - o Primary: associated with inflammatory bowel disease.
  - o Secondary: part of the IgG4 spectrum of disorders or idiopathic.
- Primary sclerosing cholangitis (PBC): strong female predilection and a strong association with antimitochondrial antibody.
  - o Liver function tests: disproportionate increases in GGT and alkaline phosphatase.
  - o Early stage: lymphocytic infiltration of portal areas, often accompanied by focal interface hepatitis.
  - o Biopsy may not be fully diagnostic until the chronic stage, when there is damage to bile ducts and with proliferation of ductules.
  - o Granulomas in half of cases.
- Overlap syndrome: clinical and histologic features of both autoimmune hepatitis and PBC.
- Nonalcoholic fatty liver disease (NAFLD): diagnosis of exclusion.
  - o Negative viral and autoimmune serologies.
  - o Negative ethanol history.
  - o Generally associated with obesity, diabetes, or a disorder of lipid metabolism.
  - o Manifestation of metabolic syndrome.
  - o Noninflammatory steatosis or steatohepatitis (NASH).
  - o NASH can develop fibrosis, and in a minority of cases, progress to cirrhosis.
  - o Separate assessments of inflammatory activity and fibrosis.
- Alcoholic liver disease: no specific histologic features, but
  - o Carbohydrate-deficient transferrin serum test may help.
  - o Kleiner and Brunt system can be used.
- Cirrhosis: final outcome of many processes, but is usually an end-stage of viral, autoimmune, or alcoholic disease.
  - o Cirrhotic nodules are regenerative, but do not reconstitute normal hepatic architecture.
- Graft-vs-host disease and hepatic allograft rejection: acute and chronic forms.
  - o Chronic GVHD and chronic biliary rejection: both have attack on biliary epithelium, with loss of bile ducts.

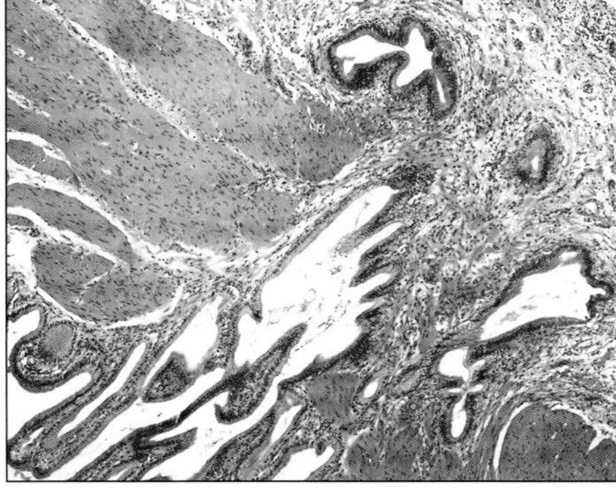

i25.1 A Rokitansky-Aschoff sinus of the gallbladder. Note the deep invaginations, through the muscularis propria, and into the serosa. The glandular structures in the serosa, if not connected to a Rokitansky-Aschoff sinus in the plane of section under examination, may appear as ducts of Luschka.

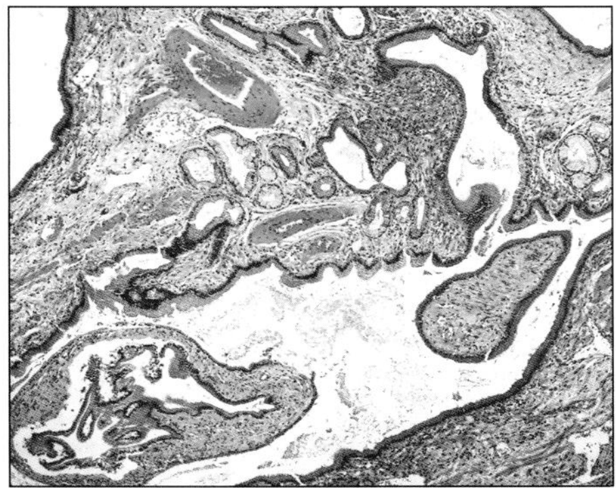

i25.2 A so-called adenomyoma of the gallbladder. There is no neoplastic process here, simply a complex intermingling of epithelium derived from Rokitansky-Aschoff sinuses and stroma.

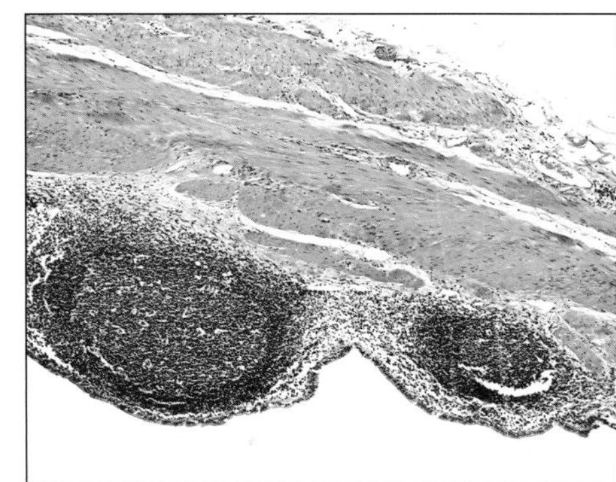

i25.3 Follicular cholecystitis

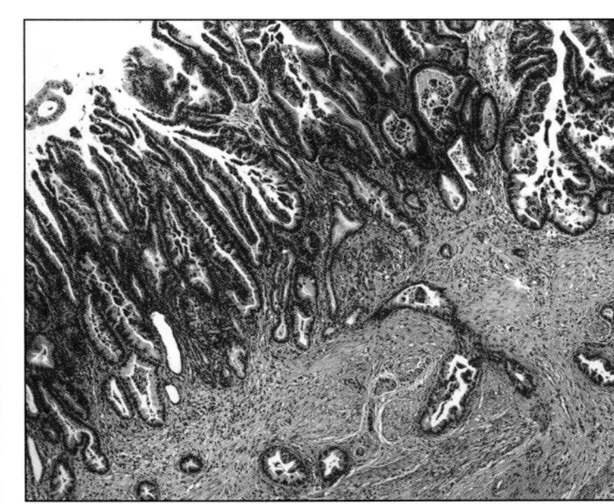

i25.4 A superficially invasive adenocarcinoma of the gallbladder, discovered incidentally in a gallbladder removed for cholelithiasis.

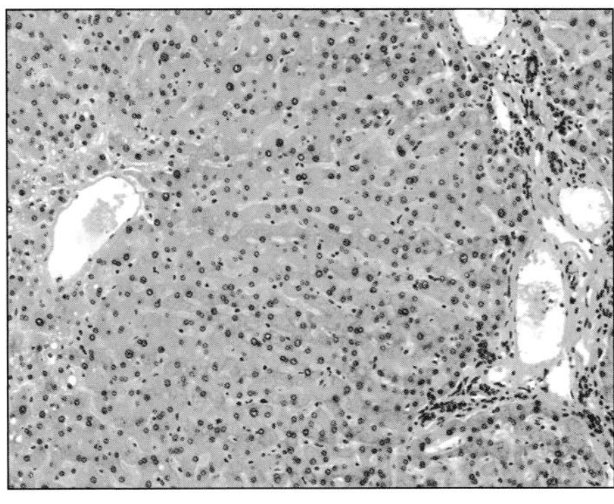

i25.5 Normal hepatic lobule. The portal area (right) contains bile ducts and branches of both the portal vein and the hepatic artery. Blood percolates through the sinusoids from right to left, and leaves the lobule through the central vein (left). The bile made by hepatocytes goes in the other direction, percolating in biliary channels of increasing caliber to leave the lobule through the bile ducts, best seen in the upper right.

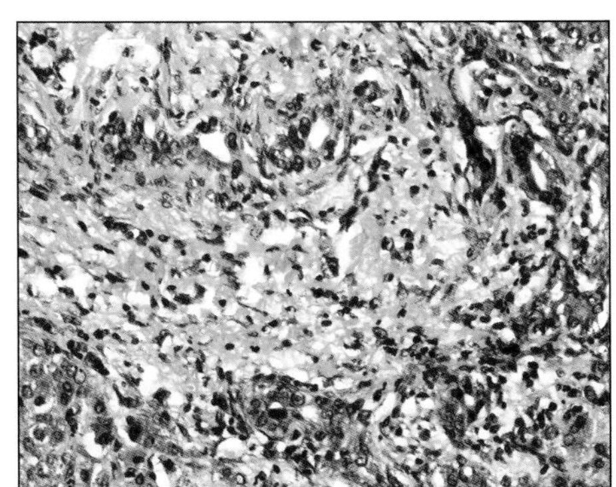

i25.6 Changes in the liver seen in large duct obstruction or extrahepatic atresia. There is cholestasis, evident in this photograph as small brown collections of bile, acute inflammation, best seen in the lower right, and a proliferation of bile ducts.

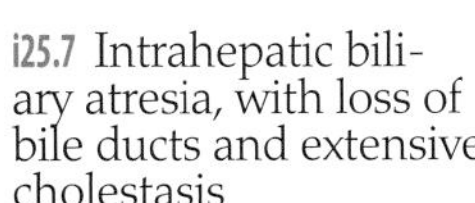

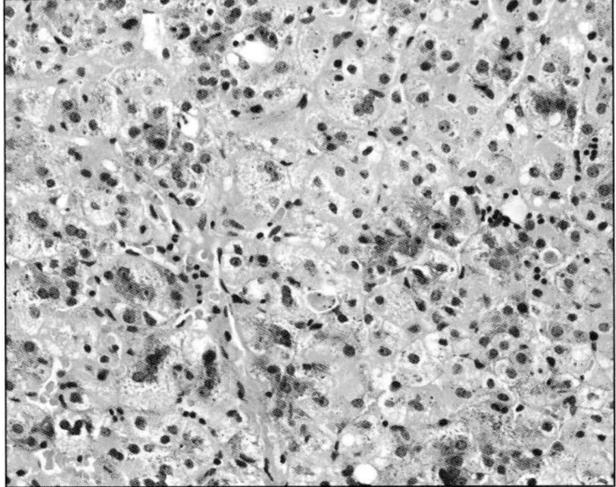

i25.7 Intrahepatic biliary atresia, with loss of bile ducts and extensive cholestasis

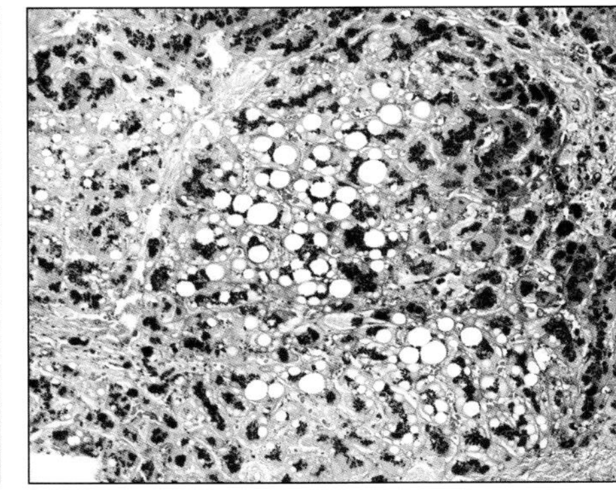

i25.8 An iron stain (Prussian blue) demonstrating hepatic iron overload. Iron overload syndrome is not synonymous with hereditary hemochromatosis, as there are other causes of iron deposition and not all cases of hereditary hemochromatosis, especially if diagnosed and treated, necessarily have significant iron deposition.

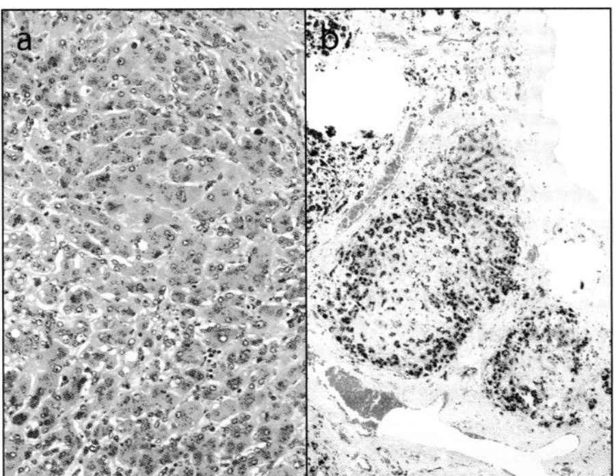

i25.9 Hereditary hemochromatosis. **a** is an H&E stain in which the iron is evident as subtle golden pigment within hepatocytes. **b** is an iron stain that not only highlights the degree of iron deposition, but also demonstrates nodules of hepatocytes, indicating cirrhosis.

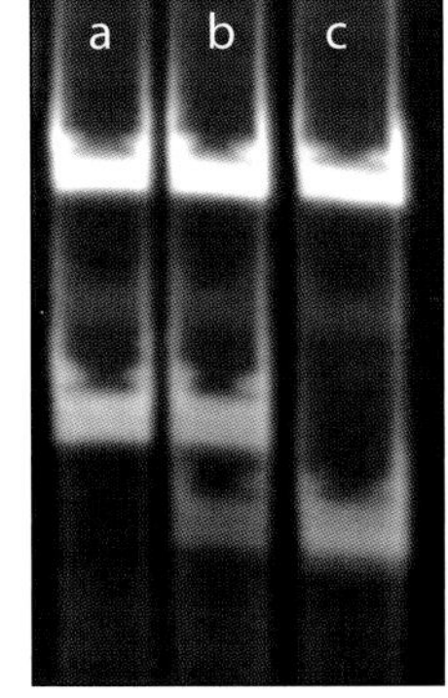

i25.10 A 393 base pair (bp) fragment of the *HFE* gene that includes nucleotide position 845 (variations of which cause the C282Y mutation) is amplified. Amplicons are digested with a restriction enzyme. **a** In the normal patient, the result is fragments of 247 bp above and 146 bp below it. **b-c** The larger fragment is maintained in the abnormal, but the 146 bp fragment is not generated. Rather, restriction cleavage results in 2 small fragments of 117 bp and 29 bp (which runs off of the gel and is not seen). **b** Sample from a heterozygous patient has bands at 247, 146, and 117 bp. **c** is from a patient who is homozygous for hereditary hemochromatosis; 247 bp fragment is retained, but the 146 bp is absent and a 117 bp band is seen.

ISBN 978-089189-5886

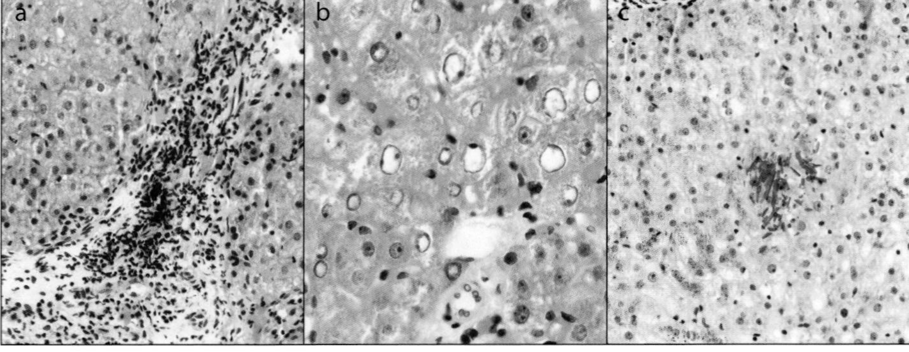

i25.11 Wilson disease. **a** demonstrates increased lymphocytes in the portal area. **b** demonstrates cytoplasmic invagination into nuclei, causing pronounced nuclear clearing. Neither of these findings is at all specific for Wilson disease. **c** is a copper stain, formerly useful in the diagnosis of Wilson disease, but seldom necessary or employed now.

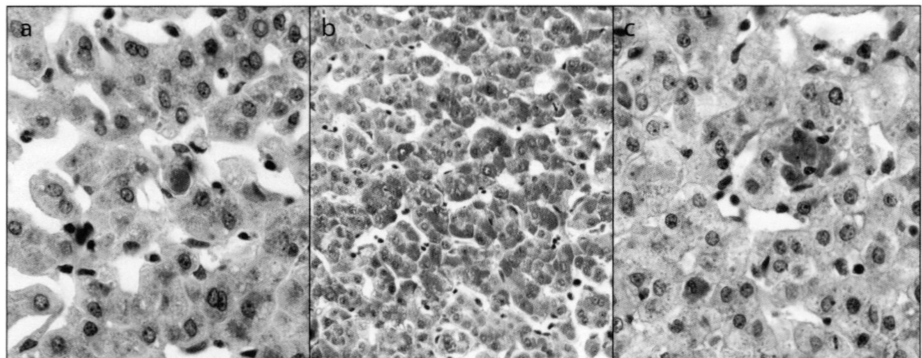

i25.12 α-1-antitrypsin deficiency. **a** is an H&E stain demonstrating a globule of the protein, evident as a red intracellular inclusion. **b** is a PAS stain without diastase. The α-1-antitrypsin globules cannot be seen because of all the glycogen. **c** is a PAS stain after thorough diastase digestion to remove the glycogen, demonstrating the α-1-antitrypsin inclusions in the cytoplasm.

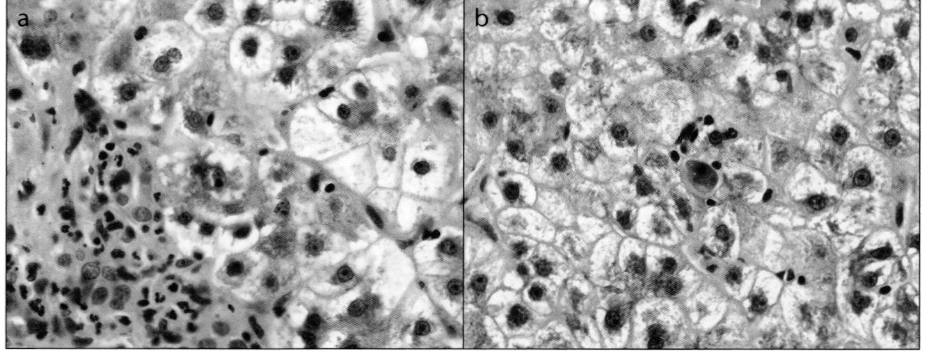

i25.13 a-b Acute hepatitis. Although acute inflammatory cells are seen in the lower left, the most important histologic finding is actually the intercellular edema (ballooning degeneration) of the hepatocytes and the disruption of the normal lobular architecture. Contrast to the orderly appearance seen in i25.5. **b** again demonstrates extensive intracellular edema and also demonstrates a Councilman body in the center. Whereas Mallory bodies are collections of intermediate filaments in the cytoplasm of viable cells, a Councilman body is an entire necrotic hepatocyte (note the pyknotic nucleus, confirming that it is a complete cell).

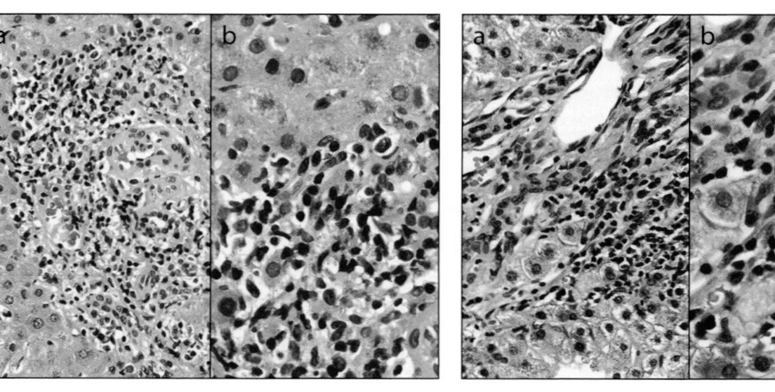

i25.14 a Chronic hepatitis in which the lymphocytes in the portal area have not spilled over into the adjacent parenchyma **b** A higher-power view of the same case as in i25.14a, confirming the sharp boundary between the expanded portal area and the limiting plate

i25.15 a Chronic hepatitis in which the lymphocytes have spilled over from the portal area into the adjacent hepatocytes **b** A higher-power view of the same case as in i25.15a, illustrating the intermingling of lymphocytes that have left the portal area with hepatocytes from the limiting plate, resulting in interface hepatitis

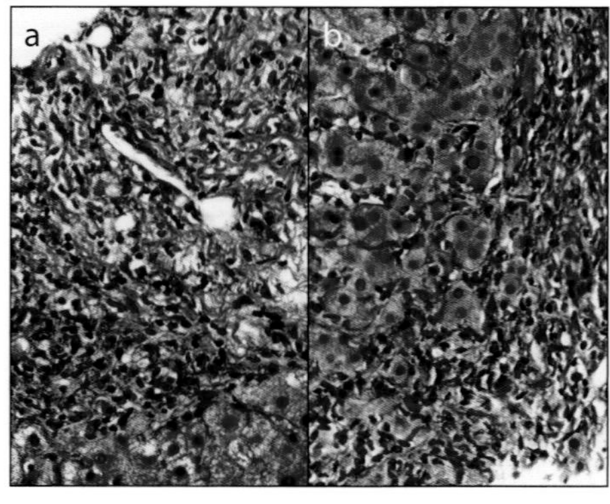

i25.16 a A trichrome stain shows a sharp division between an expanded portal area and the adjacent hepatocytes in mild chronic hepatitis **b** A trichrome stain highlighting interface hepatitis in a more serious case of chronic hepatitis. Both collagen and lymphocytes in the portal area intermingle with hepatocytes; the boundary of the portal area is indistinct and poorly defined.

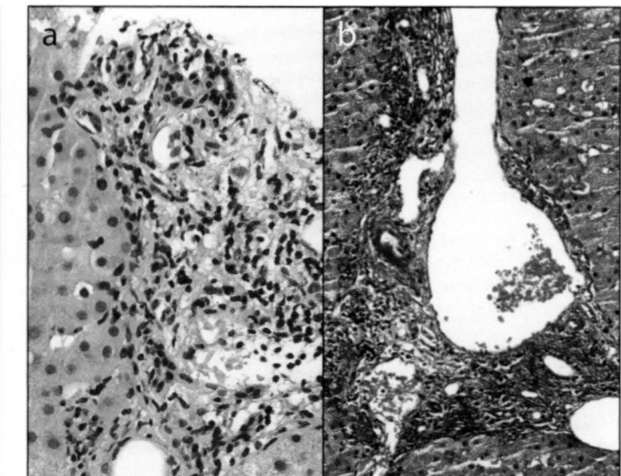

i25.17 a Chronic hepatitis of Scheuer grade 1-2, with general respect for the limiting plate and only a small focus of interface hepatitis in the lower center **b** The same case as i25.17a, with a Scheuer stage 1-2, demonstrating focal encroachment by fibrous tissue upon the limiting plate on the left

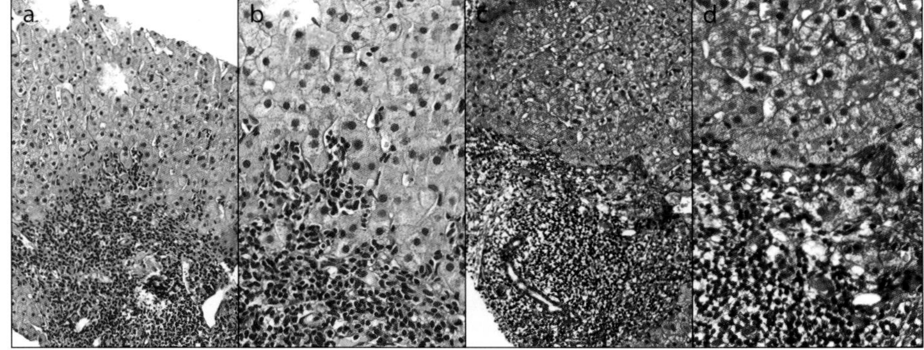

i25.18 a-b A low-power and high-power view of a chronic hepatitis of Scheuer grade 2, with focal, but obvious interface hepatitis

c-d A trichrome stain of the same case, illustrating that fibrous tissue has accompanied the lymphocytes into the limiting plate, Scheuer stage 2

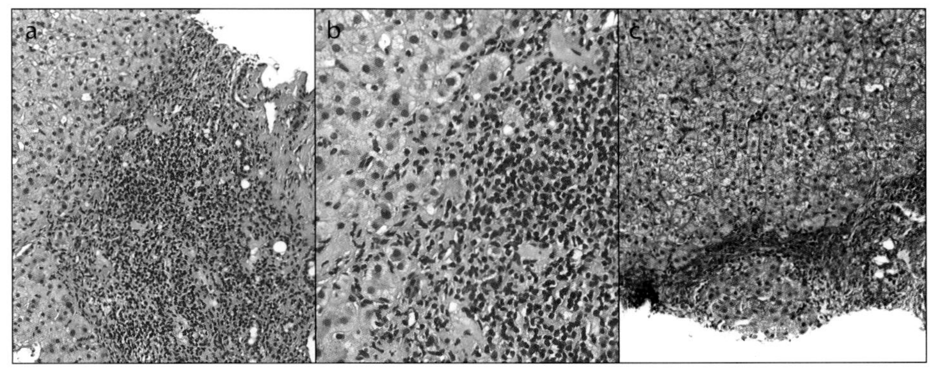

i25.19 a-b Low and high-power views of a Scheuer grade 2-3, with extensive interface hepatitis

c Chronic hepatitis of Scheuer stage 3 (bridging fibrosis). There is a small demarcated nodule of hepatocytes at the bottom, but this was the exception in this case and the fibrosis was short of cirrhosis. However, under the 2012 proposal by the International Liver Pathology Study Group, this would still be called advanced stage.

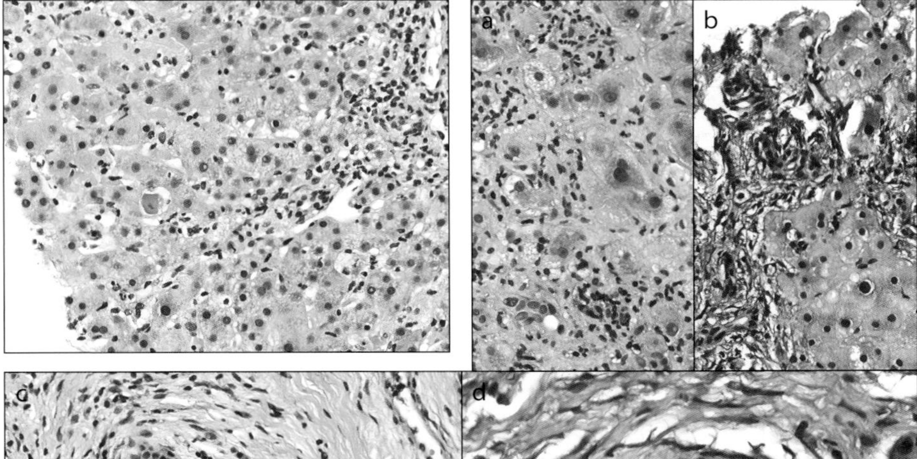

i25.20 Chronic hepatitis with a Councilman body to the left of center, illustrating ongoing acute activity

i25.21 Primary sclerosing cholangitis (PSC). These illustrations come from 3 separate cases of PSC, all in patients with a history of ulcerative colitis.
a Acute inflammation in a case of extrahepatic PSC
b Fibrosis with numerous cholangioles in a case of PSC

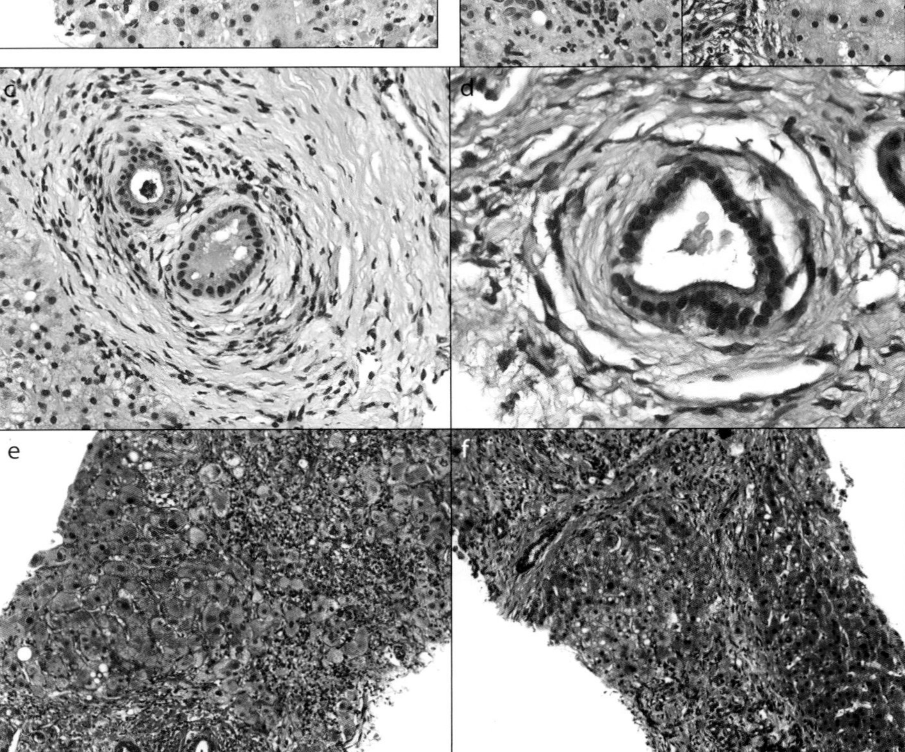

c-d "Onionskin" periductal fibrosis, a characteristic form of fibrosis that is suggestive of PSC

e A trichrome stain in PSC, illustrating severe encroachment upon the limiting plate

f Overt cirrhosis in PSC

ISBN 978-089189-5886

i25.22 Aspects of primary biliary cirrhosis (PBC). All are from patients with antimitochondrial antibodies.
a Early PBC. There is little interface hepatitis and relatively unaffected bile ducts. At this early stage, the diagnosis is not clear.
b Early stage PBC, but the epithelioid histiocytes in the portal area suggest the diagnosis even though the bile ducts have not yet been attacked.
c Early stage PBC with a well defined granuloma. The bile ducts, at the bottom of the photograph, demonstrate minimal lymphocytic infiltration, but are otherwise unaffected.
d-e Disorganized biliary epithelium in well developed PBC. The slightly larger nuclei belong to epithelial cells that do not form well defined ducts.
f Late stage PBC with dropout of bile ducts
g An AE1 immunohistochemical stain highlighting biliary epithelium but not staining hepatocytes or lymphocytes. This stain demonstrates one unremarkable bile duct and several cholangioles at the bottom of the portal area.
h A trichrome stain in a relatively early stage of PBC, a Scheuer stage 2
i A trichrome stain in a more advanced stage of PBC
j Late stage PBC with cirrhosis that is obvious even on H&E examination

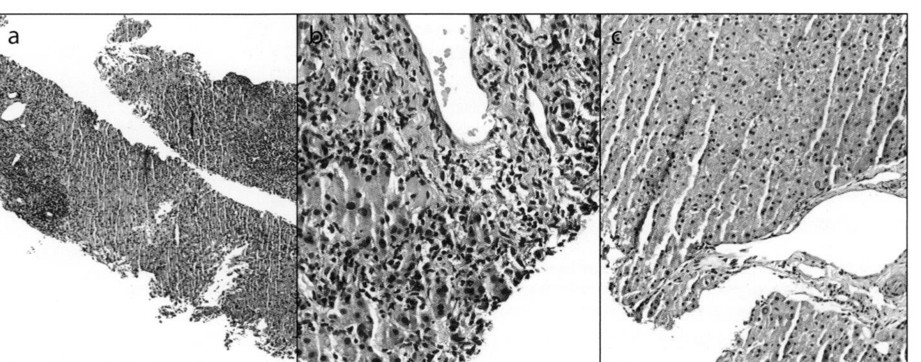

i25.23 **a** A low-power view of autoimmune hepatitis
b Extensive interface hepatitis in autoimmune hepatitis. A bile duct is visible left of center. This patient had negative viral serologies, a negative antimitochondrial antibody, and a strongly positive antinuclear antibody. Note the resemblance to chronic hepatitis of other etiologies.
c The same patient 18 months after treatment for autoimmune hepatitis, with substantial improvement

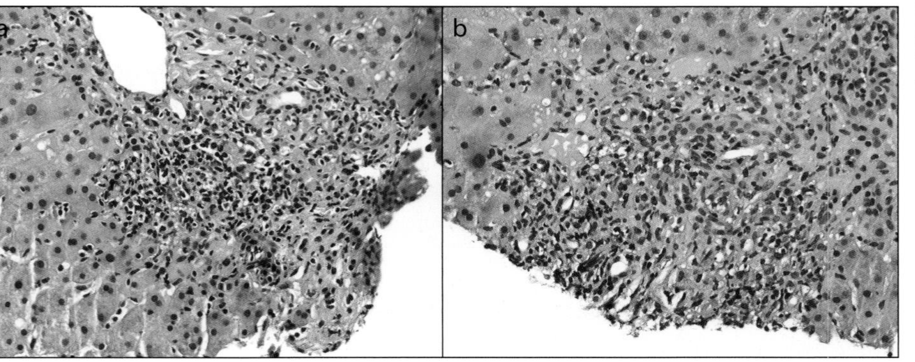

i25.24 Overlap syndrome with features of both autoimmune hepatitis and PBC.
a illustrates autoimmune hepatitis, with a relatively intact bile duct and extensive interface hepatitis, as would be seen in chronic hepatitis of other etiologies.
b, from the same biopsy, illustrates disorganized biliary epithelium, as would be seen in PBC.

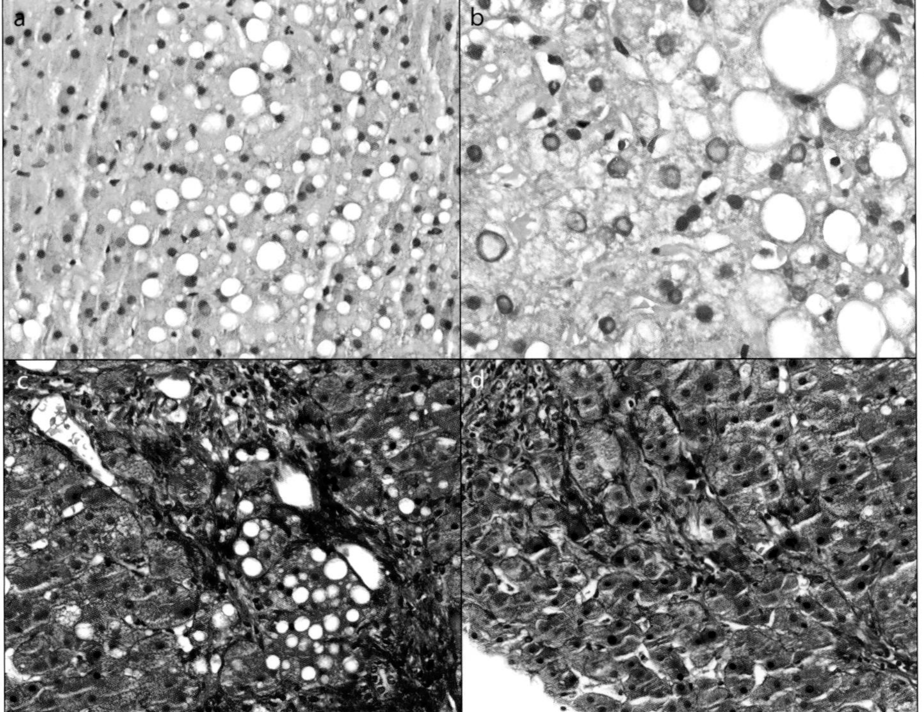

i25.25 Findings that are more commonly seen in ethanol consumption or nonalcoholic fatty liver disease.
a depicts lobular steatosis.

b depicts cytoplasmic invagination into hepatocyte nuclei (so called glycogenation of nuclei).

c and **d** illustrate fibrosis in the lobules rather than in or emanating from a portal area. Ethanol and other hepatotoxic exogenous agents, and NAFLD may engender lobular fibrosis.

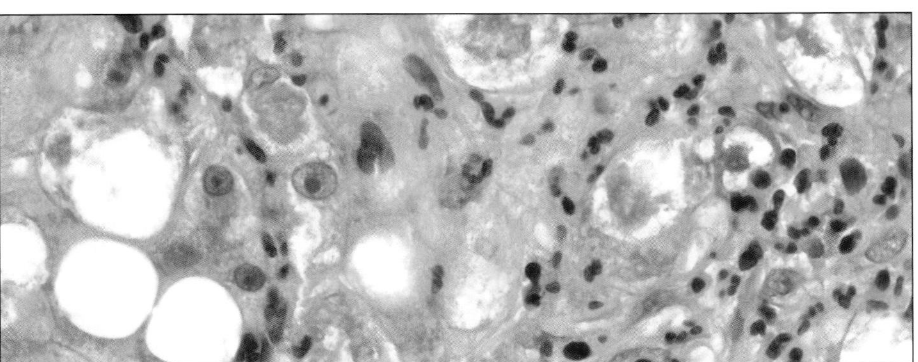

i25.26 Acute hepatitis secondary to ethanol consumption. Numerous Mallory bodies are seen, though these are not specific for ethanol.

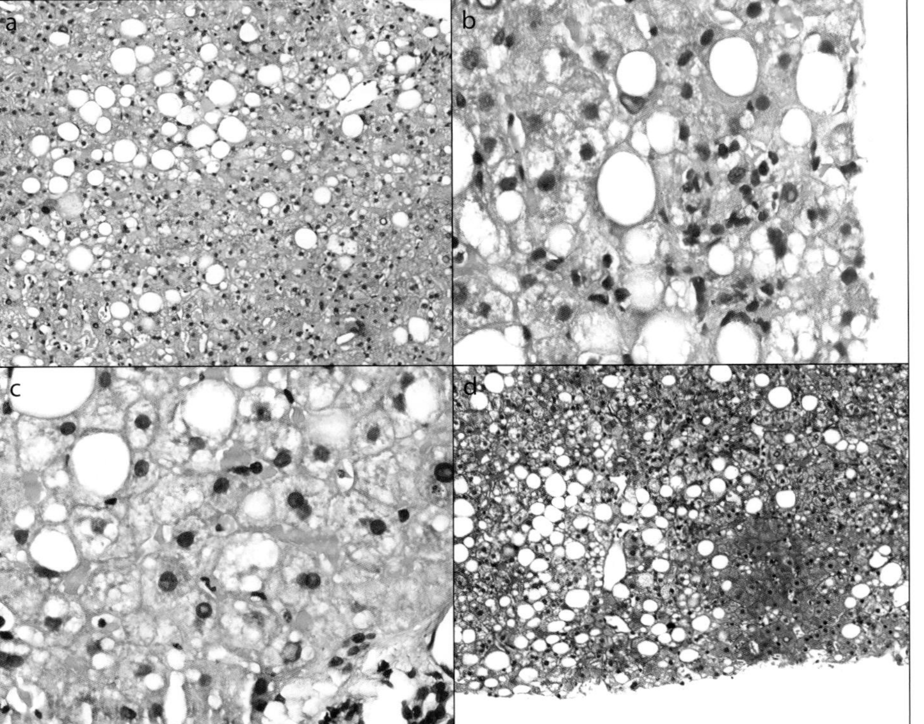

i25.27 **a-d** illustrate the use of the Kleiner and Brunt scoring systems for NAFLD.
a is steatosis involving between 33-66% of hepatocytes, for a score of 2.

b illustrates a focus of lobular inflammation, relatively rare in this case, for a score of 1.

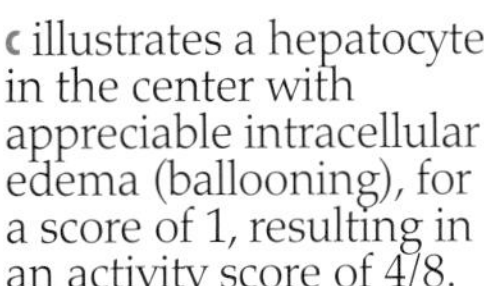

c illustrates a hepatocyte in the center with appreciable intracellular edema (ballooning), for a score of 1, resulting in an activity score of 4/8.

d demonstrates a small amount of lobular fibrosis, for a score of 1, resulting in a global score of 5/12.

ISBN 978-089189-5886

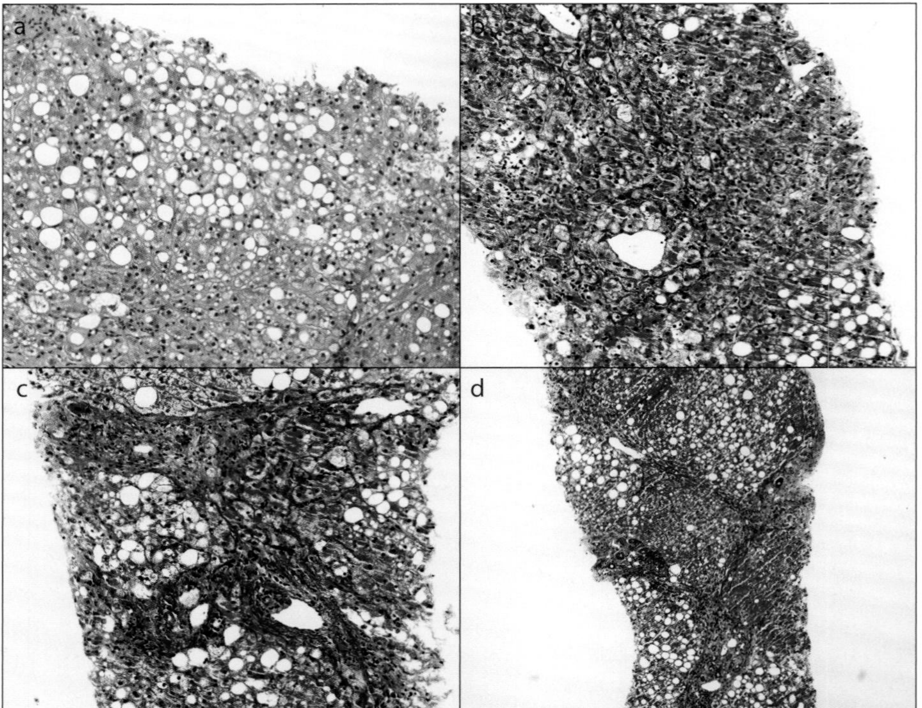

i25.28 **a** Another case of NAFLD, with an initial H&E impression similar to the case depicted in the images in i25.27. However, **b** illustrates extensive lobular fibrosis. **c** Both periportal and lobular areas are involved **d** demonstrates advanced stage fibrosis.

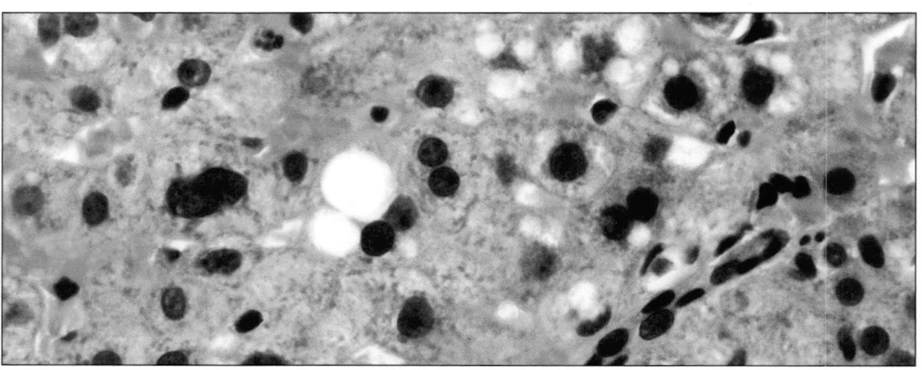

i25.29 A liver biopsy from a patient taking methotrexate for psoriasis. This is a Roenigk scale 1, with only mild steatosis and no fibrosis.

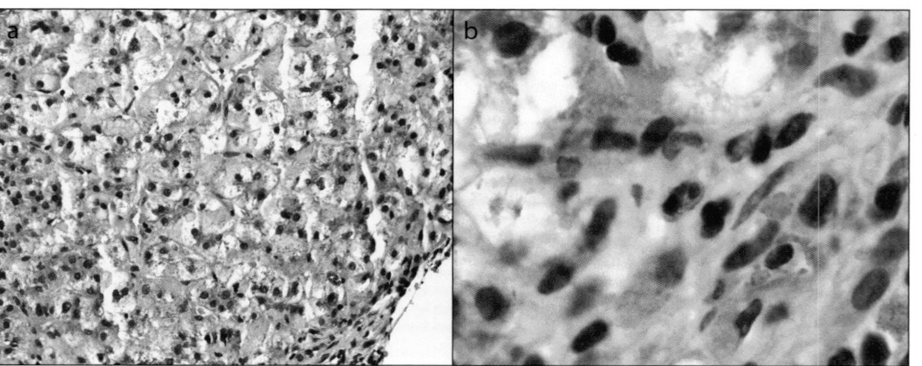

i25.30 **a** Neonatal hepatitis with severe lobular disarray **b** The same case as in i25.30a, with 2 nucleated erythrocytes seen in the center

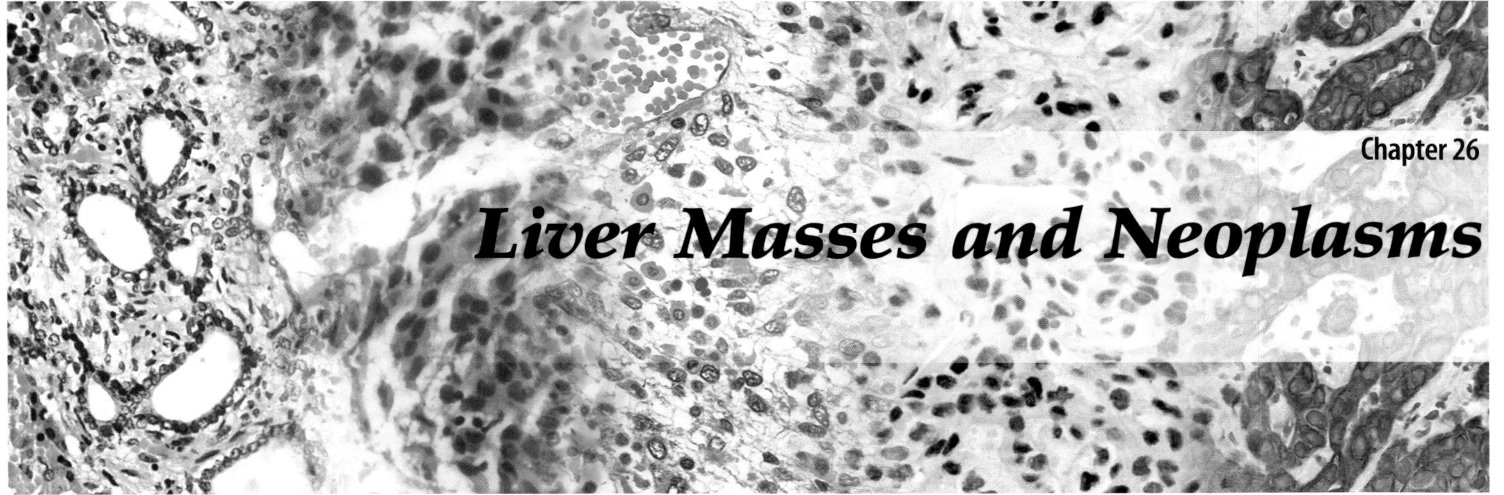

Benign Hepatic Masses

Autosomal dominant polycystic disease of the liver, also called adult type, is characterized by cysts of variable size, diffusely scattered throughout the liver. These cysts are lined by cuboidal epithelium i26.1 and are thought to arise from the biliary epithelium, but they do not communicate with the biliary tree [PMID3875218]. 70-90% of these patients also have polycystic kidneys, and the renal cysts are usually the greater clinical problem. Biliary hamartomas are commonly associated.

Polycystic kidney disease is discussed in more detail in Chapter 35, but 85% of cases of autosomal dominant polycystic renal disease are associated with a mutation in the *PKD1* gene on chromosome 16, which codes for a transmembrane protein called polycystin-1 [PMID17429048, PMID17975706]. The remaining 15% of cases are associated with a mutation in *PKD2* on chromosome 4, which codes for an integral membrane protein called polycystin-2 [PMID17975706].

Autosomal recessive cystic disease is caused by a mutation in the *PKHD1* gene [PMID16887426]. The protein products of the *PKD1*, *PKD2*, and *PKHD1* genes, and their actions, are considered more fully in Chapter 35. The hepatic manifestations of autosomal recessive renal cystic disease include cysts that are smaller than those in autosomal dominant polycystic disease i26.2, but the most serious hepatic manifestation of autosomal recessive renal cystic disease is congenital hepatic fibrosis i26.3 accompanied by portal hypertension [PMID20138815].

Another cause of hepatic cysts is Caroli disease, which is ectasia of bile ducts, often associated with fibrosis i26.4. Peliosis is multiple blood filled cysts, and is associated with chronic disease, immunodeficiency, and certain drugs (especially anabolic steroids). Depending on the cause, these cysts may or may not have an endothelial lining [PMID15734106].

An echinococcal (hydatid) cyst of the liver, caused by the dog heartworm *Dirofilaria immitis*, should be suspected if the lining of a cyst is very simple and nonepithelial, if it is hyalinized i26.5a, or if there is amorphous brown-gray material i26.5b. Rarely, parts of the organism may be seen i26.5c.

There is disagreement as to whether a bile duct hamartoma (also called a Meyenburg complex) is the same as a bile duct adenoma. Those who think these are different entities point out that hamartomas are often multiple, the glands therein are often dilated and more likely to contain inspissated bile i26.6a, while a bile duct adenoma consists of small glands without bile i26.6b. Whatever terminology is used, the multifocality of bile duct hamartomas can simulate metastatic carcinoma.

Mesenchymal hamartomas are relatively common in children and are composed of bland, embryonic-appearing stroma with edema or myxoid change and benign ducts that may undergo progressive dilatation from fluid accumulation i26.7a, i26.7b.

Focal nodular hyperplasia (FNH) is typically associated with a distinct central area of fibrosis, ramifications of which divide the nodule into smaller nodules i26.8. However, some cases, especially small lesions, may not have significant fibrosis [PMID10584697]. FNH is usually found in younger women and is often associated with a vascular malformation. While FNH may be multinodular, it is usually a single mass and never involves >1 lobe. FNH lacks normal architecture, though bile ducts, often with inflammatory cells, are haphazardly distributed in the fibrous tissue and there is often a ductular proliferation at the periphery of the fibrous bands. The fibrous tissue may also contain abnormally large vessels. FNH resembles a nodule of cirrhosis unless it is known that there is a single or, at most, a few nodules.

In contrast to FNH, nodular regenerative hyperplasia (NRH) is characterized by many small nodules, usually 1-4 mm in diameter, with little fibrous tissue between the nodules i26.9. Portal areas, if present, are indistinct. Because of the large number of diffusely distributed nodules, NRH may grossly resemble cirrhosis, but it is distinguished from cirrhosis by the essential absence of fibrous tissue. NRH is associated with a number of entities, such as autoimmune disorders, vasculitis, cardiac disorders, and certain drugs. The pathogenesis of NRH is unclear, but it may be a regenerative response to ischemia [PMID9252144]. Portal hypertension may be a contributing factor [PMID20075739], and in turn, NRH may obstruct blood flow and can be a cause of portal hypertension.

The individual hepatocytes in hepatic adenomas are unremarkable and there may even be a trabecular arrangement, resulting in an appreciable resemblance to normal liver i26.10a, i26.10b. The nuclei in hepatic adenomas, like those of normal liver tissue, may demonstrate focal mild enlargement, but they will not have the generalized enlargement that is seen in most hepatocellular carcinomas (HCCs). Nucleoli are generally inconspicuous and mitoses are virtually absent [PMID17239484, PMID16610069]. Adenomas often have fibrous septae, but these do not have portal areas or bile ducts i26.10c. Hemorrhage can occur from the vessels in the fibrous septae, often requiring surgical intervention. More than any other benign process in the liver, hepatic adenomas are associated with oral contraceptives. Indeed, so strong is the connection with steroid hormones that the few cases in men are associated with the use of anabolic steroids [PMID15849280].

It is difficult to differentiate between adenoma, FNH, and NRH solely on the basis of architecture, because all 3 entities have distorted, if any, portal areas. The distinction rests on the extent of involvement and the presence or absence of fibrous tissue. If the process is diffuse, it is either cirrhosis or NRH, depending on whether or not there is associated fibrous tissue. If there is 1 or a small number of benign nodules, it is FNH or adenoma, depending mostly on the presence or absence of a central fibrous area and on the presence or absence of a history of oral contraceptives.

Hepatocyte Dysplasia

There is growing agreement that HCCs arise from premalignant nodules [PMID15757804], but the nature of these nodules remains a matter of controversy. Some feel that the precancerous lesion is a nodule that is primarily characterized by abnormalities in *architecture*, such as thickened trabeculae i26.11a or disordered growth i26.11b. Such nodules are sometimes called adenomatous hyperplasia. Others feel that the precancerous lesion is abnormalities of *individual cells* (hepatocyte dysplasia), as is the case for squamous and adenocarcinomas. Many studies, from many modalities, including morphometry and DNA studies, have been inconclusive in this matter. To further confuse the issue, 2 types of dysplasia are reported. Large cell dysplasia shows generalized nuclear enlargement i26.12a [PMID16982109], while small cell dysplasia is characterized by a generally smaller nuclear size, but with a substantial decrease in the amount of cytoplasm, resulting in significantly greater nucleus to cytoplasmic ratio and increased nuclear density i26.12b [PMID15698394]. Moreover, these 2 processes are often found together, making it difficult to determine which of them came first. Until this matter is clarified, it seems prudent to report any of these findings, along with a comment on the controversy and uncertain significance. If any of these possibly premalignant processes are identified on a needle biopsy of discrete mass, a well differentiated HCC cannot be excluded without examination of the entire mass. One should also be aware of any area of the biopsy that stands out, or appears to form a micronodule within the biopsy, even if it is not diagnostic of HCC i26.13.

Hepatocellular Carcinoma (HCC) on Core Biopsy

A poorly differentiated HCC is characterized by generalized nuclear enlargement, pleomorphism, prominent nucleoli, and distorted architecture i26.14, but even in these situations, it is important to verify the malignant cells as hepatocellular because metastatic carcinoma may nearly perfectly simulate a HCC and mislead even experienced observers.

In contrast, identifying a well differentiated HCC on biopsy material is notoriously difficult because it is not immediately clear that there is a neoplasm. In addressing this question, it is important to first demonstrate the hepatocellular nature of the cells. If immunohistochemical stains performed on a biopsy of a distinct liver mass disclose an epithelial, as opposed to hepatocellular process, the diagnosis of metastatic carcinoma or cholangiocarcinoma is secure even if the H&E differential diagnosis was benign hepatocytes vs well differentiated HCC.

Once the hepatocellular nature is established, a distinct mass suggests, but does not prove a well differentiated HCC, because of the possibility of a benign hepatic mass (eg, an adenoma, FNH, or even a cirrhotic nodule) and the possibility that benign tissue adjacent to the target area was retrieved. The findings of nuclear atypia, high nucleus to cytoplasmic ratio, and thickened trabeculae are the most helpful clues to a well differentiated HCC i26.15 [PMID15831273]. Highlighting endothelial cells with CD34 may also help in identifying distorted architecture or thickened trabeculae. Often, caution is the better part of valor in these situations.

Immunohistochemical staining for glypican-3 is reported to be stronger in HCCs than in normal liver or in nonhepatic neoplasms, and can be helpful in identifying well differentiated HCC in a biopsy of an hepatic mass [PMID17063081, PMID19212669]. A negative stain is not informative, as HCCs may be negative. The principal difficulty with this marker is that any inflammatory condition, especially hepatitis C, will also likely result in a positive glypican-3 [PMID17949778]. More data are needed to determine the role of glypican-3, but at this writing, a positive result in the absence of hepatitis suggests a dysplastic nodule or a carcinoma. Help in this difficult area may be forthcoming from molecular biology. Compared to normal liver or adenomas, 93% of HCC have abnormalities of chromosomes 1 or 8, detectable by FISH [PMID15322490].

There are several variants of HCC, all of which can be challenging in a core biopsy if they are well differentiated, but 2 variants in particular can be diagnostically difficult. The fibrosis is more arranged in fibrous bands alternating with tumor cells, resulting in a "layered" appearance i26.16a. The individual cells in the fibrolamellar HCC are polygonal, quite large, with distinct cytoplasmic borders, vesicular nuclei, and prominent nucleoli i26.16b. The principal differential diagnosis for the fibrolamellar HCC is the sclerosing (desmoplastic) form of HCC. The fibrolamellar HCC usually occurs in younger patients in noncirrhotic livers. The fibrosis in the sclerosing HCC is more haphazard, without layering, and the individual cells are smaller and less polygonal i26.17a, i26.17b. The fibrolamellar HCC has a better prognosis than other forms.

The second particularly challenging form of HCC is the clear cell variant i26.18a. The clear cell type of HCC can have deceptively bland nuclei i26.18b and may be difficult to recognize as a malignancy. Moreover, even if successfully identified as malignant, it may resemble a metastatic renal or adrenal carcinoma. The first order of business in addressing a clear cell mass of the liver is to verify hepatic origin and to exclude a metastatic renal or adrenal carcinoma by immunohistochemistry.

The Clearly Malignant Biopsy of a Liver Mass: Hepatocellular Carcinoma or Another Tumor Type?

An equally challenging question of a different type arises when examining a biopsy of a clearly malignant neoplasm, and addressing the question of HCC vs cholangiocarcinoma or metastatic adenocarcinoma. A Klatskin tumor is a cholangiocarcinoma of the hepatic duct or a major branch, occurring in the hilum of the liver, usually with desmoplasia and considerable glandular differentiation [PMID15019927], but most cholangiocarcinomas are intrahepatic and radiographically indistinguishable from a HCC or a metastatic lesion.

Historically, the presence of cytoplasmic mucin suggested an adenocarcinoma (ie, cholangiocarcinoma or metastatic adenocarcinoma), while a negative mucin stain pointed to a HCC. This remains a simple and effective initial test, but it has largely been replaced by immunohistochemical stains. The major immunohistochemical tests are cytokeratins 7 and 20. HCC are negative for CK7 and 20. The only adenocarcinomas that are commonly negative for both CK7 and 20 are those of renal, adrenal, and prostatic origin. Cholangiocarcinomas are also negative for CK20, but are positive for CK7. Metastatic colon adenocarcinomas, always a consideration in liver tumors, are usually negative for CK7 and positive for CK20.

Additional immunohistochemical stains may point to a HCC. Canalicular staining (ie, confined to the surface of the cell membrane such that it highlights the sharp boundary between 2 adjacent hepatocytes) for CD10 stains 68% of HCC, but no other types of malignancies that are commonly found in this location [PMID11688465]. The antibody Hep (also called hepatocyte monoclonal antibody or HepPar1) is directed against hepatocyte mitochondria and stains >90% of benign and malignant liver tissues, but it also stains about 5-15% of metastatic carcinomas from a number of sites, including gastric, pancreatic, and lung [PMID11836703, PMID15491968]. Arginase-1 has been reported to have a sensitivity and specificity that are both superior to Hep [PMID20661013].

About 70% of HCCs will stain positively for carcinoembryonic antigen (CEA) in a canalicular pattern if polyclonal antibodies are used (polyclonal antisera refers to a group of antibodies that are directed to different epitopes of the same antigen) [PMID12170084]. In evaluating a CEA immunohistochemical stain, one must be careful of false positives caused by nonneoplastic hepatocytes or luminal staining of adenocarcinomas. Only a minority of HCC will stain for α fetoprotein or α-1-antitrypsin, but such staining, if found, is a strong point for hepatic origin of the neoplasm. i26.19a-f illustrate useful immunohistochemical stains that suggest a primary HCC over a cholangiocarcinoma or a metastatic carcinoma.

Useful information can also be obtained from immunohistochemical results that point away from HCC. AE-1 and EMA stain cholangiocarcinomas and most metastatic carcinomas, but is rare in HCC i26.20a-c [PMID7539881, PMID2466290]. MOC31 [PMID12481008] and claudin-4 [PMID16439986] also stain cholangiocarcinomas and metastatic carcinomas, but not HCC.

To my mind, considering sensitivity, specificity, and ease of interpretation, a panel consisting of cytokeratins 7 and 20, Hep, AE-1, and EMA seems appropriate for first line immunohistochemical testing to distinguish between an HCC on the one hand from a cholangiocarcinoma or a metastatic carcinoma on the other, but these stains are not perfect. A sizable minority of neoplasms of the breast and lung, for example, may express cytokeratin 20 as well as cytokeratin 7 i26.21a-c. A sizable minority of HCC may not express Hep, or may focally express AE1 or EMA. If the overall results of this panel favor a cholangiocarcinoma or a metastatic carcinoma, we encounter the challenge of differentiating a primary cholangiocarcinoma from a metastatic carcinoma. On H&E, this is nearly impossible. Dysplasia in adjacent bile ducts suggests a cholangiocarcinoma. Because 10-30% of patients with primary sclerosing cholangitis will develop cholangiocarcinoma, the presence of that condition suggests a bile duct tumor, but immunohistochemical stains are essential, and a second panel might furnish additional information to distinguish between a primary cholangiocarcinoma and a metastatic tumor, and if the latter, suggest a primary site.

Among carcinomas in the liver that are positive for cytokeratin 7 and usually negative for cytokeratin 20, immunohistochemical demonstration of Her2 overexpression i26.22a, or staining for gross cystic disease fluid protein 15 (GCDFP-15) or mammaglobin i26.22b, i26.22c, strongly suggests a metastatic breast carcinoma. Staining for estrogen or progesterone receptor also suggests a breast carcinoma i26.23a, i26.23b unless a metastatic carcinoma from the endometrium or ovary is a possibility. Staining with PE-10 or napsin A suggests metastatic lung adenocarcinoma, as does staining for thyroid transcription factor-1 i26.24a, i26.24b, unless a thyroid carcinoma is under consideration. Staining for CDX2 is associated with adenocarcinomas of the lower intestinal tract. This marker is present in the vast majority of carcinomas from the duodenum to the rectum, and about 1/2 of adenocarcinomas of the esophagus and stomach. Unfortunately, CDX2 is not specific for gastrointestinal adenocarcinomas and is also found in about 1/2 of ovarian mucinous and 1/2 of pancreatobiliary adenocarcinomas, including primary cholangiocarcinomas [PMID16980943, PMID15725805]. This limits its utility in identifying a primary site or even in determining that a neoplasm is a metastasis. However, a negative CDX2 suggests that a metastasis from the colon is unlikely, and lung carcinomas do not express CDX2 [PMID12548159, PMID12604886]. CDX2 can also provide additional verification of a colon primary i26.25a-d.

Primary cholangiocarcinomas are generally positive for cytokeratin 7 and negative for cytokeratin 20. If an adenocarcinoma in the liver is positive for cytokeratin 7 and negative for cytokeratin 20, there is a good chance it is metastatic from the breast or lung, as metastatic adenocarcinoma to the liver is much more common than primary cholangiocarcinoma and cytokeratin 7+, 20– is most often seen in adenocarcinomas from the breast and lung (many ovarian carcinomas are also cytokeratin 7+, 20–, but these usually do not metastasize to the liver without a well-known history or involvement of the pelvis). Because a sizable minority of adenocarcinomas of the pancreas and upper gastrointestinal tract are also cytokeratin 7+, 20–, those sites are also included in this situation. Other immunohistochemical stains, arising from proteins uniquely or preferentially expressed by other neoplasms, may also be helpful, but in many cases, they are not. Breast carcinomas are often negative for GCDFP-15, mammaglobin, estrogen or progesterone receptor, and Her2, and lung adenocarcinomas may be negative for TTF-1, napsin A, and PE-10. While CA19.9 is associated with pancreatic and hepatobiliary carcinomas, it is far from specific [PMID21577374]. In these cases, the diagnosis can only be, "Adenocarcinoma. Diagnostic possibilities include primary cholangiocarcinoma and metastases from the lung, breast, upper gastrointestinal tract, or pancreas." Clinical and radiographic correlation is required before a primary site can be found or a primary cholangiocarcinoma can be assumed. i26.26a-f illustrate 2 such cases.

The relatively rare cases in which a squamous carcinoma metastasizes to the liver can generally be identified by staining for p63 and cytokeratins 5/6, both of which are characteristic of squamous carcinoma and rarely seen in adenocarcinoma i26.27a-c.

Nonepithelial Primary Liver Neoplasms

Simple hemangiomas are relatively common in the liver, but this organ is also the site of several more complex vascular neoplasms, the terminology for which, like those in soft tissue, can be confusing. In the liver, we again encounter the perplexing term "hemangioendothelioma." An *infantile* hemangioendothelioma is a very cellular hemangioma that occurs in the liver in children, usually infants i26.28. Infantile hemangioendotheliomas are sometimes divided into type 1 and type 2 forms. The type 1 form is accepted as a benign, cellular hemangioma. The terms "type 1 infantile hemangioendothelioma," "juvenile hemangioma," "juvenile hemangioendothelioma," and "cellular hemangioma" are essentially synonymous terms in pediatric hepatic vascular proliferations. The nature of the type 2 infantile hemangioendothelioma remains controversial. Type 2 infantile hemangioendotheliomas have increased endothelial cellularity and irregularly shaped vascular channels, with more variable and hyperchromatic endothelial nuclei. They are partially unencapsulated and mitotically active [PMID20857525]. For these reasons, many now regard them as low-grade angiosarcomas [PMID19321270], but their biologic potential is unclear, and if this diagnosis is made, a comment suggesting uncertain malignant potential is appropriate.

Whatever terminology and conception one subscribes to, the difficulty with infantile hemangioendotheliomas is that they tend to be multiple and they often cause shunting of blood. The difficulty with these tumors, even those of type 2, is not overtly malignant behavior, but high output cardiac failure secondary to shunting [PMID2685411]. Solitary infantile hemangioendotheliomas may be resected, but multiple lesions, even if clearly benign, may require transplantation.

The *epithelioid* hemangioendothelioma is distinct from the infantile hemangioendothelioma and from the epithelioid hemangioma (angiolymphoid hyperplasia with eosinophilia. The individual cells in an epithelioid hemangioendothelioma have nuclear atypia, often have cytoplasmic vacuolization i26.29a, i26.29b, and may have intranuclear vacuoles secondary to cytoplasmic invaginations. The epithelioid hemangioendothelioma infiltrates into the hepatic parenchyma and is accompanied by sclerosis that simulates a sclerosing carcinoma i26.29c. It often forms multiple masses that may clinically simulate metastases. Further confusing the situation is that 15-40% of epithelioid hemangioendotheliomas are focally keratin positive [PMID19492891]. Although sclerosing, these neoplasms often demonstrates a zonal pattern, with sclerosis in the center, a myxoid matrix towards the periphery, and more cellularity at the periphery i26.29d, i26.29e. The more cellular and less sclerotic areas may resemble a cellular hemangioma, so vascular liver tumors should be liberally sampled from multiple areas in an effort to find sclerotic or myxoid areas that may suggest that what appears to be a cellular hemangioma is actually an epithelioid hemangioendothelioma.

Likewise, any sclerosing tumor that is suspicious for a carcinoma should be well sampled, looking for subtle indicators of vascular differentiation, such as septated vacuoles and nuclei directly facing each other. It is wise to employ immunohistochemical stains in any sclerosing tumor in the liver. If such stains confirm vascular origin, an epithelioid hemangioendothelioma is likely.

The clinical course of the epithelioid hemangioendothelioma is unpredictable, but some cases behave as a low-grade angiosarcoma and it is reasonable designate them as such in the report, with a comment on its unusual features and alternative nomenclatures.

Well differentiated angiosarcomas in the liver, as in other sites, may form recognizable blood vessels i26.30a. Clues that a well differentiated angiosarcoma is present include a subtle increase in the number of endothelial cells and mild nuclear atypia. In any site, well differentiated angiosarcomas may use existing structures as scaffolding and may not form a distinct mass. In many sites, the neoplastic cells run along collagen fibers. In the liver, they may proliferate alongside hepatocytes i26.30b. Immunohistochemistry is often required for the diagnosis of angiosarcoma, and the epithelioid variety may be keratin positive in about 1/3 of cases [PMID9630175].

The undifferentiated (embryonal) sarcoma of the liver occurs in children and is characterized by undifferentiated mesenchymal cells that push aside any normal structures i26.31a. The nuclear pleomorphism i26.31b distinguishes this entity from a mesenchymal hamartoma. In addition to vimentin expression, there is variable immunohistochemical positivity for muscle markers [PMID18926232], causing some belief that this tumor may be a type of rhabdomyosarcoma, but at this time, it is best regarded as a distinct entity.

HCC may occur in young children, but the most common malignant liver tumor in this age group is the hepatoblastoma. There are numerous types of hepatoblastoma, including several variants of epithelial types i26.32a, i26.32b and a mixed epithelial-mesenchymal. Heterologous elements may be seen [PMID7809507].

The γ-δ lymphoma is a peripheral T-cell lymphoma, primarily involving the liver and the spleen, with a sinusoidal pattern. It usually negative for CD4 and CD8 and often associated with hemophagocytic syndrome. This entity is discussed in greater detail in Chapter 9 and illustrated in i9.14.

Core Points for Liver Masses and Neoplasms

- Autosomal dominant (adult type) polycystic disease: most also have polycystic kidneys, which are usually of greater concern.
  - o 85% of cases secondary to a mutation in the *PKD1* gene, which encodes for the transmembrane protein polycystin-1.
  - o Remaining cases are caused by a mutation in *PKD2*, which encodes for polycystin-2.
- Autosomal recessive polycystic disease: small liver cysts
  - o Congenital hepatic fibrosis is the much more serious manifestation.
- Bile duct hamartomas (Meyenburg complexes) and bile duct adenomas: may be indistinguishable in many cases.
- Mesenchymal hamartomas: common pediatric liver masses.
  - o Embryonic-appearing stroma, with edema or myxoid change, and benign ducts.
- Focal nodular hyperplasia (FNH): central fibrosis and lobules
  - o May be bile ducts in fibrous tissue, but no normal hepatic architecture.
- Nodular regenerative hyperplasia (NRH) has many nodules
  - o May grossly resemble cirrhosis, but lacks fibrous tissue.
- Hepatic adenomas: normal trabecular pattern of hepatocytes, but no normal portal areas or bile ducts.
- Hepatic dysplasia: controversy as to whether important changes are in architecture, such as thickened trabeculae or disordered growth, or in individual cells.
- Well differentiated hepatocellular carcinoma (HCC) on biopsy: first verify hepatocellular origin
  - o Then look for: generalized nuclear atypia, a widespread increase in nucleus to cytoplasmic ratio, and thickened trabeculae.
  - o A distinct mass favors a HCC if target sampled and FNH, adenoma, and a cirrhotic nodule excluded.
- If a biopsy is clearly malignant: nature of the cells can often be elucidated by IHC.
  - o Cytokeratins 7 and 20 are an excellent starting point, as HCC usually negative for both and staining for either suggests a primary cholangiocarcinoma or a metastatic neoplasm.
  - o Additional stains are AE-1 and EMA, which stain most cholangiocarcinomas and metastatic carcinomas, but not HCCs.
  - o Staining for Hep (Hep par 1), CD10, and CEA suggests a hepatocellular carcinoma
  - o If IHC excludes an HCC, the differentiation of cholangiocarcinoma from a metastatic neoplasm usually requires clinical/historical/radiographic grounds, but
  - o Staining for GCDFP-15, mammaglobin, napsin A, or CDX2 may help.
- Infantile hemangioendothelioma: cellular hemangioma in the liver of young children.
- Epithelioid hemangioendothelioma: vascular neoplasm of low-grade malignancy
  - o May be keratin positive and sclerotic
  - o May be multiple masses.
  - o May simulate carcinoma.
- Well differentiated angiosarcoma: an increased number of endothelial cells or failure to form well defined vascular channels may be more helpful than nuclear atypia or a distinct mass.
- Undifferentiated (embryonal) sarcoma: primary pediatric liver sarcoma.
- γ-δ T-cell lymphoma should be suspected if there is a T-cell lymphoma that involves the spleen and liver more than lymph nodes.
- Hepatoblastoma: occurs in young children
  - o Several types
  - o Occasionally contains heterologous elements.
  - o Purely epithelial forms may simulate a hepatocellular carcinoma.

ISBN 978-089189-5886

i26.1 Autosomal dominant (adult type) polycystic disease of the liver with cysts of variable size, but generally large, lined by biliary epithelium

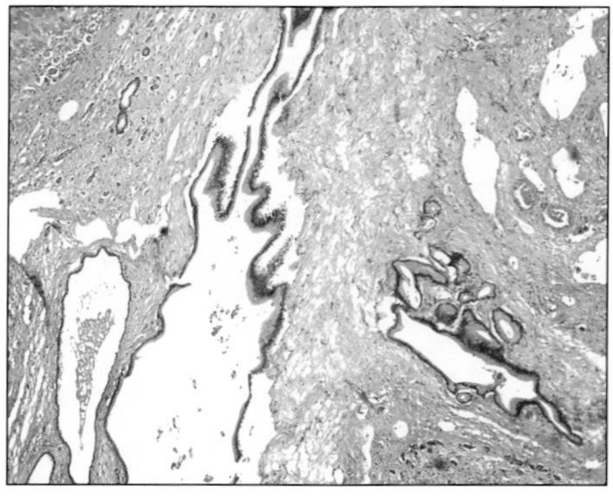

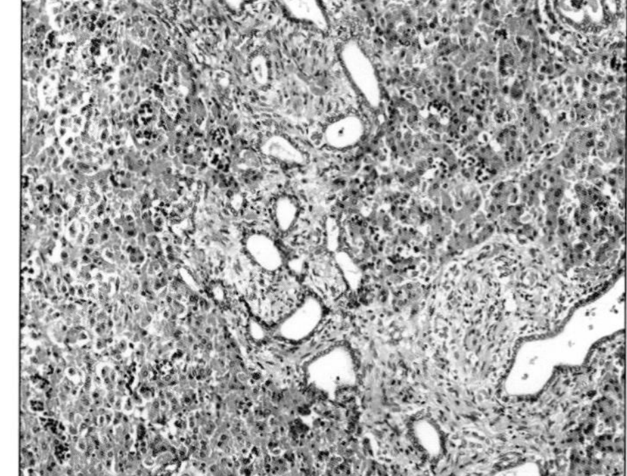

i26.2 Autosomal recessive polycystic disease of the liver, with smaller cysts

i26.3 Congenital hepatic fibrosis accompanying autosomal recessive polycystic disease

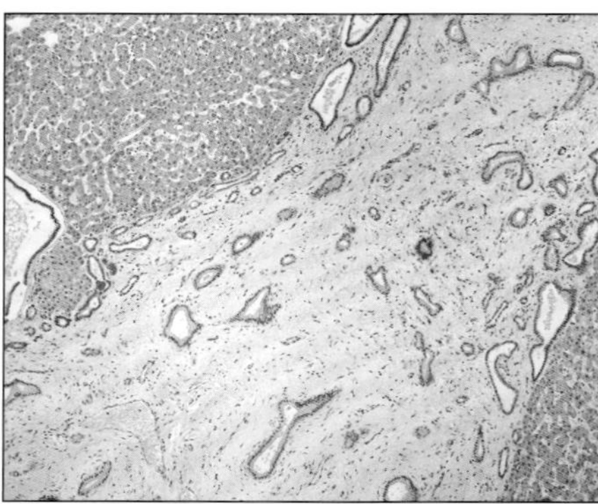

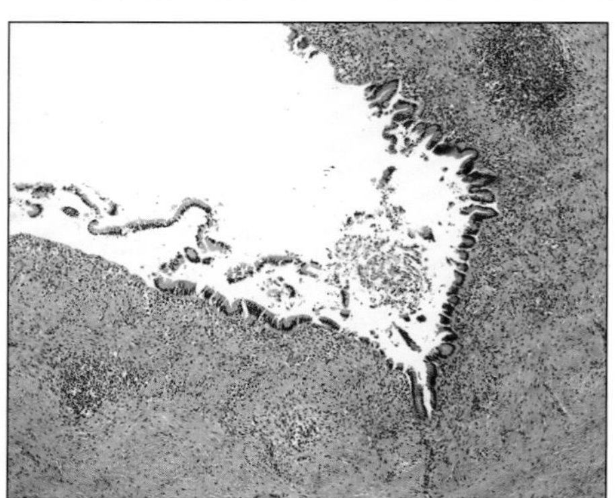

i26.4 Caroli disease (ectasia of the bile ducts)

i26.5 An echinococcal (hydatid) cyst of the liver. Note the absence of epithelium in the lining. The lining may be distinctly **a** eosinophilic, or **b** amorphous.

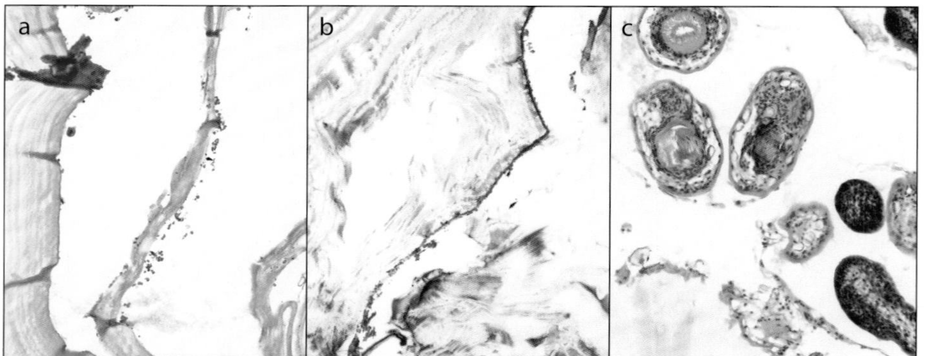

c shows parts of the *Dirofilaria immitus* organism

i26.6 **a** A bile duct hamartoma, with dilated bile ducts, some of which contain bile **b** A bile duct adenoma, with smaller glands than a hamartoma

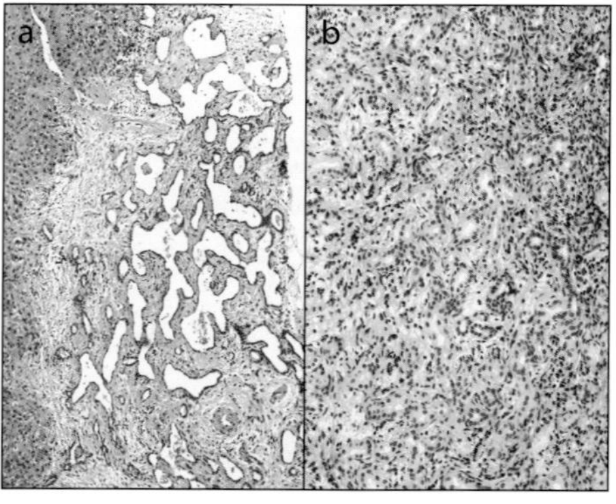

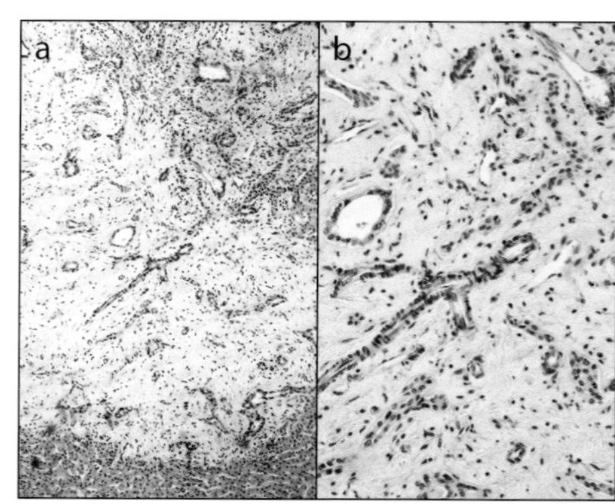

i26.7 **a** A mesenchymal hamartoma with expanded stroma that is edematous and myxoid **b** A higher-power view of the same case as in i26.7a, illustrating the benign nature of the stroma.

i26.8 Focal nodular hyperplasia. The central fibrous band that is characteristic of this entity enters this field at the lower right.

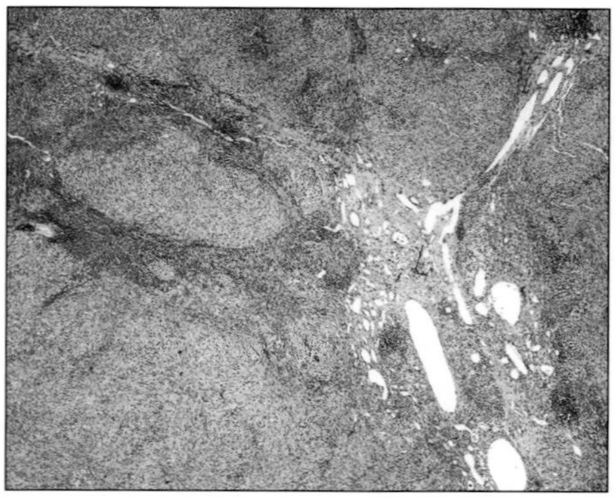

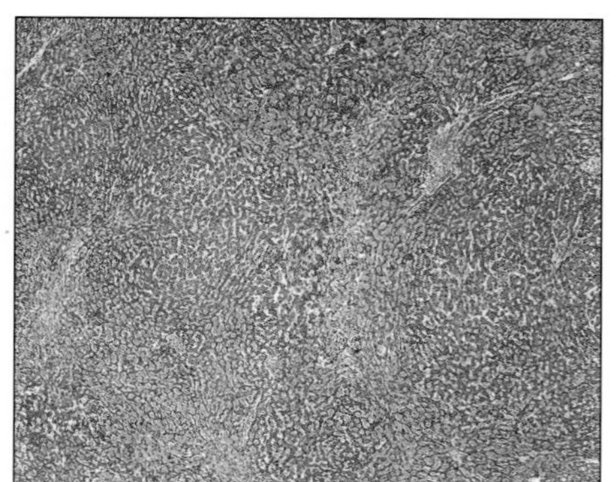

i26.9 Nodular regenerative hyperplasia. 2 small, subtle nodules of hepatocytes are seen, without significant fibrous tissue between them.

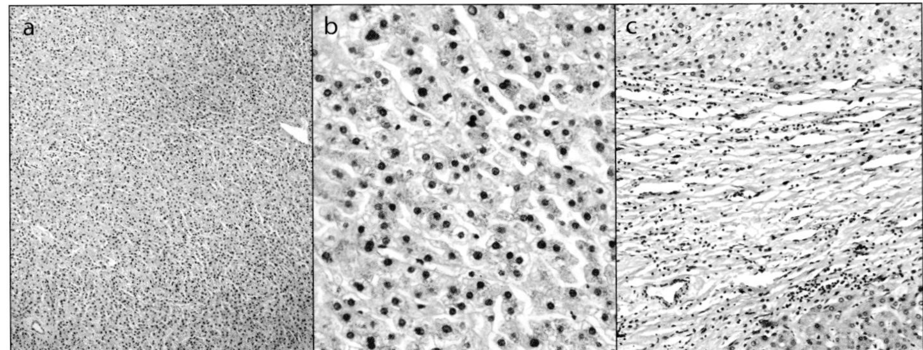

i26.10 **a** A hepatic adenoma. Note the monotonous uniformity of the hepatocytes, without normal architecture or portal areas.
b A high-power view of the same case as in i26.10a, highlighting the small, uniform nuclei
c Fibrous septa within a hepatic adenoma. This is not a portal area because it does not contain bile ducts.

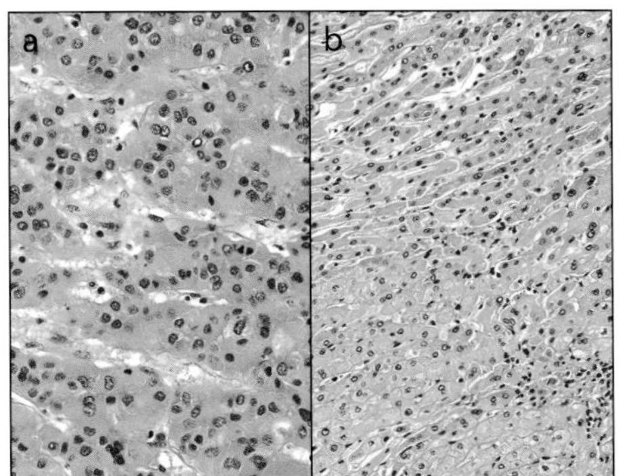

i26.11 **a** Thickened hepatic plates; insufficient for the diagnosis of hepatocellular carcinoma, but may be premalignant.
b Disordered hepatocyte architecture in the lower portion; normal trabecular architecture in the upper portion. The lack of distinct trabeculae in the lower half is insufficient for the diagnosis of malignancy but may be premalignant.

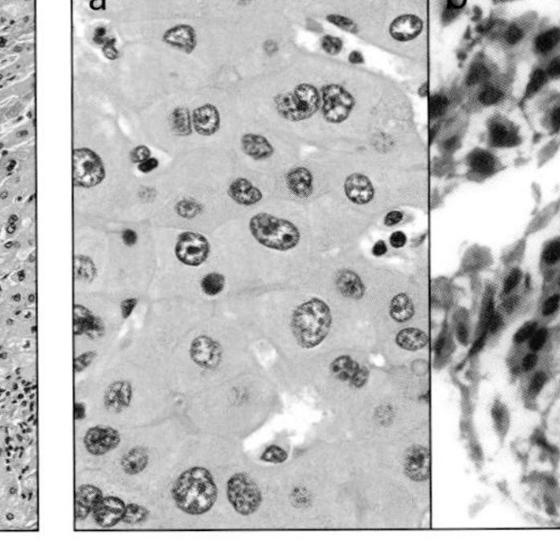

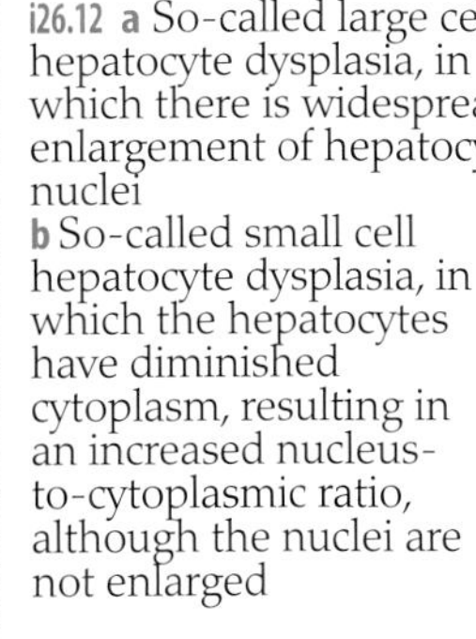

i26.12 **a** So-called large cell hepatocyte dysplasia, in which there is widespread enlargement of hepatocyte nuclei
b So-called small cell hepatocyte dysplasia, in which the hepatocytes have diminished cytoplasm, resulting in an increased nucleus-to-cytoplasmic ratio, although the nuclei are not enlarged

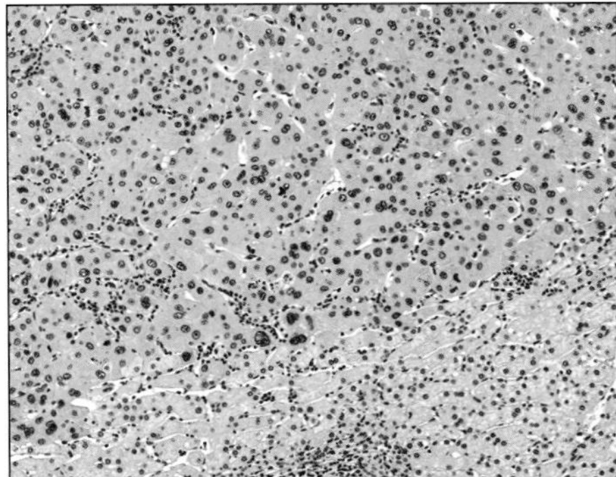

i26.13 A worrisome nodule within a liver biopsy that stands out from the normal liver in the lower portion

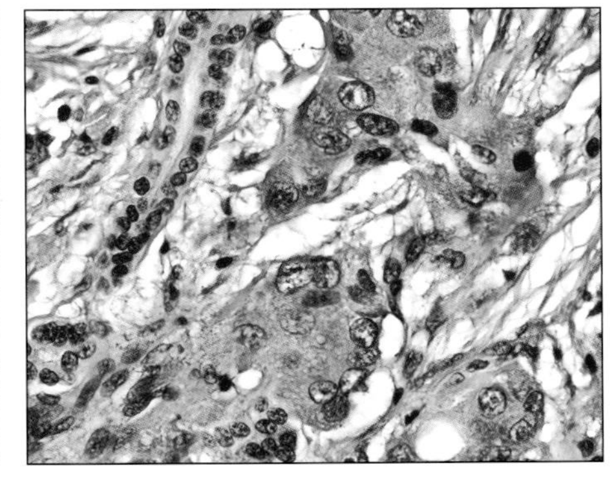

i26.14 A hepatocellular carcinoma characterized by severe nuclear atypia and disordered growth

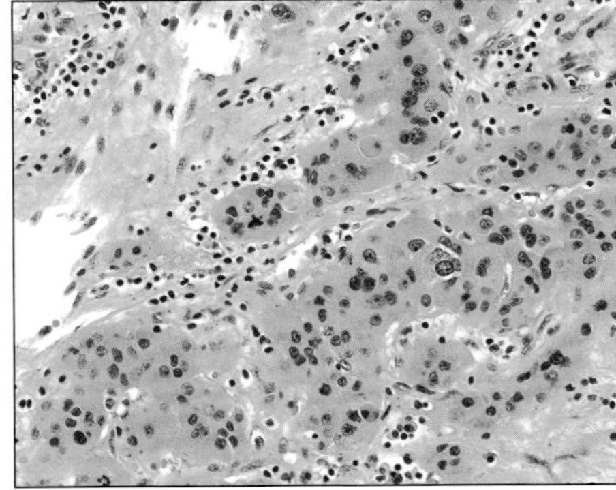

i26.15 A well differentiated hepatocellular carcinoma characterized in this field by sharply thickened trabeculae

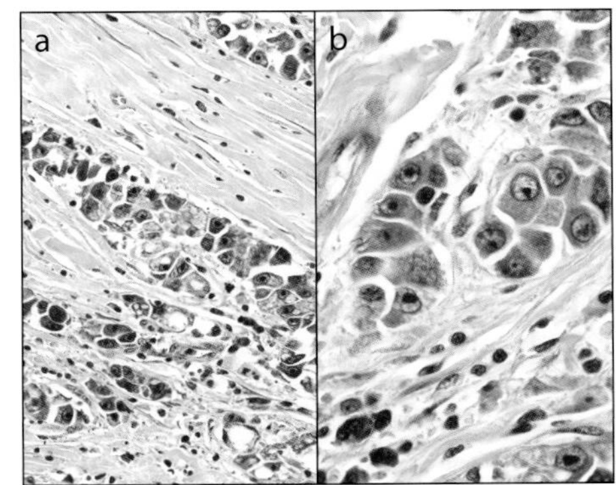

i26.16 **a** The fibrolamellar variant of HCC. Note the "layering" of fibrous tissue and neoplastic hepatocytes.
b A fibrolamellar HCC illustrating the enlarged neoplastic hepatocytes with a polygonal shape, distinct cytoplasmic boundaries, open chromatin pattern, and prominent nucleoli

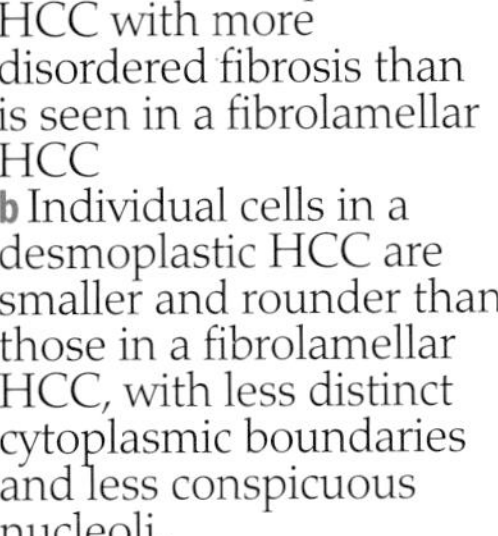

i26.17 **a** A desmoplastic HCC with more disordered fibrosis than is seen in a fibrolamellar HCC
b Individual cells in a desmoplastic HCC are smaller and rounder than those in a fibrolamellar HCC, with less distinct cytoplasmic boundaries and less conspicuous nucleoli.

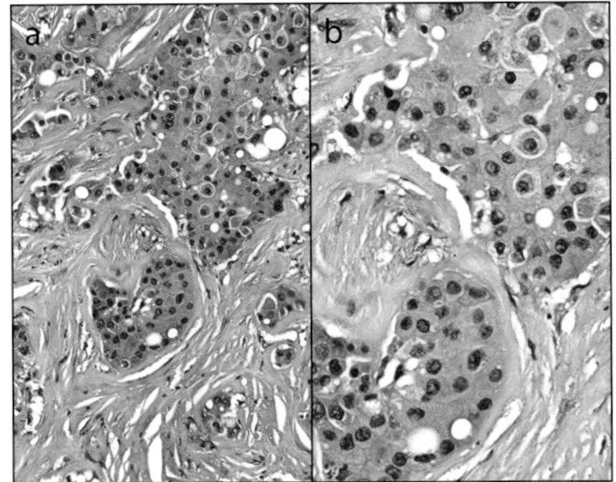

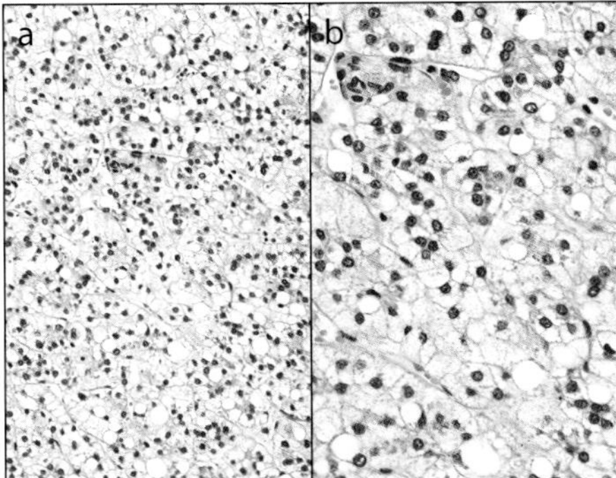

i26.18 **a** The clear cell variant of HCC. Note the striking similarity to a renal cell carcinoma or an adrenal neoplasm.
b A higher-power view of the same image as in i26.18a, highlighting the relative nuclear uniformity and abundant clear cytoplasm

ISBN 978-089189-5886

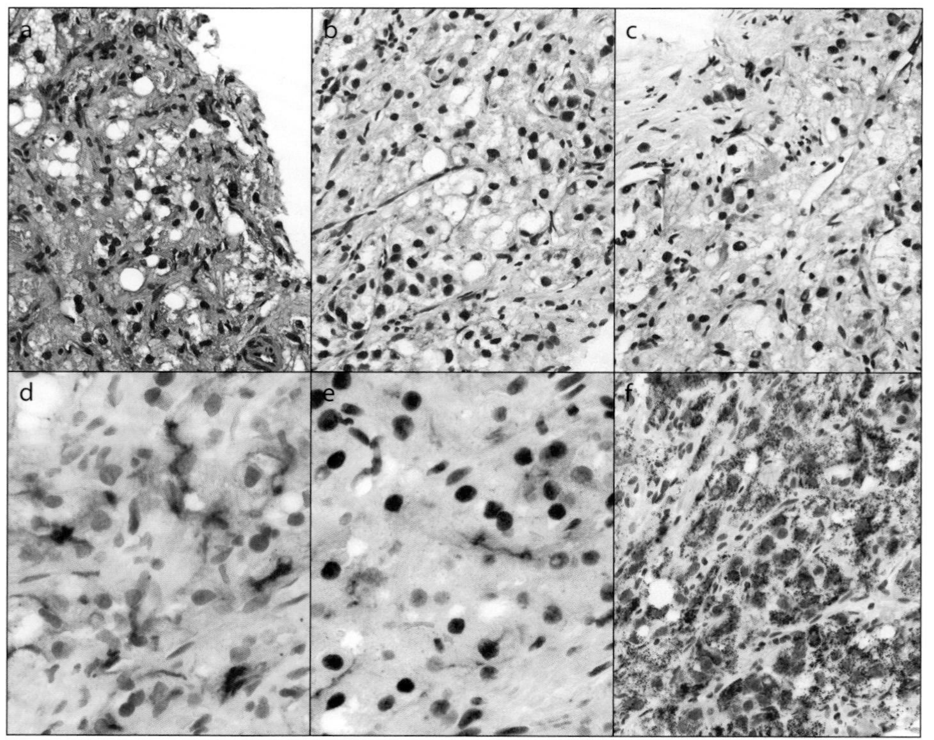

i26.19 a-c These images illustrate some of the immunohistochemical stains that can suggest a primary HCC over a cholangiocarcinoma or a metastatic carcinoma.
a An H&E stain of a malignant neoplasm in the liver
b A negative cytokeratin 7 stain for this neoplasm
c A negative cytokeratin 20 stain. Negativity for cytokeratins 7 and 20 is consistent with a primary hepatocellular carcinoma, but is also seen in a cholangiocarcinoma and a significant minority of metastatic carcinomas.
d A CD10 stain demonstrating positivity in the spaces between hepatocytes, characteristic of a primary hepatocellular carcinoma
e Stain for CEA using a polyclonal reagent, staining in a canalicular pattern between hepatocytes, again suggesting a primary hepatocellular carcinoma
f Staining for the antibody Hep (HepPar1), suggesting a primary hepatocellular carcinoma. The combination of immunohistochemical stains illustrated in i26.19a-f secure a diagnosis of primary HCC.

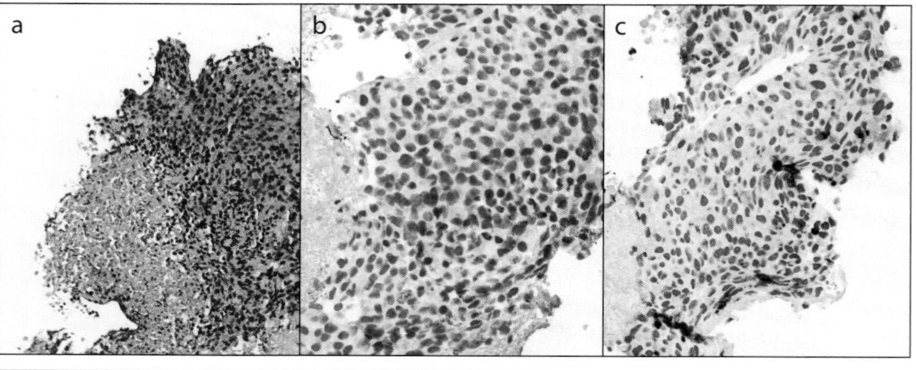

i26.20 a Another malignant neoplasm in the liver, negative for cytokeratins 7 and 20. This double-negativity suggests HCC because isolated hepatic metastases of occult carcinomas from the prostate, kidney, or adrenal are unusual.
b An epithelial membrane antigen immunohistochemical stain of the same case as in i26.20a. The negativity further suggests a primary HCC, as most cholangiocarcinoma or metastatic carcinomas will stain for EMA.
c An α fetoprotein stain on the same case as in i26.20a. The focal positivity strongly suggests a primary HCC.

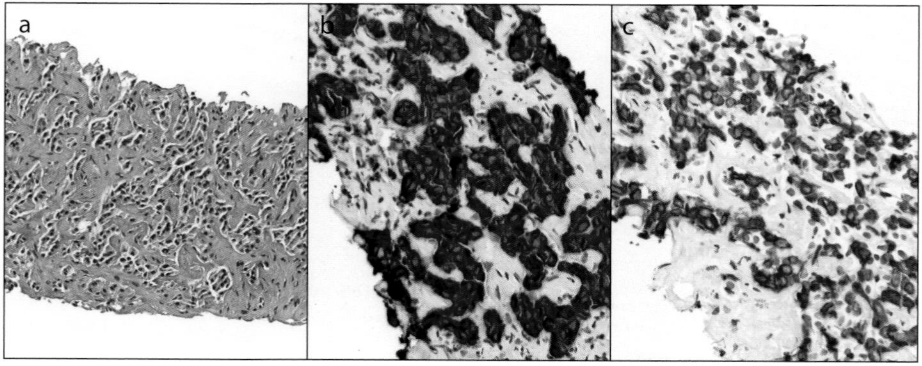

i26.21 a A metastatic breast carcinoma to the liver
b The same case as in i26.21a, staining positively for cytokeratin 7, as would be expected for metastatic carcinomas from the breast, lung, and a few other sites, but not expected in primary HCC
c The same case, however, also stained positively for cytokeratin 20, illustrating that the presence of cytokeratin 20 does not completely exclude neoplasms of the lung or breast.

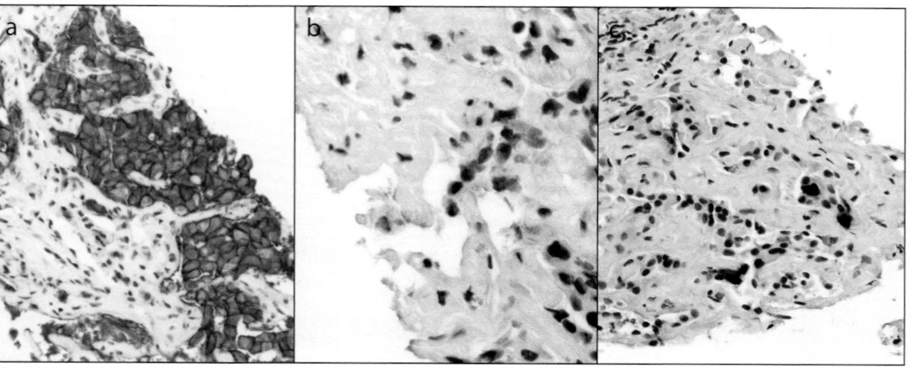

i26.22 The images in i26.22a-b illustrate some additional stains that strongly suggest a breast primary.
a A stain demonstrating Her-2 overexpression
b-c Focal staining for GCDFP-15 and mammaglobin, respectively

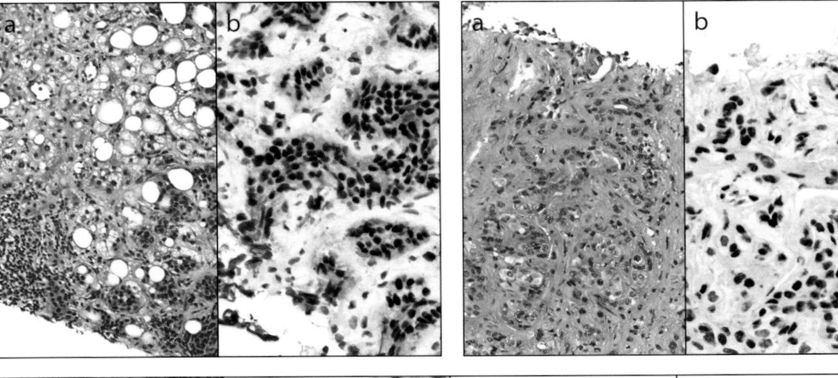

i26.23 a-b Another malignant neoplasm in the liver, staining positively for estrogen receptor, strongly suggesting a breast primary

i26.24 a-b A malignant neoplasm in the liver staining for TTF-1, suggesting a lung primary

i26.25 a A carcinoma in the liver. The tall columnar cells suggest a colon primary. This is verified by **b** a negative cytokeratin 7, **c** a positive cytokeratin 20, and **d** a positive CDX2.

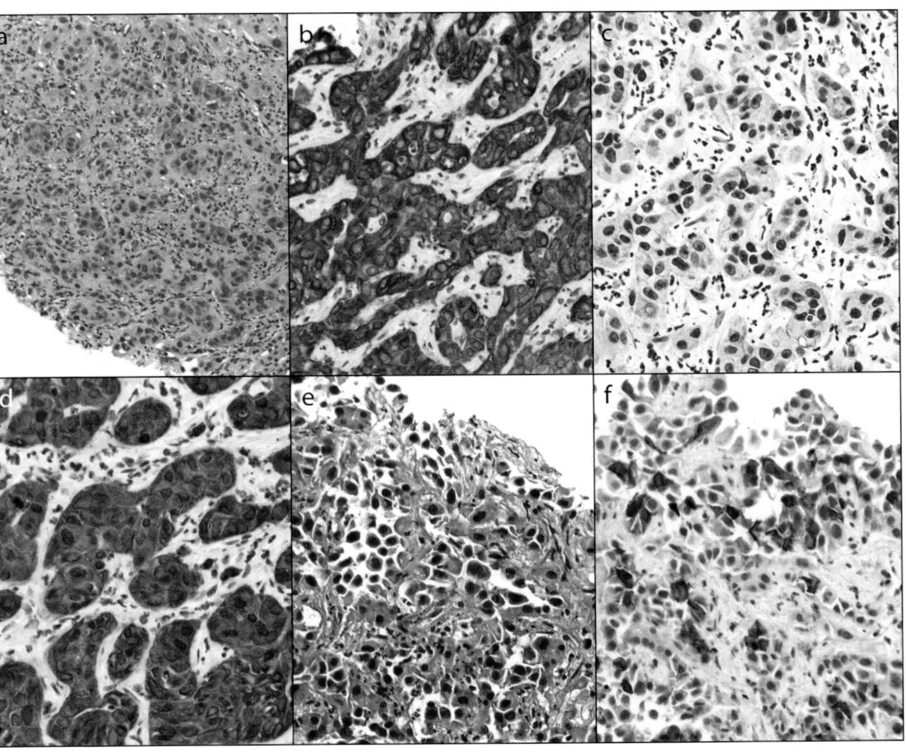

i26.26 The case illustrated in **a-d** demonstrates **a** a malignant neoplasm in the liver that is **b** positive for cytokeratin 7, **c** negative for cytokeratin 20, and **d** positive for epithelial membrane antigen. The positivity for cytokeratin 7 and EMA effectively exclude a primary HCC. Most such cases will be metastases from the breast or the lung, but cholangiocarcinomas and metastases from other sites, especially the upper gastrointestinal tract and the pancreas, may show a similar staining pattern. This case was negative for any markers that would suggest a specific primary site, and all that could be said was, "Adenocarcinoma. Diagnostic possibilities include primary cholangiocarcinoma and metastases from the lung, breast, upper gastrointestinal tract, or pancreas."

e Another poorly differentiated neoplasm of the liver which was positive for CK7+, CK20–, positive for epithelial membrane antigen, and negative for all markers suggesting lung or breast, as in the case illustrated in i26.26a-d. **f** The case in i26.26e was positive for CA19.9. CA19.9 positivity can be seen in a variety of neoplasms, but is most associated with carcinomas of the pancreas and biliary epithelium. This patient had a pancreatic mass.

i26.27 a A poorly differentiated malignant neoplasm in the liver **b** The same case as in i26.27a, illustrating positivity for cytokeratins 5 and 6

c The same case as in i26.27a, illustrating positivity for p63. Staining for both cytokeratins 5 & 6 and p63 strongly suggests a metastatic squamous carcinoma.

ISBN 978-089189-5886

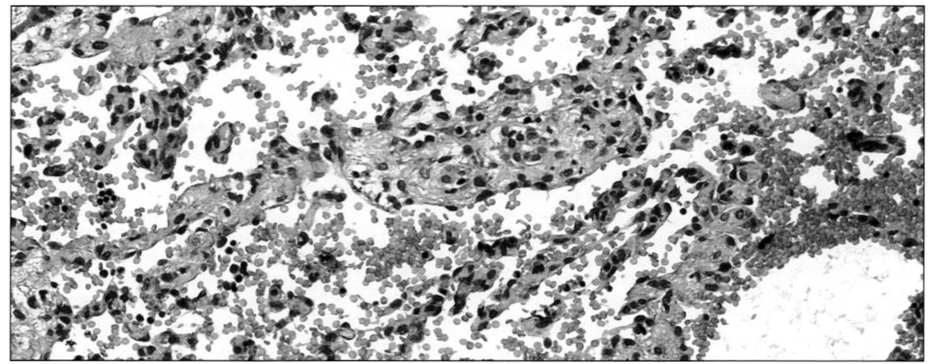

i26.28 An infantile hemangioendothelioma in a young child

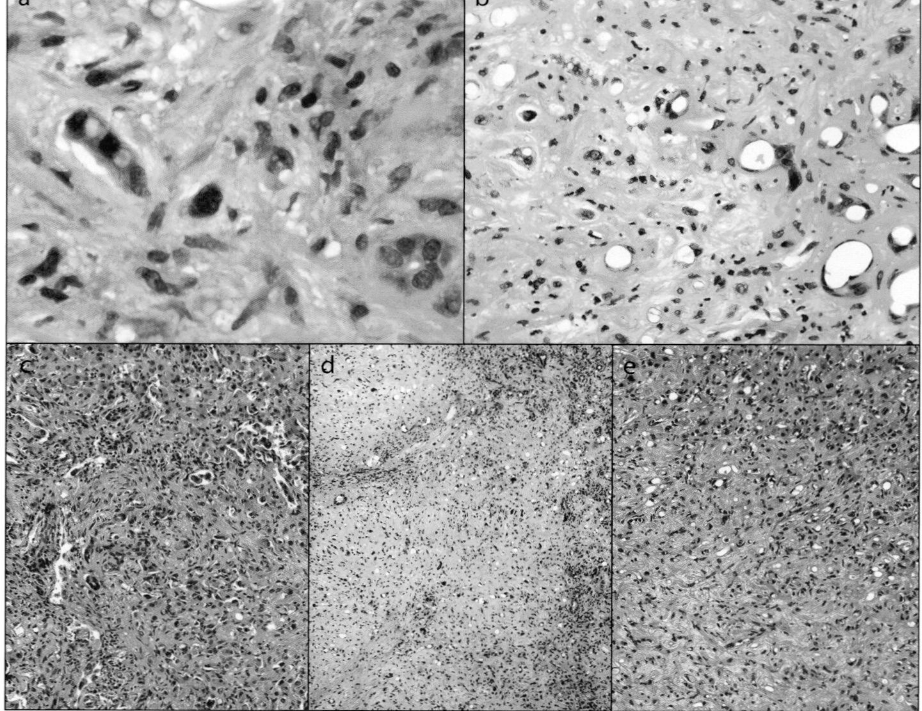

i26.29 a A close view of the cells of an epithelioid hemangioendothelioma, illustrating nuclear atypia and cytoplasmic vacuolization

b Another epithelioid hemangioendothelioma illustrating the nuclear atypia, vacuolization, and stroma that varies from myxoid to sclerotic

c An epithelioid hemangioendothelioma with appreciable cellularity in the upper portion of the photograph and more sclerotic stroma in the lower portion

d A low-power view of an epithelioid hemangioendothelioma illustrating the variability of the stroma; some areas are myxoid, some areas are sclerotic, and some areas are cellular.

e An epithelioid hemangioendothelioma with myxoid stroma in the lower portion and more cellularity in the upper portion

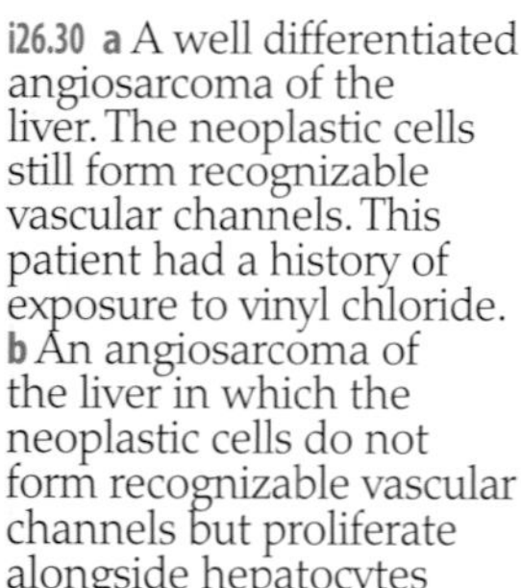

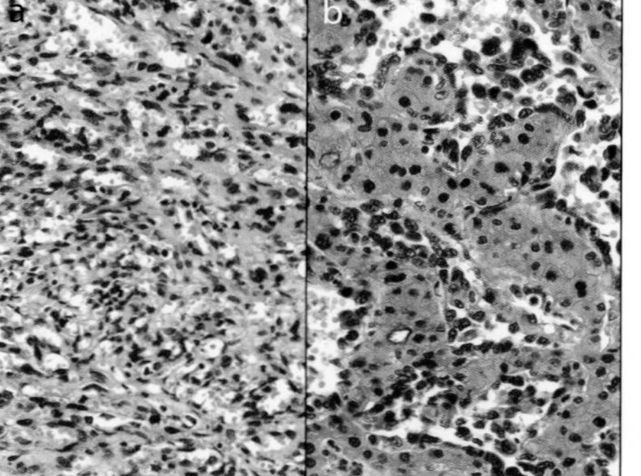

i26.30 a A well differentiated angiosarcoma of the liver. The neoplastic cells still form recognizable vascular channels. This patient had a history of exposure to vinyl chloride.
b An angiosarcoma of the liver in which the neoplastic cells do not form recognizable vascular channels but proliferate alongside hepatocytes

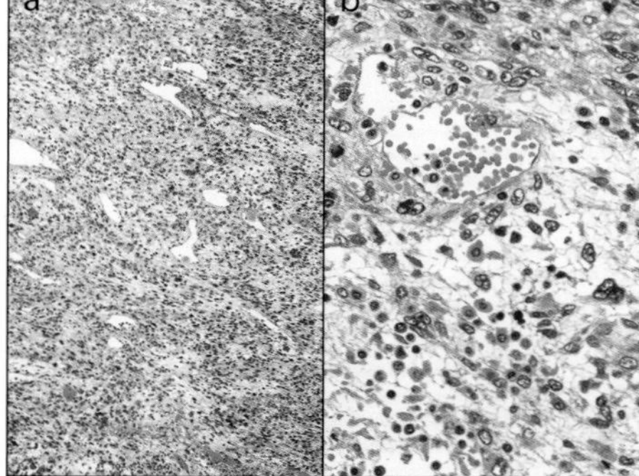

i26.31 a A low-power view of an undifferentiated sarcoma of the liver, a pediatric neoplasm characterized by undifferentiated mesenchymal cells
b A higher-power view of the same case as in i26.31a, illustrating the nuclear pleomorphism, in sharp contrast to the benign nuclei of a mesenchymal hamartoma

i26.32 a-b 2 examples of a pure epithelial variant of a hepatoblastoma. Note the absence of bile ducts and the similarity to a well differentiated hepatocellular carcinoma.

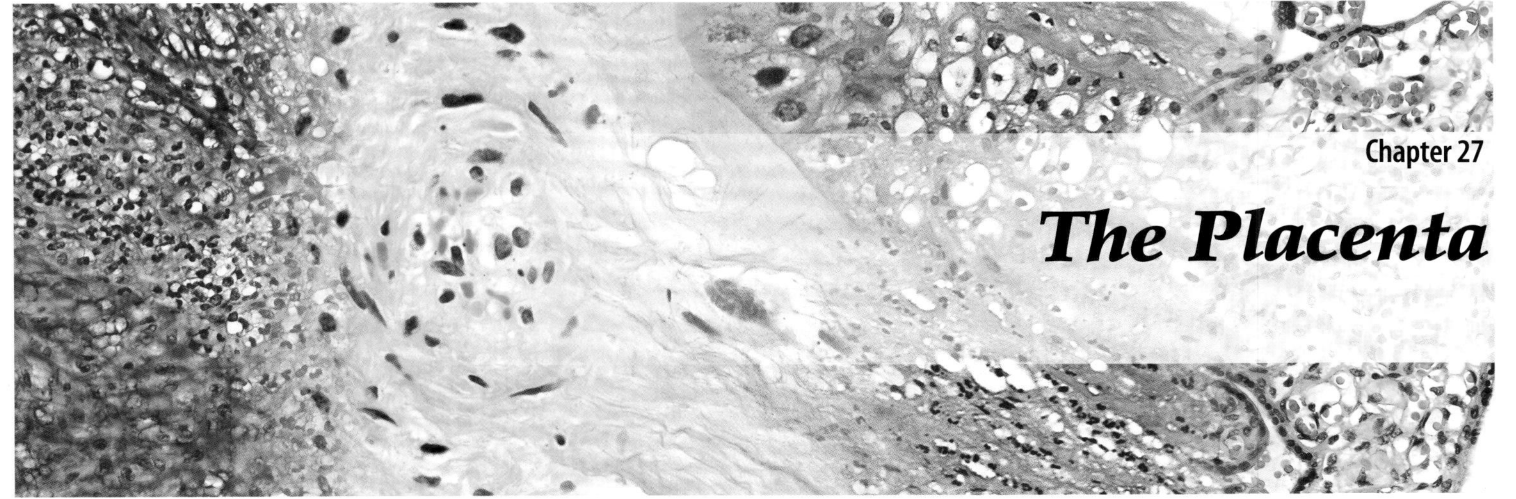

Chapter 27

The Placenta

Development of the Placenta

Following fertilization, the morula, a solid ball of 16 cells, develops by day 3. The morula develops into the blastocyst, a larger, hollow ball containing about 100 cells, by day 4 [Larsen ISBN978-0443065835]. The blastocyst is usually the structure that implants, the earlier stages having been traversed during transit in the fallopian tube. Within the blastocyst, there is a collection of cells called the inner cell mass f27.1. It has been shown in mice that any cell from the inner cell mass is capable of developing into any cell in the body, and this is also suspected in humans. When people speak of "embryonic stem cells," they are usually referring to the cells of the inner cell mass.

4 extraembryonic membranes—the amnion, the yolk sac, the allantois, and the chorion—surround the embryo f27.2 [Larsen ISBN978-0443065835]. The embryo and all extraembryonic membranes except the chorion, the outermost, develop from the inner cell mass. The chorion and placenta develop from the surrounding cells, the outer cell mass [Larsen ISBN978-0443065835, Strachan ISBN978-0815341499].

The amnion immediately surrounds the embryo. Amnions are found in many animals, including reptiles. Their original purpose was to provide a watertight environment so the animal could breed on land. The yolk sac is exterior to the amnion, and in nonmammals, its yolk is the source of nourishment for the embryo, but this function is diminished in mammals because the placenta provides nutrition. The yolk sac forms a cavity on the opposite side of the embryo from the amniotic cavity. Part of the yolk sac becomes the hindgut, and in this sense it is not entirely extraembryonic. The allantois arises as an outpouching of the hindgut. In nonmammals, it provides for gas diffusion and removal of wastes, but in mammals, because of placental development, the allantois becomes the umbilical cord. After birth, the umbilical cord becomes the urachus, and then persists as the medial umbilical ligament.

The first step in the development of the embryo from the inner cell mass is the formation of 3 layers—the ectoderm, mesoderm, and endoderm—in a process called gastrulation. Gastrulation depends on cell migration and is the key event in embryogenesis because by converting a sphere into a multilayered disk, it makes possible all subsequent development.

The chorion is the outermost membrane and is the only source of trophoblasts. Until approximately 2 weeks of gestation, when villi begin to form from the chorion, the primitive trophoblast is called a previllous trophoblast. After the formation of villi, previllous trophoblasts become either villous

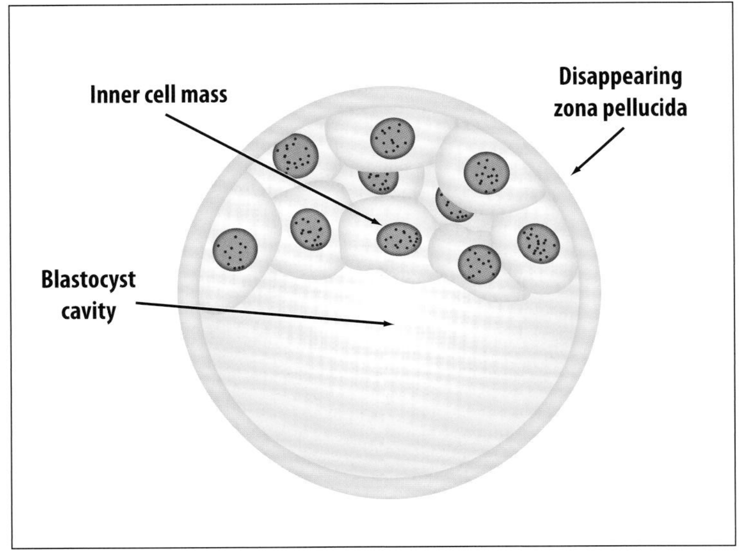

f27.1 Blastocyst

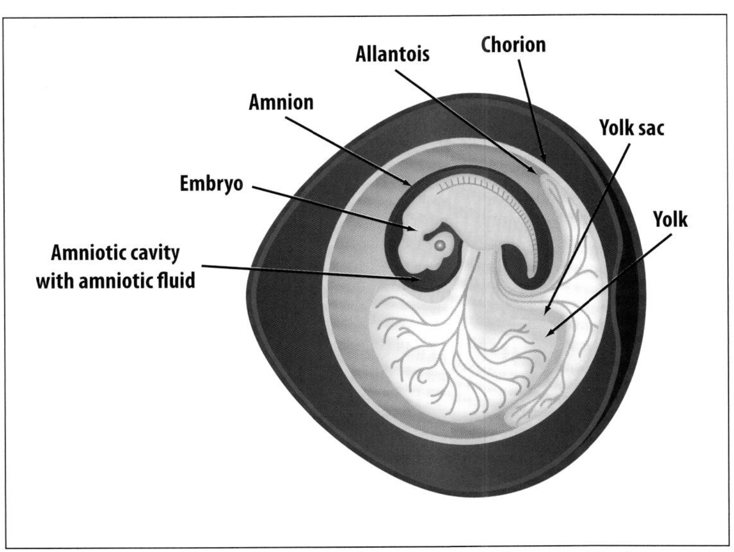

f27.2 4 extraembryonic membranes—the amnion, the yolk sac, the allantois, and the chorion, perhaps at two different times, one illustrating the fusion of the chorion and amnion

ISBN 978-089189-5886

trophoblasts or extravillous trophoblasts. Additional differentiation of the villous trophoblasts results in 3 types of trophoblasts that are associated with the villi—the cytotrophoblast, the syncytiotrophoblast, and the intermediate trophoblast. Cytotrophoblasts give rise to both syncytiotrophoblasts and intermediate trophoblasts, and are the ultimate precursor trophoblasts [PMID17397906]. The cytotrophoblast is a relatively small cell. The syncytiotrophoblast is a large, multinucleated cell formed from the fusion and continued differentiation of the cytotrophoblasts i27.1. The intermediate trophoblast has morphologic features between those of the other 2 types of villous trophoblasts. It is larger than the cytotrophoblast, with more abundant cytoplasm, but smaller than the syncytiotrophoblast and mononucleated. Cytotrophoblasts and syncytiotrophoblasts are restricted to the villi, while intermediate trophoblasts may be found in villi or in extravillous sites.

At 4 weeks gestation, the amnion and chorion are separated by the extraembryonic coelom, a residue of the space within the blastocyst, and the chorion is completely covered by villi on the side facing away from the amnion. Later, the chorion and amnion will fuse, obliterating the extraembryonic coelom. After this fusion, the joined membranes are lined by a thin layer of epithelium from the amnion on the side facing away from the villi. Immediately beneath this epithelium is a thin layer of amniotic connective tissue. The chorion consists only of connective tissue, with blood vessels and a layer of intermediate trophoblasts i27.2.

Only villi that contact endometrium will mature, and as they do so, they develop into the chorionic frondosum (placental disk). Those villi that do not contact the endometrium will atrophy, and that portion of the fused amnion/chorion, now bare, is the chorion laeve, which will become the free membranes of the developed placenta. Placenta membranacea occurs when these villi do not atrophy. In placenta membranacea, the distinction between the chorionic frondosum and chorion laeve is lost, resulting in a thin placenta with little or no free membranes, and an increased risk of hemorrhage.

The intermediate trophoblast is larger than the cytotrophoblast and, unlike the cytotrophoblast, it may be villous or extravillous. The intermediate trophoblast has also been called an "X cell," but this terminology is out of favor because it was unclear and the populations of trophoblastic cells are better understood now. When in a villus, intermediate trophoblasts are often found in a trophoblastic column, a large collection of trophoblasts on one side of the villus. Many intermediate trophoblasts in the column will migrate from the villi to become extravillous intermediate trophoblasts, of which there are 2 types. Some intermediate trophoblasts will infiltrate into the myometrium to become implantation site extravillous intermediate trophoblasts, while others become extravillous intermediate trophoblast of the chorionic type on the free membranes [PMID10374778]. This leaves 3 varieties of intermediate trophoblasts—villous, extravillous implantation site, and extravillous chorionic type—but this discussion will be concerned only with the 2 types of extravillous intermediate trophoblasts, as those intermediate trophoblasts in the trophoblastic column of the villi appear to be precursor cells for both types of extravillous intermediate trophoblasts.

Some implantation site intermediate trophoblasts invade maternal blood vessels and establish the maternal-fetal circulation. These may be spindle shaped and resemble smooth muscle cells. The intermediate trophoblasts in the implantation site can also fuse to form multinucleated cells that are called syncytiotrophoblastic giant cells. These are distinct from syncytiotrophoblasts, which form from the fusion of cytotrophoblasts. The function of extravillous intermediate trophoblast of the chorionic type, found in the chorion laeve, is not known.

Distinguishing between cytotrophoblasts and intermediate trophoblasts is difficult, as the immunohistochemical profiles overlap. Although human placental lactogen (HPL) is commonly used to distinguish between cytotrophoblasts and intermediate trophoblasts, it is of relatively low sensitivity in detecting the latter cells. Human chorionic gonadotropin (HCG) stains cytotrophoblasts and syncytiotrophoblasts, but may also stain intermediate trophoblasts before the second trimester. A subclass of HLA antigens, HLA-G, is associated with intermediate trophoblasts and can be helpful in their identification [PMID12131159]. A panel of HPL, HLA-G, epithelial membrane antigen (EMA), and CD146 (Mel-CAM) is more sensitive in distinguishing cytotrophoblasts from intermediate trophoblasts, since all of these markers are more likely to be positive in intermediate trophoblasts than in cytotrophoblasts [PMID1694585].

The 2 types of extravillous intermediate trophoblasts have slightly different immunophenotypes. Like those from the implantation site, chorionic type intermediate trophoblasts may or may not be positive for HPL, but if positive, the staining is usually weaker than for implantation site intermediate trophoblasts. Compared to implantation site intermediate trophoblasts, chorionic type intermediate trophoblasts are more strongly positive for EMA and less positive for CD146 (Mel-CAM) [PMID10374778].

Villi are initially poorly vascularized and edematous. As the placenta matures, the villi become much smaller and less edematous, and develop large numbers of capillaries. The formation of capillaries in the periphery of the villus is particularly critical to normal placental development, as it is only through peripheral capillaries that gas exchange can take place. The number of cytotrophoblasts decreases with time, and they are hardly identifiable in the term placenta, while the number of syncytiotrophoblasts increases. The latter cell type often forms minute clusters, called syncycial knots.

In the term placenta, primary stem villi are large and contain large vessels with media and adventitia. Secondary (or intermediate) stem villi have both large vessels and capillaries and give rise to the terminal villi that, when fully mature, contain only capillaries i27.3.

Gross Examination of the Placenta

The placenta consists of 3 primary elements—the umbilical cord, the placental disk, and the membranes. The umbilical cord normally consists of 3 vessels, 2 arteries, and 1 vein. These are designated relative to the fetus, so the vein brings oxygenated blood to the fetus and the arteries carry deoxygenated blood away from the fetus. The length and diameter of the cord should be described, and mention should be made of the number of vessels, whether or not there are any twists or knots (and if so, whether or not they appear gentle and nonconstrictive of blood flow or tight and likely to constrict the vessels). The insertion point of the cord should be described as central, off-center, marginal (formerly called battledore), or on the membranes themselves rather than on the disk (velamentous). The normal-term umbilical cord is between 50 and 60 cm, but detached portions of the cord may be separately received, and in some cases, not all of the cord is sent to the laboratory. The 3 vessels of the umbilical cord may not be evident at its insertion point, so the cord should be sampled 4.0 cm or more from its insertion point if the section is intended to clarify the number of vessels. There is an approximately 10-fold increase in chromosomal abnormalities and a 3-fold increase in other congenital anomalies in 2-vessel (ie, single artery) umbilical cords [PMID14726810].

The top of the placental disk is the fetal surface, which is covered by a fused amnion-chorion and upon which are the fetal vessels formed from tributaries of the umbilical vein or vessels that will coalesce into the umbilical arteries. The lower portion of the disk, which implanted into the endometrium, is the maternal surface. The maternal surface consists of cotyledons, each of which arises from a single branch of an umbilical artery and can be seen grossly [Lewis ISBN0-443-07586-7]. Some use the terms "cotyledon" and "lobule" synonymously, while others restrict the term "lobule" for a smaller unit that cannot be seen grossly.

The gross evaluation of the placental disk should include comments on its weight, shape, dimensions, degree of trauma and intactness, insertion of the membranes, vessels on the fetal surface, subchorionic hemorrhage or fibrin deposition, presence of a hematoma on the maternal surface, presence and location of infarcts (and if any, an estimate should be made of the percentage of placental volume that is infarcted), and presence of accessory lobes [PMID18708423].

There is substantial disagreement in the literature regarding placental weights, so the fetal-to-placental-weight ratio often has little meaning. Among other variables, the placental weight is dependent on when the cord was clamped. It is reasonable to use about 500 g as the mean weight for a term placenta, with a standard deviation of about 100 g, provided the placenta is received fresh, has been drained of blood, and the weight of the umbilical cord is not counted. Rough, but reasonable expected weights for preterm placentas are as follows [Lewis ISBN0-443-07586-7]:

- 24 weeks: 182 g, +/–45 g
- 30 weeks: 285 g, +/–70 g
- 34 weeks: 362 g
- 37-40 weeks: 450-500 g

The color and degree of transparency of the membranes should be described. Acute chorioamnionitis may be suspected if the membranes are opaque instead of translucent. A statement made as to whether the membranes insert into the margins of the disk, or short of the margins. The latter situation results in placental tissue that is not covered by membranes, called extrachorial placenta. There are 2 forms of extrachorial placenta. The circummarginate form of extrachorial placenta is a simple situation in which the membranes do not extend to the margin of the placental disk, but are not folded over on themselves. In the circumvallate form, the membranes fold back on themselves at the site of attachment on the disk. Historically, the circummarginate form has been considered relatively innocuous, while the circumvallate form has been associated with abortion, membrane rupture, hemorrhage, and prematurity [PMID18226129].

The diagnosis of meconium staining is usually best made by the obstetrician, who sees the placenta in its pristine state and can correlate its appearance with the clinical situation, but the pathologist is occasionally called upon to assist in this determination. Acute meconium staining imparts a green tinge to the membranes and can generally be washed off. This occurs at birth and is usually insignificant. On the other hand, brown membranes whose color is refractory to washing suggest chronic meconium staining, which is more likely to be significant. Finding meconium within macrophages indicates that the staining occurred at least several hours prior to delivery and is therefore more likely to be significant. Large numbers of such macrophages indicate passage 6-12 hours before delivery. Meconium macrophages may be much more difficult to find than the gross appearance would suggest. The best place to look for them is in the free membranes, beneath the epithelial lining i27.4.

Meconium passage may lead to the meconium aspiration syndrome, a life-threatening condition characterized by both the physical blocking of the airways by meconium and inflammation of the bronchial mucosa by meconium [PMID19381312]. Another concern with chronic meconium staining is that some of the components of meconium diffuse into the blood vessel wall and cause vasoconstriction, which in severe cases can lead to hypoxia. On the other hand, hypoxia also is a cause of meconium staining, and the association of meconium and hypoxia is somewhat of a "chicken and egg" question [PMID10612363].

Microscopic Examination of the Placenta

Infection of the placenta can occur via an ascending pathway from the vagina and cervix, or hematogenously via maternal blood. Most bacteria are transmitted via an ascending pathway, though *Treponema pallidum* [PMID9738997] and *Listeria monocytogenes* [PMID8767708] are transmitted hematogenously in most cases. Viruses and toxoplasma are usually conveyed hematogenously. Experimental work suggests that ascending infection tends to cause chorioamnionitis, while hematogenous infection is more likely to cause villitis [PMID119050]. Premature rupture of the membranes sharply predisposes to fetal/placental infection. Ascending infection may be well tolerated by the fetus, but is responsible for 30-40% of premature births. The most common and serious bacterial infection during pregnancy is caused by Group B *Streptococcus* [PMID17765489].

In chorioamnionitis of the free membranes i27.5, some have advocated a comment on whether the neutrophils are only in the chorion, the outer part of the fused chorion-amnion that contains trophoblastic cells or, also in the amnion, the inner portion of the fused membrane that consists of the lining cells and the immediately adjacent stroma because neutrophils invade the chorion first and then progress to the amnion. In this nomenclature, chorionitis is the stage 1 chorioamnionitis,

ISBN 978-089189-5886

inflammation that has extended into the amnion is stage 2 chorioamnionitis, and necrosis of the fused membranes is considered a stage 3 chorioamnionitis [PMID19046766]. This is a fundamentally sound concept, but much more important than the location of the neutrophils in the membranes is whether or not the inflammation has extended to the umbilical cord and whether or not there is any vasculitis.

"Funisitis" is a nonspecific term referring to general inflammation of the umbilical cord. Any funisitis is always potentially significant because the neutrophils are of fetal origin, but the inflammation is more likely to be significant if the vessels of the cord are inflamed. In this case, the diagnosis of umbilical cord vasculitis should be made i27.6. If there is no vasculitis, the report should specifically state that there is funisitis without vasculitis. Vasculitis of the vessels on the placental disk i27.7 is also potentially significant because the neutrophils are of fetal origin, as opposed to the maternal origin of simple chorioamnionitis [PMID15451193]. However, even if there is funisitis or vasculitis, the clinical situation determines if the inflammation is significant or not.

Acute placental ischemia is said to be characterized by a greater density of villi (because ischemia results in diminished intervillous blood flow, which permits the villi to get closer together), a reduction in the size or number of villi, and by more syncycial knots than would be expected from the gestational age (a feature of so-called accelerated maturation), but in my experience, acute placental ischemia is difficult to appreciate unless there is an acute infarct i27.8. Acute infarcts may be grossly soft and have a darker red-brown color. Infarcts in preterm placentas are of concern, but those in term placentas, especially if small, are relatively common and less likely to be significant [Lewis ISBN0-443-07586-7]. Many feel that a peripheral infarct is of less concern than one that is centrally located. Although some fibrin in the placental disk is a normal finding, large amounts should elicit a search for infarct or ischemic damage.

Grossly, older infarcts, indicative of previous or chronic ischemia, are usually firmer than acute infarcts. The key microscopic feature of chronic ischemia is widespread sclerosis of villi. Chronic ischemia is often idiopathic, but is seen in preeclampsia or pregnancy-induced hypertension [PMID17883125]. Only clinical correlation can secure a diagnosis of eclampsia or preeclampsia, but about 1/2 of patients with preeclampsia have acute atherosis, a subendothelial deposition of lipid-laden macrophages [PMID15702369].

"Villous dysmaturity" is a term used to indicate a significant discrepancy between the appearance of the villi and the clinical dates. Diminished villous maturation is characterized by increased villus size, decreased numbers of capillaries, failure of the villus to develop peripheral capillaries, diminished syncytial knots, and persistence of cytotrophoblasts i27.9a, i27.9b. Villous immaturity can be seen in diabetes, hydrops fetalis (the accumulation of fluid in the fetus), or fetal macrosomia.

Accelerated maturation is much more difficult to appreciate. Increased syncytial knots are the most reliable indicator of accelerated maturation, but even this criterion is notoriously subjective. If successfully identified, accelerated maturation is associated with ischemia, autoimmune disorders, fetal demise, or rarely, diabetes.

Hemorrhagic endovasculitis (HEV; also called hemorrhagic endovasculopathy or obliterative vasculopathy) is the sloughing of endothelial cells in vessels on or near the fetal surface, followed by incorporation of red cells into the wall of an artery i27.10, occasionally with erythrocyte fragmentation and fibrin microthrombi. While there has been some feeling that HEV may result from reflex arterial spasm after delivery and may not have significance if there is no inflammation and necrosis of the vascular wall, most believe that HEV is a type of fetal thrombotic vasculopathy, and can and should be diagnosed if there are fibrin microthrombi, damage to endothelial cells, or destruction of fetal erythrocytes [PMID8606341]. When HEV is defined in this manner, it is associated with other conditions, such as chronic villitis, villous erythroblastosis, meconium staining, and maternal hypertension, and is of potential clinical significance [PMID11825110]. However, fibrin microthrombi that are rare or restricted to the vicinity of the maternal surface are likely to be secondary to separation of the placenta from the endometrium at the time of delivery and of little significance.

The maternal floor infarct is morphologically characterized by an approximately 1/2 cm. band of tissue degeneration and fibrin deposition in the placental base, near the maternal surface. There may be some infarction, but usually fibrin deposition is the major finding i27.11a, i27.11b, and many cases have no infarction, making the term largely a misnomer. Maternal floor infarct is associated with a significantly increased risk of subsequent reproductive failure and these patients virtually always have intrauterine growth retardation (IUGR) [PMID8210775].

A *chorangioma* is a placental hemangioma, is a distinct mass, without villi i27.12, and is usually without significance. *Chorangiosis* is a generalized increase in the number of villous capillaries and is not a distinct mass i27.13. Even allowing for a capillary being counted more than once if it passes through the plane of section multiple times, a normal-term villus rarely has >10 capillary cross sections. Chorangiosis can be suspected if multiple villi in multiple areas average >10 capillaries. The precise criteria, established by Altshuler in 1984 [PMID6546343], are a minimum of 10 villi, each with 10 or more separate capillaries, from 10 or more areas dispersed throughout the placenta and from foci that are not infarcted. If well documented in this manner, chorangiosis is associated with fetal morbidity and mortality, and probably indicates hypoxia [PMID19489958].

The diagnosis of acute placental abruption requires clinical correlation and cannot be made by the pathologist alone [PMID19897298], but it can be suspected if there is copious blood on the maternal surface, indenting it. In chronic abruption, there may be maternal surface fibrin deposits and hemosiderin macrophages [PMID19897298].

There should be only occasional nucleated erythrocytes in the blood or in the placenta of normal-term infants. More than 1 per high-power field in the placental vessels is associated with diminished villous vascularity and chronic villitis [PMID18614199].

Whereas acute inflammation of the placenta is usually found in the membranes or in the blood vessels, chronic inflammation is primarily seen in the villi. Chronic villitis is found in many infections, such as syphilis, toxoplasmosis, and some viruses, but is idiopathic in most cases [PMID10419804].

Chronic villitis requires the presence of lymphocytes, plasma cells, or macrophages in the villi i27.14. The diagnosis can be suspected by increased villous cellularity on low-power examination, but increased cellularity alone does not establish chronic villitis, as many or all of the cells may be endothelial or fibrocytes. A common error is to make the diagnosis of chronic villitis too quickly at low power, upon seeing hypercellularity, without properly identifying the cell types.

Because the chorion is the sole source of trophoblasts, and because in a dichorionic, diamniotic twin placenta the chorion, with its trophoblasts, has extended into the dividing membrane, such a twin placenta will have trophoblasts in the dividing membrane. In monochorionic, diamniotic twin placentas, the chorion does not extend into the dividing membrane. These have only amniotic tissue in the dividing membrane and, therefore, no trophoblasts. For this reason, any trophoblasts at all in a section from the dividing membrane indicate a dichorionic placenta i27.15. Monozygotic (identical) twins may arise from monochorionic or dichorionic placentas, but dizygotic (fraternal) twins only arise from a dichorionic placenta. Monochorionic placentas must give rise to identical twins, whereas dichorionic placentas can give rise to either type of twin:

Monochorionic, diamniotic placenta→monozygotic twins

Dichorionic, diamniotic placenta→monozygotic or dizygotic twins

Monochorionic twin placentas always have interplacental anastomoses of varying significance, leading to some degree of twin-twin transfusion syndrome (TTTS), though this is usually mild. In contrast, such anastomoses are very rare in dichorionic twin placentas.

What Constitutes Products of Conception?

A major problem in surgical pathology is to secure a diagnosis of products of conception in tissue derived from the uterine cavity, because doing so effectively excludes an ectopic pregnancy. Historically, the presence of villi has been required for the firm diagnosis of products of conception and is still the gold standard, but for all practical purposes, the presence of trophoblasts also secures the diagnosis of products of conception. To my mind, the presence of syncytiotrophoblasts on H&E study secures a diagnosis of an intrauterine pregnancy to reasonable certainty, even in the absence of villi, as there is nothing in the normal endometrium that is likely to be confused with these cells.

On the other hand, decidual cells of endometrial stromal origin may closely resemble mononuclear trophoblasts. All trophoblasts are keratin positive, unlike decidual cells, but care must be taken not to misinterpret any trapped endometrial glands, which will also be keratin positive, as mononuclear trophoblasts. It is wise to perform additional immunohistochemical stains that will highlight trophoblasts and not endometrial epithelium. Because of the absence of villi, it is likely that any mononuclear trophoblasts seen will be of the intermediate type, and therefore any immunohistochemical staining beyond keratin can be directed at them. HPL stains only about 60% of intermediate trophoblasts, but its presence suggests the presence of trophoblasts. HCG, though associated with cytotrophoblasts and syncytiotrophoblasts, also stains most intermediate trophoblasts. Other good markers are EMA, HLA-G, and Mel-CAM [PMID18251570]. Not every trophoblast will stain for all of these markers, but in concert, they provide the necessary supplementation to a keratin stain. Overall, HLA-G and HCG are excellent supplements to a keratin stain [PMID19145204].

While the identification of trophoblasts provides reasonable assurance of an intrauterine pregnancy in most cases, there is limited experience and imperfect sensitivity and specificity of the stains described above. Therefore, in practice, the time-honored presence of chorionic villi remains the best assurance that a pregnancy is intrauterine. If the diagnosis of products of conception is reached by the identification of trophoblasts, I recommend a comment that products of conception are favored based on the probable presence of trophoblasts, but that in the absence of chorionic villi, certainty is <100%. Finally, if intermediate trophoblasts are identified, a placental site nodule (discussed in Chapter 28) should be excluded before a presumptive diagnosis of a current intrauterine pregnancy is made.

A final remark on the examination of placentas is that the pathologist should not comment on the potential effect of placental abnormalities on the long-term prognosis of the infant. This is not only sound policy from a medicolegal viewpoint, but also from a purely patient-care viewpoint. No one can currently prognosticate the development of a child from the findings in the placenta, and needless anxiety will be caused to all parties by any such attempt. The pathologist's job is to document findings in the placenta, not to predict the future.

Testing in Pregnancy

Elevated serum levels of HCG and inhibin A are associated with Down syndrome, as are diminished levels of estriol, α fetoprotein (αFP), and pregnancy-associated plasma protein A (PAPP-A; a zinc-binding enzyme). Maternal serum testing is begun in the first trimester, along with ultrasound assessment of nuchal translucency [PMID18236423]. In the second trimester, serum testing is frequently repeated, though only repeat PAPP testing appears significantly beneficial [PMID20624355]. Testing for αFP, HCG, and estriol is called triple testing, and the addition of serum inhibin A is quadruple screening.

Elevated αFP levels are associated with open neural tube defects (the neural tube gives rise to the central nervous system and the retina).

These tests notwithstanding, there is still a role for the acquisition of fetal cells in some pregnancies. Fetal cells can be obtained from amniocentesis or chorionic villus sampling, after which they can be analyzed directly or after culture. Cord blood and products of conception are also acceptable fetal tissues. Chorionic villus sampling is more complicated than amniocentesis, and does not yield fluid upon which biochemical studies may be performed, but it does allow faster results of chromosome studies. An ever-present danger in any sampling of fetal tissue is contamination by maternal cells, and it is always necessary to obtain maternal blood or buccal cells and perform a concurrent examination of maternal DNA, with comparison of results to those obtained from the apparent fetal source [PMID21227389].

Conventional culture and karyotyping takes 2 weeks or more, but a variety of rapid fluorescent or PCR techniques have been developed to decrease turnaround time in chromosomal

ISBN 978-089189-5886

studies of amniotic fluid or chorionic villi [PMID20889556]. An exciting unfolding methodology is the acquisition and analysis of cell free fetal nucleic acid from maternal plasma, which obviates the small risk of miscarriage that is inescapable in amniocentesis or chorionic villus sampling. At this writing, this technique has successfully identified fetal gender, rhesus D status, and trisomy 21 [PMID21075065].

Core Points for the Placenta

- Blastocyst: hollow ball of about 100 cells.
    - Contains inner and outer cell masses.
    - Embryo develops from the inner cell mass while the chorion and placenta develop from the outer cell mass.
- Gastrulation: development of 3 layers
- Villi adjacent to the uterine cavity develop into the placental disk, while others atrophy.
    - Villi are initially large and poorly vascularized.
    - With maturation, they become smaller and develop peripheral capillaries.
    - Cytotrophoblasts decrease in number, while syncytiotrophoblasts increase and form syncycial knots.
- Gross placental examination: Insertion of the membranes, any compromise of blood flow in the cord, and the intactness and focal masses or infarcts of the disk.
- Acute placental abruption: clinical diagnosis, though copious blood on the maternal surface, indenting the cotyledons, is supportive.
- Infections: bacterial usually ascending from the vagina, viral usually hematogenous.
    - Group B *Streptococcus* is the most common potentially serious infection.
    - Acute inflammation of the placenta usually occurs in the membranes or in the blood vessels.
    - Acute inflammation restricted to the membranes is likely of maternal origin, but inflammation of the umbilical cord or of blood vessels is likely of fetal origin.
    - Chronic inflammation is primarily manifest as chronic villitis.
- Chronic placental ischemia: sclerotic villi
    - Usually easier to appreciate than acute ischemia unless there is an acute infarct.
- Maternal floor infarct: degeneration and fibrin deposition in the placental base, usually without substantial infarction.
    - Associated with intrauterine growth retardation.
- Twin placentas: any trophoblasts in the dividing membrane indicate a dichorionic placenta.
    - Such a placenta may give rise to either identical or fraternal twins, but monochorionic twin placentas can give rise only to identical twins.
- Acquisition of cell free fetal nucleic acid from maternal plasma may obviate the need for tissue sampling by either amniocentesis or chorionic villus sampling.

i27.1 The large number of syncytiotrophoblasts that are found in full-term placentas. Because these arise from the fusion of cytotrophoblasts, cytotrophoblasts are rarely seen and difficult to identify in full-term placentas.

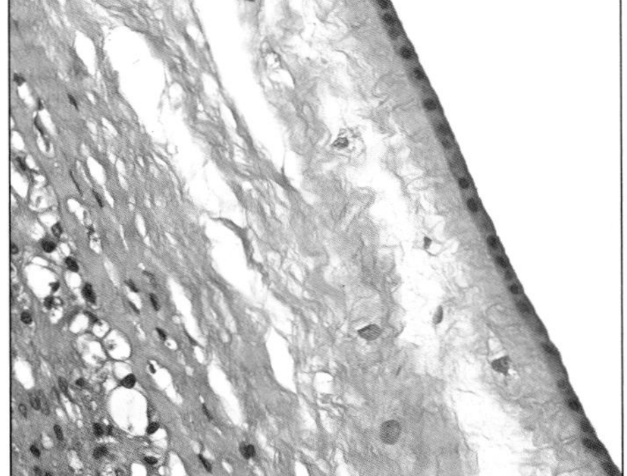

i27.2 A fused amnion-chorion. The amnion is at the upper right and is lined by a single layer of epithelium. The chorion is at the lower left and contains trophoblastic cells (intermediate trophoblasts).

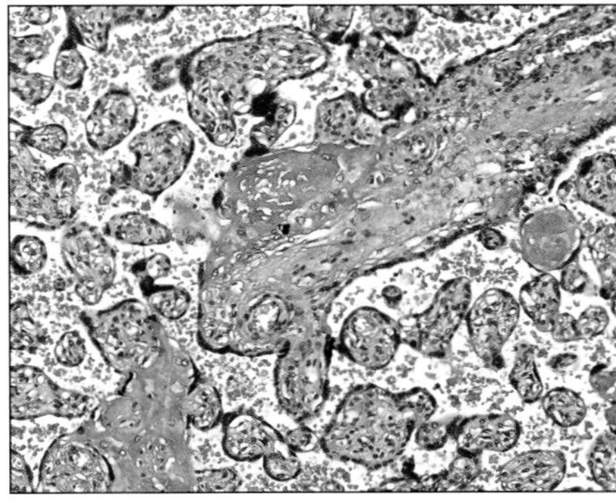

i27.3 A secondary stem villus giving rise to a terminal villus

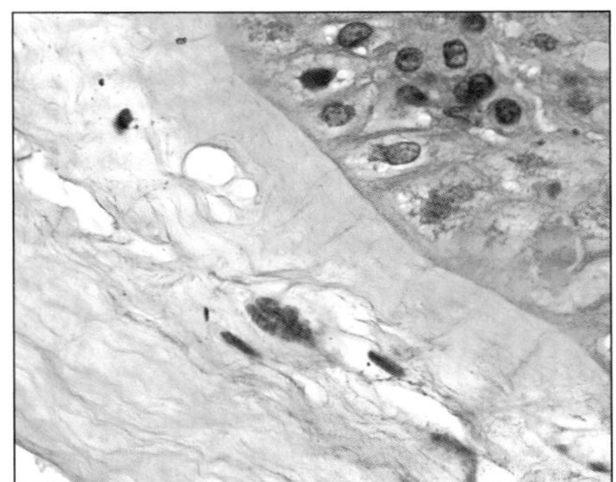

i27.4 A meconium-stained macrophage in the membrane

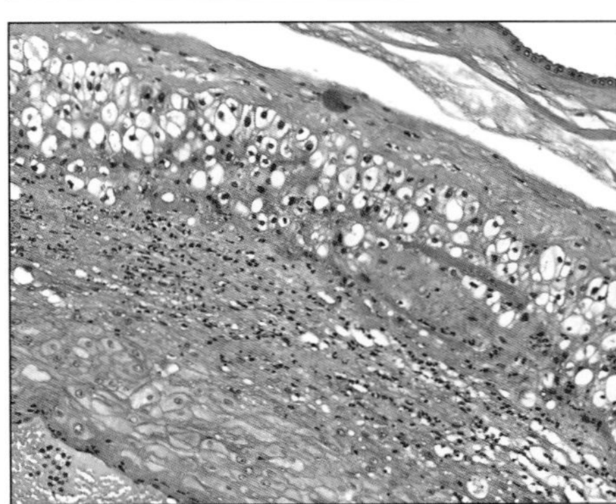

i27.5 Acute chorioamnionitis of the free membranes

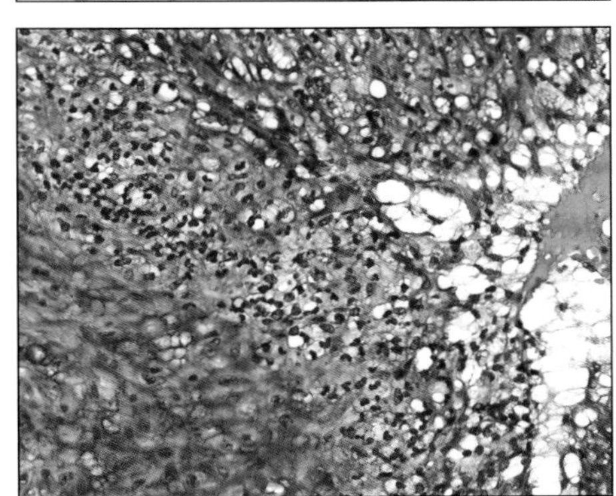

i27.6 The same case as in i27.5, demonstrating acute vasculitis of the vessels of the umbilical cord

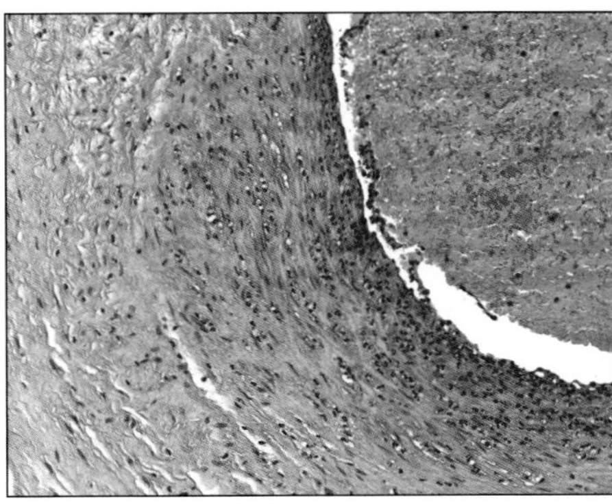

i27.7 The same case as in i27.5, demonstrating acute vasculitis of a smaller blood vessel on the placental disc

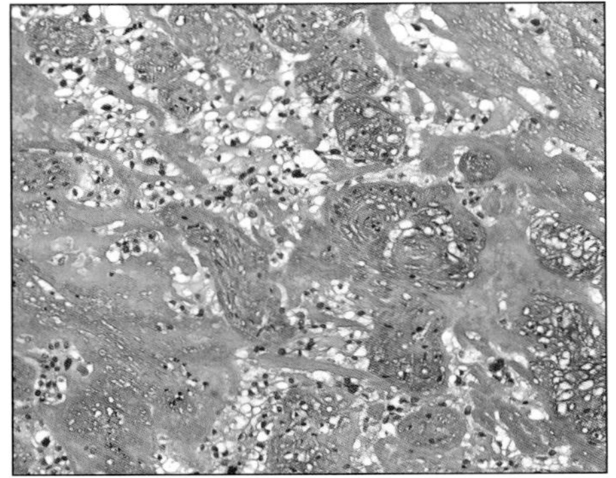

i27.8 An acute placental infarct. The villi are evident as "ghosts," with loss of the trophoblastic lining.

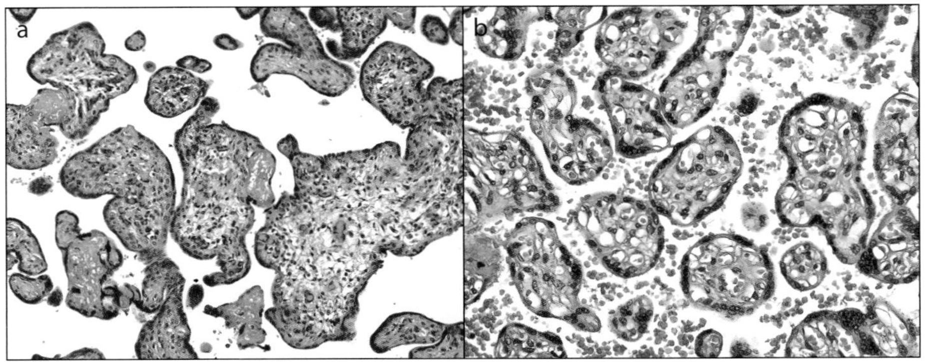

i27.9 The villi of **a** an immature placenta contrasted with those of **b** a mature placenta. In the immature placenta, the villi are not only larger, but their capillaries tend to be centrally located. The mature villi in **b** are smaller and their capillaries are disproportionately located on the periphery, facilitating gas exchange.

ISBN 978-089189-5886

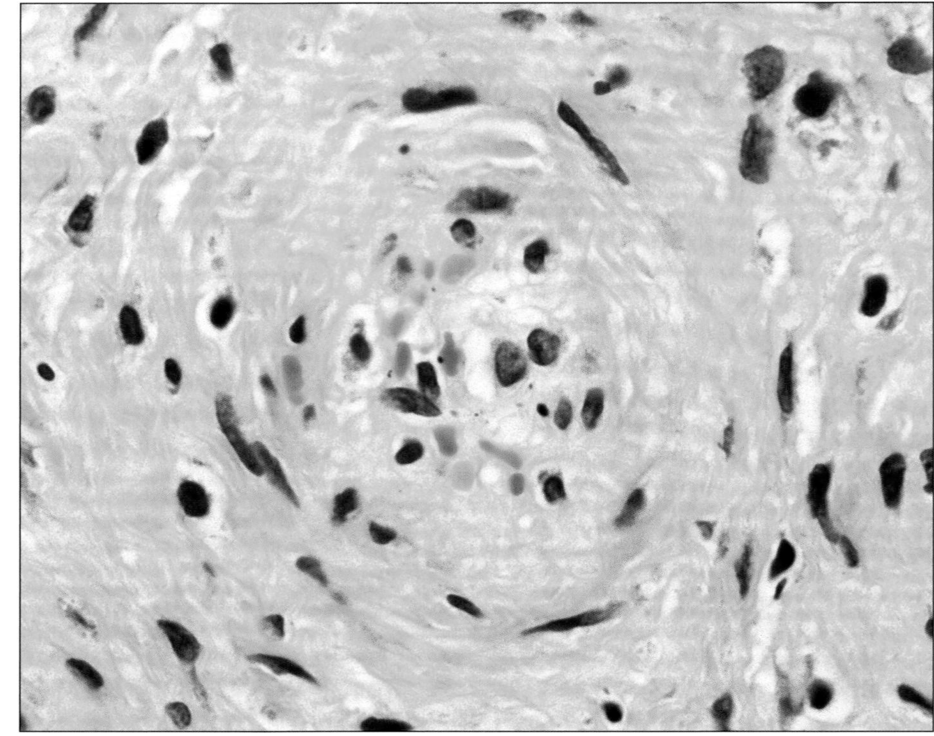

i27.10 Hemorrhagic endovasculitis, with sloughing of endothelial cells into the lumen and penetration of erythrocytes into the wall of the vessel, diminishing the caliber of the lumen and the demarcation between the lumen and the wall

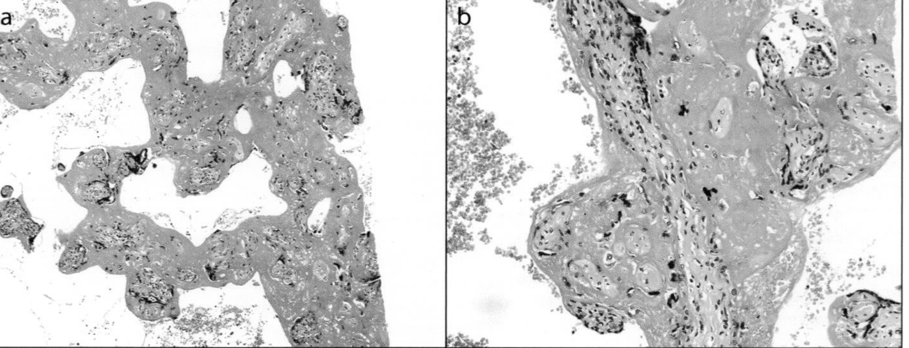

i27.11 **a** A maternal floor infarct. This low-power view is from the maternal surface and illustrates villi that are enveloped by fibrin.

b A higher-power view of the same case as in i27.11a, highlighting the extensive fibrin deposition around the villi

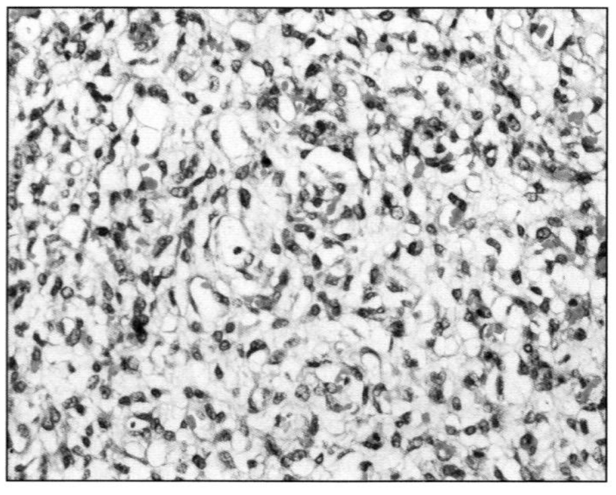

i27.12 A chorangioma. Note the absence of villi. The appearance is that of a benign, cellular capillary hemangioma of other sites.

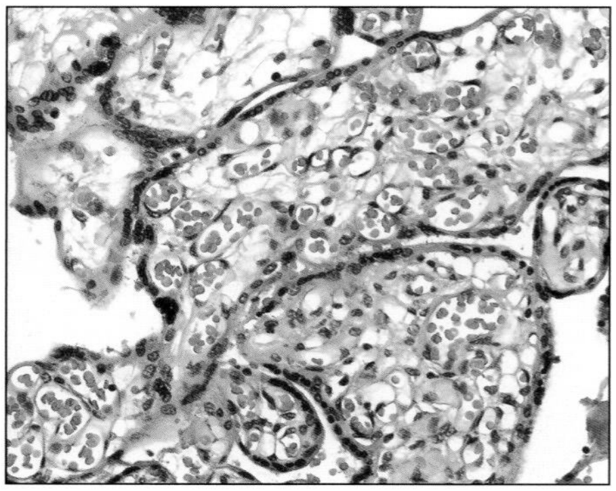

i27.13 Chorangiosis. Note that there are still villi, in contrast to a chorangioma, but they contain an increased number of capillaries.

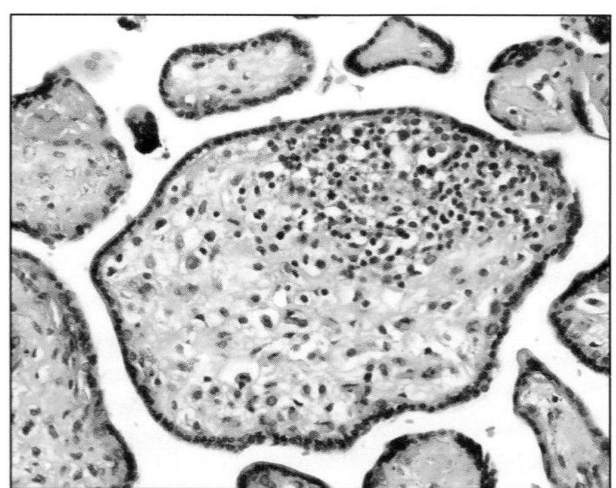

i27.14 Chronic villitis

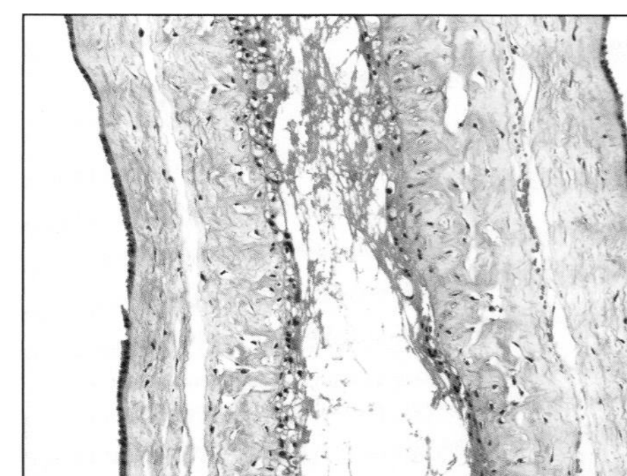

i27.15 A twin placenta which is dichorionic, diamniotic, as indicated by the presence of trophoblasts in this dividing membrane

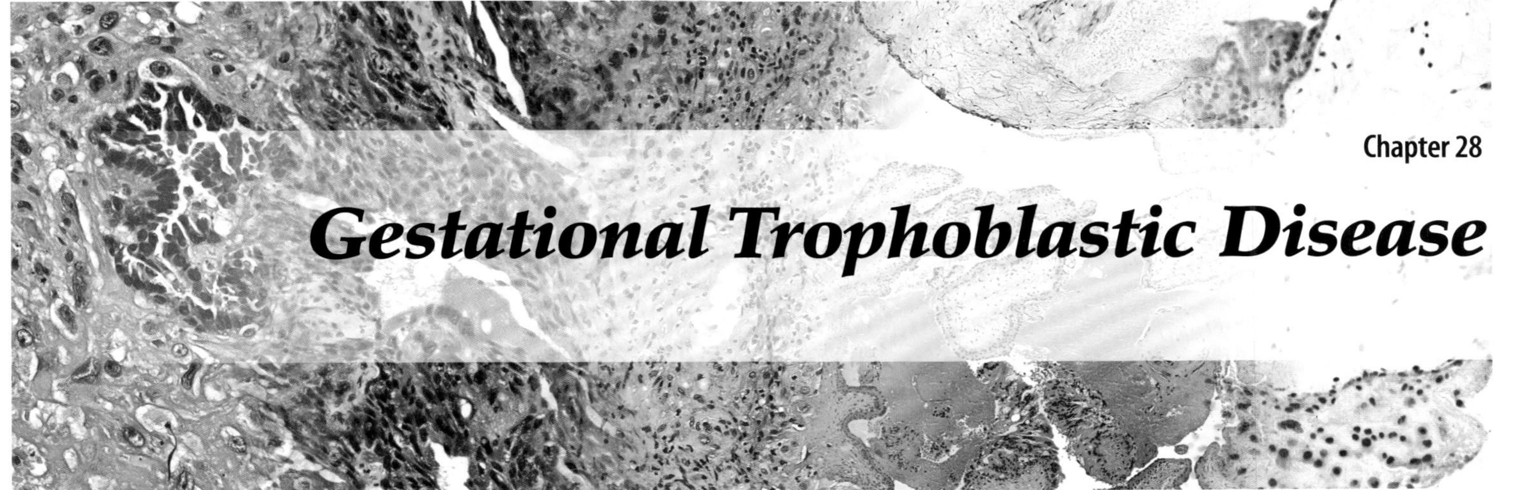

Chapter 28

Gestational Trophoblastic Disease

Gestational trophoblastic diseases can be broadly divided into 2 categories: those that form villi and those that do not. Those that form villi include the hydropic abortus, the complete hydatidiform mole, the partial hydatidiform mole, and the invasive mole. Those that normally have no villi include the placental site nodule, the exaggerated placental site, the placental site trophoblastic tumor (PSTT), the epithelioid trophoblastic tumor (ETT), and choriocarcinoma, though the last of these are often intimately associated with villi that are not actually part of the basic process [PMID18251570].

A complete hydatidiform mole is defined morphologically as the formation of nonneoplastic abnormal villi without fetal tissue. Complete hydatidiform moles have appreciable edema of essentially all villi. The edema is often accentuated in the center of the villus, resulting in a central area called a cistern, which has only fluid and no tissue i28.1a. Cisterns are not usually seen in ordinary hydropic degeneration. The trophoblasts in a mole are hyperplastic and atypical i28.1b, i28.1c. The hyperplasia is circumferential i28.1d, in contrast to the proliferation that predominately emanates from 1 pole of the villus in nonmolar pregnancies.

Complete moles are defined developmentally by origin entirely from male DNA without any contribution of maternal DNA. They are an example of uniparental diploidy [PMID7740315]. Most complete moles are 46,XX and form from the fertilization of an ovum without a nucleus, or with a nonfunctional nucleus, by a single sperm that carries an X chromosome, followed by replication of that genome into a 46,XX and cellular proliferation. The remaining complete moles are also androgenic but are formed from the fertilization of an ovum without a functioning nucleus by 2 separate sperm. These rare cases caused by dispermy may be 46,XX or 46,XY, but 46,YY is not seen and is presumably nonviable [PMID15677707].

An early complete mole may have subtle changes and can be difficult to distinguish from a nonmolar pregnancy, especially a blighted ovum or a hydropic abortus. Villous edema is prominent in a hydropic abortion i28.2a, and cisterns may be absent in early complete moles. The villi in hydropic abortions may have focal trophoblastic hyperplasia and atypia i28.2b, and these features may be mild in early moles, again causing histologic overlap. It is occasionally possible to diagnose an early mole by ultrasonography before the histologic changes are fully evident, and the pathologist may trail the obstetrician in the diagnosis.

p57kip2 (commonly called p57) is a protein that is paternally imprinted (ie, derived entirely from the maternal allele; see Chapter 47 for a discussion of imprinting) and is therefore not expressed in complete moles. Antibodies to it stain cytotrophoblasts, syncytiotrophoblasts, and villous stromal cells in normal placentas, hydropic placentas i28.3a, and partial moles, but this staining is lost in complete moles because they are purely derived from paternal DNA i28.3b [PMID11688455, PMID12514787]. Interestingly, however, intermediate trophoblasts in a complete mole may stain for p57 [PMID12514787]. Again taking advantage of the absence of maternal DNA in complete moles, it is occasionally possible to make the diagnosis by demonstrating that maternal DNA and villous DNA are mutually exclusive [PMID21704275].

An invasive mole (ie, a complete mole that invades into the myometrium) i28.4 can be suspected when human chorionic gonadotropin (HCG) levels fail to fall after evacuation. An invasive mole may be self-limiting but can cause significant bleeding, sometimes requiring a hysterectomy. The diagnosis of invasive mole can only be made with confidence upon examination of a hysterectomy. Other considerations in the diagnosis of an invasive mole include a persistent mole that is not invasive and the entities placenta accreta, placenta increta, and placenta percreta. The last 3 entities refer to the invasion of normal placental tissue to a deeper degree than usual. "Placenta accreta" refers to the invasion of normal placental tissue completely through the endometrium to the junction of the endometrium and myometrium, while "placenta increta" refers to myometrial invasion. Placenta percreta invades through the myometrium and into the serosa.

The most serious entity in the differential diagnosis of an invasive mole is a gestational choriocarcinoma. 1-2% of complete hydatidiform moles will develop into a gestational choriocarcinoma [Benirschke ISBN-13978-0387267388].

A partial hydatidiform mole is morphologically defined as the formation of nonneoplastic abnormal villi in the presence of some amount of fetal tissue, though a normal fetus is not present. The histologic changes of complete and partial hydatidiform moles are similar. They are more generalized and more pronounced in a complete mole, but there is overlap, and it is very difficult to determine morphologic differences on H&E examination. Both complete and partial moles have appreciable villous edema, and either may have central cistern formation i28.5a. A complete mole has generalized edema of all villi, while a partial mole usually may have a mixture of edematous and normal villi i28.5b. Both complete and partial moles will have trophoblastic hyperplasia and atypia i28.5c, and in either entity the hyperplasia may be circumferential.

Partial moles have 2 sets of chromosomes of paternal origin and 1 haploid maternal set, resulting in triploidy. Fertilization of 1 ovum by 2 sperm, called dispermy, is the most common cause of triploidy, and partial moles are developmentally defined by diandric triploidy (which is not to be confused with the uniparental diploidy of a complete mole; in both cases, the paternal DNA is abnormally doubled, but in the diandric triploidy of partial moles, there is also a maternal contribution). Products of conception that are diploid cannot be a partial mole and products of conception that are both diploid and express p57 cannot be any type of mole.

Just as the distinction of a complete mole from a hydropic abortus may be challenging and require a p57 immunohistochemical stain, so the distinction of a complete mole from a partial mole may also be difficult. Once it has been established that a mole is present, the simplest method of distinction is to find fetal tissue **i28.5d**, as this indicates a partial mole. Nucleated erythrocytes in the villous vessels fill this function. If fetal tissue cannot be found, ploidy studies can distinguish between the 2 types of mole because complete moles are diploid and partial moles are triploid [PMID17365825]. p57 is also useful in distinguishing between complete and partial moles. Because 2/3 of the DNA in partial moles is of paternal origin, p57 expression is diminished relative to normal villi but not altogether absent, as is the case in complete moles, so once the diagnosis of a mole is established, any p57 expression suggests a partial mole **i28.5e** [PMID12823708]. If the differential diagnosis is between a complete and a partial mole, p57 staining may occasionally obviate the need for the much more complex ploidy analysis.

Abnormalities of Intermediate Trophoblasts

With the exception of the choriocarcinoma, all of the entities in gestational trophoblastic disease that do not form villi arise from intermediate trophoblasts. To understand these entities, we must first recall that the intermediate trophoblasts of the villous column become either implantation site or chorionic intermediate trophoblasts, which have different immunohistochemical characteristics [PMID17613426, PMID17498600]. Secondly, it is helpful to recognize that the phrase "placental site" refers to implantation site intermediate trophoblasts. The placental site *nodule* is the simplest proliferation of intermediate trophoblasts. The *exaggerated* placental site is more complex than the nodule. The placental site trophoblastic *tumor* and the epithelioid trophoblastic *tumor* are the most complex lesions of intermediate trophoblasts.

The implantation site begins with the infiltration of trophoblasts into the endometrium, followed by the formation of villi **i28.6a**, **i28.6b**. A placental site nodule (also called plaque) is a microscopic, incidental finding. It is characterized by intermediate trophoblasts, often vacuolated, in a hyaline, fibrin, or cartilaginous-appearing matrix. Placental site nodules are superficial and well circumscribed. They are not necessarily associated with a current pregnancy and may be a retained placental site from a previous pregnancy or from a gestation that never developed. Although composed of intermediate trophoblasts, they are only weakly positive for human placental lactogen (HPL) and CD146 (Mel-CAM), which normally strongly stain implantation site intermediate trophoblasts, and they are also positive for placental alkaline phosphatase and p63 [PMID19700941], which do not normally stain implantation site intermediate trophoblasts. Placental site nodules are positive for cytokeratin 18 and α-inhibin [PMID10374778]. These results suggest that the placental site nodule is a lesion of intermediate trophoblasts from the chorion laeve.

An exaggerated placental site is a benign nonneoplastic lesion in which an increased number of implantation site intermediate trophoblasts infiltrate the myometrium. It is more cellular and more obvious than a placental site nodule **i28.7**, and because it is always related to a current pregnancy, it may associated with villi, in contrast to a placental site nodule, though these villi are not a part of the tumor. Whereas the placental site nodule is believed to arise from chorionic-type intermediate trophoblasts, the immunophenotype of the cells in an exaggerated placental site is that of implantation site intermediate trophoblasts, with strong and diffuse positivity for HPL [PMID15498215] and Mel-CAM [PMID8804361].

The PSTT, formally called a syncytioma, is a true neoplasm of implantation site intermediate trophoblasts. Rare giant cells may be seen in a PSTT, but they are less common than in a choriocarcinoma. Because these giant cells form from fusion of implantation site intermediate trophoblasts, they stain for HPL and Mel-CAM, as is the case for the much more numerous mononucleated cells [PMID8804361, PMID17397906]. In contrast to the giant cells of a choriocarcinoma, they stain weakly if at all for HCG. The PSTT, like the exaggerated placental site, develops from implantation site intermediate trophoblasts and appears to be the neoplastic counterpart of the latter entity [PMID10374778], but it is a distinct mass with an alarming appearance. It is also more cellular **i28.8a** and often invades blood vessels **i28.8b**. Necrosis is frequent **i28.8c**. The PSTT also has much more mitotic activity than an exaggerated placental site. Ki-67 will label no >5% of cells in an exaggerated placental site, in contrast to almost no cells in a placental site nodule [PMID15498215], and in contrast to 10% or more in the PSTT [PMID9445130].

The PSTT can resemble a carcinoma if the cells are polyhedral or form concentric structures **i28.8d**, or an epithelioid leiomyosarcoma if the cells are spindled **i28.8e**. In these situations, immunohistochemistry is needed to correctly identify the cells as intermediate trophoblasts. While there are slight differences in immunohistochemical profiles of implantation site and chorionic intermediate trophoblasts, both are generally positive for HPL, HLA-G, CD10, HCG, and Mel-CAM [PMID10374778, PMID12131159, PMID15948127, PMID19145204]. Both types of intermediate trophoblasts are also usually positive for keratin and epithelial membrane antigen, creating the hazard of an erroneous diagnosis of carcinoma if a complete immunohistochemical panel is not performed. In addition to the above panel of immunohistochemical stains, negativity for estrogen and progesterone receptors is useful in excluding carcinomas of the endometrium, and a negative P16INK4a (p16) helps to exclude cervical carcinoma. The presence of any villi at all requires the exclusion of a mole with exuberant trophoblastic hyperplasia before the diagnosis of a neoplasm of intermediate trophoblasts is entertained. The PSTT is usually treated with hysterectomy and chemotherapy and usually responds well but may be aggressive, and is generally more troublesome than a choriocarcinoma [PMID16246400].

The ETT is a very rare neoplasm thought to be derived from intermediate trophoblasts from the chorion leave [PMID18820674], and is likely the neoplastic counterpart of the placental site nodule [PMID10374778]. The cells of the ETT may have eosinophilic, clear, or "glassy" cytoplasm, resembling squamous cells **i28.9**. The ETT is more circumscribed than the PSTT, with less tendency to invade blood vessels. The ETT is immunohistochemically similar to the placental site nodule, with positivity for p63, keratin, and α inhibin, and with inconsistent expression of HCG, HPL, PLAP, and Mel-CAM [PMID17149967]. Like the PSTT, the ETT may express keratin and EMA, but a complete immunohistochemical panel will permit distinction from both carcinoma and PSTT if the initial differential diagnosis is properly constructed. Because of the rarity of the ETT and the lack of long-term followup, its clinical course cannot be well predicted, but at this time, it appears to be capable of either a benign or malignant course [PMID18720920].

Choriocarcinoma

Choriocarcinomas consist of a dimorphic population of syncytiotrophoblasts and a mononuclear component that is usually cytotrophoblasts i28.10a, i28.10b. Although it does not form chorionic villi, a gestational choriocarcinoma may be so intimately associated with nonneoplastic villi that the villi appear to be an integral component of the tumor i28.10c.

Gestational choriocarcinomas are unique tumors because they contain DNA that is not from the patient. 50% of gestational choriocarcinomas develop from a complete mole [PMID1967548], and therefore consists entirely of DNA from another person. Even in the 50% of gestational choriocarcinomas that do not develop from moles, half of the DNA is foreign.

It is now understood that choriocarcinomas may stain for HPL and most tumors of intermediate trophoblasts will stain to at least some extent for HCG. Indeed, there is sufficient similarity in the immunohistochemical profiles of choriocarcinomas and tumors of intermediate trophoblasts that the 2 often cannot be distinguished by immunohistochemistry, and there are mixed trophoblastic neoplasms with characteristics of both intermediate trophoblastic tumors and choriocarcinoma [PMID19145204].

Some cases of choriocarcinoma have few syncytiotrophoblasts and demonstrate a nearly uniform population of mononuclear cells, especially if there has been treatment i28.11a-c. An absence of the characteristic dimorphic population and the immunohistochemical overlap with tumor of intermediate trophoblasts can make the diagnosis of choriocarcinoma challenging and cause it to greatly resemble a neoplasm of intermediate trophoblasts.

Because a hydatidiform mole often has an exuberant proliferation of very atypical trophoblasts that are not necessarily associated with villi, and because villi in some complete moles can be surprisingly rare, an exuberant trophoblastic hyperplasia in a complete mole can be misinterpreted as a gestational trophoblastic neoplasm. In these situations, it is wise to submit the entire specimen. If submission of the entire specimen discloses any villi, the proliferation of trophoblasts, even if exuberant and overwhelmingly unassociated with any villi, is best regarded as a complete hydatidiform mole i28.12a, i28.12b. Even if no villi can be found, neoplasia is not assured and the best working diagnosis in these cases is persistent trophoblastic disease (PTD) [PMID20055562]. PTD is a clinical diagnosis, based on the history of a problematic trophoblastic proliferation and a persistent or rising HCG, encompassing an invasive mole and a gestational choriocarcinoma [PMID17365825]. To make a confident diagnosis of gestational choriocarcinoma, there needs to be a significant proliferation of well-preserved atypical trophoblasts without any villi in either of 2 tissue samples obtained at different times, with persistent or rising serum HCG levels. A high proliferation index, as evidenced by a Ki-67 as high as 70%, in this second sampling, suggests a choriocarcinoma over a persistent mole [PMID9445130]. Having made an initial diagnosis of probable complete mole with exuberant trophoblastic hyperplasia, the pathologist does not again play a major role until rising HCG levels have been documented, the clinical diagnosis of PTD has been made, and a second tissue sampling is obtained.

Core Points for Gestational Trophoblastic Disease

- Gestational trophoblastic diseases: those that form villi and that do not.
- Villi-forming—hydropic abortus, complete and partial hydatidiform moles, and invasive mole.
- Complete hydatidiform mole: diploid, androgenic, no fetal tissue.
  - Edematous villi, often with central cistern formation, with trophoblastic hyperplasia and atypia.
  - Early moles: subtle. With improved ultrasonography, the clinician often suggests the diagnosis.
  - Paternally imprinted protein p57 is not present in complete moles because of their androgenic lineage.
- The trophoblastic hyperplasia in a complete mole can simulate a neoplasm, especially if villi are decreased or indistinct, or there are areas of hyperplasia that are not associated with villi.
  - If suspect neoplasm, submit the remainder of the specimen. If any villi, likely a complete mole with exuberant trophoblastic hyperplasia.
  - If no villi are found and HCG does not fall, a tentative diagnosis of persistent trophoblastic disease is wise.
  - Only if HCG does not decrease or rises and a second sampling shows no villi, with well preserved, atypical trophoblasts should a choriocarcinoma be diagnosed.
- An invasive mole is suggested by persistent or rising HCG levels after a secure diagnosis of a complete mole, but
  - Hysterectomy is needed for a definitive diagnosis.
- Partial mole: triploid, contains DNA from both parents, has fetal tissue.
  - Also has edematous villi, often with central cistern formation, with trophoblastic hyperplasia and atypia, but
  - Histologic changes of a partial mole are less generalized and pronounced than a complete mole.
  - Some admixed normal villi.
  - Ploidy determination may assist in the diagnosis of a partial mole.
- No formation of villi—choriocarcinoma, placental site nodule, exaggerated placental site, placental site trophoblastic tumor, and epithelioid trophoblastic tumor.
- Choriocarcinomas: do not form villi, but those of gestational origin are likely to be associated with nonneoplastic villi.
  - Dimorphic population of cytotrophoblasts and syncytiotrophoblasts, but
  - May have few syncytiotrophoblasts and appear monomorphic.
- Other gestational trophoblastic diseases that do not form villi arise from intermediate trophoblasts.
  - Placental site nodule (plaque): incidental finding.
  - Exaggerated placental site: nonneoplastic proliferation of implantation site intermediate trophoblasts.
  - Placental site trophoblastic tumor: neoplasm of implantation site intermediate trophoblasts
    - Necrosis and vascular invasion
    - Can resemble a carcinoma or an epithelioid leiomyosarcoma.

ISBN 978-089189-5886

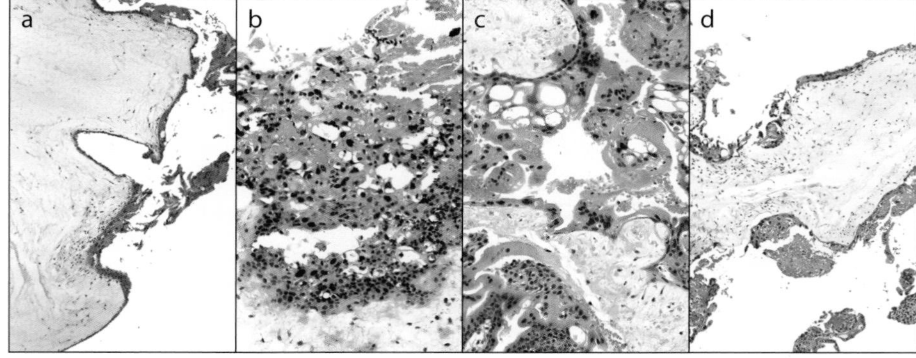

i28.1 **a** The pronounced villous edema in a complete hydatidiform mole, with central cistern formation
b-c The extensive trophoblastic hyperplasia and atypia that are seen in hydatidiform moles
d Circumferential trophoblastic hyperplasia in a complete mole

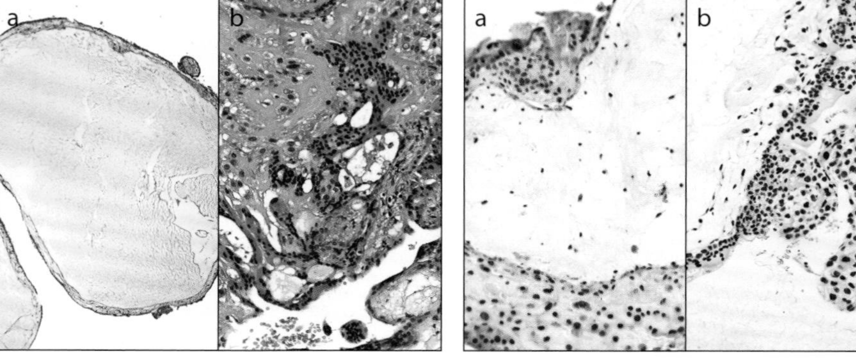

i28.2 **a** The edema in a hydropic abortion. Although the edema is extensive, there is no central cistern formation.
b Trophoblastic hyperplasia and atypia in a hydropic abortion, focally approaching that seen in hydatidiform moles

i28.3 **a** A hydropic abortion with a positive stain for p57
b A negative stain for p57 in a complete hydatidiform mole

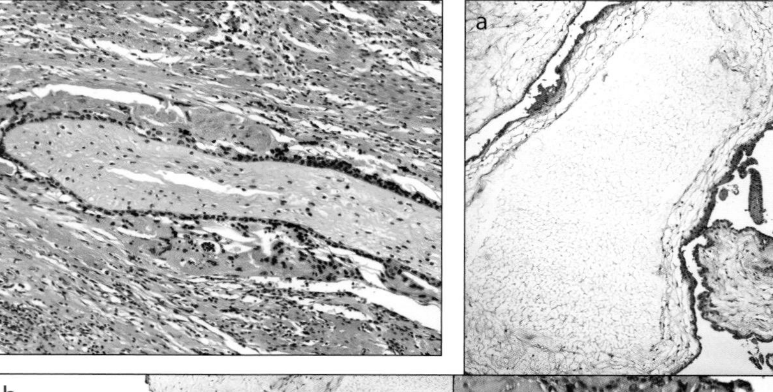

i28.4 An invasive mole. This villus, which is surrounded on all sides by myometrium, demonstrates circumferential trophoblastic hyperplasia and atypia, most evident in the lower portion of the photograph.

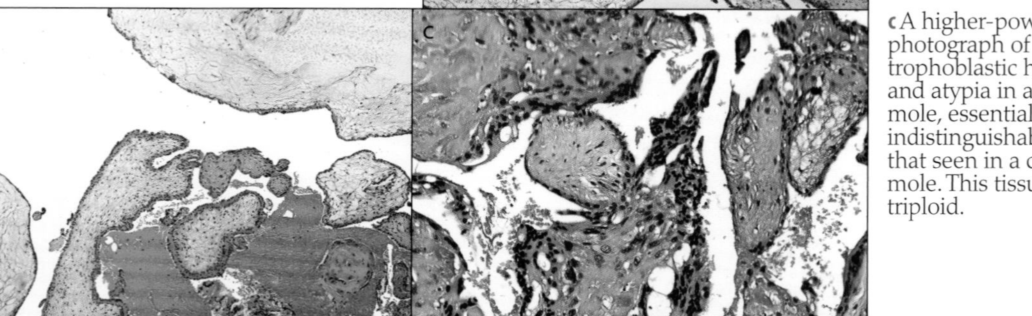

i28.5 **a** A partial hydatidiform mole, again with extensive villous edema and cistern formation. While some villi are completely indistinguishable from a complete mole, in a partial mole, there are usually smaller, less affected villi, as seen here on the right.
b Another partial mole with extensive edema in the villus in the upper portion of the photograph. Edema is less pronounced in the villi in the lower portion, but there is trophoblastic hyperplasia and atypia.
c A higher-power photograph of the trophoblastic hyperplasia and atypia in a partial mole, essentially indistinguishable from that seen in a complete mole. This tissue was triploid.

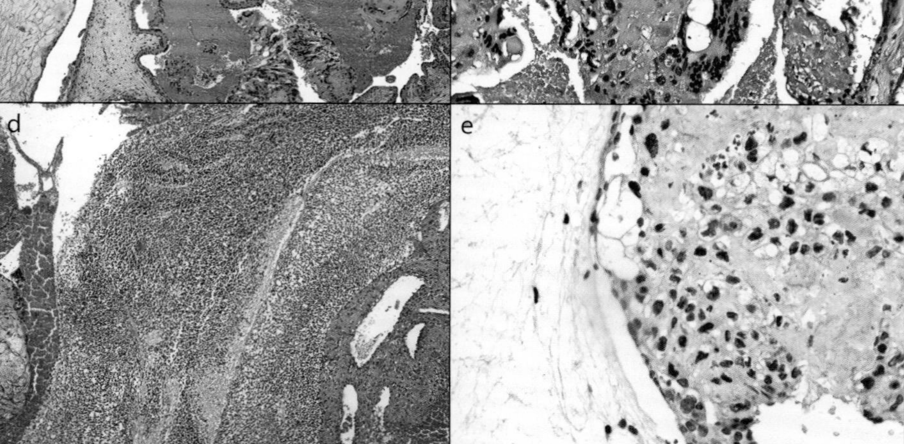

d Poorly preserved fetal tissue in a molar pregnancy, identifying the process as a partial mole
e p57 staining in a partial mole with more positive cells than in a complete mole, but fewer than in normal trophoblasts

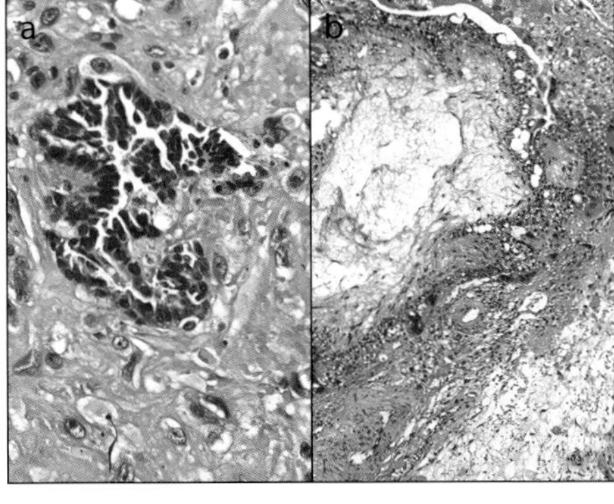

i28.6 a An early implantation site with intermediate trophoblasts infiltrating. This is from an ectopic pregnancy in a fallopian tube.
b A later implantation site, with villi beginning to form. This is also from an ectopic pregnancy in a fallopian tube.

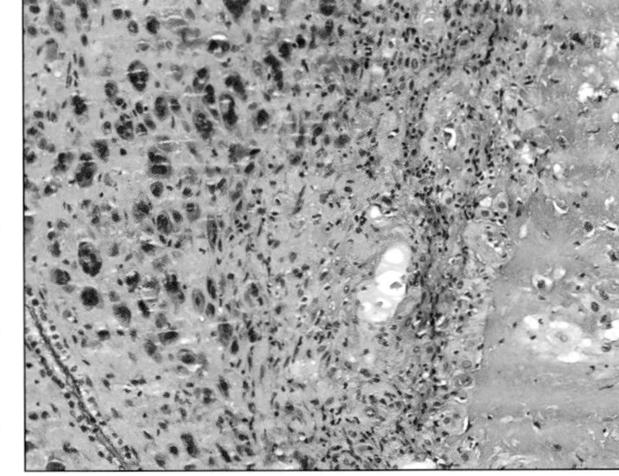

i28.7 An exaggerated placental site with hyperplasia of intermediate trophoblast

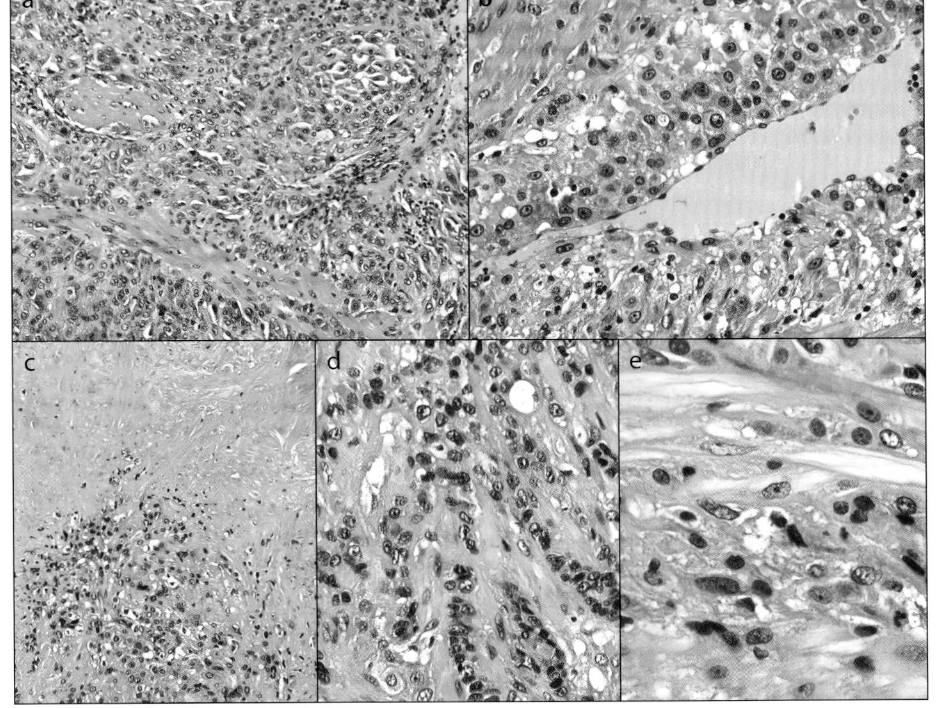

i28.8 a A placental site trophoblastic tumor (PSTT). The PSTTs illustrated in i28.8 were strongly positive for HPL and weakly positive for HCG.
b Vascular invasion in a PSTT
c Necrosis in a PSTT
d A PSTT simulating a carcinoma
e A PSTT composed primarily of spindle cells, simulating a sarcoma

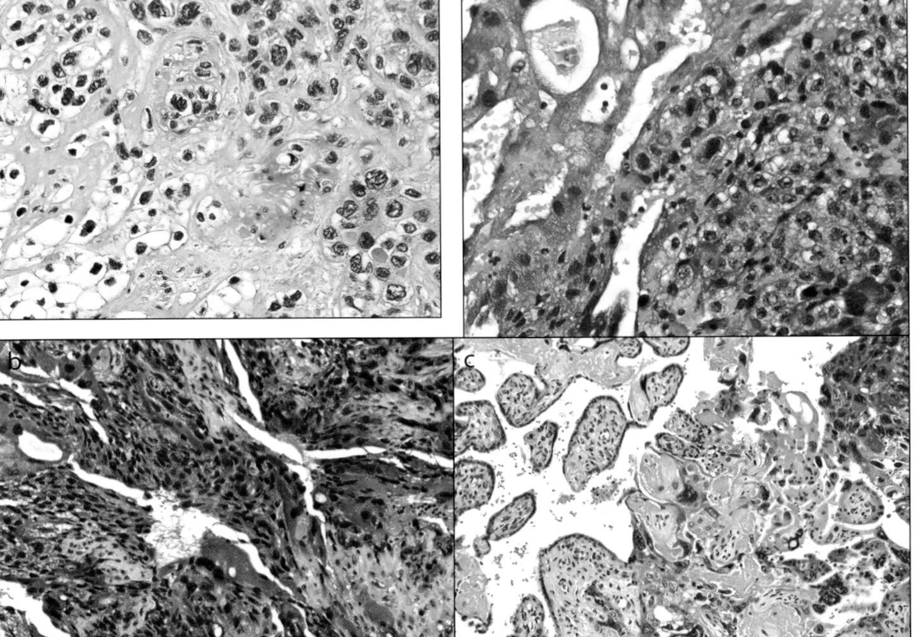

i28.9 An epithelioid trophoblastic tumor with some neoplastic cells having eosinophilic cytoplasm and others having clear cytoplasm. This neoplasm was positive for placental alkaline phosphatase, keratin, epithelial membrane antigen, HCG and weakly positive for HPL and Mel-CAM.

i28.10 a The dimorphic population that is characteristic of a choriocarcinoma
b Myometrial invasion by both cell types in a gestational choriocarcinoma
c A gestational choriocarcinoma intimately associated with nonneoplastic villi

ISBN 978-089189-5886

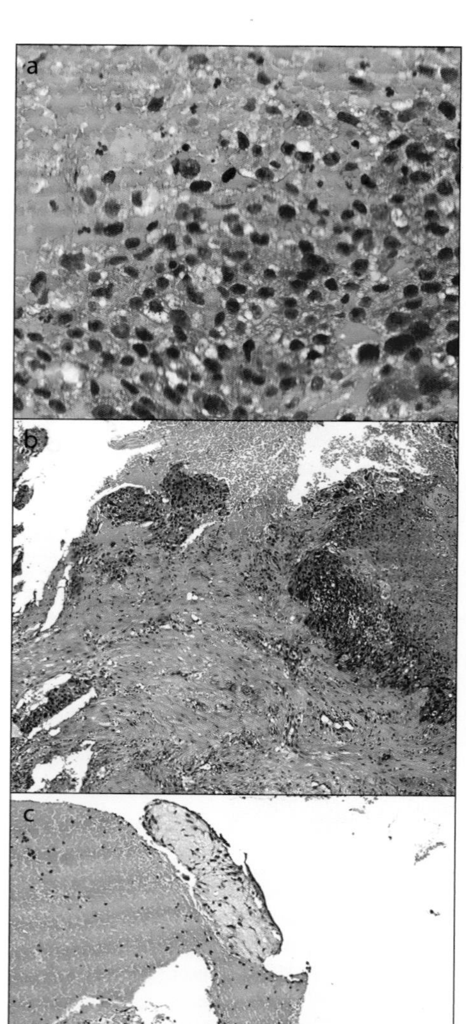

i28.11 **a** A gestational neoplasm of uncertain etiology because there is a monomorphic population of neoplastic cells

b The same case as in i28.11a, again illustrating a monomorphic population of cells, thereby engendering a wide differential diagnosis. Note the lymphatic invasion at the left.

c The same case as in i28.11a with a villus. Although the villus is nonneoplastic, its presence suggests this neoplasm is a choriocarcinoma until proven otherwise.

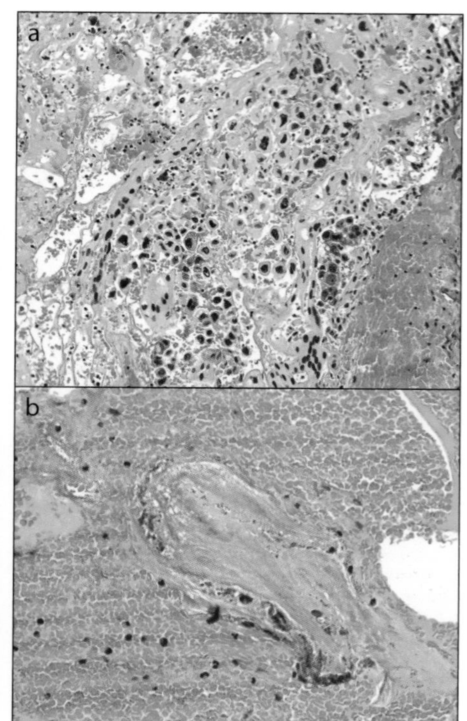

i28.12 **a** An apparent neoplastic process occurring in pregnancy. There is extensive trophoblastic atypia without villi.

b However, extensive additional sampling of the case illustrated in i28.12a eventually identified a rare villus, identifying the process as a hydatidiform mole. This patient was given a diagnosis of persistent trophoblastic disease. Her HCGs decreased to normal levels without additional therapy.

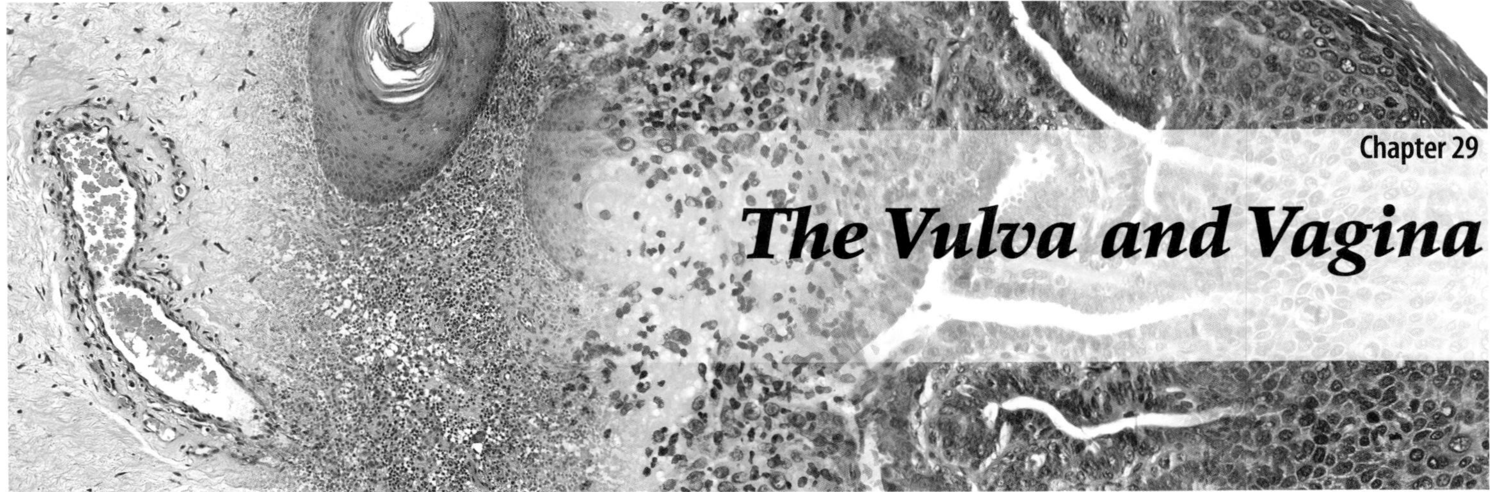

Chapter 29

The Vulva and Vagina

Benign Cysts of the Vulva and Vagina

The common benign cysts in the vagina and vulva are those derived from Bartholin glands or Gartner duct. Bartholin cysts occur primarily in the vulva, usually in young women, and are the most common symptomatic cysts in this area. They may also occur in the vagina [PMID18390079]. Normally, Bartholin glands are lined by columnar epithelium proximally, transitional epithelium in the mid portion, and squamous epithelium near the termination of the duct in the vestibule, the space between the labia minora. However, there is often variability and intermingling, and the epithelium of Bartholin duct cysts in any given specimen is variable i29.1a, i29.1b.

Gartner duct cysts are also called mesonephric cysts because they are remnants of the mesonephric (Wolffian) duct (mesonephric ducts are discussed in Chapter 34). They occur mostly in the vagina, but can occur in the vulva, and are usually lined by a single layer of cuboidal epithelium i29.2a, sometimes with amorphous eosinophilic material in the lumen, as may be seen in any mesonephric remnant i29.2b.

Other, much rarer cysts of the vulva and vagina include simple epidermal inclusion cysts and those caused by endometriosis. In the neonate, the hymenal cyst and Skene duct cysts (also called paraurethral cysts) may be encountered.

Inflammatory/Infectious Processes of the Vulva and Vagina

There are 2 abnormalities of the pilosebaceous unit that commonly occur in the vulva. Fox-Fordyce is a chronic pruritic eruption in sites that have apocrine glands. It occurs mostly in young adults and is characterized by an obstruction of a hair follicle by a keratin plug. Because apocrine glands open into the follicle, they are occluded and may rupture, but the pilosebaceous unit is otherwise preserved [PMID19712275].

Hidradenitis suppurativa is a more serious process that destroys the entire pilosebaceous unit, along with apocrine glands i29.3, and can be disfiguring. It occurs most commonly in the axilla, but also in the vulvar area [PMID19682181]. Some feel that a suppurative inflammation of the apocrine glands is the primary event in hidradenitis suppurativa, while others favor an occlusive folliculitis as the initiating process, with secondary destruction of the pilosebaceous unit and apocrine glands.

Other than herpes i29.4 and HPV-associated vulvar intraepithelial neoplasia (discussed subsequently), there are 4 major sexually transmitted diseases of the vulva: syphilis, granuloma inguinale, chancroid, and lymphogranuloma venereum [PMID737918]. The lesion of primary syphilis is the chancre, which is a painless ulcer i29.5a in which the pathogenic spirochetes may be demonstrated. The lesion of secondary syphilis is condyloma latum, papules that appear 3-6 weeks after the chancre. They are highly contagious and histologically demonstrate healing of the ulcer with vacuolar change at the dermal-epidermal junction and dermal plasma cells i29.5b, perhaps with acute inflammation i29.5c. There may also be epidermal hyperplasia without ulceration.

Granuloma inguinale is caused by *Calymmatobacterium granulomatis*. It initially presents with painless papules, followed by ulceration, extensive epidermal hyperplasia, granulation tissue, and a mixed inflammatory infiltrate containing plasma cells and vacuolated macrophages. The macrophages contain bipolar granules called Donovan bodies, the gram-negative bacteria that cause the disease. Donovan bodies are seen better in a Giemsa or Warthin-Starry stain.

Chancroid is a sexually transmitted disease caused by *Haemophilus ducreyi*. It begins as a pustule, usually on the vestibule, followed by a painful ulcer and enlarged inguinal lymph nodes.

Lymphogranuloma venereum is caused by *Chlamydia trachomatis*, some serotypes of which are associated with sexually transmitted oculogenital disease. Lymphogranuloma venereum begins as a small papule or ulcer, often on the posterior vulva, followed by swollen inguinal lymph nodes with necrotizing granulomas.

Vulvar vestibulitis syndrome is not sexually transmitted. It is a focal chronic inflammation of the vulva with considerable pain. It occurs in young women and is of unclear pathogenesis.

The major infections of the vagina include *Trichomonas*, *Candida*, and *Gardnerella vaginalis*. Bacterial vaginosis occurs when the vaginal pH is >4.5 and *Lactobacillus* is replaced by other species, such as *Bacteroides* and *Gardnerella* [PMID2645843].

Benign Neoplasms of the Vulva

The hidradenoma papilliferum, a benign adnexal neoplasm of apocrine derivation, occurs in the vulva of middle aged and older women. It is well circumscribed, with a papillary architecture and a cystic central area i29.6a-c.

The most important mesenchymal neoplasm of the vulva is the angiomyxoma. Superficial angiomyxomas in nongenital sites generally run an entirely benign course. By contrast, angiomyxomas of the vulvar region or pelvic soft tissues, while histologically identical to their superficial counterparts, are more likely to be in a deeper location, locally aggressive, and recurrent. These vulvar masses are often called aggressive angiomyxomas. Many blood vessels in an aggressive angiomyxoma are thin-walled i29.7a, but an occasional vessel will have a small amount of muscle. The stroma is myxoid, with small cells with uniform, spindled nuclei i29.7b. The cells of an angiomyxoma have myofibroblastic properties and are focally positive for actin. The differential diagnosis is that of myxoid tumors and includes myxoma, neurofibroma, myxoid smooth muscle tumors, spindle cell lipoma, myxoid undifferentiated pleomorphic sarcoma/malignant fibrous histiocytoma, myxoid liposarcoma, rhabdomyosarcoma, and angiomyofibroblastoma.

The angiomyofibroblastoma has substantial morphologic similarity to the angiomyxoma, and is likely related to the latter entity [PMID9023551]. Many cases cannot be definitively placed in either category, but the angiomyofibroblastoma often has somewhat higher cellularity, with alternating hypercellular and hypocellular areas i29.8a, i29.8b. It also tends to be more circumscribed than the aggressive angiomyxoma and has less tendency to recur [PMID19430941].

Although most fibroepithelial polyps of the lower female genital tract are clearly innocuous, a few exhibit worrisome cellularity, many mitotic figures, and pleomorphism, causing considerable similarity to a sarcoma. Except for the young girl, in whom an embryonal rhabdomyosarcoma (sarcoma botryoides) is a consideration, it is wise to be conservative in the interpretation of cellular polypoid masses in this area [PMID10680891].

Vulvar and Vaginal Intraepithelial Neoplasia (VIN and VAIN)

Vulvar and vaginal intraepithelial neoplasia (VIN and VAIN, respectively) are graded on a scale of 1-3, by the same criteria as for other body sites. Bowenoid papulosis occurs in the vulva and like true carcinoma-directed alteration of epithelial maturation, is associated with HPV types 16,18,31, and 33, but appears to be a separate entity that is less likely to progress [PMID7951618]. Because it is impossible to differentiate these processes with certainty, they are conflated under VIN. The mild nuclear atypia and slightly diminished maturation that is characteristic of VIN 1 is illustrated in i29.9a and i29.9b. i29.9c illustrates the more significant changes in VIN 2. i29.9d-f depict the nearly complete loss of maturation in VIN 3.

A condyloma is an exophytic manifestation of VIN, usually VIN 1, though higher grade condylomas may rarely be encountered, and any condyloma should be assessed for areas of higher grade VIN or microinvasive squamous carcinoma. A condyloma is more architecturally complex and acanthotic than a papilloma or skin tag. Because verrucas are rare in the genital region, the principal differential diagnosis of a condyloma is a seborrheic keratosis. Relative to a seborrheic keratosis, a condyloma usually has more epithelial hyperplasia, a more endophytic pattern to this hyperplasia, a less basaloid appearance, and often with focal viral cytopathic effect in the form of perinuclear haloes i29.10a, i29.10b. However, there are cases in which the histologic features are suggestive of a condyloma but not fully diagnostic i29.11, and the clinical situation is often more informative, in which case the pathologist may diagnose, "Epithelial hyperplasia consistent with condyloma is clinically appropriate." This allows the clinician to make the final diagnosis and avoids mistakenly labeling a patient with a sexually transmitted condition when she may simply have a seborrheic keratosis.

More problematic is an unusual type of VIN that is called the differentiated (also called keratinizing or simplex) type. Differentiated VIN can be subtle and its recognition is subject to interobserver variation. Whereas the usual VIN is characterized by diminished maturation at all levels, differentiated VIN demonstrates dyskeratotic cells within the epidermis, indicative of premature keratinization, enlarged keratinocytes, parakeratosis, elongation of rete pegs, and keratin pearls i29.12 [PMID10716158]. Differentiated VIN is characterized by *disordered* rather than *diminished* maturation. A clue to this type of VIN is the presence of well developed, "hard" intracellular keratin. This type of VIN is conventionally considered to be high-grade, despite the maturation and relatively innocuous initial appearance, because it is often found in association with invasive carcinoma and if found on a biopsy, an assiduous search for microinvasion is warranted in the ensuing resection.

Differentiated VIN may be a precursor to keratinizing squamous cell carcinoma [PMID16538050]. Differentiated VIN and keratinizing squamous cell carcinoma of the vulva are usually negative for HPV and P16INK4a (p16), whereas conventional VIN and nonkeratinizing squamous carcinoma are positive for these markers [PMID15213596, PMID15910611].

The diagnostic criteria for intraepithelial neoplasia (dysplasia) in the vagina parallel those of the vulva and other sites. Grade 1 VAIN is illustrated in i29.13a, grade 2 in i29.13b, and grade 3/CIS in i29.13c. High-grade VAIN of the keratinizing (differentiated) type is shown in i29.13d.

Lichen sclerosus et atrophicus (usually called lichen sclerosus or LS&A) is not a form of VIN, but is presented here because it often clinically simulates VIN and because there is some thought that it may predispose to VIN [PMID9744309]. In lichen sclerosus, there is often basal cell vacuolization i29.14a, but the major changes take place in the dermis, where there is a peculiar eosinophilic homogenization of the dermal collagen, myxoid deposition, or ectatic capillaries i29.14a-c. The epidermis may be atrophic, as the name implies, but may also be hyperplastic. In either case, significant atypia is lacking or the diagnosis becomes VIN, which should be excluded before the diagnosis of lichen sclerosus is made. Significant staining for the proliferation marker Ki-67 above the basal layer or appreciable staining for p53 suggests a VIN [PMID17714682]. Occasional cases will have overlapping features of LS&A and VIN i29.14d.

Vulvar Carcinoma

Conventional vulvar squamous cell carcinoma is not discussed because it is rarely diagnostically challenging. The depth of invasion of any invasive vulvar carcinoma should be reported. "Microinvasive" generally refers to 0.5 cm (5 mm) or less, though not all use the term in precisely the same way [PMID6389601].

As is the case for the larynx and esophagus, the basaloid type of squamous cell carcinoma may occur in the vulva, and as in other sites, clues to its presence include areas of conventional squamous carcinoma or squamous carcinoma in situ. The common basal cell carcinoma is rare in this location, and before such a diagnosis is made, close scrutiny should exclude foci of high nuclear grade, increased mitotic activity, or squamous carcinoma in situ, any of which favor a diagnosis of squamous carcinoma. Adenoid cystic carcinoma may rarely occur in the vulva and must be excluded in any basaloid neoplasm. The verrucous carcinoma occurs in the vulvar area and can be addressed as discussed in Chapters 12 and 39.

Glandular Cells in the Vagina

Adenosis is the presence of endocervical **i29.15a** or endometrial **i29.5b** epithelium, without stroma, in the vagina after birth [PMID9764164]. Although the association of diethylstilbestrol (DES), vaginal adenosis, and adenocarcinoma (especially clear cell adenocarcinoma) has received considerable attention [PMID6537153], there are other causes of glandular cells in the vagina, including mesonephric remnants, endometriosis, and endosalpingiosis. Indeed, now that DES has been withdrawn, these other causes are more common and fortunately, do not have the association with adenocarcinoma that was characteristic of DES-induced adenosis.

Mesonephric remnants are located deep in the lateral vaginal wall and are lined by cuboidal cells that are generally nonciliated and nonmucinous. They have dense eosinophilic secretions and may be associated with a Gartner duct, also a mesonephric remnant. Endometriosis and endosalpingiosis are discussed in Chapter 34. The glandular epithelium in endometriosis is typically associated with endometrial stroma or hemosiderin macrophages, though not all 3 components may be present. In difficult cases, a CD10 immunohistochemical stain highlights endometrial stromal cells. Endosalpingiosis is characterized by the presence of isolated benign glands with ciliated epithelium. Although glandular cells of endocervical or endometrial origin may undergo tubal metaplasia and demonstrate cilia, the diagnosis of endosalpingiosis can be favored if the location is appropriate, there is ciliated epithelium, and there is no endometrial stroma or macrophages.

Core Points for the Vulva and the Vagina

- Bartholin duct cyst: most common cyst of the vulva.
- Gartner duct (mesonephric) cyst: vagina or vulva.
- Fox-Fordyce: pruritic, caused by keratin plugging of the follicle that obstructs the apocrine glands.
- Hidradenitis suppurativa destroys the entire pilosebaceous unit.
- Sexually transmitted diseases of the vulva: HPV-associated VIN, herpes, syphilis, granuloma inguinale, chancroid, lymphogranuloma venereum.
- Major infections of the vagina: trichomonas, candida, and *Gardnerella vaginalis*.
- Hidradenoma papilliferum: benign adnexal neoplasm, papillary and cystic.
- Aggressive angiomyxoma and the angiomyofibroblastoma: related, with myofibroblastic differentiation, myxoid stroma, and a tendency to recur.
- Lichen sclerosus: often has basal cell vacuolization, eosinophilic homogenization of the dermal collage, myxoid deposition, or dilated capillaries.
    - Vulvar intraepithelial neoplasia (VIN) should be excluded.
- Vulvar and vaginal intraepithelial neoplasia (VIN and VAIN) are assessed as in other sites, but
    - Differentiated (or simplex) type of VIN may have a maturation that is falsely reassuring.
    - Evident by disordered maturation, with dyskeratotic cells, rather than diminished maturation.
    - Despite maturation, considered high-grade and is associated with invasive squamous carcinoma, especially of the keratinizing type.
- Basaloid squamous cell carcinoma: may be deceptively bland.
    - Search for more conventional squamous carcinoma or squamous carcinoma in situ.
    - If not found, need IHC to identify squamous nature.
- Adenosis: presence of endocervical or endometrial epithelium without stroma in the vagina.
    - Less common now that diethylstilbestrol has been withdrawn
    - Usually secondary to endometriosis or mesonephric remnants.
    - CD10 stain highlights endometrial stromal cells.
    - Mesonephric remnants: lined by cuboidal cells and typically contain dense eosinophilic secretions.
    - Should be suspected if there is a Gartner duct cyst.

ISBN 978-089189-5886

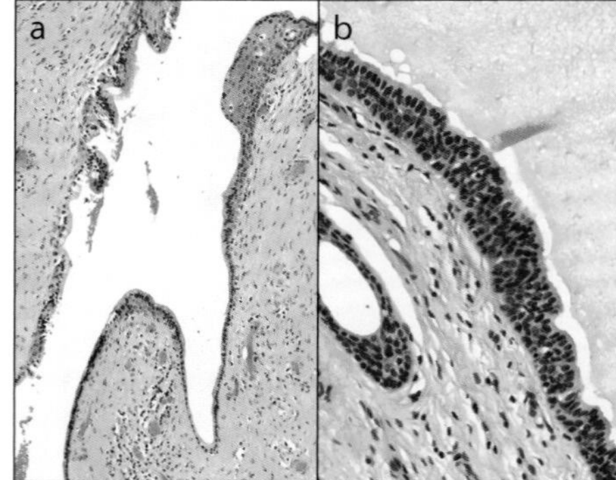

i29.1 a Bartholin duct cyst illustrating the variable lining, sometimes in immediately adjacent areas, that is characteristic **b** Transitional epithelial lining in a Bartholin duct cyst

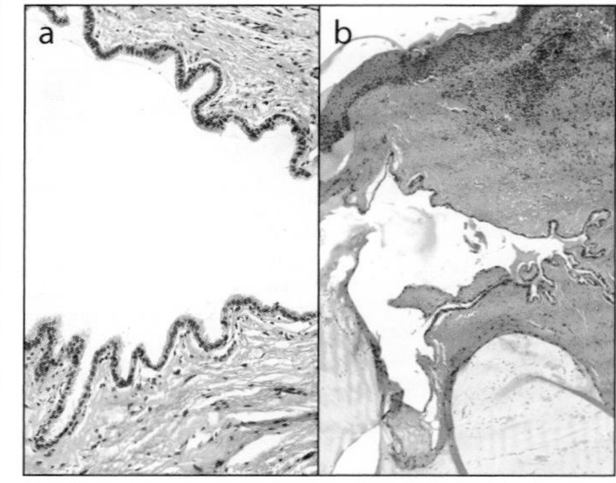

i29.2 a A Gartner duct cyst in the vagina. Note the simple cuboidal lining. **b** A Gartner duct cyst with amorphous eosinophilic material in the lumen, characteristic not only of this entity, but also of other mesonephric remnants

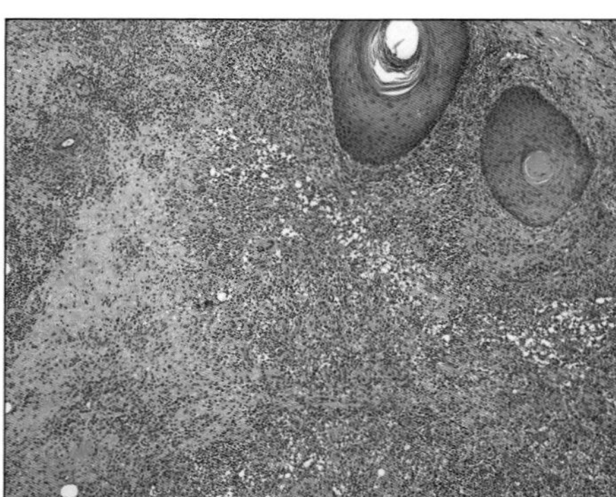

i29.3 Hidradenitis suppurativa. 2 pilosebaceous units are almost completely destroyed by the inflammatory process.

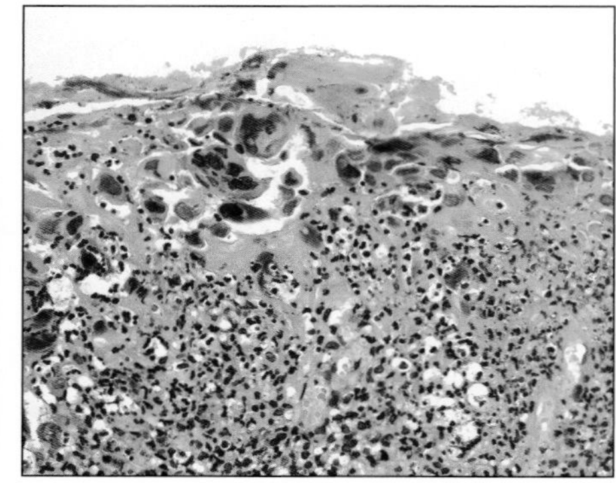

i29.4 Herpetic infection in the vulva

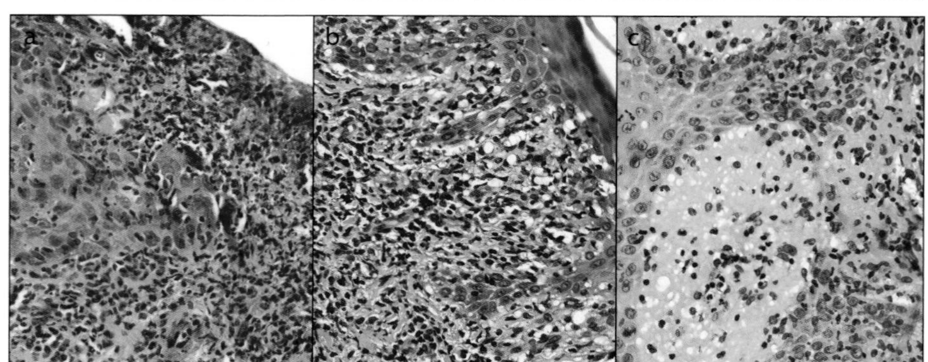

i29.5 a A chancre, the ulcerating lesion in primary syphilis **b** Condyloma latum in secondary syphilis, with vacuolar change at the dermal-epidermal junction and occasional dermal plasma cells **c** Condyloma latum with acute inflammation

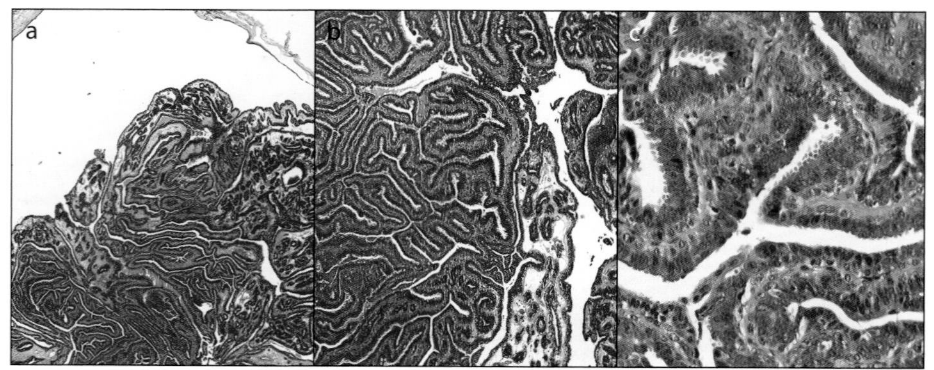

i29.6 a A hidradenoma papilliferum of the vulva, illustrating the circumscription and central cystic area **b** A hidradenoma papilliferum, illustrating the papillary architecture **c** The innocuous nuclei of a hidradenoma papilliferum. Myoepithelial cells may be discerned and there is faint "decapitation secretion" suggestive of apocrine origin.

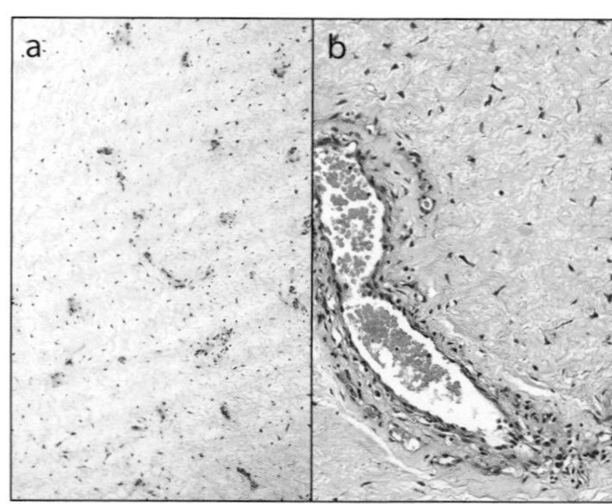

i29.7 a The thin-walled vessels and paucicellular myxoid stroma of a vulvar aggressive angiomyxoma **b** A slightly thicker vessel in an aggressive angiomyxoma. The nuclei within the myxoid areas are very small and uniform.

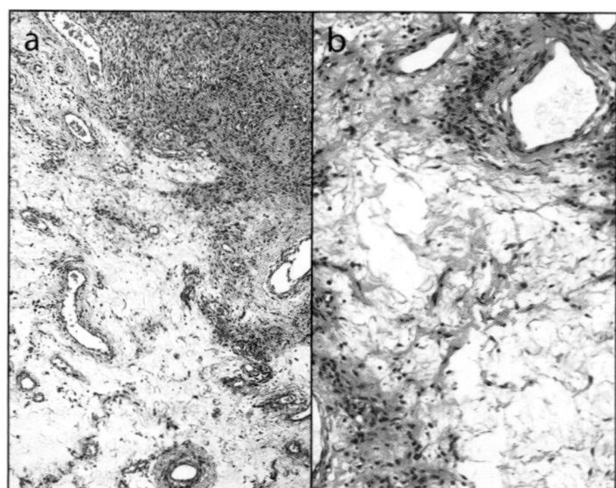

i29.8 a-b An angiomyofibroblastoma, illustrating the alternating areas of greater and lesser cellularity within a myxoid stroma that is indistinguishable from that in an aggressive angiomyxoma

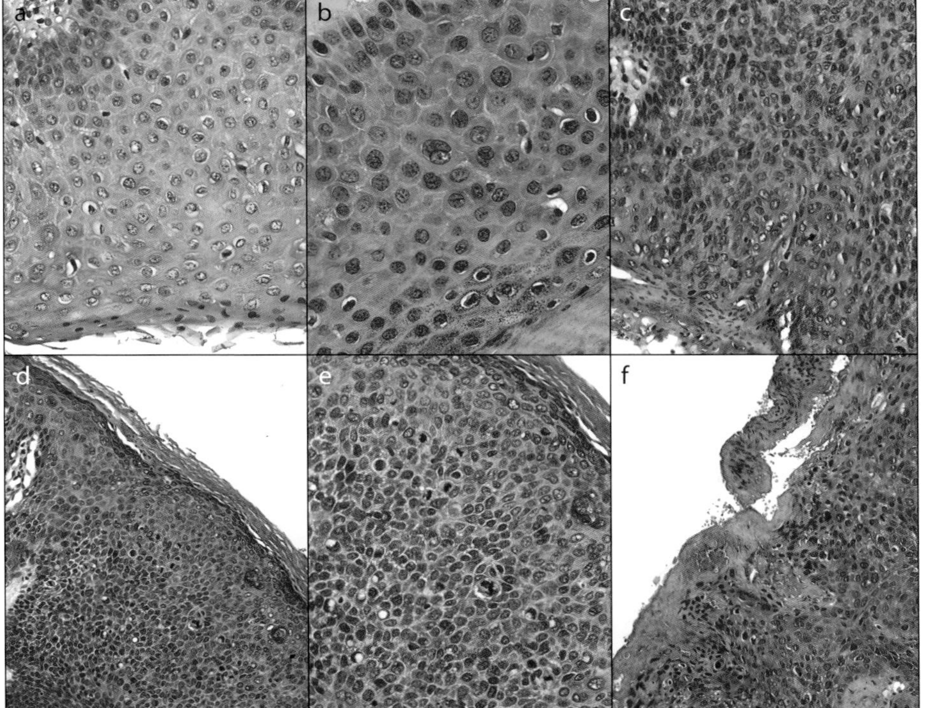

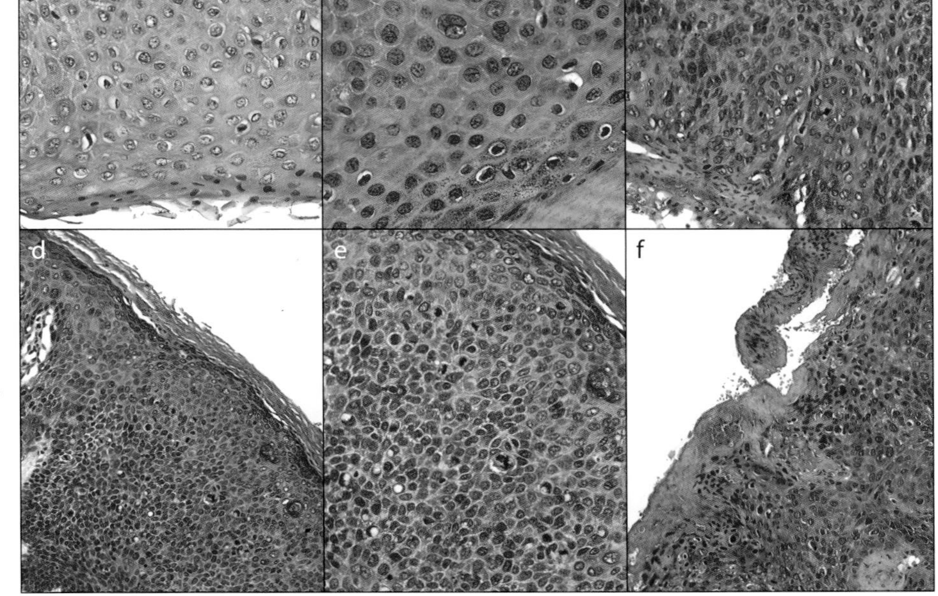

i29.9 Vulvar intraepithelial neoplasia (VIN).
a and **b** depict VIN 1, with slightly diminished maturation and small perinuclear haloes. Note the absence of mitoses above the basal layer.

c depicts VIN 2, with sharply reduced maturation.

d illustrates the complete loss of maturation of VIN 3. **e** is a higher power view of the same case as in i29.9d. Note the numerous mitotic figures well above the basal layer. The mitosis in the center appears tripolar.

f is another case of VIN 3, which is partially of the differentiated type, with premature keratinization.

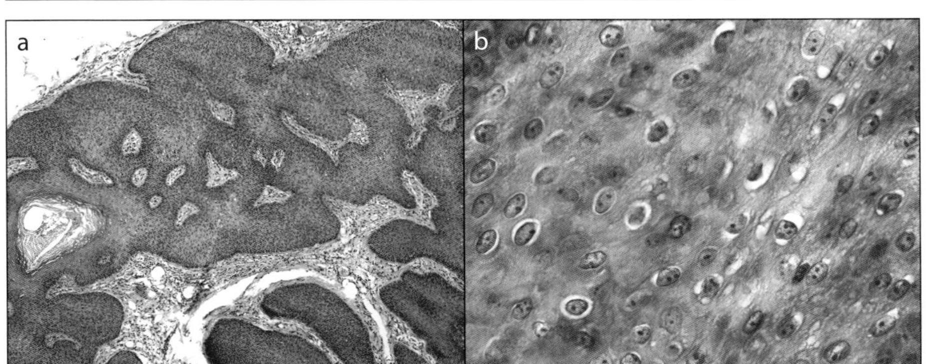

i29.10 **a** A condyloma of the vulva. Note the endophytic pattern of epithelial hyperplasia.

b A higher-power view of the same case as in i29.10a, illustrating the slight nuclear enlargement and perinuclear haloes

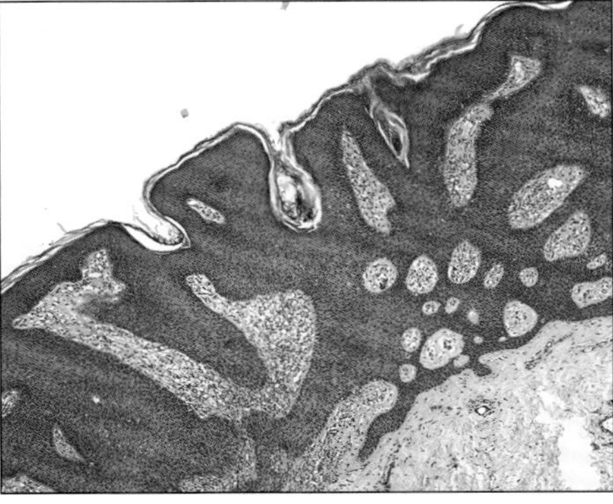

i29.11 Epithelial hyperplasia of the vulva which is equivocal for a fully-developed condyloma. The changes are similar to, but not as pronounced as those of i29.10.

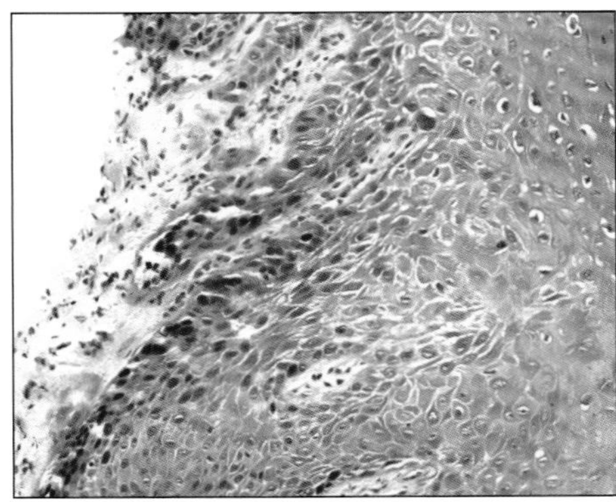

i29.12 Differentiated VIN, with premature and disordered keratinization

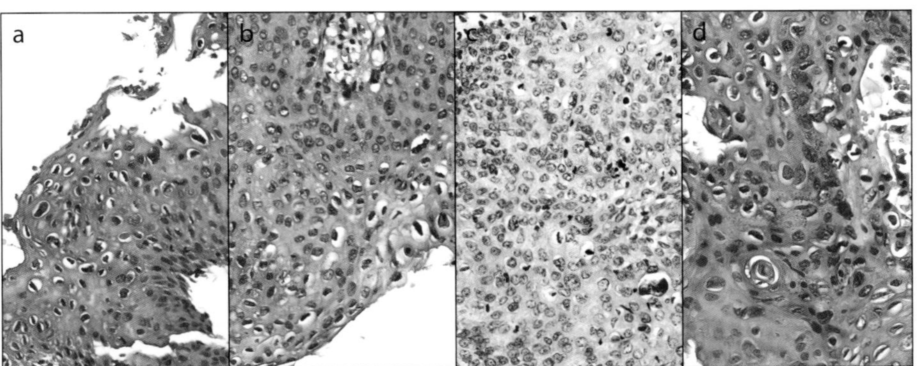

i29.13 **a** Vaginal intraepithelial neoplasia (VAIN), grade 1
b VAIN, grade 2, with significantly diminished maturation. This case is partially of the differentiated type, with a few dyskeratotic cells.

c VAIN, grade 3, with complete absence of maturation and transmural atypia
d High-grade VAIN of the differentiated type, with premature keratinization. This is a high-grade VAIN despite the presence of some maturation.

ISBN 978-089189-5886

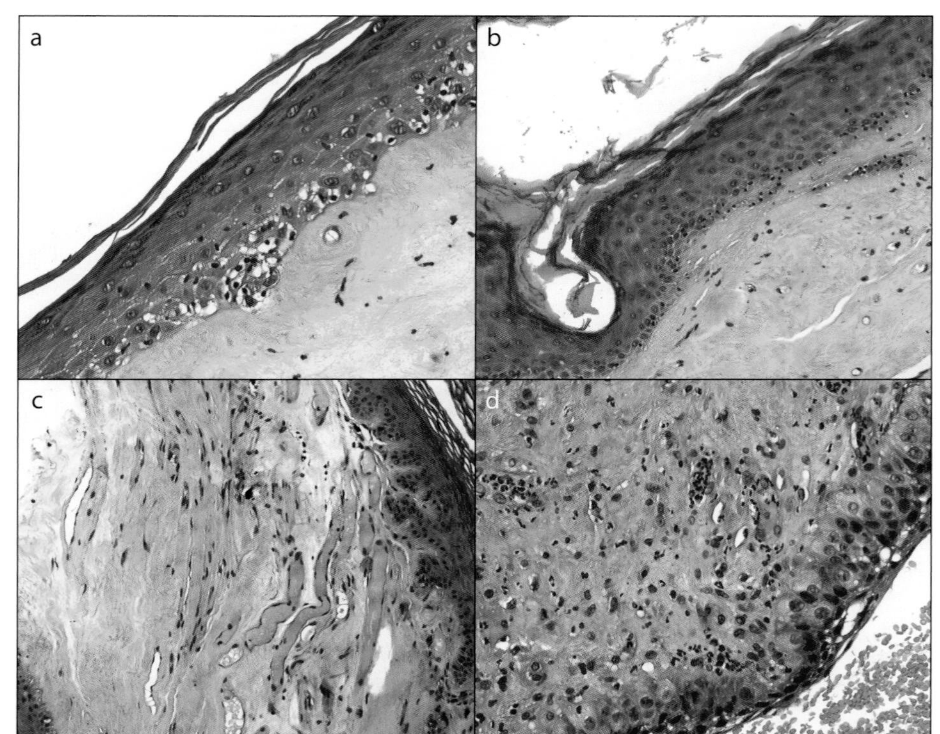

i29.14 **a** Lichen sclerosus et atrophicus (LS&A), with loss of the basal layer and vacuolar change at the dermal-epidermal junction. There is eosinophilic homogenization of the dermis.

b LS&A with an intact basal layer and characteristic dermal changes

c Dilated capillaries that occasionally seen in LS&A

d A case that has features of both LS&A and VIN. The acute inflammation suggests superimposed trauma or friction, making analysis of the epithelial atypia difficult.

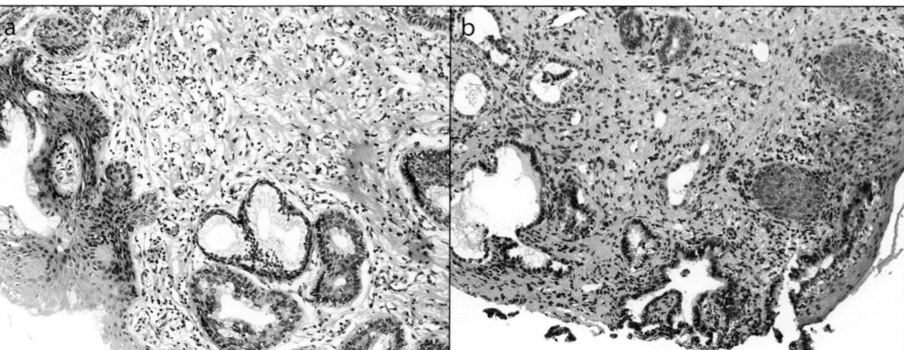

i29.15 **a** Vaginal adenosis of the endocervical type **b** Vaginal adenosis of the endometrial type

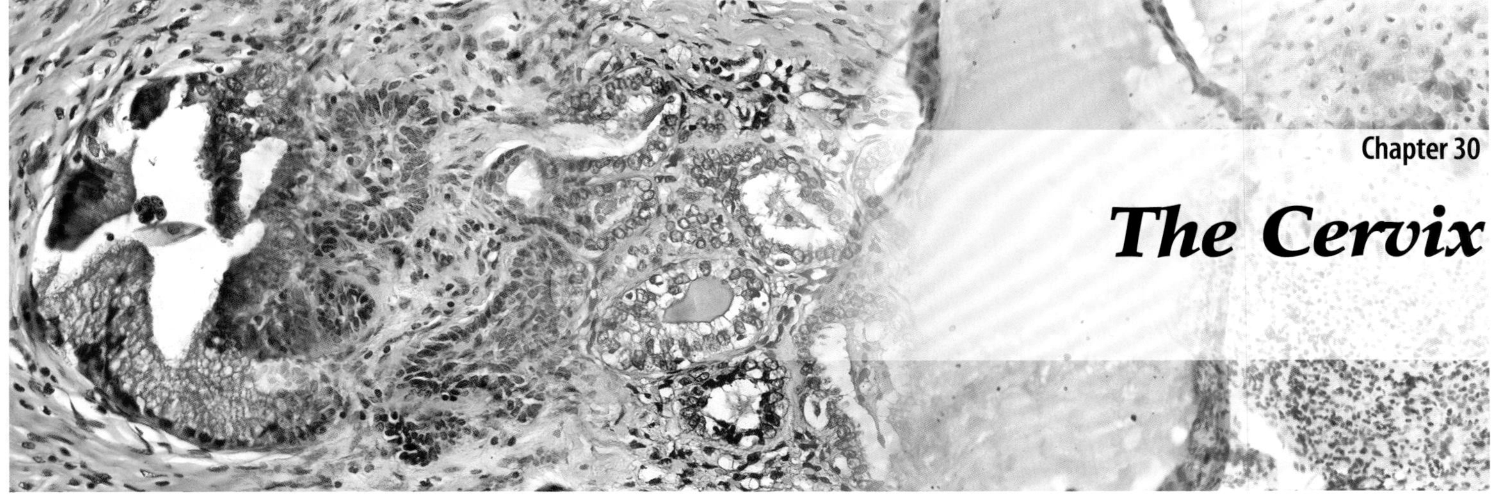

Chapter 30
The Cervix

Cervical Intraepithelial Neoplasia

The wonderful concept of in situ carcinoma, in which a cancer begins as a localized disorder of differentiation, began with the work of Dr Papanicolaou in the uterine cervix. After establishing the staining method that bears his name and describing the changes in a vaginal smear that occur during the menstrual cycle [Papanicolaou 1933], Dr Papanicolaou went on to outline how the method could screen for cervical cancer [PMID18746585], and along the way, he showed that the primary changes in a malignant cell occur in the nucleus. Since then, arguably more work has been done in the pathogenesis of cervical carcinoma than in any other type of malignancy, and the concept of in situ carcinoma has been extended to a variety of tissue types.

It is now well established, largely from the work of Harald zur Hausen [PMID183728], that the human papillomavirus (HPV) is a major contributor to cervical carcinoma and its precursors, and a vaccine to the virus promises to sharply diminish the incidence of the disease. 15 types of HPV are currently recognized as high risk (16, 18, 31, 33, 35, 39, 45, 51, 52, 56, 58, 59, 68, 73, and 82), and 3 additional types are probably high risk (26, 53, 66) [PMID12571259]. The mechanism by which HPV leads to cervical carcinoma is considered in Chapter 46. Here, we will consider only the morphology of cervical intraepithelial neoplasia (CIN).

The initial terminology for disordered maturation of the cervical squamous epithelium was "dysplasia." Subsequently, some observers adopted the cervical intraepithelial neoplasia terminology to indicate that these disorders were neoplasms (ie, clonal proliferations) despite the absence of invasion. In the CIN nomenclature, CIN 1 is equivalent to mild dysplasia, CIN 2 with moderate dysplasia, and CIN 3 conflates severe dysplasia and carcinoma in situ because these entities are indistinguishable, both morphologically and in biologic potential. Since the introduction of the CIN nomenclature, the term "intraepithelial neoplasia" has been extended to other tissues.

As in the skin, the normal cervical epithelium has a basal layer that is characterized by cells with a small amount of cytoplasm and uniform nuclei i30.1a. As mitoses occur in this layer, some daughter cells move upward, while others remain behind as new basal cells. The epithelium begins to mature in the intermediate layers, gradually acquiring more cytoplasm and a smaller nucleus until, in the superficial cells, the nucleus becomes pyknotic (ie, minute, with no demarcation of chromatin and parachromatin, because it is about to be extruded), and the cell contains abundant eosinophilic cytoplasm. Mitoses are rare above the basal layer, and are generally confined to the lowermost 1 or 2 cell layers i30.1b. Even without squamous metaplasia, there is often slight intermingling of ectocervical and endocervical epithelia, with some extension of the former into glands i30.1c.

CIN is characterized both by a constellation changes, including delayed maturation, wherein the basal layer extends upward and the epithelium gets a "late start" in maturation, and by an incomplete or disordered maturation, wherein the superficial cells at the surface do not have a normal appearance because full maturation is never attained. The superficial cells do not undergo nuclear pyknosis, but rather retain viable nuclei that are larger than normal and have discernible chromatin and parachromatin. The diagnosis of CIN 1 is made from a synthesis of the appearance of the lower and upper portions of the ectocervical epithelium. The lower portion has a basaloid appearance and mitotic activity above the normal basal 1-2 cell layers and the superficial cells, because of incomplete progression to pyknosis, have larger nuclei than would be expected. Roughly speaking, in CIN 1, the lower 1/3 of the epithelium is homogeneous and does not demonstrate any maturation. Mitoses are found throughout the lower 1/3. Only at the beginning of the second 1/3 or at about the halfway point does maturation commence i30.2. The intermediate cells have basal features, such as minimal cytoplasm and mitoses, which are normally not seen in that level of epithelium. Not all of which are present in every sample, making the diagnosis a gestalt based on the overall findings. In particular, mitoses are variable and are surprisingly rare in some cases of obvious CIN. Appreciable numbers of mitoses that are clearly above the basal layer almost always mean CIN i30.3, but the reverse is not true: Mitotic figures in the higher levels of the epithelium, evident on H&E examination, may not be seen in all cases of CIN, though a proliferation marker, such as Ki-67, will reveal proliferation in higher layers.

In CIN 2, maturation is further delayed. Even the second 1/3 is affected, so that maturation does not begin until the lower portion of the upper 1/3, resulting in a surface epithelium with minimal maturation i30.4a-c.

In CIN 3, there is essentially no maturation at all and the top and bottom of the epithelium appear nearly identical **i30.5a**. Mitoses are often found at high levels **i30.5b**. In CIN 3, maturation, if present at all, is limited to the upper 1 or 2 cell layers.

CIN, an ectocervical process, may extend into endocervical glands **i30.6**. Unless the surface component is visible, this may cause confusion as to whether the process is fundamentally ectocervical or endocervical. Particular confusion is likely to occur in Pap smears, where it can be virtually impossible to determine if an atypical epithelial cell is of ectocervical or endocervical origin. Many Pap smears reported as atypical glandular cells are actually glandular extension of CIN or atypical ectocervical cells.

Although this basic understanding is universally accepted, and cervical biopsies are one of the most commonly encountered specimens in surgical pathology, there remains considerable subjectivity in assessing cervical biopsies for CIN. Interobserver variation is greatest for CIN 2 [PMID19864243].

HPV cytopathic effect (formerly called koilocytic atypia) is usually seen in the upper layers and is a helpful feature provided that it is correctly identified and properly understood. HPV cytopathic effect is often misconstrued as simply the presence of a perinuclear clearing, but is in fact a combination of a distinct, well-formed circumferential perinuclear halo that is more sharply defined than the clear cytoplasm that results from the cell's high glycogen content and a nucleus that is too large for the level of epithelium (seen in **i30.2** and specifically shown in **i30.7a**, **i30.7b**. Perinuclear clearing alone never suffices for a diagnosis of CIN. In addition to the partial clearing that results from glycogen, perinuclear clearing is commonly seen in an inflammatory background.

In addition to nuclear enlargement and evidence of HPV, there may be other features in the upper levels of the epithelium in CIN 1 and 2, such as binucleation and dyskeratotic cells (ie, cells with intracellular keratinization) **i30.8a**, **i30.8b**. Dyskeratotic cells may indicate a differentiated CIN, similar to the differentiated VIN that occurs in the vulva or penis. In all of these locations, because dysplastic cells make keratin and show some maturation, it is easy to overlook what is actually a high-grade intraepithelial neoplasia because we are accustomed to looking for decreased maturation in any intraepithelial neoplasia. As is the case for the vulva, it is wise to respect and report dyskeratotic cells in the epithelium.

Irregular nuclear membranes and irregularly distributed chromatin are occasionally helpful in diagnosing CIN, but in my experience, are of limited value in biopsy interpretation and of only slightly more value in Pap smear interpretation.

There are 4 commonly encountered conditions that simulate CIN [PMID19415947]. These are simple hyperplasia, reactive atypia, squamous metaplasia, and atrophy. Although dysplastic epithelium may also be hyperplastic, especially in a condyloma, simple epithelial hyperplasia, with or without papillomatosis, may occur in any site in the female genital tract and does not constitute intraepithelial neoplasia. In a condyloma, there will be other features of CIN in addition to the epithelial thickness. In hyperplasia, maturation begins and ends normally and there are no other features to suggest CIN. Apparent hyperplasia may be caused by tangential sectioning **i30.9a**, **i30.9b**.

Reactive (reparative) atypia may demonstrate initially disturbing nuclear enlargement and what appears to be reduced maturation but usually occurs in a milieu of acute inflammation **i30.10a**. Adding to the difficulty is that there may be perinuclear haloes **i30.10b**. One of the most disturbing features in a reactive atypia is prominent nucleoli **i30.10c**, but if the observer subtracts out the nucleoli in the mind's eye, the appearance of the cells is much less alarming. Actually, prominent nucleoli are *not* a feature of CIN. Indeed, their presence in a clearly noninvasive biopsy, especially with concomitant acute inflammation, is a point against CIN, and their presence in an obvious CIN suggests invasive carcinoma.

Squamous metaplasia of endocervical epithelium has a uniform appearance that leads to an initially alarming appearance due to an apparent lack of maturation. The cells at the bottom of a cluster of metaplastic cells look the same as those at the top of the cluster. CIN may indeed arise in metaplastic epithelium, but uncomplicated squamous metaplasia differs from CIN in having a moderate amount of cytoplasm at all levels, no nuclear atypia, and minimal mitotic activity **i30.11a**. If one sets aside the apparent maturational delay, there are no features to suggest CIN. Helpful features in identifying squamous metaplasia are that the cells often have a slightly polygonal contour and fit together in a pattern reminiscent of a jigsaw puzzle **i30.11b**, and the problematic area is often in close proximity to glandular epithelium.

By definition, atrophy has no maturation and is therefore easily confused with CIN, indeed with CIN 3. However, other than the lack of maturation, atrophy has no features of CIN. Importantly, mitoses are minimal in atrophy and are found only in the basal layer. If one subtracts the lack of maturation, there will be no features to suggest CIN **i30.12a**, **i30.12b**. Also, elsewhere, there is likely to be a focus of unequivocal atrophy that does not simulate CIN **i30.12c**.

Each of these 4 mimics of CIN has only 1 feature that is alarming—epithelial thickness in hyperplasia, nucleoli in reactive atypia, and diminished maturation in squamous metaplasia and atrophy. In each of these situations, the imaginary removal of that one characteristic will help prevent a misinterpretation. This reinforces that CIN should never be diagnosed from a single feature.

There are 2 less commonly encountered conditions that may simulate CIN: transitional cell metaplasia and immature metaplasia [PMID10757336]. Transitional cell metaplasia is a rare entity that differs from atrophy by its greater thickness, from CIN 3 by its lack of mitotic activity, and from squamous metaplasia by the transitional appearance of the cells, resembling those from the bladder [PMID9158674, PMID20085511].

Immature metaplasia (formerly called immature condyloma) is a proliferation of ectocervical epithelium, often in a papillary configuration (it is sometimes called papillary immature metaplasia), that may simulate high-grade CIN. Immature metaplasia may have perinuclear clearing, but it is associated with HPV types 6 and 11 rather than high-risk HPV types, and it has much lower expression of Ki-67 than a papillary CIN or squamous carcinoma. [PMID11748359] One should be cautious in making the diagnosis of a high-grade CIN in a papillary architecture.

Nevertheless, there are cases that are equivocal for CIN. One of many such commonly encountered cases is shown in i30.13. In those cases that are equivocal for dysplasia, one can describe the findings and comment on the inability to diagnose or to exclude CIN. Options at that time include following the patient, repeat biopsy, or additional testing on the biopsy. Helpful additional tests include high-risk HPV genome, the proliferation marker Ki-67, and p16.

In cases in which a biopsy is equivocal for CIN, demonstration of HPV of a high-risk type favors a diagnosis of CIN, though the association of HPV and CIN is far from invariant and HPV cannot be demonstrated in 23% of cases of CIN 1, 16% of cases of CIN 2, and 6% of cases of CIN 3 [PMID20592555]. Moreover, not everyone who acquires HPV will necessarily develop CIN. It should also be remembered that despite the propensity for HPV to be multicentric and persistent, in most cases of high-risk HPV-associated CIN, the virus is ultimately cleared if there has been effective treatment [PMID21173650].

HPV is often tested by the hybrid capture technique on the same vial that is used for the Pap smear. Hybrid capture technology uses RNA probes (called riboprobes), which hybridize to the viral DNA target. The hybrids are then immobilized by monoclonal antibody that only binds the DNA:RNA hybrid. Detection is by a second monoclonal antibody that contain a chromogen, usually alkaline phosphatase, which binds the antibodies used to capture the DNA:RNA hybrid.

HPV can also be detected on paraffin processed tissue by immunohistochemistry (usually directed to the major capsid protein) or by in situ hybridization. Because many laboratories perform an HPV test on a vial taken for a Pap smear only if the interpretation is atypical squamous cells, and not if it is CIN, if a biopsy taken to confirm a Pap smear diagnosis of CIN is equivocal, HPV testing may not have been performed and may need to be obtained from a paraffin block, in which case immunohistochemistry or in situ hybridization are the only options.

Immunohistochemical staining for Ki-67, which highlights cells in or committed to mitosis, may reveal mitotic activity (or a cell's commitment thereto) that is not evident on H&E examination. Ki-67 staining in the intermediate or superficial layers suggests CIN over a reactive or atrophic process, while staining restricted to the basal layer favors a mimic of CIN. Ki-67 shows progressively greater staining of the upper portions of the epithelium in CINs of increasing severity.

Additionally helpful is nuclear staining for p16 [PMID17365826]. As discussed in Chapter 46, HPV causes the production of p16, which inhibits the normal regulatory function of the product of the *RB* tumor suppressor gene. p16 is diffusely (not focally) expressed by the vast majority of cases of CIN and invasive carcinomas, and is generally absent in processes that are not CIN. Positivity is generally limited to the lower epithelium in CIN 1 but extends upward in high-grade CIN. CIN expresses both p16 and Ki-67 more diffusely and at higher levels of the epithelium than its mimics [PMID17824788].

In my experience, most false-positive diagnoses of CIN occur in cases where there appears to be diminished maturation, but that in which suprabasal mitoses, high-risk HPV genome, and p16 are all absent i30.14a-d. The diagnosis of CIN, and certainly the diagnosis of high-grade CIN, should be questioned if neither increased mitoses nor high-risk HPV genome or p16 can be demonstrated. Insisting on at least 2 of these findings will prevent overdiagnosis in most problematic cases. The images in i30.15 illustrate a subtle case of CIN 1 that is identified by the demonstration of suprabasal staining for Ki-67, a positive stain for p16, and a positive test for high-risk HPV genome by hybrid capture.

A false positive is particular prone to arise in middle-aged women who have had negative Pap smears and who suddenly have a smear interpreted as a CIN. These patients are generally too young to have atrophy of the cervical epithelium, a common mimic of CIN seen in older patients, and indeed, biopsy often shows maturation and appears to confirm a CIN. Without question, many of these cases are legitimate occasions of late-onset CIN, but it has been my experience that some of them are false positives that are detected when a complete workup fails to demonstrate HPV by immunohistochemistry or in situ hybridization, p16 is negative, and Ki-67 shows only basal mitotic activity. Despite the apparent CIN found on both the Pap smear and the biopsy, by the currently accepted immunohistochemical and molecular criteria, CIN cannot be verified.

Women with CIN who are over the age of 30 are less likely to have demonstrable high-risk HPV [PMID20592555], but even in that age group, about 2/3 are positive [PMID19894254]. I recommend that in middle-aged patients who do not have a history of CIN, even an apparently obvious biopsy with CIN be questioned unless at least 1 of the following 3 confirmatory findings is present: demonstration of high-risk HPV genome by any technique, proliferation above the basal layer, verified either by mitotic figures or by Ki-67 immunohistochemical staining, or the presence of p16.

Developments in molecular pathology have led to the development of additional ancillary tests that may prove beneficial. ProExC, a collection of antibodies to topoisomerase IIα and minichromosome maintenance 2 proteins, is positive in the vast majority of cases of high-grade ectocervical and endocervical intraepithelial neoplasia and nearly uniformly negative in reactive processes [PMID19952938].

A potentially important finding is that the enzyme telomerase, which repairs the ends of chromosomes and is generally absent in normal cells and present in some cancer cells, is expressed in high-grade cervical intraepithelial neoplasia and invasive carcinoma, but not in normal cervical epithelium or low-grade CIN. Telomerase is composed of both protein and RNA. The RNA component is encoded by the gene *TERC*, amplification of which can be identified in high-grade CIN and invasive carcinoma by FISH on the same fluid from which the Pap smear is made, furnishing a potentially important new means of detection [PMID20864639].

The Pap Smear

The Pap smear presents both a unique opportunity and a frustrating challenge in pathology. It is an opportunity to identify patients who are at risk of cervical carcinoma, and the advent of screening has unquestionably saved tens of thousands of lives. On the other hand, the Pap smear requires that a full assessment of maturation of the epithelium be made from the appearance of the most superficial 1 or 2 cells layers that

ISBN 978-089189-5886

are recovered for examination. Fortunately, the incomplete maturation of the superficial layers is usually detectable in a Pap smear. Superficial cells that have larger nuclei with a distinction between chromatin and parachromatin rather than the expected pyknotic nuclei, or that have nuclear hyperchromasia, binucleation, dyskeratosis, or HPV cytopathic effect permit the Pap smear diagnosis of most cases of CIN 1 **i30.16**. In CIN 2, the above findings are more pronounced **i30.17**. There may be a complete absence of superficial cells, because of the more severe maturational delay. In CIN 3, where the maturational delay is full-thickness, the basaloid cells extend to the surface and can be directly detected as cells with a very high nucleus-to-cytoplasmic ratio **i30.18**.

Current Pap smear terminology uses the term "squamous intraepithelial lesion" (SIL) rather than CIN. Low-grade SIL equates to CIN 1. High-grade SIL encompasses both CIN 2 (moderate dysplasia) and CIN 3 (severe dysplasia/carcinoma in situ). SIL terminology was adopted because in a Pap smear, where the full thickness of the epithelium cannot be assessed, it is difficult to distinguish CIN 2 from CIN 3.

The current convention for premalignant squamous abnormalities on a Pap smear is governed by the Bethesda 2001 system [PMID15504231] and is as follows:

1. Atypical squamous cells (ASC)
   A. Of undetermined significance (ASC-US)
   B. Cannot exclude a high-grade SIL (ASC-H)
2. Low-grade SIL (L SIL or LGSIL)
3. High-grade SIL (H SIL or HGSIL)

It is important to note, and to be sure that clinicians understand, that ASCUS cases may be reactive, low-grade SIL, or high-grade SIL. In Pap smears, there are some cases for which a distinction of reactive atypia from high-grade SIL is not possible. The traditional recommendation for ASCUS Pap smear results is that the patient have a repeat Pap smear in a year and if there are 2 such results, colposcopy and biopsy are often done. However, it may be better to proceed to colposcopy and biopsy after 1 ASCUS result [PMID21917680].

Because of the great (but not invariable) association of CIN with HPV, the demonstration of high-risk HPV genome in an ASC case makes it very likely that it is a CIN. For this reason, the current recommendation of the American College of Obstetricians and Gynecologists is that HPV testing be undertaken immediately upon the finding of any ASC smear, even if all previous smears have been normal. Indeed, many are beginning to believe that cervical cancer screening should take the form of screening for high-risk HPV, with cytology reserved for the positive cases. The primary advantages of HPV testing as a potential screening technique are greater reproducibility and objectivity, and potentially, more practical use in developing countries because results can be obtained more quickly and by less trained personnel than is the case for a Pap smear. Moreover, testing for HPV alone is more sensitive than cytology in the detection of high-grade CIN [PMID18364502]. p16 has also been shown to be of value in liquid based Pap smear material, but at this time, HPV testing on liquid-based cytology preparations is more sensitive than p16 testing [PMID18232003].

An ongoing controversy in Pap smear examinations is the form that quality control should take. 10% random rescreening has long been a standard, but has added minimal value [PMID8834084]. Some have advocated an immediate rescreen of all negative cases [PMID16719853]. Still others have advocated the seeding of positive cases into those that are immediately rescreened [PMID18618517]. Yet another approach has been to rapidly prescreen some cases before they are subjected to a full examination [PMID19711473].

An evolving frontier in Pap smear examination is automation. In the 1990s, the Food and Drug Administration approved automated rescreening of Pap smears that had already been manually screened. Currently, there are 2 FDA-approved instruments for automated primary Pap smear screening. The first of these is based on the ThinPrep system (Hologic), in which the entire slide is screened and the 22 most problematic fields are projected to a microscope for examination by the cytotechnologist. The second system is based on SurePath (Becton-Dickinson) and screens the entire slide and assigns a likelihood of a significant process. If the system concludes that there is no likelihood of a significant process, manual reexamination by a cytotechnologist is not mandatory but is typically performed in a significant percentage of such cases. Any other conclusion by the system mandates a manual review. These 2 systems are collectively referred to as "image-guided" Pap smear screening. The Becton-Dickinson system has been shown to have a higher sensitivity than purely manual screening for the detection of SILs, especially those of high-grade [PMID19846820], but its complete role has not yet been defined, and there is concern that the increased cytotechnologist workloads that are permitted in computer-assisted screening negate the benefit [PMID20151428].

Invasive Squamous Cell Carcinoma of the Cervix

Invasion squamous carcinoma should be suspected if there is an uneven interface of the epithelial cells with the stroma, including a scalloped border, pseudoglandular structures, or confluent clusters of epithelial cells without intervening stroma **i30.19a**. Even if each cluster has an even interface with the stroma, a large number of them, with coalescence, suggests invasion, with the caveat to be sure the sectioning is not tangential. In equivocal situations, stromal desmoplasia **i30.19b** suggests invasion. Caution is indicated in the diagnosis of invasion in situations where the epithelial-stroma interface is obscured by inflammation. Cervical squamous carcinoma, like squamous carcinomas from other sites, is negative for cytokeratin 20, but whereas other squamous carcinomas are also negative for cytokeratin 7, those from the cervix are positive for CK7 in almost 90% of cases [PMID7524976]. Microinvasion is defined by the Society of Gynecologic Oncologists as a carcinoma that invades to a depth of 0.3 cm (3 mm) or less and does not have lymphatic invasion [PMID14599856].

The demonstration of a disrupted basement membrane is helpful in identifying microinvasive foci [PMID6348406], but as is the case in other sites, disruption of the basement membrane is not specific for microinvasion because it can also be focally disrupted without invasion, especially if there is inflammation at the junction [PMID2659627], nor does apparent continuity of a basement membrane exclude invasion because neoplastic cells may make basement membrane material, as is the case in other sites [PMID2437505]. Despite these caveats, I have found basement membrane staining, either by PAS or an immunohistochemical stain for collagen type 4, to be generally useful in identifying foci of microinvasion in problematic situations.

The basaloid type of squamous carcinoma occurs in the cervix, but only rarely. Much more common is the so-called adenoid basal carcinoma, which is much less aggressive. The adenoid basal carcinoma consists of small islands of basaloid cells i30.20a, with focal pseudoglandular or squamous differentiation. It has low-grade nuclei i30.20b, no areas of classic invasive squamous carcinoma, and an appearance which resembles basalosquamous carcinoma of the skin. The adenoid basal carcinoma has a high association with SILs i30.20c [PMID15712186]. Before making the diagnosis of adenoid basal carcinoma, any foci of classic invasive squamous carcinoma must be excluded, as any such component negates the indolent behavior of the adenoid basal carcinoma and conveys the prognosis of conventional squamous carcinoma.

Because its behavior is relatively indolent, some have proposed the term "adenoid basal epithelioma" instead of adenoid basal carcinoma [PMID15712186]. To my mind, the term "epithelioma" is likely to cause more confusion than clarification. I recommend continuing with the term "adenoid basal carcinoma," but to avoid confusion since the terminology among several different forms of carcinoma is similar, I also recommend a comment that this is a much less aggressive neoplasm that is not to be confused with the conventional squamous carcinoma, the basaloid type of squamous carcinoma or the adenoid cystic carcinoma, and that careful examination of the specimen has excluded any component of these other types of neoplasms.

Adenoid cystic adenocarcinoma must also be excluded before diagnosing adenoid basal carcinoma. Verrucous, papillary, and condylomatous variants of squamous carcinoma may occur in the cervix. These forms of squamous carcinoma are discussed in Chapter 39.

Endocervical Lesions

In the 2001 Bethesda system, the previous category of "atypical glandular cells of undetermined significance" (AGUS) is eliminated and replaced by the term "atypical glandular cells" (AGC), though in practice, "AGUS" is still commonly used. In the AGC nomenclature, an attempt is initially made to classify the atypical glandular cells as endocervical, endometrial, or not otherwise specified (NOS). Then an attempt is made at a more precise diagnosis, such as "favor neoplastic." Endocervical adenocarcinoma in situ and adenocarcinoma, NOS, are accepted diagnostic opinions. Thus, examples of AGC comments may include the following:

- AGC, probably endocervical, favor neoplastic
- AGC, probably endometrial, favor neoplastic
- AGC, endocervical adenocarcinoma in situ
- AGC, NOS (origin unclear, no opinion on neoplastic vs nonneoplastic)
- AGC, NOS, adenocarcinoma (malignant cells identified, but origin unclear)

A comment may also be made that endometrial cells are seen in a patient who is 40 or older [PMID15504231].

The terminology of intraepithelial neoplasia is not as well established in the endocervix as in the ectocervix, and the older term "dysplasia" continues to predominate.

Atypical glandular cells and atypical squamous cells may be nearly indistinguishable on a Pap smear because there is no opportunity to assess the architectural context of an atypical cell i30.21a-c. p63 expression can be helpful in these cases because its presence indicates squamous origin [PMID17173320], though in practice, the finding of atypical cells of either apparent glandular or squamous origin requires histologic followup, which will be the final arbiter of histogenesis.

Endocervical dysplasia, like the more familiar ectocervical dysplasia, is also associated with HPV [PMID19387129], and reflex testing of HPV in atypical glandular cells on Pap smears has been advocated because those AGC that are associated with HPV are more likely to be significant [PMID18548530]. Another reason to perform HPV testing in AGC cases is that distinguishing AGC from a squamous process can be difficult, even with p63 immunohistochemistry. If a subsequent biopsy demonstrates that the AGC are actually of squamous origin and is equivocal for CIN, the HPV status of the original cytology specimen will be important.

On biopsy or resection material, low-grade endocervical dysplasia is recognized by nuclear enlargement with crowding, but with minimal stratification and with retention of mucinous cytoplasm, resulting in an appearance that is similar to a colonic adenomatous polyp i30.22a-c. High-grade endocervical dysplasia has full-thickness nuclear stratification, mitoses, and less cytoplasm [PMID10757337], roughly resembling a colonic polyp with high-grade dysplasia i30.23a-c. It is likely futile to attempt to distinguish high-grade endocervical dysplasia from endocervical adenocarcinoma in situ (AIS). Recognizing that mitotic activity and stratification are reliable criteria in the differentiation of reactive atypia from endocervical dysplasia, a scoring system has been proposed whereby foci are graded on a scale of 0-3 for stratification and 0-3 for nuclear atypia. Then the 2 most active glands are assessed for mitoses or apoptosis, with <0.5 figures per gland being 1, up to 3 figures per gland receiving a score of 2, and >3 figures per gland being 3. These 3 criteria are added and a total score of 0-3 indicates reactive atypia, 4-5 endocervical dysplasia, and 6-9 AIS [PMID12657929].

Invasive endocervical adenocarcinoma is diagnosed by the same criteria as adenocarcinomas in other sites, including nuclear atypia i30.24a, haphazard infiltration i30.24b, and a stromal reaction i30.24c.

The minimal deviation adenocarcinoma (formerly called adenoma malignum) deserves special comment because it can be extremely difficult to identify. The glands are haphazardly distributed and deeply infiltrative i30.25a, i30.25b. Many nuclei are normal, but there is usually focal mild nuclear enlargement, and one of the best ways to make this diagnosis is to identify associated endocervical adenocarcinoma of a more conventional appearance. In the absence of an area of conventional adenocarcinoma, important diagnostic features include glands with an irregular outline, stromal desmoplasia i30.25c, perineural or vascular invasion, positivity for CEA, and an infiltrative pattern [PMID2764221], though a cone or a hysterectomy

ISBN 978-089189-5886

may be needed to establish infiltration [PMID12207781]. However, HPV and p16 staining are unlikely to help, as these are less reliably found in minimal deviation adenocarcinoma than in the more common type of endocervical adenocarcinoma [PMID20727021]. Despite the deceptively bland nuclei, minimal deviation adenocarcinoma of the cervix is often aggressive [PMID20451906].

There are a number of benign mimics of invasive endocervical adenocarcinoma. Mesonephric remnants deserve special mention, as they are readily confused with an invasive adenocarcinoma. Mesonephric remnants may or may not have a lobular pattern i30.26a, but the glands contain eosinophilic material, an important diagnostic clue. Nuclei are generally bland, but may show focal enlargement that overlaps with some nuclei in a minimal deviation adenocarcinoma i30.26b. However, even if there is not a distinct lobular pattern and there is mild nuclear enlargement, there is no true infiltrative pattern and a study of the entire lesion and the overall milieu will secure the correct diagnosis.

Microglandular hyperplasia is characterized by small, crowded glands that may simulate adenocarcinoma because of increased epithelial cellularity, but there is no infiltration and the nuclei are small, uniform, and basal i30.27a, i30.27b. Tunnel clusters are invaginations of endocervical glands into the stroma, simulating invasive adenocarcinoma. They appear as a well demarcated collection of dilated glands with only minimal nuclear atypia i30.28a [PMID2206083]. They are believed to form from mucosal involution and are filled with amphophilic mucin rather than the eosinophilic secretions that are characteristic of mesonephric remnants i30.28b. In all of these mimics, the key to the correct diagnosis is attention to the atypical nuclei that are at least focally present in endocervical adenocarcinoma but which are absent in the mimics.

In difficult cases, immunohistochemical stains may help. In addition to HPV, Ki-67, p16, and CEA expression are all increased in dysplastic endocervical epithelium relative to normal endocervical epithelium, and increased further in endocervical adenocarcinoma in situ [PMID17197900]. p16 is rarely expressed in normal endocervical epithelium, but may be expressed in dysplastic or neoplastic endocervical processes. While the utility of p16 in endocervical processes appears less than for ectocervical processes, a positive p16 in a problematic endocervical lesion is likely to be significant [PMID16462152]. Likewise, an obvious glandular process that is p16 positive will likely be of endocervical, rather than endometrial, origin. It is also likely that p16 will also be of benefit in distinguishing metastatic adenocarcinomas of endocervical origin from those of other sources.

An algorithm has been offered whereby convincing positivity for CEA and also for either Ki-67 or p53 secures a diagnosis of an AIS or invasive adenocarcinoma over a benign mimic [PMID9071723]. On the other hand, cyclin D1 (bcl-1) is generally strongly positive in reactive endocervical lesions, but weakly positive or negative in AIS or invasive endocervical adenocarcinoma [PMID20062011].

It is occasionally difficult even in a cone or resection to determine if a cervical carcinoma is of squamous or glandular origin (and the 2 types may occur together). In these unusual cases, immunohistochemical staining for p63 staining may help, as it is positive in squamous carcinomas and the squamous portion of adenosquamous carcinomas, but weak or negative in adenocarcinomas [PMID19700941].

HPV and p16 positivity suggest an endocervical origin for a metastatic adenocarcinoma of unknown primary. CDX2, generally used to identify adenocarcinomas of the lower gastrointestinal tract, also stains about half of endocervical adenocarcinomas [PMID18753946]. Confusion with an intestinal primary can usually be avoided by the concomitant presence of p16 and CK7.

Core Points for the Cervix

- Concept of in situ carcinoma, effective screening, and cancer vaccine all arose in the cervix.
- PAP smear: enormous triumph, challenges are quality control, integration of immunohistochemical and/or molecular testing, and the role of automation.
- Cervical intraepithelial neoplasia (CIN): delayed, disordered, or incomplete maturation.
    - o Interobserver variation greatest in distinction of CIN 1 from a mimic of CIN and in the distinction of CIN 2 from CIN 1 and CIN 3.
- 4 processes commonly simulate CIN: simple hyperplasia, reactive atypia, squamous metaplasia, and atrophy.
    - o Demonstration of high-risk HPV genome favors CIN Because the prevalence of HPV infection is high, this finding alone does not secure a diagnosis of CIN.
    - o Mitotic activity above the basal layer, perhaps identified by Ki-67 stain, favors CIN, as does staining for p16.
    - o Caution indicated if at least one of these additional findings cannot be demonstrated.
- Differentiated CIN: as in the vulva, deceptively complete, but disordered maturation with dyskeratotic cells.
- Invasion squamous carcinoma: stromal desmoplasia, atypical epithelial cells with a jagged or irregular interface with the stroma, coalescence of clusters of epithelial cells.
- Adenoid basal carcinoma: more common than basaloid squamous carcinoma.
    - o Less aggressive, often associated with CIN.
- Atypical glandular cells on Pap smear may resemble atypical squamous cells.
- Endocervical dysplasia is also associated with HPV
- Low-grade endocervical dysplasia: modest nuclear enlargement and crowding
    - o Retain mucinous cytoplasm, and there is little stratification
    - o Appearance similar to a common colonic adenomatous polyp.
- High-grade endocervical dysplasia: larger nuclei with less cytoplasm, as well as full-thickness nuclear stratification and numerous mitoses
    - o Appearance suggestive of a colonic adenomatous polyp with high-grade dysplasia.
- Reflex testing of HPV in atypical glandular cells on PAP smears is reasonable.

- In problematic endocervical process, HPV, Ki-67, and p16 expression favors dysplasia, as is the case for ectocervical processes.
- Benign mimics of invasive endocervical adenocarcinoma: mesonephric remnants and microglandular hyperplasia.
  - o Mesonephric remnants: innocuous nuclei and eosinophilic intraglandular material.
  - o Microglandular hyperplasia: are small and crowded glands, but
  - o Nuclei are small and basally oriented, with no infiltration.
- Minimal deviation adenocarcinoma (formerly called adenoma malignum): combination of slight nuclear enlargement, glands that are deeply and randomly distributed in the stroma, glands that are irregularly shaped, and areas of more conventional endocervical adenocarcinoma.
  - o May require a cone or hysterectomy for detection.
- Endocervical adenocarcinomas and ectocervical squamous carcinomas may occasionally resemble each other and may occur together
  - o Positive p63 staining suggests squamous origin.

ISBN 978-089189-5886

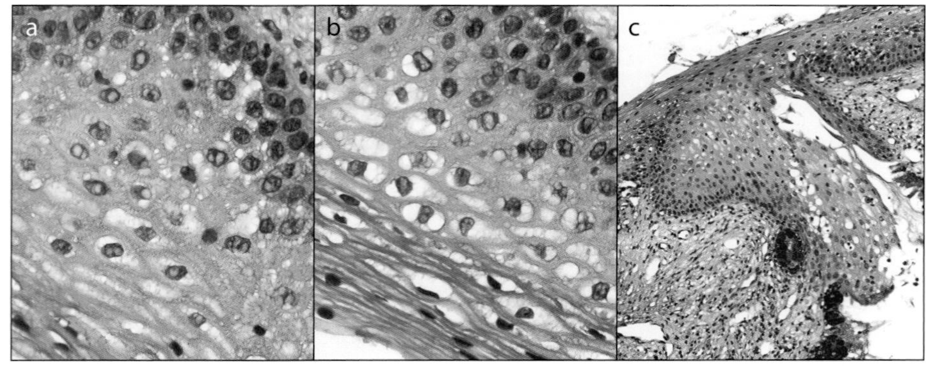

i30.1 **a** Normal ectocervical epithelium with a basal layer, the cells of which have minimal cytoplasm, in the upper right. Maturation is towards the lower left. The cells acquire more cytoplasm during maturation but do not overtly keratinize. At the luminal surface, the nuclei are pyknotic. **b** Another view of normal ectocervical epithelium. Note that perinuclear halos may be seen in normal epithelium. Some of the perinuclear clearing is secondary to glycogen, but some is not. **c** Extension of normal ectocervical epithelium into an endocervical gland. This is neither dysplasia nor squamous metaplasia.

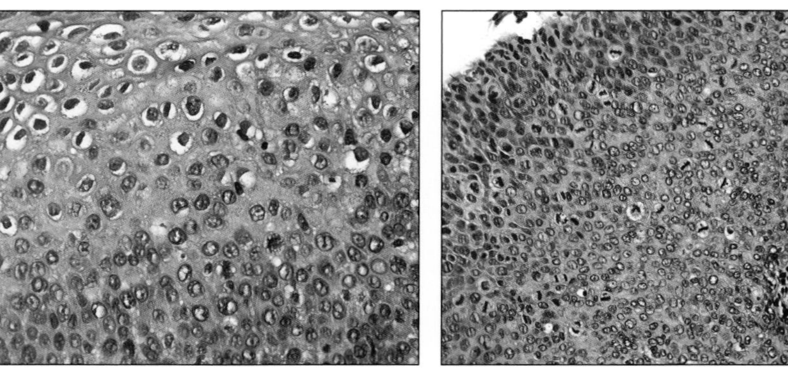

i30.2 CIN 1 (mild ectocervical dysplasia). Note that the basal layer extends upward for approximately 1/3 the thickness of the epithelium. There are 2 mitotic figures in the upper portion of the augmented basal layer. Maturation is reasonably complete but not totally so, and most nuclei do not achieve complete pyknosis. Perinuclear halos are prominent and are associated with mild nuclear atypia.

i30.3 Large numbers of mitotic figures well above the basal layer in the upper left in a case of high-grade CIN

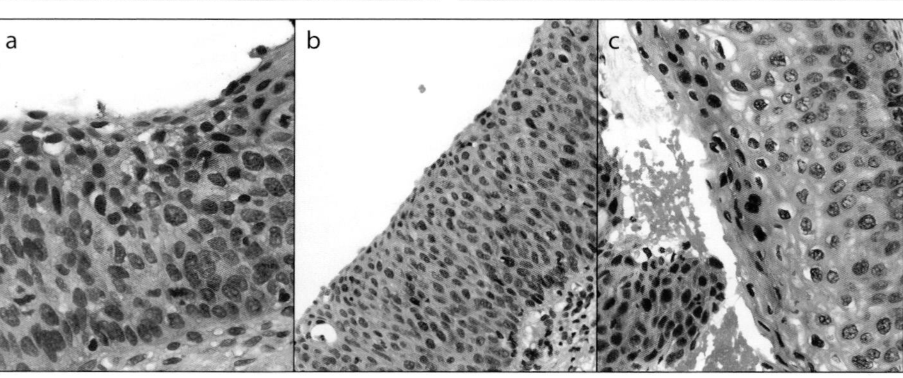

i30.4 **a-c** These 3 images illustrate high-grade CIN. Because all 3 cases either illustrate some degree of maturation or have minimal mitotic activity above the basal layer, a good argument can be made that these 3 cases are all CIN 2. On the other hand, any or all could be regarded as CIN 3. Interobserver variation is greatest for cases that are often regarded as CIN 2.

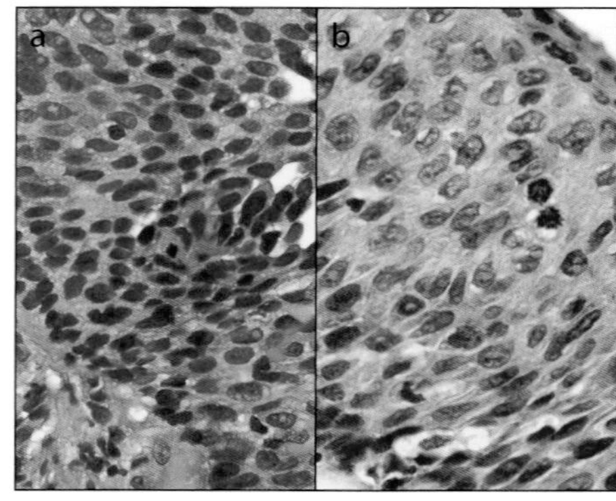

i30.5 **a** CIN 3, with no maturation at all
b CIN 3, with extremely little maturation and 2 high mitotic figures

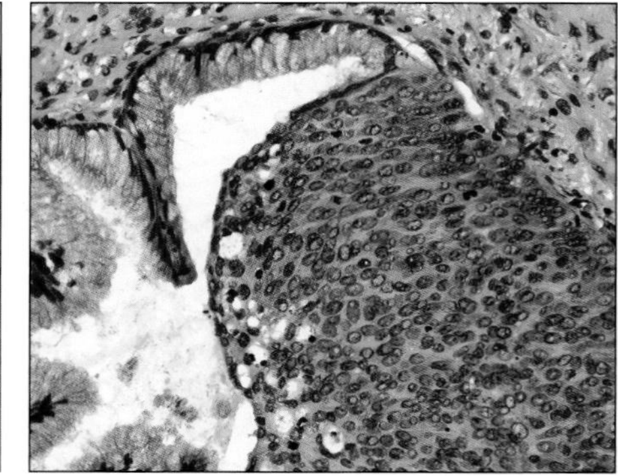

i30.6 High-grade CIN extending into an endocervical gland. Note the nuclear atypia, crowding, and mitotic activity relative to i30.1c.

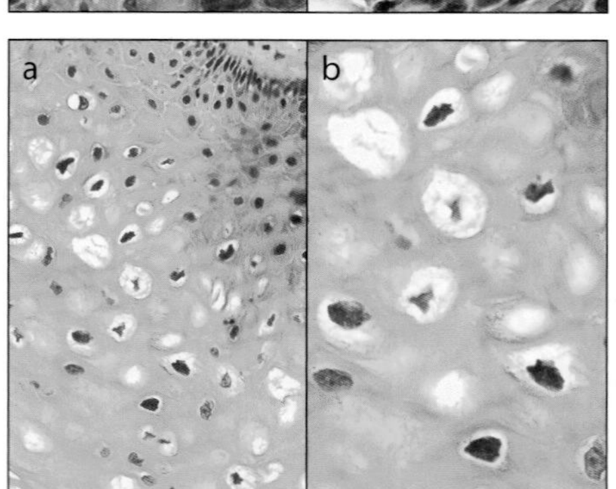

i30.7 **a-b** HPV cytopathic effect (koilocytic atypia). Note the enlarged, hyperchromatic, and irregularly shaped nuclei, which are required for this diagnosis and would separate this entity from simple perinuclear halos such as those seen in i30.1b.

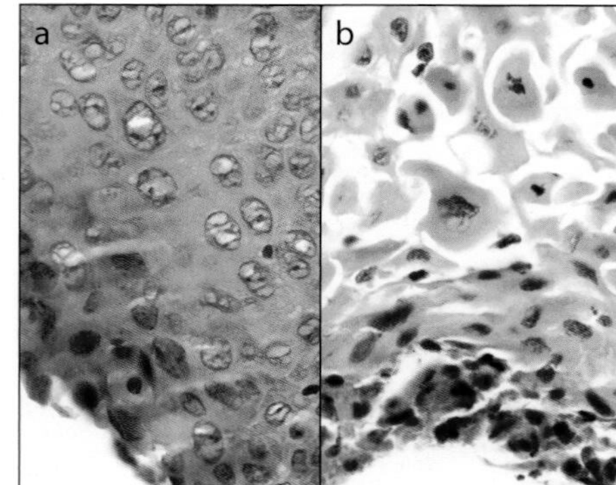

i30.8 **a** A cervical biopsy with mild atypia, but with a dyskeratotic cell. Cases of this nature may be a subtle differentiated CIN. **b** Differentiated CIN in endocervical curettings

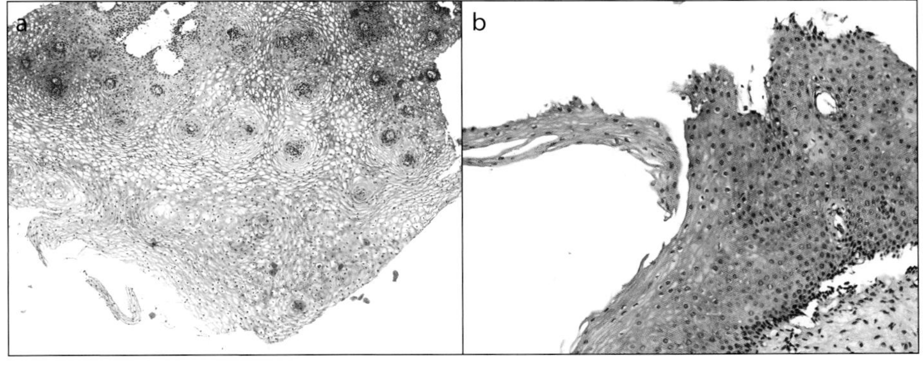

i30.9 **a** Artifactual ectocervical hyperplasia caused by tangential sectioning

b A cervical biopsy which appears, in the upper right, to demonstrate diminished maturation and nuclear atypia. However, the detached fragment on the left likely folded over this area in vivo, in which case the epithelium is slightly hyperplastic but not dysplastic, and there is normal maturation.

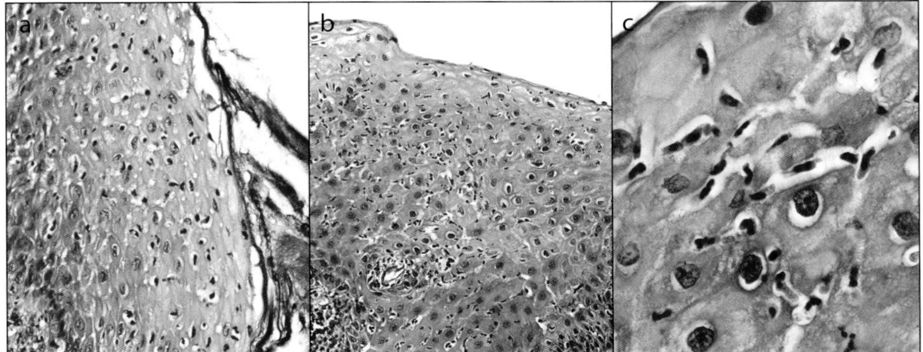

i30.10 **a-b** Cervical biopsies with ectocervical atypia, worrisome for CIN 1, but with an acutely inflamed background

c A higher-power view of the same case as in i30.10b illustrating a prominent nucleolus and distinct perinuclear halo that can be additionally worrisome

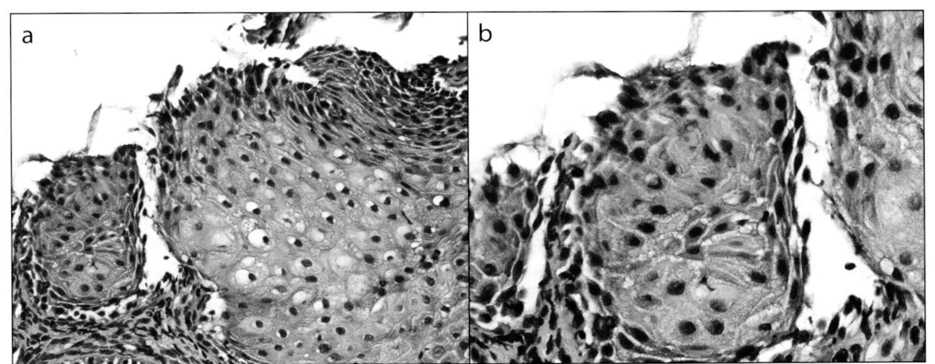

i30.11 **a** Squamous metaplasia simulating CIN because of an apparent lack of maturation

b A higher-power view of the same case as in i30.11a, illustrating the "jigsaw" manner in which the problematic cells fit together. Intercellular bridges can be seen.

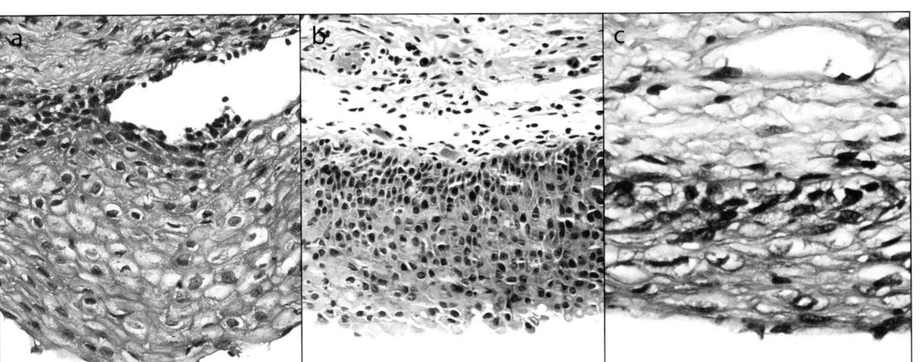

i30.12 **a** Cervical atrophy simulating CIN because of an apparent lack of maturation
b Another case of cervical atrophy with atypia augmented by prolapse and chronic irritation. The area immediately adjacent to this focus on one side was hyperkeratotic, but not suspicious for CIN.

c The same case as in i30.12b, with a focus of uncomplicated atrophy adjacent to the problematic area

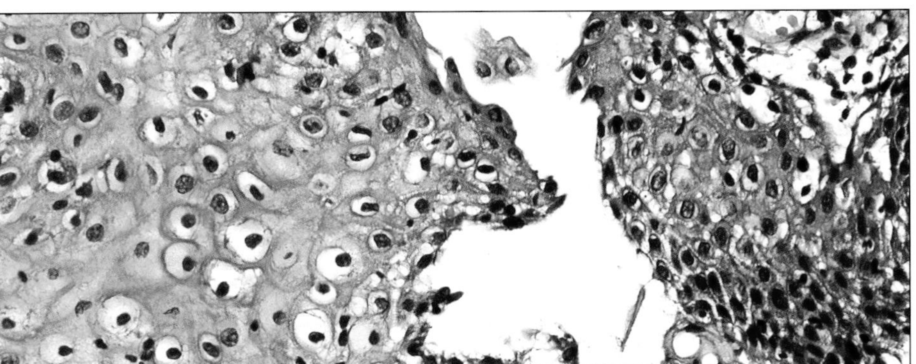

i30.13 An example of a cervical biopsy that is equivocal for CIN

ISBN 978-089189-5886

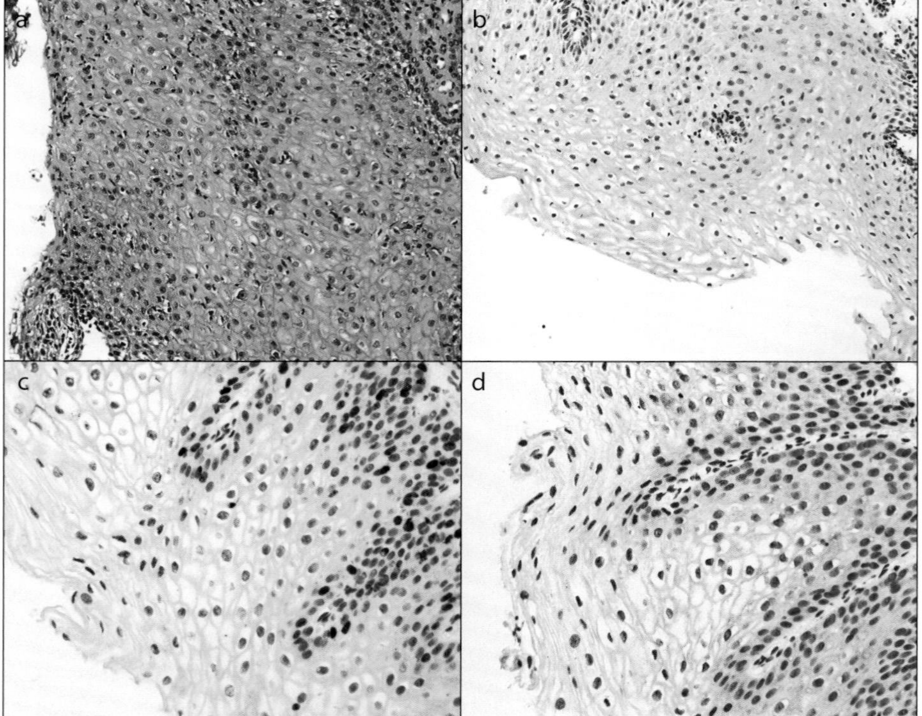

i30.14 **a** A cervical biopsy with mild atypia and a very rare dyskeratotic cell, but an acutely inflamed background, again equivocal for CIN 1.

b The same case as in i30.14a, with a negative immunohistochemical stain for high-risk HPV types

c The same case stained for Ki-67, illustrating positivity only in the basal layer

d The same case staining negatively for p16. These 3 stains exclude CIN in this case.

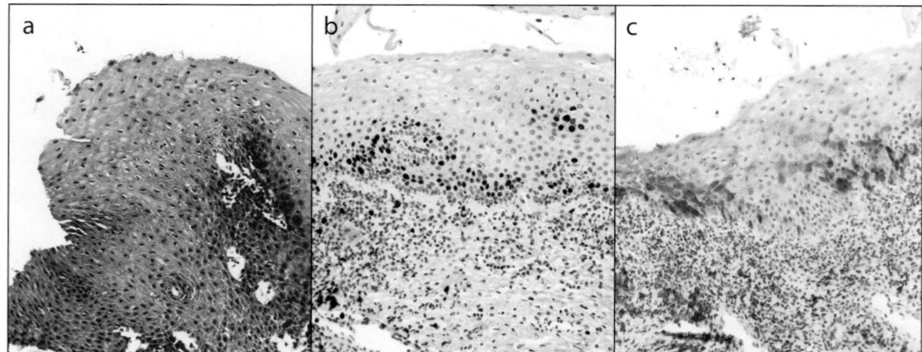

i30.15 **a** Another case equivocal for CIN 1. This case was positive for HPV by the hybrid capture method and also demonstrated focal suprabasal staining for Ki-67

b and **c** positive staining for p63, confirming the presence of a subtle CIN 1.

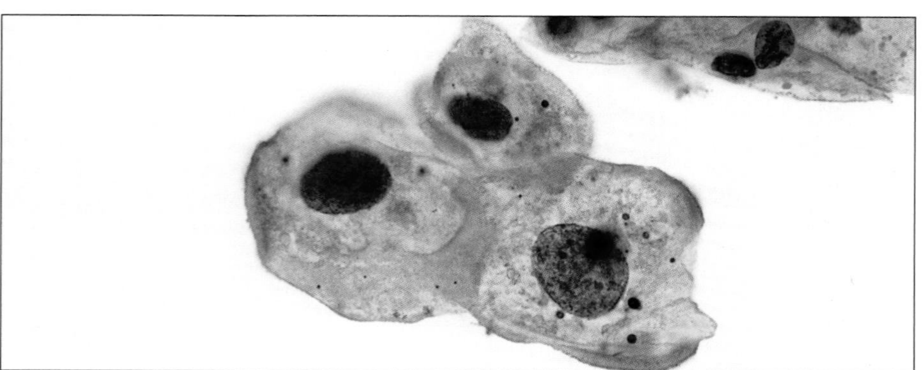

i30.16 Mild dysplasia, CIN 1, LSIL. Perhaps unexpectedly, the largest nuclei occur in mild dysplasia; however, cytoplasm is relatively abundant. Therefore, the N/C ratio, a measure of cell maturity, is low.

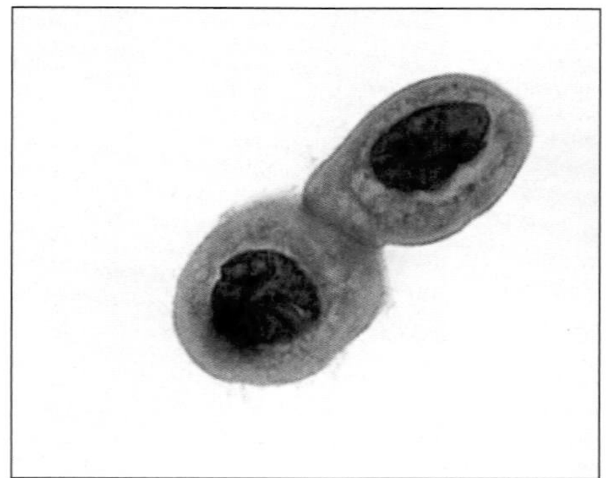

i30.17 CIN 2, HSIL.

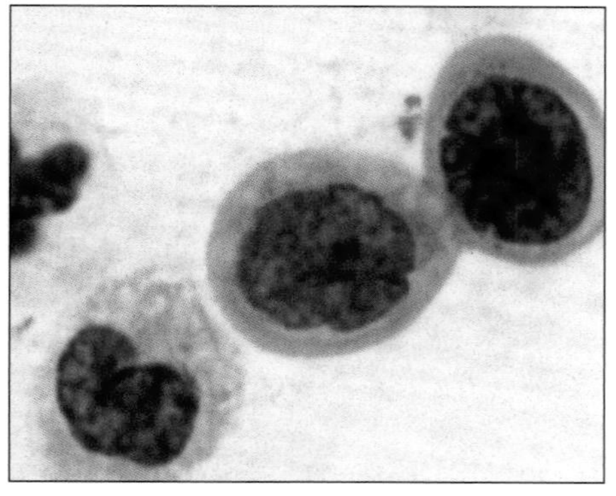

i30.18 Severe dysplasia, CIN 3, HSIL. High-grade dysplastic cells can be small, and difficult to spot, and difficult to interpret once spotted. They can mimic ordinary immature squamous metaplasia or even histiocytes.

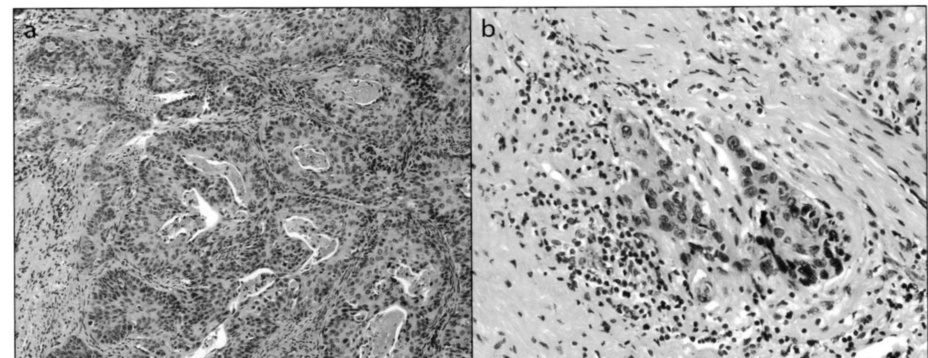

i30.19 **a** Invasive squamous cell carcinoma of the cervix with confluent clusters of neoplastic squamous cells

b Invasive squamous cell carcinoma of the cervix with irregularly shaped clusters of cells and stromal desmoplasia

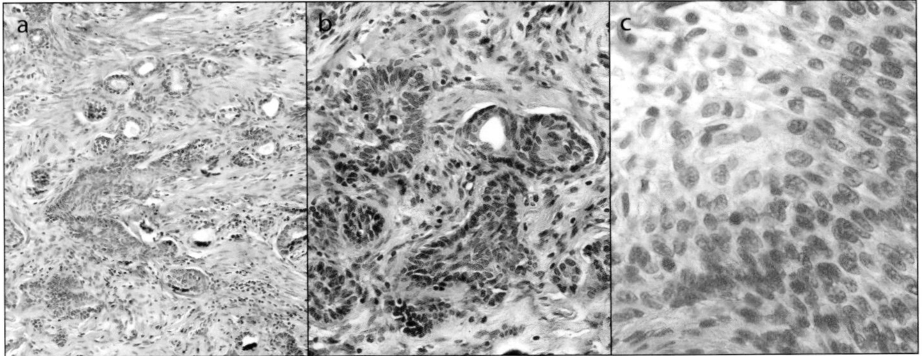

i30.20 **a** Adenoid basal carcinoma of the cervix with small clusters of tumor cells with a basaloid appearance
b A higher-power view of the same case as in i30.20a, illustrating the low nuclear grade and the occasional pseudoglandular structures

c A high-grade CIN associated with the adenoid basal carcinoma illustrated in i30.20a and i30.20b

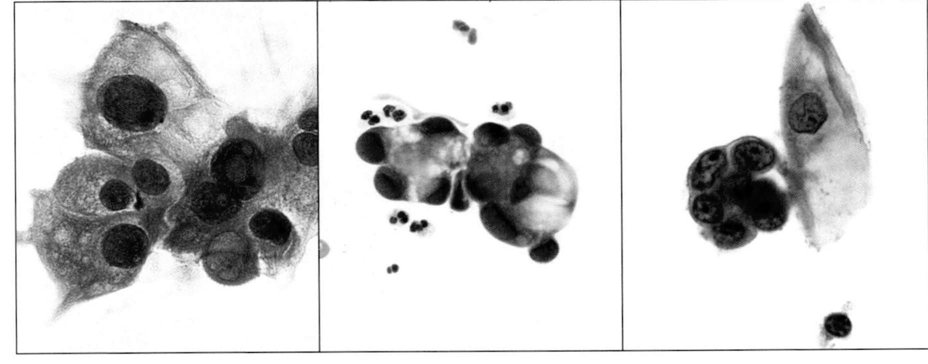

i30.21 Atypical glandular cells and atypical squamous cells may be nearly indistinguishable on a Pap smear because there is no opportunity to assess the architectural context of an atypical cell.

i30.22 **a-c** 2 different cases of low-grade endocervical dysplasia. Note the obvious nuclear enlargement and diminution of cytoplasm (this being particularly evident in **b** and **c**, where the process involves some, but not all of the gland), but at the same time, the nuclei are not strikingly pleomorphic and nuclear stratification is relatively minimal.

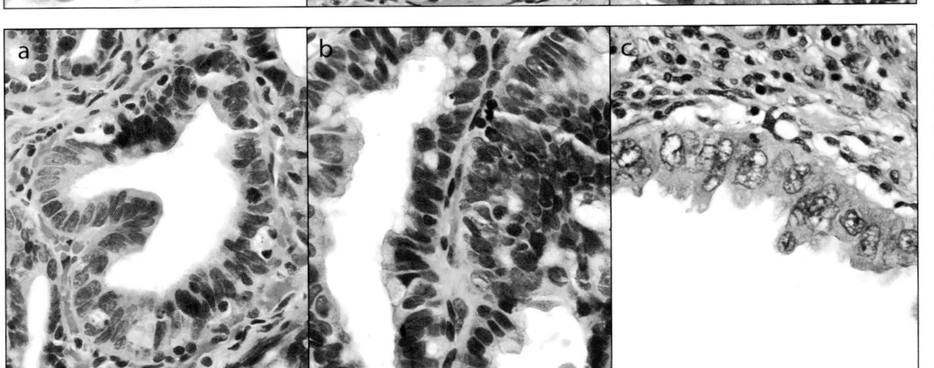

i30.23 **a-c** High-grade endocervical dysplasia/adenocarcinoma in situ. There is extensive nuclear enlargement, variability, and stratification.

Particularly in **c**, there is a vesicular chromatin pattern reminiscent of that seen in colonic adenomatous polyps with high-grade dysplasia.

ISBN 978-089189-5886

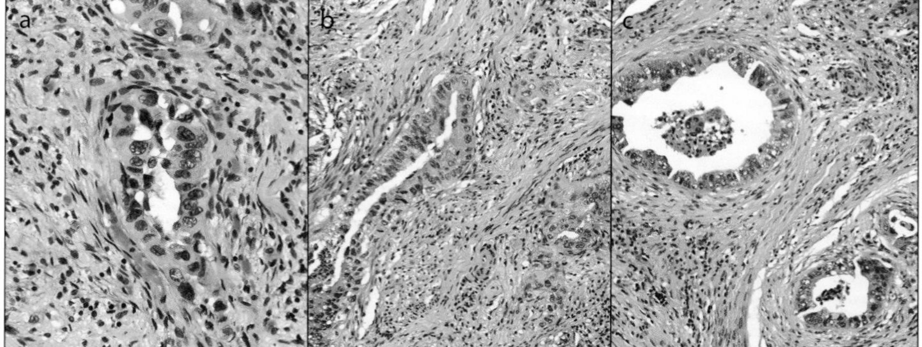

i30.24 **a** Nuclear pleomorphism in an invasive endocervical adenocarcinoma
b An invasive endocervical adenocarcinoma with complete loss of normal architecture and a haphazard infiltration
c Stromal desmoplasia surrounding 2 glands in invasive endocervical adenocarcinoma

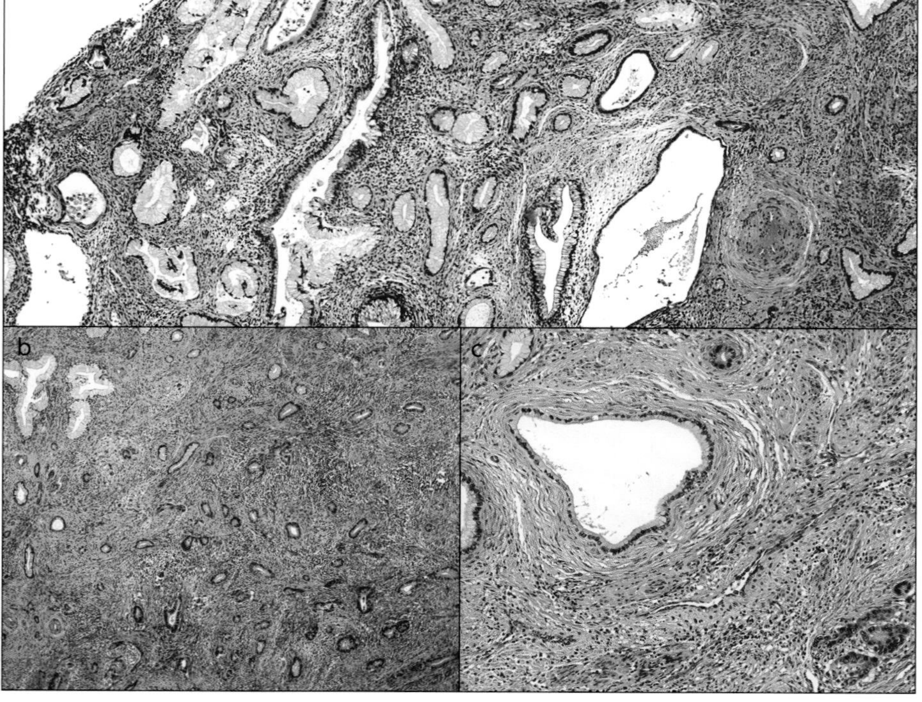

i30.25 **a** Minimal deviation adenocarcinoma of the endocervix. The endocervical epithelium near the surface, at the upper left, appears unremarkable. At the mid and lower right portions of the photograph, smaller glands can be discerned.
b The same case as in i30.25a. This field is immediately below the field photographed in i30.25a and illustrates that the small gland that were seen in i30.25a continue to infiltrate deeply into the wall of the cervix. Note the loss of a lobular pattern.
c A high-power view of minimal deviation adenocarcinoma. All of the epithelial structures in this photograph are neoplastic, but those at the upper left have a nearly normal appearance, causing this entity to be easily missed if it is not closely examined in its entirety. Note the irregular outline of the large gland in the upper left and the stromal desmoplasia surrounding it. These features, plus its very deep location within the wall, suggest the diagnosis. However, as is typical of this entity, smaller glands that are more clearly malignant are adjacent to the benign-appearing gland. Attention to deep penetration, a stromal reaction, and associated glands that are clearly atypical are the keys to diagnosis.

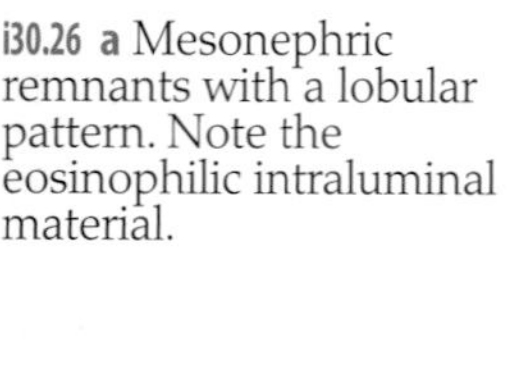

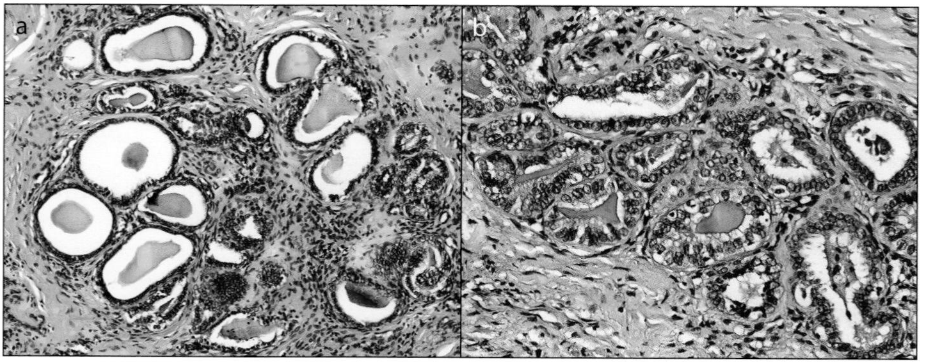

i30.26 **a** Mesonephric remnants with a lobular pattern. Note the eosinophilic intraluminal material.
b Mesonephric remnants with mild nuclear atypia that may overlap that seen in a minimal deviation adenocarcinoma. The eosinophilic intraluminal material and the vaguely lobular pattern are helpful, but in an out of context comparison, these glands may resemble those found in minimal deviation adenocarcinoma.

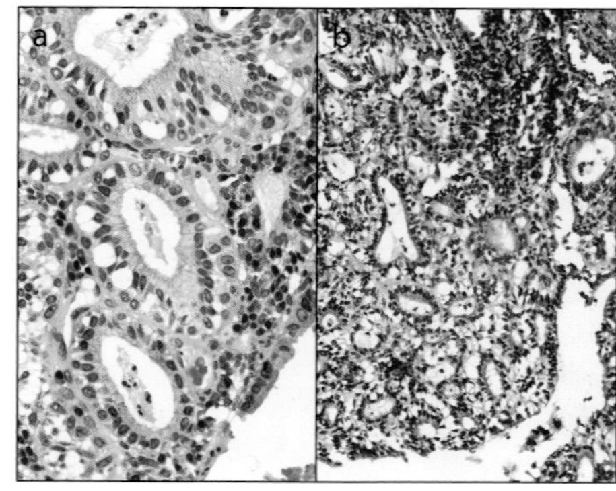

i30.27 **a** Microglandular hyperplasia in a cervical biopsy. The glands are very crowded, but the nuclei are small, basal, and uniform.
b Microglandular hyperplasia in endocervical curettings

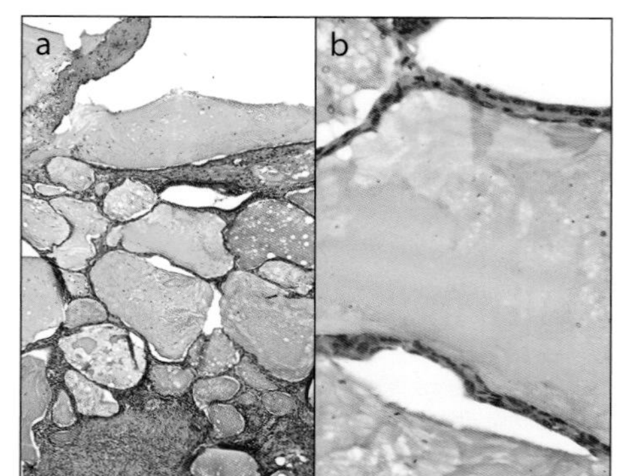

i30.28 **a** Tunnel clusters consisting of numerous dilated glands, generally close to the surface
b A higher-power view of the same case as in i30.28a, illustrating the very innocuous nuclei and the amphophilic mucinous material

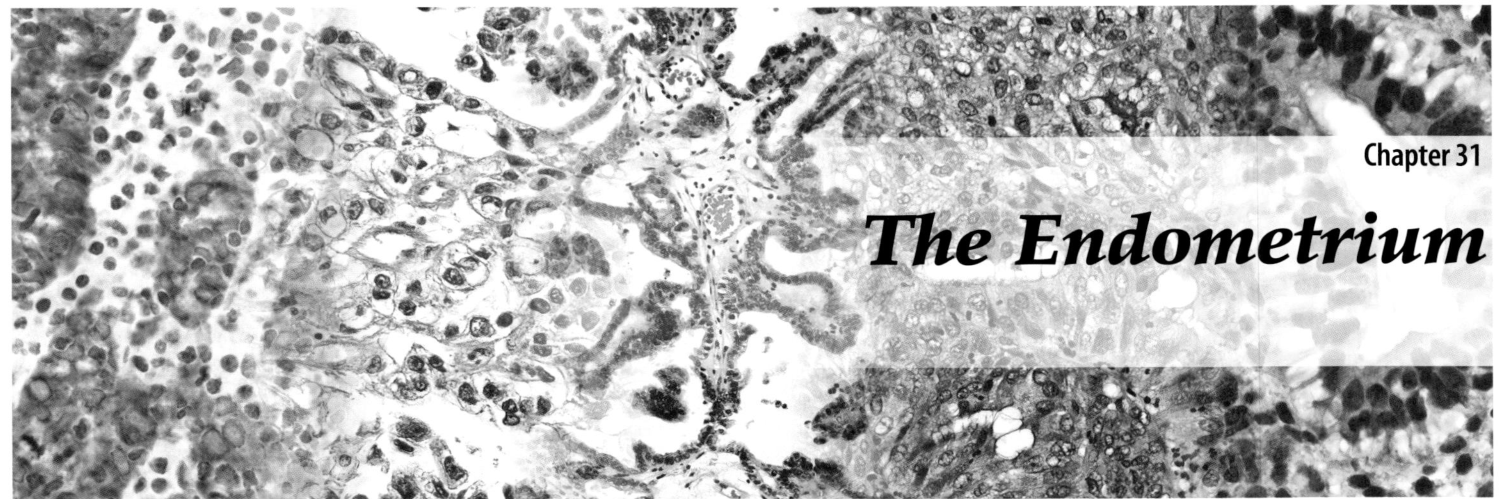

Normal Histology and Dating

The normal endometrium consists of a basal layer that does not cycle and a more superficial cycling layer. The ratio of glands to stroma in the normal proliferative endometrium is approximately 1 (ie, about equal volumes are occupied by glandular or stromal tissue).

The appearance of the endometrium is often modified by exogenous hormones, but classically, normal proliferative glands are straight, small, and round i31.1. Their nuclei are pseudostratified and mitoses are readily seen i31.2. Proliferative phase stromal cells have minimal cytoplasm and occasional mitoses. It is rarely productive to attempt any specific dating of proliferative endometrium because clinically important abnormalities of dating concern the secretory phase. Normal proliferative glands have both pseudostratification and mitoses. Weakly proliferative glands may have slightly pseudostratified nuclei, but no mitoses to speak of i31.3a, while atrophic endometrium has neither pseudostratification nor mitoses, and often cystically dilated glands i31.3b [PMID15280405].

Dating of secretory endometrium is important in the diagnosis and treatment of some patients with infertility. Dating can be based on the days since onset of bleeding (day 1 of the menstrual cycle) or can be given as postovulatory days (eg, a sample can be designated as day 24 or postovulatory day 10).

The criteria used to date endometria were published in 1950 [PMID1155504]. Early secretory endometrium may still have occasional mitoses and pseudostratification. The earliest well defined secretory change is subnuclear vacuoles i31.4, but the designation of a sample as early secretory (with the implication that the patient has ovulated) requires distinct, well defined vacuoles in the majority of glands. The presence of occasional subnuclear vacuoles is often misconstrued as early secretory change but does not assure ovulation. Only if the vacuoles are distinct, subnuclear, and are found in the majority of glands should ovulation and secretory phase be assumed. Interval endometrium is a late proliferative endometrium in which there is focal subnuclear vacuolization.

Cytoplasmic vacuoles assume a luminal position (ie, the nuclei move to a basal position, with the vacuoles above them) by postovulatory day 4 and are essentially absent by postovulatory day 6. Whereas proliferative glands are straight, reminiscent of test tubes in a rack, endometrial glands become slightly coiled in the midsecretory period i31.5 and become increasingly coiled in the later secretory stages. Likewise, secretions become evident in the midsecretory period and become progressively more apparent. Instead of the pseudostratification that characterizes the proliferative phase, the glandular nuclei in the mid – and late secretory phase are basal i31.6. During the secretory phase, the arterioles become more coiled (hence, the designation of spiral arterioles) and their walls become thicker.

Stromal cells in the secretory phase acquire progressively more cytoplasm until pseudodecidualization becomes evident on about postovulatory day 10. Pseudodecidualization commences around spiral arterioles i31.7, making these more prominent. The secretory phase stroma also contains granular lymphocytes (formerly thought to be neutrophils), which are CD3–, CD56+ natural killer cells whose precise function is not known, but which are apparently concerned with regulation of implantation [PMID18716934].

In late secretory endometrium, the stroma begins to break up i31.8. During the very late secretory phase, neutrophils begin to enter the endometrium i31.9. Menstrual endometrium is characterized by fragmentation and degeneration in a background of acute inflammation i31.10a, with pyknotic nuclei and fibrin thrombi i31.10b. Residual secretory changes may be evident i31.10c, but are often inconspicuous because of degeneration.

These criteria remain valid, though more recent studies have shown that the most commonly used criteria are not as temporally distinct as was commonly believed and there is considerable interobserver variation in dating, especially in assessing subnuclear vacuoles and pseudodecidual change, making these criteria less clinically useful than is typically appreciated [PMID15136099].

The basal layer of the endometrium does not cycle completely and is therefore not suitable for dating. Basal endometrium typically has a densely cellular stroma. Another clue to its presence in an endometrial sample is that since it does not cycle, the glands of the basal portion are always weakly proliferative, even when a secretory appearance might be expected or other glands in the sample appear different i31.11.

Ideally, dating of the endometrium is performed on a fragment that affords a full-thickness view, but this is often not possible in biopsy and curettage samples. In these samples, optimal dating is done on fragments that are lined by surface

ISBN 978-089189-5886

epithelium, as these fragments have the greatest likelihood of complete cycling.

The common pitfalls in dating endometrium are dating samples that have been exposed to exogenous hormones, the use of fragments from the basal portion, and the dating of fragments that are from a polyp. The changes of exogenous hormones are discussed in the next section. The classic changes of a polyp are disorganized glands that are often dilated, a fibrotic stroma, and prominent arterioles that have thicker walls than would be seen at any time in the normal endometrium i31.12. Like basal endometrium, a polyp does not cycle completely and cannot be properly dated.

In addition to an assessment of ovulation and dating, the pathologist is often asked to assess an endometrial sample for dyssynchrony (ie, temporally uneven response to endogenous hormones). Most examples of dyssynchronous endometrium are secondary to exogenous hormones or polyps, but in the rare cases in which there are significant temporal differences in the sample and hormones and polyps are excluded, there may be clinical relevance in the evaluation of dysfunctional uterine bleeding (DUB) or fertility.

Some question if luteal phase defect (also called inadequate luteal phase) is a true entity [PMID15550332]. If it exists, it is defined as a >3-day disparity between the clinical and histologic dates, usually in conjunction with uneven maturation in different areas of the biopsy and a gland-stroma dyssynchrony. Before this diagnosis is made, there should be 2 biopsies obtained at different times during the luteal phase, with assurance that neither biopsy contains basal endometrium or a polyp and that the patient is not on exogenous hormones. There is substantial interobserver variation in the diagnosis of luteal phase defect and the unavoidable subjectivity in dating has likely caused some false positive diagnoses.

In theory, a persistent corpus luteum can be diagnosed by inappropriate progesterone affect in a biopsy taken during the proliferative phase, but again, there is substantial variation among observers, and most such patients are on exogenous hormones.

The Effect of Exogenous Hormones on the Endometrium

Many endometrial samplings that come to the pathologists for DUB involve tissue that has been subjected to exogenous hormones because hormonal treatment is usually given before tissue sampling. The histologic changes caused by oral contraceptives of either a mixed estrogen/progesterone or pure progesterone type are basically similar because in the combined preparations, the changes are fundamentally from the progesterone. The histologic appearance depends on whether the hormones are sequential or combined, and the length of time the patient has been exposed, but in the most common preparations, at the early stages, both glands and stroma may show secretory changes. However, the glands quickly lose their responsiveness to progesterone, and by the time of biopsy, they have a proliferative appearance, while the stroma shows the pseudodecidualization that is characteristic of progesterone effect i31.13a [PMID10757339]. In addition to the gland-stroma dyssynchrony, there is also often a dyssynchrony among individual glands. Glands may have an overall proliferative appearance, but also have small cytoplasmic vacuoles i31.13b.

Estrogen replacement therapy (ERT) has become controversial, and its use is declining. In most patients on ERT, the histologic effects are usually minimal, but the endometrium may be more proliferative than might be expected from the patient's age, and there is some risk of hyperplasia.

As discussed in Chapter 4, estrogen receptor blockade is used in premenopausal patients with estrogen receptor positive breast cancers, while aromatase inhibitors are used in most postmenopausal patients. The histologic effects of either receptor blockade or aromatase inhibitors on the endometrium are usually minimal.

Danazol is a testosterone analogue that is androgenic and antiendometrial, and is occasionally used in the treatment of endometriosis and leiomyomas. The long-term effect of danazol on the endometrium is atrophy [PMID17636649].

Progesterone receptor modulators may also be used to treat leiomyomas or endometriosis. Like oral contraceptives, they may cause dyssynchrony in endometrial biopsies. Mifepristone (RU486) is a progesterone receptor antagonist used for pregnancy interruptions [PMID20102310]. Biopsies show reduced progesterone effect in both glands and stroma [PMID14668004].

Phytoestrogens are plant compounds not yet in widespread clinical use, but which may have beneficial affects both in endometrial carcinoma and bone density [PMID20347861].

Endometritis

Many of the cells previously thought to be neutrophils in the late secretory phase are now known to be granular lymphocytes. Significant numbers of neutrophils are uncommon in the endometrium except during menstruation. The diagnosis of acute endometritis has traditionally been made when there are microabscesses or destruction of glands in endometria that are not menstrual. Now, many feel that the diagnosis can be made by the presence of significant numbers of neutrophils, just as in any other body site, provided that the tissue is not menstrual, the putative neutrophils have been properly identified, and the diagnosis is clinically appropriate i31.14.

Because lymphocytes are normally found in the endometrium and plasma cells have historically been regarded as the only cell type not normally found at any time during the menstrual cycle, the latter cell has traditionally been regarded as both necessary and sufficient for the diagnosis of chronic endometritis—the diagnosis cannot be made without plasma cells, and a single such cell secures the diagnosis. It is now understood that plasma cells are indeed an indication of chronic endometritis in the proper clinical context and are generally required for the diagnosis, especially if there is stromal fibrosis i31.15. But plasma cells are not independently diagnostic of chronic endometritis and are also found other conditions, including disordered endometrium and stromal breakdown secondary to anovulation or hormonal imbalance [PMID17188330]. Moreover, occasional endometrial plasma cells may not be associated with any major clinical findings and may have no significance. If the patient does not have a clinically symptomatic inflammatory condition, occasional plasma cells are unlikely to indicate a significant inflammatory process [PMID15763793, PMID19952932].

If chronic endometritis is a clinical concern, such that identifying plasma cells is likely to have clinical implications, their identification can be assisted by an immunohistochemical stain for syndecan-1 (CD138), a cell surface proteoglycan found on plasma cells and some epithelial cells, since these cells can be easily missed on H&E [PMID15335255]. However, in such a situation, care must be taken to ensure that any plasma cells found are not from the endocervix, and even if endometrial origin is assured, a rare plasma cell in an otherwise unremarkable endometrium is no longer necessarily considered significant.

It is now believed that eosinophils are another cell type that is not generally found in the normal endometrium, and their presence may suggest chronic endometritis in the proper clinical context. In one study, 72% of cases in which plasma cells were identified by immunohistochemistry also had eosinophils [PMID19801162], but neither of these cell types necessarily implies a clinically significant chronic endometritis.

While lymphocytes are certainly commonly found in the endometrium, clearly increased numbers of them, with epithelial infiltration or lymphoid follicles, especially in the presence of a fibrotic stroma and a compatible clinical presentation, can establish the diagnosis without plasma cells, or at least elicit a search for plasma cells by immunohistochemistry for CD138, and in such cases, even a rare plasma cell secures a diagnosis of chronic endometritis.

Chronic endometritis, if properly diagnosed, is a manifestation of pelvic inflammatory disease (PID). Classically, about 1/4 of cases of chronic endometritis are associated with *Chlamydia*, and texts have suggested that *Chlamydia* should be particularly suspected in cases with follicular lymphoid hyperplasia, However, a PCR study found almost no cases of chronic endometritis that were caused by this organism [PMID8892595], underscoring that histology is of little value in elucidating the etiology in most cases of chronic endometritis.

The Endometrium in Dysfunctional Uterine Bleeding

About half of perimenopausal women undergoing endometrial biopsy for DUB will have a dyssynchronous or difficult to date endometrium by the usual criteria [PMID10515672]. Fortunately, dating is not a concern in these situations.

In 2011, the International Federation of Gynecology and Obstetrics (FIGO) designated 9 causes of DUB (which they call abnormal uterine bleeding). The first 4 causes are structural (ie, can be visualized by radiographic methods or histopathology) and are given by the acronym PALM—polyp, adenomyosis, leiomyoma, malignancy and hyperplasia. The last 5 abnormalities are nonstructural and are given by the acronym COEIN—coagulopathy, ovulatory dysfunction, endometrial, iatrogenic, and not yet classified [PMID21345435].

In common practice, the most common cause of DUB that is not related to hyperplasia, neoplasia, inflammation, polyp formation, or adenomyosis is hormonal imbalance, usually from unopposed or incompletely opposed estrogen. DUB is usually indicative of anovulatory or irregularly ovulatory cycles, and is often manifest in the endometrial biopsy in 1 of 2 ways [PMID14581820, PMID8979202]. The first pattern is a breakup of the tissue in the absence of menstruation, with clumps of stroma, as the endometrium breaks down without receiving progesterone stimulation i31.16. This glandular and stromal breakdown is sometimes called breakthrough bleeding. Although the breaking up causes some similarity to menstrual endometrium, the key difference is that the glands in menstruation have more acute inflammation, and often have secretory changes, since the secretory phase has just been completed, but in this form of DUB, acute inflammation is minimal unless there is a superimposed acute endometritis, and the glands show no evidence of any secretory effect.

The second pattern seen in incompletely opposed estrogen is disordered proliferative endometrium. Disordered proliferative endometrium has a normal 1:1 gland to stroma ratio and is in no way hyperplastic. The glands are lined by pseudostratified epithelium with mitotic activity, just as in the normal proliferative endometrium. The only difference is that gland development is not uniform, causing some glands to have a distorted outline and contour i31.17a, i31.17b. For example, some glands are cystically dilated while are weakly proliferative. Disordered proliferative endometrium simply consists of glands that have an unusual contour, reflecting dyssynchronous growth. It is generally advisable to diagnose disordered proliferative endometrium with caution in the presence of a polyp, as glandular distortion is a feature of polyps i31.17c.

Endometrial Metaplasia

There are numerous forms of metaplasia in the endometrium [PMID7212146, PMID21126963], including squamous, eosinophilic (in which the cytoplasm acquires a deep pink color), ciliated (or tubal), mucinous, clear cell, and papillary syncytial metaplasia. Squamous metaplasia results in morules, balls of benign squamous cells i31.18 that if florid, may mimic a squamous carcinoma or a squamous component of an adenocarcinoma i31.18b. Eosinophilic metaplasia causes the endometrium to resemble apocrine metaplasia of the breast i31.19. Ciliated metaplasia causes the epithelium to resemble that of the fallopian tube and is associated with slight nuclear enlargement i31.20. It is customary to regard the presence of cilia as metaplasia, but because the epithelia of the uterus and fallopian tube are not perfectly demarcated and may slightly intermingle, it is unclear if this is a true metaplasia (ie, a change in the type of epithelium after birth). Clear cell metaplasia, if pronounced, may rarely cause a resemblance to clear cell carcinoma.

Papillary syncytial metaplasia (not to be confused with papillary immature metaplasia of the cervix) is the most complex of the endometrial metaplasias. It is characterized by a papillary process, without fibrovascular cores, and endometrial epithelium that often has eosinophilic cytoplasm or squamous differentiation i31.21. The name derives from the frequent squamous metaplasia associated with the papillations.

Endometrial Hyperplasia

Endometrial hyperplasia is the endometrial counterpart to the intraepithelial neoplasia that occurs in many sites. Although some may accept a rare case of secretory hyperplasia, for all practical purposes, any hyperplasia must occur in a proliferative endometrium, as the sequence of

ISBN 978-089189-5886

hyperplasia⊠carcinoma is driven by estrogen. Endometrial hyperplasia can be manifest as either a glandular crowding or as nuclear atypia. It is now agreed that the latter finding is more important, and the World Health Organizaton (WHO) classification reflects this [Tavassoli ISBN978-9283224129].

Simple hyperplasia can be diagnosed when the gland to stroma ratio exceeds the normal 1:1, but not markedly, there is no outpouching or infolding of the epithelium, and no nuclear atypia i31.22a-c. Simple hyperplasia may resemble disordered proliferative endometrium and may be found in association with the latter entity.

Appreciable glandular crowding, resulting in a gland to stroma ratio of 3:1 or greater, combined with outpouching or infolding of the epithelium, establishes the diagnosis of complex (also called adenomatous) hyperplasia i31.23a, i31.23b. In uncomplicated complex hyperplasia, the glandular nuclei are only slightly larger than those of normal glands and maintain the same mild degree of chromatin clumping. As is the case for glandular nuclei in normal endometrium, they are usually somewhat elongated, without vesicular chromatin, and without large nucleoli. There may be mild nuclear stratification in complex hyperplasia, but this is also seen in normal proliferative endometrium. Likewise, there may be slight nuclear enlargement relative to normal endometrium, but these findings do not indicate atypical hyperplasia. The chromatin in complex hyperplasia, like that in the normal proliferative gland, has little demarcation of chromatin and parachromatin i31.23c.

Although complex hyperplasia does not carry the same degree of significance as atypical hyperplasia, it may be accompanied by foci of atypical hyperplasia or even adenocarcinoma, that have not been sampled. Moreover, the natural history of endometrial hyperplasia has not been completely clarified and interobserver reproducibility is poor in the assessment of nuclear atypia in hyperplasia [PMID18347507]. For this reason, when complex hyperplasia is encountered, it is prudent to comment that a more significant process cannot be excluded.

A common problem is that endometrial polyps often have mild glandular crowding i31.24a, i31.24b, the significance of which cannot be assessed because there is no way of knowing if the crowding is confined to the polyp, in which case no further therapy may be needed, or if it is also found in other areas.

The addition of nuclear atypia to the histologic picture of complex hyperplasia allows the diagnosis of atypical hyperplasia, also called complex (or adenomatous) hyperplasia with atypia. In atypical hyperplasia, the ratio of glands to stroma is 3:1 or greater, as is the case for complex hyperplasia, but the nuclei are larger and more pleomorphic, with a more vesicular chromatin pattern and occasional nucleoli i31.25a-d [PMID19098463]. Roughly speaking, the nuclei in atypical hyperplasia should resemble those in a colonic adenomatous polyp with severe dysplasia, demonstrating once again the general principle that in many sites, adenocarcinoma-directed dysplasia is characterized by glandular cells with enlarged nuclei, a vesicular chromatin pattern, and at least focally prominent nucleoli. 50% of patients who receive a diagnosis of atypical hyperplasia on biopsy or curettage will have carcinoma on hysterectomy [PMID19285814], making a comment that a more significant process cannot be excluded essential.

Very rarely, one will encounter endometria that have severely atypical nuclei, but lack the increased gland-to-stroma ratio, infoldings, and outpouchings of a complex hyperplasia. These endometria appear to have "skipped" a stage and progressed directly to atypical hyperplasia. In these rare and problematic situations, a diagnosis of endometrial atypia of uncertain malignant potential seems prudent. Likewise, one may rarely encounter a situation in which there is no significant nuclear atypia, but there is more worrisome and pronounced glandular crowding and architectural distortion than is seen in most cases of complex hyperplasia. Although there is no uniform consensus on these rare cases, again, the designation of uncertain malignant potential seems reasonable.

Recognizing that it is nuclear appearance and not architecture that carries malignant potential, and further recognizing that atypical hyperplasia and adenocarcinoma are nearly impossible to distinguish on a biopsy or curetting, a 2-tiered system has been proposed. In this system, simple and complex hyperplasia are combined if there is no atypia because increased glandular density, with epithelial budding and outpouchings, does not independently confer significant malignant potential. Atypical hyperplasia and well differentiated adenocarcinoma are combined because of their similar histologic appearance and biologic potential. This simpler 2-tiered system is in fundamental agreement with the WHO classification and has been shown to be more reproducible among observers [PMID18580308]. However, it is unclear if it offers any advantages over the existing system if both the pathologist and the clinician understand that the important breakpoint occurs with the diagnosis of atypical hyperplasia, not complex hyperplasia. The other difficulty with a 2-tiered system is that some feel that complex hyperplasia without atypia, though clearly not as significant as atypical hyperplasia, represents a further step in the progression towards carcinoma and should not be conflated with simple hyperplasia, which is clearly innocuous. There is also some support for the terminology of endometrial intraepithelial neoplasia (EIN) for premalignant endometrial conditions, reflecting the growing preference for the term "intraepithelial neoplasia" for preinvasive lesions in a variety of body sites, but this nomenclature has not been generally adopted [PMID18726114].

Endometrial Adenocarcinoma

The common form of endometrial adenocarcinoma is the endometrioid form, leading to the confusing and seemingly redundant designation of endometrioid endometrial adenocarcinoma or endometrial adenocarcinoma of the endometrioid type. This type of endometrial adenocarcinoma can be diagnosed when there is atypical hyperplasia and either a desmoplastic stromal reaction i31.26a or a confluent crowding of glands without intervening stroma i31.26b [Tavassoli ISBN978-9283224129, PMID15944963]. It is generally not productive to make a diagnosis of endometrial adenocarcinoma in situ. There will be unavoidable cases in which it is not possible on biopsy or curettage material to definitively distinguish between an atypical hyperplasia and an endometrial adenocarcinoma. In these cases, I recommend reporting the findings as "atypical hyperplasia/cannot exclude adenocarcinoma," and defer the definitive diagnosis until hysterectomy. Although young patients with atypical hyperplasia, or even a well differentiated carcinoma, may rarely be managed with progestational agents for a sufficient time to permit childbearing, these are exceptional and temporary situations, and a hysterectomy will generally follow the diagnosis of either atypical hyperplasia or well differentiated carcinoma, obviating the need for a definitive distinction on limited material. Even in cases where progestational agents are temporarily used to permit childbearing, the distinction between atypical hyperplasia and well differentiated adenocarcinoma is unlikely to influence that therapy.

The FIGO system of classification of endometrial adenocarcinomas was developed in 1988, last revised in 2009, and now includes staging criteria as well as grading guidelines [PMIS99047115, PMID21508690]. In a FIGO grade 1 carcinoma, 95% or more of the neoplastic cells are engaged in obvious gland formation, and no more than 5% of the neoplastic cells have another growth pattern, such as solid. Grade 2 carcinomas have between 6 and 50% of the tumor in a solid growth pattern i31.27. Care should be taken not to consider areas of squamous metaplasia as solid areas, as these cells are not neoplastic. A grade 3 tumor occurs if >50% of the neoplastic cells fail to form glands i31.28. FIGO allows for an increase of 1 grade (ie, FIGO 2 to FIGO 3) for "notable nuclear atypia" i31.29.

Some have advocated replacing the 3-tiered FIGO system with a 2-tiered, low-grade-high-grade classification in which a high-grade adenocarcinoma must have 2 of the following 3 features: >50% solid areas, infiltrative growth pattern, and necrosis [PMID10976693]. This binary classification system is potentially more reproducible and may prove to be of benefit, but it is not currently in general use.

An extreme paucity of glands or a very high nuclear grade requires the exclusion of a fundamentally different type of carcinoma, such as a neuroendocrine carcinoma, by immunohistochemical stains. Poorly differentiated adenocarcinomas may demonstrate areas in which there is virtually a small cell carcinoma appearance, and if a neuroendocrine component is identified by immunohistochemistry, the report should document the presence of both patterns.

In endometrial adenocarcinomas, the presence or absence of endocervical involvement and the depth of myometrial invasion must be documented. Assessing invasion of the myometrium can be difficult because the normal endometrial-myometrial junction is irregular. Consequently, a noninvasive carcinoma may appear invasive because tumor cells are found below the apparent endometrial-myometrial junction. A basement membrane stain, such as PAS or an immunohistochemical stain for laminin or collagen type 4 may help in difficult cases.

Another problem is that endometrial carcinomas may involve areas of adenomyosis, thus appearing deep in the myometrium, but this does not constitute invasion. When carcinoma involves a focus of adenomyosis, there will be normal endometrial stroma intermingled with the atypical epithelial cells i31.30, whereas stroma is absent in true invasion i31.31. In addition, though the myometrium may have a hyperplastic response around a focus of adenomyosis, a true desmoplastic (ie, densely fibrotic) reaction around a problematic focus suggests invasive carcinoma [PMID17413976]. In questionable situations, it is reasonable to favor a greater degree of invasion in high-grade carcinomas and a lesser degree of invasion in low-grade carcinomas.

There are different conventions for reporting the depth and degree of myometrial invasion. The FIGO staging uses the inner and outer half, while others divide the myometrium into thirds. Still others report the depth in millimeters. It is probably wise to report depth in millimeters, as well as percent of myometrial thickness. This allows the reader of the report to quickly understand the situation, whatever system he or she may be accustomed to.

Although the molecular changes in the progression of hyperplasia to carcinoma are not well described, loss of immunohistochemical staining for the product of the tumor suppressor gene *PTEN* is associated with hyperplasia and there is further loss of staining in carcinoma [PMID19930726]. However, neither the sensitivity nor specificity of this stain is sufficient for clinical utility.

Microsatellite instability (MSI), though associated with colon carcinomas in hereditary nonpolyposis colon cancer syndrome (Lynch syndrome), is also found in approximately 25% of endometrial adenocarcinomas, and 40-60% of patients with Lynch syndrome will develop an endometrial carcinoma [PMID19659756]. As discussed in Chapter 46, excellent immunohistochemical surrogate testing can be performed, primarily with antibodies to DNA mismatch repair enzymes, such as MLH1 and MSH2. Loss of nuclear staining is good evidence of MSI [PMID17460459]. Immunohistochemistry for mismatch repair enzymes should be considered in high-grade endometrial adenocarcinomas that occur in younger women [PMID19898223].

Unusual Types of Endometrial Adenocarcinoma

There are a number of unusual forms of endometrial adenocarcinoma [Tavassoli ISBN978-9283224129, PMID19078929, PMID15096727] but only a few are discussed here. The term "malignant mixed Mullerian tumor" is falling out of favor, and these neoplasms are better referred to as carcinosarcoma or, even better, as carcinoma with metaplastic features or carcinoma with sarcomatous metaplasia. In most cases, evidence of both epithelial and mesenchymal components is apparent on H&E study i31.32a. Occasionally, these neoplasms may have a paucity of epithelial elements and may initially appear to be a pure sarcoma i31.32b, but the golden rule of sarcomas in organs applies—an apparent sarcoma in an organ is much more likely to be a sarcomatoid carcinoma than a true sarcoma. Evidence of both epithelial and mesenchymal differentiation is required for the diagnosis. Vimentin positivity is the rule and is supportive of the diagnosis, but because endometrial adenocarcinomas of the usual type are usually vimentin positive [PMID16648864], the identification of this protein does not establish a diagnosis of carcinosarcoma. In addition to the epithelial component, there must also be areas that, if removed from the tumor under study, have an appearance that would normally be diagnostic of sarcoma. Heterologous elements are often seen i31.32c, and their presence in conjunction with an epithelial component is essentially diagnostic.

The uterine papillary serous carcinoma (UPSC) has papillations with well developed fibrovascular cores **i31.33a**. The nuclei are of high grade **i31.33b**, and there is often tufting of nuclei, resulting in small mini-papillations **i31.33c**, **i31.33d**. This tumor is always high grade and aggressive [PMID18928665]. UPSC is morphologically indistinguishable from ovarian serous carcinoma. While primary ovarian serous carcinomas are reported to be positive for WT1 in about 90% of cases, and primary endometrial serous carcinomas are negative in 80% of cases [PMID14764054], the 2 neoplasms are essentially also indistinguishable by immunohistochemistry. The diagnosis of uterine UPSC is based on the finding of normal ovaries, and therefore requires either an operative or radiographic assessment.

Otherwise routine endometrioid carcinomas may have a focal papillary component that simulates a UPSC [PMID15096727], but the diagnosis of UPSC requires that the papillary pattern and high nuclear grade are major features. The differential diagnosis of UPSC includes a metastatic ovarian serous carcinoma and a primary villoglandular adenocarcinoma of the endometrium. Villoglandular carcinoma is a variant of common (endometrioid) carcinoma and is usually well differentiated [PMID9808130]. It has delicate fibrovascular cores, rather than the well developed, broad fibrous stalks of UPSC **i31.34a**, and low-grade nuclei, without tufting **i31.34b**.

Like the UPSC, the clear cell carcinoma is always a high-grade neoplasm. Like its ovarian counterpart, it may have several morphologies, and the cytoplasm may be clear or faintly eosinophilic **i31.35a**. In some, but not all cases, many of the nuclei are apically located, as if about to be extruded (so-called hobnail nuclei) **i31.35b**. Many cases of apparent clear cell carcinoma of the endometrium are actually endometrioid (usual) carcinomas with clear cytoplasm [PMID15096727]. In these cases, liberal sampling will usually disclose areas of classic endometrioid appearance. Squamous metaplasia suggests an endometrioid carcinoma.

At the other end of the spectrum from UPSC and clear cell carcinoma, secretory carcinoma is a form of endometrioid carcinoma, with cytoplasmic vacuoles (often subnuclear), causing a resemblance to benign secretory endometrium, that is always low grade [PMID11981113]. Secretory carcinoma is grade 1 by definition and should not be diagnosed even in the presence of extensive cytoplasmic vacuolization if the neoplasm is not well differentiated.

Only the glandular component is malignant in the adenocarcinoma with squamous metaplasia (formerly called adenoacanthoma), which tends to be low grade **i31.36**. In contrast, both components are malignant in the rare, true adenosquamous carcinoma, which tends to be of high grade **i31.37**.

Primary mucinous adenocarcinoma or the endometrium may occur, but many such cases will be a mucinous carcinoma extending upward from the endocervix. Before making the diagnosis of primary mucinous adenocarcinoma of the endometrium in biopsy or curettage material, where the endocervix cannot be examined, it is wise to look for associated endometrial hyperplasia or carcinoma of the more routine type. In difficult situations, one can simply report the presence of a mucinous carcinoma and comment that the primary site can be either endometrium or endocervix. As is the case for the atypical hyperplasia/carcinoma difficulty, a hysterectomy will usually follow and the patient will be well served if a statement concerning the primary site is postponed until then.

Even in a hysterectomy, it may occasionally be difficult to determine if a carcinoma is of endometrial or endocervical origin, in which case it is helpful to recall that most endometrial carcinomas are positive for estrogen and progesterone receptors [PMID16122180], while endocervical adenocarcinomas are usually negative. Whereas almost all endometrial carcinomas are vimentin positive, this protein is rare in endocervical carcinomas. Most endocervical carcinomas stain for CEA, but only a minority of endometrial carcinomas will do so [PMID11781516]. 2/3 of endocervical carcinomas are positive for human papillomavirus, whereas endometrial carcinomas are negative. Diffuse p16 expression is a point for endocervical origin [PMID16462152]. The 5 images in **i31.38** illustrate the identification of a poorly differentiated adenocarcinoma in a cone biopsy as being of endocervical origin.

In pelvic washings or peritoneal fluid obtained at the time of resection of endometrial carcinoma, tumor cells may be very difficult to distinguish from mesothelial cells. As is the case in the pleura, immunohistochemical stains are invaluable. As discussed in Chapter 17, staining of any problematic cells with thrombomodulin, calretinin, cytokeratins 5 and 6, and WT1 suggests mesothelial origin, while staining for adenocarcinoma-associated antigens, especially Bg-8 and B72.3, suggest carcinoma. In addition, the antibody AR-3 stains many endometrial carcinomas, without staining mesothelial cells, and can therefore add to sensitivity of peritoneal washings [PMID10680892].

Endometrial Stromal Proliferations

Differentiating an endometrial stromal tumor from a uterine smooth muscle neoplasm can be problematic. Both endometrial stromal neoplasms and smooth muscle neoplasms may be actin and desmin positive, but traditionally in the uterus, desmin positivity, unless minimal and focal, tends to warrant the classification of a problematic neoplasm as a smooth muscle tumor. H-caldesmon is a smooth muscle marker and is felt by some to be more specific for muscle than actin or desmin [PMID11257619]. CD10 stains essentially all endometrial stromal sarcomas and 20% of leiomyomas. CD10, desmin, and h-caldesmon can be employed as a panel in problematic situations **i31.39a-d** [PMID11914617]. Another marker is oxytocin receptor, which stains muscle and not endometrial stroma [PMID14576480]. If the situation cannot be clarified, it is usually considered an endometrial stromal tumor. One situation in which this distinction is particularly important is that endometrial stromal tumors that infiltrate the myometrium or vessels are malignant, while smooth muscle tumors may infiltrate the myometrium or vessels and still be benign (eg, infiltrating leiomyoma and intravenous leiomyomatosis; discussed in Chapter 32).

Once endometrial stromal histogenesis is assured, endometrial stromal proliferations are divided into benign nodules, low-grade sarcomas, and high-grade sarcomas [Tavassoli ISBN978-9283224129, PMID17365823, PMID17347285]. An endometrial stromal nodule usually has fewer than 10 mitoses per 10 high-power fields (HPFs) and has pushing margins rather than true infiltration i31.39a. Before making this diagnosis, a focus of adenomyosis must be excluded, as some such foci will have so few glands that they appear to be purely stromal. Extensive levels may help by revealing a rare gland.

Once it is established that a proliferation is of endometrial stromal origin and is not adenomyosis, the low-grade endometrial stromal sarcoma has relatively uniform nuclei and is usually mitotically active, with between 10 and 15 mitotic figures per 10 HPFs. Lymphatic or vascular invasion may occur i31.40a, but one may not be fortunate enough to observe this, in which case the key diagnostic feature of the low-grade endometrial stromal sarcoma is its infiltrative borders i31.40b.

The high-grade endometrial stromal sarcoma is perhaps better referred to as an undifferentiated uterine sarcoma or an undifferentiated endometrial sarcoma and is characterized by large numbers of mitoses, invasion, vascular invasion, nuclear pleomorphism, and abnormal mitotic figures i31.41.

Both an endometrial adenofibroma and an adenosarcoma are recognized. Both of these entities have benign glands, but the adenosarcoma is distinguished from the adenofibroma by nuclear atypia in the stroma, stromal hypercellularity (which is particularly evident around glands), and stromal mitoses (>4 mitotic figures per 10 HPFs). Adenosarcomas have an indolent behavior, with recurrence in about 1/4 of cases and only rare metastases [PMID20179434].

In very rare cases, immunohistochemical staining may reveal 2 clearly distinct populations of cells. If this happens, and if each population occupies at least 1/3 of the tumor, the designation of combined smooth muscle-stromal tumor may be used [PMID1710807].

A final point about endometrial stromal tumors is that they may occasionally occur outside of the uterus, such as in a focus of endometriosis [PMID19333789]. The same diagnostic criteria apply, except that because of the exceptionally low probability of a uterine smooth muscle tumor outside of the uterus, the presence of even double positivity for both actin and desmin positivity is still acceptable for the diagnosis of an endometrial stromal tumor in an extrauterine site. The presence of an occasional benign gland in a focus of endometriosis with atypical stroma precludes the diagnosis of a pure stromal sarcoma, but an adenosarcoma is still possible, though diagnosis is usually only made in the uterus.

Core Points for Endometrium

- Dating endometrium: Criteria largely unchanged, but avoid dating fragments from a polyp, from the basal portion of the endometrium, or when the patient has been exposed to exogenous hormones.
  - Exogenous hormones: Usually, glands are weakly proliferative/atrophic, stroma is pseudodecidualized.
- Chronic endometritis: part of pelvic inflammatory disease.
  - Should not be diagnosed simply on the presence of an occasional plasma cell.
  - Plasma cells should be present in substantial numbers and in conjunction with a compatible clinical picture.
  - Obvious lymphocytic attack on glands and stromal fibrosis are additional indicators.
- Dysfunctional uterine bleeding: may have no histologic correlate.
  - Occasionally associated with fragmentation and clumps of stroma, without a menstrual phase, or
  - Disordered proliferative endometrium, in which the glands have distorted contours.
- Simple hyperplasia: modest increase in the normal 1:1 gland-to-stroma ratio without outpouching or infolding of epithelium.
- Complex (adenomatous) hyperplasia: gland-to-stroma ratio of approximately 3:1 with outpouchings and infoldings of epithelium.
- Atypical hyperplasia: significant enlargement or variation of nuclei, especially with a vesicular chromatin pattern and nucleoli.
  - On biopsy and curettage material, often impossible to differentiate atypical hyperplasia from endometrial adenocarcinoma and cannot exclude possibility of carcinoma, even if complex hyperplasia without atypia.
  - When hyperplasia identified on a biopsy or curettage, comment that a more significant process cannot be excluded.
- Endometrial adenocarcinoma: atypical hyperplasia accompanied by significant glandular crowding
  - No intervening stroma or with a desmoplastic stroma.
  - FIGO grading system primarily based on architecture.
    - FIGO 2 carcinoma: 6% of the tumor cells have a solid growth pattern. Do not count squamous metaplasia.
    - FIGO 3 carcinoma: >50% of neoplastic cells do not form glands.
    - Elevation of one grade for "notable nuclear atypia".
  - Describe endocervical involvement and depth of invasion into the myometrium, both as percentage of the thickness of the wall and in millimeters.
  - Involvement of adenomyosis is not invasion.
- 3 endometrial adenocarcinomas are always high-grade: uterine papillary serous carcinoma (UPSC), clear cell carcinoma, and metaplastic carcinoma.
- Villoglandular carcinoma: low-grade mimic of UPSC.
  - Less nuclear pleomorphism and more delicate fibrovascular cores than UPSC.
- IHC may be needed to determine if an adenocarcinoma is of endometrial or endocervical origin.
- Endometrial stromal proliferations: benign stromal nodules, low-grade sarcomas, or high-grade sarcomas.
  - Stromal nodule: well circumscribed, few mitosis.
    - Exclude a gland-poor focus of adenomyosis and a low-grade sarcoma.
  - Low-grade stroma sarcoma: infiltrative.
    - May also have mitotic activity or invade lymphatics.
  - High-grade stromal sarcoma (undifferentiated uterine sarcoma or undifferentiated endometrial sarcoma): appreciable invasion and mitotic activity
    - Often with vascular invasion.
  - IHC may be needed to differentiate an endometrial stromal proliferation from a smooth muscle neoplasm.

ISBN 978-089189-5886

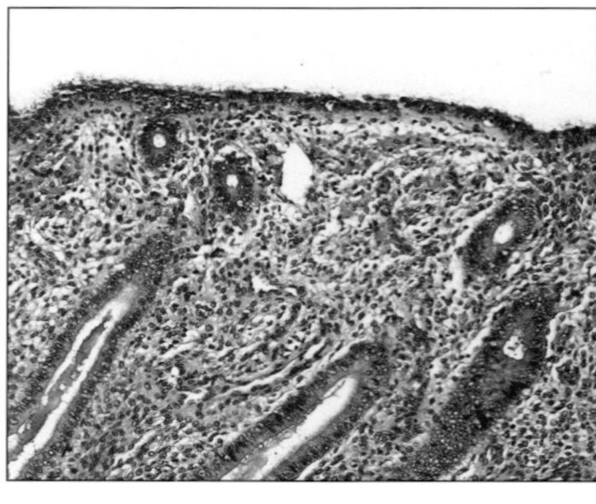

i31.1 Normal proliferative endometrium, with straight, unbranched gland and minimal intraluminal secretions

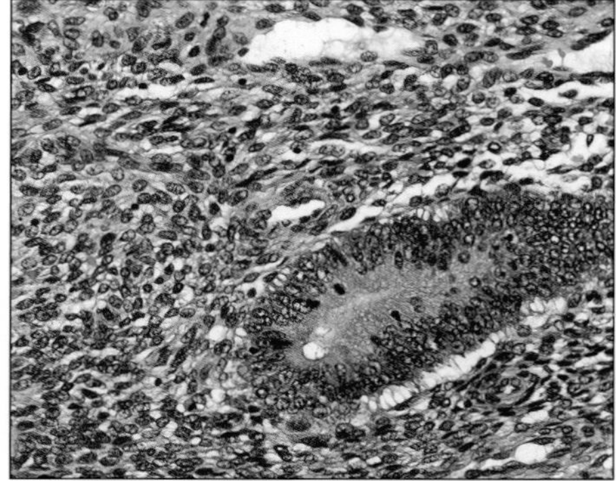

i31.2 A cross section of a normal proliferative gland, demonstrating pseudostratification and mitotic activity

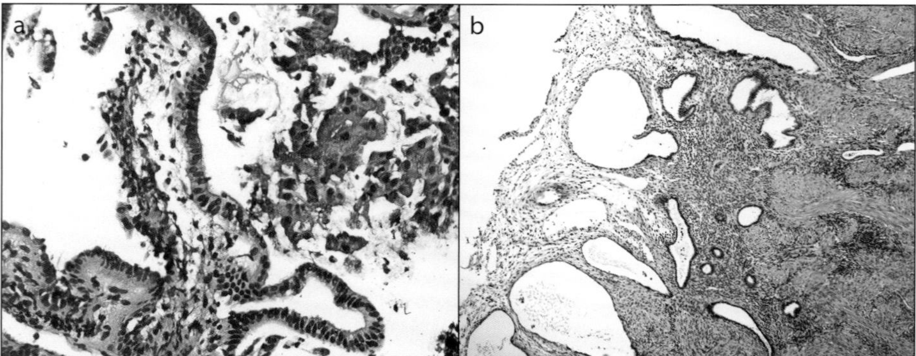

i31.3 **a** Weakly proliferative endometrium with little pseudostratification and no mitotic activity

b Atrophic endometrium with dilated glands

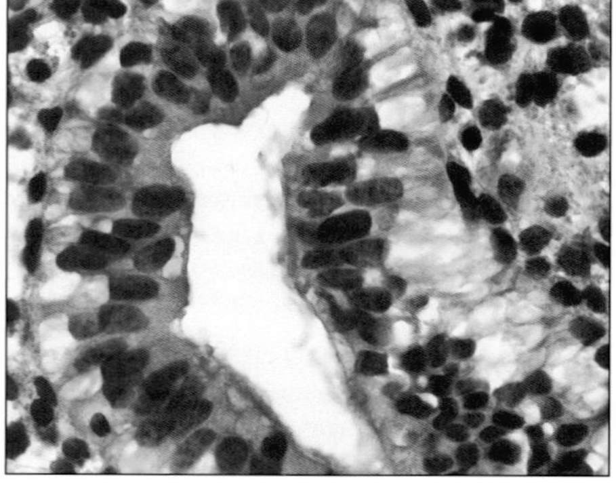

i31.4 Early secretory endometrium with well defined, prominent subnuclear vacuoles

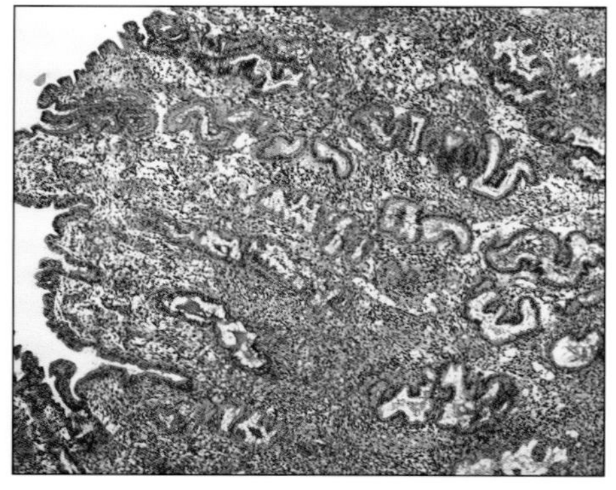

i31.5 Midsecretory endometrium, approximately postovulatory day 10, with coiled glands, intraluminal secretions, and abundant cytoplasm in the stromal cells (pseudodecidualization)

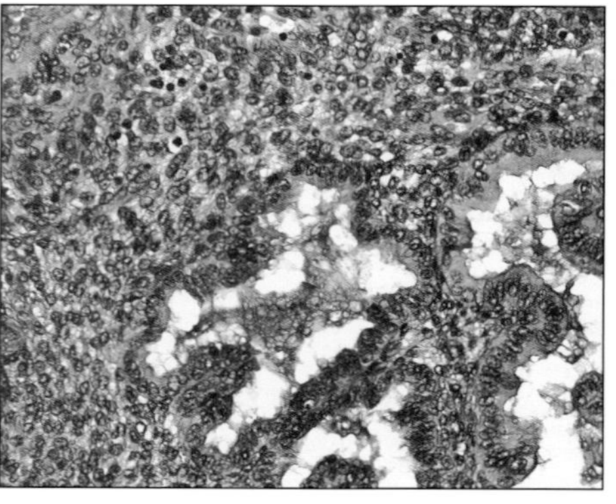

i31.6 A higher-power view of the same case as in i31.5, highlighting the coiled configuration secretory glands, the basally oriented nuclei, and the cytoplasm of the pseudodecidualized stromal cells

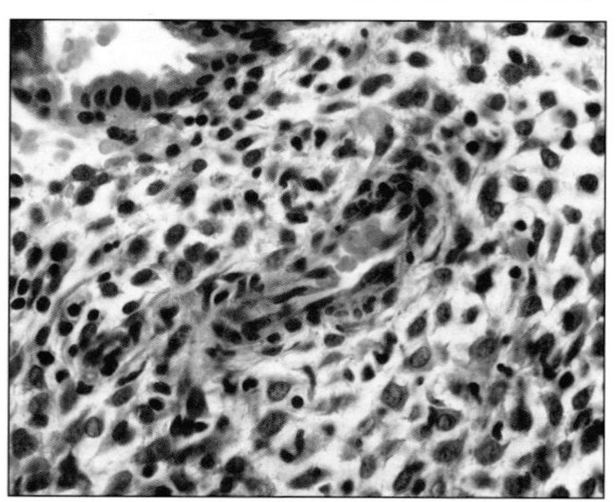

i31.7 A spiral arteriole with incipient pseudodecidualization occurring in the surrounding stromal cells

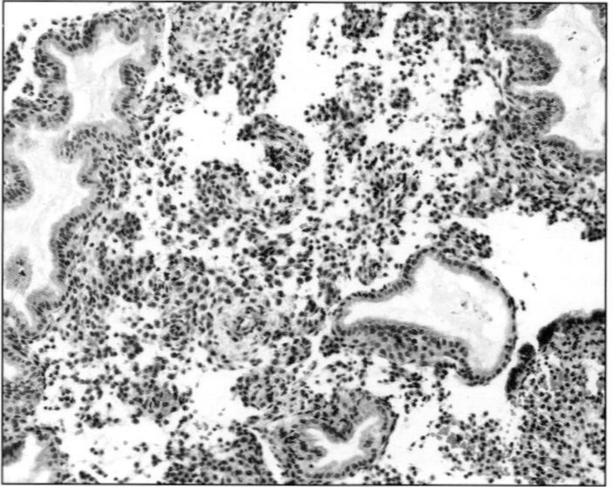

i31.8 Late secretory endometrium beginning to break up, with clumps of stroma

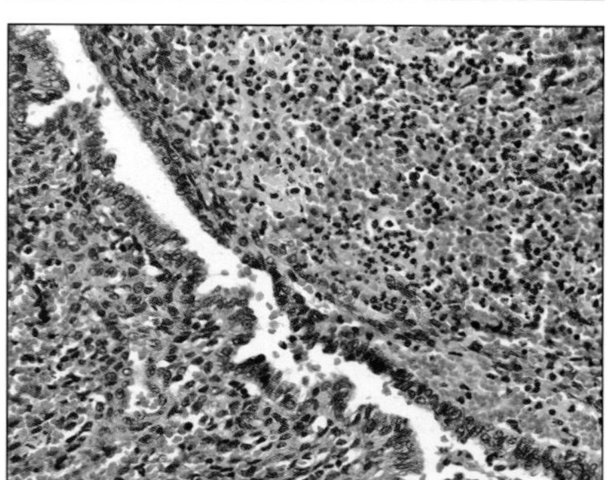

i31.9 Neutrophils in late secretory endometrium

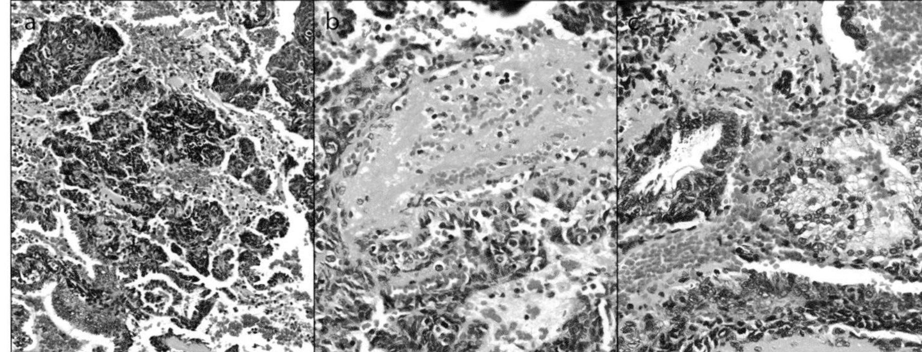

i31.10 **a** Menstrual endometrium with breakup and clumps of stroma
b Menstrual endometrium with fibrin thrombi
c Menstrual endometrium with a small amount of residual secretory endometrium

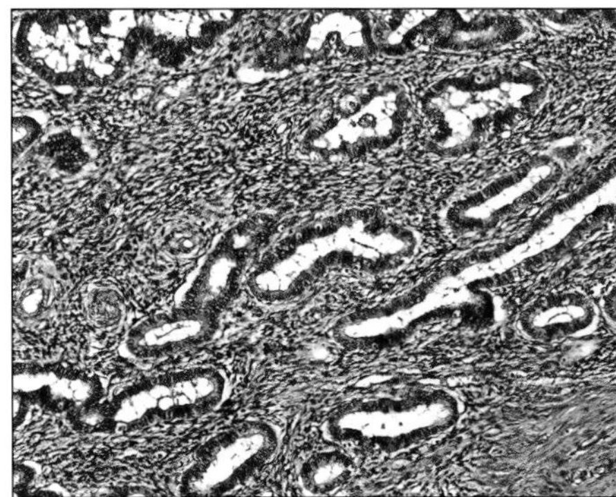

i31.11 Basal endometrium with a cellular stroma and glands that always appear proliferative, at any time in the cycle

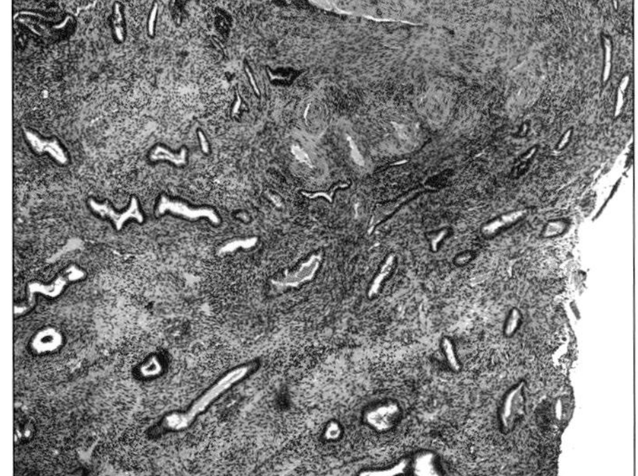

i31.12 An endometrial polyp with fibrous stroma and prominent arterioles, seen in the upper right

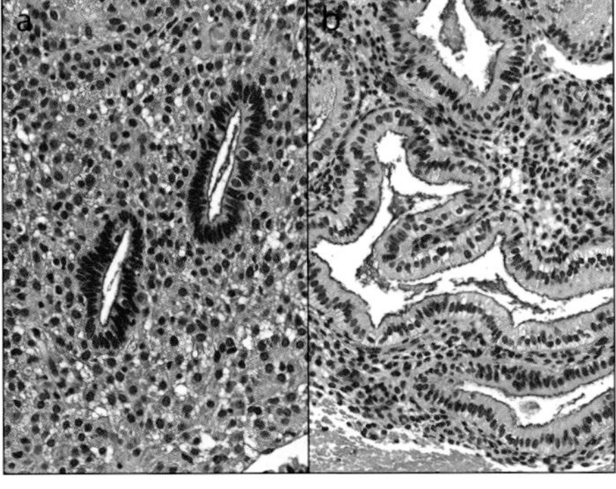

i31.13 **a** Weakly proliferative glands in a pseudodecidualized stroma, the most common morphology of the endometrium in exogenous hormones
b Another example of exogenous hormones with dyssynchrony within individual glands. The glands have delicate subnuclear vacuolization, but the vacuoles are not well enough developed for an early secretory endometrium.

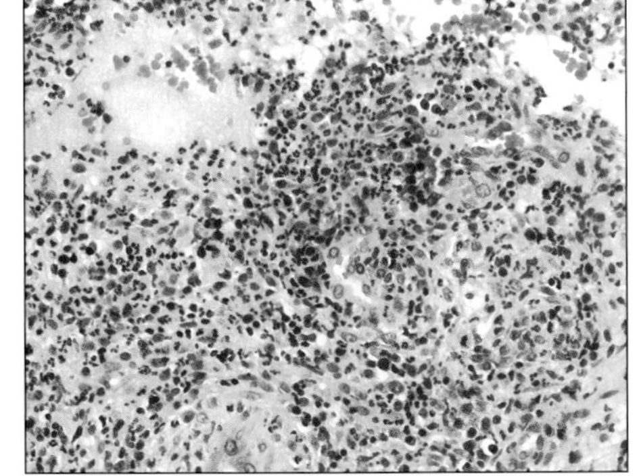

i31.14 Acute endometritis. While neutrophils are a normal part of the menstrual cycle during the late secretory phase, this endometrium has abundant neutrophilic infiltration, damaging the glands, without the breakup that is characteristic of late secretory and menstrual endometrium.

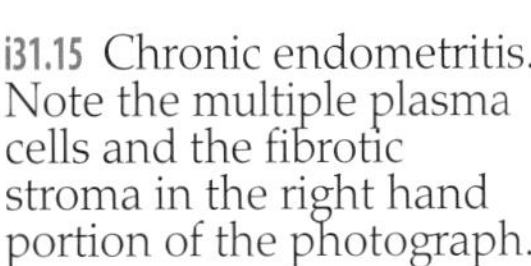

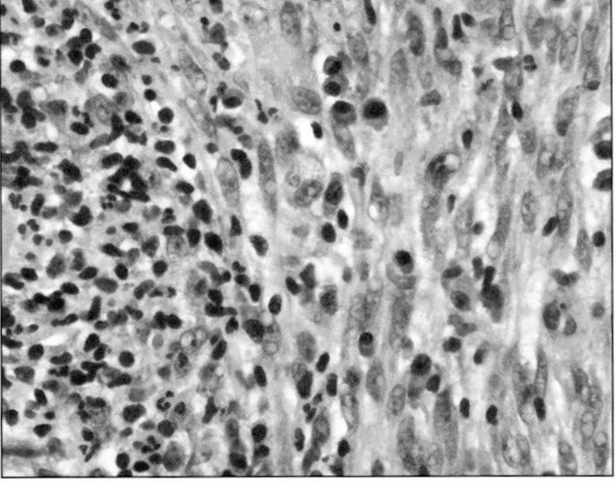

i31.15 Chronic endometritis. Note the multiple plasma cells and the fibrotic stroma in the right hand portion of the photograph.

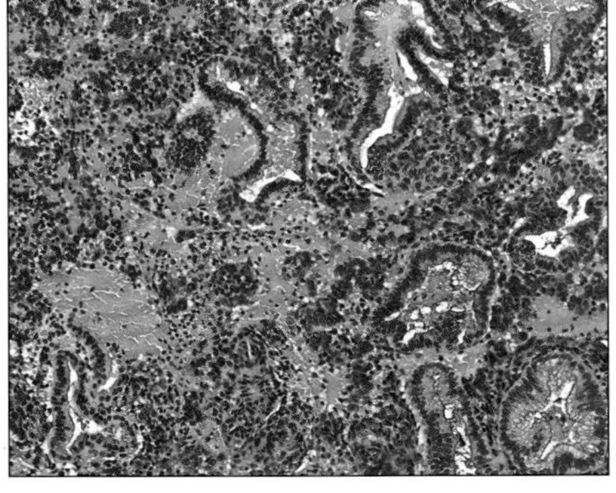

i31.16 Dysfunctional uterine bleeding secondary to incompletely opposed estrogen. This endometrium is breaking down without having passed through a secretory phase. While breakup is also seen in menstrual endometrium, this endometrium has fewer neutrophils, fewer thrombi, and less evident secretory change in the glands than would be expected in normal menstrual endometrium.

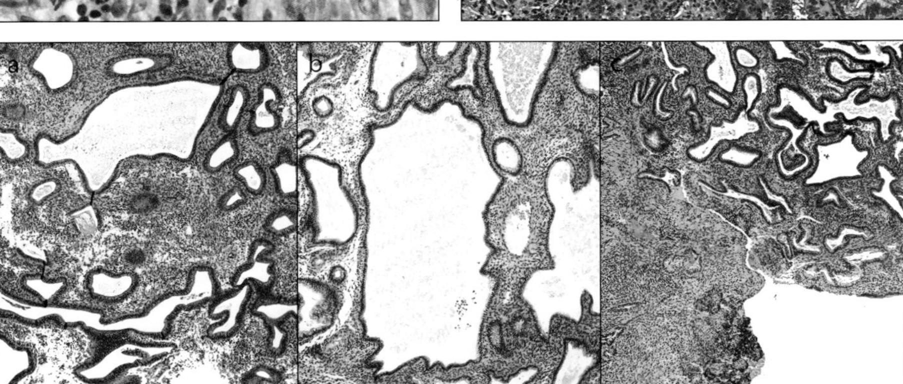

i31.17 **a-b** Disordered proliferative endometrium. The gland-to-stroma ratio is normal at approximately 1:1, but the glands are dilated and have distorted contours instead of the expected sharply defined tubular outlines.
c An endometrial polyp associated with disordered proliferative endometrium

ISBN 978-089189-5886

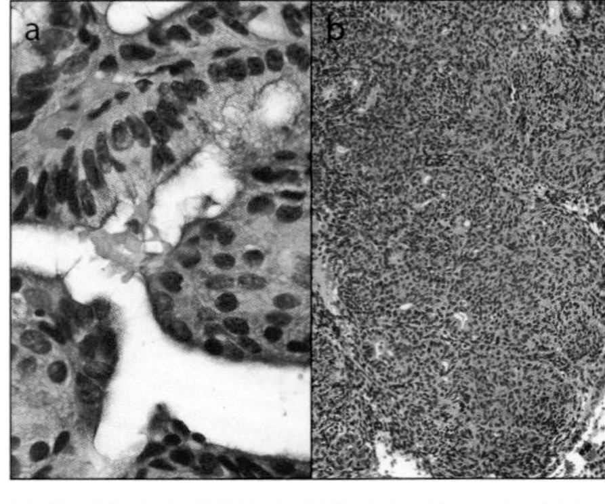

i31.18 **a** Squamous metaplasia in proliferative endometrium (morule formation)
b Florid squamous metaplasia, resulting in a small mass that stands out from the remaining specimen

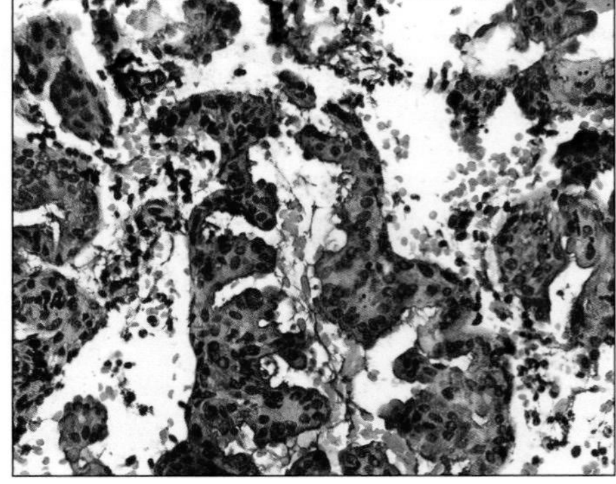

i31.19 Eosinophilic metaplasia in which the individual cells have an increased amount of sharply eosinophilic cytoplasm

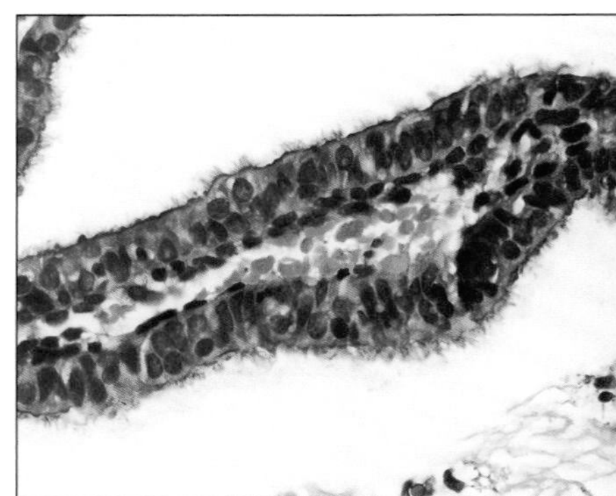

i31.20 Ciliated or tubule metaplasia. Note the prominent cilia.

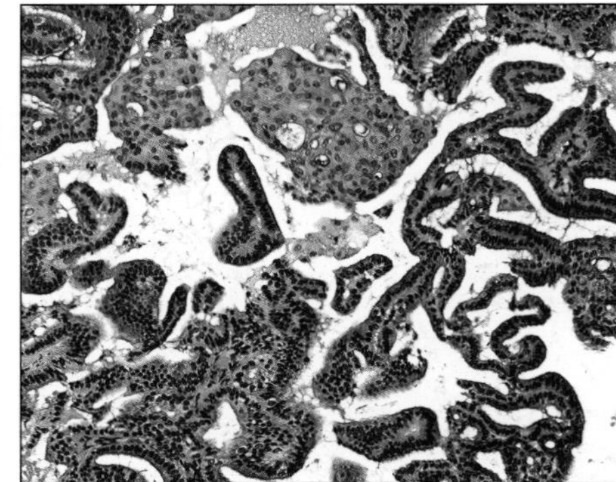

i31.21 Papillary syncytial metaplasia. There are small micropapillations, without well defined cores, associated with squamous metaplasia. Eosinophilic metaplasia is also commonly seen.

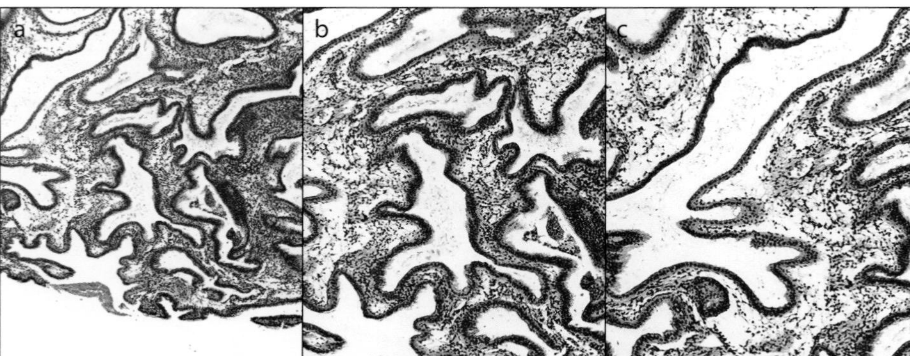

i31.22 **a-c** Simple hyperplasia in which the gland-to-stroma ratio is increased, but the amount of epithelium is not increased within individual glands. The glands have outpouchings or infoldings only because of their distorted contour. There is no epithelial hyperplasia.

The appearance is similar to disordered proliferative endometrium except that the gland-to-stroma ratio is slightly higher.

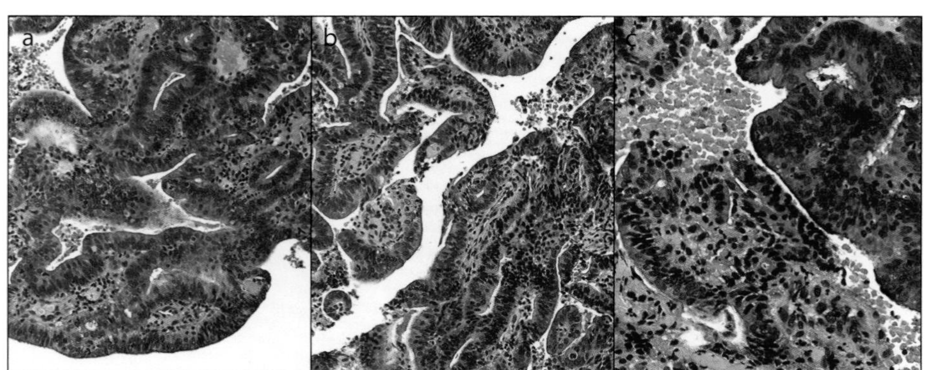

i31.23 **a-b** Complex hyperplasia in which the gland-to-stroma ratio is increased and there is epithelial hyperplasia within individual gland.

c Complex hyperplasia on the upper right contrasted with normal endometrium on the lower left. The nuclei in the hyperplastic endometrium are only slightly larger than the normal nuclei, and like normal nuclei, have little distinction between chromatin and parachromatin.

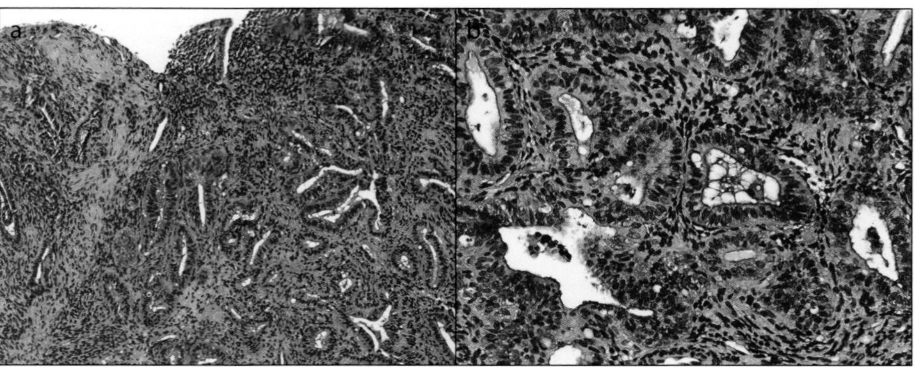

i31.24 **a-b** Glandular crowding and focal complex hyperplasia are occasionally encountered in endometrial polyps.

i31.25 a-b Atypical hyperplasia on the left contrasted with complex hyperplasia on the right. In atypical hyperplasia, the nuclei are significantly enlarged and have a vesicular chromatin pattern, often with nucleoli.

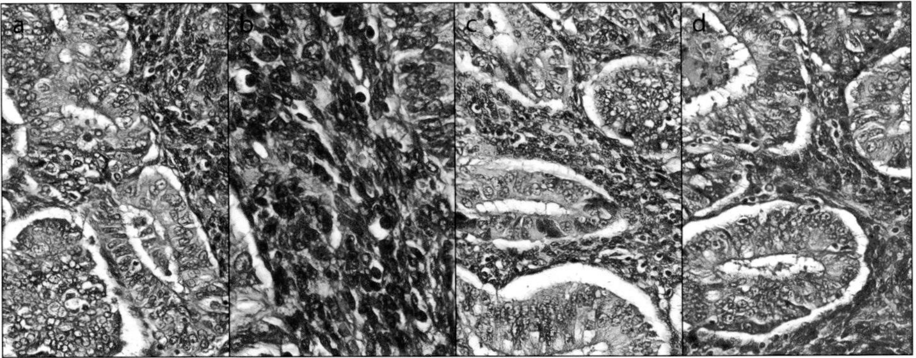

c-d Atypical hyperplasia in which the glands are separated by normal endometrial stroma.

i31.26 a The glands fulfill the criteria for atypical hyperplasia, but are not separated by normal endometrial stroma. Rather, they are separated by an abnormal fibrous stroma, an indication of well differentiated adenocarcinoma.
b Atypical glands are mostly confluent, with no stroma between them except for very thin fibrovascular tissue, another indication of adenocarcinoma

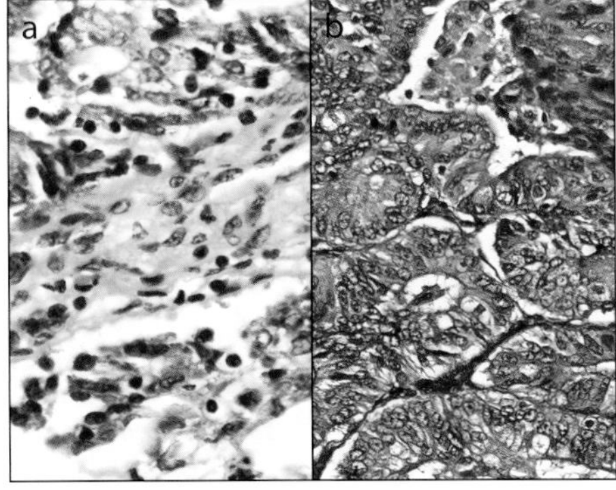

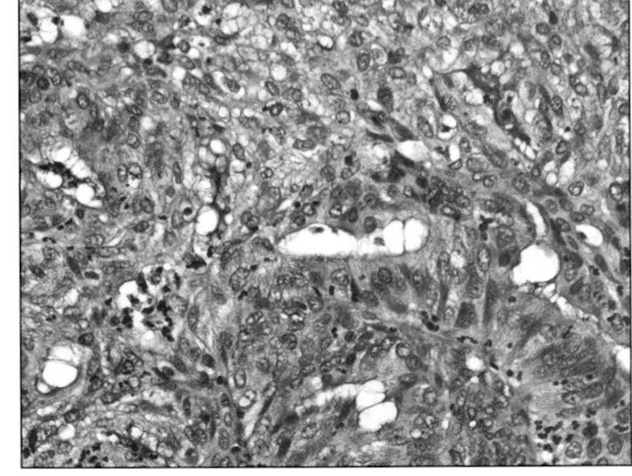

i31.27 A moderately differentiated (FIGO 2) endometrial adenocarcinoma. The neoplastic epithelium in the lower portion forms distinct glands while that in the upper portion does not.

i31.28 A poorly differentiated (FIGO 3) adenocarcinoma in which >50% of the neoplastic cells do not participate in discernible gland formation

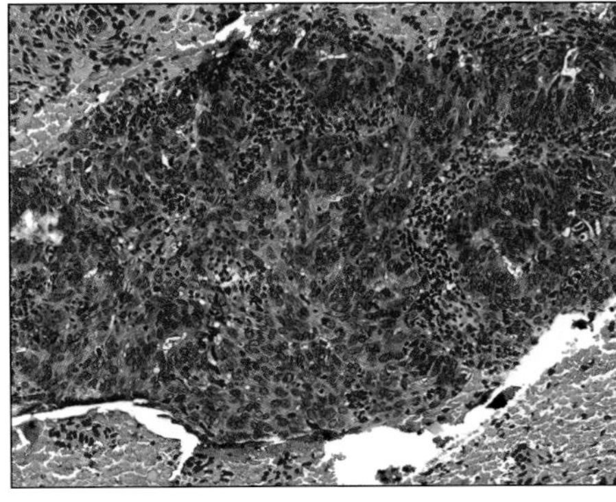

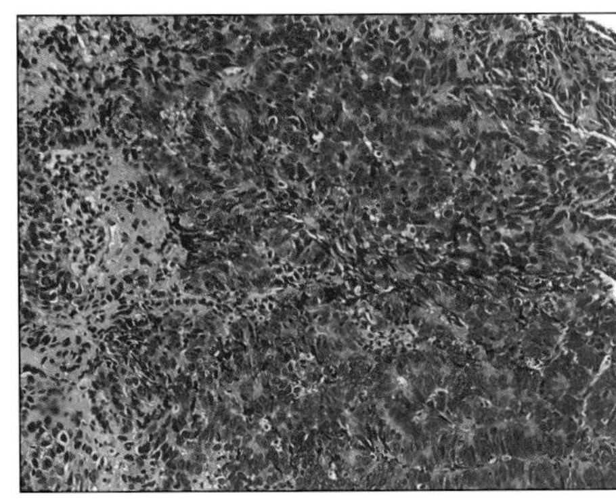

i31.29 A FIGO 3 endometrial adenocarcinoma in which gland formation is identified in 50% of the epithelium, but nuclear pleomorphism is extensive

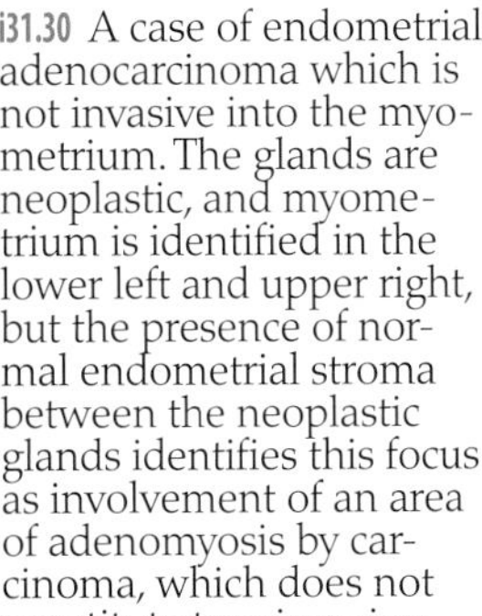

i31.30 A case of endometrial adenocarcinoma which is not invasive into the myometrium. The glands are neoplastic, and myometrium is identified in the lower left and upper right, but the presence of normal endometrial stroma between the neoplastic glands identifies this focus as involvement of an area of adenomyosis by carcinoma, which does not constitute true invasion.

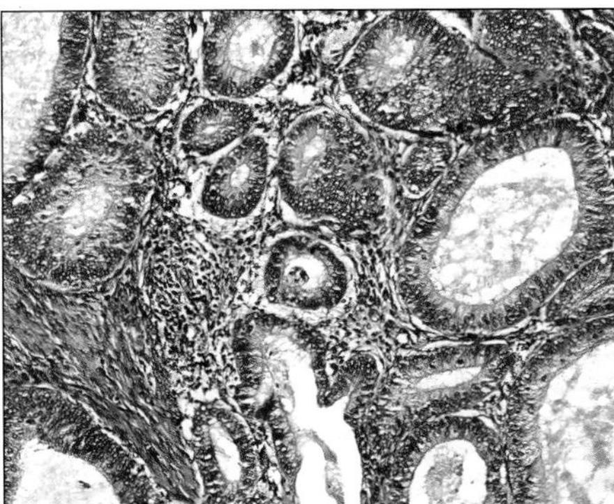

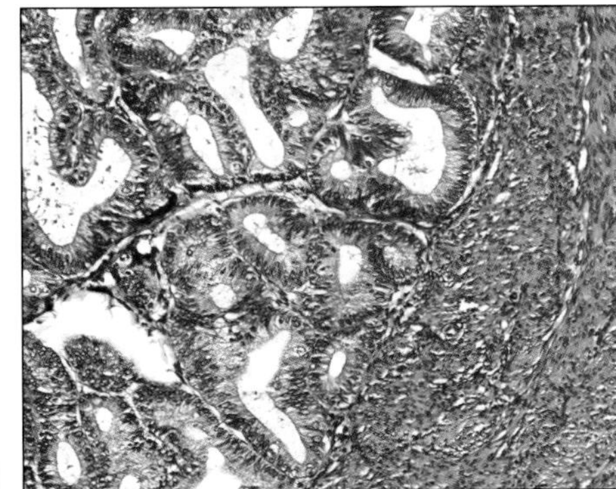

i31.31 Well differentiated endometrial adenocarcinoma invasive into myometrium. In contrast to i31.30, the glands are not separated by normal endometrial stroma.

i31.32 a A carcinoma of the endometrium with sarcomatous metaplasia. Several glands can be identified.
b A carcinoma with sarcomatous metaplasia in which there is a proliferation of spindle cells with an indistinct epithelial component

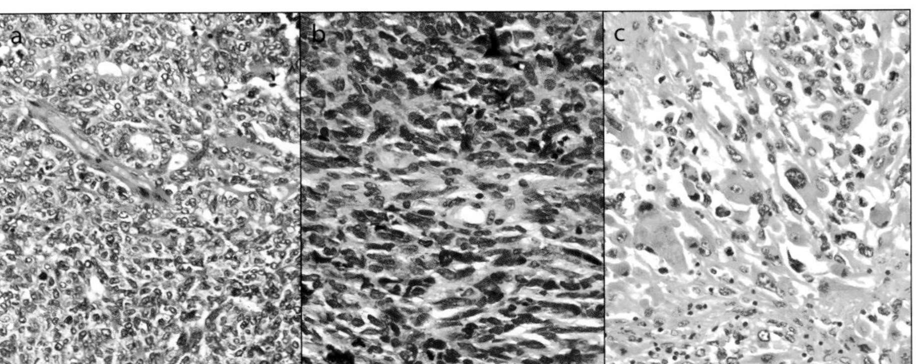

c Heterologous elements, demonstrating muscle differentiation, in a carcinoma with sarcomatous metaplasia

ISBN 978-089189-5886

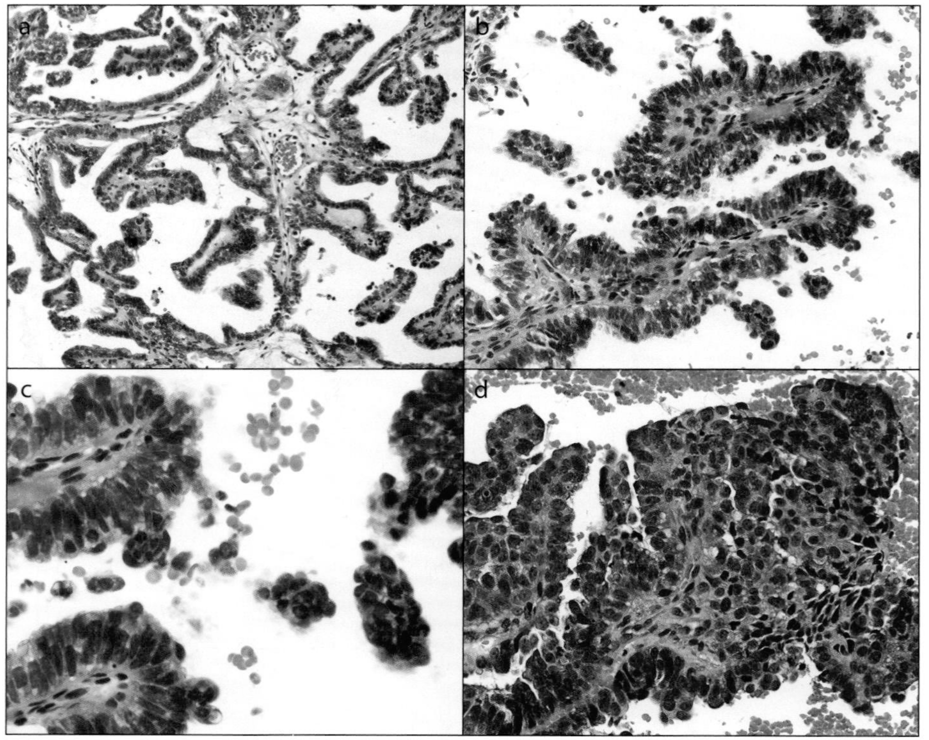

i31.33 **a** A low-power view of uterine papillary serous carcinoma (UPSC). Note the well developed broad fibrovascular cores.

b A higher-power view of UPSC, illustrating the well developed fibrovascular cores, the high nuclear grade, and the extensive epithelial cellularity resulting in microtufts

c-d The high nuclear grade, intense cellular crowding, and microtufts of UPSC

i31.34 **a** Villoglandular adenocarcinoma with very thin fibrovascular cores, in contrast to UPSC

b A higher-power view of the same case as in i31.34a, highlighting the very subtle cores, the lower nuclear grade relative to UPSC, and the absence of microtufts

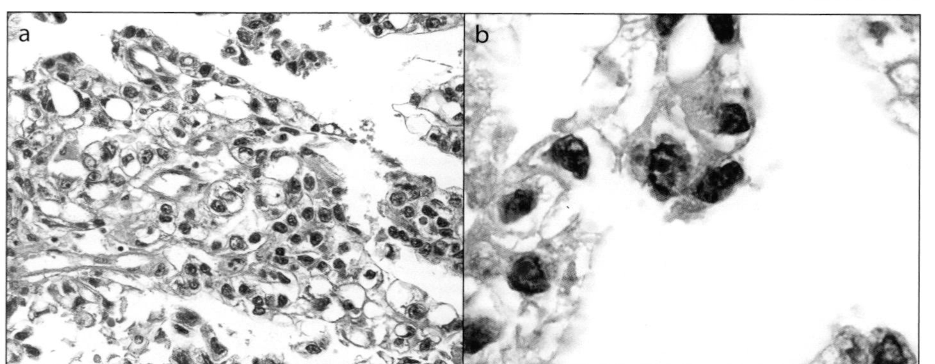

i31.35 **a** Clear cell adenocarcinoma of the endometrium

b Clear cell adenocarcinoma with apical (hobnail) nuclei

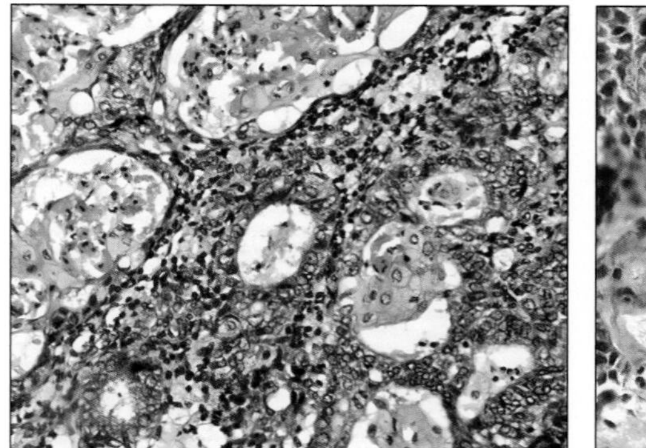

i31.36 A low-grade endometrial adenocarcinoma with squamous metaplasia. Note the innocuous appearance of the squamous epithelium.

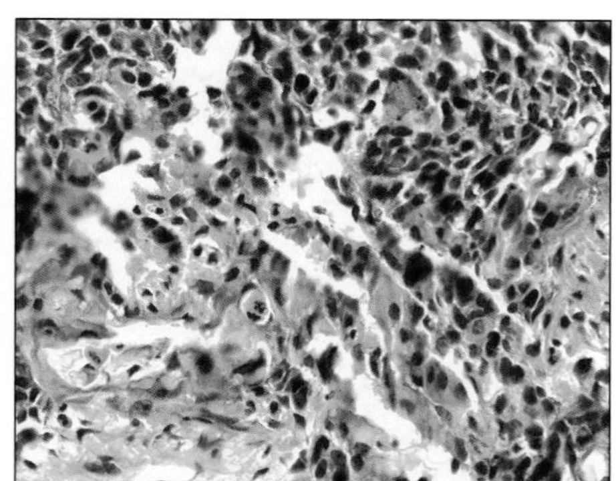

i31.37 An adenosquamous carcinoma of the endometrium. Note the high-grade appearance of the glandular components at the top and bottom as well as the malignant appearance of the squamous component in the middle.

i31.38 **a** A poorly differentiated adenocarcinoma encountered in a cervical cone

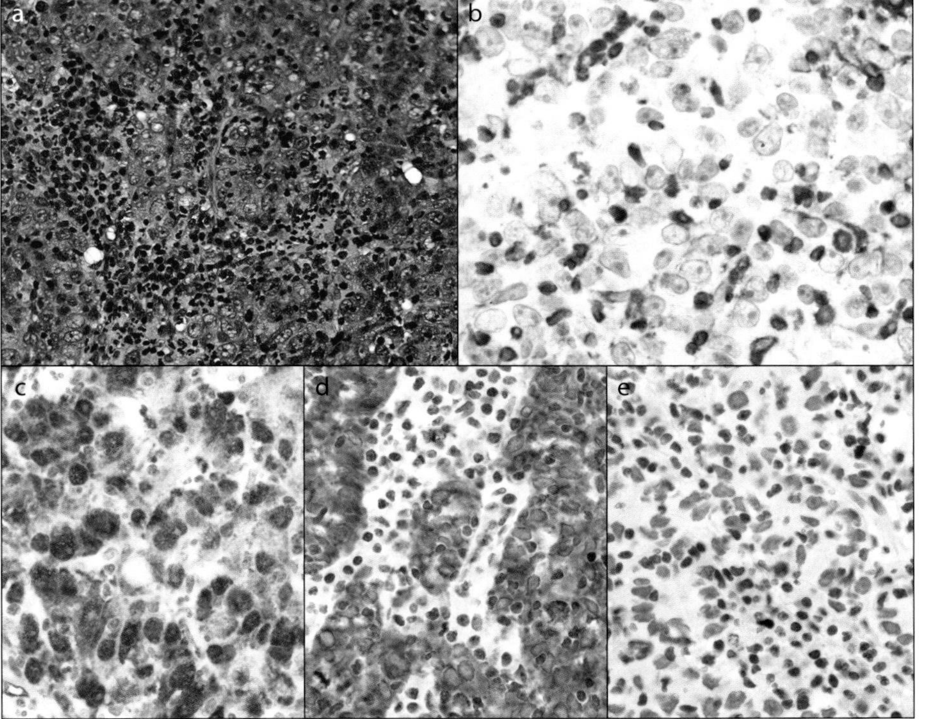

b A vimentin stain of the case illustrated in i31.38a. There is some staining of stromal cells, but the neoplastic cells are negative.

c Positive staining of the case for p16 in the neoplastic cells

d Positive staining for carcinoembryonic antigen **e** Negative stain for estrogen receptor. These 4 immunohistochemical stains identify the carcinoma as being of endocervical, not endometrial origin.

i31.39 **a** A cellular proliferation in the center and on the right, which is well demarcated from the normal myometrium on the left

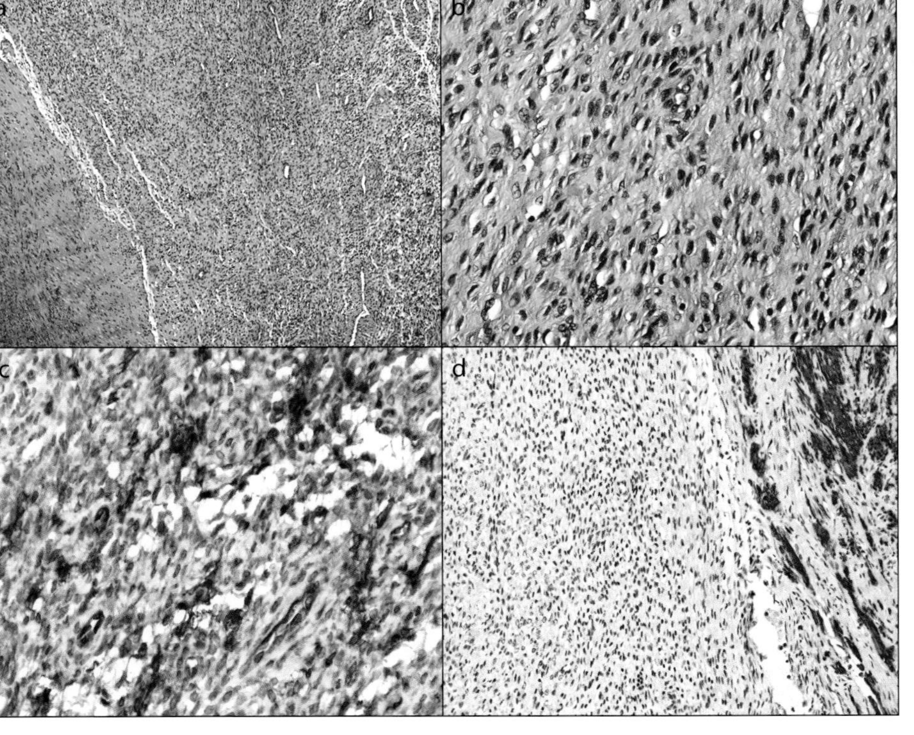

b A higher-power view of the proliferation demonstrating relative nuclear uniformity and eosinophilic cytoplasm that suggests the possibility of a smooth muscle tumor

c A positive CD10 stain of the proliferation

d A negative h-caldesmon stain. The proliferation is on the left and the normal myometrium, which stains positively, is on the right. The CD10 and h-caldesmon stains identify the proliferation as being of endometrial stromal origin, not a smooth muscle tumor. The sharp demarcation from the myometrium identifies the process as a simple endometrial stromal nodule.

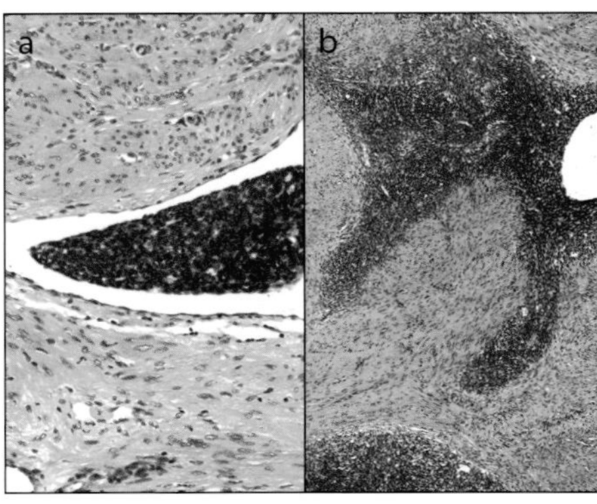

i31.40 **a** A low-grade endometrial stromal sarcoma with lymphatic invasion **b** A low-grade endometrial stromal sarcoma with infiltration into the myometrium. Compared to the sharp demarcation in i31.39a. Note the relative nuclear uniformity, underscoring that the diagnosis of a low-grade endometrial stromal sarcoma is made by infiltration or lymphatic invasion.

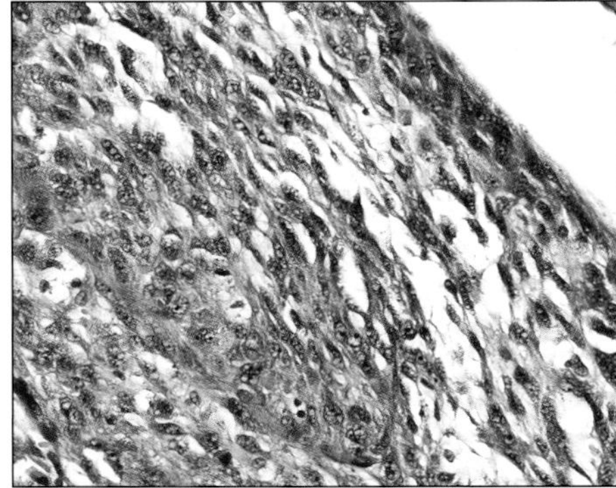

i31.41 A high-grade endometrial stromal sarcoma with nuclear pleomorphism. This nodule has invaded a lymphatic space

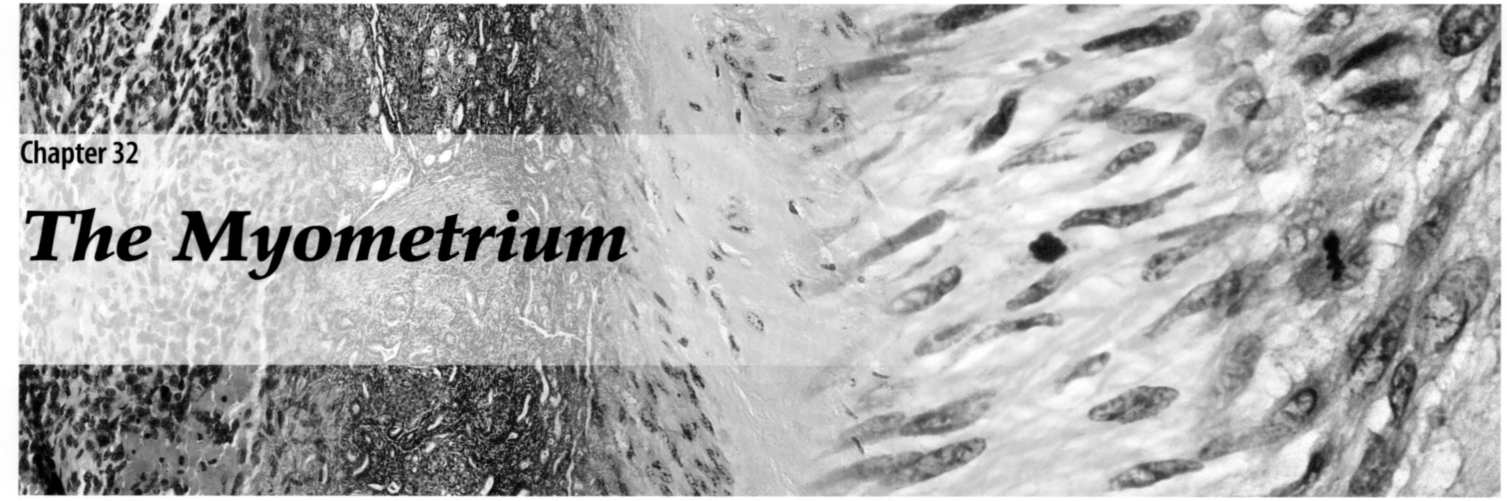

Chapter 32

The Myometrium

Adenomyosis

Adenomyosis is the occurrence of both endometrial glands and stroma within the myometrium. The diagnosis of adenomyosis is subjective, with substantial interobserver variation [PMID18681999], particularly in cases of so-called superficial adenomyosis, in large part because of the histologic uncertainty of the location of the normal endometrial-myometrial junction. Although there is no universal standard, most accept the presence of both endometrial glands and stroma 2.5 mm or more below the apparent endometrial-myometrial junction as indicative of adenomyosis [PMID19797011]. Because the endometrial tissue in adenomyosis does cycle, it usually appears proliferative at all times i32.1.

An adenomyoma is a discrete manifestation of adenomyosis. Other than uncertainty stemming from the location of the endometrial-myometrial junction, simple adenomyomas are rarely a problem, but the atypical polypoid adenomyoma, described in 1981 [PMID7282995], is a polypoid expression of adenomyosis i32.2a, i32.2b that is characterized by appreciable glandular atypia that may simulate malignancy i32.2c. In difficult cases, a helpful feature is that the glandular component of the atypical polypoid adenomyoma has extensive squamous metaplasia (morule formation) in about 90% of cases i32.2d [PMID8540600]. An atypical polypoid adenomyoma of low malignant potential has been described [PMID8540600].

Uterine Smooth Muscle Neoplasms

Uterine smooth muscle tumors remain a problematic and subjective area in pathology. The old criterion of relying solely on mitoses is no longer employed, and the thinking of Bell, Kempson, and Hendrickson [PMID8179071], which assesses a tumor based on its mitoses, atypia, and necrosis is becoming standard.

We will consider each of these 3 criteria separately, beginning with mitoses. There are 4 considerations in counting mitoses: where to count, how much to count, verifying that the fields of view are comparable, and verifying that the object is a true mitotic figure. As was mentioned in the counting of mitotic figures in breast neoplasms, mitoses often vary considerably in different areas of a tumor. Interobserver variation can be diminished by selecting the most active areas and counting >1 set of 10 high-power fields (HPFs). It is assumed that the linear field of view of most medical microscopes on the 40× objective is approximately 0.5 mm, resulting in a surface area of approximately 0.2 mm^2. The criteria for a mitotic figure are discussed in Chapter 2, but a common pitfall is to mistake a karyorrhectic nucleus for a mitosis i32.3a, i32.3b.

The nuclear atypia referred to in the system of Bell et al must be generalized to have significance, as it has long been known that benign leiomyoma may have very alarming focal atypia (the so-called symplastic leiomyoma i32.4. The decision as to whether or not there is significant nuclear atypia in myometrial lesions is best made at low power.

Necrosis is quite common in leiomyomas, and the necrosis that constitutes an indication of malignancy is a particular type that is sometimes referred to as "coagulative necrosis," as opposed to the "hyalinizing" type of necrosis that is typically seen in leiomyomas. One of the few criticisms that can be offered for the work of Bell et al is that the terms "hyalinizing necrosis" and "coagulative necrosis" are somewhat confusing. Hyalinizing necrosis is a gradual transition from the viable to the necrotic with a zone of eosinophilic collagen or granulation tissue between i32.5a, i32.5b. By contrast, coagulative tumor necrosis is an abrupt transition between necrotic and well-preserved cells, without an intervening zone of collagen. Individual necrotic cells appear as "ghosts" and are immediately adjacent to viable cells i32.6. Reflecting the fact that these "ghost" cells are not typical of hyaline necrosis, it has been proposed that the term "coagulative necrosis" be replaced with "tumor cell necrosis" [PMID9042296]. Another helpful feature is that in leiomyosarcomas with necrosis, many of the viable cells are near a vessel. In practice, however, there are cases in which it is difficult to determine which type of necrosis is present.

With the criteria of mitoses, atypia, and necrosis clarified, we now consider the usual spindle cell type of uterine smooth muscle tumor. As a general rule, most such tumors are malignant if any 2 of the following 3 criteria are fulfilled: widespread atypia, 10 or more mitoses per 10 HPFs, or tumor cell (coagulative) necrosis. For example, such tumors with both *widespread* atypia i32.7 and a significant amount of tumor cell necrosis are malignant without any mitoses. Tumors with 10 or more mitoses/10 HPFs and diffuse atypia are malignant without necrosis.

If neither tumor cell necrosis nor significant atypia is present, there is controversy as to how many mitoses make the tumor malignant. All agree that up to 5 mitoses/10 HPFs is benign if there are no other problematic features. In smooth muscle tumors of the usual type, the study of Bell et al found no deaths from bland, nonnecrotic tumors even with up to 20 mitoses/10 HPFs. Accordingly, they call these mitotically active leiomyomas, with the qualification that experience is limited. Others prefer the designation of uncertain malignant potential (UMP) if mitoses are >5/10 HPFs, and certainly if they exceed 10/10 HPFs, and feel that a tumor lacking necrosis or generalized atypia can be considered malignant if mitoses exceed 20 per 10 HPFs. Likewise, there is no consensus on the identification of an atypical mitotic figure, but it seems prudent to either designate an otherwise unremarkable tumor with an atypical mitosis as UMP or to comment that experience is limited.

Another area in which experience is limited is in those tumors that have tumor cell necrosis or appreciable nuclear atypia, but only focally. Focal nuclear atypia or tumor cell necrosis does not have the same significance as the diffuse presence of these features, and a diagnosis of leiomyoma appears appropriate, but again, a comment on limited experience or a designation of UMP is prudent. It may be that some prognostic information will emerge in smooth muscle tumors of uncertain malignant potential from immunohistochemical staining for p16, p53, and Ki-67 [PMID19734847].

Smooth muscle tumors with myxoid stroma, even focally i32.8, are more likely to be malignant. Even with no atypia and no tumor cell necrosis, myxoid tumors may still be malignant if they have 2 mitotic figures per 10 HPFs. Likewise, a myxoid tumor with any atypia or any necrosis, even without mitoses, is likely a myxoid leiomyosarcoma i32.9 [PMID18384211]. Whereas 2 of the 3 criteria of atypia, mitoses, and necrosis are generally needed for a malignant diagnosis, myxoid smooth muscle tumors are considered malignant with only 1 criterion, and if that criterion is mitotic activity, the threshold for a sarcoma diagnosis is only 2 per 10 HPFs [PMID18384211].

Whereas the interface of the tumor and the normal smooth muscle is generally not important in evaluating the malignant potential of smooth muscle tumors because leiomyomas may be infiltrative, myometrial infiltration is characteristic of myxoid leiomyosarcomas and is of concern i32.10. Although infiltration alone does not make any smooth muscle tumor—even a myxoid one—malignant, this finding indicates a higher probability of malignancy in a myxoid smooth muscle tumor and warrants additional sampling.

A similar situation exists in smooth muscle tumors with epithelioid differentiation. Although experience is somewhat limited, without atypia, necrosis, or mitoses i32.11, epithelioid smooth muscle tumors can safely be regarded as leiomyomas. But it is likely that >5 mitotic figures per 10 HPFs indicates a malignant lesion, even if there is no tumor cell necrosis or atypia, and any degree of atypia or necrosis in the presence of such a mitotic count secures the diagnosis of epithelioid leiomyosarcoma i32.12 [PMID18384211]. Epithelioid smooth muscle tumors may occasionally have some expression of keratin, which should not be interpreted as an indication of a carcinoma [PMID11914617].

A very unusual form of uterine smooth muscle neoplasm is intravenous leiomyomatosis (IVL), in which leiomyomas grow within vascular lumens and are surrounded by endothelial cells i32.13. Although these may rarely extend into pelvic vessels beyond the uterus and may rarely recur after hysterectomy, IVL generally follows an innocuous course and is well treated by resection [PMID20179432].

A rare tumor that may masquerade as a smooth muscle tumor, and which should be considered in unusual uterine neoplasms, is the perivascular epithelioid cell tumor (PEComa) [PMID19391667, PMID19604538]. In addition to the uterine PEComa, other examples of this rare tumor include the angiomyolipoma, clear cell myomelanocytic tumors (which occur predominantly in the falciform ligament), sugar tumor of the lung, and lymphangioleiomyoma. PEComas may stain for muscle markers such as actin, but they also tend to be positive for melanocytic markers, such as HMB-45, HMB-50, and Melan-A. They are negative for S100 and keratin. Particularly helpful is that uterine PEComas, like those of other sites, are positive for CD1a [PMID18251780], whereas uterine smooth muscle tumors are negative [PMID18995203].

Core Points for Myometrium

- Adenomyosis: subjective, but presence of endometrial glands and stroma 2.5 mm or more below the apparent endometrial-myometrial junction is prudent.
- Atypical polypoid adenomyoma: unusual form of adenomysosis.
  - May have sufficient glandular atypia to resemble a carcinoma.
- Smooth muscle tumors: assessed on the basis of mitoses, generalized nuclear atypia, and necrosis.
  - Necrosis must be of the "tumor cell" or "coagulative" type
    - Sharp transition from ghost-like necrotic cells to well-preserved cells, without intervening collagen fibers (typical of the more common and innocuous "hyalinizing" of necrosis)
- Sarcoma likely if 2 of the following 3 criteria: widespread atypia, 10 or more mitoses per 10 HPFs, or tumor cell necrosis.
- Smooth muscle neoplasms without atypia or necrosis: up to 20 mitoses/10 HPF generally designated as mitotically active leiomyomas.
  - Some prefer the designation of smooth muscle tumors of uncertain malignant potential (UMP).
- Myxoid and epithelioid smooth muscle tumors: special cases, more likely to be malignant.

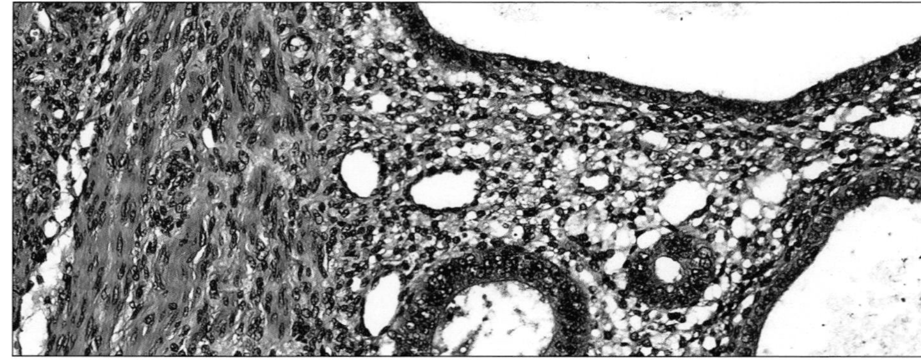

i32.1 Adenomyosis. This focus contains both endometrial glands and stroma and is found deep within the myometrium. Note the proliferative appearance of the glands and the stroma, because adenomyotic foci do not cycle.

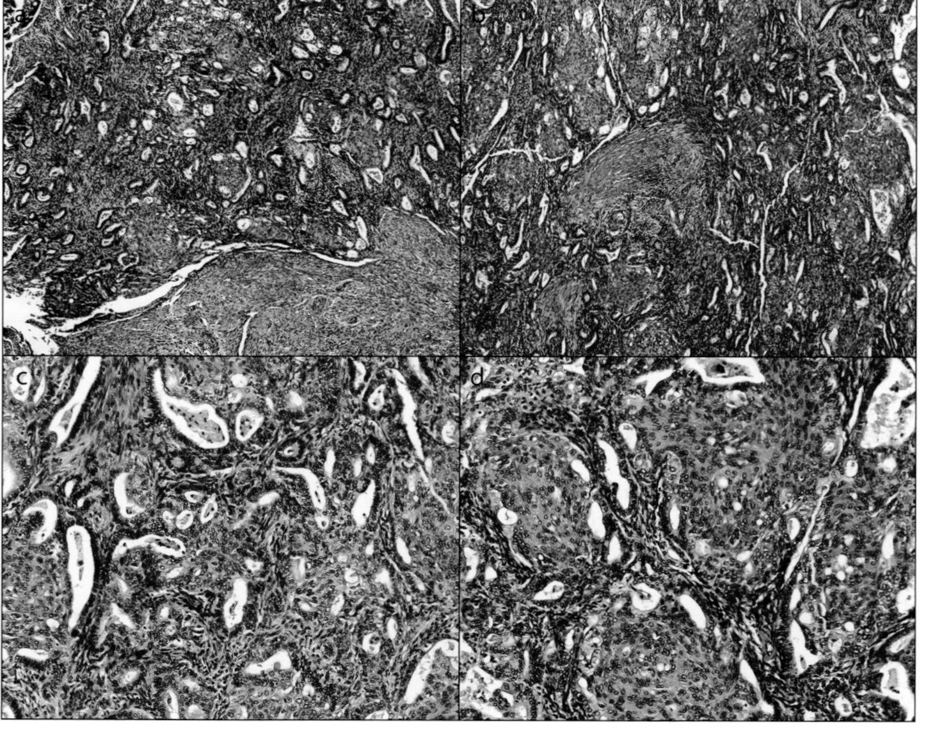

i32.2 **a** An atypical polypoid adenomyoma. This low-power view illustrates the polypoid architecture.

b A higher-power view illustrating a small amount of myometrium. Myometrium may be relatively rare in an atypical polypoid adenomyoma, but will be found somewhere.

c Glandular crowding in an atypical polypoid adenomyoma, causing concern for a well differentiated carcinoma. Note the foci of squamous metaplasia on the right and on the left.

d Squamous metaplasia in an atypical polypoid adenomyoma

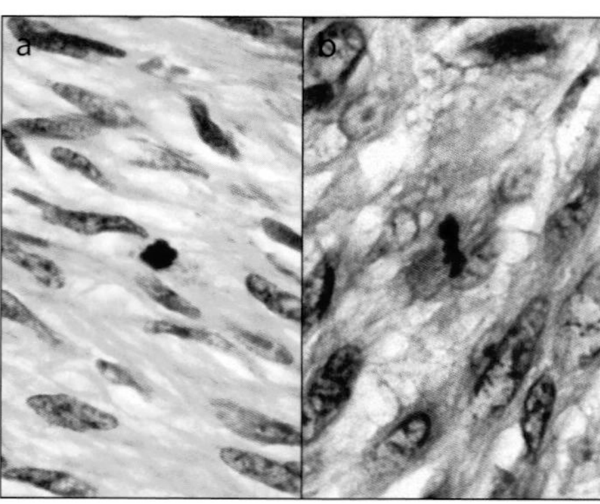

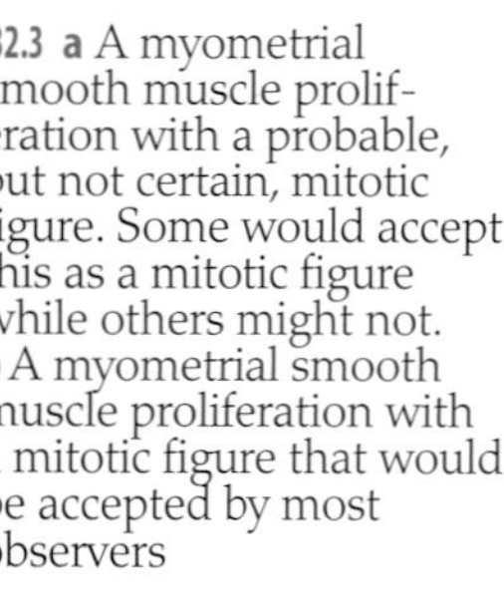

i32.3 **a** A myometrial smooth muscle proliferation with a probable, but not certain, mitotic figure. Some would accept this as a mitotic figure while others might not. **b** A myometrial smooth muscle proliferation with a mitotic figure that would be accepted by most observers

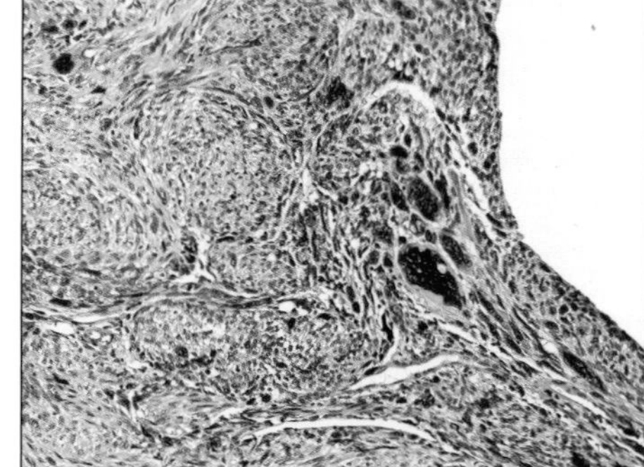

i32.4 A bizarre (symplastic) leiomyoma. While some of the nuclei are extraordinarily atypical, note that most of the nuclei appear innocuous.

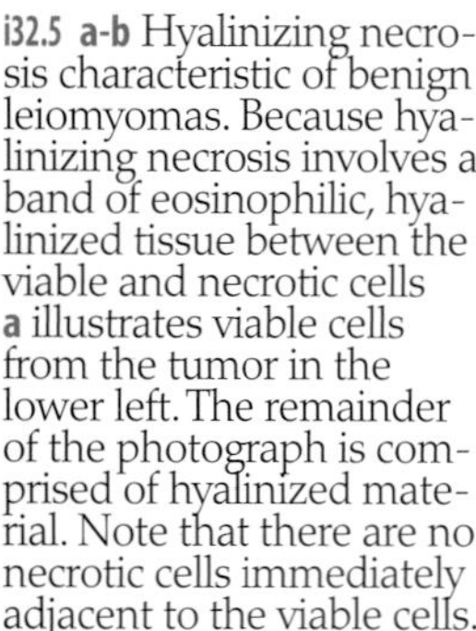

i32.5 **a-b** Hyalinizing necrosis characteristic of benign leiomyomas. Because hyalinizing necrosis involves a band of eosinophilic, hyalinized tissue between the viable and necrotic cells **a** illustrates viable cells from the tumor in the lower left. The remainder of the photograph is comprised of hyalinized material. Note that there are no necrotic cells immediately adjacent to the viable cells.

b is a continuation of the field illustrated in i32.5a. In the upper right, necrotic myocytes are seen. The 2 images together illustrate the broad transition zone between the necrotic and the viable muscle cells, and underscore that they are not immediately adjacent to each other.

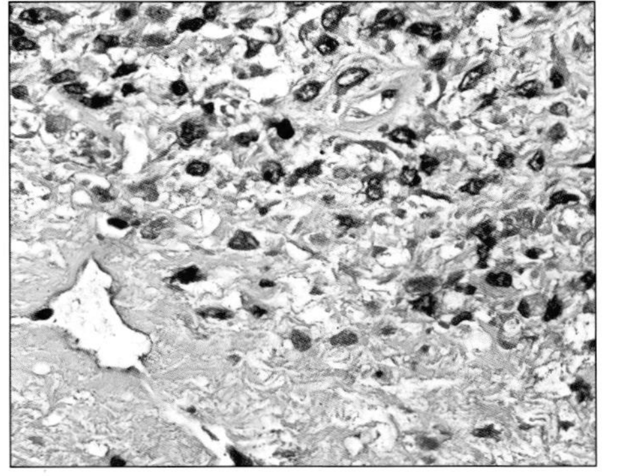

i32.6 The coagulative type necrosis seen in a leiomyosarcoma. Note that the necrotic cells, as shown by barely discernible nuclei, are immediately adjacent to viable tumor cells, with no transition or hyalinized area between them.

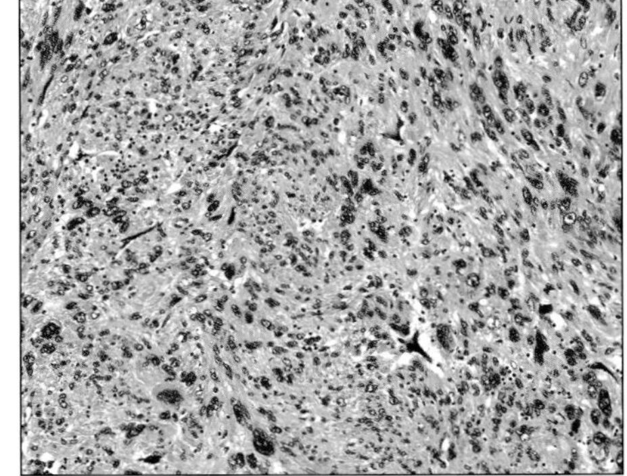

i32.7 The nuclear atypia of a leiomyosarcoma. Note that it is generalized and readily discernible at low power, in contrast to the bizarre leiomyoma shown in i32.4.

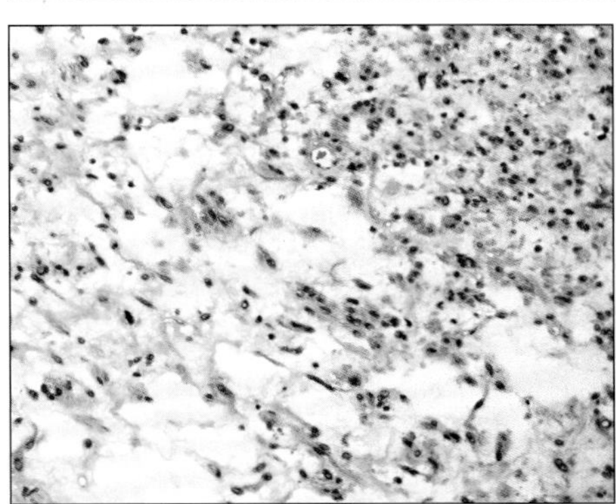

i32.8 A myxoid leiomyoma. Tumor has no necrosis, nuclear atypia, or mitotic activity.

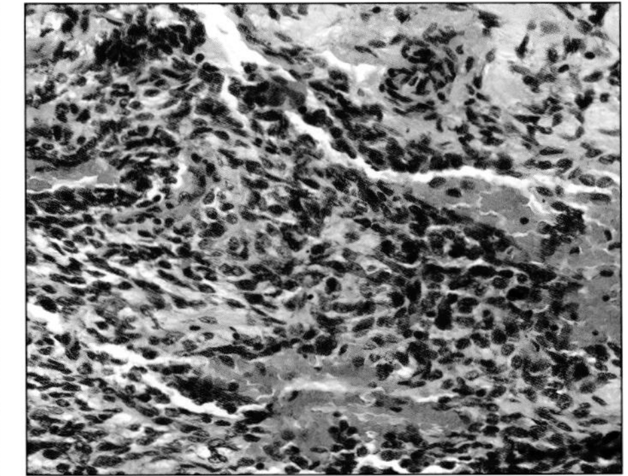

i32.9 A myxoid leiomyosarcoma. There is myxoid change in the upper right. In contrast to the case depicted in i32.8, there is nuclear atypia and hypercellularity. The atypia would be insufficient for a diagnosis of leiomyosarcoma in most situations but suffices in a myxoid smooth muscle tumor.

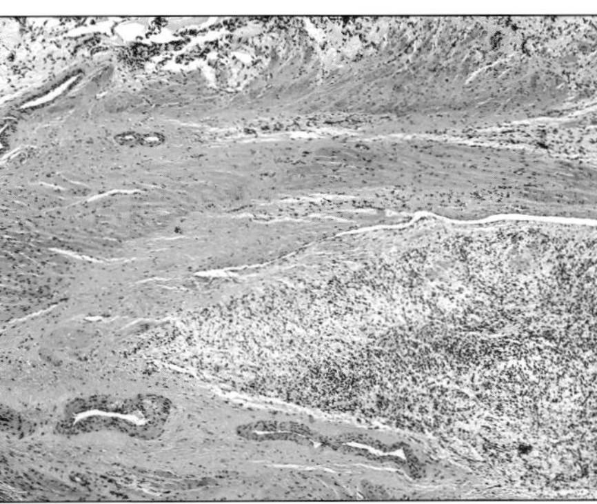

i32.10 A myxoid smooth muscle tumor that is infiltrating into the normal myometrium. Infiltration is not a criterion of malignancy in smooth muscle tumors, and even in myxoid smooth muscle tumors, it is not independently diagnostic of malignancy, but is of concern.

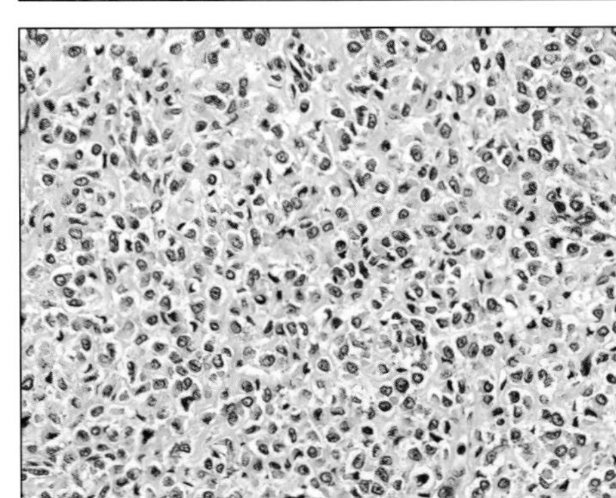

i32.11 An epithelioid leiomyoma. This neoplasm did not have significant nuclear atypia, necrosis, or mitotic activity.

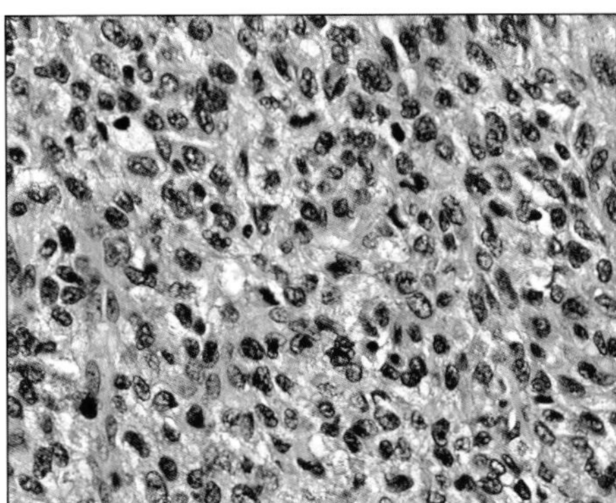

i32.12 Another epithelioid smooth muscle neoplasm with nuclear atypia and at least 1 probable mitotic figure in the center, suggesting a diagnosis of epithelioid leiomyosarcoma.

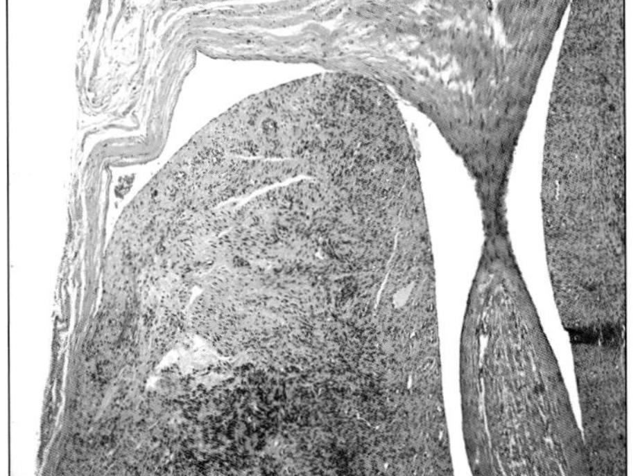

i32.13 Intravenous leiomyomatosis. A leiomyoma has grown into a lymphatic space on the left. There is also a leiomyoma in a lymphatic channel on the right.

ISBN 978-089189-5886

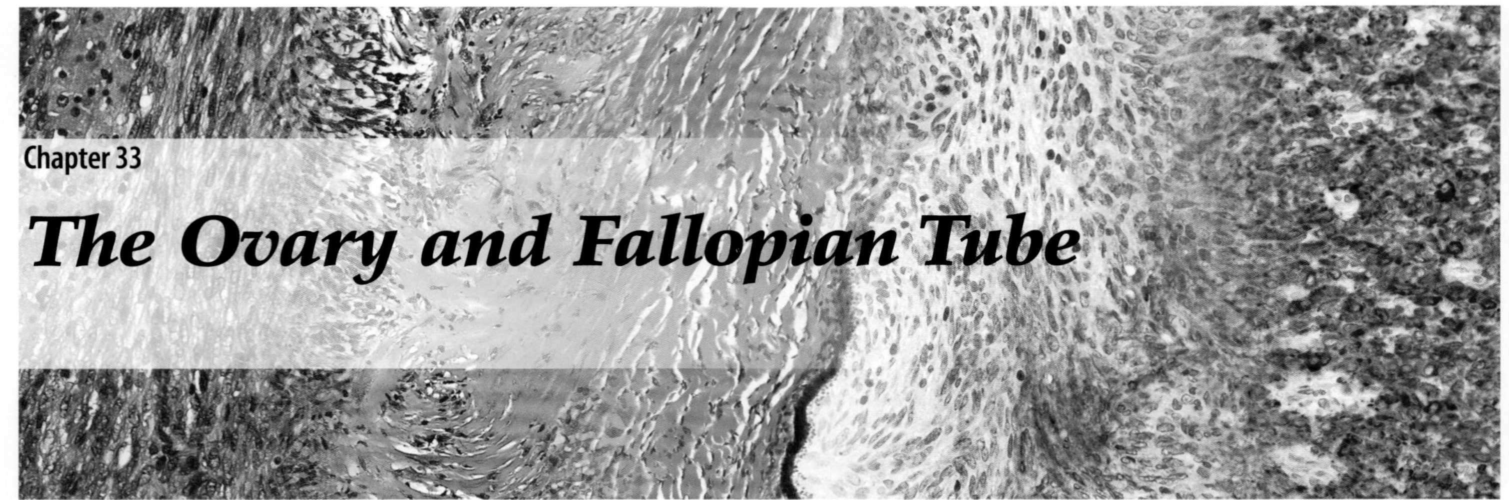

Chapter 33

The Ovary and Fallopian Tube

Normal Function and Histology

The ovum goes through a remarkable maturation process. The primary oocyte enters meiosis I during fetal life. Progress resumes only at ovulation. When meiosis I is completed, asymmetric cytoplasmic division produces a secondary oocyte and a polar body. The secondary oocyte proceeds as far as metaphase of meiosis II, but maturation is again arrested. Only upon fertilization is meiosis completed. If this happens, the products are a zygote and a second polar body.

The primary oocyte, awaiting completion of meiosis I, is contained within a primordial follicle. As the primary oocyte matures, the primordial follicle enlarges into a recognizable follicular cyst, which has an inner layer of granulosa cells and an outer layer of theca interna cells. Either of these cell layers may become luteinized, but the granulosa layer is only luteinized after puberty. The corpus luteum is lined predominantly by granulosa cells, with occasional wedge-shaped clusters of smaller luteinized theca cells peripherally.

Premature ovarian failure is amenorrhea in a patient under 40 with low estrogen and high levels of gonadotropins (ie, the low estrogen is not caused by a pituitary problem). Known causes of premature ovarian failure include genetic mutations and autoimmune oophoritis. The genetic causes are further divided into errors of metabolism, abnormalities that lead to premature follicle depletion (true premature menopause), or resistant ovary syndrome (where the ovaries do not respond to gonadotropins, probably because of a defect in receptors for FSH or LH). Autoimmune oophoritis is rare, but antibodies to granulosa and theca cells have been found [PMID19465673, PMID19461434].

Nonneoplastic Stromal Processes

There is a primary endometrial stromal sarcoma of the ovary, but this tumor is very rare and most such cases are metastatic from the endometrium. Comments here will be limited to nonneoplastic process in the ovarian stroma.

The most common ovarian stromal process is endometriosis. As is the case elsewhere, well developed endometriosis has a triad of features—endometrial glands, endometrial stroma, and hemosiderin-laden macrophage i33.1a—but the difficulty, as elsewhere, is that very often 1 or more of these features is not well seen, and there are many situations in which only a presumptive diagnosis of endometriosis can be made. In questionable cases—of which there are many—CD10 positivity in the stroma adjacent to the lining of the cyst points to endometriosis, as it stains endometrial but not ovarian stroma i33.1b, i33.1c [PMID15236994]. Even with a CD10 stain, however, some cases cannot be definitively resolved and can only be regarded as suspicious for endometriosis i33.1d, i33.1e.

The principal differential diagnosis is the follicular cyst and the simple inclusion cyst (the normal ovarian stroma is punctuated by invaginations of surface epithelium). Generally, a normal follicular cyst is lined by multiple layers of cells, whereas endometriosis is lined by only 1 or 2 layers, but there are situations in which a follicular cyst may have an attenuated lining. An additional difficulty is that ovarian stromal cells adjacent to a follicular cyst may simulate endometrial stroma cells, in which case a CD10 stain is helpful. Endometriosis may have atypical nuclei, or it may form a bulky or polypoid mass, simulating a neoplasm [PMID17592255]. Although endometriotic foci do not undergo complete cycling, they may demonstrate mild pseudodecidual reaction.

There are 6 pregnancy-associated conditions of the ovary: the large luteinized solitary follicle cyst of pregnancy and puerperium, the pregnancy luteoma, hilus cell hyperplasia, hyperreactio luteinalis, intrafollicular granulosa cell proliferations, and ectopic decidua in pregnancy-associated conditions [PMID8463033]. The large luteinized solitary follicle cyst of pregnancy and puerperium may present as an adnexal mass and may have bizarre nuclei i33.2. The pregnancy luteoma is a solid mass of luteinized cells i33.3. There is virilization of mother and infant in about 25% of cases. Pregnancy luteomas are essentially indistinguishable histologically from steroid cell tumors, which are discussed and illustrated subsequently. Unless crystals of Reinke are found (indicating a Leydig cell tumor, a type of steroid cell tumor), such masses in pregnant patients should be considered pregnancy luteomas. In hilus cell hyperplasia, the individual cells resemble those of a pregnancy luteoma, but there are multiple nodules, each of which is <2 mm, in contrast to the single, larger pregnancy luteoma.

Hyperreactio luteinalis is characterized by multiple cysts in both ovaries and high maternal HCG levels [PMID12621799]. Some of these cysts are corpus lutea, while others are not i33.4a. Hyperreactio luteinalis may occur with normal or abnormal pregnancies and may be virilizing. There is usually stromal luteinization i33.4b, which may be pronounced enough to cause confusion with a pregnancy luteoma, though the latter is more discrete. All of these conditions involute after pregnancy.

Stromal hyperthecosis shares some features with the pregnancy-associated conditions, but patients with stromal hyperthecosis are not usually pregnant. Stromal hyperthecosis is an extensive luteinization occurring in a background of stromal hyperplasia. Stromal hyperthecosis is usually more diffuse than a pregnancy luteoma or a steroid cell tumor, and typically involves both ovaries **i33.5**. The ovaries are often yellow, with clusters of luteinized cells throughout the stroma. A thecoma should be excluded before making the diagnosis of stromal hyperthecosis. Although there may be occasional cysts in stromal hyperthecosis, unlike hyperreactio luteinalis, these are not a primary feature. There may be some stromal sclerosis in stromal hyperthecosis, which suggests to some that polycystic ovary disease, stromal hyperplasia, and stromal hyperthecosis may be part of a continuum [PMID7033852].

The diagnosis of polycystic ovary disease requires clinical correlation. Corpora lutea and corpora albicans are generally absent, and there is a fibrotic, hypocellular superficial ovarian cortex overlying multiple follicular cysts **i33.6**. However, there may some luteinization and up to 30% of patients may have a corpus luteum. Most of these patients can achieve normal cycles with medication [PMID18339252].

Massive ovarian edema can grossly appear to be a neoplasm and even microscopically must be differentiated from a myxoma (unlike a myxoma, it is not a distinct mass).

Epithelial Ovarian Neoplasms

The 3 major classes of primary ovarian tumors are epithelial (sometimes called surface epithelial), sex cord-stromal, and germ cell. Epithelial tumors include serous, mucinous, endometrioid, Brenner, and clear cell tumors. Sex cord-stromal tumors include granulosa, thecoma/fibroma, Sertoli/Leydig, and steroid cell tumors. Germ cell tumors encompass the dysgerminoma, embryonal carcinoma, yolk sac tumor, choriocarcinoma, and teratoma.

The epithelial neoplasms are the simplest and the most similar to neoplasms in other body sites. The origin of ovarian surface epithelial tumors was a matter of controversy until the advent of immunohistochemical stains. A mesothelial origin was originally favored, but this view is no longer held because the immunohistochemical properties of these tumors are quite different from those of mesotheliomas.

Serous and Mucinous Epithelial Neoplasms

Serous and mucinous cystadenomas are common, and rarely difficult to recognize. They are simple cysts, without solid areas, and are lined by 1-2 layers of simple cuboidal epithelium. Associated fibrosis is indicated in the nomenclature (eg, adenofibroma and cystadenofibromas) **i33.7**. Mucinous cystadenomas may be filled with a more mucinous fluid than their serous counterparts, but the distinction is made on the basis of the epithelium, not the nature of the fluid. Mucinous neoplasms are lined by epithelial cells with distinctly mucinous cytoplasmic vacuoles rather than the dispersed mucin in serous adenomas **i33.8**.

The malignant counterparts of these adenomas are much more problematic. Either serous or mucinous carcinoma may have a papillary or a cystic component that is reflected in the nomenclature (eg, papillary serous carcinoma, mucinous cystadenocarcinoma). When such tumors are exophytic, the word "surface" is added to the tumor designation (eg, serous surface papillary carcinoma).

As is the case for adenomas, examination of the epithelial lining, not the nature of the fluid, makes the distinction between a serous and a mucinous carcinoma because necrosis can simulate mucinous fluid. Mucinous tumors have cells with obvious cytoplasmic mucin, sometimes demarcated into a sharply defined vacuole **i33.9**. In contrast, serous carcinomas have cytoplasmic mucin that is subtle and dispersed **i33.10**. In cases in which it is not clear if the process is serous or mucinous, immunohistochemical stains may help. Both serous and mucinous ovarian carcinomas are usually positive for cytokeratin 7, but in contrast to serous tumors of the ovary, about 1/2 of mucinous tumors are also positive for CK20 and CDX2, and they are often positive for CEA [PMID18776815], an immunohistochemical profile that resembles metastatic colon carcinoma, underscoring the need to clinically exclude a metastatic colon carcinoma when a mucinous ovarian carcinoma is found.

The psammoma carcinoma (psammocarcinoma) is a low-grade serous ovarian carcinoma that may be diagnostically challenging because there are few actual tumor cells [PMID16051342]. Most of the sample is fibrous tissue with psammoma bodies, laminated concretions of calcium and iron **i33.11a**, and malignant cells are identified only after an assiduous search **i33.11b**. If malignant cells are not found, a benign diagnosis is in order, as psammoma bodies alone are insufficient for the diagnosis of neoplasia. In a situation where psammoma bodies are prominent but neoplasia cannot be documented, serial serum CA125 levels may be indicated, and increased or rising levels suggest a neoplasm.

Epithelial Tumors of Low Malignant Potential

Serous and mucinous ovarian carcinomas have a peculiar ability to exhibit marked cellularity and architectural complexity without invading the stroma. These are called low malignant potential (LMP) or borderline *tumors* (or *neoplasms*). They should not be called LMP "adenomas" or "carcinomas" because the use of these terms, even in conjunction with the phrase "low malignant potential," conveys greater certainty about the potential of the process than actually exist. Rarely, an LMP tumor of the endometrioid type, resembling complex hyperplasia of the endometrium, may be encountered, but the LMP neoplasms are generally restricted to serous and mucinous types. Some believe that the LMP category is not appropriate and that all serous or mucinous neoplasms can be classified as benign or malignant, but the traditional view is presented first.

ISBN 978-089189-5886

Serous LMP Neoplasms

The cellularity and complex, often papillary architecture of serous LMP tumors initially suggests invasion. There may be micropapillations or microtufts without stroma i33.12, but cellularity and architectural complexity do not imply a fully-malignant carcinoma. For that diagnosis there must be invasion [PMID15297961, PMID15761465], based on the usual criteria, such as stromal desmoplasia, irregularly shaped clusters of tumor cells, single tumor cell infiltration, etc. Care must be taken not to misinterpret invaginations of epithelium in an LMP neoplasm as stromal invasion i33.13.

Almost 25% of serous LMP tumors will have local lymph node involvement [PMID19898226], underscoring that these are not clearly benign neoplasm for which a nonaggressive course is assured and suggesting that even LMP patients may need pelvic lymphadenectomy for optimal staging.

Attempts have been made to identify a subgroup of LMP neoplasms that might behave more aggressively than the usual LMP tumor. For example, some believe that serous LMP neoplasms which have micropapillary, solid, or cribriform architecture should be considered full carcinomas, while others remain skeptical. Some believe that cribriform and micropapillary serous LMP tumors are more aggressive than routine LMP tumors, but still should be in the LMP category [PMID12218569]. The suggestion has been made that serous LMP tumors with widespread micropapillary architecture have a greater recurrence potential and should be retained in the LMP category but separately designated from other serous LMP tumors [PMID11979089]. The important point is that these architectural features require a thorough search for unequivocal invasion and should be mentioned, along with a discussion of the controversy. Likewise, some believe that high nuclear grade excludes a noninvasive serous tumor from the LMP category and mandates a diagnosis of frank carcinoma, while others maintain that invasion is required for a full carcinoma diagnosis.

Another area of controversy in serous LMP tumors concerns microinvasion. By definition, LMP tumors are noninvasive, but about 10% of serous LMP tumors will have foci of microinvasion, defined as <3 mm (0.3 cm) i33.14. There is usually no stromal reaction in these microinvasive foci, but occasionally there may be stromal fibrosis, myxoid change, or inflammation. Extensive levels are often needed to distinguish between microinvasion and epithelial invaginations that simulate microinvasion. In cases where microinvasion is proven, the prognosis remains that of a purely LMP tumor [PMID2318481, PMID17001150], and the finding is of unclear clinical significance but should elicit a thorough search for a greater degree of invasion. The extent of microinvasion is also potentially important and should be mentioned.

Peritoneal implants are relatively common in serous LMP neoplasm and can be disconcerting. Most recognize 3 types of implants that may be associated with these tumors [PMID15761465]:

1. Noninvasive epithelial. These are usually papillary and have abundant epithelial cellularity. There is no desmoplasia or invasion, and the focus appears to sit on top of the stroma or to reside in a well demarcated invagination i33.15.
2. Noninvasive desmoplastic. These have a few epithelial cells but consists primary of fibrous tissue. The area of desmoplasia again sits on the surface or is well demarcated. Noninvasive implants of either the epithelial or desmoplastic type do not lessen the prognosis unless there is epithelial atypia, in which case they should be considered equivalent to invasive implants.
3. Invasive. These have a combination of appreciable cellularity and a stromal reaction i33.16. There is usually more atypia than in the other types of implants, and either a micropapillary architecture or clusters of epithelial cells surrounded by a cleft suggest invasion. But the key feature is that the area of desmoplasia blends in with the stroma and is not demarcated. These are the most serious type of implant, and the only type that lessens survival. Indeed, it has been proposed that the category of serous LMP be discarded, since those serous LMP tumors that do not have a micropapillary architecture and are confined to the ovary or give rise to noninvasive implants behave as adenomas, while those that either have a micropapillary architecture or give rise to invasive implants behave as carcinomas [PMID12413931]. Because invasive implants are prognostically serious, it has been proposed that the term "implant" not be used if there is invasion, but rather that these foci be designated invasive "well differentiated serous carcinoma" [PMID11257616].

Mucinous LMP Neoplasms

As is the case for their serous counterparts, mucinous LMP neoplasms may have increased cellularity on the surface but little or no invasion i33.17. The issues of micropapillary, solid, and cribriform features are not usually considered in mucinous LMP tumors in the way that they are for serous. Rather, mucinous LMP tumors are divided into endocervical and intestinal types, a designation not used in fully invasive mucinous carcinomas. 85% of mucinous LMP tumors are of the intestinal type, with goblet cells and nuclear stratification, while 15% are of the endocervical type, with dispersed mucin and basal nuclei [PMID15761465]. But it is not settled if even this distinction has prognostic significance.

Mucinous LMP tumors may have microinvasion (<3 mm), as for serous LMP, and may have implants that are essentially the same as for serous LMP tumors. Historically, the most common form of implant in mucinous LMP tumors is pseudomyxoma peritonei. "Pseudomyxoma peritonei" is a clinical term, discussed more fully in Chapter 34, referring to gelatinous deposits within the peritoneal cavity. Typically, the deposits in pseudomyxoma peritonei consist predominantly pools of mucin and contain few, if any, epithelial cells i33.18. However, it is now known that most cases of pseudomyxoma peritonei, even in the presence of a known ovarian mucinous LMP tumor, are from an appendiceal mucocele or neoplasm [PMID17511804]. Indeed, many have moved to the opinion that the category of mucinous LMP be discarded, as those ovarian LMP mucinous tumors that remain confined to the ovary have an excellent prognosis, and those that supposedly give rise to pseudomyxoma peritonei are actually cases of an appendiceal process. Others favor retaining the concept of mucinous LMP neoplasm with the understanding that an appendiceal process must be excluded if pseudomyxoma peritonei is found [PMID10472378]. This opinion permits rare cases of pseudomyxoma peritonei to be secondary to an ovarian mucinous LMP tumor, as some investigators believe that not all cases of pseudomyxoma peritonei derive from the appendix [PMID21970481]. In any event, there is agreement that the appendix should be examined before any pseudomyoma peritonei is ascribed to an ovarian process, even if there is a history of a mucinous LMP tumor.

In summary, the entire concept of LMP ovarian neoplasms is questioned, and there is evidence that those of the serous type are either adenomas if they do not give rise to invasive implants and carcinomas if they do, while those of mucinous origin are adenomas and there is an appendiceal process if there is pseudomyxoma peritonei. To the extent that the concept of an ovarian LMP neoplasm remains viable, its fully developed description entails the type (serous, mucinous, or rarely, endometrioid), architecture (micropapillary, solid, cribriform, etc) if serous, subtype (endocervical or intestinal) if mucinous, presence or absence of microinvasion, and analysis of implants, if any, with discussion of the presence and significance of any invasion of an implant, and the need to examine the appendix in *all* cases of pseudomyxoma peritonei.

Endometrioid Adenocarcinoma of the Ovary

Although usually similar in appearance to the typical form of endometrial adenocarcinoma, ovarian endometrioid carcinomas i33.19a may be challenging because they may have a number of morphologies and can resemble other types of ovarian neoplasms, especially if high grade. Endometrioid carcinomas may have papillary areas and resemble serous papillary carcinomas. It is unclear if such areas are part of the spectrum of endometrioid carcinomas or represent a mixed neoplasm, but in either case, such areas imply an aggressive course and require liberal sampling to fully understand the neoplasm [PMID8017563]. An endometrioid carcinoma should be considered in any ovarian tumor with a focal papillary pattern, especially if there is an endometrioid appearance in the nonpapillary areas. Also, papillations whose cores are long and thin favor an endometrioid carcinoma.

Endometrioid carcinomas may resemble mucinous carcinomas, but in contrast to the latter neoplasm, has less obvious intracellular mucin, less extracellular mucin, and fewer goblet cells. Concomitant endometriosis in nonneoplastic ovarian tissue favors endometrioid carcinoma, as this type and clear cell carcinoma are found in higher frequencies in patients with endometriosis [PMID12658347]. Any foci of squamous metaplasia in a poorly differentiated ovarian carcinoma suggest the endometrioid type i33.19b.

There is also a secretory variant of endometrioid carcinoma that can resemble clear cell carcinoma [PMID17667544], but there are often areas that have a more typical appearance for endometrioid appearance. Also, in the secretory type of endometrioid carcinoma, there is usually some nuclear stratification, which is not typically a feature of clear cell carcinomas, and there may be foci of squamous metaplasia.

In 15-20% of cases of endometrioid carcinoma of the ovary, there is a coexisting endometrioid carcinoma of the endometrium [PMID15492758]. In these cases, the relationship of the 2 tumors is not clear, but the important point is that the diagnosis of an endometrioid carcinoma in either the ovary or the endometrium requires the exclusion of a similar neoplasm in the other site. Endometrioid carcinomas of the ovary and endometrium have nearly identical immunohistochemical profiles. If endometrial sampling reveals a concomitant endometrial carcinoma, it may be difficult to determine if there are synchronous primaries or if one is a metastasis, and if the latter, which was the primary.

Primary Ovarian Adenocarcinoma vs Metastatic Adenocarcinoma

Invasive epithelial carcinomas of the serous, mucinous, and endometrioid types may all resemble metastatic adenocarcinoma. 65% of metastatic tumors to the ovary are bilateral but so are many cases of primary ovarian mucinous adenocarcinomas. Metastatic carcinomas often have focal necrosis, poor differentiation, bilaterality, a small ovary, disproportionate surface involvement, and multiple discrete nodules. Most colon carcinomas are positive for cytokeratin 20 and negative for cytokeratin 7. Most ovarian carcinomas are the reverse, though most ovarian mucinous carcinomas are positive for both CK7 and CK 20. Positivity for CA125, ER, and PR favors an ovarian primary, while CEA and CDX2 staining favor colonic origin. Again, primary ovarian mucinous adenocarcinomas are an exception, as approximately half of them will stain for CDX2, but a negative CDX2 suggests an ovarian primary over a colonic metastasis. Positivity for MUC2 suggests colonic origin [PMID19926591]. A potential pitfall in the use of immunohistochemical stains in these situations is that many primary ovarian endometrioid and mucinous adenocarcinomas may be positive for p16, a marker otherwise suggestive of cervical carcinoma [PMID18156969].

At the end of the day, poorly differentiated serous, mucinous, and endometrioid carcinomas of the ovary can all resemble metastatic adenocarcinoma from the gastrointestinal tract or the endometrium. For this reason, I recommend a comment that a metastatic tumor, especially from the endometrium, stomach, or colon, be ruled out in any ovarian carcinoma of these types. If a tumor is found in the stomach or colon, it is probably the primary. If these sites are all negative in an ovarian mucinous carcinoma whose morphology or immunohistochemical profile suggests that it is metastatic, the appendix should be removed. Ovarian mucinous tumors are usually cytokeratin 7 positive, while appendiceal tumors usually follow the colonic pattern of being CK7 negative, but this is not foolproof, and the appendix is a common primary site of mucinous neoplasms that are metastatic to the ovary that often escapes detection by conventional endoscopic and radiographic techniques.

ISBN 978-089189-5886

Other Ovarian Epithelial Neoplasms

There are many patterns of clear cell carcinoma, including solid (the most common) i33.20, tubular, papillary, oxyphilic, and trabecular [Tavassoli ISBN978-9283224129]. Because the characteristic clear cytoplasm and apical (hobnail) nuclei are not always present, this is the surface epithelial tumor that is most often confused with germ cell tumors. Like all ovarian epithelial carcinomas, clear cell carcinomas occur predominantly in postmenopausal patients, while germ cell tumors tend to occur in younger patients. If an ovarian tumor resembles a germ cell tumor, but the patient is postmenopausal, a variant of a clear cell carcinoma should be considered. Relative to dysgerminomas, clear cell carcinomas have polyhedral cells with eccentric nuclei, sharp cell boundaries, and fewer lymphocytes, as opposed to the rounded cells with central nuclei of dysgerminomas. Relative to yolk sac tumor, the papillations of clear cell carcinoma often have a hyalinized core, and the nuclei are generally less pleomorphic. The immunohistochemical profile of germ cell tumors is discussed subsequently, but epithelial tumors such as clear cell carcinomas stain for keratin and epithelial membrane antigen (EMA), and are negative for placental alkaline phosphatase (PLAP).

Poorly differentiated clear cell carcinomas may also resemble high-grade serous, endometrioid, or mucinous carcinomas. If liberal sampling fails to clarify the tumor, immunohistochemistry may help. Clear cell carcinomas of the ovary are generally positive for cytokeratin 7, high molecular weight keratin, CEA, Leu-M1 (CD15), p53, and CA-125, and are negative for cytokeratin 20 [PMID11444201], estrogen receptor and WT1, markers that are positive in most serous carcinomas [PMID18830127].

Finally, a metastatic renal/adrenal cell carcinoma should be excluded before making the diagnosis of clear cell carcinoma, and again, immunohistochemistry is valuable. Most renal cell carcinomas are negative for cytokeratin 7 and 20, and usually positive for RCC.

Brenner tumors are considered a type of surface tumor, though many are thought to be derived from entrapped epithelium. Brenner tumors have clusters of transitional-type epithelium dispersed throughout the tumor, and they also have a fibrous stroma. A Brenner tumor should be excluded when there are small clusters of bland cells in a stroma that is more cellular than normal ovarian stroma i33.21a. The LMP Brenner tumor (also called a proliferating Brenner tumor) is a more florid proliferation, with larger nests of cells and often with areas that resemble a low-grade, noninvasive papillary urothelial neoplasm of the bladder i33.21b [PMID4005815].

Malignant Brenner tumors are rare, and by definition, have some areas that are recognizable as benign or LMP Brenner tumor i33.21c. In contrast, the very rare pure urothelial (transitional cell) carcinoma of the ovary does not have any areas of benign or LMP Brenner component [PMID8463036]. I recommend that the diagnosis of a pure ovarian urothelial carcinoma be accompanied by a comment that a bladder tumor should be clinically excluded.

Sex Cord-Stromal Neoplasms

In development, the coelomic epithelium lines the coelom, the major body cavity, and the developing abdominal organs. This epithelium becomes the peritoneum. In the 5th week of development, the coelomic epithelium and the mesenchymal tissue beneath it proliferate to form the gonadal ridges. In the 6th week, primordial germ cells migrate into the gonadal ridges [Larsen ISBN978-0443065835]. Continued proliferation of the coelomic epithelium and adjacent mesenchymal tissue surrounds the germ cells, forming the primary sex cords, the structures that precede the development of the male or female gonads [Larsen ISBN978-0443065835].

In the female embryo, the primary sex cords degenerate and will form tissue that becomes the hilum of the ovary, but secondary sex cords form in much the same way, by proliferation of the coelomic epithelium. The secondary sex cords surround the primordial germ cells, forming the ovarian follicles [Larsen ISBN978-0443065835].

Sex cord-stromal tumors originate from the remnants of these secondary sex cords or from the ovarian stroma, not from epithelium. The most common such tumor is the granulosa cell tumor. The adult type of granulosa cell tumor is a low-grade malignancy, with recurrence potential but no significant metastatic potential [PMID12637488]. 75% are estrogenic [PMID9443026]. There are numerous patterns, the most familiar of which is a microfollicular pattern with pseudoglandular structures called Call-Exner bodies, that are often filled with eosinophilic basement membrane material i33.22.

There is a macrofollicular pattern of the adult granulosa cell tumor, and there are other patterns that are not follicular, each of which carries its own differential diagnosis. For example, the trabecular pattern has ribbons that may resemble metastatic lobular carcinoma or a low-grade neuroendocrine (carcinoid) tumor. There is also a diffuse or solid pattern of granulosa cell tumor that may resemble a small cell carcinoma. The insular pattern is characterized by clusters of tumor cells.

The nuclei of adult granulosa cell tumors have deep grooves, the so-called "coffee bean" nuclei, but this feature is less important than in times past because immunohistochemical stains provide a more reliable means of differentiating the granulosa cell tumor from its many mimics. α-inhibin is a good stain for the entire class of sex cord-stromal tumors [PMID15502809]. Granulosa cell tumors are inhibin positive and EMA negative i33.23a, i33.23b, whereas epithelial tumors (primary or metastatic) are the reverse. Melan-A may also stain sex cord stromal tumors. Calretinin also stains virtually all of the tumors in this class but also stains 22% of epithelial neoplasms [PMID12409724]. CD56 stains most tumors of the sex cord-stromal class and is helpful in separating these tumors from epithelial neoplasms [PMID17581419], but it also stains neuroendocrine neoplasms, so chromogranin and synaptophysin should be shown to be negative before a positive CD56 is taken as evidence of a granulosa cell tumor.

The juvenile granulosa cell tumor is a cellular neoplasm whose cells have abundant eosinophilic cytoplasm and whose nuclei lack the grooves that are seen in the adult form i33.24. The juvenile granulosa cell tumor often forms irregularly shaped follicles that are intermediate in size between the Call-Exner bodies and the macrofollicles of the adult variety

[PMID6465418]. Unlike adult granulosa cell tumors, where the contents of the follicles are derived from the basement membrane, the follicles of a juvenile granulosa cell tumor contain acidic mucopolysaccharides [PMID2910225]. The juvenile granulosa cell tumor has a brisk mitotic rate, and some cases may have appreciable nuclear pleomorphism [PMID15502809]. These neoplasms can be misinterpreted as a germ cell tumor or as a thecoma or steroid tumor if they are of the solid type. Like the adult granulosa cell tumor, the juvenile variety is inhibin positive [PMID15502809].

The sclerosing stromal tumor occurs mostly in young people, is usually estrogenic, and consists of lobules of tumor cells separated by hyalinized connective tissues and areas of edema. The lobules consist of round cells with clear cytoplasm, admixed with spindle cells, and contain ectatic vessels [PMID19071970]. An apparent fibroma/thecoma in a young person should prompt exclusion of a sclerosing stromal tumor, as should any fibrotic, paucicellular areas or any ectatic vessels. Massive ovarian edema must also be excluded before the diagnosis of sclerosing stromal tumor is made, as edema is a prominent component of this tumor.

Sertoli cell tumors are usually estrogenic. Pure Sertoli cell tumors are rare in the ovary and most such cases will have a Leydig cell component if closely studied. Although many feel that the Leydig component is nonneoplastic, its presence should prompt a diagnosis of Sertoli-Leydig cell tumor rather than Sertoli cell tumor. The cytoplasm is usually lightly eosinophilic, but rarely is foamy (in the so-called lipid-rich variant).

The Sertoli-Leydig cell tumor also has a variety of patterns, often in the same tumor [PMID3911780]. A tubular pattern is common, especially in well differentiated tumors. A well differentiated Sertoli-Leydig cell tumor consists of well defined tubules, lined by Sertoli cells, with Leydig cells in the stroma **i33.25**. In a moderately differentiated Sertoli-Leydig tumor, the Sertoli and Leydig cells are intermingled without distinct tubule formation. There is often a trabecular pattern and there may be hypocellular areas, resulting in a vague nodularity. Poorly differentiated Sertoli Leydig cell tumors are diffuse sheets, without any pattern, often resembling a sarcoma.

Sertoli-Leydig cell tumors can resemble granulosa cell tumors, neuroendocrine tumors, dysgerminomas, or metastatic tumors. Sertoli-Leydig cell tumors are positive for keratins, but negative for EMA. They are usually positive for inhibin, CD99, and vimentin. Calretinin positivity is also usually found, but this is a less sensitive and less useful stain. Atypia, mitoses, and necrosis suggest malignancy [PMID15644771]. A Sertoli-Leydig tumor should be considered for any apparent dysgerminoma or granulosa cell tumor that is not quite "right," for any tumor with a neuroendocrine appearance for which immunohistochemical stains for chromogranin or synaptophysin are negative, or for any apparent metastatic carcinoma that is keratin positive but EMA negative.

Heterologous elements may be seen in Sertoli-Leydig cell tumors [PMID7139537, PMID7139538], especially if they are poorly differentiated, so it is wise not to diagnose a teratoma in the presence of a Sertoli-Leydig component. The heterologous elements are usually limited to mesodermal or endodermal elements, and are predominantly gastrointestinal epithelium or immature muscle or cartilage. Heterologous elements in Sertoli-Leydig cell tumors are virtually never ectodermal [PMID15502809]. On the other hand, a teratoma will almost always have ectodermal elements, such as skin, respiratory, or neuro tissue, the presence of which points to a teratoma over a Sertoli-Leydig cell tumor. A Sertoli-Leydig tumor with heterologous elements should be excluded in any apparent teratoma without an ectodermal component. In such situations, care should be taken to ensure that apparent teratomatous liver tissue is not actually clusters of Leydig cells.

The sex cord tumor with annular tubules is characterized by cells with pale cytoplasm which form tubules, some of which are surrounded by fibrous tissue. Some tubules are simple, while others are complex. There is a variable amount of fibrous tissue between the tubules [PMID15502809].

Another major class of ovarian sex cord-stromal tumors is steroid cell tumors (formerly called lipid cell tumors), of which there are 3 types [PMID17883070]. These types are all essentially indistinguishable histologically and consist of cells with uniform, round nuclei, often with small nucleoli, and cytoplasm that is abundant and eosinophilic **i33.26a** or focally clear **i33.26b**. The first type of steroid cell tumor is the stomal luteoma. A stromal luteoma is a nodule that is least 0.5 cm, usually occurring in a background of stromal hyperthecosis. These are often estrogenic and are essentially indistinguishable from the pregnancy luteoma except for the history. By convention, in pregnant patients, the diagnosis of pregnancy luteoma is given priority over a steroid cell tumor. The other types of steroid cell tumor are the Leydig cell tumor and the steroid cell tumor, not otherwise specified (NOS). Both of these are discrete masses not occurring in a background of hyperthecosis, are usually androgenic, and are essentially indistinguishable from each other unless crystals of Reinke, the hallmark of the Leydig cell tumor [PMID17284120], are found, though a hilar location and an older patient favor a Leydig cell tumor, while another location or a younger patient suggest a steroid cell tumor, NOS. The differential diagnosis of a steroid tumor includes a luteinized fibroma/thecoma, an extensively luteinized granulosa cell tumor, and a lipid rich Sertoli cell tumor. Because the cytoplasm in a steroid tumor may be clear as well as eosinophilic, tumors with clear cytoplasm, such as clear cell carcinoma and metastatic renal cell carcinoma, should also be excluded.

Ovarian fibromas consist of small fibroblastic cells, with a slightly collagenous background. Often, some cells have slightly more cytoplasm and may contain steroids (thecoma component) **i33.27**. It is not necessary to perform a fat stain to identify the lipid-containing cells and a diagnosis of fibroma/thecoma serves the patient quite well. If the thecoma component is pronounced, the neoplasm may resemble stromal hyperthecosis (but it will be a more obvious mass) or a steroid cell tumor.

Ovarian fibromatosis may have extensive cellularity or may be paucicellular, with a collagenous stroma. It can be nearly indistinguishable from a fibroma, except that fibromatosis envelops normal structures, while a fibroma displaces them and is more likely to be a discrete mass. Mitoses should be counted in any fibrous ovarian lesion to exclude a fibrosarcoma. Previously, it was thought that ovarian fibrous tumors with as few as 3 mitoses/10 HPF are fibrosarcomas, but a 2006 study showed that even with increased cellularity and mitoses exceeding 4/10 HPF, most such tumors behaved

ISBN 978-089189-5886

in a benign manner [PMID16861962]. Although more followup is needed, it appears that considerably more mitotic activity can be accepted than has been thought. The key criterion is nuclear pleomorphism, not mitotic activity.

A closing comment on ovarian tumors of the sex cord-stromal type is that because of the many types of tumors in this class, their variable appearance, and their similarity to tumors of other types, keratin, EMA, inhibin, chromogranin, and synaptophysin stains should be considered in any apparent stromal tumor that is unusual.

Ovarian Germ Cell Tumors

Germ cell tumors develop from the actual ovum and its immediately accompanying cells. While some germ cell tumors (yolk sac and embryonal) are more aggressive than others (eg, dysgerminoma, the ovarian counterpart to the testicular seminoma), the prognosis is generally excellent for stage 1 disease for any type of germ cell tumor, and with the advent of cisplatin therapy, is good for higher stages even in the more aggressive forms. Because germ cell tumors typically young women, fertility is often an issue, but reproductive function can usually be preserved [PMID18378402].

Because of the similarity in the development of male and female gonadal structures, this class of ovarian tumors is quite similar to those found in the testis. Germ cell tumors, including the immunohistochemical staining patterns of the various types, are discussed more fully in Chapter 38. The exception to this similarity is the ovarian teratoma, and comments here will be limited to this neoplasm.

Like complete hydatidiform moles, ovarian teratomas are an example of uniparental diploidy, but whereas hydatidiform moles arise from 2 *paternal* genomes, without maternal input, ovarian teratomas arise from 2 *maternal* genomes, without paternal input. Like most complete hydatidiform moles, ovarian teratomas are usually 46,XX. They can arise from a variety of processes, usually from a defective meiosis and proliferation of a single ovum [PMID2220805], analogous to the way in which most complete hydatidiform moles arise from the duplication of a single sperm that carries an X chromosome, after fertilization of an ovum without a functioning nucleus.

Most ovarian mature teratomas are cystic and primarily ectodermal. These are commonly called dermoid cysts because skin and adnexal structures predominate i33.28a, though a wide variety of tissue types are often seen. A dermoid is simply a type of mature teratoma. In the ovary, the presence of immature tissue is the determining factor in the metastatic potential of teratomas [PMID1260722], though there is some feeling that immaturity is better tolerated in children. This is in contrast to testicular teratomas, where the age of the patient—specifically the prepubertal or postpubertal status—not the presence or absence of immaturity, is the important consideration [PMID15761467].

Ovarian immature teratomas are graded on a scale of 1 to 3, based on the amount of immature tissue. A potential mistake in evaluating ovarian teratomas that are not simple dermoid cysts is to interpret fetal tissue as immature. Although fetal tissue is immature, it does not constitute sufficient immaturity for the diagnosis of immature teratoma. The diagnosis of an immature component requires that the tissue be *embryonic* [PMID15782074]. For example, if brain tissue is present, a simple collection of glial cells i33.28b does not constitute immaturity, even though the fully mature brain does not have such collections. For the diagnosis of immature teratoma, the glial cells must have 1 or more of the following embryonic characteristics: they form rosettes or tubules i33.28c, they are mitotically active, they form a solid mass, they have the appearance of neuroblasts, or they have an appearance of a glioma. Perhaps the term "embryonic teratoma" would be better than "immature teratoma," but we will not see the nomenclature change in our lifetimes.

Although grading of immaturity can be based on any embryonic tissue, in practice, grading is usually based on neural tissue because this is the easiest to identify and quantify. Grade 1 tumors have an amount of immature neural tissue that is <1 low-power field. Grade 2 tumors have immature neural tissue that occupies more than 1, but fewer than 4 low-power fields in any slide. Grade 3 tumors have a >4 low-power fields of immature tissue [PMID1260722]. Because the clinical breakpoint appears to be between grade 1 immaturity on the one hand, and grades 2 and 3 on the other (ie, a small amount of immaturity is well tolerated), and because of the large amount of interobserver variability in the 3-tiered system, a 2-tiered system has been proposed [PMID7814189].

Another potential error is to misinterpret a frankly malignant component of another type of germ cell tumor as immature tissue. The 2 most common examples of this involve unusual variants of yolk sac tumor. The hepatoid type of yolk sac tumor can be misinterpreted as immature liver and the well differentiated glandular type of yolk sac tumor as immature lung. These are potentially serious errors because a frankly malignant component, such as a yolk sac tumor, conveys a much more aggressive course than simple immaturity, especially if immaturity is focal [PMID9737245].

The struma ovarii is a type of teratoma consisting completely or primarily of thyroid tissue. This term is used only when thyroid tissue occupies most or all of the tumor. Occasional foci of thyroid tissue may be found in common teratomas. The thyroid tissue may be difficult to recognize if it has a trabecular rather than follicular pattern, and a thyroglobulin stain may be required. A strumal carcinoid consists of carcinoid tumor associated with thyroid tissue i33.29. Some, but not all, believe that pure ovarian carcinoid tumors are also a type of monodermal teratoma.

The choriocarcinoma is discussed in Chapters 28 and 38, and is therefore omitted here, except to mention 2 points. First, the finding of a choriocarcinoma in a woman in either the ovary or the uterus requires that such a tumor be excluded in the other site (ie, that a metastasis be ruled out). Second, the presence of multinucleated giant cells alone does not establish the diagnosis of choriocarcinoma. Virtually any germ cell tumor may have occasional giant cells that are composed of fusion of mononuclear cells. Indeed, most germ cell tumors with scattered giant cells are not choriocarcinomas.

Unusual Ovarian Neoplasms

The ovarian small cell carcinoma, hypercalcemic type, is an undifferentiated carcinoma that is usually associated with hypercalcemia. Morphologically, the cells of the primary ovarian small cell carcinoma, hypercalcemic type, may be slightly larger than the usual small cell carcinoma, often have a moderate amount of eosinophilic cytoplasm i33.30, and may rarely contain a small amount of cytoplasmic mucin. They may form cords or follicles. Immunohistochemically, this neoplasm, like the pulmonary small cell carcinoma, may be negative for chromogranin and synaptophysin, but it usually reacts with CD10 and WT1, while the lung small cell carcinoma does not. In addition, thyroid transcription factor 1 stains most pulmonary small cell carcinoma, but not the ovarian tumor [PMID17727473]. Radiographic studies, especially the presence or absence of a lung mass, remain important in the differentiation of this tumor from a pulmonary small cell carcinoma.

The ovarian small cell carcinoma, hypercalcemic type, can also resemble an adult or juvenile granulosa cell tumor. The nuclei of the ovarian small cell carcinoma, hypercalcemic type, are darker and more pleomorphic than adult granulosa cell tumors, and they do not have the grooves that are characteristic of the latter tumor. But they may resemble the nuclei of juvenile granulosa cell tumors, and inhibin may be required for a diagnosis. In contrast to stromal tumors, ovarian small cell carcinomas usually react with EMA and keratins, but not with inhibin [PMID9475192]. The clinical situation is also helpful in distinguishing this tumor from granulosa cell tumors. In addition to hypercalcemia, absence of estrogenic effects or the presence of metastases suggest a small cell carcinoma, hypercalcemic type, over a granulosa cell tumor.

The gonadoblastoma is a mixture of a sex cord-stromal tumor with a germ cell tumor. It is often calcified and is almost always found in patients with gonadal dysgenesis. The germ cell component is usually seminomatous, while the sex cord-stromal component usually has Sertoli differentiation. A gynandroblastoma is a combination of a Sertoli-stromal cell tumor and a granulosa-stromal cell tumor.

The Fallopian Tube

Nonneoplastic Conditions of the Fallopian Tube

Moving from the uterus outward, the portions of the fallopian tube are the isthmus, ampulla, and infundibulum, the site of the fimbriae. The commonly seen paratubal cysts (hydatids of Morgagni) are Mullerian remnants (the Mullerian and secondary Mullerian systems are discussed in Chapter 34.

Inflammation of the fallopian tube is commonly seen and is a component of pelvic inflammatory disease. Severe acute salpingitis often involves the ovary as well, resulting in a tubo-ovarian abscess (TOA). Lesser degrees of inflammation, or the healed stage of a TOA, often result in tubo-ovarian adhesions. Another indication of a healed salpingitis is fusion of plicae within the lumen. The reactive epithelial atypia resulting from severe salpingitis can be quite alarming and simulate carcinoma i33.31. The occasional presence of cilia is very reassuring in problematic cases and essentially mandates a benign diagnosis unless the evidence is overwhelming.

Endometrial tissue may extend into the proximal fallopian tube (isthmus), so endometriosis is usually not diagnosed in this part of the fallopian tube unless there is a compelling histologic picture, with a generous amount of endometrial glands and stroma in the wall of the tube, away from the lumen.

Salpingitis isthmica nodosa (SIN) consists of glandular epithelium that is connected to the lumen. They appear as separate glands in the wall i33.32, but are simple diverticula. The pathogenesis is unclear. Unlike vasitis nodosum, SIN is not clearly linked to previous surgery, trauma, or obstruction. SIN may predispose to infertility or ectopic pregnancies. Because SIN occurs primarily in the isthmus, where endometrial stroma may extend into the fallopian tube, the glands of SIN may be surrounded by endometrial type stroma, making distinction from endometriosis difficult. It is conventional to lean away from the diagnosis of endometriosis in the presence of salpingitis isthmica nodosum, especially in the isthmus, unless there are foci of endometriosis elsewhere.

Neoplasms of the Fallopian Tube

The fallopian tube is rarely the site of a primary malignancy. The most common type, accounting for half of all primary carcinomas of the fallopian tube, is a serous papillary adenocarcinoma that is morphologically identical to its ovarian counterpart. Most of the remaining carcinomas of the fallopian tube are of the endometrioid type [PMID17365827]. Prophylactic salpingo-oophorectomy in cases where a mutation in either *BRCA1* or *BRCA2* is present has identified an early stage of primary serous carcinoma of the fallopian tube, mostly in the fimbriae, that had previously escaped detection. These are tentatively called tubal intraepithelial carcinoma (TIC) or serous tubal intraepithelial carcinoma (STIC) i33.33. 5-7% of patients undergoing prophylactic salpingo-oophorectomy will be found to have TIC [PMID20567141]. Indeed, as discussed further in Chapter 34, the fallopian tube may be an undetected source for metastatic serous adenocarcinoma or for a primary peritoneal carcinoma when the ovary is found to be negative [PMID17456833].

Female adnexal tumor of probable Wolffian origin (FATWO) is usually found within the broad ligament, or hanging from it, but may rarely be attached to the fallopian tube. A mesonephric (Wolffian) origin is suspected because there are mesonephric remnants in the broad ligaments (which are folds of peritoneum). There are numerous microscopic patterns, such as diffuse, tubular, cystic, and sieve-like i33.34 [PMID16800270]. These patterns may have a low-power resemblance to such entities such as yolk sac tumor and Sertoli cell tumor, but on closer study, the nuclei appear innocuous. Although the FATWO is rare, it should be suspected in any tumor that is confined to the area in or around the broad ligament.

ISBN 978-089189-5886

Core Points for the Ovary and Fallopian Tube

- Ovarian endometriosis: classic triad of endometrial glands, endometrial stroma, and hemosiderin-laden macrophages may be indistinct
  - IHC for CD10 may be needed to identify endometrial stroma.
- 6 pregnancy-associated conditions of the ovary—the large luteinized solitary follicle cyst of pregnancy and puerperium, the pregnancy luteoma, hyperreactio luteinalis, hilus cell hyperplasia, intrafollicular granulosa cell proliferations, and ectopic decidua in pregnancy.
- Stromal hyperthecosis: stromal hyperplasia and luteinization.
- Polycystic ovary disease: multiple follicular cysts, generally without corpora lutea or corpora albicans, since ovulation is limited.
  - But many patients can ovulate with medical assistance.
  - Fibrotic, hypocellular cortex overlies cysts.
- 3 major classes of primary ovarian tumors: epithelial, sex cord-stromal, and germ cell. Serous and mucinous adenomas are common.
- Serous and mucinous adenocarcinomas: most common ovarian malignancies.
  - Examination of the epithelial lining distinguishes between them.
- Low malignant potential (LMP or borderline) neoplasms: greater cellularity and complexity than adenomas, without invasion.
  - Serous LMP tumors: may have local lymph node involvement or peritoneal implants.
    - 3 types of implants are commonly seen in serous LMP tumors: noninvasive epithelial, noninvasive desmoplastic, and invasive.
  - Mucinous LMP tumors: endocervical and intestinal types.
- LMP tumors controversial because:
  - Mucinous LMP tumors and pseudomyxoma peritonei are almost always secondary to an appendiceal process.
  - Serous LMP tumors behave well even if implants if implant is not invasive.
  - Behave aggressively if there are invasive implants.
- Other ovarian epithelial neoplasms: endometrioid carcinomas, clear cell carcinomas, Brenner tumors.
- Endometrioid carcinomas: may have papillary areas that resemble a serous papillary carcinoma.
  - Search for squamous metaplasia or areas of more classic endometrioid carcinoma.
  - 15-20% of cases have concomitant endometrioid carcinoma of the endometrium.
- Any serous, mucinous, and endometrioid carcinoma may resemble metastatic adenocarcinoma.
  - IHC can help, but wise to clinically exclude a coexisting neoplasm of the gastrointestinal tract, appendix, or endometrium.
- Sex cord-stromal tumors: originate from remnants of secondary sex cords or from the ovarian stroma, not from epithelium.
  - Stain for inhibin.
  - Adult granulosa cell tumor is most common.
    - Low-grade malignancy, most common pattern is microfollicular, with Call-Exner bodies.
  - Juvenile granulosa cell tumor: cellular, irregularly shaped follicles, nuclei without the grooves that are seen in the adult form.
- Sertoli-Leydig tumor: consider when a neoplasm does fit clearly into another category.
  - May contain heterologous elements, usually only of mesenchymal origin.
- Steroid cell tumors (formerly called lipid cell tumor): 3 types, all similar.
- Germ cell tumors: develop from the ovum or the cells immediately surrounding it.
  - Stains for placental alkaline phosphatase (PLAP).
- Ovarian teratomas: example of uniparental diploidy
  - But whereas hydatidiform moles arise from two paternal genomes, ovarian teratomas arise from two maternal genomes.
  - Most are cystic, fully mature, and primarily ectodermal (dermoid cysts).
  - Even if more complex, overt malignancy is rare, greater danger is immaturity.
  - Immaturity usually graded 1-3 on neural tissue.
  - Consider only embryonic tissue, not fetal tissue.
  - Pitfall: misinterpreting malignant tissue of another type as immature tissue (eg, a yolk sac component as immature liver or lung).
- Salpingitis isthmica nodosa: diverticula of the epithelium, may simulate invasive carcinoma.
- Carcinomas of fallopian tube: usually similar to ovarian serous carcinomas.

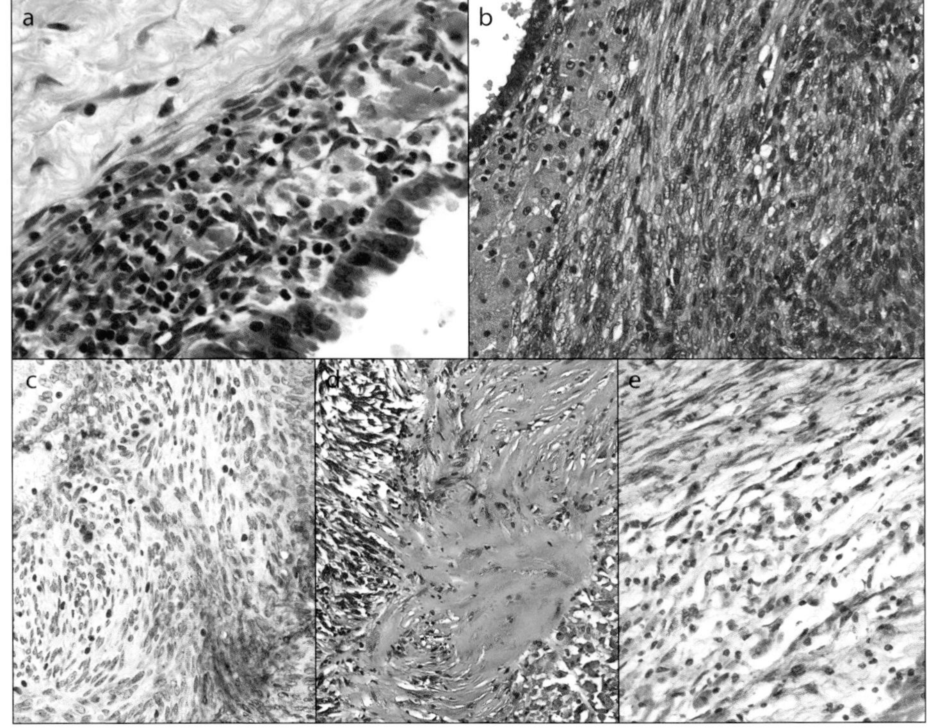

i33.1 **a** Ovarian endometriosis. Beneath an endometrial lining, hemosiderin macrophages are seen in the upper right and endometrial stroma in the lower left.

b An ovarian cyst demonstrating, from left to right, probable endometrial epithelium, hemosiderin macrophages, and probable endometrial stroma

c A CD10 stain on the same case, with a few positive cells, permitting a presumptive diagnosis of endometriosis

d A hemorrhagic cyst of the ovary with numerous hemosiderin macrophages. The stroma is suspicious for endometriosis.

e A negative CD10 stain on this cyst. The case remains suspicious for endometriosis because CD10 is not perfectly sensitive for endometrial stroma, but a secure diagnosis cannot be achieved.

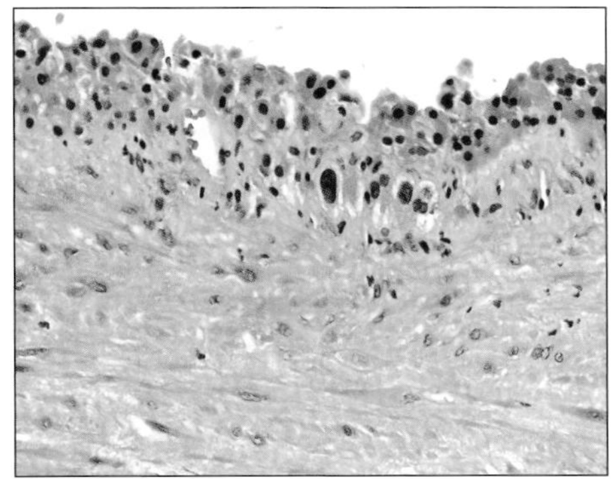

i33.2 A large luteinized solitary follicle cyst pregnancy, with isolated atypical cells in the lining

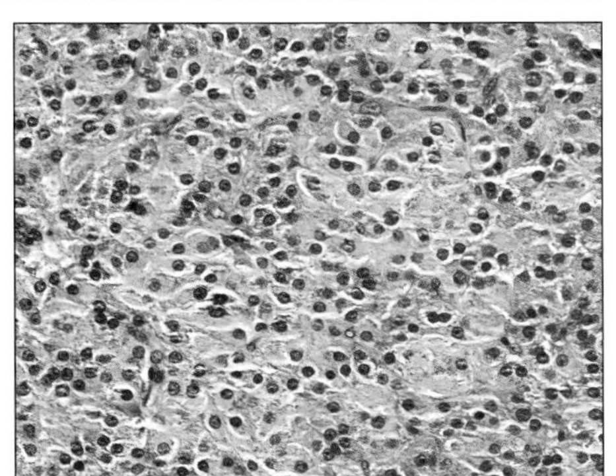

i33.3 A pregnancy luteoma. Note the essential histologic identity to steroid cell tumors.

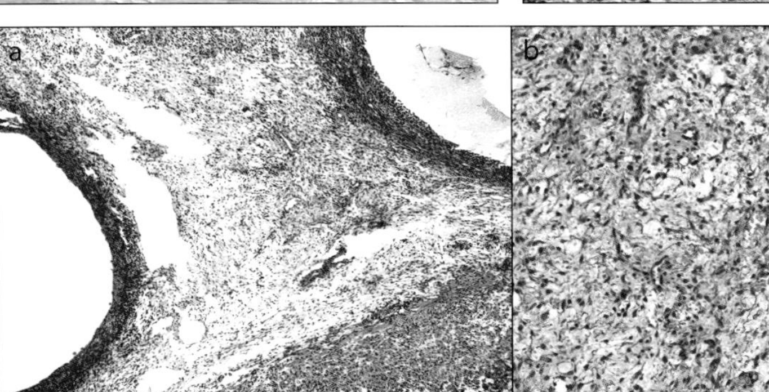

i33.4 **a** Hyperreactio luteinalis with several cysts, one of which is a corpus luteum

b Stromal luteinization in hyperreactio luteinalis

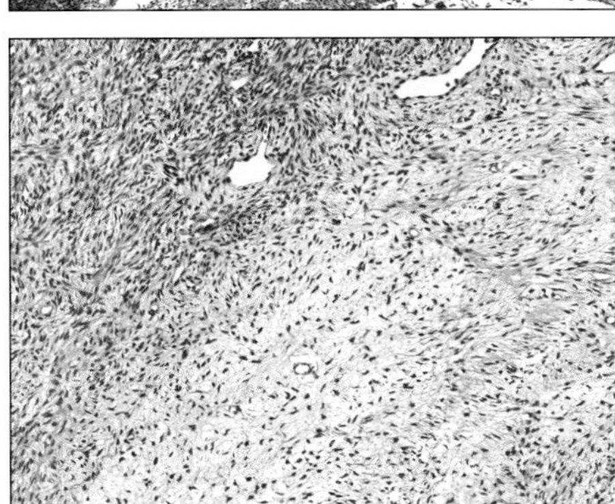

i33.5 Stromal hyperthecosis with a cluster of luteinized stromal cells in the center and a slightly fibrotic stroma in the upper left

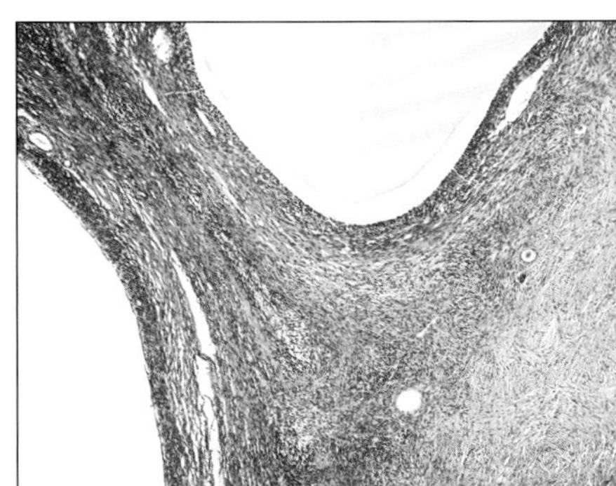

i33.6 Polycystic ovary. There are 2 follicular cysts, without luteinization, separated from the surface by a slightly fibrotic ovarian cortex.

ISBN 978-089189-5886

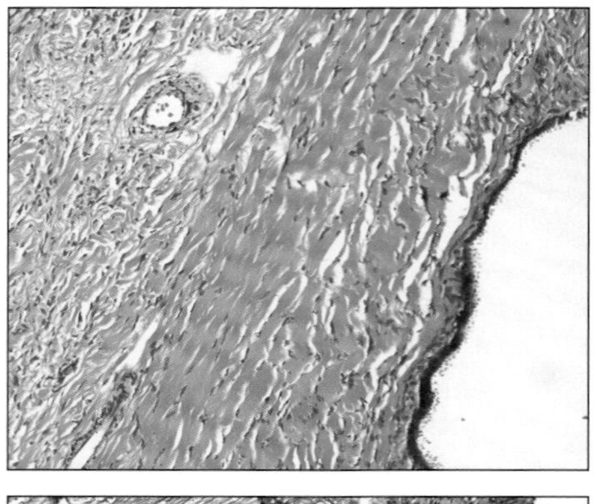

i33.7 A serous cystadenofibroma of the ovary

i33.8 A mucinous adenoma of the ovary

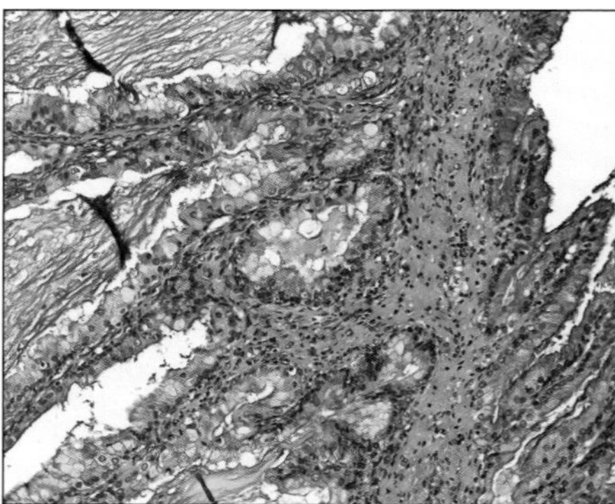

i33.9 A mucinous carcinoma of the ovary. Note the abundant, well defined cytoplasmic mucin in both this case and in the adenoma in i33.8.

i33.10 A serous adenocarcinoma of the ovary. Although an adenocarcinoma, cytoplasmic mucin is inconspicuous.

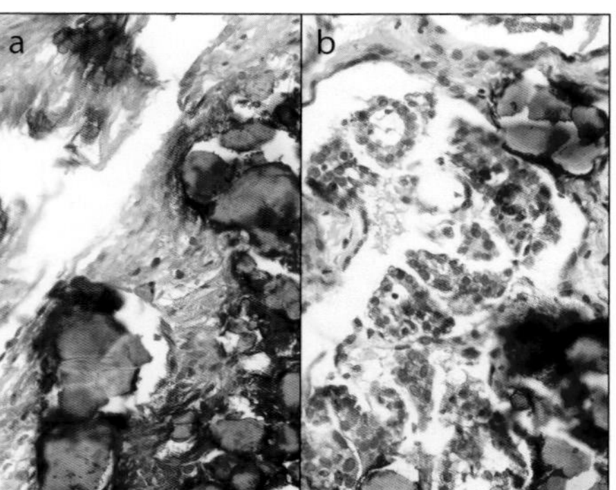

i33.11 **a** Large numbers of psammoma bodies on the surface of an ovary, not diagnostic of malignancy **b** Elsewhere in the same ovary, however, a serous carcinoma is present.

i33.12 A serous low malignant potential (LMP) ovarian neoplasm. Despite the extensive cellularity, there is no invasion.

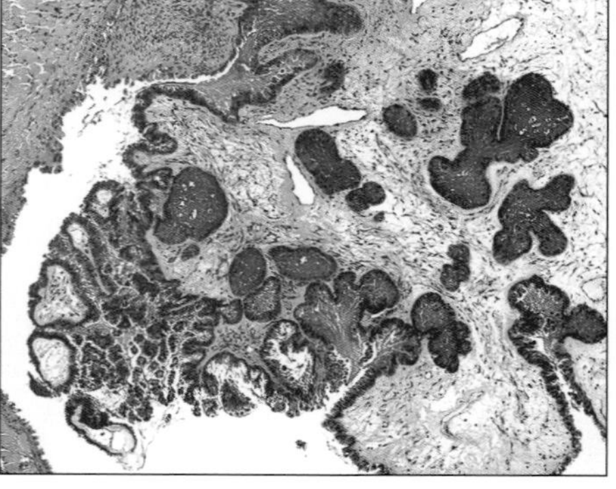

i33.13 Another serous LMP in which invagination of the neoplastic epithelium from the surface simulates invasion.

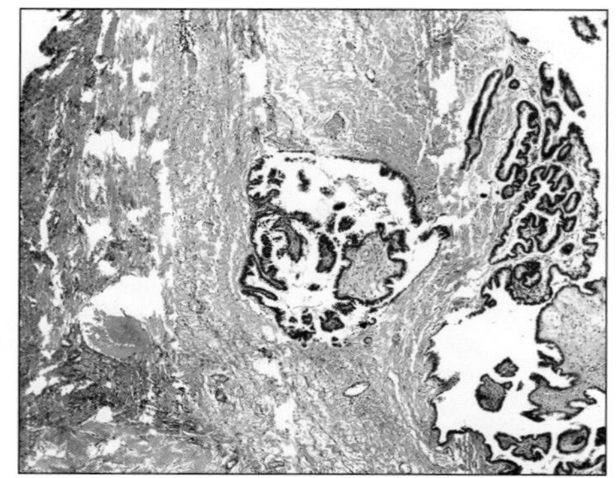

i33.14 A serous LMP tumor with microinvasion

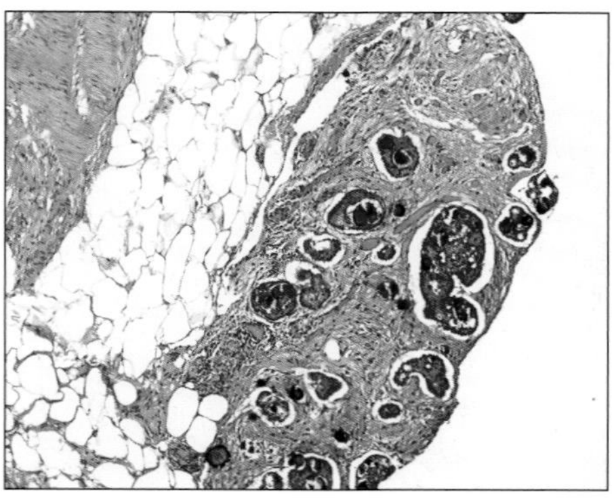

i33.15 A noninvasive omental implant in a patient with a history of a serous LMP ovarian neoplasm

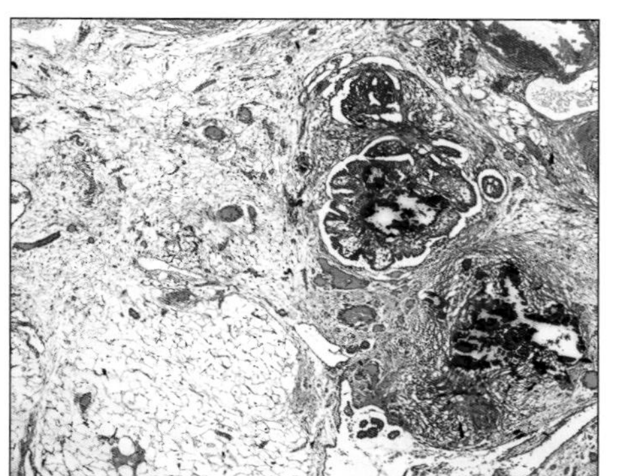

i33.16 An invasive omental implant. Both neoplastic cells and psammoma bodies are found in the interior, and there is a stromal reaction.

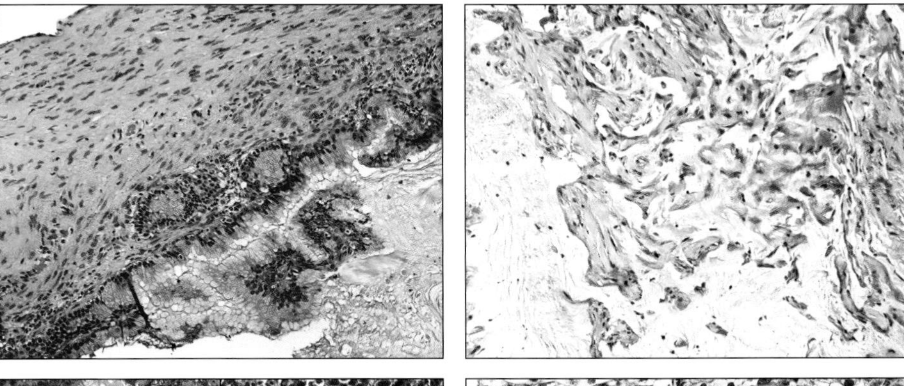

i33.17 A mucinous LMP neoplasm of the ovary

i33.18 Pseudomyxoma peritonei in which there are pools of mucin in this omental biopsy. Epithelial cellularity is minimal and sometimes requires a keratin stain.

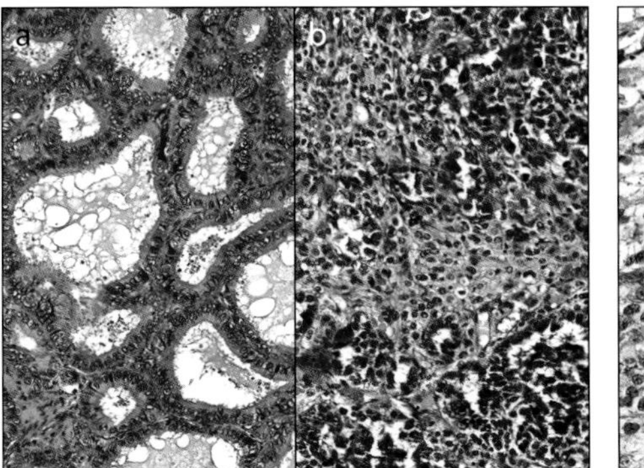

i33.19 **a** An endometrioid carcinoma of the ovary. Note the similarity to a FIGO 1 adenocarcinoma of the endometrium (see i31.26b. **b** A poorly differentiated ovarian adenocarcinoma, the endometrioid nature of which is suggested by the squamous metaplasia in the center

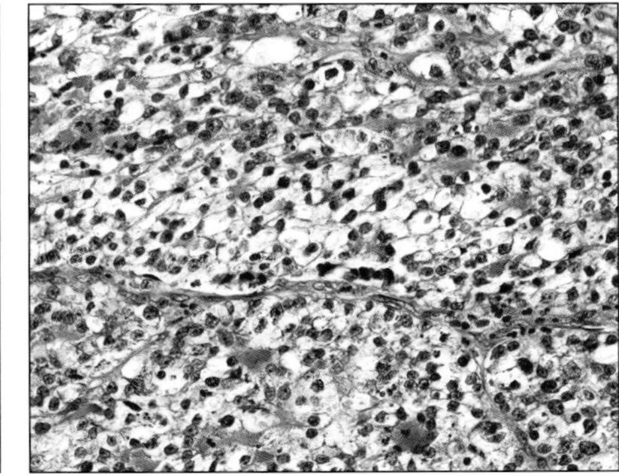

i33.20 A classic, solid variant of clear cell carcinoma of the ovary

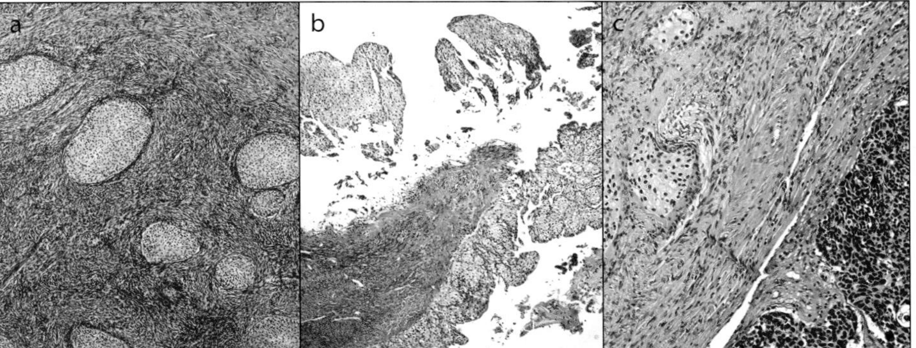

i33.21 **a** A Brenner tumor of the ovary. Note the relatively small clusters of urothelial-like epithelium and a cellular stroma that surrounds these clusters and that is sharply demarcated from the normal, less cellular ovarian stroma. **b** An LMP Brenner tumor, resembling a low-grade noninvasive papillary urothelial carcinoma of the bladder. Other areas of this tumor were not papillary, but had much larger clusters of neoplastic cells than are seen in i33.21a. **c** A malignant Brenner tumor is seen on the right. The nature of the malignancy is identified by the benign Brenner tumor on the left.

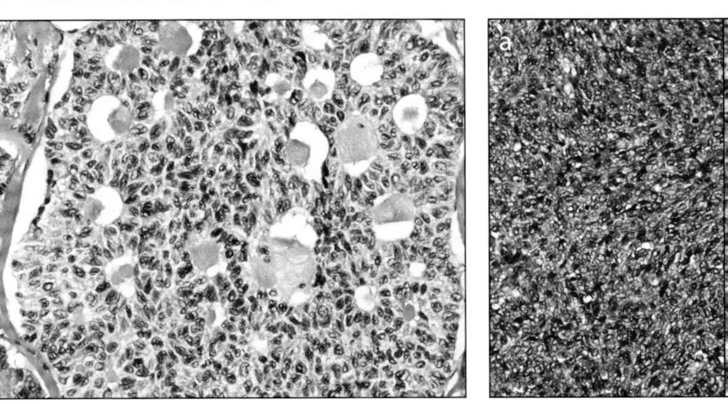

i33.22 A common, microfollicular variant of adult granulosa cell tumor with Call-Exner bodies. Note the eosinophilic material within the lumens and the irregular nuclear membranes, with frequent and prominent grooves.

i33.23 **a** A solid granulosa cell tumor that was negative for epithelial membrane antigen and placental alkaline phosphatase **b** The same neoplasm staining positively for inhibin

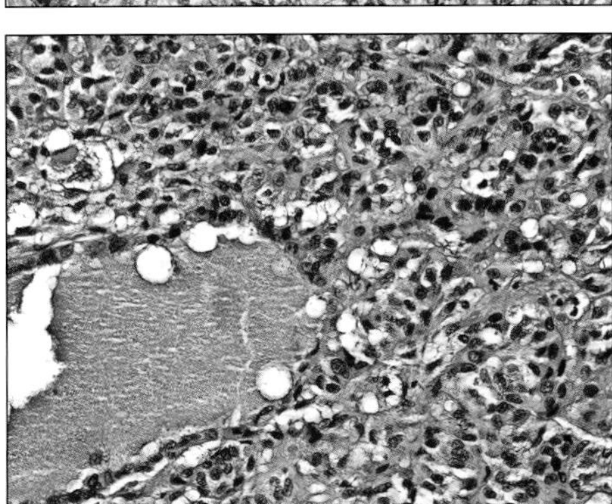

i33.24 A juvenile granulosa cell tumor with large cells containing abundant eosinophilic cytoplasm. Note that nuclear grooves are inconspicuous and that the follicle is distinct from the Call-Exner body of the adult granulosa cell tumor.

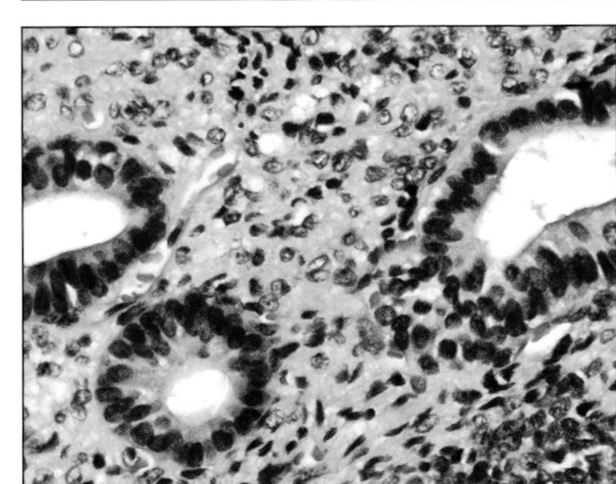

i33.25 A well differentiated Sertoli-Leydig cell tumor with Leydig cells interspersed between well defined tubules formed by the Sertoli component

ISBN 978-089189-5886

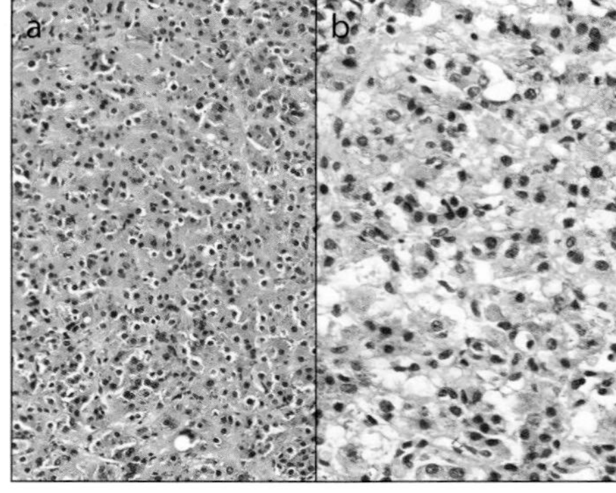

i33.26 A steroid cell tumor, with **a** eosinophilic and **b** focally clear cytoplasm. Note essentially identical appearance to a pregnancy luteoma i33.3.

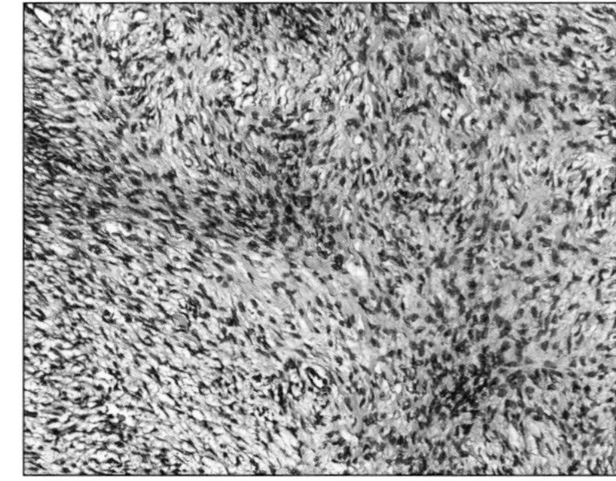

i33.27 An ovarian fibroma/thecoma. Some cells are fibroblasts, associated with collagen, and others have a moderate amount of clear cytoplasm.

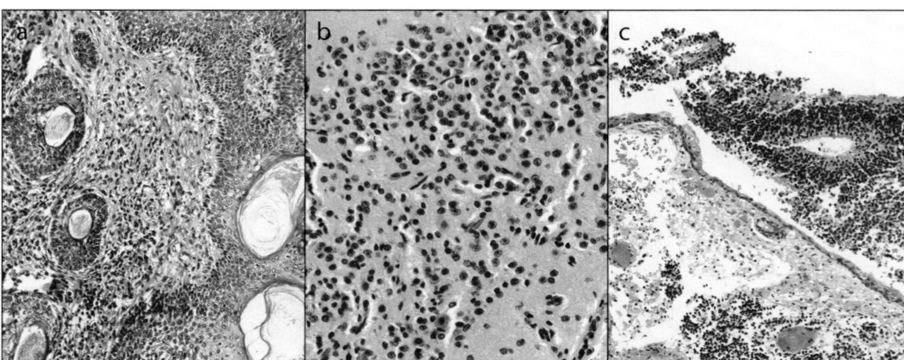

i33.28 **a** A commonly encountered mature cystic teratoma with cutaneous adnexal structures (dermoid cyst) **b** A mature teratoma with a cluster of glial cells in brain tissue **c** An immature teratoma with rosette formation

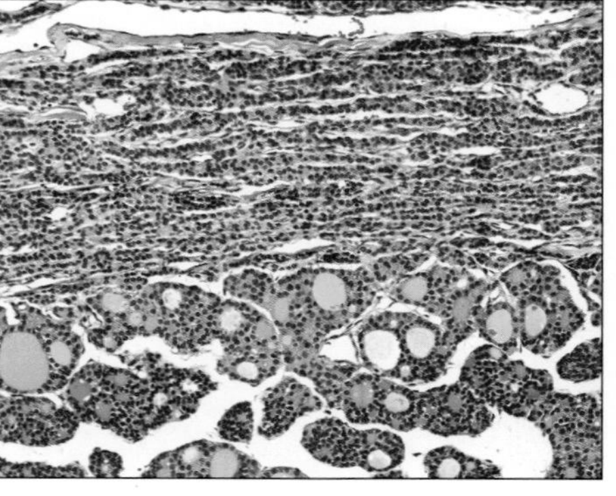

i33.29 Strumal carcinoid, with thyroid tissue on the bottom and a carcinoid tumor on the top

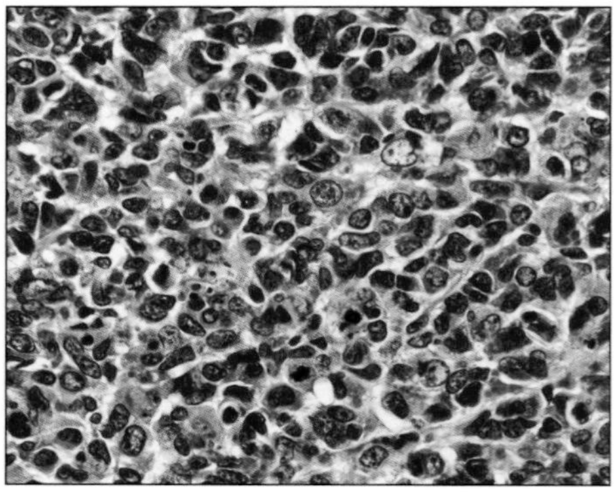

i33.30 An ovarian small cell carcinoma, hypercalcemic type. The neoplasm is similar to small cell carcinomas in other sites, but some cells are larger, with more cytoplasm.

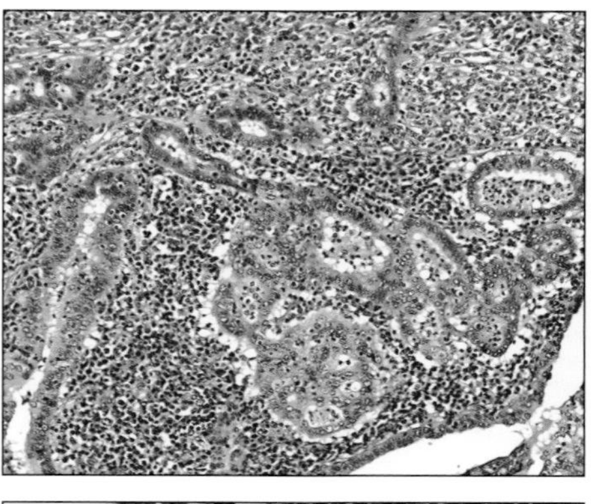

i33.31 Severe acute and chronic salpingitis simulating carcinoma. Clues to a benign diagnosis in such cases include absence of invasion into the wall, severe inflammation, and the occasional presence of cilia.

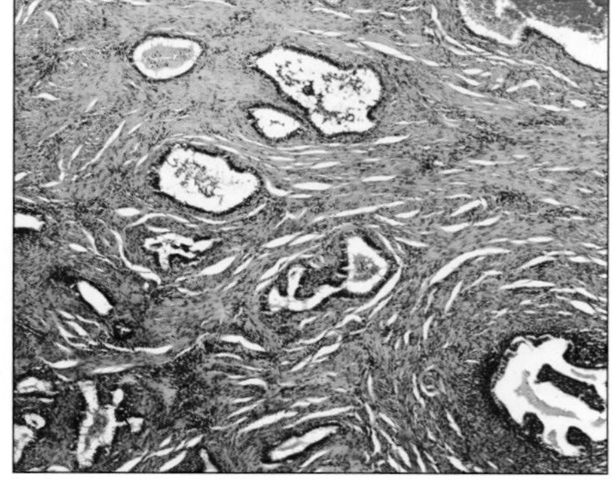

i33.32 Salpingitis isthmica nodosa. The lumen of the fallopian tube is in the lower right.

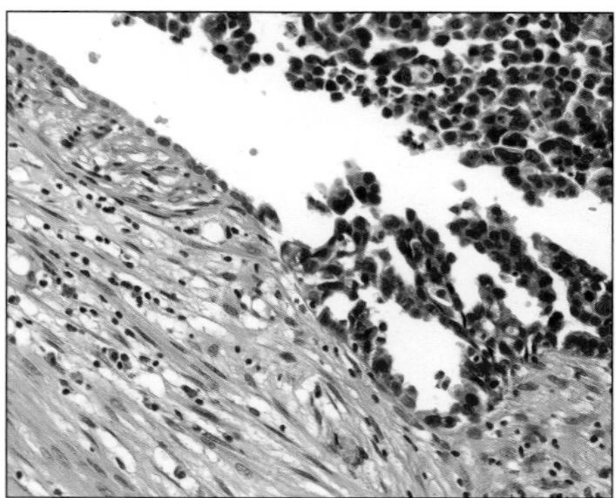

i33.33 A poorly differentiated serous carcinoma primary in the fallopian tube. This photograph shows tubal intraepithelial neoplasia in the lower portion. This patient did not have a BRCA abnormality.

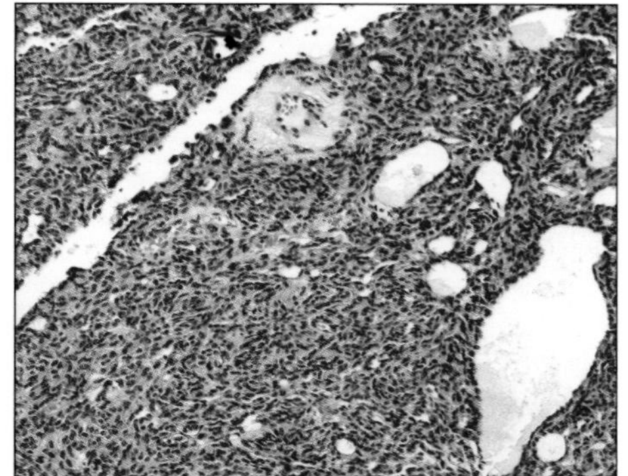

i33.34 A female adnexal tumor of probable Wolffian origin (FATWO), sieve-like pattern, in the broad ligament. There is s resemblance to a yolk sac tumor, but the nuclei are innocuous.

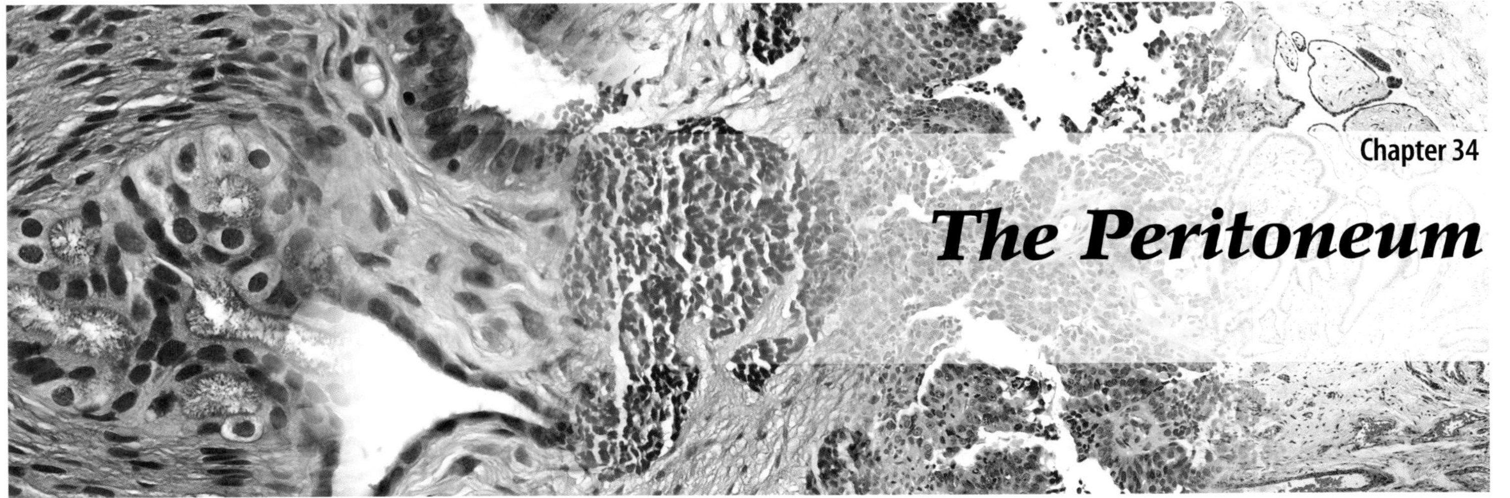

Chapter 34 The Peritoneum

The Normal Serosa, Reactive Fibrosis, and Inclusion Cysts

Serosal surfaces, such as the pleura and the peritoneum, consist of a mesothelial lining and a thin underlying layer of connective tissue. The mesothelium is a modified epithelium whose developmental and immunohistochemical properties differ from usual epithelium.

Sclerosing peritonitis is a fibrosclerosing disorder that may be related to sclerosing mesenteritis, retroperitoneal fibrosis, sclerosing mediastinitis, and sclerosing cholangitis. Infection and malignancy are occasional culprits and must be excluded [PMID9606807], but other cases are manifestations of the IgG4-associated sclerosing disorders. The principal differential diagnosis is with solitary fibrous tumor (SFT), discussed below.

Peritoneal inclusion cysts typically occur in the peritoneal cavity of young women. They may be either unilocular or multilocular i34.1. The multilocular cysts were formerly called multicystic peritoneal mesothelioma, but these are not true neoplasms, though they must be differentiated from cystic mesotheliomas and multilocular cystic lymphangiomas. Peritoneal inclusion cysts may have focal nuclear atypia, but the gross appearance, the lack of generalized nuclear atypia, and most important, the lack of invasion prevent an overdiagnosis [PMID19386139].

Mesothelioma and Mesothelial Hyperplasia

The differentiation of mesothelial processes from metastatic adenocarcinoma in the peritoneum can be done as in the pleura, and is discussed in Chapter 17. Likewise, the types of and diagnosis of malignant mesotheliomas are discussed in Chapter 17.

Here, we discuss a number of benign mesothelial proliferations that are more common in the peritoneum [PMID1759060]. There are many patterns of mesothelial hyperplasia, including solid, trabecular, tubular, papillary, and tubulopapillary. All of these have an epithelial rather than fibrous appearance, and most cases of "benign mesothelioma of the epithelial type" are better regarded as mesothelial hyperplasia.

Once mesothelial origin has been established, distinguishing any form of mesothelial hyperplasia from malignant mesothelioma of the epithelial type can be difficult in biopsy material. The clinical and radiographic findings are helpful in making this differentiation, as processes that are large or show radiographic evidence of invasion are more likely to be malignant, while benign mesothelial proliferations are small (<2.0 cm), localized, and radiographically well demarcated. Mesothelial hyperplasia generally has blander nuclei and a simpler architecture than an epithelial mesothelioma [PMID17044190]. Desmoplasia, if present, suggests malignancy, but is not always seen in a biopsy of malignant mesothelioma. It has been reported that cells of diffuse malignant mesothelioma tend to stain more intensely for epithelial membrane antigen (EMA), p53, and glucose transport protein-1 than hyperplastic mesothelial cells, while the latter are more likely to stain for desmin [PMID20209622], but the clinical utility of this is unclear.

As in the pleura, the only pathway to certainty in diagnosing a malignant mesothelial process in biopsy material is to prove invasion [PMID16253023]. Care should be taken not to regard entrapment of mesothelial cells secondary to specimen acquisition as invasion. Factors favoring entrapment include detached clusters of cells, fibrin, inflammation, and small fragments that are lined by mesothelium on both sides. If invasion is not unequivocal, a comment should be made that clinical correlation is needed to exclude malignancy because the biopsy may not have captured an invasive focus.

Papillary mesothelial hyperplasia must also be distinguished from low malignant potential (LMP) serous tumors that are from the ovary or are primary in the peritoneum. This may require immunohistochemical stains, but the history and clinical presentation are helpful. Columnar cells and psammoma bodies favor epithelial origin (ie, an LMP tumor) over mesothelial.

Well differentiated papillary mesotheliomas are very rare and usually occur in the peritoneum of younger women. They may be single or multiple. They are considered LMP neoplasms because recurrence is rare and deaths are not expected [PMID22024662]. Well differentiated papillary mesothelioma resembles papillary mesothelial hyperplasia i34.2 but tends to have more prominent fibrous cores. Despite the possibility of slightly greater potential in the well differentiated papillary mesothelioma, these entities can be confused without compromising patient care, as long as they are successfully distinguished from a malignant mesothelioma and from adenocarcinoma.

The SFT (also called localized fibrous tumor) is discussed and illustrated in more detail in Chapter 17 because it is more common in the pleura, but the morphology and immunohistochemical characteristics of the SFT in the peritoneum match those of its pleural counterpart. Just as most cases of benign epithelial-type mesothelioma are now considered mesothelial hyperplasia, so most cases of benign fibrous mesothelioma are now considered to be SFT. SFT is considered to arise from submesotheial fibroblasts and not from the actual mesothelium because they are negative for cytokeratin. SFTs have alternating areas of greater and lesser cellularity and

ISBN 978-089189-5886

a hemangiopericytoma-like vascular pattern (thin-walled, dilated, branching vessels; see i17.19, i17.20. As in the case of epithelial mesothelial proliferations, clinical and radiographic correlation is helpful in determining malignancy, but invasion is the essential finding in the pathologic diagnosis of a malignant SFT in a biopsy. Even if the biopsy suggests a benign SFT, it is prudent to comment that the biopsy may not have captured an invasive focus and that if there is clinical or radiographic evidence of invasion, a malignant SFT is not excluded.

The true sarcomatous mesothelioma and the malignant SFT are both rare. Because mesothelial markers are weak or absent in sarcomatous mesothelioma, these 2 entities are difficult to distinguish from each other. Keratin, which is focally positive in sarcomatous mesotheliomas, and CD31, characteristic of SFT, may help, but the more important distinction is sarcomatous mesothelioma and malignant SFT on the one hand from a metastatic desmoplastic carcinoma on the other [PMID21043818].

Pseudomyxoma Peritonei

As discussed in Chapter 33 and illustrated in i33.18, "pseudomyxoma peritonei" is a clinical term referring to mucinous deposits within the peritoneal cavity, often with few or no epithelial cells. The vast majority of cases of pseudomyxoma peritonei are derived from mucinous neoplasms or mucoceles of the appendix [PMID17511804], and many question if any significant number of these cases are of ovarian origin even when a mucinous ovarian neoplasm has been documented, but historically, mucinous ovarian neoplasms are a cause of pseudomyxoma peritonei. Even with our new understanding, the ovaries and the gastrointestinal tract still require investigation in cases of pseudomyxoma peritonei if the appendix is found to be normal. In any event, these deposits should prompt great concern for carcinoma unless it can be shown that the pools of mucin are completely acellular and a full workup fails to demonstrate a mucinous neoplasm.

The Secondary Müllerian System

During development, the primitive kidney is formed from the mesonephros (the final kidney is formed from the metanephros). The mesonephric (Wolffian) ducts are part of the mesonephros and, in the male embryo, develop into the epididymis, the vas deferens, the seminal vesicles, and the ejaculatory duct (but not the testes).

The Müllerian (also called paramesonephric) ducts develop beside the mesonephric ducts. The Müllerian system regresses in male embryos under the influence of Müllerian inhibiting substance produced by Sertoli cells. In the female embryo, the absence of testosterone causes the mesonephric ducts to regress, though mesonephric remnants may occasionally be encountered, especially in the vagina and cervix. The Müllerian ducts give rise to the main structures of the female genital system—fallopian tubes, uterus, cervix, proximal vagina, and the surface epithelium of the ovaries, but not the ovaries themselves [Larsen ISBN978-0443065835]. These structures are called primary Müllerian structures. This common Müllerian origin has led to the suggestion that serous tumors of the ovary, serous tumors of the fallopian tube, and the primary peritoneal carcinoma all arise from the Müllerian system and are fundamentally the same entity [PMID19038766].

Within the primary Müllerian structures, there may be a slight mixing of epithelial types, so that one may encounter epithelial cells in one site that are more commonly seen in another site. For example, endocervical or endometrial cells epithelial cells are occasionally ciliated and epithelial cells in the fallopian tube may be mucinous. By convention, these are called metaplasias (implying a change) but are probably better regarded as congenital variants of normal.

The mesothelium of the lower abdomen and the pelvis (including the subjacent mesenchyme) has a somewhat similar potential to the primary Müllerian tissue because of its proximity to the Müllerian ducts. This tissue is called the secondary Müllerian system, a term first used by Lauchlan [PMID4614139]. Lesions developing in this area from the secondary Müllerian system include endometriosis, endosalpingiosis, endocervicosis, primary peritoneal carcinoma, transitional cell metaplasia (outside of the ovary, prostate, and anus), and peritoneal decidual reaction. Some include disseminated peritoneal leiomyomatosis in this category. Secondary Müllerian processes occur almost exclusively in women. The pathogenesis of these entities has never been clarified. Some have favored an actual migration of cells while others have favored an in situ metaplasia of cells. A diffusible factor from the primary Müllerian structures during development may someday be implicated.

The most common entity in the secondary Müllerian system is endometriosis. As discussed in Chapter 33 and illustrated in i33.1, the epithelium of an endometriotic cyst may be attenuated and difficult to recognize, in which case the proper diagnosis rests on identifying endometrial stroma. Quite frequently, even this is lost and replaced by granulation tissue, in which case only a presumptive diagnosis of endometriosis can be made [PMID17592255]. In difficult cases, CD10 positivity may help establish the diagnosis of endometriosis by highlighting endometrial stromal cells. Exuberant endometriosis may simulate carcinoma, particularly on frozen section. Patients who are on progestational agents or who have been treatec for endometriosis may have implants with pseudodecidua change in the stroma and atrophic epithelium, reminiscen of exogenous hormone affect in endometrial samplings i34.3.

Endosalpingiosis has a more restricted location than endo metriosis and tends to occur on the pelvic peritoneum coverin the uterus, fallopian tubes, ovaries, cul-de-sac, and within para aortic lymph nodes [PMID5805528], though it has been reported i other locations, such as the bladder and the serosa of the bowe Endosalpingiosis is rare inside an organ. In addition to an appro priate location, the diagnosis of endosalpingiosis requires a absence of endometrial stroma. Some cells will be ciliated i34. but others may not be, and the presence of cilia does not rul out endometriosis. In addition to endometriosis, the differentia diagnosis of endosalpingiosis also includes mesonephric rem nants, serous carcinomas of LMP, and mesothelial hyperplasia.

Endocervicosis, the presence of benign glands of the endc cervical type in the peritoneum, peritoneal decidual reactior in which there is a decidual reaction in the submesotheli stroma of the peritoneum in the pregnant or postpartu patient, and primary serosal mucinous neoplasms, are a very rare manifestations of secondary Müllerian processes.

The most serious and perplexing of the neoplasms arisin from the secondary Müllerian system is the primary peritone carcinoma (formerly called by a variety of names, includin serous surface carcinoma). This unusual neoplasm was fir reported by Swerdlow in 1959 [PMID13606191]. Like other entities the secondary Müllerian system, these almost always (but n always!) occur in women. The primary peritoneal carcinoma is a serous adenocarcinoma whose morphology matches that of a serous carcinoma of the ovary i34.5 [PMID8406199]. The diagnosis of primary peritoneal carcinoma has 3 sequential requirements. First, immunohistochemistry is needed to exclude a mesothelial proliferation. The panel employed and its interpretation are the same as for adenocarcinoma vs mesothelioma.

Second, the immunohistochemical characteristics of the neoplasm must be consistent with a primary peritoneal carcinoma. The immunohistochemical characteristics of this rare neoplasm are essentially identical to ovarian serous tumor, with positivity for keratin, EMA, CA-125, estrogen receptor, and B72.3, and negativity for calretinin, thrombomodulin, cytokeratin 5/6, and vimentin [PMID19897383].

Once the carcinomatous nature of the cells has been established by immunohistochemistry, and the findings are consistent with an ovarian serous neoplasm or a primary peritoneal carcinoma, the third requirement for the diagnosis of primary peritoneal carcinoma is the exclusion of a specific site of origin. Specifically, the ovaries must be shown to be normal, to contain tumor only on the surface [PMID9644683], or with focal microinvasion to a depth not exceeding 5 mm (0.5 cm) [PMID8406199]. This means that the definitive diagnosis of primary peritoneal carcinoma requires not only an immunohistochemical characterization of the neoplastic cells, but also a laparoscopy to ensure that there is no distinct primary source and, in particular, that the ovaries are not the culprit, as the absence or minimal nature of ovarian involvement is the key distinguishing feature between the primary peritoneal carcinoma and an ovarian carcinoma.

While the origin of many of these tumors remains elusive, the advent of prophylactic salpingo-oophorectomy for *BRCA1/2* mutations has revealed a surprising number of very early serous carcinomas of the fallopian tube, especially of the fimbriae, and some cases of primary peritoneal carcinoma may be of fallopian tube origin [PMID17456833]. There is also a primary LMP peritoneal serous tumor whose morphology and immunohistochemical characteristics match those of LMP serous ovarian tumors.

Müllerian glands within lymph nodes may be seen in some women, especially in pelvic or paraaortic lymph nodes, though they have been reported elsewhere [PMID7668944, PMID11781525]. The glands tend to be at the periphery of the node, either in the capsule, or in the superficial cortex between lymphoid follicles. Caution is recommended in situations in which glands are found only in these locations and not in the interior of the node or in the sinuses. Other clues to the benign nature of the glands are the lack of atypia and possibly, occasional ciliated cells. Nevertheless, there can be difficult situations, particularly on frozen section or in situations where one is addressing a possible nodal metastasis from a known ovarian serous tumor.

Unusual Peritoneal Neoplasms

Of the many unusual processes that occur in the peritoneum, only 2 will be mentioned here. The desmoplastic small round cell tumor (DSRCT) affects young men and is often in the mesentery, pelvis, or peritoneum [PMID18191563]. It usually has a low-power appearance similar to a cutaneous cylindroma, with small blue cells forming nests in a desmoplastic stroma i34.6a. The appearance of the individual cells is similar to that seen in a Ewing/PNET [PMID16945240]. Actually, the DSRCT has a translocation that is similar to that found in Ewing/PNET. Both tumors have a translocation involving the *EWS* gene on chromosome 22 i34.6b. In Ewing/PNET, the partner is usually the *FLI-1* gene on the long arm of chromosome 11 (11q), whereas in DSRCT, the *EWS* gene is fused to the *WT1* gene on the short arm of chromosome 11 (11p) [PMID19936782]. Thus, immunohistochemical staining for the WT1 protein can separate DSRCT from Ewing/PNET, provided that Wilms tumor, which is also positive for WT1, is excluded [PMID10843285]. DSRCT is negative for the FLI-1 protein. Like Ewing/PNET, desmoplastic small round tumors may express keratin, especially CAM 5.2 (low molecular weight), and vimentin. In contrast to Ewing/PNET, only about 20% of DSRCT are CD99 positive. Unlike Ewing/PNET, they may also express desmin, often in a perinuclear dot pattern, though other muscle markers are usually negative. Some investigators believe that the DSRCT is derived from mesothelioblasts.

Multiple peritoneal nodules of bland smooth muscles suggest disseminated peritoneal leiomyomatosis i34.7, which occurs in young women, almost always during pregnancy, and typically regresses spontaneously after pregnancy. Some consider this to be to be a metaplasia of submesothelial mesenchymal cells, while others favor an origin from the secondary Müllerian system, but it is agreed that the nodules are synchronous primary processes [PMID8604458]. They are not metastases and, in all probability, are not neoplasms.

Core Points for the Peritoneum

- A biopsy of a mesothelial process cannot be considered diagnostically malignant without invasion.
- Mesothelial hyperplasia: account for most cases previously called benign epithelial mesothelioma.
  - Small, well demarcated, and not invasive.
  - If papillary, must be distinguished from low malignant potential serous tumors of the ovary
  - IHC often needed.
  - If papillary, very similar to well differentiated papillary mesothelioma (very rare and usually occurs in peritoneum of younger women)
- Secondary Müllerian system: the mesothelium of the lower abdomen and the pelvis.
- Lesions nearly unique to women: endometriosis, endosalpingiosis, endocervicosis, primary peritoneal carcinoma, transitional cell metaplasia, and peritoneal decidual reaction.
  - Endometriosis: most common.
    - CD10 stain for endometrial stroma may help.
  - Primary peritoneal carcinoma: must be distinguished from metastatic ovarian carcinoma. This requires:
    - IHC to confirm the carcinomatous nature of the process.
    - Demonstration that ovaries and other possible primary sites are either free of tumor or are minimally involved.
    - Some cases are of fallopian tube origin.
  - Müllerian glands within lymph nodes may be seen in some women in the pelvic or para-aortic area, and may cause confusion, especially on frozen section.
- Desmoplastic small round cell tumor (DSRCT): young men often in the mesentery, pelvis, or peritoneum.
  - Clusters of small blue cells in a desmoplastic stroma.
  - *EWS/WT1* translocation.
- Disseminated peritoneal leiomyomatosis: multiple nodules of bland smooth muscle in peritoneum of young women
  - Usually during pregnancy and usually regresses

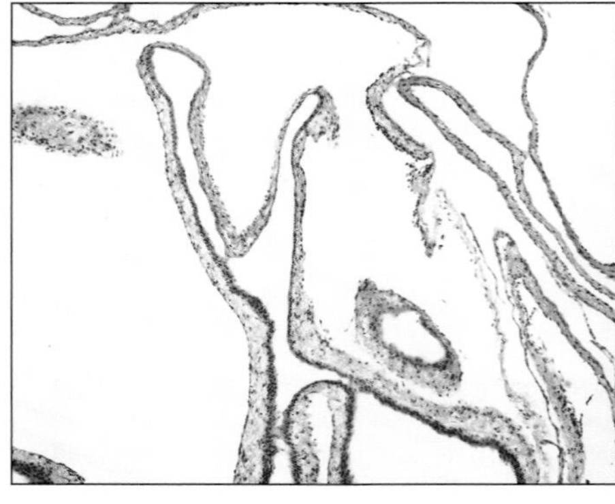

i34.1 Peritoneal inclusion cysts (formerly called multicystic peritoneal mesothelioma)

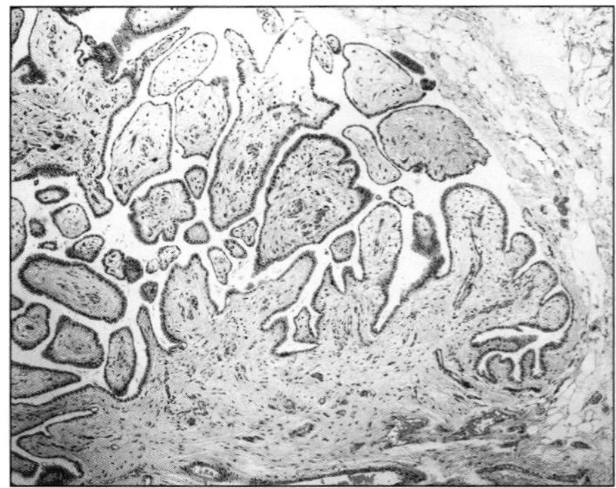

i34.2 A small mesothelial proliferation that can be regarded as either papillary mesothelial hyperplasia or a well differentiated papillary mesothelioma

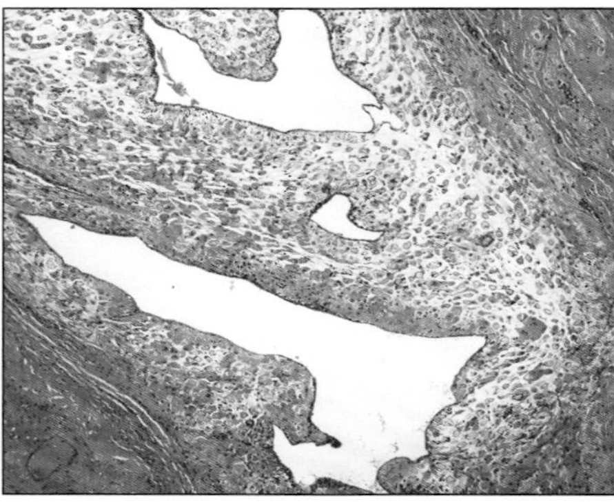

i34.3 Endometriosis in a patient who is receiving exogenous progesterone, causing pseudodecidual change in the stroma and atrophy of the glands

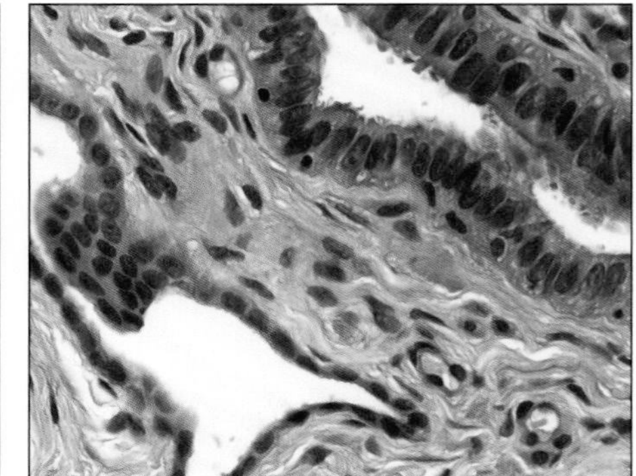

i34.4 Endosalpingiosis of the serosa. There is fallopian tube-like epithelium, with cilia, in the upper right, contrasted with the mesothelial lining of the lower left. Note the complete absence of any stroma that could be regarded as being of endometrial origin.

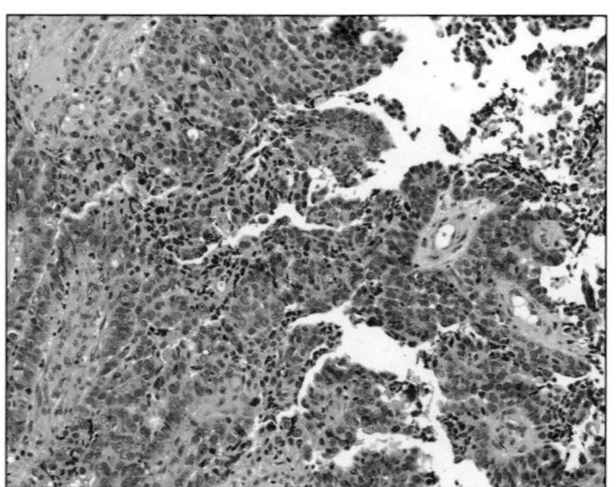

i34.5 A primary peritoneal carcinoma. Note the essentially identical appearance to a primary ovarian serous carcinoma and to a uterine papillary serous carcinoma.

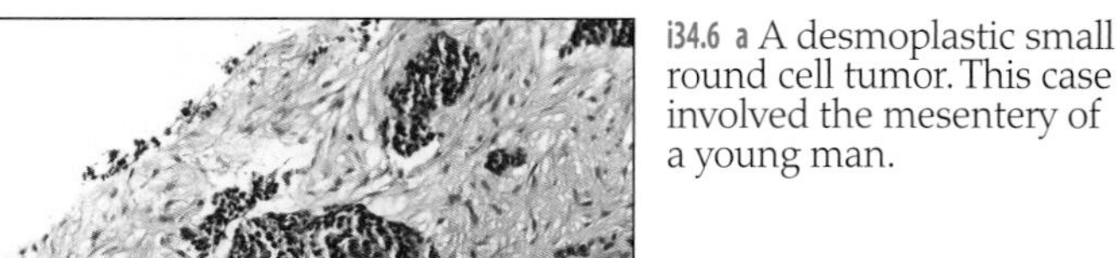

i34.6 a A desmoplastic small round cell tumor. This case involved the mesentery of a young man.

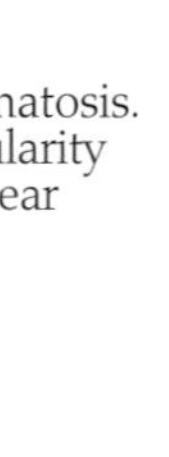

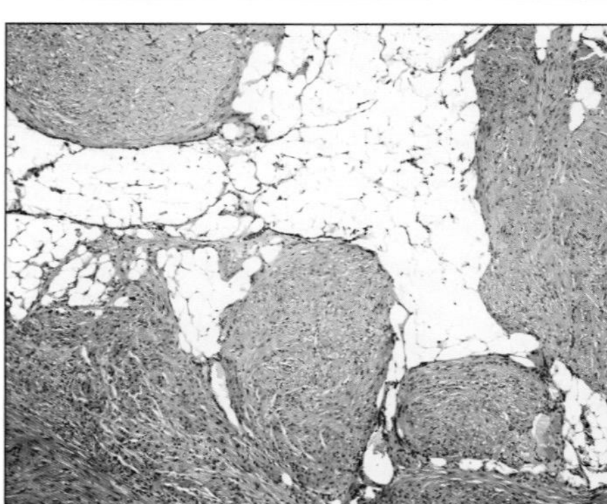

i34.7 Disseminated peritoneal leiomyomatosis. Note the multinodularity and the lack of nuclear atypia.

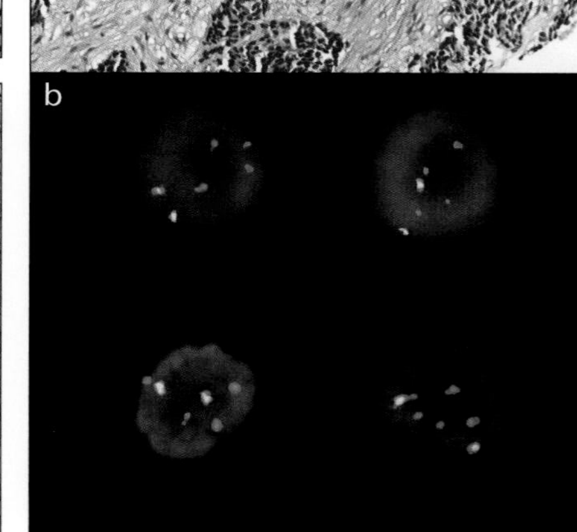

b Break apart FISH study for *EWSR1* in a desmoplastic small round cell tumor showing a variant signal pattern with 2 intact genes fluorescing as fused yellow signals and 2 disrupted genes with split red and green signals. This often corresponds to tumor tetraploidy on metaphase spreads.

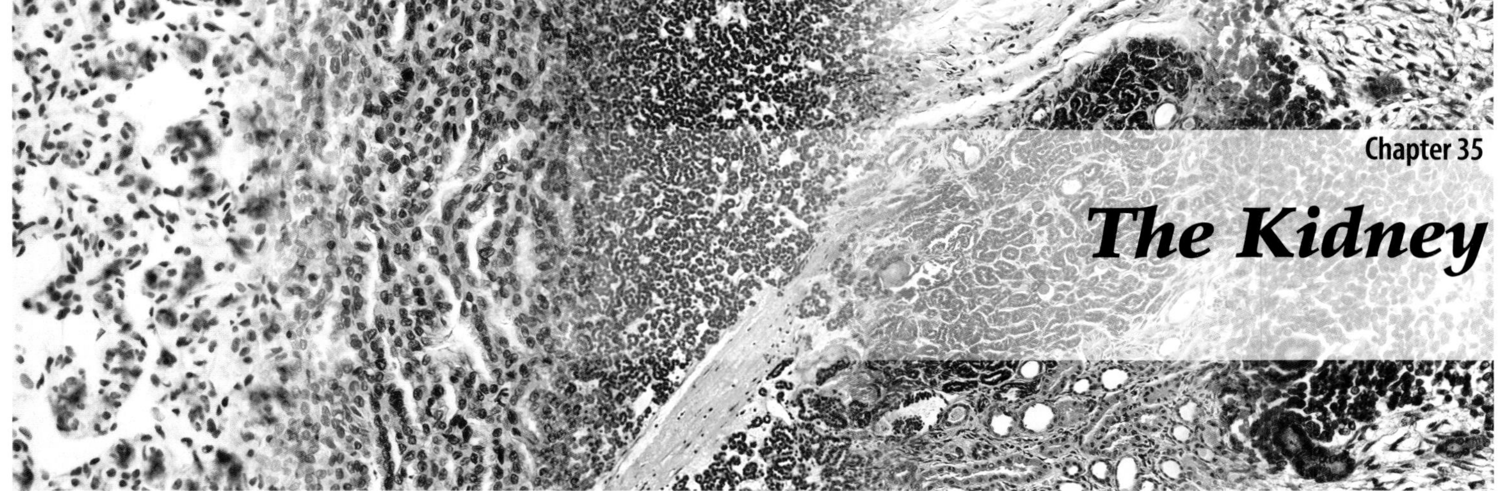

Nonneoplastic Conditions

Congenital Disorders

Few older classifications have stood the test of time as well as the Potter system of renal cystic disease [PMID4478964], which recognized 4 types of renal cystic conditions. Potter type I is the autosomal recessive form of polycystic kidney disease and is often associated with congenital hepatic fibrosis i26.3. Potter type II is cystic dysplasia, in which, unlike the other 3 forms, the kidneys are architecturally abnormal from the beginning and have no significant amount of normally functioning renal tissue. Potter type III is autosomal dominant polycystic kidney disease (ADPKD) and is associated with hepatic cysts (but not with hepatic fibrosis), often with cysts of the pancreas and ovary, and often with hypertension. Type IV renal cystic disease is thought to be secondary to obstruction. There are also a number of forms of acquired renal cystic disease that may be morphologically indistinguishable from autosomal dominant polycystic disease and have an unclear pathogenesis [PMID16462154].

ADPKD (so-called adult type) results from defects in either the *PKD1* gene on 16p13.3 (85% of cases) or *PKD2* gene on 4q21 (15% of cases) [PMID17429048, PMID19879844]. In the normal state, polycystin 1, a transmembrane protein, and polycystin 2, an integral membrane protein, are found in cilia of renal tubular cells. Urine flow in the developing nephron causes motion of cilia in tubular cells. Ciliary motion signals cells to stop dividing and initiate the next phase of development, which is to position intracytoplasmic proteins in an apical-basal arrangement that will permit the resorption of solutes from the urine at the apical end of the cell, their transportation through the cytoplasm, and their return to the bloodstream at the basal portion of the cell. In ADPKD, defects in one of the polycystin proteins cause the cell to fail to sense the flow of urine, so they do not continue their differentiation [PMID19879844]. The result is continued, disordered proliferation, with dilatation of a portion of the nephron that usually becomes disconnected from the glomerular filtrate i35.1.

In autosomal recessive polycystic kidney disease (ARPKD), the responsible gene is *PKHD1* (polycystic kidney and hepatic disease 1), located on 6p12 [PMID19879844, PMID17975706]. *PKHD1* encodes the protein fibrocystin/polyductin (FPC). Like the polycystin proteins, FPC is found in the cilia of renal tubules [PMID18156813]. The precise function of FPC is not clear, but it is part of the same complex as polycystin-2 and appears to work with polycystin-1 and polycystin-2 in the modulation of cell processes that permit normal functioning of the tubular or biliary cell [PMID18235088].

Vascular Changes in the Kidney

In 1934, Harry Goldblatt established an animal model of hypertension based on stenosis of the renal artery [PMID19870251], pioneering work that led to the discovery of the renin-angiotensin system. While atherosclerosis is the most common cause of renal artery stenosis, renal artery dysplasia, a collection of developmental disorders, causes renal artery stenosis and hypertension by the same mechanism as observed by Goldblatt, and is surgically correctable (other causes of surgically correctable hypertension include pheochromocytoma, coarctation of the aorta, Cushing syndrome, Conn syndrome, and a renin-secreting juxtaglomerular cell tumor). The most common form of renal artery dysplasia is medial fibroplasia, most often found in younger women, in which areas of constricting medial fibrosis alternate with areas of muscle atrophy that cause thinning of the wall and minute aneurysms, resulting in a multinodularity that produces a characteristic "string of beads" angiographic appearance.

In systemic hypertension, renal vessels have the same vascular changes that are seen elsewhere, and may also have fibrous intimal thickening or hyaline change of arteriole walls i35.2.

Chronic Pyelonephritis

Chronic pyelonephritis is not simply the presence of lymphocytes, as its name might suggest, but is diagnosed by the following constellation of findings [Weiss ISBN978-0781747509]:

- A history of multiple urinary tract infections, clinically from the upper tract
- Gross findings of calyceal, and pelvic deformities
- Chronic interstitial inflammation
- Scarring (which needs to be differentiated from vascular scars caused by arterial disease)

Because the diagnosis of chronic pyelonephritis requires this constellation of findings, it can only be suspected, not definitively diagnosed, in a small renal biopsy **i35.3**. The etiology of chronic pyelonephritis is probably reflux [PMID18775677], and in many publications, the terms "chronic pyelonephritis" and "reflux nephropathy" are used interchangeably.

There are several unusual forms of chronic pyelonephritis. Segmental hypoplasia (formerly called Ask-Upmark) simulates a developmental anomaly but is usually caused by localized reflux. Malakoplakia is a proliferation of macrophages thought to be secondary to defective intracellular bacterial killing [PMID14709516]. It may have Michaelis-Gutman bodies, laminated concretions of calcium and iron [Weiss ISBN978-0781747509]. Xanthogranulomatous pyelonephritis occurs in immunocompetent patients and is secondary to obstruction from a large calculus and consequent infection, usually from *Proteus mirabilis, Escherichia coli, Staphylococcus aureus,* or *Klebsiella, Pseudomonas,* or *Enterobacter* species. There is a mixed infiltrate of cells, including copious macrophages, mixed with giant cells and acute inflammatory) cells **i35.14** [PMID21526966]. Both xanthogranulomatous pyelonephritis and malakoplakia can be mistaken for a clear cell renal cell carcinoma (RCC).

Other Commonly Encountered Nonneoplastic Renal Conditions

No attempt will be made here to cover the full range of glomerulonephridites, but the general pathologist is likely to encounter the diabetic kidney. In diabetic nephropathy, there may be changes in the renal vessels and thickening of the tubular basement membrane, mirroring similar vascular and basement membrane changes systemically, but the major changes occur in the glomerulus. In the glomerulus, both capsular drop and fibrin cap are depositions of serum protein. In capsular drop, the deposition is between the parietal epithelial cell and Bowman capsule. In fibrin cap, the protein deposits occur between the glomerular endothelium and basement membrane. This is in contrast to the mesangial thickening of glomerulosclerosis. The most immediately pathognomonic lesion in diabetic glomerular disease is nodular glomerulosclerosis (Kimmelstiel-Wilson), in which there are homogenized eosinophilic deposits **i35.4** [PMID1397774]. Unless there is a clear history of diabetes, amyloidosis should be excluded before a diagnosis of nodular glomerulosclerosis is made.

Another situation that is commonly encountered is the myeloma kidney. The most common condition encountered in the myeloma kidney is amyloid deposition, the characteristics of which are similar to those of amyloid deposition in other sites. The other 2 commonly encountered renal findings in myeloma are light chain disease and cast nephropathy [PMID19229815]. In light chain disease, light chains are deposited in the mesangium and in the glomerular and tubular basement membranes. These deposits may be crystalline. In myeloma cast nephropathy, casts containing light chains are found in the tubules and collecting system. These casts are often laminated and associated with a giant cell reaction **i35.5** [Silva ISBN 978-0893521431].

End stage renal disease can be caused by a variety of disorders, usually either diabetes or hypertension, and is characterized by significant changes in all 3 of the main components of the kidney—the glomeruli, the tubules, and the interstitium. There is advanced global glomerulosclerosis, tubular atrophy, and interstitial fibrosis. A lymphocytic infiltrate is frequently seen.

The Thrombotic Microangiopathy Conditions

Hemolytic uremic syndrome (HUS) and thrombotic thrombocytopenic purpura (TTP) are often lumped together as TTP-HUS or called the thrombotic microangiopathy conditions. Fragmentation of erythrocytes is common, resulting in schistocytes. End organ damage stems from obstruction of capillaries by the damaged erythrocytes. HUS and TTP may be microscopically indistinguishable from each other. To the extent that a distinction is possible, it is made clinically—HUS is the preferred diagnosis in pediatric cases which result from *Shiga* toxin–producing bacteria and primarily involve diarrhea and renal failure. Food poisoning from *E coli* O157 is a common culprit in HUS. TTP is the favored diagnosis in adult cases, those stemming from pregnancy, or those with significant central nervous system involvement [PMID21240869]. Although both of these conditions are different from DIC, there are overlapping features and they may be difficult to differentiate from that condition. Very low platelet counts (<20,000) suggest TTP-HUS more than DIC [PMID20154285]. TTP is associated with mutations in and lower activity of the enzyme ADAMTS13, which cleaves von Willebrand factor, while in HUS, there are often mutations of complement genes [PMID20539230].

The Kidney in Transplantation

The kidney follows the general rule in transplantation pathology that hyperacute and acute vascular rejection are primarily humoral, while acute cellular rejection tends to involve an attack on epithelium. Hyperacute and acute vascular (also called acute humoral) rejection are thankfully very rare now. Hyperacute rejection is usually evident within hours and is characterized by fibrin microthrombi, while acute vascular rejection takes 2 weeks or more to develop. In milder forms of acute vascular rejection, there are inflammatory cells in the subendothelial space (endarteritis or subintimal vasculitis). In more severe forms, there is acute vasculitis and there may be fibrinoid necrosis [PMID11856785]. Donor-specific antibodies and peritubular capillary C4d deposition are characteristic of acute humoral rejection [PMID10505698]. Because humoral rejection is not as amenable to therapy as cellular rejection, its diagnosis carries significant clinical implications. The thrombotic microangiopathy conditions, such as HUS and TTP, must be excluded before diagnosing hyperacute or acute vascular rejection, as these conditions may have fibrin microthrombi and fibrinoid necrosis of the vessel wall.

Acute renal transplant glomerulopathy occurs in 5-25% of transplant cases. Acute renal transplant glomerulopathy is characterized by mesangial expansion with thickening of the capillary walls, often with a pale zone in the center of the basement membrane (so-called tram-tracking) [PMID19590229]. Because these changes can resemble membranoproliferative glomerulonephritis, immunofluorescence may be needed for the diagnosis. Although transplant glomerulopathy is distinct from acute humoral rejection, it has also been associated with donor-specific antibodies and deposition of C4d in peritubular capillaries in some cases, suggesting that chronic damage to endothelial cells from humoral immunity may contribute to its development [PMID19590229]. Possibly, transplant glomerulopathy is an example of chronic humoral rejection, a new category of rejection recognized in 2001 and characterized by donor-specific antibodies, deposition of C4d in glomerular or tubular capillaries, interstitial fibrosis, tubular atrophy, and intimal thickening of vessels [PMID19001815].

Most cases of acute rejection are caused by cell mediated immunity (cellular rejection) and are directed against the tubules (tubulitis). Nonspecific chronic inflammation should not be overinterpreted as rejection—the diagnosis of acute cellular rejection requires a clearly directed attack on the tubules i35.6. The infiltrate may start in the interstitium, but tubules are the ultimate target [Nádasdy ISBN978-0443077845]. Acute cellular rejection is mild if <1/3 of the parenchyma shows changes, moderate if between 1/3 and 2/3 show changes, and severe if >2/3 of the parenchyma is affected. Glomeruli are usually not affected or show only minimal changes in acute cellular rejection.

Posttransplant lymphoproliferative disorder (PTLD) [Swerdlow ISBN978-9283224310], discussed in Chapter 8, should be excluded in the diagnosis of acute cellular rejection. In acute cellular rejection, the lymphocytes are T cells, whereas in PTLD, B cells usually constitute the primary lymphocyte population and Epstein Barr virus is usually present. Tubulitis and intimal inflammation suggest acute cellular rejection, but can also be seen in PTLD. The presence of nuclear atypia and a mass effect strongly suggest PTLD [PMID8840949].

There are no good clinical or laboratory signs of chronic renal rejection, though it is usually accompanied by a rising serum creatinine level. In chronic rejection, there is chronic inflammation and thickening of the intima of the blood vessels, with interstitial fibrosis and tubular atrophy i35.7 [PMID16534463]. Active tubulitis is absent unless there is superimposed acute rejection.

Other than steroids, drugs to fight rejection fall fundamentally into 2 classes. The first group consists of drugs that inhibit DNA synthesis, such as cyclophosphamide and mycophenolate (CellCept). The second group consists of drugs that inhibit T-cell activation, such as cyclosporine, tacrolimus (formerly called FK506), and the rapamycins. Cyclosporine and tacrolimus inhibit the enzyme calcineurin, so that the protein NFAT is never dephosphorylated and therefore cannot enter the nucleus and modulate transcription [PMID15041303]. The rapamycins, the parent compound of which is rapamycin (Rapamune or Sirolimus), also inhibit T cells, by binding to and inhibiting a serine/threonine kinase that initiates a series of reactions that modulate protein turnover and transcription [PMID12878853, PMID17635837, PMID20420793]. The rapamycins are also being investigated for possible antineoplastic properties. Azothioprine (Imuran) is a purine analog that acts in both manners, inhibiting DNA synthesis and also inhibiting the CD28 costimulatory signal that is critical to T-cell activation [PMID16908341].

Because the pathways of T-cell activation, discussed in Chapter 7, are long and complex, there are theoretically many places to intervene in the rejection process. Monoclonal antibodies to some of the critical proteins involved in the activation cascade have occasionally been used to treat or prevent rejection, as they have been in some autoimmune disorders. At this writing, success has been limited, but hopes are high.

Cyclosporine and tacrolimus may cause changes in arterioles, principally a hyalinization of the walls and occasionally a mucoid subendothelial thickening, but obliterative intimal hyperplasia is rare. Patchy interstitial fibrosis and tubular atrophy are commonly seen, but the renal parenchyma is relatively spared and care should be taken not to overinterpret the vascular changes caused by immunosuppressive agents as rejection. An acute reaction to these drugs may occasionally occur and is characterized by vacuolization of tubular epithelium.

As is always the case in the use of immunosuppressive agents, opportunistic infections may occur. In addition to the opportunistic agents commonly encountered elsewhere, polyomavirus is commonly seen in transplanted kidneys and can be suspected if intranuclear inclusions are seen in tubular cells in urine cytology. Much more sensitive molecular testing is available [PMID21325560].

Benign Renal Neoplasms

Although not all accept the existence of a true renal cell adenoma, most support that diagnosis provided that the mass has papillary or tubulo-papillary architecture, has no clear cells, no areas resembling a chromophobe or collecting duct carcinoma, and is <0.5 cm (5 mm). The size stipulation of 0.5 cm does not apply to oncocytomas or metanephric adenomas [PMID18846240]. The renal adenoma may resemble a very small papillary RCC (discussed in the next section), but it should not resemble any other type of RCC.

Angiomyolipomas have varying proportions of smooth muscle, sometimes with an epithelioid morphology, adipose tissue, and vasculature i35.8a. Although the precise histogenesis of these neoplasms is not settled, they appear to be members of the unusual family of neoplasms called perivascular epithelioid cell tumor (PEComa), as are lymphangioleiomyomatosis, the sugar tumor of the lung, and rhabdomyoma. All of these neoplasm are reactive with HMB-45 and usually also with HMB-50 [PMID19604538, PMID19391667] and CD1a [PMID18251780]. In addition, angiomyolipomas may also be positive for CD117 (c-kit) or Melan-A/MART-1.

The angiomyolipoma may have a number of appearances, based largely on the morphology of the muscle cells, which may have a variable and very atypical appearance. If the muscle component predominates and has an epithelioid morphology i35.8b, an oncocytoma, a RCC, and a chromophobe carcinoma must be excluded [PMID11958671]. If spindled muscle cells predominate, a leiomyoma or a leiomyosarcoma enters the differential diagnosis. Some cases may even resemble a sarcomatoid RCC, a urothelial carcinoma, or a collecting duct carcinoma. It is prudent to consider an angiomyolipoma for any unusual renal tumor, and if immunohistochemical stains are performed, to include HMB-45, CD1a, and muscle markers. Rare malignant angiomyolipomas are encountered, but the vast majority behaves in a benign manner.

ISBN 978-089189-5886

The mesoblastic nephroma is almost exclusively a tumor of infancy. Adult mesoblastic nephromas are more likely fibromatosis, inflammatory myofibroblastic tumor, or a smooth muscle tumor. The classic appearance of a mesoblastic nephroma is a bland stromal proliferation that resembles fibromatosis or a leiomyoma [PMID2544507]. Immunohistochemical stains confirm a myofibroblastic origin, with focal actin staining [PMID2544507]. There may be some epithelial elements i35.9, but these are likely entrapped. There is a more cellular variant of the mesoblastic nephroma that may have numerous mitoses and simulate a fibrosarcoma. These are often locally invasive, but they are nonmetastasizing, and nephrectomy is curative.

The cystic nephroma is a multiloculated lesion that is benign and lined by cuboidal epithelium i35.10a [PMID2544253]. Some believe that a cystic nephroma may have some solid areas and that an ovarian-like stroma is often seen i35.10b. Others believe that a cystic nephroma should have minimal solid areas, and that any appreciable solid areas are more consistent with a diagnosis of mixed epithelial-stromal tumor. In either case, the important differential diagnosis is a multilocular cystic RCC. Clear cytoplasm favors a carcinoma, while ovarian-like stroma favors a benign process. The stroma in a cystic nephroma is often positive for estrogen and progesterone receptors [PMID17873894], and if such staining is demonstrated in questionable cases, the balance is tipped away from a carcinoma.

The mixed epithelial-stromal renal tumor (MEST) is a rare renal neoplasm that generally behaves in a benign fashion. These often have cysts lined by benign-appearing cuboidal cells in a bland stroma that may resemble ovarian stroma, causing a great resemblance to the cystic nephroma [PMID16390243]. The distinction of a MEST from a cystic nephroma is further complicated by the fact that the stromal cells in the MEST, like those in a cystic nephroma, may also be positive for estrogen and progesterone receptors [PMID19722760]. Some have suggested that the MEST and the cystic nephroma are slightly different manifestations of the same entity [PMID17414095, PMID18971776, PMID18006141]. The MEST occurs primarily in premenopausal women, and the stromal component may also express actin, desmin, and CD10. To my mind, these 3 markers must be immunohistochemically demonstrated before a diagnosis of MEST can be made in lieu of a diagnosis of cystic nephroma, if in fact, these are separate entities. In any event, the important point is not to miss a cystic (also called multicystic or multilocular) clear cell renal carcinoma. The cystic RCC has deceptively bland nuclei and simulates a cystic nephroma. Cells with clear cytoplasm in the septae favors a cystic RCC i35.11a, i35.11b, while ovarian-type stroma or positivity for estrogen or progesterone receptors suggests a nephroma.

The metanephric adenoma resembles a florid adenosis or a tubular adenoma of the breast or a well circumscribed, benign-appearing epithelial/tubule-forming Wilms tumor i35.12 [PMID7573669, PMID7755148]. A metanephric adenoma should be suspected if there is a small or circumscribed mass that appears to be a Wilms tumor in a child or a papillary RCC in an adult. A metanephric adenoma is likely to be circumscribed. α-methylacyl-coenzyme A racemase (αMACR) is much more likely to be positive in papillary RCC than in a metanephric adenoma. CD57 positivity favors a metanephric adenoma [PMID16424894]. An immunohistochemical stain for WT1 can be employed if the differential diagnosis is between metanephric adenoma and an epithelial/tubular Wilms tumor. Metanephric adenomas may be focally positive for WT1, but strong and diffuse positivity is the rule in Wilms tumor [PMID16424894].

Nephrogenic rests are small collections of "Wilms-like" cells. The diagnosis of nephrogenic rests is usually made in a child for whom there has been a nephrectomy for Wilms, whereas metanephric adenoma is usually diagnosed in adults. In addition, nephrogenic rests are distinguished from metanephric adenomas either by their tiny size i35.13 or by the admixture of normal tissue, though large or coalescing nephrogenic rests (nephroblastomatosis) can resemble a metanephric adenoma or even a Wilms tumor. The principal significance of nephrogenic rests is that their presence in a kidney removed for Wilms indicates an increased risk for Wilms in the remaining kidney [PMID2156243].

Oncocytomas are benign, but are discussed with malignant neoplasms because they invariably cause concern form malignancy.

Malignant Renal Neoplasms

Only a few comments will be made about conventional (clear cell) RCC because they are commonly encountered, rarely diagnostically difficult, and well treated in numerous other texts. RCC may have a trabecular, solid, or acinar pattern. The cystic form is discussed above. Rarely, they have cells with granular rather than clear cytoplasm. Many RCC have 3p– [PMID8370620, PMID1671759]. In addition to an overall assessment of differentiation, the Fuhrman nuclear grading system [PMID7180965], based on nuclear diameter, shape, and the prominence of nucleoli, is sometimes used to grade the nuclei on a scale of 1-4, though combining Fuhrman grades 1 and 2, resulting in a 2-tiered nuclear grading system, has been proposed [PMID20804473].

Xanthogranulomatous pyelonephritis i35.14 and malakoplakia may resemble clear cell RCC, but both of these entities consists of macrophages whose cytoplasm is foamy rather than simply clear, lack the arborizing vascular pattern of an RCC, have a mixture of other types of inflammatory cells, and are keratin negative, CD68 positive, provided that care is taken to exclude entrapped epithelial cells.

Conventional RCC, especially if high-grade and with sarcomatous metaplasia (so-called sarcomatoid variant) i35.15, may simulate urothelial carcinoma, in which case extensive sampling may be needed. Expression of cytokeratins 7 or 20, high molecular weight keratin CK903 (also called 34βE-12), or CEA favor a urothelial carcinoma over a RCC.

Although oncocytomas usually run a benign course, they are included in this discussion of malignant renal neoplasms because they are easily confused with malignant tumors and even if the diagnosis is secure, such patients must be followed closely for recurrence. First described by Zippel in the German literature in 1942, oncocytomas did not become generally known until a 1976 study of 13 cases [PMID975006]. Grossly, oncocytomas are dark brown rather than yellow, the general color of a RCC. There is usually a central band of fibrous tissue in an oncocytoma. They are circumscribed, occasionally with a small group of cells that trail off slightly into the stroma. Their cells have abundant eosinophilic, granular cytoplasm **i35.16**. They have generally uniform nuclei, though they may have small clusters of pleomorphic and hyperchromatic nuclei (oncoblasts). They do not have necrosis and there is only a very rare mitosis.

The papillary (Chromophil) RCC was first described in full in 1976 [PMID1000477]. The papillary renal carcinoma usually has trisomy of chromosomes 7, 16, and 17, as well as loss of chromosome Y [PMID8370620, PMID1671759]. Papillary renal carcinomas may have distinct fibrovascular cores, with large neoplastic cells (type 2 papillary RCC) **i35.17a**, **i35.17b**. But fibrovascular cores may be compressed or indistinct, resulting in a trabecular appearance, often accompanied by neoplastic cells that are small, with uniform nuclei and minimal cytoplasm (type 1 papillary RCC) **i35.18** [PMID9195569]. A type 1 papillary carcinoma should be excluded in any renal tumor that has a trabecular pattern or is composed of small cells with minimal cytoplasm. The prognosis of type I papillary RCCs is often more favorable, but this may be because they tend to present with a lower stage [PMID17275070]. Macrophages are common in papillary renal carcinoma **i35.19** and psammoma bodies and neutrophils may occasionally be seen. Because conventional RCCs may have focal papillary areas, there should be adequate sampling and either a predominance of a papillary architecture or a characteristic cytogenetic anomaly before the diagnosis of papillary RCC is made.

The chromophobe RCC was well described in 1985 [PMID2859694]. It has losses of chromosomes 1 and Y, and often of other chromosomes as well [PMID8816891]. Grossly, chromophobe RCCs are beige or tan rather than yellow. The growth pattern is solid with sharply defined cell borders. There is perinuclear clearing and indented nuclear membranes **i35.20a**, **i35.20b**. Many chromophobe carcinomas have cytoplasmic iron that stains with Hale colloidal iron stain. 1/2 of cases have calcification. The eosinophilic variant, in which the cells have denser eosinophilic cytoplasm, also has perinuclear clearing but the nuclei are not as indented **i35.20c**. The eosinophilic variant of chromophobe carcinoma should be considered whenever a lesion appears to be a granular RCC or an oncocytoma.

RCCs with predominantly granular cytoplasm, the oncoctyoma, and chromophobe carcinoma (especially its eosinophilic variant) can all have a similar appearance. Cytogenetic studies can be very helpful in the distinction, but at this writing, are rarely possible since the question is not apparent until after the tissue has been fixed in formalin. FISH is the only option for cytogenetic studies in formalin fixed tissue and one is dependent on an appropriate probe being commercially available.

Chromophobe carcinomas differ from the oncocytoma in the perinuclear clearing and in having more frequent mitoses. In general, oncocytomas have more abundant cytoplasm, and it is more deeply pink and granular than even the eosinophilic type of chromphobe carcinoma. Also, many eosinophilic chromophobe carcinomas will have areas of more classic chromophobe carcinoma somewhere. Oncocytomas are generally well circumscribed (only a minute focus of loss of circumscription is permitted in the diagnosis), in contrast to chromophobe carcinomas and granular RCC. A distinct mahogany brown gross appearance favors an oncocytoma, as does circumscription.

Immunohistochemical studies are useful in the precise diagnosis of renal tumors but should generally be performed only in cases where the tumor has been resected, and generous sampling has failed to secure a firm diagnosis. In biopsy material of a renal mass, if there is an oncocytic process, it is wise to comment that a precise diagnosis requires a resection. There are no immunohistochemical or cytogenetic studies that supersede a thorough sampling and an appreciation of the tumor's overall architecture, circumscription, and areas of variability. Moreover, the results of immunohistochemical studies are not entirely concordant, and it is clear that immunohistochemistry is not a "magic bullet" in distinguishing these forms of carcinoma. But they can be of great help, and a few general statements can be made [PMID15848735, PMID19926310, PMID16512599].

The monoclonal antibody RCC (also called RCCMa) stains about 90% of conventional and papillary RCCs. It stains about 1/2 of chromophobe carcinomas and 25% of sarcomatoid carcinomas in 1 report, but no cases of either in another report. Oncocytomas are negative for RCC. CD10 stains 90-100% of conventional and papillary RCCs, but also 30-40% of chromophobe carcinomas or oncocytomas and is therefore less specific [PMID17683191]. Paxillin consistently stains chromophobe carcinomas and oncocytomas, but only rarely stains conventional, papillary, or collecting duct carcinomas. Conventional RCC are negative for β defensin-1 and parvalbumin in 96% of cases, and positive for vimentin in 83% of cases, while chromophobe carcinomas and oncocytomas stain in a reverse pattern—they are almost uniformly positive for β defensin-1 and parvalbumin and negative for vimentin [PMID12548166]. CD117 is negative in virtually all conventional RCC, but positive in a membranous pattern in most cases of chromophobe carcinoma or oncocytoma. The most practical panel in distinguishing conventional RCC of either the granular or clear cell type on the one hand from a chromophobe carcinoma or oncocytoma on the other hand is RCC, vimentin, and CD117. The former tumors are RCC+, vimentin+, CD117–, while chromophobe carcinomas and oncocytomas tend to stain RCC–, vimentin–, CD117+ [PMID17683191].

Once a conventional RCC has been excluded and the differential diagnosis is between a chromophobe carcinoma and an oncocytoma, effective stains are cytokeratin 7, epithelial cell adhesion molecule (EpCAM), claudin-7, and Pax-2. CK7 stains most chromophobe carcinomas, but no conventional RCCs. CK7 expression in oncocytomas is weaker and more focal than in chromophobe carcinomas [PMID12047768]. EpCAM strongly stains all chromophobe carcinomas, but only 29% of oncocytomas, and with weaker staining [PMID17683191]. Pax-2 stains virtually all oncocytomas and only 10% of chromophobe carcinomas [PMID18941400]. Chromophobe carcinomas are negative for cytokeratin 20 and CD15, whereas about 1/2 of oncocytomas exhibit weak positivity [PMID16512599]. CD63 is reported to stain both oncocytomas and the eosinophilic variant of chromophobe carcinoma, but with an apical location in the former and diffuse staining in the latter [PMID16133362].

About 1/3 of renal oncocytomas have overexpression of the cyclin D1 protein by immunohistochemistry (nuclear staining), and of these, about 1/2 have evidence of a translocation of the *BCL-1* (*CCND1*) gene that codes for this protein. These findings are not seen in chromophobe carcinomas, making their presence reasonably specific, but not sensitive in the detection of oncocytomas [PMID19386349].

Identification of papillary RCCs by immunohistochemistry is more problematic and less specific. Most papillary carcinomas have a little CK7 staining, whereas conventional RCC does not [PMID16512599], but p504S (αMACR) is useful, as it stains virtually all papillary RCCs in the cytoplasm, but only 25% of conventional RCCs, 15% of oncocytomas, and no chromophobe carcinomas [PMID16512599].

The antibody RCC is less useful in assessing metastatic tumors because the sensitivity drops to about 67% and a number of other metastatic tumors will stain for RCC. The incidence of staining ranges from nearly 100% for the very rare metastatic parathyroid carcinoma to about 15-35% for adenocarcinomas of the breast, colon, prostate, lung, and ovary [PMID17721277]. PAX-2 is more effective than RCC in identifying metastatic RCC, staining approximately 85% of such cases [PMID18685487]. Still, positivity of a metastatic carcinoma for RCC **i35.21a**, **i35.21b** suggests renal origin until proven otherwise.

The collecting duct carcinoma entered surgical pathology as a distinct entity in 1986 [PMID3542784]. It has high-grade nuclei with appreciable stromal desmoplasia **i35.22a**, **i35.22b** and occurs in the medulla. Collecting duct carcinomas may be tubular or papillary and can resemble high-grade conventional RCC, papillary carcinomas, or urothelial carcinomas. The collecting duct carcinoma should be suspected if the nuclei are of high grade, the tumor is medullary, or if there is appreciable stromal desmoplasia. The principal differential diagnosis is a high-grade urothelial carcinoma, and the distinction between these 2 entities is difficult because both their H&E appearance and their immunohistochemical characteristics overlap.

The medullary carcinoma, described in 1995 [PMID7528470], occurs in the renal medulla of young African American patients and is associated with sickle cell disease. The medullary carcinoma is aggressive, has an appearance that is similar to a collecting duct carcinoma, with high-grade nuclei and stromal desmoplasia **i35.23**, and may be a variant of the latter neoplasm.

Urothelial (formerly called transitional cell) carcinomas occur in the renal pelvis and ureter. Since these have the same characteristics as their bladder counterparts, they are discussed in Chapter 36. Poorly differentiated urothelial carcinoma may resemble poorly differentiated RCC, especially of the collecting duct or medullary type. Urothelial carcinoma is positive for p63 and CK7, whereas all forms of RCC, including collecting duct and medullary carcinoma, are negative [PMID22260386].

Wilms tumor (nephroblastoma) usually has a triphasic morphology: blastema (immature small blue cells), mesenchymal (usually immature myxoid or spindle stroma, but sometimes mature or heterologous tissues), and epithelial (usually tubules, but sometimes glomerular structures). **i35.24a** demonstrates all 3 components. Occasional cases have only 1 or 2 of these components, resulting in a large array of possible morphologies [Murphy ISBN978-1881041887, PMID10463275]. The principal entities in the differential diagnosis of Wilms are the metanephric adenoma and a carcinoid tumor.

Anaplasia in Wilms tumor as defined by the National Wilms Tumor Study consists of a triad of all of the following 3 findings: abnormal mitotic figures, 3-fold variation in nuclear size among cells of the same type (ie, blastema cells as compared to other blastema cells or epithelial cells as compared to other epithelial cells; mesenchymal or heterologous tissue should not be used in comparison of nuclear size, and blastema cells should not be compared with cells from an epithelial component), and hyperchromasia of the enlarged nuclei **i35.24b-d** [PMID2844645]. Variation in nuclear size should be generalized, not focal. If the changes are focal, or all 3 criteria are not fulfilled, the more appropriate interpretation is focal anaplasia, which is much less significant [PMID8827069].

As is the case elsewhere, care must be taken not to confuse normal morphologic variations of mitotic figures with abnormal figures. Abnormal mitotic figures are tripolar or multipolar (ie, having more than the 2 poles that characterize the normal anaphase mitosis), and for a part of the mitotic figure to be considered a pole, it must be at least as long as a normal mitotic figure [PMID18528701]. Generalized anaplasia is usually seen in slightly older children and has traditionally portended a more aggressive course, though many patients with anaplasia do well [PMID2984344].

Clear cell sarcoma of the kidney (not to be confused with the clear cell sarcoma of soft tissue) occurs in the same age group as Wilms tumor, and the latter tumor is the principal mimic. The cells of a clear cell sarcoma of the kidney may have lightly eosinophilic rather than completely clear cytoplasm. Nuclei have mild pleomorphism with small nucleoli, and cell borders are indistinct **i35.25**. The stroma typically has fine fibrovascular septae. Relative to a Wilms tumor, the margins are infiltrative, and the tumor is more mitotically active [PMID10632483].

The rhabdoid tumor is a high-grade renal neoplasm that occurs in infants [PMID7275104]. The nucleus is typically pushed to the periphery by aggregates of vimentin intermediate filaments and has vesicular chromatin and a prominent nucleolus **i35.26**. In addition to vimentin, rhabdoid tumors are often positive for keratin or epithelial membrane antigen. They may involve the renal medulla and can resemble medullary carcinoma.

RCCs are often associated with translocations or other cytogenetic abnormalities and any of the common types of RCCs may rarely occur in children, but children may get a collection of RCCs that have translocations not usually found in adult renal carcinomas. These neoplasms are called translocation carcinomas and are now recognized as a distinct group of renal tumors. The H&E appearance of these tumors is that of a conventional adult RCC or a papillary RCC, but they are uniformly associated with a translocation, usually involving the gene on the short arm of the X chromosome that encodes the transcription factor E3 (TFE3). Less commonly, a translocation involving the gene on the short arm of chromosome 6 that encodes the transcription factor EB (TFEB) occurs [PMID15848741]. Any apparent RCC in a child should be subjected to cytogenetic or FISH studies to exclude this group of tumors. Alternatively, there is an immunohistochemical stain for TFE3 that works in paraffin-processed tissue and identifies the majority of translocation carcinomas that involve this transcription factor [PMID17667536].

Core Points for the Kidney

- Potter system of renal cystic disease: 4 types.
  - o Type I: autosomal recessive polycystic kidney disease.
    - Associated with congenital hepatic fibrosis.
    - Results from mutations in *PKHD1*, which encodes the protein fibrocystin/polyductin, found in cilia of tubular cells.
  - o Type II cysts from developmental dysplasia.
  - o Type III: autosomal dominant.
    - Mutations in the *PKD1* or *PKD2* gene, coding for polycystin 1 and 2, proteins found in cilia of tubular cells.
  - o Type IV: cystic disease may be secondary to obstruction.
- Chronic pyelonephritis: caused by reflux.
  - o History of upper urinary tract infections, calyceal and pelvic deformities, chronic interstitial inflammation, and fibrosis.
- Diabetic nephropathy: major changes are in the glomerulus.
  - o Nodular glomerulosclerosis (Kimmelstiel-Wilson).
  - o Also, vascular changes in renal vessels or a thickening of the tubular basement membrane.
- Myeloma kidney: amyloid deposition likely.
  - o May also exhibit light chain disease and cast nephropathy.
- Hemolytic uremic syndrome (HUS) and thrombotic thrombocytopenic purpura (TTP): overlap and may be histologically indistinguishable; often called TTP-HUS or thrombotic microangiopathy.
  - o HUS is generally diagnosed in children with renal failure and TTP in adults with CNS symptoms.
- Acute cellular rejection: cell mediated response that is directed against the tubules.
- Chronic rejection: chronic inflammation, thickening of vascular intima, tubular atrophy, and interstitial fibrosis.
- Benign renal neoplasms: angiomyolipoma, cystic nephroma, metanephric adenoma, nephrogenic rests.
  - o Angiomyolipoma: smooth muscle, adipose tissue, and blood vessels.
    - Members of perivascular epithelioid cell tumor family, positive for HMB-45
    - Muscle cells may be predominant and epithelioid, simulating epithelial neoplasm, or predominant and spindled, resembling leiomyoma or leiomyosarcoma
  - o Cystic nephroma: multiloculated, simple lining
    - If clear cells in lining exclude cystic RCC
  - o Metanephric adenoma: resembles a florid adenosis of the breast or a circumscribed, epithelial variant of Wilms tumor
  - o Nephrogenic rests: small collections of "Wilms-like" cells, usually diagnosed in children
- Conventional renal cell carcinoma (RCC): usually predominantly composed of clear cells.
- Oncocytomas: grossly dark brown.
  - o Abundant, granular, eosinophilic cytoplasm.
  - o Predominantly uniform nuclei, sometimes mixed with an occasional enlarged cell (oncoblasts).
  - o Circumscribed, minimal mitotic activity, no necrosis.
  - o May have central fibrosis.
- Papillary renal carcinomas: fibrovascular cores may be broad and obvious (type 2), or delicate, with smaller and more uniform nuclei (type 1).
  - o Macrophages, often with hemosiderin, common, especially in type 2.
  - o Often have trisomy of chromosomes 7, 16, and 17.
- Chromophobe carcinoma: nuclei often surrounded by a clear space and are often slightly grooved.
  - o Losses of chromosomes 1 and Y.
  - o Eosinophilic variant, in which the nuclear folding is less prominent.
- Differential diagnosis of renal neoplasms with granular cytoplasm:
  - o Oncocytoma
  - o Granular variant of conventional RCC
  - o Chromophobe carcinoma, especially its eosinophilic variant.
  - o IHC may help, but a resection is often needed for certainty,
  - o A comment to this effect on the biopsy report is wise.
  - o Even with a resection, extensive sampling and IHC often needed.
- Collecting duct carcinoma: medullary neoplasm with stromal fibrosis.
- Medullary carcinoma: patients with sickle cell disease.
- Urothelial (formerly called transitional cell) carcinomas: in renal pelvis and ureter.
- Wilms tumor (nephroblastoma): some combination of blastema (immature small blue cells), mesenchymal (usually immature myxoid or spindle stroma), and epithelial (usually tubules) components.
  - o These are not usually equally represented and one or more component may be completely absent.
  - o Anaplasia in Wilms tumor: all of the following: abnormal mitotic figures, 3-fold variation in nuclear size among cells of the same type, and hyperchromasia of the nuclei that are enlarged.
- Clear cell sarcoma and rhabdoid tumor: rare, high-grade renal tumors seen in children.
- Translocation carcinomas: occur in children.
  - o Usually involve translocations of genes that encode for transcription factors.

ISBN 978-089189-5886

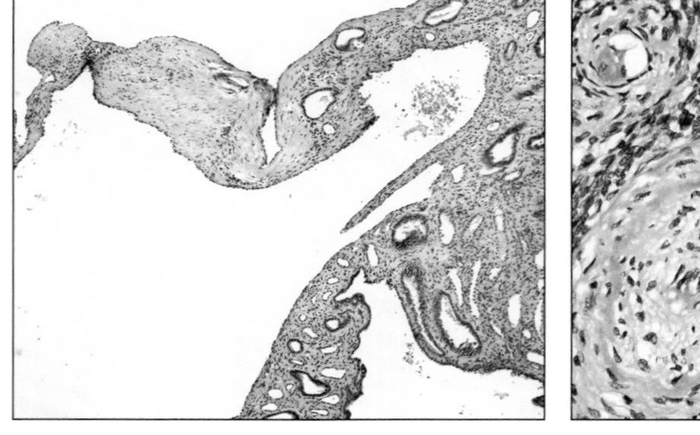

i35.1 Autosomal dominant polycystic kidney disease. The cysts are lined by tubular epithelium, but it is attenuated in many foci.

i35.2 Vascular changes in the kidney in systemic hypertension. There is intimal thickening of the arteriole on the left and hyaline change in the wall in the vessels on the right.

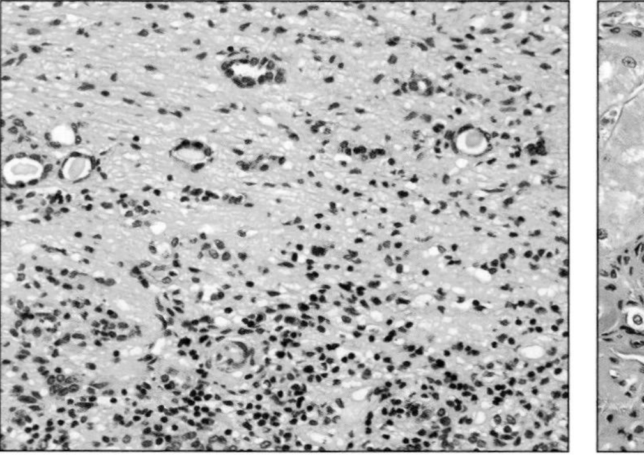

i35.3 Chronic pyelonephritis with chronic inflammation in the lower portion of the photograph and extensive interstitial fibrosis in the upper portion.

i35.4 Kimmelstiel-Wilson nodule in the glomerulus in a patient with diabetes

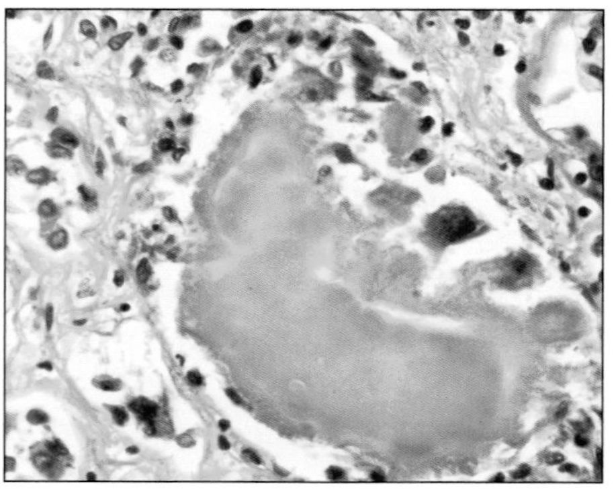

i35.5 A myeloma cast, with subtle lamination and a giant cell

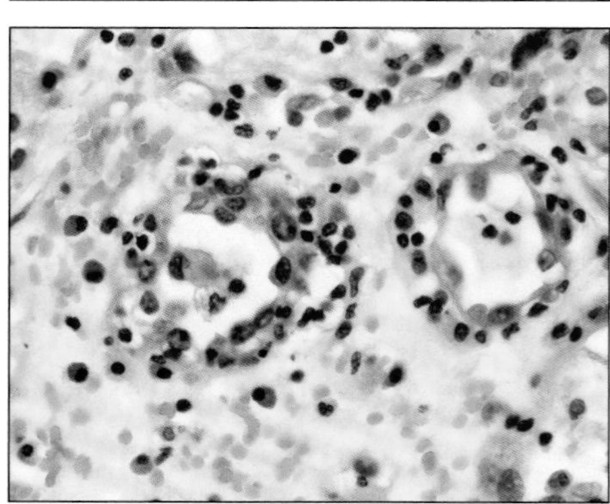

i35.6 Acute cellular rejection with lymphocytic attack on tubular epithelium

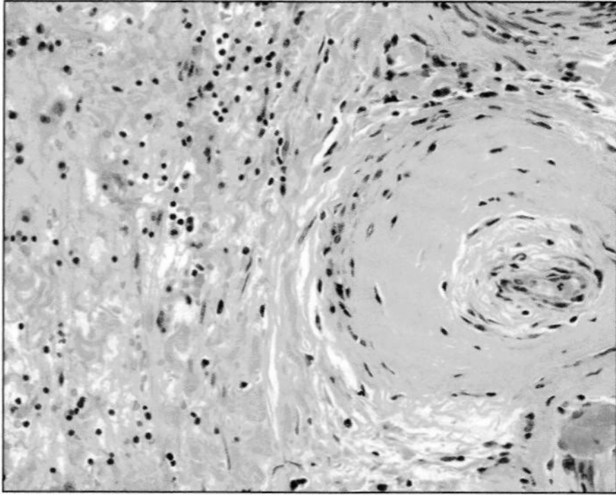

i35.7 Chronic renal allograft rejection with interstitial fibrosis and loss of tubules on the left and pronounced intimal thickening of the blood vessel on the right

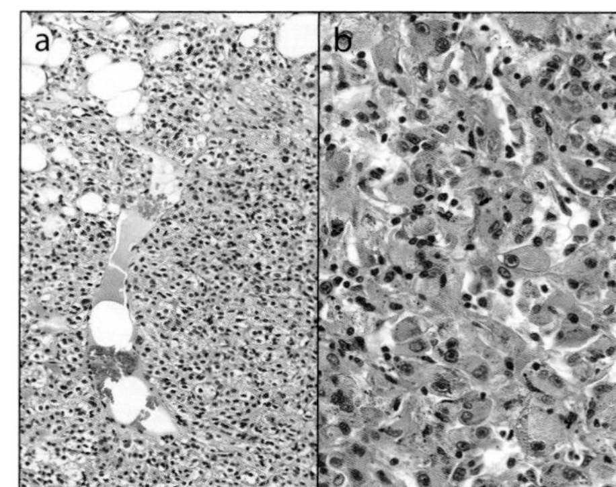

i35.8 **a** An angiomyolipoma, illustrating all 3 components of the neoplasm, although often, 1 component strongly predominates or is indistinct. In this example, the muscle cells have eosinophilic to clear cytoplasm.
b An angiomyolipoma in which the muscle component predominates and has an epithelioid morphology, causing a resemblance to an epithelial neoplasm

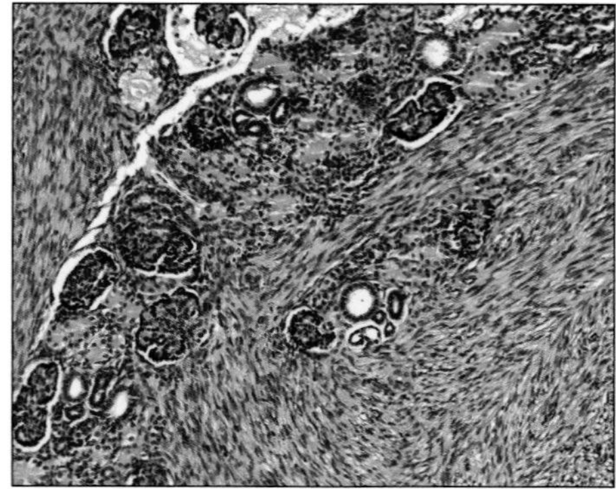

i35.9 A mesoblastic nephroma, resembling a leiomyoma. The epithelial structures are probably entrapped.

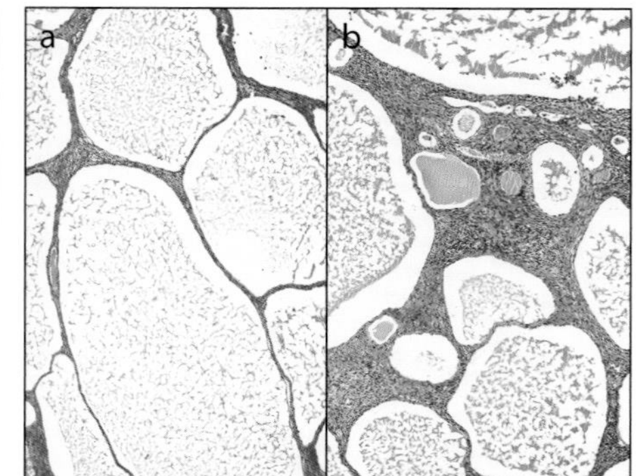

i35.10 **a** A cystic nephroma in which there is very little stroma
b A cystic nephroma in which the stroma resembles that of the ovarian cortex. Some would regard this neoplasm as a mixed epithelial-stromal renal tumor.

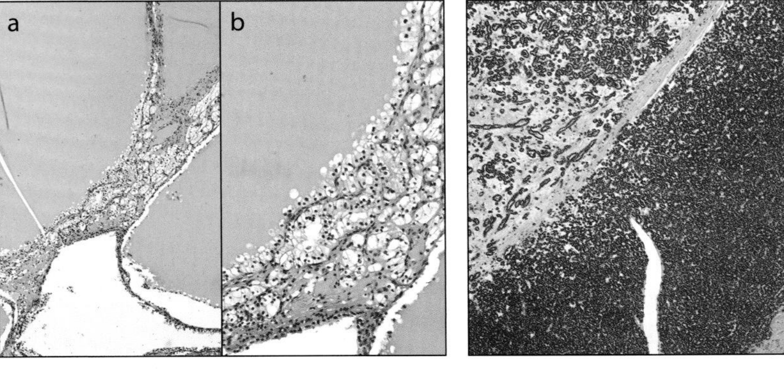

i35.11 **a** A cystic renal cell carcinoma that resembles a cystic nephroma **b** A higher-power view of the same case. Cells with clear cytoplasm in the septae in a renal cystic mass suggest a cystic renal cell carcinoma over a cystic nephroma.

i35.12 A metanephric adenoma. Note the sharp circumscription, the small cells with uniform nuclei, and the resemblance to a benign epithelial proliferation of the breast and also to Wilms tumor.

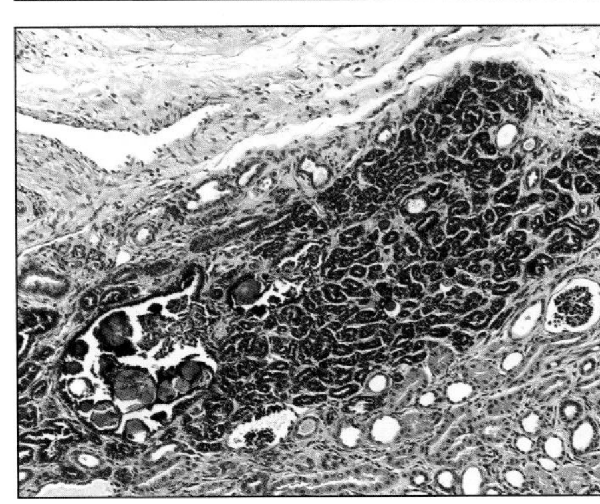

i35.13 A nephrogenic rest

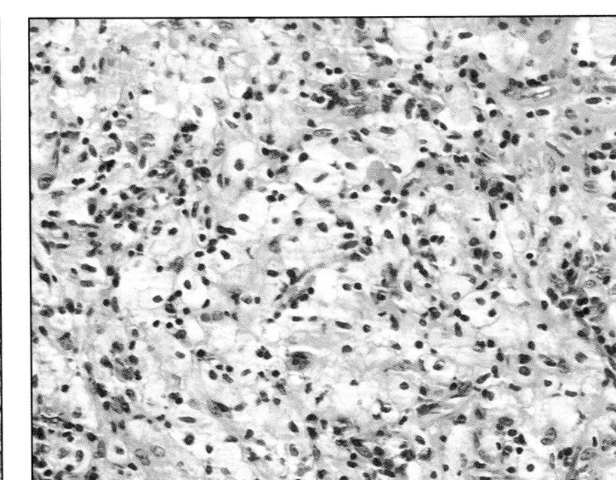

i35.14 Xanthogranulomatous pyelonephritis. It is distinguished from a clear cell renal cell carcinoma by the lack of the characteristic arborizing vascular network, the admixture of other types of inflammatory cells, and the foamy, rather than clear cytoplasm.

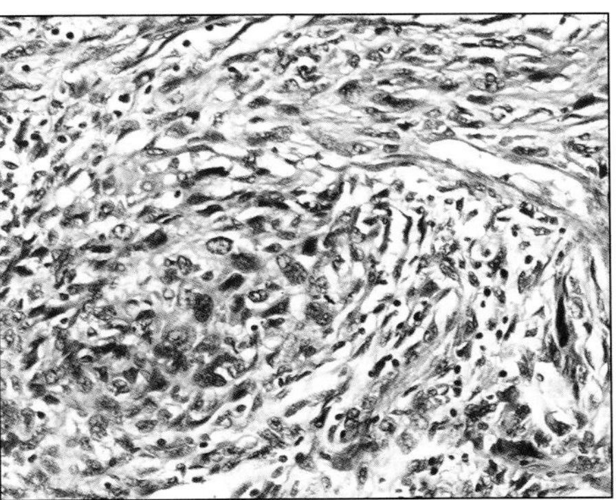

i35.15 A high-grade renal cell carcinoma with sarcomatous metaplasia (sarcomatoid carcinoma)

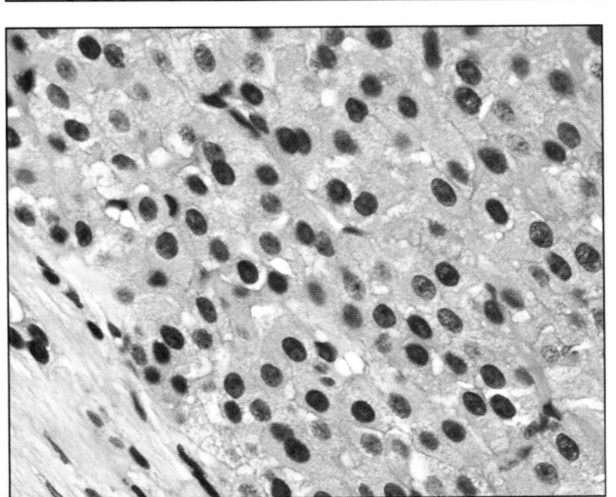

i35.16 An oncocytoma. Note the sharp circumscription, the deeply eosinophilic cytoplasm with extensive granularity, the absence of any clear cells, and the absence of any mitoses.

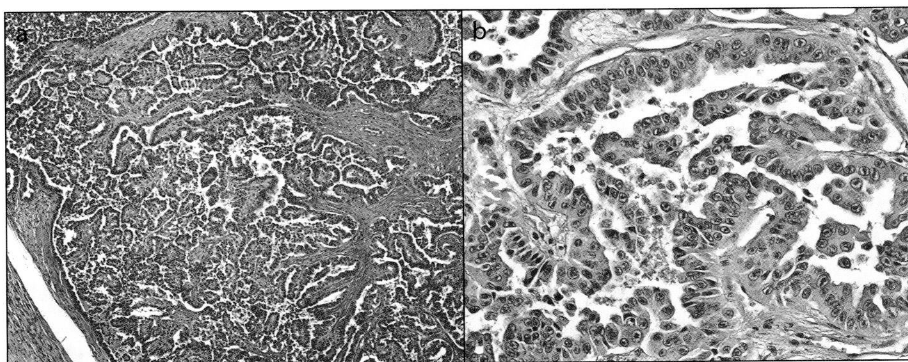

i35.17 **a** A type 2 papillary renal cell carcinoma, with distinct fibrovascular cores **b** A higher-power view of the same case as in i34.17a, illustrating that the neoplastic cells are relatively large and pleomorphic

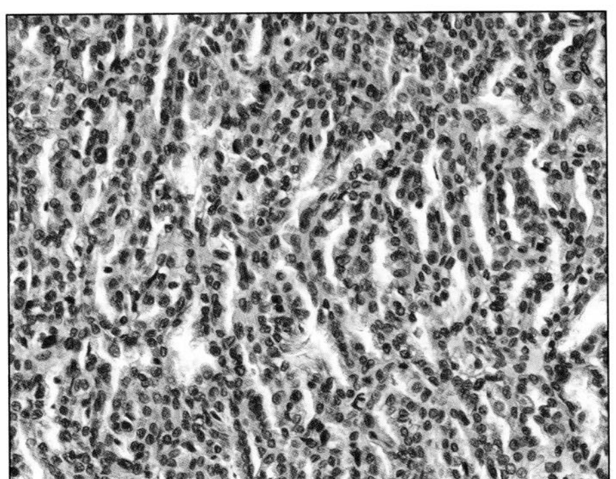

i35.18 A type 1 papillary renal cell carcinoma with subtle fibrovascular cores and much smaller, more uniform nuclei. This type of papillary renal cell carcinoma can be diagnostically challenging.

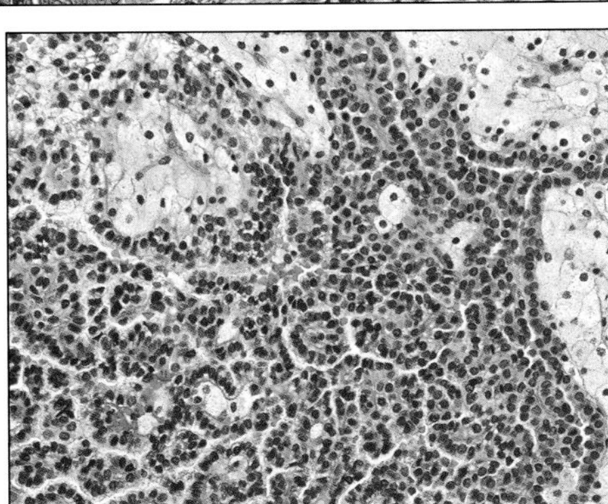

i35.19 Macrophages are common in papillary renal cell carcinoma

ISBN 978-089189-5886

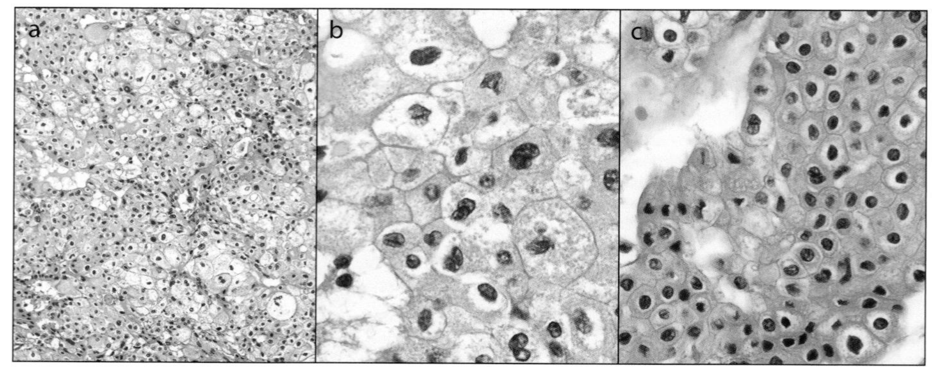

i35.20 **a** A chromophobe renal cell carcinoma. Note the distinct perinuclear clearing.
b A higher-power view of the same case as in i35.20a, highlighting the nucleus clearing, the very sharp cytoplasmic boundaries, and the uneven nuclear membrane
c The eosinophilic form of chromophobe carcinoma

i35.21 **a** A metastatic carcinoma in the retroperitoneum
b Positive staining for RCC, suggesting a metastatic renal cell carcinoma, which was the correct diagnosis

i35.22 **a** A collecting duct carcinoma. There is a tubular pattern in the upper right, with papillae to the left of center and a solid growth pattern in the lower left.
b A collecting duct carcinoma, highlighting the high nuclear grade and stromal desmoplasia

i35.23 A medullary carcinoma occurring in the renal medulla of a patient with sickle cell disease. These neoplasms have high nuclear grade and stromal desmoplasia.

i35.24 **a** A triphasic Wilms tumor, illustrating all 3 components. There is immature mesenchyme in the lower left and upper right. Running from the upper left to the lower right are immature epithelial cells (blastoma). A few tubules are also seen. This neoplasm has favorable histology because there are no abnormal mitotic figures and there are no nuclei which are significantly more chromatic or larger than their peers.

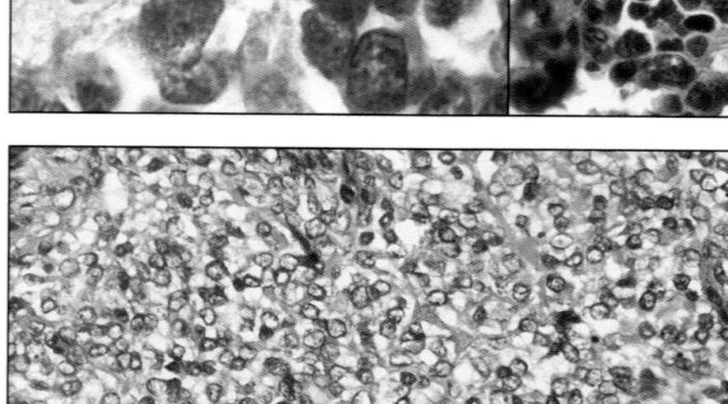

b-d The features of a Wilms tumor with unfavorable histology.
b depicts an abnormal mitotic figure.
c depicts significant nuclear enlargement and hyperchromasia of the epithelial nuclei in the center and on the right relative to those on the left, which are also neoplastic.
d depicts significant nuclear enlargement of the mesenchymal nuclei in the lower portion vs those in the upper portion, which are also neoplastic.

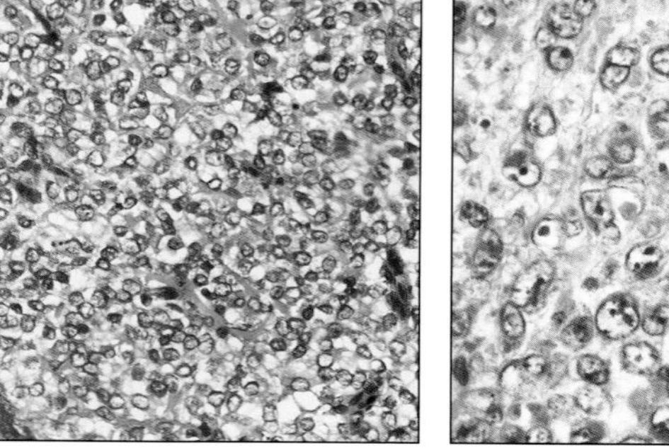

i35.25 Clear cell sarcoma of the kidney. Note the relatively uniform nuclei, the vesicular chromatin pattern, indistinct nucleoli, and fine capillaries.

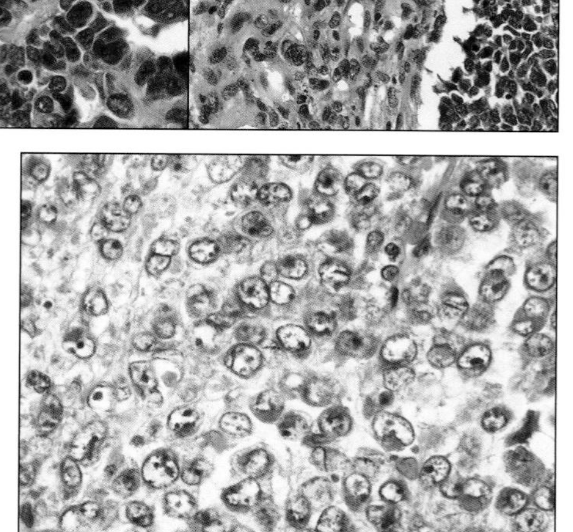

i35.26 A rhabdoid tumor. The nuclei have vesicular chromatin, but unlike those in a clear cell sarcoma of the kidney, nucleoli are prominent. In the center, many cells contain eosinophilic bodies in the cytoplasm which are on one side of the cell while the nucleus is on the other side.

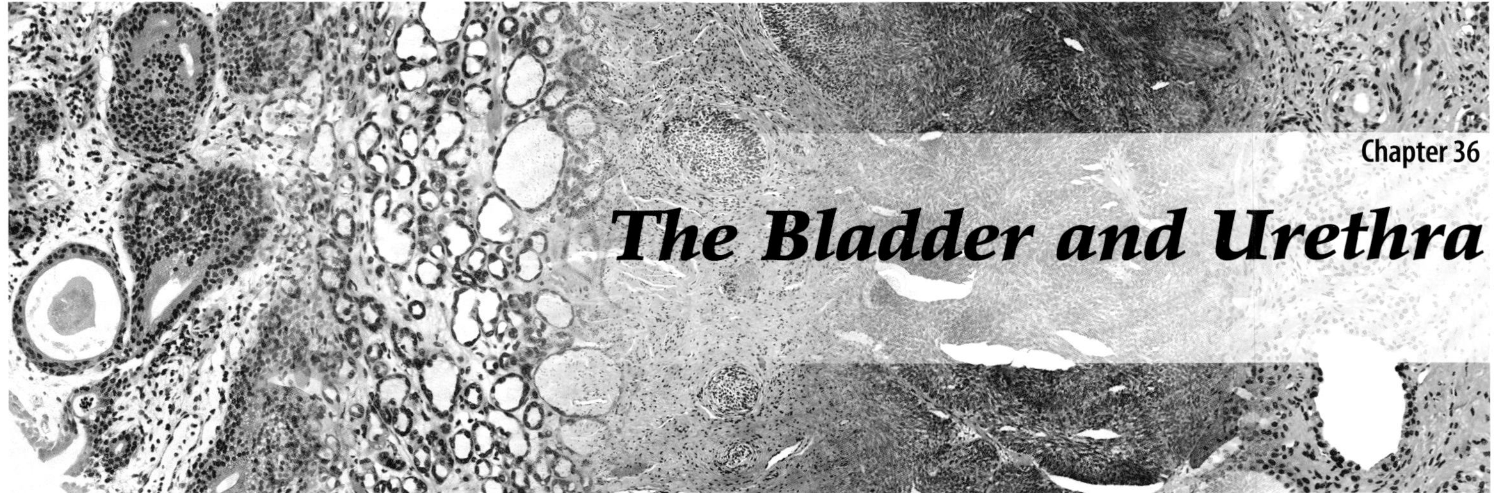

Chapter 36

The Bladder and Urethra

Inflammatory Conditions of the Bladder

Brunn nests are invaginations of the urothelium into the superficial stroma, though they may become detached from the surface i36.1. Cystitis cystica results from cystic change in Brunn nests and cystitis glandularis is glandular metaplasia of these nests i36.2.

Eosinophilic cystitis is rare and when seen, is often associated with allergic disorders or peripheral blood eosinophilia. It may have a chronic stage in which there is fibrosis and a paucity of eosinophils [PMID19195972]. As is always the case when large numbers of eosinophils are found in an organ, it is wise to check the peripheral eosinophil count and exclude a myeloproliferative neoplasm.

Interstitial cystitis was first described by Skene in 1887. It was later described by Hunner in 1915 and is still occasionally called Hunner cystitis. By definition, there are no pathogenic bacteria in interstitial cystitis, and an autoimmune etiology is suspected. Pelvic pain is very common in interstitial cystitis, and the condition is often referred to as painful bladder syndrome/interstitial cystitis. Other symptoms of interstitial cystitis include urinary urgency, frequency, and nocturia. Symptoms overlap those of many gynecologic conditions, and this entity should be excluded before definitive therapy is rendered for a presumed gynecologic disorder [PMID19793476].

Histologic changes in interstitial cystitis are variable, and no specific histologic findings are required for the diagnosis. Indeed, while cystoscopy is necessary and a biopsy is frequently performed, the diagnosis as established by the criteria of National Institute of Diabetes, Digestive and Kidney Diseases (NIDDK) [PMID3379688] can be made without tissue sampling. The diagnosis is based on the above symptoms in the absence of other explanations (ie, gynecologic abnormalities). When a biopsy is performed, the findings range from normal bladder tissue to edema, chronic inflammation, and urothelial ulceration i36.3a [PMID14641407]. Mast cells, which may be seen in small numbers in the normal bladder, are readily seen in interstitial cystitis i36.3b, though the reason for this has never been elucidated [PMID17462477]. Fibrosis may occur in chronic cases. The diagnosis of interstitial cystitis should be made with great caution, if at all, in patients who have received intravesicular therapy for urothelial carcinoma.

Hemorrhagic cystitis is often seen in patients who have had intravesicular chemotherapy with any agent or systemic chemotherapy with cyclophosphamide. In the latter case, renal excretion of metabolites damages the bladder urothelium [PMID14486208].

Benign Neoplasms and Neoplasm-Like Conditions of the Bladder and Urethra

There are a number of conditions that can simulate urothelial neoplasia in the bladder. Foremost among these are severe reactive changes in patients who have received intravesicular chemotherapy for a bladder tumor or whose bladder was in the field of radiation therapy that was targeted at another site, such as the cervix or prostate. In addition to the indispensable role of the history, a severely inflamed background or giant cells i36.4 suggests that the atypia is reactive unless the evidence for carcinoma is compelling. Stromal desmoplasia favors carcinoma, as do jagged clusters of atypical cells and demonstrable penetration of the basement membrane. As in other sites, localization of the basement membrane with a PAS or immunohistochemical stain may help, though these stains can be difficult to interpret. A reactive process should be suspected if the putative invasive clusters surround blood vessels or are associated with deposits of fibrin [PMID15223961]. In patients who have been treated for urothelial carcinoma, before concluding that there is recurrent/residual carcinoma, it is wise to compare the problematic cells to the original tumor and to favor a reactive process if there is not a good morphologic match.

The so-called inverted papilloma is a nonneoplastic reactive lesion in which a large number of endophytic aggregates of cells makes the lesion as a whole polypoid and exophytic i36.5. This entity is distinct from the family of papillary neoplastic lesions.

Other nonneoplastic entities that can simulate neoplasia include nephrogenic adenoma and postoperative spindle cell nodule [PMID19494852]. The nephrogenic adenoma (also called mesonephric adenoma or mesonephric metaplasia) is a glandular metaplasia of the bladder or urethra. It may have a complex low-power tubulo-papillary appearance that is worrisome for adenocarcinoma, but the nuclei are uniform and bland, and the cells have minimal cytoplasm i36.6. Like the metanephric adenoma in the kidney, a nephrogenic adenoma

ISBN 978-089189-5886

of the bladder must be excluded before diagnosing a small, well differentiated, well demarcated adenocarcinoma.

The postoperative spindle cell nodule usually involves the vagina, bladder, or prostatic urethra within months after a surgical procedure. It consists of a cellular proliferation of plump spindle cells that can be infiltrative and locally destructive. These nodules usually have an edematous or myxoid matrix. Mitotic figures may be frequent, but there is no significant pleomorphism. The differential diagnosis includes leiomyosarcoma and spindle cell carcinoma and can be extremely difficult if the patient does not have a known history of recent surgery. An edematous or myxoid stroma, resulting in an appearance that resembles nodular fasciitis, favors a benign diagnosis. Because the cells of a postoperative spindle cell nodule are myofibroblasts, which may have some keratin positivity, a keratin stain alone may suggest an incorrect diagnosis of carcinoma. The immunohistochemical panel in such cases should include actin and ALK, as 70% of postoperative spindle cell nodules stain for actin and almost 1/2 stain for ALK-1, suggesting that the postoperative spindle cell nodule may be a manifestation of an inflammatory myofibroblastic tumor [PMID16819319]. Rarely, a similar myxoid tumor may occur without a history of surgery, in which case it may be called a pseudosarcomatous fibromyxoid tumor, but these cases are likely an inflammatory myofibroblastic tumor.

"Urethral caruncle" is a general term for a mass near the urethral opening, almost always in postmenopausal women. The most common histologic finding is a vascular polypoid lesion with inflammatory cells and edema **i36.7**, resembling granulation tissue. Rarely a urethral caruncle will be secondary to prolapse, abscess, or neoplasm.

Urothelial Dysplasia and Carcinoma in Situ

The bladder has 2 separate and independent pathways to invasive carcinoma—flat precursor lesions of the dysplasia/carcinoma in situ (CIS) group and papillary lesions. Reflecting this, the most recent World Health Organization (WHO) classification of tumors of the urinary system includes urothelial flat lesions (flat hyperplasia, dysplasia and CIS) and papillary lesions [Eble ISBN978-9283224150]. Although by definition any noninvasive papillary carcinoma is a CIS, the pathology report should clearly distinguish this group of lesions from flat dysplasia/CIS, and must leave no doubt as to which of the 2 potential precursors of invasive is identified.

DNA studies have verified the long-held histologic observation that there are 2 pathways to invasive bladder carcinoma. Flat CIS and invasive carcinomas often have loss of function mutations in tumor suppressor genes such as *P53*, *RB*, and *PTEN*, while noninvasive papillary neoplasms often have gain of function mutations in the oncogenes *RAS* and *FGFR3*, and may also have del(9q) [PMID18815930].

The basic concepts of flat urothelial dysplasia and CIS are similar to those encountered in other sites, though there is less standardization and interobserver agreement at every level. The following types of urothelial CIS are recognized: large cell pleomorphic **i36.8a**, large cell nonpleomorphic **i36.8b**, small cell, and clinging **i36.8c**, in which there is only 1 or 2 layers of atypical cells [PMID11224606]. A small amount of maturation, including the presence of umbrella cells, does not preclude a high-grade dysplasia/CIS. Any of these forms of CIS may extend into a Brunn nest without invading **i36.8d**.

CIS may also spread laterally to undermine the adjacent urothelium, so the finding of atypical cells in the lower portion of the urothelium, covered by cytologically normal urothelium, should elicit a search for CIS in the adjacent tissue. If such a focus is not found, a comment might be made that an unsampled focus of CIS cannot be excluded.

If there is difficulty in determining if urothelial atypia is reactive or CIS, it might be helpful to stain for CK20 and p53. Normal and reactive urothelium shows p53 staining that is weak, focal, and basal. CK20 reactivity in normal or reactive urothelium is largely restricted to the superficial layer. In contrast, CIS shows diffuse p53 reactivity in 57% of cases and diffuse and significant CK20 reactivity throughout the urothelium in 81% of cases [PMID11474293]. p16 is reported to stain normal or reactive urothelium weakly but to stain CIS much more strongly, particularly in the nucleus [PMID18234280]. IMP3, like p16, first came to attention in differentiating cervical dysplasia from reactive epithelium, but also has potential in urothelium. About 1/2 of cases of high-grade urothelial dysplasia will express IMP3, while only 5% of low-grade dysplasia cases and 1% of reactive urothelium [PMID18547613].

Papillary Urothelial Lesions

Cystitis may have a polypoid presentation that can simulate a papillary neoplasm. Papillary cystitis generally demonstrates fronds that are broader and less architecturally complex, with less branching. The papillations are usually less cellular and frequently edematous [PMID18379418]. A background of cystitis suggests that a problematic papillary lesion is more likely reactive. In the urethra, the simple fibroepithelial polyp may simulate a papillary neoplasm.

The nomenclature of noninvasive urothelial papillary neoplasms has undergone appreciable metamorphosis over the years. After years of nearly universal belief that any papillary lesion in the bladder was a carcinoma, the simple papilloma was eventually recognized [PMID10570437]. Papillary lesions are broadly subdivided into benign (papilloma and inverted papilloma), papillary urothelial neoplasm of low malignant potential (PUNLMP), and noninvasive papillary urothelial carcinoma (low or high grade).

A urothelial papilloma can be diagnosed if the lesion is absolutely normal in both its architecture and nuclear appearance, with normal orientation, evenly spaced nuclei, a normal umbrella cell layer, and no atypia. I recommend the use of the term "papilloma" in a completely bland lesion in a young person who may apply for health or life insurance. Otherwise, beginning the classification of noninvasive papillary urothelial lesions with papillary neoplasm of low malignant potential does the patient no harm, initiates appropriate surveillance, and makes the system more reproducible.

The PUNLMP (the word "carcinoma" is not used for low malignant potential lesions) has increased thickness of the urothelium with very mild nuclear atypia. Nuclei are evenly spaced and there is no crowding **i36.9a** [PMID9850170].

If there is any cellular crowding, uneven spacing of nuclei, or any nuclear pleomorphism, the lesion is best designated as a noninvasive low-grade papillary urothelial carcinoma **i36.9b**.

Extensive pleomorphism and hyperchromasia, and an essential absence of orientation are the hallmarks of a high-grade papillary lesion i36.9c. The diagnosis of intermediate-grade noninvasive papillary carcinoma remains reasonable, though these are often classed with the high-grade lesions because the recurrence potential for intermediate-grade lesions is similar to that of the high-grade lesions. I recommend a 2-tier low-grade/high-grade system for the noninvasive papillary carcinomas because of greater reproducibility. A 2-tiered system for noninvasive papillary carcinomas, in conjunction with omission of the term "papilloma," transforms an overall 5-tiered system for papillary urothelial lesions into a much more reproducible 3-tiered system (low malignant potential neoplasm, low-grade carcinoma, and high-grade carcinoma).

Invasive Urothelial (Transitional Cell) Carcinoma

The term "urothelial carcinoma" has largely replaced "transitional cell carcinoma" (TCC), though either term is acceptable. Little will be said about the usual invasive urothelial carcinoma, since it is rarely a challenge and is well treated in other works, but 4 points regarding invasion are in order. First, it may occasionally be difficult to determine if a neoplasm is invasive or not, especially if there is tangential sectioning. In such cases, a jagged stroma-epithelial interface, a disrupted basement membrane, increased nuclear atypia, or a stromal desmoplastic reaction favor the diagnosis of invasion. Also, clusters with clear spaces around them are suspicious because microinvasive foci may have retraction artifact of the stroma [PMID18815930]. In cases that cannot be resolved in this manner, immunohistochemical stains for the basement membrane (collagen type 4 or laminin) may help, or it might be prudent to simply comment that focal superficial invasion cannot be excluded.

Second, because it is now accepted (after long controversy) that the bladder does have a wispy, discontinuous muscularis mucosa [PMID3631381, PMID9882808], carcinoma in association with thin wisps of muscle, although indicative of invasion, does not indicate invasion of the muscularis propria. The muscularis mucosa is often easy to distinguish from the much denser muscularis propria, but there are cases, especially in small biopsies, when it is difficult to determine if a carcinoma has invaded the muscularis propria or simply the muscularis mucosa. It is wise to equivocate in these situations, though it has been reported that antibodies to smoothelin show stronger staining for the muscularis propria than for the muscularis mucosa [PMID20636795].

Third, it should be remembered that the normal lamina propria may contain adipose tissue [PMID7879346], so invasion into fat does not prove invasion through or even into the muscularis propria.

Fourth, "microinvasion" has been defined both as 5 mm or less and as 2 mm or less [PMID9298882], and is therefore a term that is likely to confuse the clinician. The central requirement is that invasion of the muscularis propria be identified if possible.

Immunohistochemistry may help identify urothelial carcinoma in metastatic sites. Most urothelial carcinomas are positive for both cytokeratins 7 and 20. Uroplakin III is reasonably specific for urothelium, but only stains about 1/2 of urothelial carcinomas [PMID12502922]. Indeed, positivity diminishes in progressively less differentiated urothelial carcinomas [PMID18313120]. In the absence of uroplakin III, expression of thrombomodulin, high molecular weight keratin, and cytokeratin 20 suggests urothelial origin of a poorly differentiated carcinoma [PMID12502922].

Unusual types of Urothelial Carcinoma

Rare forms of urothelial carcinoma, attesting to the ability of urothelium to differentiate along divergent lines, include micropapillary, lymphoepithelioma-like, clear cell, osteoclast-rich, lipoid cell, rhabdoid, sarcomatoid (carcinoma with sarcomatous metaplasia), and plasmacytoid types [PMID19494856, PMID19178589]. In addition, there are 3 forms of urothelial carcinoma that may be difficult for the pathologist to appreciate as primary bladder tumors—pure squamous carcinoma, pure adenocarcinoma, and small cell carcinoma.

The micropapillary variant of urothelial carcinoma consists of small clusters of cells, with subtle fibrovascular cores, that are often surrounded by a clear space that is an artifact of fixation and processing. It may resemble an ovarian serous adenocarcinoma and is aggressive [PMID7977945].

The lymphoepithelioma-like variant of urothelial carcinoma consists of sheets of poorly differentiated cells accompanied by a dense infiltrate of lymphocytes and plasma cells, resulting in an appearance nearly indistinguishable from the lymphoepithelioma of the nasopharynx (see i15.14a). Immunohistochemistry may be needed to exclude a large cell lymphoma.

Because urothelium is, as its former name implies, "transitional," both frankly squamous and glandular carcinomas may occur. Before making the diagnosis of primary adenocarcinoma of the bladder, a metastasis or extension, such as from the prostate, should be excluded. A urachal carcinoma must also be excluded. In development, the urachus extends from the dome of the bladder to the umbilicus. Its involution results in the median umbilical ligament. Any residual epithelium in the median umbilical ligament is called a urachal remnant. Urachal carcinoma is an adenocarcinoma that may involve the dome of the bladder, but it is not truly a bladder neoplasm since it arises from urachal remnants in the bladder wall, not from the urothelium or the bladder stroma. While it is possible that there may be benign, intact overlying urothelium or benign urachal remnants adjacent to the carcinoma, providing a clue to the origin, in practice it is likely that a urachal carcinoma will efface the overlying urothelium and obliterate any residual urachal remnants, so the diagnosis depends heavily on location. Most adenocarcinomas in the dome of the bladder or that extend toward the umbilicus will be of urachal origin. The urachal adenocarcinoma is treated by a partial cystectomy involving the dome and extending to and including umbilicus.

As is always the case for small cell carcinomas, the imperative is to exclude a metastasis from another site, especially the lung. While nothing within the pathologist's purview replaces clinical correlation, generous sampling of a primary bladder small cell carcinoma often reveals small areas of greater differentiation, identifying the tumor as primary in that site.

ISBN 978-089189-5886

Subtle Forms of Urothelial Carcinoma

There are 4 subtypes of urothelial carcinoma that may be cytologically bland and diagnostically difficult [PMID19494856, PMID9179971]. All of these subtle forms of invasive urothelial carcinoma resemble well-known benign entities, and in all of these types, important points are to look for areas of more typical carcinoma in other locations and look for evidence of invasion, either in the form of a stromal reaction or by finding epithelium in a location that is too deep for normal anatomic structures.

The urothelial carcinoma with tubules may look deceptively bland, with tubules lined by relatively unremarkable urothelium. It may resemble a nephrogenic adenoma. Clues to the neoplastic nature of the process are a urothelial lining (instead of glandular, as in a nephrogenic adenoma), a stromal reaction, and infiltration.

The nested urothelial carcinoma consists of rounded clusters of bland tumor cells. It resembles florid Brunn nests but may also resemble nephrogenic adenoma or inverted papilloma. Normal Brunn nests are generally larger than those of nested urothelial carcinoma, and are of more uniform size. They are evenly spaced, not overly crowded, have frequent cystic change, may have some glandular differentiation, and lack an infiltrative pattern. Most importantly, Brunn nests are not found in the muscularis propria. In contrast, nested urothelial carcinoma has smaller nests that are close together, more variability in size and spacing, an infiltrative pattern, and perhaps a stromal reaction. There is usually focal nuclear atypia somewhere in a nested carcinoma, with a slightly larger overall cell size, and about 2/3 of cases have a small focus of classic urothelial carcinoma somewhere. The most obvious clue to this diagnosis is apparent Brunn nests that are in the muscularis propria **i36.10a**, **i36.10b** [PMID19800100].

In my experience, a paraganglioma, which rarely occurs in the bladder, can simulate a nested variant of urothelial carcinoma and should be excluded before making the latter diagnosis.

Microcystic urothelial carcinoma resembles florid cystitis glandularis or cystitis cystica. Again, the key diagnostic features are evidence of invasion **i36.11** or a stromal reaction, and there is usually some degree of nuclear atypia and variation in the size and shape of the nests.

Urothelial carcinoma with an endophytic growth pattern (inverted urothelial carcinoma) resembles an inverted papilloma but differs from the benign entity in the greater extent of the proliferation, subtle nuclear atypia, focal infiltration, and an appearance reminiscent of a verrucous carcinoma, or in areas of more typical carcinoma elsewhere [PMID9298882].

Screening for Urothelial Carcinoma

Urothelial carcinoma is currently the fifth leading cause of cancer death in the United States and is frustratingly difficult to detect by screening. Urine cytology has excellent specificity but suffers from poor sensitivity, missing approximately 70% of all cases and up to 90% of low-grade lesions. Still, because of its ease of collection and examination, and because of its excellent specificity, urine cytology continues to have an important role in screening. Because urine is relatively toxic to cells (in contrast to effusions), exfoliated tumor cells that have been in suspension overnight are unlikely to have sufficient preservation of detail for optimal study. For this reason, I recommend that the patient empty the bladder in the morning, hydrate, and submit a subsequent specimen for cytology.

Early attempts to supplement or replace voided urine cytology in patients with hematuria or abnormal urinalysis included searching for cytokeratins that might be shed by bladder tumors and a latex agglutination reaction for basement membrane complexes that were associated with urothelial neoplasia (bladder tumor antigen).

There is hope that patients can be screened for bladder carcinoma by DNA testing. For example, many carcinomas of the bladder are associated with increases in the numbers of chromosomes 3, 7, and 17, or with a deletion of 9p21 [PMID15790699]. Vysis markets a FISH test, called UroVysion, which contains DNA probes for these 4 abnormalities. Testing is performed on a pellet from a voided specimen and employs chromosome enumeration probes, which hybridize to the α DNA that is near the centromeres (α DNA and chromosome enumerator probes are discussed in Chapter 45). 4 different probes, 1 for each abnormality to be screened for, are each attached to a different fluorescent compound. At least 2 abnormalities must be detected to have clinical significance. Because tetraploidy is normal in bladder mucosa, there must be true aneuploidy, not simple tetraploidy, for chromosomes 3, 7, or 17 to be considered abnormal. The Federal Drug Administration has approved this test both for initial diagnosis and monitoring for recurrence, and it has been shown to be more sensitive than cytology [PMID18724101]. However, it is less specific [PMID1732550], an overall cost/benefit advantage remains to be proven, and the sensitivity and specificity of UroVysion is not sufficient to obviate the need for cystoscopy with washings or biopsies in patients with persistent hematuria, abnormal urinalysis, or atypical cells in voided urine cytology [PMID19347824].

The ImmunoCyt assay (Diagnocure Inc, Quebec, Canada) is a fluorescent test that uses 3 monoclonal antibodies to detect antigens that are associated with urothelial neoplasia (1 for each of 2 mucins and 1 for a high-molecular-weight glycosylated carcinoembryonic antigen). Compared to UroVysion, ImmunoCyt is reported to have a higher sensitivity, but a lower specificity in the detection of low-grade urothelial neoplasms [PMID19365828].

Both UroVysion and ImmunoCyt have a higher sensitivity than urine cytology and a higher negative predictive value. However, both require special equipment and specially trained personnel. They also have more false positives than cytology and are more expensive. Most importantly, neither test is a replacement for cystoscopy with washings or biopsies. It has been a pleasure watching supplementary testing develop in this important area, but at this writing, we have not progressed sufficiently to replace the time-honored algorithm of abnormal cells in a voided urine or clinical findings triggering cystoscopy, with washing or biopsies.

Core Points for the Bladder and the Urethra

- Interstitial cystitis: urgency, frequency, nocturia, pelvic pain.
  - No specific histologic changes, but chronic inflammation, often with mast cells.
- Urethral caruncle is a polypoid mass near the urethral opening in older women, usually resembling granulation tissue.
- Benign simulators of malignancy: reactive changes.
  - Cystitis or in patients who have received intravesicular chemotherapy or radiation therapy.
  - Inverted papilloma, nephrogenic adenoma, and post-operative spindle cell nodule.
- 2 separate pathways to invasive carcinoma: flat precursor lesions and papillary lesions.
  - Multiple forms of urothelial carcinoma in situ. Maturation does not exclude urothelial dysplasia/CIS.
  - Multiple forms of papillary lesions.
- Indicators of invasion: jagged stroma-epithelial interface, increased nuclear atypia, stromal desmoplasia, discontinuity of the basement membrane.
- Pitfall: bladder has a thin muscularis mucosa, so intermingling of tumor with muscle does not prove invasion into the muscularis propria.
- Pitfall: lamina propria has adipose tissue, so intermingling of tumor with fat does not prove transmural invasion.
- Rare forms of urothelial carcinoma: micropapillary, lymphoepithelioma-like, clear cell, osteoclast-rich, lipoid cell, rhabdoid, sarcomatoid, and plasmacytoid types.
- Pure squamous carcinoma, pure adenocarcinoma, and small cell carcinoma are also rare forms that may not appear to be bladder primaries.
- 4 subtypes of urothelial carcinoma that are subtle: urothelial carcinoma with tubules, the nested urothelial carcinoma, the microcystic urothelial carcinoma, and the urothelial carcinoma with an endophytic growth pattern (inverted urothelial carcinoma).
  - Clues in these subtle forms are the identification of areas of more classic carcinoma and evidence of invasion, such as infiltration and stromal fibrosis.
  - Presence of seemingly innocuous collections of urothelium deep within the wall.
- Screening for urothelial neoplasia: urine cytology has poor sensitivity.
  - Fluorescent techniques based on chromosomal abnormalities or abnormal antigens in carcinoma are promising, but not proven.
  - Require special equipment, trained personnel, and generate false positives.
  - None obviates the need for cystoscopy, with washings or biopsies.

ISBN 978-089189-5886

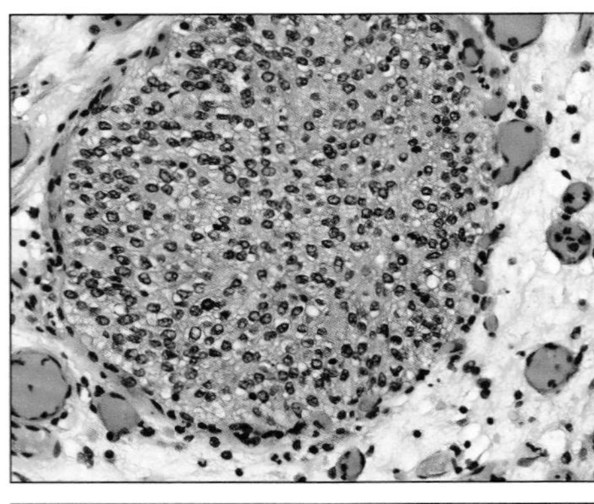

i36.1 A Brunn nest

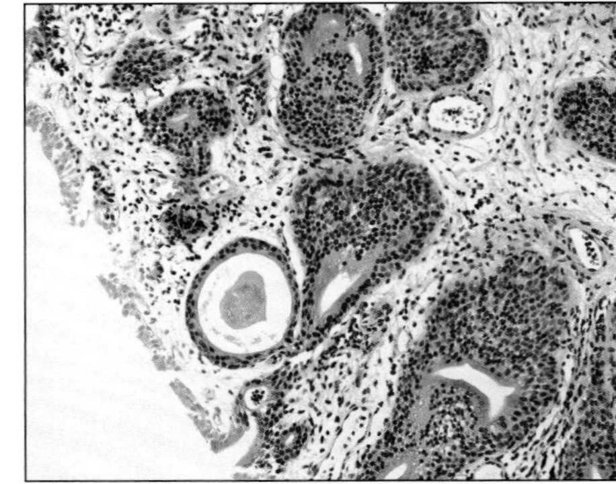

i36.2 Normal bladder mucosa with 2 Brunn nests in the upper right, cystitis cystica in the lower left, and cystitis glandularis in the center

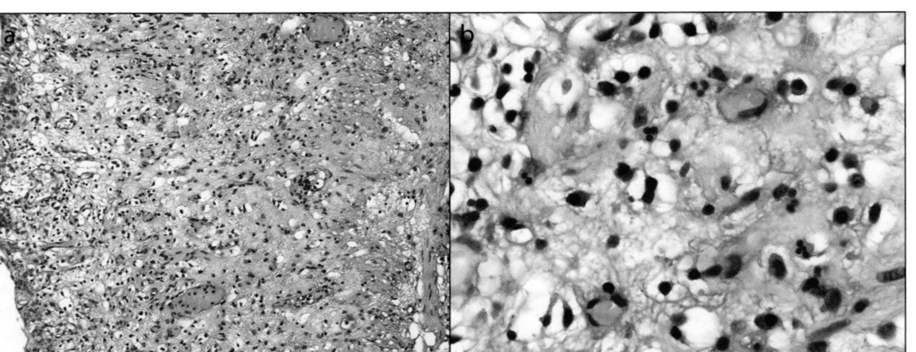

i36.3 **a** Interstitial cystitis, with ulceration of the urothelium, acute and chronic inflammation in the stroma, and stromal edema

b Mast cells in interstitial cystitis

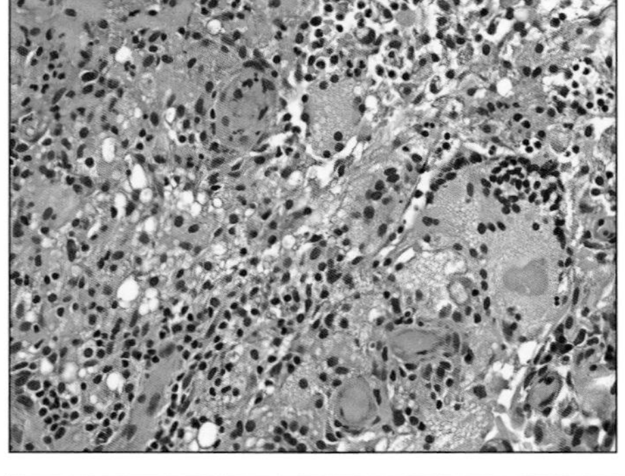

i36.4 A bladder biopsy in which BCG has been previously employed for urothelial carcinoma. The urothelium is often completely denuded in these cases, as it is here, but may be atypical if present. The stroma demonstrates acute and chronic inflammation, with giant cells. Occasionally, there is an overt granulomatous response in the stroma.

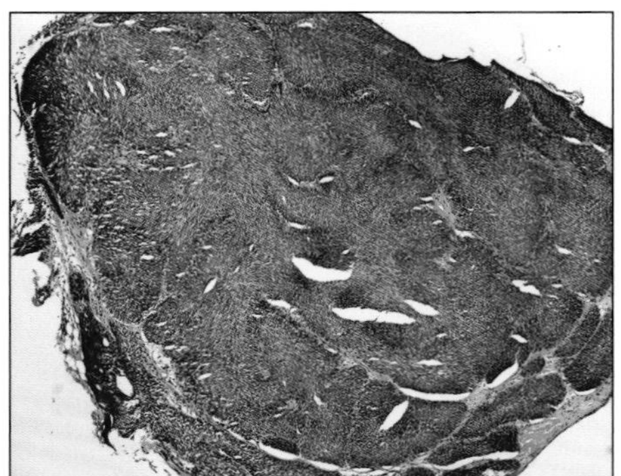

i36.5 An inverted papilloma of the bladder. The lesion as a whole is exophytic, but it consists of clusters of urothelial cells that appear to grow in an endophytic manner.

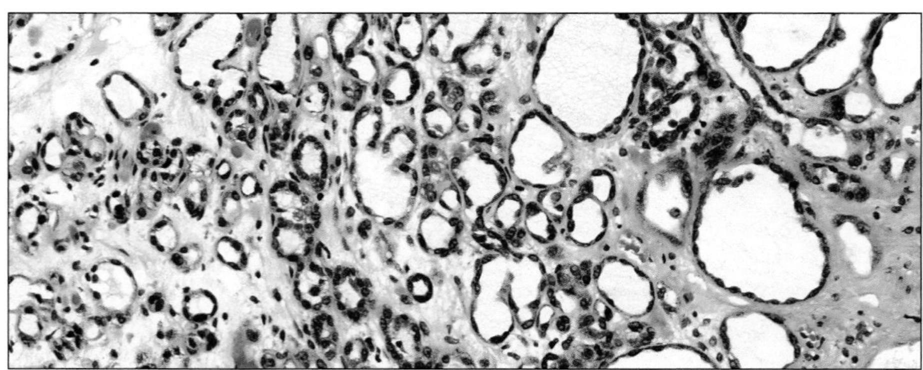

i36.6 A nephrogenic adenoma of the bladder, which initially appears to be an adenocarcinoma, but the nuclei are small and uniform. Note the almost complete absence of cytoplasm.

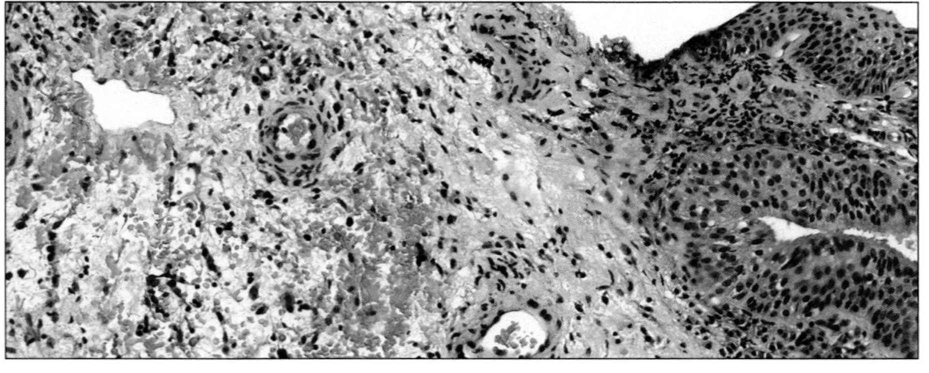

i36.7 A urethral caruncle. On the right, the surface epithelium is stratified squamous while underneath it, there is a transition from urothelial (formerly called transitional) lining to squamous. This transition is normal in the distal urethra. There is ulceration with acute and chronic inflammation, edema, and vascularity in the stroma.

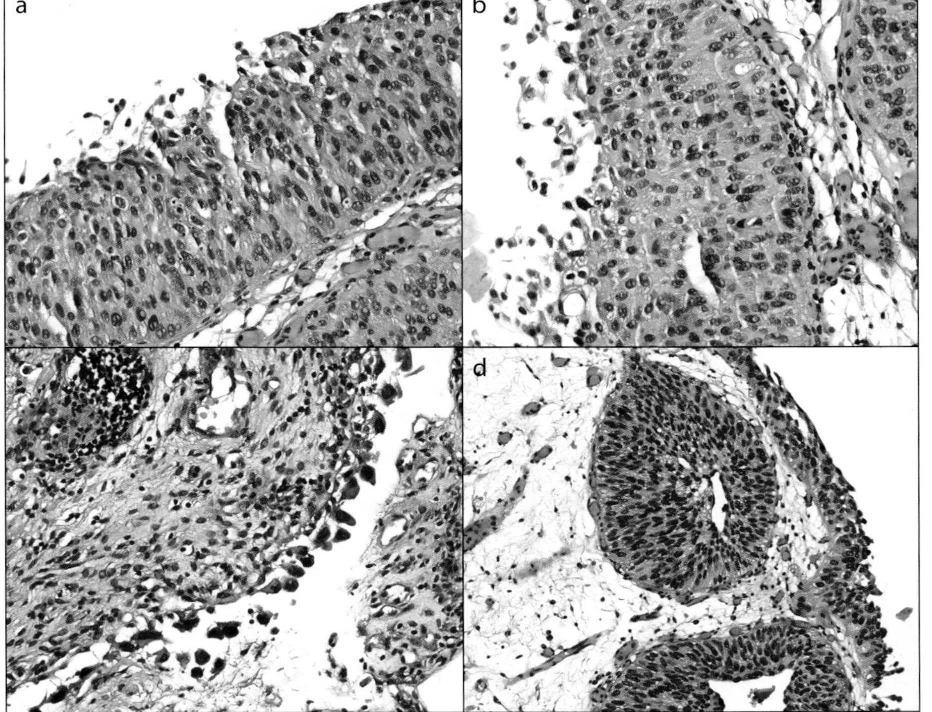

i36.8 **a** The large cell pleomorphic variant of urothelial carcinoma in situ. Pleomorphic cells extend throughout the urothelium.

b The large cell nonpleomorphic variant of urothelial carcinoma in situ. Admittedly, it is a judgment call as to whether a particular manifestation of large cell carcinoma in situ is pleomorphic or nonpleomorphic.

c The so-called "clinging" form of urothelial carcinoma in situ. Although the urothelium is very thin, with only 1 cell layer in many places, there is severe nuclear atypia.

d Extension of carcinoma in situ into a Brunn nest. Note the nuclear atypia in the Brunn nest, as contrasted with i36.1.

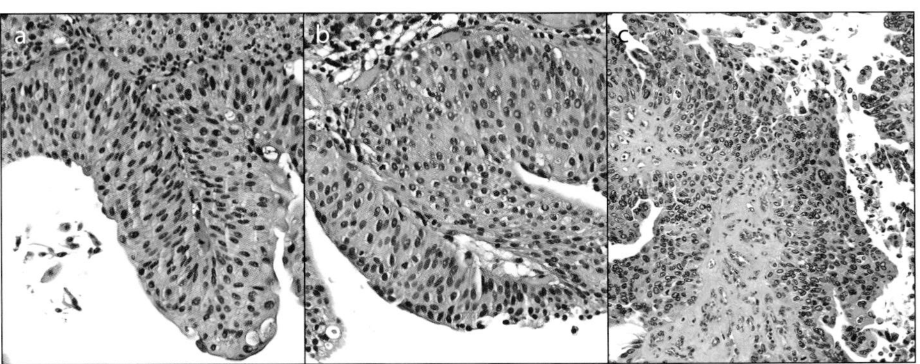

i36.9 **a** A papillary urothelial neoplasm of low malignant potential. The nuclei are small and uniform, with abundant cytoplasm, and essential retention of polarity and orientation.

b A low-grade papillary urothelial carcinoma. Compared to i36.9a, the nuclei are slightly larger, with slightly less cytoplasm, and arranged in a less orderly manner. **c** A high-grade papillary urothelial carcinoma

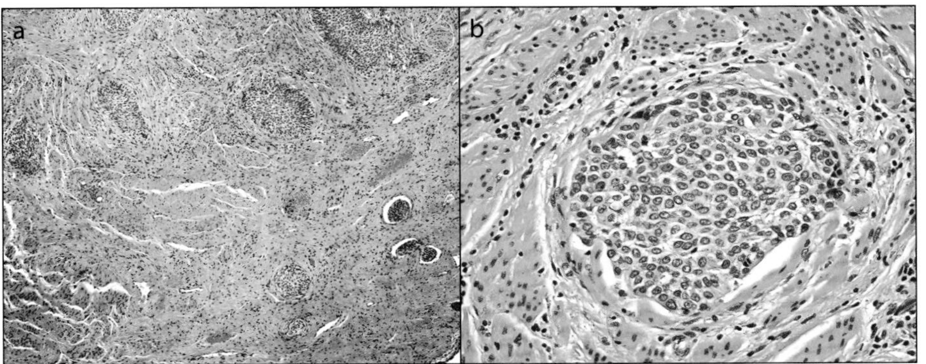

i36.10 **a** The nested variant of invasive urothelial carcinoma. The urothelial surface is seen in the lower right. Innocuous-appearing clusters of cells are seen in the bladder wall, but they infiltrate too deeply for Brunn nests.

b A higher-power view of a cluster of neoplastic cells from the case in i36.10a. The individual cells do not appear alarming, and the cluster that they form is round, but this cluster is deep within the muscularis propria.

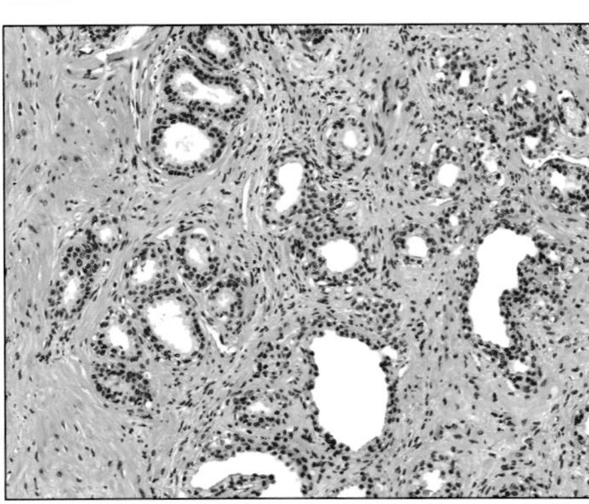

i36.11 Microcystic urothelial carcinoma. Note the resemblance to benign cystitis cystic or cystitis glandularis, but these clusters are deep within the muscularis propria.

ISBN 978-089189-5886

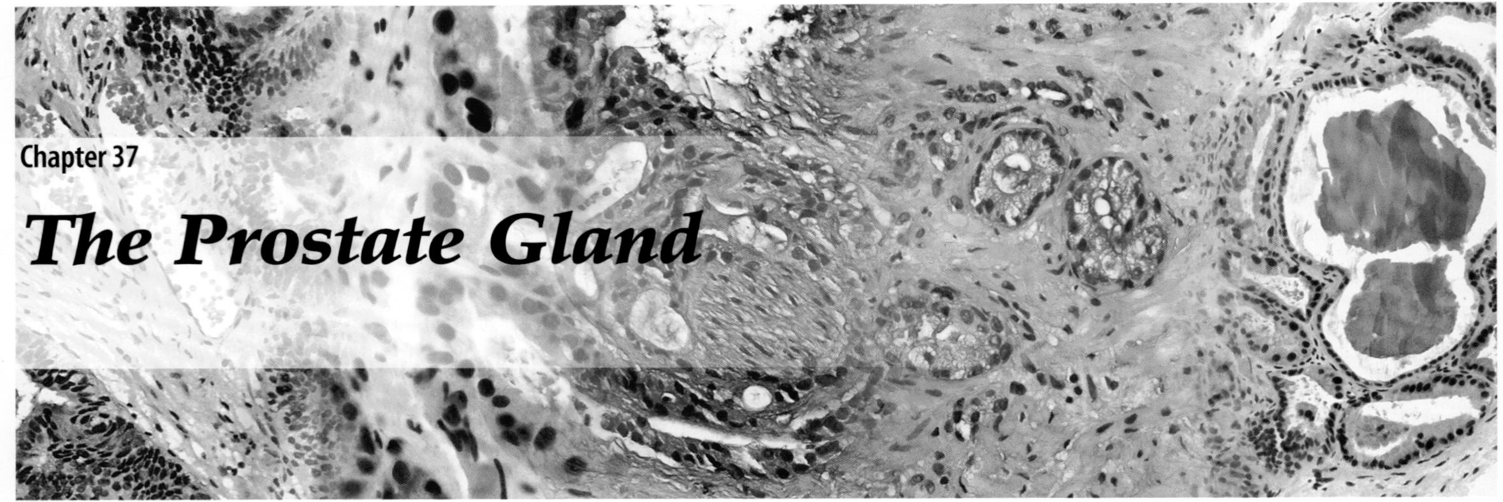

Chapter 37

The Prostate Gland

Prostate Cancer Screening

No other organ in the body has proved as frustrating as the prostate in the early detection of malignancy. The prostate specific antigen (PSA) test is the mainstay of early detection, but suffers from poor sensitivity and specificity. Indeed, in 2008, the United States Preventive Services Task Force (USPSTF) recommended that routine PSA screening not be performed in men over the age of 75 because in this age group, there are more difficulties and expense in screening and acting on elevated PSA levels than there is benefit in early detection of this usually indolent cancer [PMID18678845]. Also in 2008, the American Academy of Preventive Medicine recommended against general PSA screening [PMID18201648]. In 2012, the USPSTF went further, recommending "against PSA-based screaning for prostate cancer regardless of age" [PMID22315362]. Predictably, these recommendations were quickly attacked, and the matter remains hotly debated. At this writing, both the American Urological Association and the American Cancer Society continue to recommend PSA screening for all men over age 50 whose life expectancy is considered to be 10 years or more.

Prostate cancer screening illustrates the more general problem that on the one hand, early detection of cancer is crucial, but on the other hand, the diagnosis and treatment of cancer is unnecessary and potentially counterproductive if the disease will not limit longevity or curtail quality of life. Such "overdiagnosis" not only causes unnecessary treatment, but also needless patient anxiety. In the years ahead, we will need to balance the proven benefits of screening and the early diagnosis it affords, with the risks of overtreating incidental, inconsequential cancers [PMID20413742].

A variety of attempts have been made to "tweak" the PSA [PMID19860930], but these have been disappointing. The PSA density, also called the PSA index, is the serum PSA divided by the volume of the gland as determined by ultrasound. Some have advocated this measurement, the theory being that carcinoma produces more PSA per gram of tissue than does BPH [PMID19928413]. Another approach relies on the fact that most PSA in serum is complexed to α-1-antichymotrypsin, and that benign prostate tissue tends to produce more free (uncomplexed) PSA, while prostate carcinoma tends to produce PSA in complexed form [PMID19778292].

There have been some suggestions for both an age-adjusted and a race-adjusted normal range for PSA [PMID16093978]. It seems to be "common sense" that younger men should have a lower PSA, and that African-Americans, in whom prostate carcinoma is more prevalent, should be followed more aggressively for the same PSA value. However, many are now moving away from this idea, and the issue remains unsettled.

Attention has turned to early detection by alternative serum markers. α-methylacyl-coenzyme A racemase, which is very helpful as an immunohistochemical stain in tissue samples (where it is often called p504S), has disappointing sensitivity and specificity as a serum marker [PMID16143040].

Another approach uses predictive autoantibodies, which are autoantibodies that may or may not be pathogenic, but which appear with early disease or even years before its onset [PMID16177248]. Still another approach, called the uPM3 test, uses nucleic acid sequence-based amplification (discussed in Chapter 45) to look for the mRNA of prostate cancer antigen 3 (PCA3), a gene that is overexpressed in prostate carcinoma, in the urine [PMID15302485]. PCA3 urine assay has been shown to be more specific than either total or free PSA in prostate cancer screening, but it is slightly less sensitive. Unlike PSA, urine levels of PCA3 are not dependent on the volume of the gland and will hopefully lead to fewer false positives from benign hyperplasia. While promising, PCA3 is far from ideal and seems likely to supplement, rather than replace, PSA [PMID20230386, PMID20619529].

Attempts to detect early prostate carcinoma by radiographic modalities have also been frustrating. Transrectal ultrasound is commonly used, but is limited in its ability to identify areas for biopsy. Indeed, even when the entire gland is available for gross examination, there is still very poor sensitivity and specificity in locating a carcinoma. Can we expect an imaging modality to be superior to gross examination?

The poor specificity of serum PSA and the poor sensitivity of radiographic methods makes the early detection of prostate carcinoma intensely challenging. Because of the unique ability of MRI to image soft tissue, attention has naturally turned to this modality [PMID22261768], but experience is limited. At this time, one of the best uses of MRI in the detection of prostate cancer is to increase the yield of repeat biopsy in patients with previously negative biopsies and rising PSA levels [PMID22192873].

The Prostate Biopsy

The normal prostate gland consists of lobules i37.1 whose acini contain 2 layers of cells—a readily seen, relatively round cell near the lumen, and a less conspicuous, spindled basal cell between the round cell and the basement membrane i37.2. Importantly, the spindled, basal layer is lost in carcinoma, and verification of its loss is critical in establishing a malignant diagnosis in difficult cases.

In addition to nonspecific acute and chronic prostatitis, granulomatous prostatitis is relatively common. The cause of granulomatous prostatitis is usually unknown, but it is associated with previous transurethral resection and the use of BCG for bladder carcinomas, and some cases may be an autoimmune reaction to prostatic secretions [PMID17092284]. Infectious agents are rarely found.

Squamous and transitional metaplasia i37.3 are relatively common in the prostate, though the latter may be a consequence of normal intermingling of epithelium rather than a true change from one type to another. The benign prostatic urethral polyp is a metaplastic process containing benign prostatic glands covered by both transitional and prostatic epithelium.

The postoperative spindle cell nodule, discussed in Chapter 36, may rarely be seen in the prostate if a recent surgical procedure (such as a TURP) has been performed. Because this is a proliferation of spindle cells, it is unlikely to be confused with adenocarcinoma, but it can resemble a urothelial carcinoma invading into the prostate.

Transrectal prostate biopsy, like the elevated serum PSA levels that often engender it, suffers from a high false-negative rate because there is no good means to locate the best area to biopsy. Likewise, there is poor correlation between apparent benign hyperplasia on needle biopsy and on resected prostates, and it is probably not worthwhile diagnosing hyperplasia on biopsy. With rare exceptions, the detection of cancer is the sole purpose of the prostate biopsy.

In most prostate carcinomas, there are small glands that infiltrate between the benign glands i37.4. The individual tumor cell in most prostatic carcinomas typically has a moderately enlarged nucleus with a prominent nucleolus, and a moderate amount of cytoplasm that is more amphophilic than that of the normal prostatic epithelial cell. A good way to appreciate the nuclear features that suggest carcinoma is to compare a problematic focus with adjacent, clearly benign glands i37.5. Unlike most carcinomas, nuclear pleomorphism is not a major feature in prostatic carcinomas, and the appearance of individual tumor cells remains relatively constant even in high-grade carcinomas. What changes is the architectural pattern. Therefore, unlike most carcinomas, those of the prostate are not given a nuclear grade.

Likewise, though prostatic carcinomas have more mitotic activity than benign prostatic tissue, and mitoses suggest a carcinoma in a problematic situation, there is no firm evidence that the number of mitoses increases with the grade of the tumor, so something akin to the Bloom-Richardson system used in breast carcinomas, employing a combination of gland formation, mitoses, and nuclear pleomorphism, is not appropriate in the prostate. This unusual feature of prostate carcinoma is the basis of the Gleason grading system, which is purely architectural. The Gleason grading system was introduced in 1966 [PMID5948714], was refined in 1974 [PMID11905924], and remains valuable in large part because with occasional exceptions, lessening degrees of differentiation in prostate carcinoma are manifest in architecture rather than nuclear grade.

A Gleason grade (or pattern) 1 carcinoma has small round glands without obvious infiltration. Because infiltration is a key feature in most cases of prostate carcinoma, a Gleason grade 1 carcinoma can only be diagnosed by its enlarged nuclei, prominent nucleoli, and amphophilic cytoplasm. Most cases diagnosed as Gleason 1 carcinoma on needle biopsy are actually examples of adenosis or prostatic intraductal neoplasia (PIN; both discussed subsequently) or will be accompanied by areas of higher grade on a resection.

For all practical purposes, a Gleason grade 2 carcinoma is the lowest grade that can be detected on a biopsy, and even here, immunohistochemical stains are often needed. In a Gleason grade 2, a small amount of infiltration is apparent, with intervening stroma between the neoplastic glands. The minimal infiltration is still sufficient to see that the focus is not perfectly rounded and circumscribed. The individual glands maintain a rounded contour and are of relatively unchanged and uniform size i37.6.

A Gleason grade 3 has obvious infiltration i37.7 and also has glands that have a more variable appearance, with loss of a rounded contour i37.8. The key feature in a Gleason grade 4 carcinoma is confluence of neoplastic glands. A majority of the tumor should be in the form of glands that have fused with adjacent glands i37.9. Neoplastic glands that have a cribriform appearance are very likely to be of grade 4.

In a Gleason grade 5 carcinoma, most of the tumor exists in solid sheets, with little or no glandular differentiation i37.10. Necrosis of neoplastic epithelium, though not specifically a criterion in the Gleason system, suggests grade 5. Signet ring cells i37.11 suggest a Gleason grade 5.

The only difficulty with the Gleason system is that there is some variability between observers, primarily concerning grades 3 and 4. Much of this is unavoidable, but a number of publications have attempted to reduce this [PMID19886716]. Caution is recommended in making the diagnosis of a prostatic carcinoma of Gleason grade 2 or less on a biopsy. If the diagnosis of carcinoma is secure on a biopsy, it is very likely to be a higher grade than 2 on prostatectomy. At the other extreme, care should be taken in assigning a grade of 4. A grade of 4 is sometimes inappropriately assigned to what in fact is a cellular grade 3. A true grade 4 has some confluence of the glands.

The 2 most common grades are added for the Gleason score, with the predominant grade listed first. For example, a carcinoma that is 70% grade 3 and 30% grade 4 is said to have a Gleason score of 3 + 4 = 7, while one that is 70% grade 4 and 30% grade 3 is a score of 4 + 3 = 7. Most use the term "pattern" or "grade" for a single Gleason number, and the term "score" or "sum" for the total. However, some might use the term "grade" for the sum, so one should not be confused by a phrase like "Gleason grade 3 + 3 = 6." For clarity, I recommend the word "grade" for a single number and the word "score" for the sum of 2 grades.

ISBN 978-089189-5886

In 2005, the Gleason grading system underwent a major revision. The fundamental concepts were not changed, but an effort was made to obtain greater interobserver agreement and to obtain greater agreement between Gleason scores obtained on needle biopsies and those obtained after prostatectomy. The main points of agreement at this conference, and the refinements that have arisen from it, are as follows [PMID17111167]:

Gleason score 2 + 2 is very rare and should be reported with caution and only after exclusion of benign mimics.

Of those carcinomas with a Gleason score of 7, those with a major grade of 3 (3 + 4 = 7; called 7a) are less aggressive than those with a major grade of 4 (4 + 3 = 7; called 7b). Indeed, 7a/7b may be a major prognostic breakpoint.

A tertiary grade should be commented on if it is of higher grade than either the primary or secondary grades.

Clearly, a definitive assessment of the appropriate Gleason score, like staging, must await a prostatectomy and may never be forthcoming in patients treated nonsurgically, but the modified Gleason system applied to biopsies has somewhat improved interobserver agreement, especially when the highest grade, regardless of extent, is reported as the primary grade of the tumor [PMID20006878]. It has also led to better correlation with scoring on prostatectomies [PMID19793829] and better correlation with clinical stage [PMID19283673].

Since the 2005 conference, the identification of a very small high-grade tertiary focus has been additionally advocated, especially if it is a grade of 5 [PMID16600733, PMID17674043]. For example, a carcinoma that consists of 50% grade 3, 40% grade 4, and 10% grade 5 would be scored as 3 + 4 = 7 in the traditional system, but 3 + 5 = 8 in the modified system. However, inconstant implementation of this recommendation and implementation in different ways (such as reporting the above example as 3 + 5 = 8 by some, but as 3 + 4 = 7, with a comment on a small focus of grade 5 by others) remain causes of differences of opinion in Gleason scoring.

If a secondary component is both less than the primary component and is <5% of the total tumor, it can be ignored and the primary number reported twice. For example, a secondary component of 3 that occupies <5% of a tumor that is otherwise a grade 4 can be reported as 4 + 4 = 8. However, if the minor component is of a higher grade, it should be reported, even if it is <5% (eg, a tumor that is almost all Gleason grade 3 with only 1 or 2% grade 4 is a 3 + 4 = 7, not a 3 + 3 = 6) [PMID17674043, PMID18550106].

While the Gleason score is never a complete prognostic indicator, 5 prognostic groups can be discerned from the score: 4 and less, 5 and 6, 3 + 4 = 7 (7a), 4 + 3 = 7 (7b), and 8-10 [PMID18550106]. Because there is a prognostic breakpoint between a 6 and a 7, one should be particularly careful in the identification of a grade of 4 as either a major or minor grade.

A variety of proposals have been suggested in positive biopsies to report the amount of carcinoma, but there is no consensus on the need for indicating the amount of tumor or how to do so. Many pathologists report the number of positive biopsies, the percentage of biopsy length involved, or the cumulative linear extent of tumor on the biopsies. In view of the frequent multicentricity of prostate carcinoma and the inability to assess the remainder of the gland, it is not clear that attempting to quantitate the amount of carcinoma in the biopsy adds meaningful information. Indeed, for carcinomas of low Gleason score, there seems little correlation between prognosis and tumor volume as assessed on a *prostatectomy* [PMID17826492], so how can we expect useful information to come from an estimate of tumor volume on a *biopsy*? With all due respect to the very meritorious desire to be thorough, I believe the pathologist should focus on placing prostate biopsies in 1 of 3 categories: positive (at all, in any amount), negative, and indeterminate. For positive biopsies, the next step will depend on the patient's age, comorbidities, and preference, not on an estimate of tumor volume from the biopsy. To the extent that an estimate of tumor volume is important, it can be far more accurately estimated in a prostatectomy than in a biopsy. For those patients who are treated with another modality, a staging assessment by clinical and radiographic means and serial PSA determinations after treatment are more important prognostic indicators than an estimate of tumor volume.

True perineural invasion requires immediate proximity of tumor and nerve fibers in a nearly circumferential manner i37.12. Anything less may be simple proximity of tumor and nerve. Historically, some have regarded perineural invasion as invasion of lymphatic vessels that accompany nerves, while others have regarded it simply as spread of tumor along a plane of least resistance. Neither of these viewpoints has been proven, and there is now evidence that perineural invasion is a distinct and true invasion of the perineurium [PMID19484787]. Benign glands may rarely appear to invade the perineural space.

True perineural invasion, if unequivocally demonstrated, is a compelling point for a malignant diagnosis, but its significance as an independent prognostic factor is unclear and hotly debated. Because high Gleason score, positive resection margins, and perineural invasion tend to be found together, it is very difficult to study perineural invasion as an independent variable. While perineural invasion is a prognostic indicator in many types of cancer [PMID19484787], definitive evidence that perineural invasion is an independent prognostic factor in the prostate has not been forthcoming [PMID18500264].

There are several variants of prostatic adenocarcinoma. In the foamy (or xanthomatous) cell variant, the nuclear features are subtle. In addition to the abundant foamy cytoplasm, the imperatives in the diagnosis are infiltration and certainty that the cells are epithelial and not macrophages, using immunohistochemical stains if needed [PMID11342773]. The rare mucinous carcinoma, with abundant mucinous cytoplasm [PMID15072909], must be distinguished from 2 benign mucinous entities—mucinous metaplasia and sampling of bulbourethral glands (commonly called Cowper glands)—by nuclear appearance and presence or absence of infiltration.

The basal cell carcinoma of the prostate has nuclei with minimal cytoplasm and a basaloid appearance. There are often areas that resemble an adenoid cystic carcinoma, and there may be overlap between these entities [PMID17460452].

In contrast to the usual acinar adenocarcinoma, prostatic ductal adenocarcinoma generally has tall columnar cells with stratification, often with a papillary architecture i37.13. Prostatic ductal adenocarcinoma may resemble carcinoma of the endometrium or an endometrioid carcinoma of the ovary (hence, its former designation of prostatic endometrioid adenocarcinoma). It may also have a cribriform architecture that is difficult to distinguish from cribriforming hyperplasia or cribriforming high-grade PIN on biopsy. Attention to nuclear detail is necessary for differentiation from a cribriforming hyperplasia. The differentiation of prostatic duct adenocarcinoma from high-grade PIN depends on the demonstration of infiltration and is discussed in the section on PIN. Ductal carcinomas are often more aggressive than the more common acinar carcinomas [PMID19996627].

Mimics of Prostatic Adenocarcinoma

A number of entities may mimic acinar prostatic adenocarcinoma, including glandular hyperplasia, atrophy, basal cell hyperplasia, adenosis, seminal vesicle tissue, nephrogenic adenoma, and inflammatory conditions [PMID14976539, PMID9575372]. Of these, glandular hyperplasia and atrophy are the most common [PMID15958851]. I do not recommend the specific diagnosis of glandular hyperplasia on a biopsy because the localized focus of hyperplasia on a biopsy may not be representative of the gland as a whole, and a specific benign diagnosis may impart an unwarranted reassurance regarding a clinical finding or an elevated PSA, but the features of glandular hyperplasia on a biopsy must be recognized to avoid a misdiagnosis of carcinoma. Hyperplasia can be alarming because increased glandular density is a nearly universal feature of prostatic adenocarcinoma. However, in glandular hyperplasia, serial levels will never reveal infiltration and close study of the nuclei will show that they are not enlarged i37.14. As is always the case in pathology, the diagnosis of malignancy should not be made on a single criterion. If the glandular density is subtracted in the mind's eye, there are no features to suggest carcinoma.

Atrophy occurs when the prostatic epithelial cells have diminished cytoplasm. Although the nuclei are unchanged, the high nucleus to cytoplasmic ratio may lead to an initial perception of nuclear enlargement. The lobular pattern is maintained, but may be slightly less distinct in atrophy i37.15a. Focusing on the nuclei i37.15b, and not the nucleus-to-cytoplasmic ratio, will prevent an overdiagnosis.

In basal cell hyperplasia, there are multiple layers of basal cells instead of the usual subtle, single layer. Basal cell hyperplasia is distinguished from carcinoma by an absence of infiltration and by acini that are solid, or nearly so i37.16, whereas a single layer of cells and a well defined lumen are the rule in adenocarcinoma [PMID15948114]. Basal cell hyperplasia may have occasional nucleoli, but the nuclei are generally bland. Immunohistochemical stains, as described subsequently, may help.

Adenosis (also called atypical adenomatous hyperplasia) is a mimic of carcinoma that is characterized by closely spaced, but well circumscribed glands i37.17. Immunohistochemical stains are often needed, but there are a few clues to the presence of adenosis on H&E. Adenosis has evenly spaced glands, whereas the glands in low-grade carcinoma, even if not overtly infiltrative, are slightly unevenly spaced. In adenosis, the lobule is crowded, but still orderly. Glands that are angulated are more common in low-grade carcinoma than in adenosis. In adenosis, there is usually a gradual transition between the problematic focus and obviously benign glands, whereas the glands of low-grade carcinoma tend to be sharply and suddenly different from surrounding glands. Adenosis may have modest nuclear enlargement and small nucleoli, but should not have generalized large nucleoli. Intraluminal crystalloids (rare in benign glands) and basophilic cytoplasm favor malignancy [PMID7520673].

Seminal vesicle tissue may occasionally be captured in a prostate biopsy, in which case the closely-spaced glands i37.18a and hyperchromatic nuclei may be alarming. The cytoplasmic lipofuscin pigment that is characteristic of this tissue is helpful in preventing a misdiagnosis of prostatic carcinoma, but is neither sensitive nor specific. Seminal vesicle cells have hyperchromatic nuclei with dense chromatin and minimal nucleoli i37.18b, in contrast to the open chromatin and prominent nucleolus of prostatic carcinoma cells. In difficult cases, immunohistochemistry may help. Seminal vesicle tissue is generally negative for PSA and prostatic acid phosphatase. High molecular weight keratin stains seminal vesicle epithelium but not prostatic epithelium itself (only the basal layer of benign prostatic glands). In addition, cytokeratin 7 stains most seminal vesicle tissue but very rarely stains prostatic tissue [PMID10658909]. Also, MUC6 stains seminal vesicle epithelium but not benign or malignant prostate epithelium [PMID12657938].

The nephrogenic adenoma can also occur in the prostatic urethra and can simulate prostatic carcinoma, in which case the clues to the correct diagnosis are the lack of infiltration and the innocuous nuclei. Focal staining for PSA and PSAP may occur in nephrogenic adenoma, causing further confusion with prostatic carcinoma, but cytokeratin 7 is consistently positive in this benign mimic [PMID11395559]. In addition, PAX2, a renal transcription factor, stains nephrogenic adenomas in the prostate in a nuclear pattern and does not stain prostatic carcinomas [PMID16400326].

Immunohistochemistry of Prostatic Tissue

The one bright spot in the frustrating matter of early detection of prostatic adenocarcinoma is the excellent immunohistochemical panel that can usually distinguish carcinoma from benign lesions. The prostate is nearly unique in that there are good immunohistochemical stains that are characteristic of benign tissue and a stain that is characteristic of malignancy. While the latter stain, α-methylacyl-coA racemase (αMACR; also called p504S) is not completely sensitive or specific for carcinoma, it is closer to a "cancer antigen" than almost any other situation the pathologist is likely to encounter. We therefore have a 2-pronged, mirror-image approach to the immunohistochemical evaluation of problematic foci in prostate tissue.

In the first use of immunohistochemistry, the underlying principle is the identification of the basal epithelial layer that benign glands invariably possess to some extent and which is absent in prostatic carcinoma. High molecular weight keratin (called CK903 or 34βE12) and p63 (a nuclear stain) are good markers for prostate basal cells [PMID12218572]. Cytokeratins 5 and 6 (a single stain containing both keratins) are equally good for this purpose [PMID14502799, PMID12121235, PMID18788849]. The presence of any of these markers is strong evidence for the presence of a basal layer and should prompt a conservative diagnosis.

ISBN 978-089189-5886

In the second use of immunohistochemistry, p504S is a racemase enzyme (ie, interchanges D and L forms of a molecule) that preferentially stains the cytoplasm of cells of prostatic carcinoma or high-grade PIN. p504S has been found to stain all prostatic carcinomas strongly, while staining only a small minority of cases of adenosis, and these only focally and weakly [PMID11684956, PMID12218573]. In practice, p504S, in the right H&E context, is a strong point for a focus of invasive carcinoma or high-grade PIN.

Immunohistochemistry is especially helpful in clarifying cases in which the differential diagnosis is between adenosis and low-grade carcinoma. Adenosis retains the basal layer of epithelium, as demonstrated by staining for either high molecular weight keratin CK903 or low molecular weight keratins 5 and 6, while carcinoma does not. Carcinoma and intraductal neoplasia almost always stain for p504S, while adenosis rarely does [PMID12131160].

A convenient and useful 2-color double stain can be done on 1 section. Cytokeratins 5 and 6, highlighting the basal cells that are characteristic of benign glands are 1 color, while p504S, preferentially expressed by high-grade PIN and invasive carcinoma, is a second color **i37.19** [PMID16512601, PMID19605815]. This technique is especially valuable since many problematic foci on needle biopsy are very small and not amenable to multiple sections.

Dual-approach immunohistochemistry should resolve most cases of carcinoma vs a benign mimic, with 2 caveats. First, high-grade PIN is routinely positive for p504S, so positivity for this stain does not necessarily imply invasion. Second, not every gland in a benign mimic necessarily has a demonstrable basal layer because it is discontinuous and may not be present in that section. Occasional benign glands may fail to stain for basal cells.

Immunohistochemical staining for basement membrane (collagen type 4 and laminin) is unlikely to be contributory in prostate biopsies. While benign prostatic glands invariably make a well defined basement membrane, and the capacity to do is progressively lost in prostatic carcinoma, about 2/3 of well differentiated carcinomas will continue to express basement membrane and about 15% of Gleason grade 4 carcinoma will do so [PMID2657718].

Immunohistochemistry has elucidated an unusual lesion called sclerosing adenosis. The relationship of sclerosing adenosis to ordinary adenosis is unclear. Like ordinary adenosis, sclerosing adenosis is circumscribed, with generally bland nuclei, but the stroma is more cellular and spindled **i37.20**. An immunohistochemical feature of prostatic sclerosing adenosis, apparently unique to this lesion, is that the basal cells, in addition to their normal staining for cytokeratin 903 or low molecular weight keratins 5 and 6, also stain for S-100 and actin [PMID1711794, PMID1373581, PMID1720930]. If a focus of crowded glands demonstrates a basal layer that stains for S-100 and actin, it is likely sclerosing adenosis.

Problematic foci in a prostate biopsy that cannot be resolved with immunohistochemistry have been called atypical hyperplasia, but to avoid confusion with adenosis, a clearly benign process that is also called atypical hyperplasia or atypical adenomatous hyperplasia, a better designation is atypical small acinar proliferation (ASAP) **i37.21** [PMID10631713]. When a focus is designated as ASAP, a comment should be made that this is an equivocal biopsy and that the patient is at increased risk for the concurrent presence of carcinoma that has not been clearly captured by the biopsy and also at increased risk for the future development of carcinoma if he does not have it now. The urologist may repeat the biopsy in these cases, but it must be understood that while a positive repeat biopsy clarifies the situation, a negative repeat biopsy is not reassuring and makes no contribution to patient care.

Prostatic Intraductal Neoplasia (PIN)

As is the case in many other sites, attempts have been made to identify an early histologic manifestation of adenocarcinoma. These attempts have resulted in a general consensus that invasive carcinoma begins in the gland as PIN. Low-grade PIN has minimal nuclear enlargement or slight stratification. The cytoplasm may be basophilic and nucleoli are inconspicuous [PMID19048290]. Obvious nuclear enlargement and prominent nucleoli are the hallmark of high-grade PIN **i37.22a**. In high-grade PIN, the individual cells are indistinguishable from those in an invasive carcinoma and it is only the lack of infiltration **i37.22b** that precludes the latter diagnosis. High-grade PIN usually appears as larger glands with micropapillations, but there is also a cribriform type. In the micropapillary type of high-grade PIN, the nuclei become less atypical towards the lumen [PMID19048290].

To my mind, low-grade PIN may be worth noting in a microscopic description of comment but should not be included in the final diagnosis because it has not been established that it significantly increases the likelihood of concurrent or future invasive carcinoma, and its mention in the final diagnosis may cause unnecessary concern and confusion to the clinician and patient. High-grade PIN, on the other hand, is associated with invasive carcinoma [PMID19048290], and its presence should be indicated in the final diagnosis. A comment similar to that used for cases of ASAP may be made.

High-grade PIN of any architectural type may simulate invasive carcinoma not only on H&E, but immunohistochemically as well, since the basal layer in high-grade PIN is usually attenuated and often lost altogether [PMID19048290], and it often expresses p504S [PMID15297968]. The distinction of high-grade PIN from invasive carcinoma is particularly difficult when there are large numbers of ducts with high-grade PIN. As in other body sites, invasion can be inferred from severe crowding, with little or no intervening stroma, or from confluence of glands. Necrosis also favors invasive carcinoma.

Small glands that look malignant but are adjacent to a focus of high-grade PIN can be either infiltrating carcinoma or tangentially sectioned portions of the gland with PIN. Because both high-grade PIN and invasive carcinoma can express p504S and may not have basal cells, immunohistochemistry is not helpful. In theory, a well defined basement membrane around the problematic glands suggests tangential sectioning of the gland with PIN, but this is not a well defined approach, and in practice, the most reliable course of action is to regard a large number of atypical small glands, especially at an appreciable distance from the high-grade PIN, as most consistent with infiltrating carcinoma, while a conservative interpretation is appropriate if there are a small number of atypical glands close to a focus of high-grade PIN.

Some observers recognize the existence of a frank intraductal carcinoma of the prostate, distinguished from high-grade PIN by the complete filling of the lumen with markedly pleomorphic cells, while other regard this as an expression of high-grade PIN [PMID19048290]. In either case, this finding in a biopsy is usually associated with invasive carcinoma in a prostatectomy [PMID16980940].

The Prostate Biopsy after Treatment for Carcinoma

A variety of nonsurgical treatments are now available for prostate carcinoma, including external radiation, localized radiation therapy (brachytherapy) with radioactive iodine seeds, cryotherapy, and androgen-deprivation therapy [PMID15595340]. The newest modality of radiation therapy is a form of external beam therapy called intensity-modulated radiation therapy (IMRT). In IMRT, the linear accelerator(s) is controlled by a computer so that the dose varies and conforms more precisely to the 3-dimensional shape of the tumor [PMID20426851, PMID20535952]. IMRT not only allows every portion of the tumor to be targeted, it also permits greater avoidance of adjacent normal tissue. In IMRT, 3-dimensional CT images are used to plan treatment. Often, 2 or more beams are used in combination. At this writing, IMRT is used primarily in cancers of the prostate, head and neck, and central nervous system, though its use is growing other types of cancer.

The pathologist is occasionally called upon to determine if there is residual/recurrent carcinoma in a prostate biopsy after treatment for a previously diagnosed carcinoma has been given [PMID17128417]. The key to distinguishing between radiation therapy effects and recurrent/residual carcinoma is to insist on the same criteria in the diagnosis of carcinoma that were used in the initial diagnosis—modest nuclear enlargement, prominent nucleoli, and infiltration. A common mistake in these situations is to interpret very pleomorphic cells as carcinoma. After radiation therapy, benign cells may have striking nuclear pleomorphism i37.23. Indeed, because prostate carcinoma does not normally display significant nuclear pleomorphism, such a finding actually suggests radiation effect more than carcinoma.

Because radiation treatment will alter the appearance of nuclei but not the architectural pattern, the demonstration of invasion is indispensable in the diagnosis of carcinoma in biopsies from prostate glands that have been irradiated. If recurrent/residual carcinoma is identified, one can comment on the degree of radiation damage the neoplastic glands have sustained, as carcinoma with severe radiation change presumably lacks the metastatic potential. Viable (ie, with metastatic potential) residual prostate cancer should look essentially the same as before treatment.

In questionable cases, a characteristic of radiation change is an uneven distribution of atypia, with abnormal nuclei in a gland adjacent to normal nuclei. In viable carcinoma, one would expect all cells in a gland to show malignant features. Intraluminal crystalloids and amphophilic cytoplasm suggest carcinoma [PMID10524518]. Immunohistochemical stains may help, but if they are employed in cases that have received radiation therapy, it is doubly important to ensure that the H&E appearance is fully supportive of the diagnosis because at this writing, there have not been definitive studies on the effects, if any, of radiation therapy on antigenicity of prostatic tissue.

Androgen-deprivation therapy avoids the frank pleomorphism of radiation change but may cause the nuclei in malignant cells to become smaller, with more condensed chromatin and less conspicuous nucleoli [PMID16097140]. This can mask the characteristic nuclear changes of prostate carcinoma, so an infiltrative pattern must be carefully sought, and close study will usually disclose occasional nuclei that maintain the characteristic chromatin pattern and nucleoli of carcinoma. Cryotherapy is also available, but at this writing, the post-treatment morphology has not yet been definitively described.

A final comment on the prostate biopsy concerns the difficult situation that arises when a minute focus of carcinoma is identified in a clinical situation in which its significance is questionable. What should be done, for example, if a 70-year-old man with a PSA of 4.5 has a biopsy that discloses a minute focus of Gleason 3 + 3 = 6 carcinoma? This matter has not yet been completely clarified, and no uniform consensus has emerged, but many cancers detected by PSA screening are clinically insignificant, (ie, the patient would not have been affected if the carcinoma had been undetected) [PMID12096083], and given the indolence of most prostate carcinomas, some feel that one can adopt a "wait and see" attitude in at least some of these cases [PMID15954083].

The Radical Prostatectomy

Initially, it was thought that if pelvic node dissection preceded the prostatectomy and positive pelvic nodes were identified on frozen section, the procedure was pointless and was terminated. However, there is now evidence that positive pelvic lymph nodes should not necessarily preclude the completion of the procedure [PMID12752279, PMID10976815]. Frozen section of pelvic nodes is less sensitive in predicting their positivity than a normogram constructed from already available date such as Gleason score and PSA [PMID11992847]. Moreover, patients with small amounts of metastatic disease in pelvic nodes do reasonably well [PMID19297079]. Indeed, for serum PSA <10 and a biopsy Gleason score of 7 or less, pelvic lymph nodes may not need to be removed at all [PMID10720855].

In most situations, unless the Gleason score is 8 or higher, positive lymph nodes, while indicating a higher probability of eventual disease progression, are associated with only slightly diminished long-term survival. Some therefore believe that a radical prostatectomy should not be aborted upon the frozen section finding of positive lymph nodes unless the biopsy had a Gleason score of 8 or higher. If this line of thought is verified, it would seem to follow that there is no need to obtain a frozen section of lymph nodes if the biopsy Gleason score was 7 or less, because those patients will still benefit from radical prostatectomy even if positive lymph nodes are found on frozen section.

The gross examination of a prostatectomy is well described in a number of grossing manual and has been reviewed [PMID9037309]. The first step in the gross examination of a prostatectomy specimen is to ensure proper orientation. Discerning "up" from "down" is not always a trivial matter. Classical teaching is that the seminal vesicles are on the posterior surface, but after surgery, they may be partially detached from the prostate gland and thus ineffective in providing orientation. Even if the seminal vesicles are not disturbed, there may be sufficient distortion of the gland that they are no longer attached to a well defined posterior surface. In my experience, the surgeon should be asked to either place a Foley catheter (the upper portion of which indicates the superior surface) or denote the superior surface by a suture.

After orientation the entire gland should be inked (some prefer different colors for the left and right lobes). The important margins are the bladder neck (the proximal margin), the apex (the distal margin), the base, the posterior surface, and, to a lesser extent, the radial (so-called capsular) margins. It might be desirable to shave the bladder neck, apical, posterior, and basal surfaces prior to sectioning of the gland, then section these shaved fragments at right angles, so that there will be multiple slices from each of these 4 margins, and on each slice, the ink represents the precise location of the surgeon's cuts. The radial margins can be captured as part of the sections taken of the parenchyma and need not be separately obtained prior to sectioning.

After these margins are taken, the gland can be sectioned. The gross examination of the prostate is handicapped by the fact that carcinoma is often inconspicuous even to the experienced observer. While classical teaching is that prostate carcinomas are yellow, there are many foci that are not, and many yellow areas are benign. In assessing a prostatectomy specimen or cross sections thereof, it is helpful to look not only for a yellow color, but also for asymmetry or nodularity.

There is considerable confusion regarding the radial (so-called capsular) margins of the prostate. The capsule of the prostate is not well defined. The glandular parenchyma is covered by a thin layer of smooth muscle and collagen. The smooth muscle surrounding the glands in the parenchyma merges imperceptively with the smooth muscle of the apparent capsule, and the glands fade gradually into the covering, without a sharp line of demarcation, and come close to the external surface of the covering [Sternberg ISBN088167-6217]. Because the prostate does not have a well defined capsule, and because benign glands penetrate into the thin fibromuscular covering, the term "capsular invasion" is relatively meaningless. The 2 questions to ask are, first, "Does the tumor extend outside the prostate (extraprostatic extension)?" and, second, "Is the resection margin negative?" The first question is addressed by seeing neoplastic glands beyond the thin covering of the prostate. This is not always easy, however, because the covering is subtle and may be rendered even less clear by any fibrosis engendered by the tumor. It is helpful to follow the contour of the peripheral glandular tissue at low power and look for an alteration.

At most sites around the prostate, the surgeon can only resect 1-2 mm of adjacent soft tissue. The pathologist simply cannot expect to see the wide and clear margins that are commonly found in other body sites. This is rarely a problem, however, because while a positive margin correlates with PSA recurrence, its presence does not guarantee a biochemical recurrence [PMID18068455], and the significance of a focally positive margin as an independent prognostic indicator is unclear. A positive margin adds little long-term prognostic information to that already obtained from Gleason score and serum PSA [PMID16189146], and in fact, there appears to be no correlation between the amount of tumor found at a resection margin and subsequent PSA levels [PMID17490720]. A positive bladder neck margin has been particularly well studied and has not been shown to be an independent indicator [PMID19914651]. Radial margins of 1 mm can be reported as negative [PMID20729812]. A margin should be reported as close or equivocal only if there is nothing more than a thin fibrous membrane separating the carcinoma from the margin. Anything more than this can be reported as negative.

The neurovascular bundle runs on the posterolateral margin. This is the only place the surgeon can exercise significant discretion and take more tissue, and he can do so here only at the cost of further compromising postoperative erectile function [PMID20219562]. In most cases when this margin is positive, which would initially suggest that the neurovascular bundle should have been resected, there will be other positive margins as well [PMID10197851], in sites where the surgeon could not have taken more tissue. This suggests that if the surgeon had taken the neurovascular bundle, he still would not have removed all of the carcinoma. This is one rationale for conservative surgery—it is unlikely that an aggressive approach toward the neurovascular bundle will result in the clearance of what had been the only positive margin.

Although not a margin, the seminal vesicles should be sampled, as extension of carcinoma into them increases the stage and is a significant finding.

As mentioned in the discussion of the prostate biopsy, there is no consensus as whether or not perineural invasion is an independent prognostic indicator. Tumor volume is not a prognostic indicator unless the Gleason score is 7 or greater [PMID17826492], and in most cases, volume cannot and need not be precisely calculated, though a comment should be made as to whether the amount of tumor is minimal, moderate, or extensive.

The Transurethral Resection

TURP specimens can be quite large (up to 100 g), with a large number of fragment, and the pathologist faces a decision as to which fragments and how much tissue to submit initially, and whether or not to submit more if a small focus of carcinoma is uncovered. No consensus has emerged on these matters, but in general, the submission of fragments with yellow areas is reasonable. Because a diagnosis of stage T1a carcinoma in younger patients may result in therapy or an additional diagnostic procedure, the submission of a larger number of fragments in that age group is reasonable, while a smaller number may be submitted in older patients, for whom a less aggressive approach will be followed if carcinoma is found. A "more is better" approach to all patients may result in the "overdiagnosis" problem, alluded to earlier, in older patients.

Likewise, there are differences in the reporting of carcinoma that is found in TURP specimens. Some report the percentage of fragments that are positive, while others attempt an estimate of the total volume of tissue that is replaced by carcinoma and still others do both. As is the case for biopsies, the central question in the assessment of TURP specimens is the presence or absence of tumor. The American Joint Committee on Cancer Staging for prostate carcinoma assigns a stage of

T1a if <5% of the total volume in a TURP specimen is tumor and a T1b if >5% is tumor [Greene ISBN 0-387-95271-3], so an estimate on tumor volume may be needed for staging, but as is the case for biopsies, the immediate clinical benefit of an estimate of tumor volume is unclear, since the status of the remainder of the gland cannot be known.

Prostatic Carcinoma in Metastatic Sites

As is the case for any tumor, prostatic adenocarcinoma can be difficult to identify in a metastatic site, especially if it has undergone dedifferentiation. PSA is the best immunohistochemical stain if prostate carcinoma is suspected, but poorly differentiated or dedifferentiated carcinomas may be negative. Although only 5-10% of prostatic carcinomas are completely negative for PSA, 25% may have only focal positivity and therefore may appear negative in limited material. p504S appears to be a promising complement to PSA in possible metastatic prostate carcinoma, as does the enzyme p501S [PMID17721190].

Prevention of Prostate Carcinoma

Before we leave the huge area of prostate carcinoma, a final topic of consideration is the use of hormone therapy to lessen the chances of developing it. Testosterone is converted in some peripheral tissues, including the prostate, into the more potent form, 5α-dihydrotestosterone, by the enzyme Type 2 5α-reductase [PMID11469812]. Finasteride, originally developed to slow alopecia in men, inhibits this enzyme and was subsequently employed in benign prostatic hyperplasia. Evidence that it decreased the risk of developing carcinoma came in 2008 [PMID19249063]. Although initial reports suggested that finasteride use caused an increased number of higher-grade prostate carcinomas, a subsequent study indicated otherwise [PMID19138953]. Side effects of 5α-reductase inhibitors include erectile dysfunction, loss of libido, and gynecomastia, the last of which may persist even after cessation of the drug. If these drugs have any role in the prevention of prostate carcinoma, the dosage will also have to be addressed, as the initial studies employed relatively high doses (5 mg). At this writing, it is not clear what place, if any, these drugs will find in prevention of prostate carcinoma.

Core Points for the Prostate

- Early detection of prostate carcinoma: PSA is insensitive and nonspecific.
  - Attempts to modify PSA (rate of rise, ratio to gland size, or different normal ranges for different ages and ethnic groups), have been disappointing.
  - Alternative serum markers are promising, but not yet helpful.
- Prostatic carcinoma cells: moderately enlarged nucleus, often with a prominent nucleolus, and a moderate amount of amphophilic cytoplasm, but
  - The sine qua non of carcinoma on a biopsy is infiltration.
- Mimics of carcinoma: glandular hyperplasia, atrophy, basal cell hyperplasia, adenosis, seminal vesicle tissue, nephrogenic adenoma, transitional cell metaplasia, and inflammatory conditions.
- Basal layer retained in benign glands and lost in carcinoma or high-grade prostatic intraductal neoplasia (PIN).
  - IHC for p63 or for cytokeratins 5 & 6 highlight this layer.
  - p504S: associated with high-grade PIN or invasive carcinoma.
- Gleason system: architectural.
  - Usually, two most common Gleason grades are added to generate the Gleason score.
  - But many advocate the inclusion of a third pattern if it is of higher grade than the two predominant patterns.
- Estimations of quantity and identification of perineural invasion in biopsies: unclear importance.
- Prostatic ductal adenocarcinoma: larger ducts.
  - Resembles endometrial carcinoma.
- Low-grade PIN: slight nuclear enlargement with indistinct nucleoli.
- High-grade PIN: cells individually identical to those of invasive carcinoma.
  - But no infiltration.
- Post-treatment biopsies: cardinal criterion of residual/recurrent cancer is infiltration.
  - Benign, irradiated glands may have striking atypia.
- Prostatectomy specimens: important margins are the bladder neck, the apex, the posterior surface, and the base.
  - So-called capsular or radial margins: determine if tumor extends outside of the prostate and if the resection margin is positive or negative.
  - Widely negative margins are not possible, significance of minute foci of marginal positivity is unclear.
- Metastatic prostate carcinoma: PSA is good, but
  - Poorly differentiated prostate carcinoma may be negative, especially in small foci.
- Risk reduction: inhibiting the 5α-reductase enzyme necessary for testosterone synthesis, but
  - Utility of this is unclear, and side effects include erectile dysfunction, loss of libido, and gynecomastia, the last of which is sometimes permanent.

i37.1 Normal prostatic tissue with a well defined lobular pattern

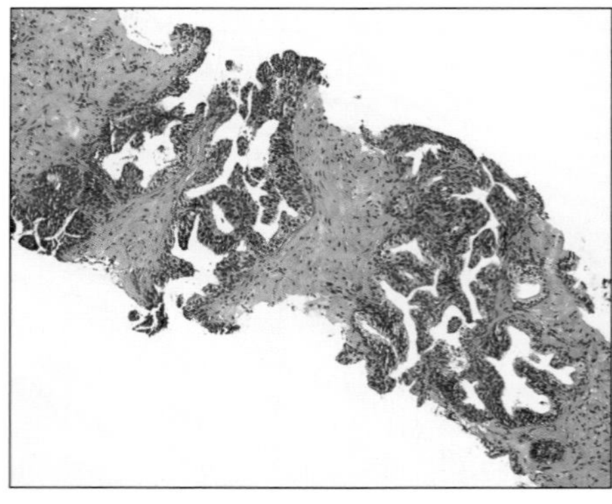

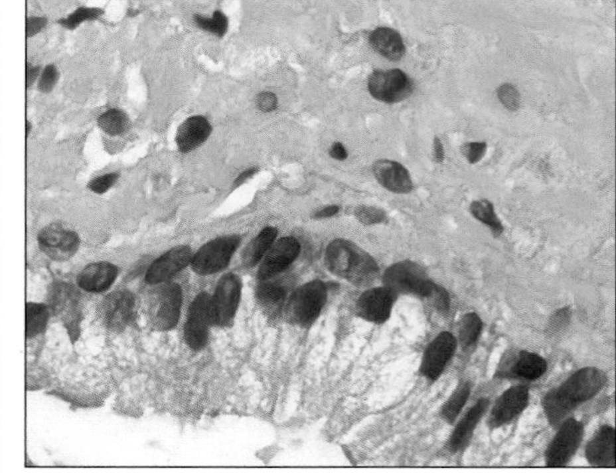

i37.2 A high-power view of the benign prostatic gland with a basal layer underneath the columnar epithelium

i37.3 So-called transitional metaplasia of the prostate

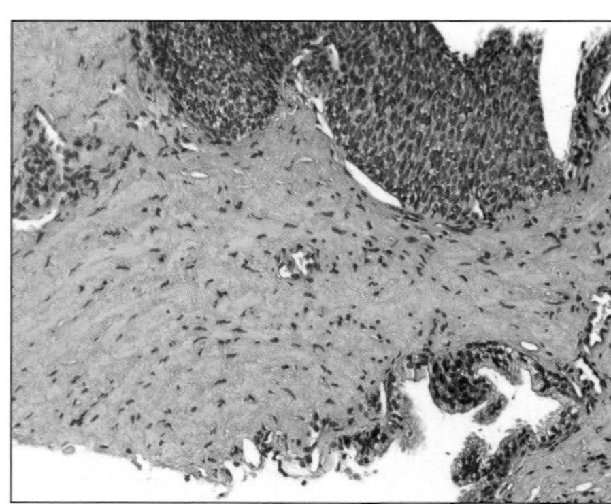

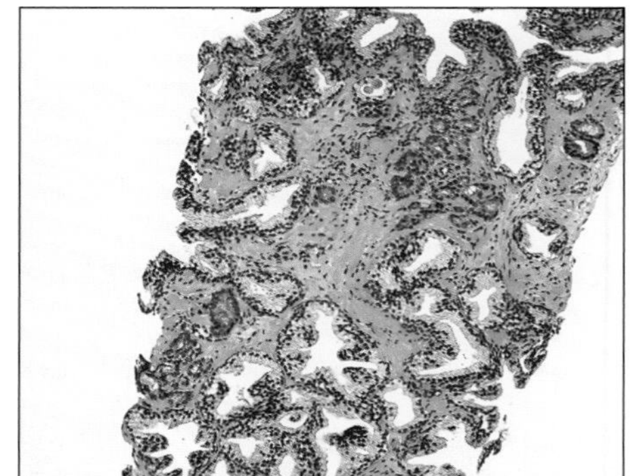

i37.4 Prostatic adenocarcinoma, evident as small glands infiltrating between the larger benign glands that constitute the lobules

i37.5 A higher-power view of prostatic adenocarcinoma in which neoplastic glands on the top are contrasted with the benign gland on the bottom. Note the slightly (but only slightly) larger nuclei, the generally small but distinct nucleoli in many of the cells, the smaller size of the glands, and the amphophilic cytoplasm in the neoplastic glands.

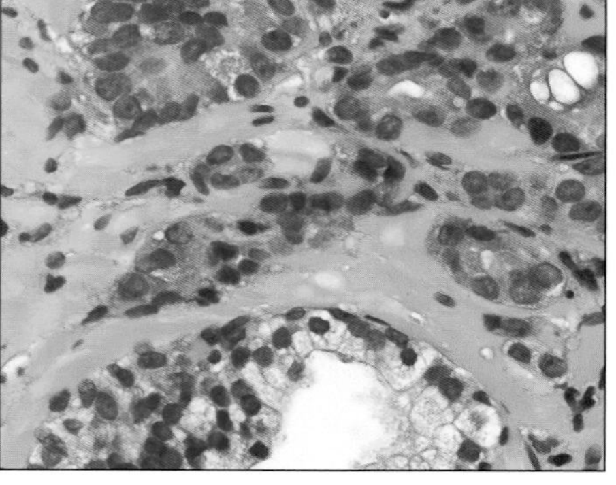

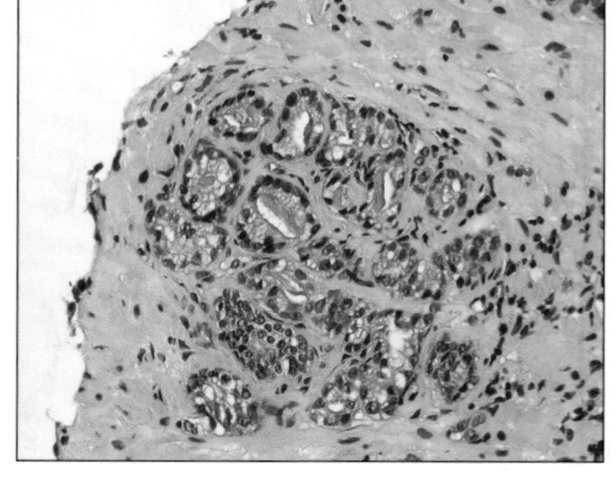

i37.6 A Gleason grade 2 prostatic adenocarcinoma. Note the lack of obvious infiltration and the general retention of a lobular appearance. Nuclei are slightly enlarged and small nucleoli are seen. Cytoplasm is amphophilic. The glands in the upper left portion may be benign. This diagnosis was verified with immunohistochemical stains.

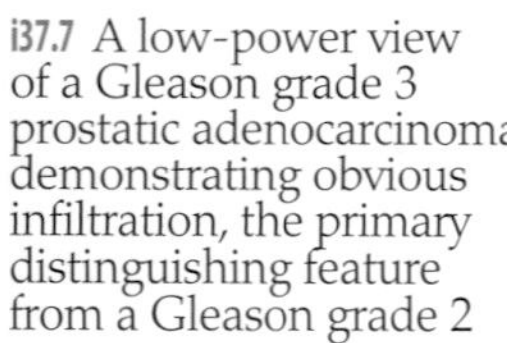

i37.7 A low-power view of a Gleason grade 3 prostatic adenocarcinoma demonstrating obvious infiltration, the primary distinguishing feature from a Gleason grade 2

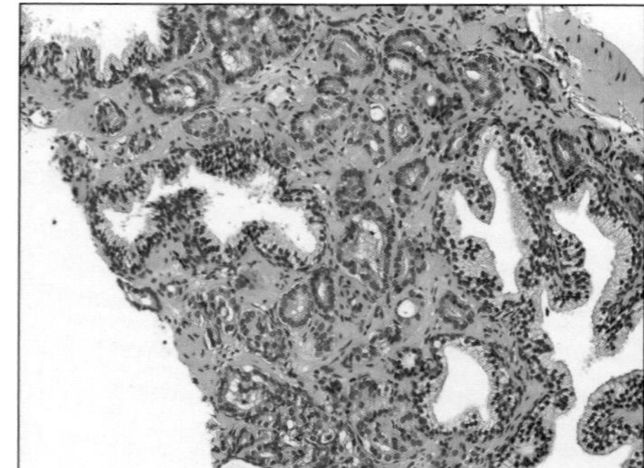

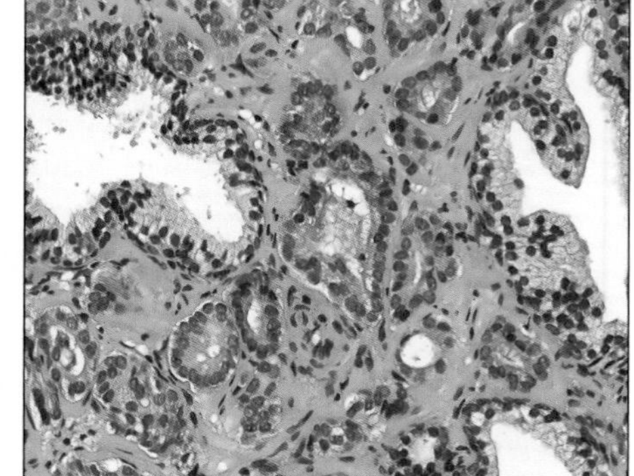

i37.8 A higher-power view of the same case as in i37.7. The gland in the center has departed from a round contour.

i37.9 A Gleason grade 4 carcinoma. Glandular differentiation is still readily apparent but the glands are confluent, without intervening stroma.

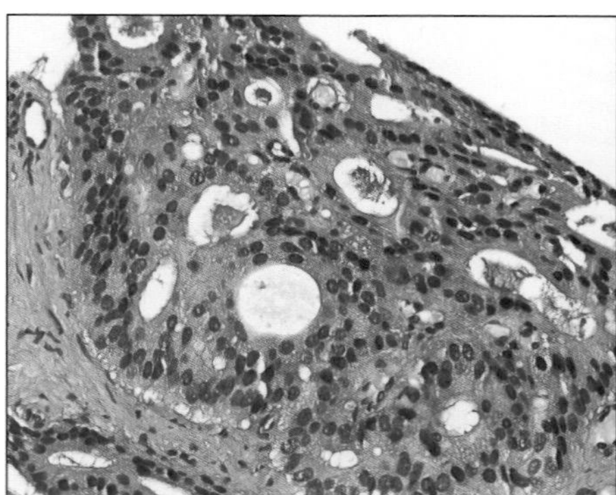

i37.10 A Gleason grade 5 prostatic adenocarcinoma in which gland formation is indistinct. Nucleoli may be slightly larger and found in a higher percentage of nuclei than in a lower-grade prostatic adenocarcinoma, but for the most part, the nuclei in this neoplasm are very similar to those in a lower grade prostatic adenocarcinoma.

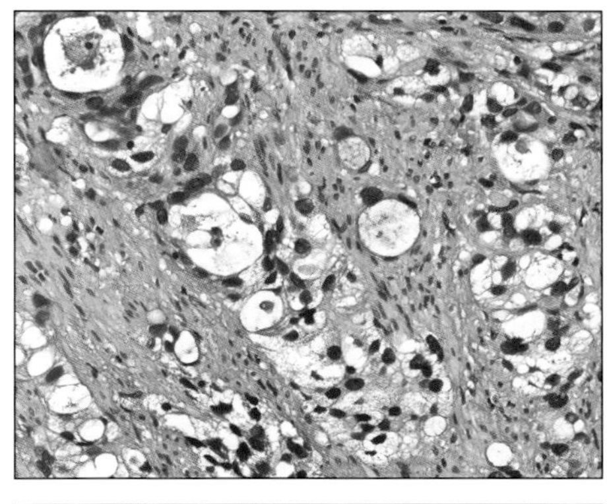

i37.11 Another view of a Gleason grade 5 carcinoma, with signet ring cells

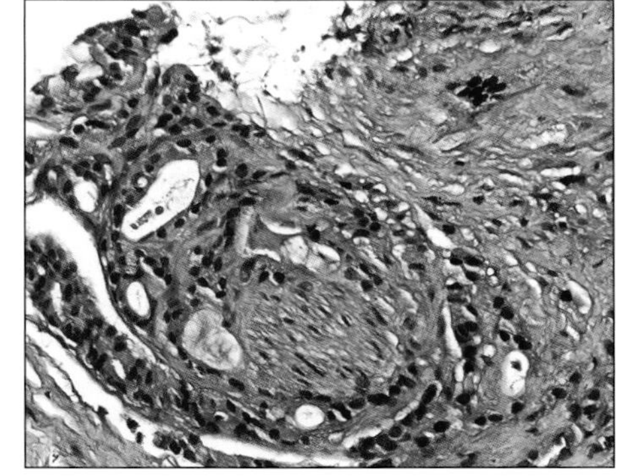

i37.12 Perineural invasion in a prostatic adenocarcinoma. Note that the neoplastic cells are immediately adjacent to the nerve and surround it essentially circumferentially.

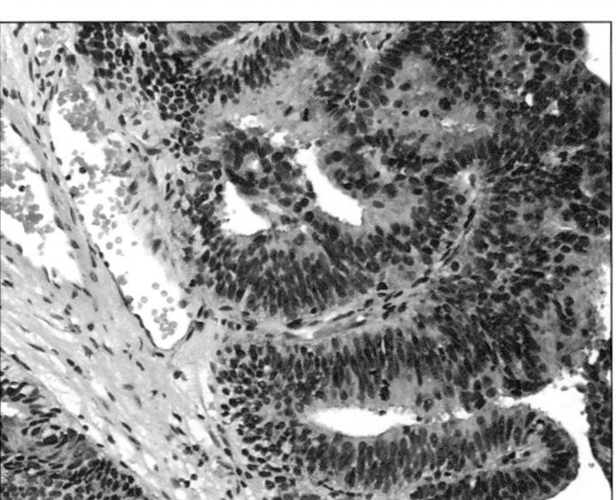

i37.13 Prostatic ductal adenocarcinoma, with tall columnar cells, stratification, and a papillary architecture

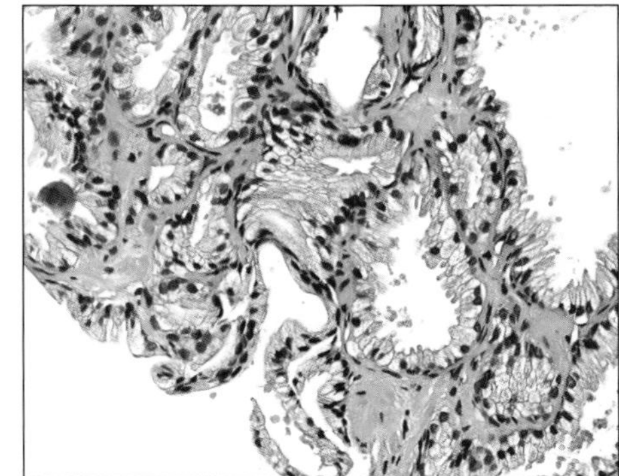

i37.14 Glandular hyperplasia in a prostate biopsy. The increase in the number of glands initially suggests infiltration, but a lobular pattern can be discerned and the individual cells are unremarkable.

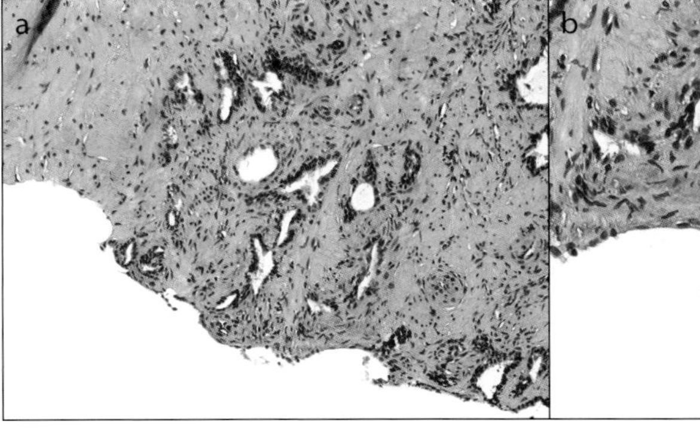

i37.15 **a** Atrophy in a prostate biopsy. The diminished amount of cytoplasm, resulting in a high nuclear to cytoplasmic ratio, is initially alarming. In addition, the lobular architecture may be less distinct in atrophy.

b A higher-power view of the same case as in i37.15a, illustrating that other than an increased nucleus-to-cytoplasmic ratio, the epithelial cells do not have the characteristics of prostatic adenocarcinoma.

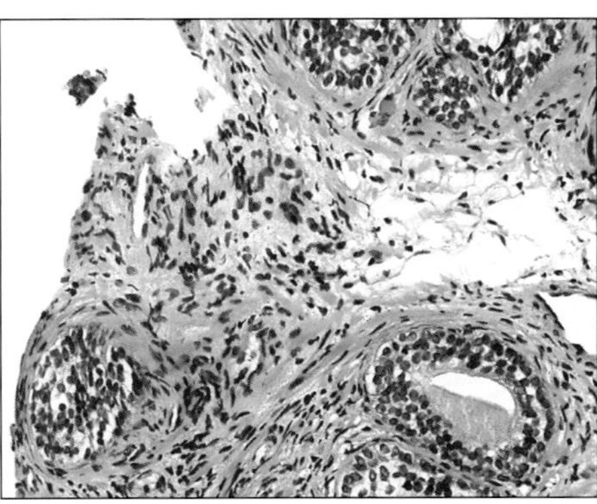

i37.16 Basal cell hyperplasia. The lumens of the glands on the left are completely filled while those of other glands are partially filled, but there is no infiltration and the individual cells are unremarkable. A single layer of cells and a well defined lumen are characteristic of carcinoma.

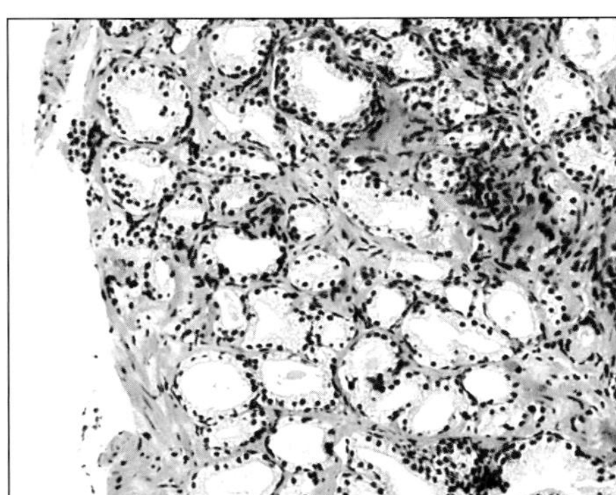

i37.17 So called adenosis of the prostate. The glands are small and closely spaced, simulating a low-grade adenocarcinoma. However, the individual cells have a normal appearance and the basal layer is demonstrable. Compare to i37.6.

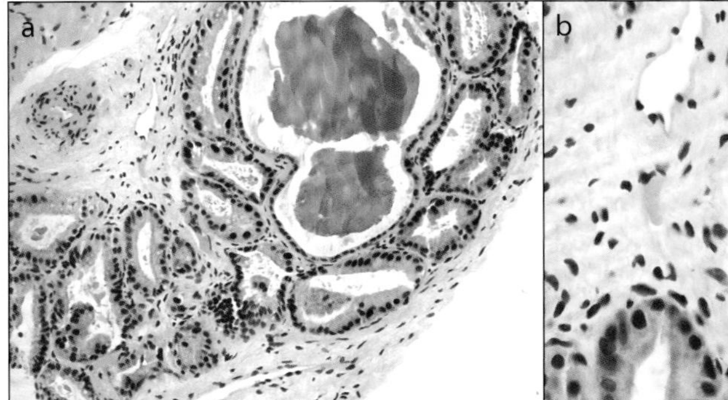

i37.18 **a** Seminal vesicle tissue. The closely spaced glands and hyperchromatic nuclei are alarming.

b A higher-power view of the same case as in i37.18a. Yellow-brown lipofuscin pigment is apparent, but more importantly, the nuclei, although very hyperchromatic, do not have the open chromatin and nucleoli that is characteristic of prostatic adenocarcinoma.

ISBN 978-089189-5886

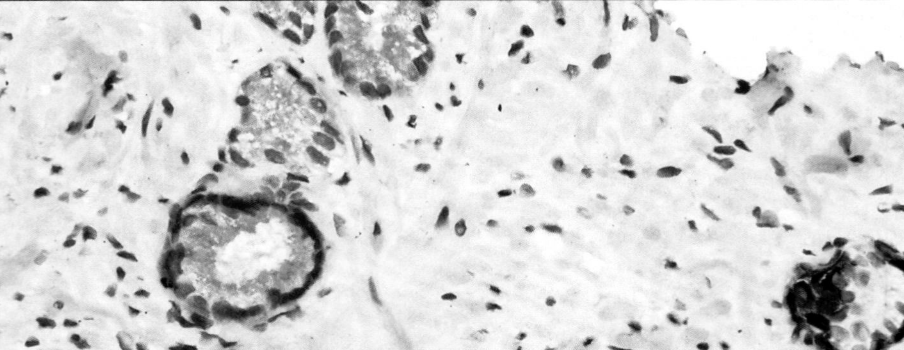

i37.19 Immunohistochemical identification of a subtle prostatic adenocarcinoma. This tissue is double stained for basal cells by high molecular weight cytokeratin, which appears brown, and for the p504S enzyme, which appears red. The gland on the right has a well defined basal layer and does not stain for p505S, indicating it is benign. The other glands lack a basal layer and also stain for p504S, indicating adenocarcinoma.

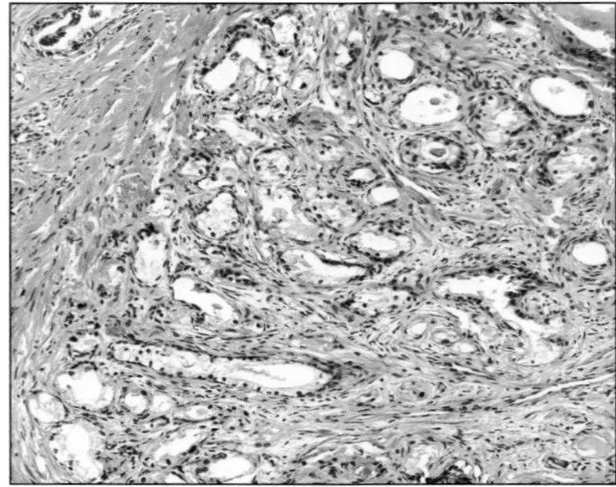

i37.20 So-called sclerosing adenosis of the prostate. The lesion is similar to adenosis i37.17 but the stroma is more cellular. The important points remain the same, that there is no infiltration and the individual cells do not have the characteristics of carcinoma.

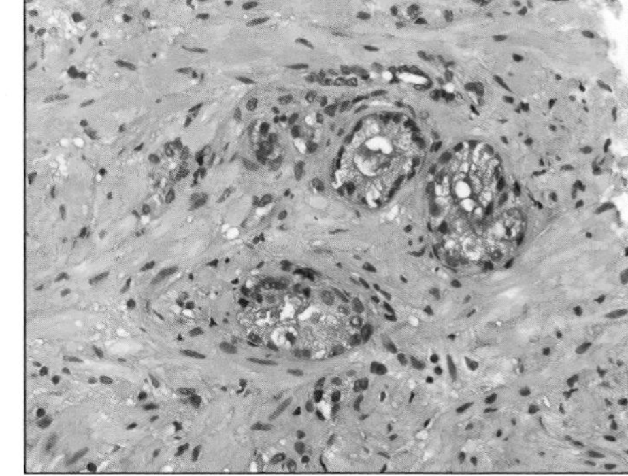

i37.21 A focus of atypical small acinar proliferation (ASAP)

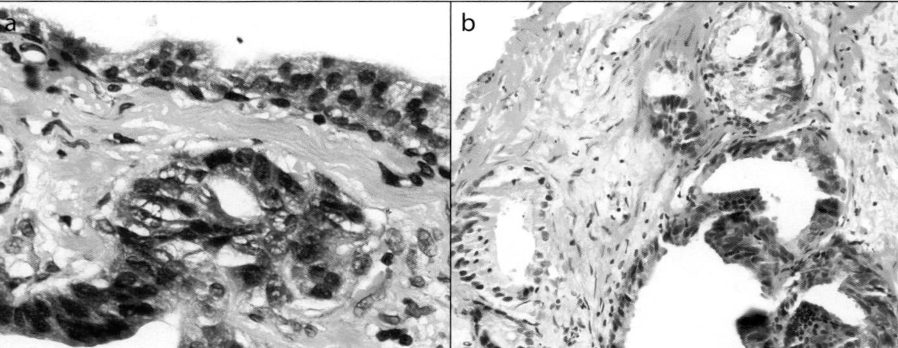

i37.22 **a** Low-grade prostatic intraductal neoplasia (PIN) is evident on top, with slight stratification of nuclei, but the individual nuclei are unremarkable. On the bottom, there is high-grade PIN with larger nuclei, an open chromatin pattern, and nucleoli. Note that the nuclei on the right are indistinguishable from those of an infiltrating carcinoma, while those of the low-grade PIN can be distinguished from those in invasive carcinoma. **b** Another example of high-grade PIN, with malignant-appearing nuclei, but no infiltration

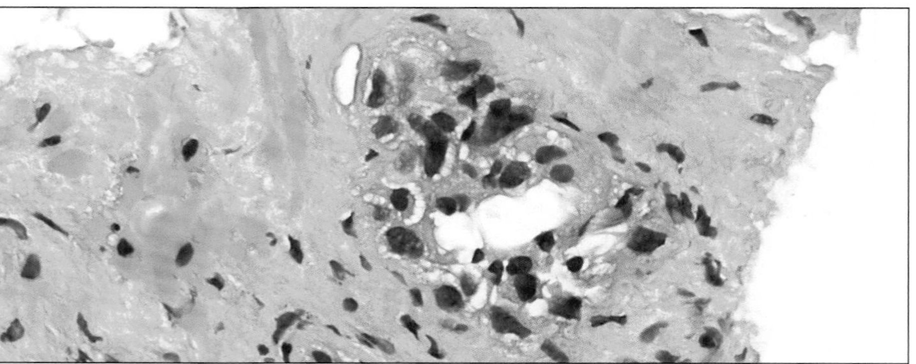

i37.23 A benign prostatic gland after radiation therapy. The nuclei are hyperchromatic and the amount of cytoplasm may be diminished, but there is no infiltration, the chromatin is coarse rather than open, and nucleoli are indistinct.

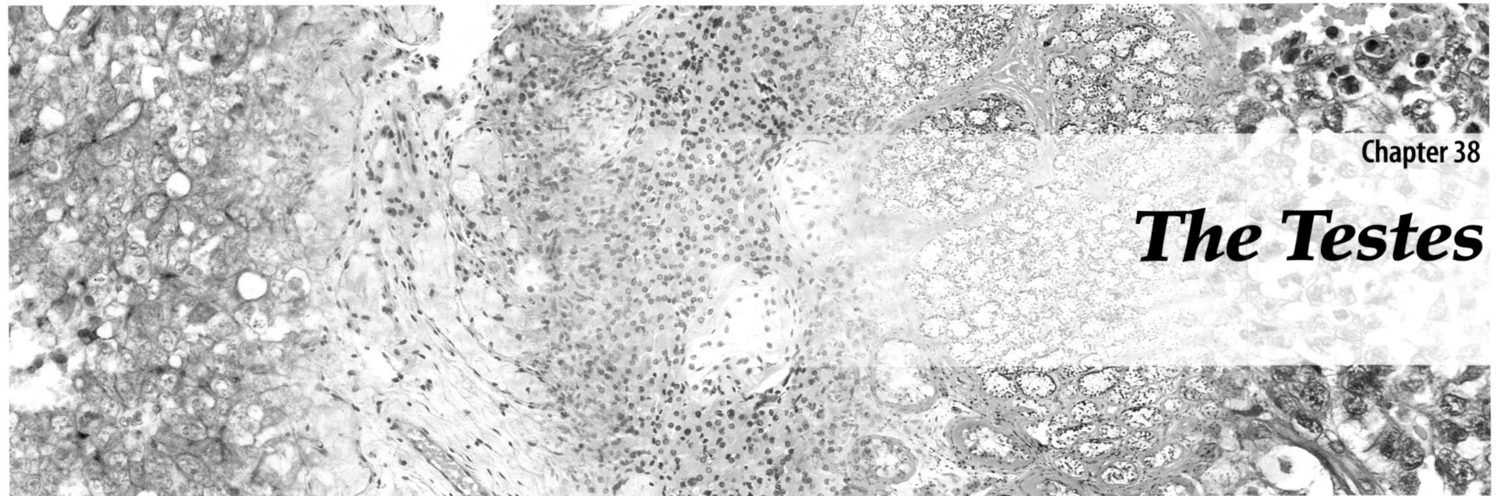

Normal Development and Structure of the Testis

The *SRY* (sex-determining region on the Y chromosome) gene on the short arm of the Y chromosome causes testicular development. The *SRY* gene product results in the development of Sertoli cells, which in turn, foster the development of both sperm and Leydig cells. Its presence, even in a 46,XX patient, will result in testes, and its absence, even in a 46,XY patient, will result in an absence of testes [PMID21062860]. A mutation or translocation of *SRY* that renders it inoperative is called sex reversal. Even with the presence of *SRY*, however, the downstream genes *SOX9* and *FGF9* must be properly activated for male development. The *WNT4* gene promotes ovarian differentiation if there is no intervention by *SRY*. Physical gender is determined by the net effect of these genes [PMID17666585].

As is the case for the female embryo, in the male embryo, a genital ridge forms and primordial sex germ cells migrate into it from the yolk sac to form the primary sex cords. Whereas the primary sex cords degenerate in the female embryo and are replaced by the secondary sex cords, in the male, the cortical region of the primary sex cords degenerate, but cells in the medullary region of the primary sex cords, responding to the *SRY* gene product and the products of genes activated by *SRY*, differentiate into Sertoli cells. Sertoli cells secrete anti-Mullerian hormone (also called Mullerian-inhibiting substance), which causes regression of Mullerian structures [Larsen ISBN978-0443065835]. The persistent Mullerian duct syndrome, which has a combination of male genitalia and a uterus, may be caused by either a defect in the gene for anti-Mullerian hormone or a defect in its receptor [Larsen ISBN978-0443065835].

By the 7th week, Sertoli cells begin to organize the testis cords, which will become the seminiferous tubules, thus beginning the development of the testis. About 2 weeks later, products from *SRY* and the genes it activates cause mesenchymal cells in the gonadal ridge to differentiate into Leydig cells, which make testosterone. Testosterone is required for the differentiation of the Wolffian (mesonephric) duct into the epididymis, vas deferens, and seminal vesicles, and also induces the development of the penis, scrotum, and prostate [Larsen ISBN978-0443065835]. In androgen insensitivity (testicular feminization), anti-Mullerian hormone secretion is normal and Mullerian structures have regressed, but there is an inability to respond to testosterone, either because of a mutation in the receptor or an impairment in the subsequent pathway [PMID19931639]. This precludes the development of male sexual structures, resulting in a phenotype that is externally female.

Spermatogonia are the primitive germ cells that have not yet entered meiosis (in contrast, female gametes begin meiosis while the individual is in utero). The primary spermatocytes have begun the first stage of meiosis and are therefore tetraploid. The secondary spermatocytes have completed the first stage of meiosis and are therefore diploid. Completion of the second stage of meiosis results in the spermatids, which then differentiate into mature sperm, largely through loss of cytoplasm [Larsen ISBN978-0443065835].

The contents of the seminiferous tubules are conveyed into the rete testis, and then into the efferent ducts. 8 to 15 efferent ducts coalesce to form the epididymis, which stores sperm and conveys them into the ejaculatory duct. The tunica albuginia is a fibrous capsule covering the testis. The tunica vaginalis is a looser tissue that covers the tunica albuginia.

Disorders of Testicular Development and Location

After birth, there are large numbers of Leydig cells in the testis, but these involute rapidly and are rare by about 4 months. The seminiferous tubules of prepubertal testes have no lumens. They contain only Sertoli cells and spermatogonia. In the cryptorchid testis in an adult, the seminiferous tubules are generally more mature than those in a prepubertal testis, with primary spermatocytes and lumens. However, there is very little, if any, complete spermatogenesis, and many of the tubules remain prepubertal in their morphology i38.1a. Collections of prepubertal tubules are called Pick adenoma because the predominance of Sertoli cells resembles a neoplasm i38.1b. Caution is indicated in the diagnosis of a Sertoli cell tumor in a cryptorchid testis. The cryptorchid testis may also have fibrosis of tubules and occasional small clusters of Leydig cells i38.1c. Cryptorchid testes occasionally present as diagnostically difficult inguinal masses because their immaturity makes recognizable testicular elements indistinct. Clusters of Leydig cells are a clue to a cryptorchid testis in an inguinal mass. Cryptorchid testes must be placed in their proper position or there will be insufficient development for fertility and a significantly increased risk for germ cell neoplasia [PMID16432987].

Klinefelter syndrome is characterized by sclerotic tubules and Leydig cell hyperplasia **i38.2a**, often with nodules of Leydig cells. The degree of fibrosis **i38.2b** and Leydig cell hyperplasia exceeds that seen in cryptorchidism. Spermatogenesis is sharply reduced but may not be totally absent [PMID2895491], but hormone supplementation may occasionally permit fertility.

Rarely, there are no germ cells at all. This is germinal cell aplasia, commonly called the Sertoli cell-only syndrome.

The Testis in Infertility

Male infertility can be pretesticular (eg, endocrine failure), testicular, or posttesticular (eg, obstruction). A microdeletion in Yq11 is the most common known genetic cause of decreased spermatogenesis, accounting for about 10% of cases [PMID19421675]. 3 regions in Yq11, *AZFa*, *AZFb*, and *AZFc* encode for proteins called azoospermia factors a, b, and c, respectively. Deletions in *AZFc* are the most common, and these patients, in contrast to those with deletions in *AZFa* or *AZFb*, may have some spermatogenesis and may be candidates for sperm recovery and intracytoplasmic sperm injection (ICSI) [PMID19896650].

Testicular biopsy can often be avoided in fertility evaluations, but is still occasionally needed to differentiate testicular failure from obstruction, and is particularly indicated if ICSI is an option. If there is a biopsy for infertility, the evaluation begins with an assessment of the architecture of the testis (ie, are seminiferous tubules present in normal numbers and are they of normal caliber; is the interstitial tissue between the tubules normal, or is it fibrotic, with an increased or decreased number of Leydig cells?). Then Sertoli cells, which support spermatogenesis and nurture each stage of the developing sperm, are identified, after which maturation of the germ cells is assessed by evaluating each stage, similar to the way in which one evaluates maturation in the bone marrow [PMID20670143]. Testicular neoplasia is a cause of male infertility and may be evident in a biopsy as intratubular germ cell neoplasia.

Nonneoplastic Conditions

Only 2 nonneoplastic conditions of the testes and paratesticular tissue will be briefly mentioned. The most common cystic lesions of the testis are the spermatocele and the hydrocele. Most spermatoceles occur in the efferent ducts or in the epididymis and are lined by its normal ciliated columnar epithelium, while most hydroceles are in the tunica vaginalis and either have no lining or are lined by mesothelial cells. If mature sperm are not seen in what is clinically felt to be a spermatocele, but the cyst is lined by ciliated columnar epithelium, it is still more likely to be a spermatocele than a hydrocele. Although the clinician will generally correctly identify the process based on its location, the pathologist should be willing to offer, and the clinician should be willing to accept, a different diagnosis if the observed lining does not match the clinical diagnosis.

Orchitis is not discussed in this work except to caution that granulomatous orchitis may resemble the unusual entity malakoplakia or, more importantly, may resemble a seminoma.

Another nonneoplastic situation that arises is verification of vas deferens tissue, with full cross-section, after a vasectomy. This is less important than verification of fallopian tube tissue after female sterilization, because the patient's sperm count can be monitored and shown to drop to undetectable levels with or without histologic verification of vas tissue, but in questionable situations, a small focus of keratin-positive cells surrounded by smooth muscle provides reasonable certainty of an effective procedure. Additional certainty can be obtained by recognizing that vas deferens epithelium also expresses CD10 [PMID19926581].

Testicular Neoplasms

Although epithelial tumors of the ovary (eg, serous, mucinous, and endometrioid neoplasms) are the most common type of tumor in that tissue, they are exceptionally rare in the testis and are not recognized as a specific class of testicular tumors. Most primary testicular neoplasms are germ cell tumors and almost all of the remainder are sex cord-stromal tumors. Both of these classes their ovarian counterparts.

The testicular neoplasm is typically received with a portion of the spermatic cord. The pathologist must assess the presence or absence of invasion of the tunica albuginia, the dense fibrous covering of the testicle, and if there is any extratesticular tumor. If there is, extension into the spermatic cord becomes a possibility. Sections of the cord can be taken before the tumor is incised to prevent artifactual spread of tumor into the cord. If the tumor has spread into the spermatic cord, it is easy to mistake spread along the fascial planes in the cord as vascular invasion, and it has been recommended that a tumor thrombus be demonstrated before vascular invasion in the cord is diagnosed [PMID18336561]. A comment should be made on whether or not there is invasion of the rete testis, because involvement by the rete testis constitutes extratesticular spread and increases the stage.

Germ Cell Neoplasms

In contrast to the ovary, germ cell tumors are the most common class of testicular neoplasms. Testicular germ cell tumors are classified essentially as it is in the ovary, except that the dysgerminoma of the ovary is called a seminoma in the testis. Like their ovarian counterparts, testicular germ cell tumors generally occur in young patients. Pure yolk sac tumors and teratomas arise in prepubertal patients. Seminomas arise in postpubertal young men and spermatocytic seminomas arise in middle-aged to older men [PMID15761466]. Other germ cell tumors include the embryonal carcinoma and the choriocarcinoma.

The seminoma is the most common testicular germ cell neoplasm to occur in pure form, but testicular germ cell tumors often occur in a mixed pattern with multiple components, one of which is usually a seminoma. Occasionally, a testicular tumor will be purely nonseminomatous. The first step in assessing a testicular mass is to determine if it is a neoplasm or a nonneoplastic process. If a neoplastic nature is confirmed, it must then be decided if the tumor is a germ cell tumor, and if so, if it is a seminoma or another type of germ cell tumor. If it is a seminoma, it must be determined if it is a pure seminoma or has nonseminomatous component, as this may influence treatment and prognosis.

In the classic pattern of a seminoma, the tumor cells are large, with abundant cytoplasm. Nuclei are large, with prominent nucleoli, but are relatively uniform. Cytoplasmic borders are sharp. Classically, cords of fibrovascular tissue, within which there are numerous lymphocytes, ramify through the tumor i38.3. The cells may occasionally infiltrate as cords or tubules. Seminomas may have rare giant cells resembling syncytiotrophoblasts. These may even be HCG positive, but the rarity of these cells and the absence of a cytotrophoblastic element oppose a diagnosis of choriocarcinoma. In addition, the nuclei of the giant cells in a seminoma are less pleomorphic than those of a choriocarcinoma, and the cells demonstrate nuclear staining for OCT3/4, as do the much more common mononuclear tumor cells, which choriocarcinoma cells do not [PMID18156809]. Seminomas usually have an aneuploid DNA content and have abnormalities of chromosome 12, such as isochromosome or amplification of 12p [PMID15761466].

Attempts to identify those seminomas that will be more aggressive have been unsuccessful. The so-called anaplastic seminoma, with more atypia and mitoses, has not proven to be more aggressive and is no longer recognized as a distinct entity. It is much more important to detect a nonseminomatous component than to attempt to recognize aggressive patterns in a pure seminoma.

Important nonneoplastic simulators of seminoma include granulomatous orchitis, malakoplakia, and collections of macrophages secondary to chemotherapy. Placental alkaline phosphatase (PLAP), in a cell membrane pattern, is a hallmark of germ cell tumors and is not expected in any of these nonneoplastic mimics. In addition, nuclear staining for OCT3/4 is an excellent marker for seminomas and embryonal carcinomas and is negative in nonneoplastic processes [PMID15223965]. Additional immunohistochemical stains, such as CD68, may identify the putative neoplastic cells as macrophages.

The major non-germ cell neoplasms that resemble a seminoma are a large cell lymphoma and a Sertoli cell tumor. The presence of intratubular germ cell neoplasia i38.4, typically found on the periphery of germ cell tumors, is not found in either lymphoma or Sertoli cell tumor and is helpful in excluding a non-germ cell origin. Lymphomas tend to occur in older patients and are often bilateral. Immunohistochemistry is also helpful. PLAP and OCT3/4 positivity are common in seminoma and not expected in lymphoma or Sertoli cell tumors. In contrast to seminomas, Sertoli cell tumors will usually be positive for epithelial membrane antigen (EMA), and about 75% will be positive for inhibin, a marker for stromal tumors that is not generally expressed by germ cell tumors. Immunohistochemical stains for lymphoid antigens can clarify any possible lymphoproliferative process.

Once a seminoma has been identified, a concomitant nonseminomatous component must be recognized because pure seminomas are often treated with radiation, which is an uncommon treatment modality in other types of testicular malignancy [PMID18156809]. In addition to morphologic differences, there are also important differences in immunohistochemical staining between seminomas and nonseminomatous germ cell tumors. These have been reviewed [PMID16512598] and are discussed in more detail subsequently, with each type of germ cell tumor, but a few comments are made here. Seminomas are negative for EMA, and are usually negative for keratins such as CAM 5.2 (a low molecular weight keratin) and AE-1/AE-3, but 1/3 may have some keratin positivity [PMID10761461]. AE-1 and AE-3 stains can be performed in all seminomas to rule out a nonseminomatous component. Negativity is reassuring regarding a nonseminomatous component, but because of the occasional positivity of seminomas for keratins, positive cases should also have some morphologic features of a nonseminomatous component, such as papillae, glands, or nuclear pleomorphism, before such a component is diagnosed. Seminomas are negative for CD30 [PMID16512598], and any foci that are unusual for a seminoma and that are CD30 positive establish the presence of a component of embryonal carcinoma. Melanoma-associated gene C2 (MAGEC2) has been reported to be nearly specific for seminoma, not staining other germ cell tumors [PMID21780320], and particularly difficult cases that stain for MAGEC2 and are negative for CD30 are likely seminoma. Most seminomas express CD117 (c-kit) in a cell membrane pattern, and its loss may suggest focus of a higher-grade germ cell tumor [PMID18297810].

The spermatocytic seminoma is a rare germ cell tumor that is not related to the classic seminoma. Patients with spermatocytic seminoma are older than most patients with germ cell neoplasms (the average age is 50-60). The typical appearance has 3 cell types. The predominant population of cells that are 15-20 μm in diameter. These often have chromatin that is clumped in an unusual manner, often described as filamentous or rope-like i38.5. There is a population of smaller cells that may be derived from degeneration of the first group. The third component consists of rare large cells, up to 100 μm in diameter, which may be multinucleated. Although fibrous tissue may be present, the fibrous septae of a classic seminoma are absent. The mitotic rate is very high, causing confusion with the so-called anaplastic seminoma. The spermatocytic seminoma is negative for keratin, but in contrast to the classic seminoma and most other germ cell tumors, it is also PLAP negative [PMID10223302]. These neoplasms generally behave in a benign manner [PMID15761466].

In embryology, the yolk sac is an extraembryonic membrane cavity on the opposite side of the trilayered embryo from the amniotic cavity. In nonmammalian development, it is the principal source of nourishment for the embryo. In mammals, where the placenta furnishes nourishment, the yolk sac becomes the hindgut, and its remnants are thought to be the source of yolk sac tumors. The pure form of testicular yolk sac tumor occurs in very young children, with a mean age of 18 months. A pure yolk sac tumor is rare in adults, but a yolk sac component is commonly seen in adult germ cell tumors. There are numerous patterns of yolk sac tumor, and most cases demonstrate >1 pattern [Eble ISBN978-9283224150]. Indeed, the occurrence of multiple patterns suggests that a yolk sac tumor should be excluded. 4 of the most commonly encountered patterns are as follows:

- Reticular (or microcystic). This is the most common form. The microcysts are formed by cytoplasmic vacuoles and small extracellular pseudoglandular spaces i38.6a.

The cytoplasm is primarily filled with glycogen, but there may be some lipid, and some cells may resemble lipoblasts. The appearance is often that of vesicles that are separated by cellular stroma, and the vesicles may demonstrate eccentric constrictions.

- Endodermal sinus. This form is characterized by Schiller-Duval (glomeruloid) bodies, which are fibrovascular cores lined by neoplastic epithelium. In contrast to the papillary form of yolk sac tumor, the fibrovascular cores are smaller i38.6b, and there is usually a component that is reticular or solid.
- Papillary. In contrast to the endodermal sinus form, papillations are the primary feature and are larger and more prominent. They may be lined by neoplastic cells with hobnail nuclei.
- Solid i38.6c. This form is likely to resemble an embryonal carcinoma, but there are usually areas with 1 of the other patterns.

Most, but not all, yolk sac tumors are α-fetoprotein (αFP) positive. Approximately 1/2 of yolk sac tumors are PLAP positive. Cytokeratin is strongly positive while EMA is usually negative [PMID16512598, PMID18045648]. Any of the patterns of a yolk sac tumor may have cytoplasmic or extracellular hyaline globules i38.6d. These occasionally can be shown to contain αFP, but in most cases consists of other proteins. The differential diagnosis of a yolk sac tumor includes a seminoma and embryonal carcinoma.

Like the yolk sac tumor, an embryonal carcinoma may have multiple patterns, but 3 are common—solid i38.7a, papillary i38.7b, and glandular. The papillary pattern may have some fibrovascular cores, causing resemblance to the papillary type of yolk sac tumor or the Schiller-Duval bodies of the endodermal sinus type of yolk sac tumor. CD30 positivity in a cell membrane pattern indicates an embryonal carcinoma i38.7c. It is also helpful to remember that the nuclei of embryonal carcinoma are usually larger and more pleomorphic than those of yolk sac tumor.

Some believe that embryonal carcinomas may have a stromal component, while others regard any neoplastic stromal tissue as a teratomatous component. For this reason, the term "teratocarcinoma," which referred to a combination of embryonal carcinoma and teratoma i38.8, is not recommended now. The term was popular before the current understanding of germ cell tumor classification and morphology. In any germ cell tumor, the components should be described, and if there is a combination of embryonal carcinoma and teratoma, the report should discuss the nature of the teratomatous component and any controversies regarding nomenclature.

Isolated syncytiotrophoblast giant cells are often present in embryonal carcinoma, as they are in seminomas, and should not be construed as a choriocarcinoma. Most germ cell tumors with scattered giant cells are not choriocarcinomas, but a germ tumor of another type with incidental giant cells.

Vascular invasion is common in embryonal carcinoma. Most embryonal carcinomas are PLAP positive. Almost all embryonal carcinomas are pan-keratin positive, and most are positive for cytokeratin 7, in contrast to seminoma. Only about 2% are positive for EMA. CD30 positivity is almost always found in embryonal carcinoma and is very helpful in its identification [PMID16512598]. CK7, AE-1/AE-3, CD-30, and CAM 5.2 are most useful in identifying an embryonal component in a mixed germ cell tumor.

In addition, OCT3/4 is a transcription factor that marks seminomas and embryonal carcinomas (both testicular and ovarian) as well or better than PLAP [PMID15223965]. OCT3/4 appears especially useful in the diagnosis of these types of tumors in nongonadal locations, particularly after chemotherapy. Additionally helpful is that Glypican 3 stains almost all yolk sac tumors and choriocarcinomas, but very few embryonal carcinomas and essentially no seminomas [PMID17122513]. Glypican 3 is more sensitive for yolk sac tumor than αFP in either the testis or the ovary [PMID20546340].

Pure testicular choriocarcinomas are rare and most such neoplasms occur as mixed germ cell tumors. Classical choriocarcinomas have a dimorphic population of tumor cells, with multinucleated cells and mononuclear cells i38.9. The mononuclear cells may be cytotrophoblasts or intermediate trophoblasts. As discussed in Chapter 27, there is substantial immunohistochemical overlap between cytotrophoblasts and intermediate trophoblasts. PLAP is positive in about 1/2 of choriocarcinomas. These neoplasms are usually positive for cytokeratin, and in contrast to other germ cell tumors, about 1/2 of choriocarcinomas are positive for EMA. As one moves from seminoma to yolk sac/embryonal to choriocarcinoma, there is increasing keratin positivity, increasing EMA positivity, and decreasing PLAP positivity [PMID16512598]. But these tumors are on a continuum, so the H&E morphology must be consistent with the diagnosis suggested by immunohistochemical stains.

The giant cells in a choriocarcinoma may be rare, resulting in a nearly uniform population of mononuclear cells, particularly in previously diagnosed choriocarcinomas that have been treated. These are diagnostically challenging situations, as the mononuclear cells are typically only weakly and focally positive for HCG, and may be completely negative. EMA positivity may be the clue that a tumor is a monophasic choriocarcinoma and not a yolk sac or embryonal carcinoma.

There are important differences between the ovarian and testicular teratomas. Whereas ovarian teratomas tend to occur in young adults, pure testicular teratomas occur mostly in children and are rare in adults. Most testicular teratomas in children consist solely of mature tissues, whereas the few teratomas in adults usually have some amount of immaturity or are mixed with other types of tumor. However, teratomas in prepubertal males, even if immature, are virtually always benign in behavior, whereas those occurring after puberty, even if pure and entirely mature, have metastatic potential. For this reason, all testicular teratomas in adults should be regarded as malignant [PMID15761467]. This is in contrast to ovarian teratomas, where it is the presence of immature tissue, not the age of the patient, that is prognostically important.

Because it is the age of the patient and not the presence of immature tissue that has the principal prognostic significance in testicular teratomas, these are not generally graded with respect to immature tissue in the way that ovarian teratomas are. More important than a comment on immaturity is a search for another type of germ cell tumor, another type of tumor arising from the teratoma (eg, primitive neuroectodermal tumor or nephroblastoma-like), and a comment on the potential of even mature testicular teratomas in adults to metastasize. The primary significance of immaturity in the adult testicular teratoma is that such foci may be confused with embryonal or yolk sac tumors. In such cases, Wilms tumor-like areas or immature mesenchyme favor an immature teratoma over a germ cell tumor of another type.

The exception to the above comments is a pure testicular dermoid. Although the relationship of testicular dermoids to mature teratomas is not completely clear, most people believe that a dermoid is defined by the absence of solid areas, the absence of intratubular germ cell neoplasia, and the presence of hair. A pure testicular dermoid, even in an adult, does not have metastatic potential [PMID19955600]. Because a dermoid is the one type of adult testicular teratoma that has no significant metastatic potential, its distinction from a mature teratoma is important in the adult testes, but not important in the ovary, where all mature ovarian teratomas have no significant metastatic potential.

The immunohistochemical staining pattern of teratomas is dependent on the component tissue. For example, they may be αFP positive if they contain liver, keratin and EMA positive in epithelial structures, etc.

A final comment on testicular germ cell tumors is that they will rarely undergo spontaneous regression after metastasis, leaving the pathologist with the conundrum of a metastatic germ cell tumor, but no apparent primary or history.

Sex Cord-Stromal Neoplasms

With the exception of the Sertoli cell tumor and the Leydig cell tumor, sex cord-stromal tumors are rare in the testes. Testicular sex cord-stromal tumors have similar morphologies and immunohistochemical staining patterns to their ovarian counterparts, and will generally stain for inhibin and, with slightly less specificity, also for calretinin [PMID15502809].

The most common type of sex cord-stromal tumor of the testis is the Leydig cell tumor. True Leydig cell tumors form a mass and displace or efface the seminiferous tubules i38.10a, i38.10b, whereas the cells in Leydig cell hyperplasia (such as is seen in Klinefelter syndrome) infiltrate between tubules. The differential diagnosis of a Leydig cell tumor includes the large-cell calcifying Sertoli cell tumor (discussed below) and the testicular nodules that occur in adrenogenital syndrome. Testicular nodules in adrenogenital syndrome are nonneoplastic and are composed of ACTH-dependent adrenal cells thought to be derived from embryologic rests. The correct diagnosis of these nodules requires knowledge of a history of adrenogenital syndrome, but clues are the young age of the patient and the fact that the nodules are usually bilateral and multifocal. The nodules will regress with therapy for the adrenogenital syndrome. Leydig cell tumors may also resemble a solid or hepatoid variety of yolk sac tumor, but will have more nuclear uniformity and more cytoplasm.

Like other tumors of sex cord-stromal class, Leydig cell tumors are positive for inhibin and calretinin, and negative for PLAP. Melan-A positivity has also been reported [PMID17041205]. 15% of Leydig cell tumors are malignant. Histologic study cannot reliably identify this subset, but the usual endocrine neoplasia warning signs apply—vascular invasion, poor circumscription, mitoses, large size, generalized nuclear atypia, and necrosis.

Pure Sertoli cell tumors are rare in the ovary, and most such cases will have a Leydig cell component, but in the testis, the opposite is true—Sertoli-Leydig cell tumors are rare, and one should suspect that the Leydig cell component of an apparent testicular Sertoli-Leydig cell tumor may be nonneoplastic [PMID15502809]. As discussed in Chapter 33, Sertoli cell tumors, with or without a Leydig cell component, can have a number of different patterns. They may form trabeculae and tubules i38.11, or they may be solid. The better differentiated examples often resemble seminomas. Sertoli cell tumors usually have smaller nuclei than a seminoma and the often clear cytoplasm that is often seen is from lipid accumulation, not from glycogen, as is the case in seminomas. In addition, seminomas are associated with intratubular germ cell neoplasia, while Sertoli cell tumors are not, but immunohistochemical characterization is often needed for the correct diagnosis. Less differentiated Sertoli cell tumors may resemble a yolk sac tumor, again requiring immunohistochemical characterization. Like other sex cord-stromal tumors, Sertoli cell tumors are PLAP negative, usually inhibin positive, and often positive for calretinin. CD99, keratin, and EMA positivity have been shown [PMID9720506]. A good rule is to consider a Sertoli cell tumor in any unusual ovarian or testicular neoplasm which has a trabecular or tubular pattern.

The large-cell calcifying Sertoli cell tumor occurs in very young men and has neoplastic cells with abundant eosinophilic cytoplasm. There may be a number of growth patterns, often with stromal calcification or ossification, and there may be large numbers of neutrophils. Multifocality and bilaterality are common [PMID15943795] and may help in the exclusion of a Leydig cell tumor. These tumors are often positive for inhibin, vimentin, calretinin, and S100 [PMID20004940].

The adult granulosa cell tumor is extraordinarily rare in the testis, but the juvenile granulosa cell tumor is encountered in infants, usually around 5 months of age [PMID18548396]. These tumors are positive for inhibin, as are their ovarian counterparts. They may resemble a yolk sac tumor, but are vimentin and inhibin positive, and cytokeratin negative.

The gonadoblastoma is a very rare neoplasm consisting of a combination of germ cell and sex cord components.

Other Testicular Neoplasms

The most common malignant testicular neoplasm that does not arise from testicular tissue is lymphoma. Lymphomas of the testis tend to be diffuse large B-cell lymphomas, and are usually positive for MUM1 and negative for bcl-6 and CD10, indicating postgerminal center phenotype [PMID16998463]. These lymphomas are discussed in detail in Chapter 8.

The most common paratesticular mass is the well differentiated liposarcoma/atypical lipoma, diagnosed as discussed in Chapter 2. Mesotheliomas are rare in the testis, but the adenomatoid tumor, which is thought to be of mesothelial derivation, is common in the epididymis. Nodular fibrous proliferation and diffuse fibrous proliferation occur in the tunica albuginia and are likely examples of inflammatory myofibroblastic tumor. A few cases of desmoplastic small round cell tumor have been reported in the paratesticular area.

ISBN 978-089189-5886

Core Points for the Testes

- *SRY* gene on the Y chromosome: encodes proteins that result in Sertoli cells, which then cause the development of sperm and Leydig cells.
- Seminiferous tubules of prepubertal testes: no lumens, contain only Sertoli cells and spermatogonia.
- Cryptorchid testis: more maturation, tubules have lumens and primary spermatocytes, but very little complete spermatogenesis.
- Klinefelter syndrome: sclerotic tubules, Leydig cell hyperplasia.
- Spermatoceles: in the efferent ducts or epididymis, lined by ciliated epithelium.
- Hydroceles: in the tunica vaginalis, mesothelial lining or none at all.
- Germ cell tumors: most common primary testicular neoplasms.
  - Positive for PLAP.
- Seminoma: most common germ cell tumor.
  - Positive for OCT3/4.
  - 1/3 are positive for keratins AE1/AE3.
  - Nonseminomatous component must be excluded by H&E examination and often by IHC.
- Embryonal carcinoma: positive for PLAP, OCT3/4, keratin, and CD30. EMA–.
- Yolk sac tumor: many patterns. Positive for PLAP and keratin, negative for EMA, CD30, and OCT3/4.
- Choriocarcinomas: PLAP positive in only half of cases. Keratin positive.
  - Unlike other germ cell tumors, 1/2 are EMA positive.
  - Multinucleated cells may be rare, in which case may be only weakly positive for HCG.
- Testicular teratomas: pure form occurs in children.
  - In prepubertal patients, virtually always benign even if there is an immature component.
  - After puberty, have metastatic potential even if entirely mature, so all testicular teratomas in adults, except for the very rare pure dermoid, should be regarded as malignant.
  - Unlike ovarian teratomas, age of patient and presence of a germ cell tumor of another type, not the presence of immature tissue, matters.
- Sex cord-stromal tumors: limited to Sertoli cell tumor and the Leydig cell tumor.
- Lymphoma: usually diffuse large B-cell lymphoma.

i38.1 a A cryptorchid testis in an adult. These seminiferous tubules have only Sertoli cells.
b A cryptorchid testis in which there is a proliferation of small seminiferous tubules containing only Sertoli cells, creating the illusion of a benign neoplasm (Pick adenoma)

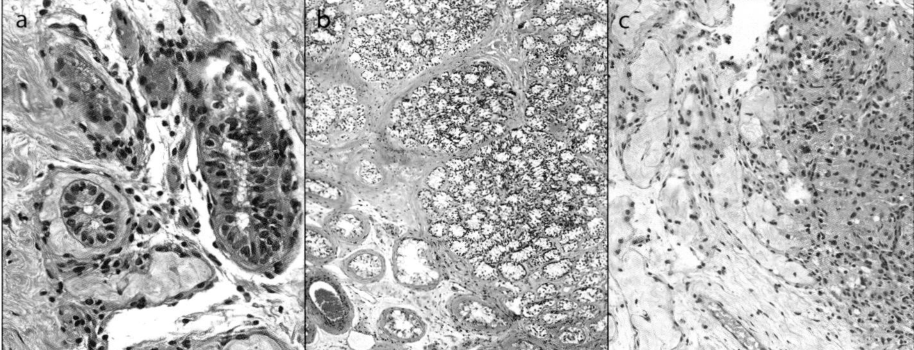

c A cryptorchid testis with Leydig cell hyperplasia on the right and fibrotic seminiferous tubules, not even containing Sertoli cells, on the left

i38.2 a Klinefelter syndrome, with extensive Leydig cell hyperplasia and atrophic tubules
b Extensive fibrosis in Klinefelter syndrome, in which tubules are completely obliterated

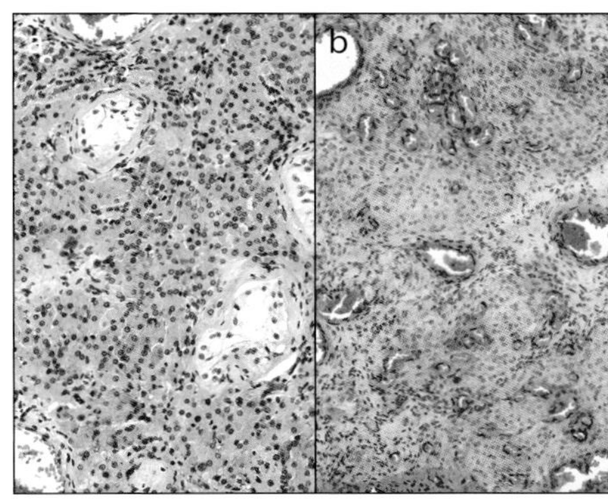

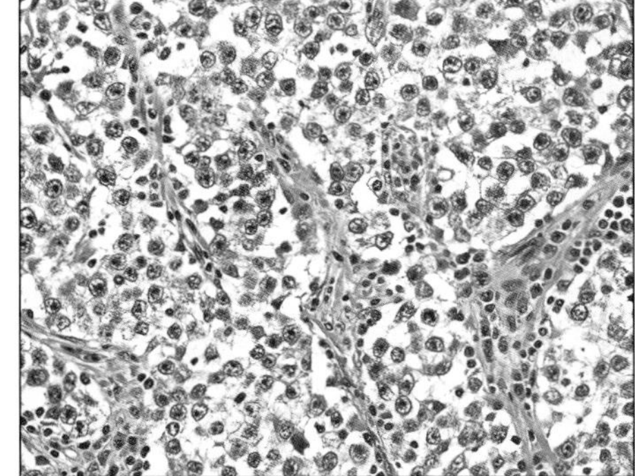

i38.3 A testicular seminoma. The neoplastic cells have large nuclei, with prominent nucleoli and are separated by fibrovascular septae that contain lymphocytes. Although the nuclei are large, they are relatively uniform. Nuclear pleomorphism is not a common feature of seminomas.

i38.4 Intratubular germ cell neoplasia. Note the numerous mitotic figures. Compare to the benign tubules containing only Sertoli cells in figure i38.1a.

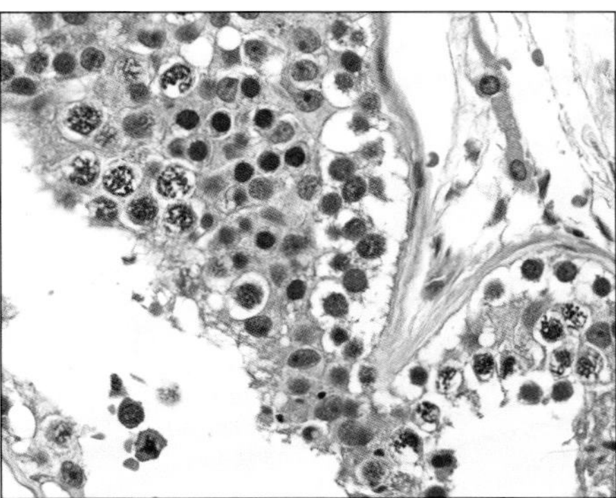

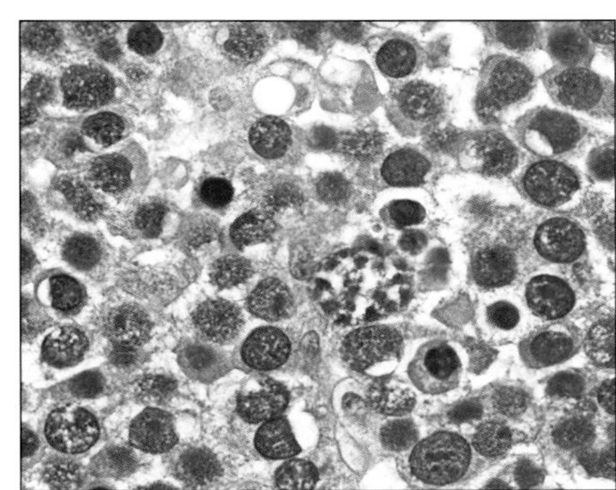

i38.5 A spermatocytic seminoma. Characteristic cell type, in the center, has very coarsely clumped chromatin.

i38.6 a A reticular variant of yolk sac tumor. There is both intracellular vacuolization and extracellular spaces.

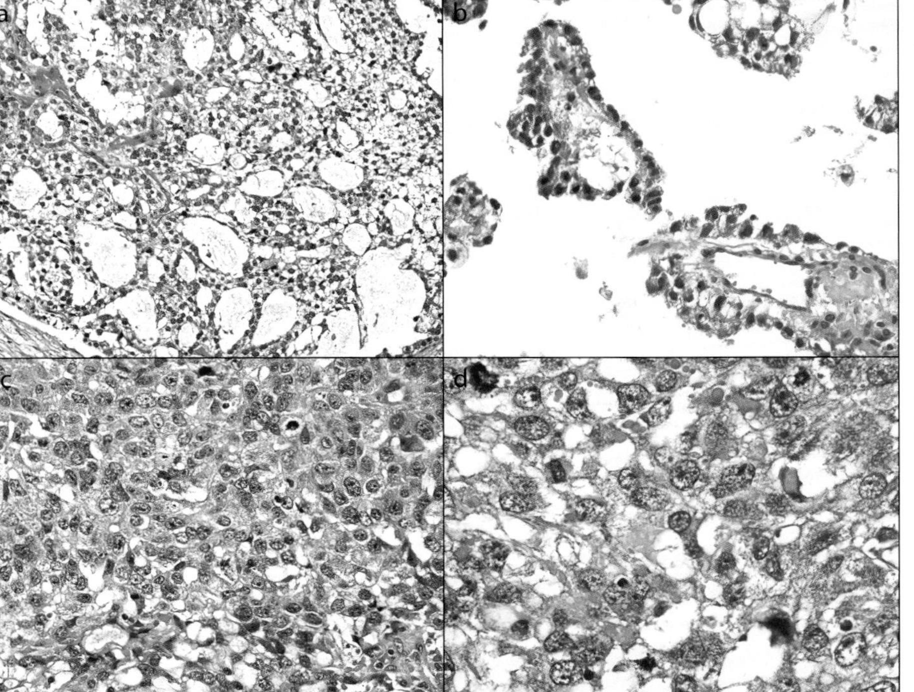

b Schiller-Duval bodies in an endodermal sinus variant of yolk sac tumor

c The solid variant of yolk sac tumor

d A yolk sac tumor in which there are numerous hyaline globules, both intracellular and extracellular. More brightly eosinophilic erythrocytes are present in the top center.

ISBN 978-089189-5886

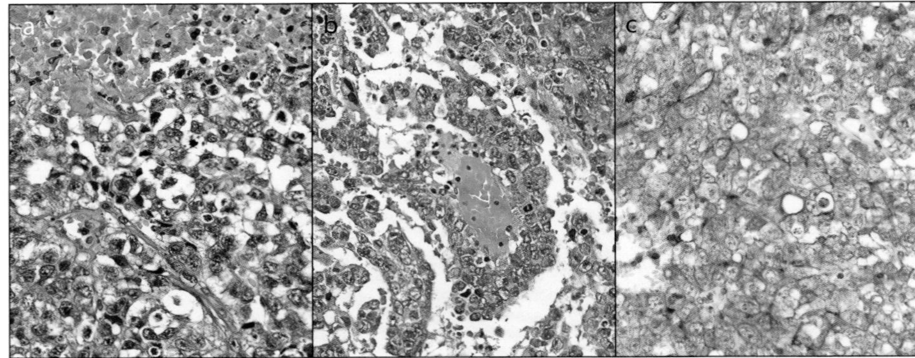

i38.7 a An embryonal carcinoma of the testis, solid pattern. Note that the nuclei are more pleomorphic than in either a seminoma or a yolk sac tumor.
b A papillary form of embryonal carcinoma

c CD30 staining in an embryonal carcinoma. This distinct and diffuse staining, cell membrane pattern, is not expected in other testicular germ cell neoplasms.

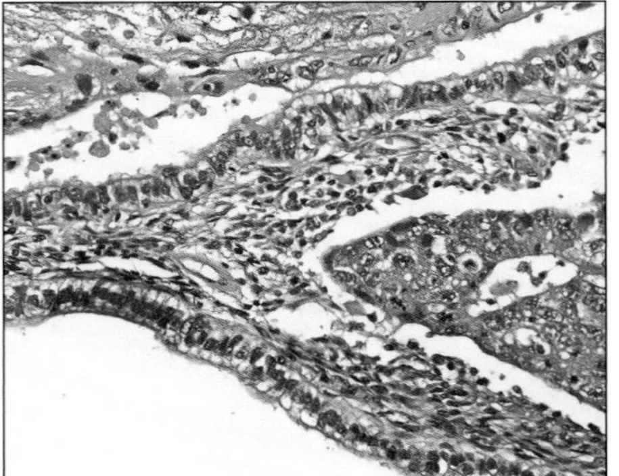

i38.8 A nonseminomatous mixed germ cell tumor with embryonal carcinoma in the center right and a mature teratoma above and below it (ciliated respiratory-type epithelium). Testicular neoplasms with this combination were formerly called teratocarcinomas.

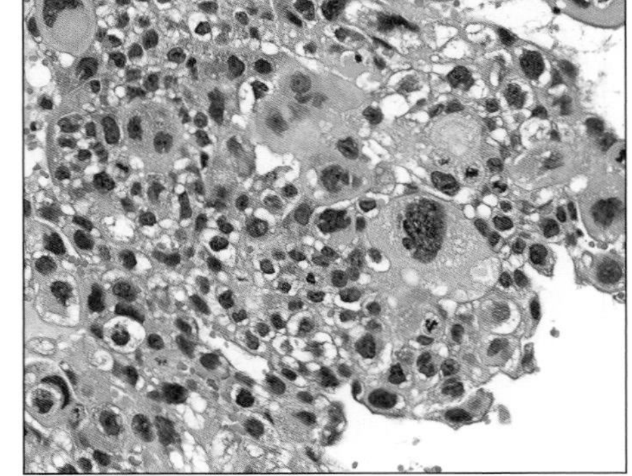

i38.9 A pure choriocarcinoma of the testis

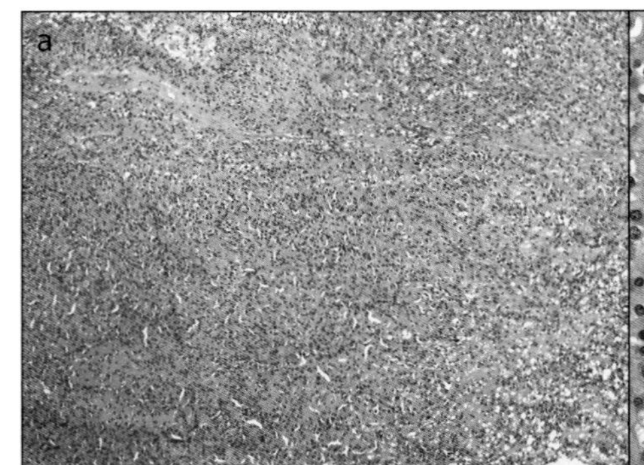

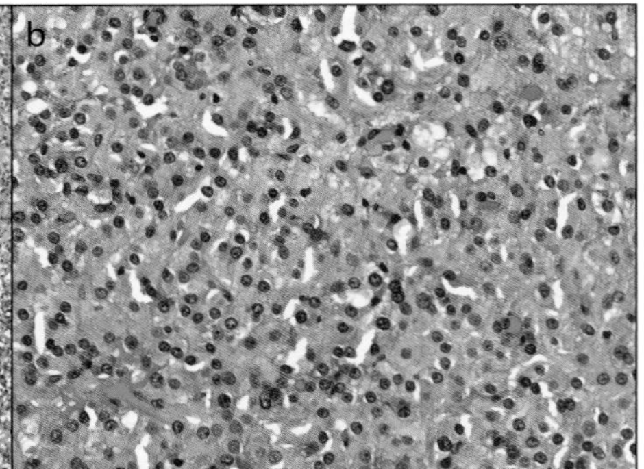

i38.10 a A Leydig cell tumor of the testis. Note that in contrast to a cryptorchid testis or Klinefelter syndrome, there is a distinct mass which has pushed aside all seminiferous tubules.

b A higher-power view of the same case as in i38.10a, illustrating the eosinophilic cytoplasm and relatively uniform nuclei that is characteristic of the entire family of steroid cell tumors, of which Leydig cell tumors are a type. Tumors of this family may also have focally clear cytoplasm.

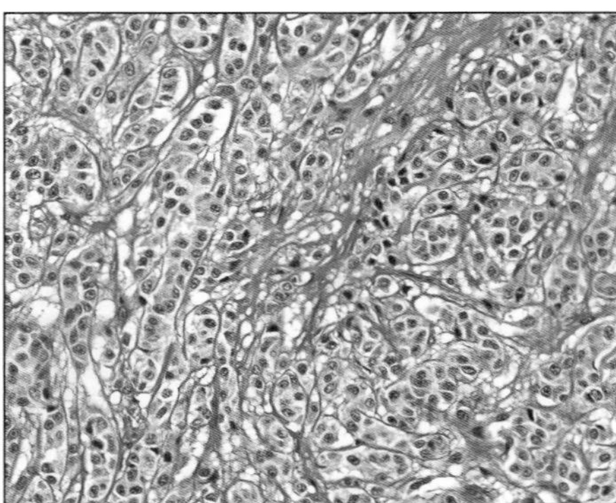

i38.11 A Sertoli cell tumor that is well differentiated, with a trabecular/tubular pattern

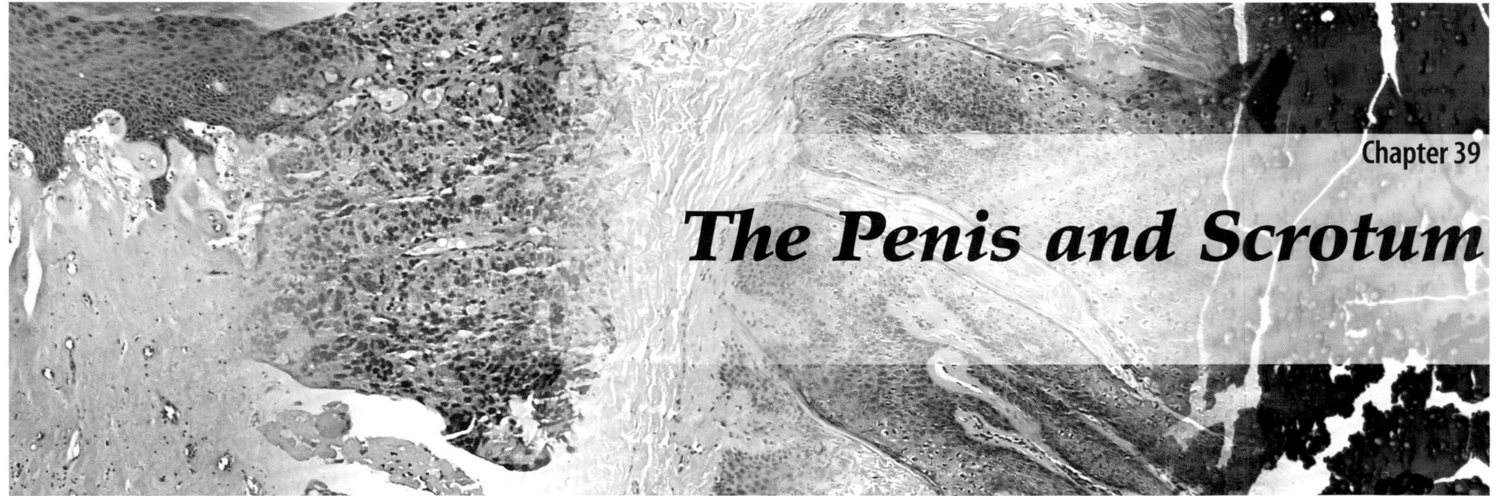

Chapter 39

The Penis and Scrotum

Normal Anatomy

The corpus spongiosum (also called the corpus cavernosum urethra) surrounds the urethra in the ventral portion of the penis. The 2 corpus cavernosa are in the dorsal aspect of the penis. The frenulum is a band of fibrous tissue on the ventral surface that attaches to the foreskin (prepuce) and helps to ensure that it surrounds the glans with an appropriate amount of tension.

Nonneoplastic Conditions

Phimosis is the inability to retract the foreskin behind the glans and is normal until about age 5. Paraphimosis is the opposite problem—a retention of the foreskin behind the glans, resulting in the constriction of the glans. Lichen sclerosus et atrophicus of the penis is called balanitis xerotica obliterans and tends to occur on the foreskin and occasionally on the glans i39.1. As is the case for the vulva, some cases of lichen sclerosus of the penis may be a precursor lesion for squamous cell carcinomas that are not associated with human papillomavirus [PMID14576478, PMID15223959, PMID11453912].

Primary noncutaneous inflammatory processes are rare in the scrotum, but in the attempt to find an etiology for unexplained granulomatous processes in this location, consideration should be given to a sperm granuloma arising from and connected to the epididymis. Idiopathic scrotal calcinosis i39.2 is a relatively common and peculiar form of cutaneous calcification that is not related to either dystrophic calcification (in necrotic tissue) or to metastatic calcification (from metabolic abnormalities). It may be related to an obliterated inclusion cyst.

The infectious diseases that occur in the penis, in large measure, parallel those in the female genital area and are discussed in more detail in Chapter 29.

Neoplasms of the Penis

The epithelium of the penis undergoes dysplastic changes similar to those in other locations, and these changes are assessed in the same way. As is the case for the vulva and the cervix, there is a keratinizing or differentiated variant of dysplasia that can be subtle because there may be substantial maturation. As in other sites, the presence of hard, refractile keratin in the epithelium is a clue to this type of dysplasia.

Approximately 1/2 of penile squamous carcinomas are of the conventional type, while the remaining half is composed of a number of variants [PMID22595011]. As is the case for the female genital area, a basaloid type of squamous carcinoma occurs in the penis. Basaloid tumors in this location are more likely to be variants of squamous carcinoma than true basal cell carcinoma. As in other sites, the diagnosis of basaloid type of squamous carcinoma can be made by identifying areas of conventional squamous cell carcinoma or squamous carcinoma in situ.

In addition to the conventional and basaloid varieties of squamous carcinoma, there are several forms of squamous carcinoma of the penis that are collectively designated as "verruciform" because they have an exophytic component. These include condylomatous (also called warty), papillary, and verrucous carcinomas. There is no universal agreement on the properties of these lesions, and there will be considerable interobserver variation in their diagnosis.

In general, condylomatous carcinoma has prominent fibrovascular cores and perinuclear clearing in its upper portion. The deeper portion resembles a common squamous cell carcinoma, with invasion and pleomorphism. The relatively innocuous appearance of the upper portion of this lesion underscores the need not to make a definitive diagnosis of a simple condyloma of the penis on a superficial biopsy without a comment that an invasive process cannot be excluded. The condylomatous carcinoma is capable of metastasis [PMID10757397].

The upper portion of a papillary carcinoma is less "warty" than a condylomatous carcinoma, with variable fibrovascular cores, moderate nuclear atypia, and no significant perinuclear clearing i39.3. The deeper portion has the appearance of a typical squamous carcinoma. The difference between the condylomatous and papillary carcinomas is the more pronounced condylomatous changes and less nuclear atypia in the surface portion in the former neoplasm. The papillary squamous carcinoma is also capable of metastasis [PMID20061934].

The verrucous carcinoma of the penis has the properties and morphology described in other locations [PMID8472225]. Its diagnosis is difficult, as it is in other sites. In contrast to the condylomatous carcinoma, the verrucous carcinoma has few, if any, fibrovascular cores in its upper portion, and true perinuclear clearing is absent. The verrucous carcinoma also differs from the condylomatous carcinoma and the papillary carcinoma in the deeper portion, which is not a typical squamous cell carcinoma, but rather has a pushing type of invasion caused by rounded nests of cells, usually with a stromal infiltrate of lymphocytes and plasma cells. The verrucous carcinoma differs from the condylomatous carcinoma and the papillary carcinoma on the surface by having no significant perinuclear clearing and fewer fibrovascular cores, and in its lower portion by having a pushing margin and a less obviously malignant appearance. Of all the types of "verrucoid" squamous carcinomas in this site, only the verrucous carcinoma has relatively bland nuclei throughout its thickness and a smooth interface between the lower epithelium and the stroma.

The giant condyloma (Buschke-Lowenstein) has a condylomatous appearance in its superficial portion but also a broad, pushing lower portion that pushes into the dermis rather than raggedly infiltrates it i39.4. Some believe that the giant condyloma is a verrucous carcinoma, while others feel that it is a distinct entity, and that the prominent perinuclear clearing and fibrovascular cores in the upper portion distinguish it from the verrucous carcinoma, while the smooth, pushing expansion into the stroma distinguishes it from a condylomatous or papillary carcinoma (ie, that it has an unusual combination of a condylomatous carcinoma appearance on the surface and a verrucous carcinoma appearance in the lower portion). To my mind, the giant condyloma can be regarded as a type of verrucous carcinoma because it is the bottom of the lesion, where it interfaces the stroma, that determines biologic potential.

These entities substantially overlap and can be confused without harm as long as there is complete removal. The important point is to recognize the inability to exclude a conventional squamous carcinoma in the unsampled lower portion when a superficial biopsy demonstrates an exophytic low-grade squamous proliferation and to recommend a complete excision of any of the lesions in this group.

Aside from those of cutaneous origin, neoplasms of the scrotum are uncommon and are primarily of smooth muscle origin.

Core Points for the Penis and the Scrotum

- Phimosis: inability to retract the foreskin.
  - Normal until about age 5.
- Paraphimosis: retention of the foreskin behind the glans.
- Balanitis xerotica obliterans (lichen sclerosus et atrophicus of the penis): on foreskin or glans.
- Idiopathic scrotal calcinosis: cutaneous calcification, accounting for many scrotal masses.
- Dysplasia and invasive carcinoma: diagnosed as in other sites.
- Verruciform types of squamous carcinoma: condylomatous, papillary, and verrucous carcinomas.
  - Precise distinction among these unlikely to be clinically important, but condylomatous and papillary carcinoma have slight metastatic potential, while verrucous carcinoma does not.
- In superficial sampling of a penile lesion with papillations, comment that invasive carcinoma cannot be excluded.

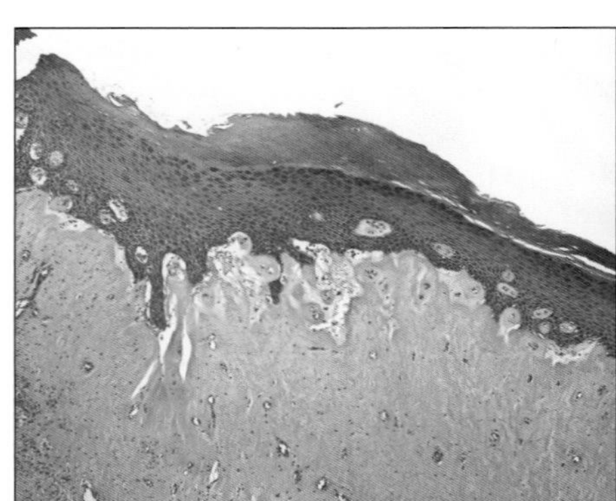

i39.1 Balanitis xerotica obliterans, the penile or foreskin counterpart to lichen sclerosus of the vulva (see i29.14. As in lichen sclerosus, there is often eosinophilic homogenization of the dermal collagen. There may be vacuolar change at the dermal-epidermal junction. The epidermis may be atrophic or hyperplastic.

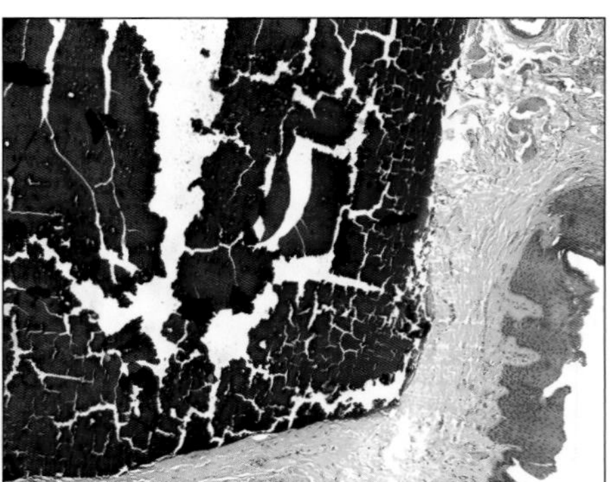

i39.2 Idiopathic scrotal calcinosis

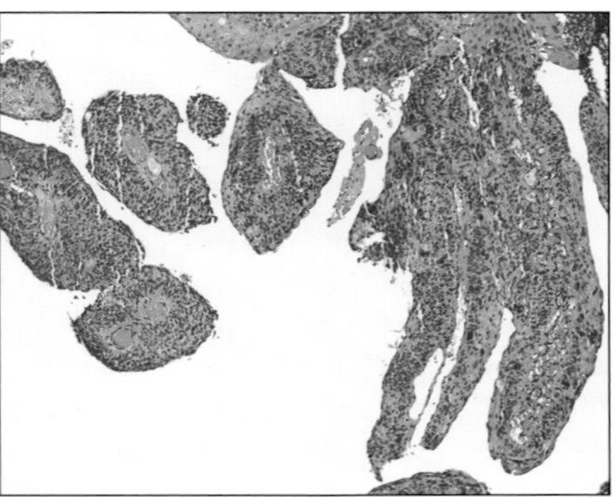

i39.3 Papillary squamous cell carcinoma of the penis. Although the exophytic portion is papillary, it is not distinctly condylomatous. In both papillary and condylomatous carcinoma, the deep portion is a squamous cell carcinoma of the usual type, but in papillary carcinoma, the exophytic portion has more nuclear atypia and less HPV cytopathic effect.

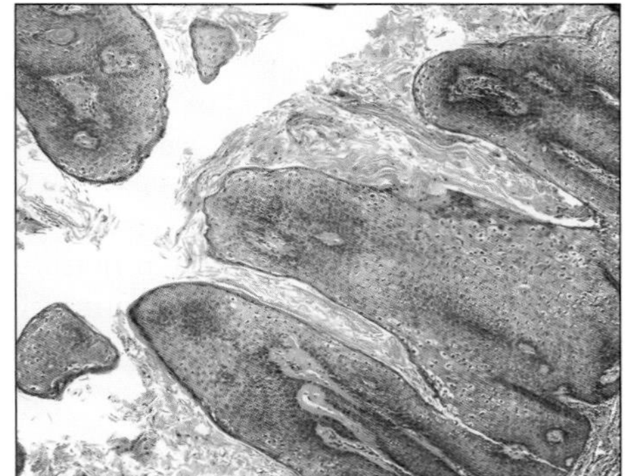

i39.4 The giant condyloma of Buschke-Lowenstein. The upper portion (shown), is indistinguishable from a simple condyloma except for the large size of the lesion and resembles the upper portion of the condylomatous carcinoma. However, the lower portion of the giant condyloma does not invade like a common squamous carcinoma, but rather pushes into the stroma as in a verrucous carcinoma.

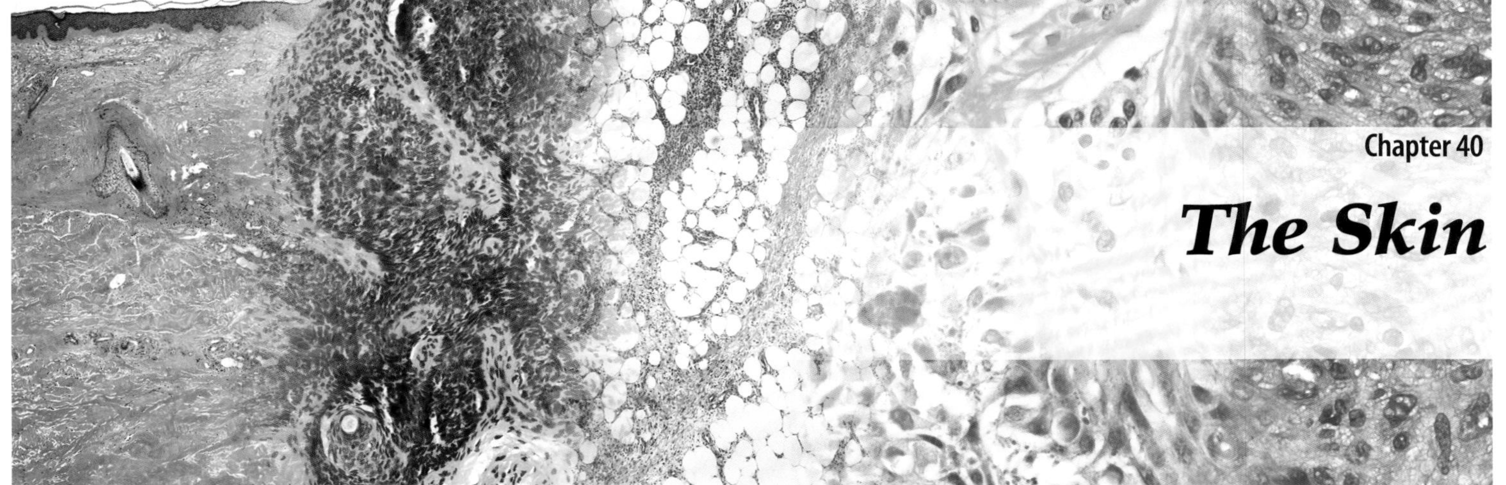

No attempt is made here to offer a thorough treatment of cutaneous disorders, which are well covered in other books, such as those of Lever [Elder ISBN978-0781773638], Farmer and Hood [Farmer ISBN978-0838580790], and Ackerman [Ackerman ISBN978-1893357259]. Here, only a few comments are offered on the most commonly encountered lesions that can cause confusion.

The subcutaneous tissue is adipose, with only thin fibrovascular septae. Although it is traditionally considered to be part of the skin, many processes in the subcutaneous tissue are actually more in the purview of soft tissue pathology than dermatopathology.

Normal Structure of the Skin

The skin consists of the thin but multilayered epidermis, the dermis, and the subcutaneous adipose tissue. In the basal layer of the epidermis, the cells have small, uniform nuclei and minimal cytoplasm. With maturation, the cells acquire more cytoplasm and the nuclei become smaller, until at the outermost portion of the epidermis, the nuclei are completely lost and there is only keratin. The spinous layer, named because the cells are connected to their neighbors by thin spinous processes, is above the basal layer. The granular layer, so named because its granular cytoplasm indicates incipient keratinization, is above the spinous layer and just below the keratin outer layer. In most sites, the epidermis completely turns over about every 28 days, making it one of the fastest regenerating tissues in the body, along with the mucosa of the gastrointestinal tract and hematopoietic cells. Periodically, epidermal cells extend into the superficial dermis in small papillae called rete pegs.

The dermis consists of a small layer of looser collagen in the upper portion, surrounding the rete pegs, called the papillary dermis. Most of the dermis consists of denser collagenous tissue called the reticular dermis i40.1. The papillary dermis invaginates into the reticular dermis to surround adnexal structures (sweat glands, sweat ducts, and hair follicles). This extension of the papillary dermis is called the adventitial or periadnexal dermis. Sebaceous glands empty into the hair follicle just above the arrector pili muscle, forming a pilosebaceous unit. Obstruction of the follicle is also likely to obstruct the gland. The base of some mature hair follicles may be in the subcutaneous tissue, but adnexal structures in the dermis are usually surrounded by adventitial dermis, not by reticular dermis. Adnexal structures also often have a small amount of adipose tissue around them.

Cutaneous Neoplasms and Masses

Benign Epidermal Hyperplasia

"Benign epidermal hyperplasia" is a general term referring to nonspecific hyperplasia of the epidermis without dysplasia. Benign epidermal hyperplasia is usually exophytic or verrucous. Seborrheic keratoses i40.2 are examples of verrucous epidermal hyperplasia. If congenital, verrucous epidermal hyperplasia can be called an epidermal nevus.

Verrucous epidermal hyperplasia may be secondary to viruses. Verruca vulgaris, the common wart, is a virus-associated epidermal hyperplasia. Early verrucas often have perinuclear clearing and obvious viral effect, but this is may be lost in older lesions, in which case the only distinguishing diagnostic features are papillomatosis, hyperplasia of the granular layer (hypergranulosis), and perhaps a bending of the rete pegs toward the center i40.3.

Condylomas are another form of virus-induced epidermal hyperplasia. In a classic condyloma, the epidermal hyperplasia is partially endophytic, there is viral cytopathic effect, and mild nuclear atypia, but there is substantial overlap with other processes, such as a verruca or a seborrheic keratosis. Molluscum contagiosum is another virus-associated epidermal hyperplasia and is characterized by a squamous proliferation within which numerous eosinophilic collections of virus particles called molluscum bodies are seen.

Lesions of the verrucous epidermal hyperplasia family may have overlapping features, and in problematic cases, a diagnosis of benign epidermal hyperplasia is usually sufficient, though a condyloma has the biologic significance of mild dysplasia.

If associated with abnormal adnexal structures, verrucous epidermal hyperplasia is a nevus sebaceous (also called organoid nevus; the word "organoid" refers to an architecture that has multiple tissue types recapitulating an organ). The appearance of a nevus sebaceous, both clinically and histologically, changes with the age of the patient. Immature hair follicles dominate in early childhood i40.4, while epidermal hyperplasia with mature sebaceous and ectopic apocrine glands is seen after puberty.

Not all forms of benign epidermal hyperplasia are verrucous. The acanthomas are a group of epidermal hyperplasias that grow inward i40.5. There are clear cell, large cell, and acantholytic acanthomas. The so-called warty dyskeratoma is a type of acantholytic acanthoma. The tumor of follicular infundibulum and the pilar sheath acanthoma are of hair follicle derivation.

Epithelial Neoplasms

A basal cell carcinoma may not be evident in the initial sections of a biopsy, so multiple levels should be considered unless there is another identifiable lesion to account for the clinical presentation. Additional levels are especially indicated if any of the following are seen on the first level: calcification, empty spaces, dermal fibrosis, or epidermal atypia in the absence of dermal sun damage [PMID10976705].

A common problem in basaloid neoplasms is the distinction of the basal cell carcinoma from other, less common basaloid neoplasms. The trichoepithelioma greatly resembles a basal cell carcinoma. Clues to its presence include papillary mesenchymal structures, basaloid cells in a frondlike arrangement, and attempts to form hair follicles i40.6a, i40.6b. A trichofolliculoma has 1 or more central follicles, which may or may not contain discernible hairs, around which are smaller vellous follicles. Expression of cytokeratin 20 favors a trichoepithelioma or trichoblastoma over BCC [PMID22112636].

A basal cell carcinoma with sebaceous differentiation (formerly called sebaceous epithelioma or sebaceoma), like any basal cell carcinoma, has minimal nuclear pleomorphism. In contrast, the rare sebaceous carcinoma has much more nuclear atypia. Most true sebaceous carcinomas occur around the eyes.

Merkel cell carcinomas are better referred to as primary cutaneous high-grade neuroendocrine carcinomas, because origin from the Merkel cell, a receptor cell found in the basal layer, has not been proven. Merkel cell carcinomas have the appearance of small cell carcinoma of the lung i40.7 and must be differentiated from a pulmonary metastasis for effective therapy. Pulmonary small cell carcinomas are positive for thyroid transcription factor-1 and negative for cytokeratin 20, while the reverse is true of Merkel cell carcinomas [PMID16625069]. In about 90% of Merkel cell carcinomas, a polyomavirus is integrated into the genome on chromosome 3 at 3p14. This integration compromises tumor suppressor activities, leading to carcinogenesis. A Merkel cell polyomavirus tumor antigen can only be detected by immunohistochemistry in 2/3 of cases but, if found, strongly suggests a Merkel cell carcinoma over a metastatic pulmonary small cell carcinoma [PMID19609205]. However, clinical correlation and radiographic examination of the chest and mediastinum remain essential.

Adnexal neoplasms are well discussed in the text by Wick and Swanson [Wick ISBN978-0891892885] and have been thoroughly reviewed [PMID16882696, PMID16882695]. An acrospiroma is a tumor of eccrine ducts. If confined to the epidermis, it is an epidermal acrospiroma. If involving both the epidermis and the dermis, it is a poroma. Poromas can resemble seborrheic keratosis, but the latter usually has a more exophytic architecture and more prominent keratin cysts than a poroma. If an acrospiroma is restricted to the dermis, it can be called a dermal acrospiroma, a dermal duct tumor, or if the cells have clear cytoplasm, a clear cell hidradenoma. In practice, these distinctions are largely academic, and a diagnosis of benign eccrine neoplasm serves the patient well i40.8.

It can be virtually impossible to distinguish a cylindroma from a spiradenoma. Indeed, both neoplasms result from a mutation in the *CYLD* gene, and some neoplasms have areas of both types [PMID21598248]. In general, the lobules of a cylindroma are irregularly shaped, like pieces in a jigsaw puzzle i40.9, whereas those of a spiradenoma tend to be rounded i40.10. In difficult situations, a lymphoid infiltrate favors a spiradenoma, as does less distinctive lobules.

Nonepithelial Neoplasms

The dermatofibroma, the dermatofibrosarcoma protuberans (DFSP), and the atypical fibroxanthoma (AFX) are related to the fibrohistiocytic family of tumors discussed in Chapter 2 but are dermal processes that are likely to be encountered and biopsied by a dermatologist and are therefore discussed here. The dermatofibroma is a superficial, benign proliferation of fibroblasts in the dermis, usually considered to be a superficial benign fibrous histiocytoma. The fibroblasts may be plump i40.11a, causing a resemblance to histiocytes, or may be small, with thin nuclei i40.11b. While dermatofibromas may be minimally infiltrative, especially on their lateral borders, where they often intermingle with collagen i40.11c, they do not infiltrate the subcutaneous adipose tissue i40.11d. Some believe that dermatofibromas are nonneoplastic reactive processes and point to their occasional spontaneous regression as evidence. But most dermatofibromas will not regress, and a neoplastic origin is generally favored.

There are numerous variants of dermatofibroma [PMID16827912], 2 of which are easy to confuse with a DFSP: the cellular dermatofibroma and the bizarre dermatofibroma. The cellular dermatofibroma i40.11e lacks significant nuclear atypia and mitoses but is primarily distinguished from the DFSP by the absence of subcutaneous invasion, whereas DFSP typically invades into the subcutaneous tissue. The dermatofibroma with rare very atypical cells, sometimes called the bizarre dermatofibroma, is distinguished from the DFSP by its confinement to the dermis.

The most common diagnostic dilemma concerning the dermatofibroma, particularly some of its variant forms, is its distinction from the DFSP. Both the dermatofibroma and the DFSP are usually composed of bland spindle cells with little pleomorphism and rare mitoses. The DFSP may have slightly more nuclear atypia and a somewhat higher mitotic activity than the dermatofibroma, but the distinction between these 2 entities resides on the presence or absence of invasion into the subcutaneous tissue, which is the hallmark of the DFSP i40.12. However, biopsies often do not include a significant amount of subcutaneous tissue, and in these situations, immunohistochemistry may be beneficial. While CD34 may stain an occasional dermatofibroma, diffuse positivity for this marker in a situation where the differential diagnosis is between a dermatofibroma and a DFSP points to the latter entity [PMID8867761]. Indeed, in cases where a DFSP occurs in deep tissue or its connection to the dermis is not apparent, CD34 positivity may be important in making the correct diagnosis and excluding other sarcomas. It must be remembered, however, that CD34 also stains solitary fibrous tumors, Kaposi sarcoma, gastrointestinal stromal tumors, and unusual lipomas, such as the pleomorphic and spindle cell types. Factor 13 stains dermatofibromas, and very few DFSP, making this is a useful additional stain in the distinction of dermatofibroma from DFSP [PMID9129699]. DFSP may also stain for bcl-2, resulting in an immunohistochemical panel for DFSP of positive for bcl-2 and CD34, and negative for factor 13, all of which are reversed in dermatofibromas.

Rare metastases of the DFSP have been noted, but the primary difference in behavior between this tumor and the dermatofibroma is the much greater propensity for local recurrence in the former if it is not widely excised. With each such recurrence, a curative procedure will require an increasingly large excision, so the prudent action is a complete excision of a DFSP upon initial diagnosis.

The AFX is a dermal tumor, generally composed of spindle cells, that has extensive nuclear pleomorphism, resembling a high-grade sarcoma **i40.13**. These are traditionally considered to be dermal manifestations of malignant fibrous histiocytomas, but some will stain positively for keratin, indicating that at least a subset of AFX is better regarded as poorly differentiated squamous cell carcinomas. AFXs are often positive for CD99 in a cell membrane pattern [PMID16972949]. There is a small metastatic potential, but local recurrence is the greater concern. The bizarre dermatofibroma may be confused with an AFX as well as with a DFSP. The important factors in the distinction of a bizarre dermatofibroma from an AFX are the more generalized nuclear atypia and greater mitotic activity in the latter neoplasm. Immunohistochemical stains, as outlined above, may be needed.

Vascular neoplasms in the skin are diagnosed essentially as in soft tissue. The great majority of vascular proliferations in the skin are benign, but the few cutaneous angiosarcomas can be subtle and are diagnosed by identifying atypia, mitotic activity, or slight crowding of the endothelial cells, or by recognizing that endothelial cells fail to form distinct vascular channels but instead infiltrate into the stroma, often along collagen fibers.

Special care should be taken in the evaluation of cutaneous vascular lesions from the breast, as the patient may have an unknown history of radiation therapy for breast carcinoma. A wide range of vascular cutaneous proliferations may occur in skin that has received radiation. Many of these are nonneoplastic postradiation vascular atypia (see **i4.72**) or cellular hemangiomas that will do well [PMID17357996], but a postradiation angiosarcoma (see **i4.73**, **i4.74**) is much more likely in these situations and must be excluded.

Urticaria pigmentosum is histologically identical to solitary mastocytoma, with large numbers of dermal mast cells, usually with eosinophils, but clinically has multiple lesions. Urticaria pigmentosum is not to be confused with simple urticaria, which may be histologically normal, since its only abnormality—edema—may be very subtle.

Amyloidosis is not a neoplastic process but may clinically simulate a neoplasm. "Amyloid" is a term applied to any protein that is deposited in a linear arrangement called antiparallel β-pleated sheet. More than 2 dozen different proteins may be deposited as amyloid, including immunoglobulins in multiple myeloma, calcitonin in thyroid medullary carcinoma, and τ protein in neurofibrillary tangles in the brain in dementia. The most common cause of amyloidosis is light chain deposition from excessive secretion by plasma cells [PMID21483018].

Amyloid is pink or gray-pink on routine H&E sections. Amyloid deposits are amorphous or waxy, and may have a cracked appearance. Amyloid usually deposits initially around small blood vessels. The traditional Congo red stain, examined under polarized light, is effective as a confirmatory technique but is technically difficult. The appearance of amyloid in H&E and Congo red is shown in thyroid medullary carcinoma (see **i6.27**, **i6.28**, **i6.29**). A thioflavin stain is easier to read and more reproducible but requires a fluorescent microscope. After amyloid is identified in the skin, it must be determined if it is a primary deposition (ie, no systemic disorder) or secondary to a systemic amyloid-depositing condition [PMID20071301].

Cutaneous Lymphoproliferative Disorders

Distinguishing benign lymphoid hyperplasias from lymphomas is as difficult in cutaneous sites as it is in other locations, and the same general rules apply. A cutaneous lymphoid infiltrate in a patient with a history of systemic lymphoma is malignant until clearly proven otherwise. A mass effect, with displacement and/or destruction of adnexal structures, suggests a lymphoma. As in other sites, reactive lymphoid infiltrates typically have a mixed population of cells, while lymphomas are often relatively monomorphic. Germinal centers, with tingible body macrophages, virtually exclude malignancy, but the observer must be sure the structure is a true germinal center and not a nodule of nodular lymphoma, and must also be wary of the possibility that there is both benign and malignant lymphoid tissue. Immunohistochemical stains are often required, and rarely, clonality studies, as described in Chapter 7, are needed.

Historically, the European Organization for the Research and Treatment of Cancer (EORTC) has proposed its own classification of cutaneous lymphomas, holding that there are sufficient differences in behavior in several entities to justify a classification different from that used by the World Health Organization (WHO) for lymphoid proliferations in other sites. After years of controversy in this matter, consensus meetings between the 2 organizations began in 2003, resulting in a joint classification system of cutaneous lymphomas published in 2005 [PMID16293178]. A good summary of and comment on this classification has also been published [PMID15692063]. The imperative in dealing with a lymphoma in the skin is to be sure it is not a cutaneous manifestation of a systemic lymphoma. If it is, then the systemic classification applies.

ISBN 978-089189-5886

Joint WHO/EORTC System for Primary Cutaneous Lymphomas

- Cutaneous T-cell and NK-cell lymphomas
- Mycosis fungoides (MF)
- MF variants and subtypes
- Folliculotropic MF
- Pagetoid reticulosis
- Granulomatous slack skin
- Sézary syndrome
- Adult T-cell leukemia/lymphoma
- Primary cutaneous CD30+ lymphoproliferative disorders
- Primary cutaneous anaplastic large cell lymphoma
- Lymphomatoid papulosis
- Subcutaneous panniculitis-like T-cell lymphoma
- Extranodal NK-/T-cell lymphoma, nasal type
- Primary cutaneous peripheral T-cell lymphoma, unspecified
- Primary cutaneous aggressive epidermotropic CD8+ T-cell lymphoma (provisional)
- Cutaneous γ/δ T-cell lymphoma (provisional)
- Primary cutaneous CD4+ small/medium-sized pleomorphic T-cell lymphoma (provisional)
- Cutaneous B-cell lymphomas
- Primary cutaneous marginal zone B-cell lymphoma
- Primary cutaneous follicle center lymphoma
- Primary cutaneous diffuse large B-cell lymphoma, leg type
- Primary cutaneous diffuse large B-cell lymphoma, other Intravascular large B-cell lymphoma
- Precursor hematologic neoplasm
- CD4+/CD56+ hematodermic neoplasm (blastic NK-cell lymphoma)

Cutaneous T-Cell Lymphoid Proliferations

Mycosis fungoides (MF) is the most common peripheral cutaneous T-cell lymphoma (PCTCL) lymphoma, accounting for about 1/2 of all cases. It is composed of CD4 positive T lymphocytes. In its early stages, MF can be very difficult to differentiate from inflammatory cutaneous conditions, even in the most experienced hands [PMID19602072]. The most helpful features are cerebriform cells singly or in small clusters in the epidermis and in the dermis. Such clusters in the epidermis are called Pautrier abscesses **i40.14**. Multiple biopsies and clinical correlation are often needed. In difficult cases, demonstration of gene rearrangement of the T-cell receptor may be necessary [PMID14671650, PMID20203005].

A folliculotropic type of MF, in which there is relative sparing of the epidermis, is recognized. Pagetoid reticulosis is a form of PCTCL with massive epidermal invasion that may be localized or generalized. If localized, it is often considered to be a form of MF, but the generalized form may not be in the MF group. Granulomatous slack skin is a very rare form of MF in which atypical CD4+ T cells are found in dermal granulomas. Sézary syndrome is a systemic manifestation of MF, with more severe skin manifestations, lymph node involvement, and circulating neoplastic cells.

Subcutaneous panniculitis-like T-cell lymphoma is a rare form of PCTCL that is often CD8 positive and that may respond well to a combination of steroids and chemotherapy [PMID18388378].

Anaplastic lymphoma and lymphomatoid papulosis are the CD30+ cutaneous lymphoproliferative disorders. Anaplastic lymphoma may be a systemic condition, as discussed in Chapter 8, or it may be restricted to the skin, in which case it is much less aggressive [PMID20669794]. 10-20% of patients with systemic anaplastic have skin involvement [PMID17511113], and the systemic form must be excluded before it is concluded that the patient has only the cutaneous form. In the skin, there is a dense dermal infiltrate of lymphocytes, sometimes extending into the subcutaneous tissue, that are usually large and atypical **i40.15a**, **i40.15b**, but as in systemic sites, small cell and monomorphic variants are recognized. Because ALK is rarely expressed in the primary cutaneous form, demonstration of CD30 positivity is critical in the diagnosis. Failure to express ALK suggests a more aggressive course in systemic anaplastic lymphoma, but this is not the case in the cutaneous form [PMID17511113].

Lymphomatoid papulosis generally has a less pronounced dermal lymphoid infiltrate than anaplastic lymphoma **i40.15c**. A dense dermal infiltrate or extension into the subcutaneous tissue is more consistent with anaplastic lymphoma. However, there is clinical and histologic overlap between these entities, and many cases cannot be placed into one or the other category and are best designated as CD30+ cutaneous lymphoproliferative disorder or lymphoid proliferations of the lymphomatoid papulosis/anaplastic lymphoma type [PMID20043512, PMID17564326]. Further supporting the association between these 2 entities is that while most cases of lymphomatoid papulosis will spontaneously regress, many cases have gene rearrangement [PMID11594579], and about 10-20% will progress to anaplastic lymphoma [PMID17124079], suggesting that lymphomatoid papulosis may be an early form of anaplastic lymphoma.

Other forms of PCTCL are more likely to be secondary to a systemic lymphoma. Adult T-cell leukemia/lymphoma (ATCL) is almost never restricted to the skin and virtually always has concomitant involvement of lymph nodes, organs, and blood.

MF and primary cutaneous CD30+ lymphoproliferative disorder are low grade, while Sézary syndrome, ATCL, and secondary involvement of the skin by systemic anaplastic lymphoma are high grade.

Precursor lesions of cutaneous T-cell lymphoma (CTCL) are semantically and histologically confusing, primarily because parapsoriasis and its variations are not clearly defined. Currently, small plaque (guttate) parapsoriasis is not considered to be neoplastic or preneoplastic. It has a superficial perivascular lymphoid infiltrate under a slightly acanthotic epidermis. There is no atypia of the lymphocytes. The histologic appearance of guttate parapsoriasis is that of a dermatitis, which it probably is [PMID17975354].

On the other hand, large plaque parapsoriasis is considered a pre-CTCL condition. In its fully developed state, large plaque parapsoriasis is characterized by epidermal thinning, a superficial perivascular and interface lymphoid infiltrate with nuclear atypia, epidermatropism, and CD4 expression in the absence of CD5 and CD7—all features of MF. Some regard large plaque parapsoriasis as early MF, an opinion supported by the finding of gene rearrangement in some cases [PMID10678699].

The joint WHO/EORTC classification lessens the controversy regarding the previously separate systems and more clearly addresses unusual entities, but many questions remain, especially in precursor lesions of CTCL and the group of CD30+ cutaneous lymphoid proliferations.

Cutaneous B-Cell Lymphoid Proliferations

Primary cutaneous B-cell lymphomas generally resemble their systemic counterparts, and can be diagnosed with the same criteria, as discussed in Chapter 8. The t(14;18) and follicular bcl-2 expression seen in most cases of systemic lymphomas of follicle center origin are usually absent in primary cutaneous follicle center lymphoma [PMID15613857]. Marginal zone lymphoma is also common in the skin and has the same characteristics as elsewhere.

There is an unusual form of B-cell cutaneous lymphoma that is clinically restricted to the leg, called primary cutaneous large B-cell lymphoma, leg type. This is a diffuse large B-cell lymphoma that is aggressive and which is likely a distinct entity [PMID20461044]. These are often treated as systemic lymphomas, even if there is no evidence of involvement of noncutaneous sites. Most cases aberrantly express both the germinal center marker bcl-6 and the postgerminal center marker MUM-1 [PMID16778825], whereas the normal lymphocyte loses its bcl-6 expression when it moves out of the germinal center and expresses MUM-1.

Melanocytic Proliferations

Nevi are often considered to be benign tumors of melanocytes, but are better thought of as hamartomas, which are nonneoplastic "overgrowths" of structures that are normally found in a site. The melanocytes in congenital nevi may surround or even infiltrate adnexal structures and often appear to infiltrate in a single file manner.

The melanocytic nuclei in the superficial portion of a benign nevus may be slightly atypical but are smaller and more uniform in the deeper portion, a process called maturation. In a melanoma, the nuclei tend not to mature but rather maintain their atypia throughout the thickness of the proliferation. Melanomas are characterized by nuclear atypia, invasion of the epidermis, increased mitotic activity, and a lack of maturation **i40.16**. However, melanomas can be very difficult to diagnose because not all of these features need be present, nor does their presence guarantee a malignant process. All of these features are commonly seen to some extent in benign pigmented lesions, and there are important considerations in the use of these criteria.

Benign melanocytic processes may have occasional extension of melanocytes into the epidermis, particularly as small groups. In most melanomas, melanocytes invade the epidermis in significant numbers, primarily as single cells. Because this results in an appearance similar to Paget disease of the nipple, this is called pagetoid invasion of the epidermis. 2 caveats must be made regarding pagetoid invasion. First, pigment in the epidermis or even in the keratin layer does not constitute pagetoid invasion and is sometimes seen in benign melanocytic lesions, especially those in sun-damaged skin. Indeed, the processes of melanocytes extend into the epidermis, so it is not surprising that benign nevi or even normal skin may have epidermal pigmentation. Although any pigment in the epidermis above a problematic melanocytic process should elicit a search for pagetoid invasion, this criterion is not met until atypical melanocytes—the whole cell, not just their processes—are found in the epidermis.

The second caveat concerning epidermal invasion is that formalin fixation often causes the cytoplasm of normal keratinocytes to contract away from the nucleus, causing the epithelial cell to resemble a melanocyte **i40.17**. One should verify that the cells involved in putative pagetoid invasion are truly melanocytes. This may require immunohistochemical stains, but it is helpful to ensure that the appearance of the nuclei of the cells in the epidermis matches that of the melanocytes in the upper dermis. Spinous connections from the cytoplasm of the putative melanocyte to adjacent cells identify it as an epithelial cell.

Mitoses are neither necessary nor sufficient for the diagnosis of melanoma and can be seen in nevi. Spitz nevi, in particular, are known to have occasional mitoses. But a large number of mitoses, especially if they are morphologically abnormal, point to a melanoma.

Gp100 (or Pmel17) is transmembrane protein necessary for the maturation of melanosomes, specifically in the maturation of stage 1 premelanosomes to stage 2 [PMID16682408, PMID16704461]. This protein, detected by the monoclonal antibody HMB-45, is present in immature or neoplastic melanocytes but not usually in mature melanocytes. Compound nevi are positive for HMB-45 in the junctional regions and minimally positive or negative in the dermal regions [PMID9242453, PMID16466507], reflecting maturation of melanocytes. Intradermal nevi are generally HMB-45 negative [PMID8506418]. Dysplastic nevi are often positive for HMB-45 [PMID2473661].

While HMB-45 is an excellent adjunct stain in the assessment of melanocytic lesions, it is not specific for melanoma because it also stains benign melanocytes that are not fully mature and often stains junctional nevi or the junctional component of compound nevi. There is no reliable panel of immunohistochemical stains that will separate a benign from a malignant melanocytic process. We are just now reaching the point where a panel of immunohistochemical stains, reflecting developments in molecular pathology, can be productively employed to assess the benign vs malignant nature of lymphoid lesions or soft tissue masses, the areas in which understanding at the molecular level is greatest. But in melanocytic proliferations, only a good interpretation of H&E stained tissue can make a diagnosis of melanoma. The principal value of immunohistochemical stains in melanomas lies in highlighting pagetoid invasion of the epidermis, identifying minute numbers of melanoma cells in sentinel lymph node examination, and in differentiating melanoma cells from other types of cells that have reparative atypia (often in a reexcision) **i40.18a**, **i40.18b**.

ISBN 978-089189-5886

Breslow introduced an absolute measurement of depth in millimeters in 1970 [PMID5477666] and, in this study, was able to recognize that melanomas with a thickness of 0.75 mm or less were associated with excellent outcomes. Even more than 40 years after Breslow's pioneering study, 0.75 mm remains a universally accepted breakpoint in prognosis. Depth measurement in millimeters is superior to Clarke leveling, which is based on boundaries in the dermis, because it is more reproducible and more clinically relevant since the dermis is of variable thickness in different body sites. For example, a Clarke level 4 melanoma (into the reticular dermis) may be much deeper on the back, where the dermis is thickest, than on the abdomen.

Many believe that melanomas should be considered low-risk if they are less than Breslow depth 0.76 mm or less. About 1.7% of melanomas of depth <0.75 mm will have nodal metastases [PMID12663722], and this number is often taken as the cutoff in determining patients who need sentinel node examination. Melanomas between 0.76 and 1.5 mm are of intermediate aggressiveness, while those >1.5 mm are high-risk.

Over the years, many prognostic factors in cutaneous melanoma in addition to depth of invasion have been considered, such as site (head and neck worse than extremities), sex (better in women than men), presence and extent of ulceration, age, and presence or absence of signs of regression (such as lymphoid reaction, fibrosis). There is continuing debate as to whether these factors are truly independent prognostic indicators or not, and many believe that absent metastases, the depth of invasion is the only clinically relevant histologic finding.

Fibrosis and a lymphoid infiltrate associated with a melanoma are considered an immune response to it and are termed "regression" **i40.19**. Regression has been considered a poor prognostic sign because the immune response that causes it only occurs after systemic exposure to the antigens of the tumor (ie, metastasis), but this has not been proven. The principal importance of regression is that it may occasionally obscure melanocytes and cause a melanoma to appear less invasive than it actually is or was at a previous time. Rarely, it may cause a melanoma to essentially disappear both clinically and histologically after a metastasis, resulting in a situation where there is metastatic melanoma without an apparent primary.

Some will factor in the Clarke level or the presence of ulceration in their prognostic algorithm or decision regarding sentinel lymph node examination. For example, Dubois et al [PMID11559220] recommend sentinel node examination if the melanoma invades to a depth of >1.0 mm and also for thinner tumors if they have either ulceration or are a Clark level 4 or higher.

There are several unusual varieties of melanoma that are diagnostically difficult [PMID16446716]. The polypoid or exophytic melanoma primarily projects above the surface, making the determination of the depth of invasion difficult. A good policy is to report a depth of invasion but to qualify that this may not have the usual meaning.

Desmoplastic melanomas may have a variety of appearances, depending on the melanocytic cellularity and density of the fibrous tissue, but they are usually spindled and may initially appear as fibromatosis, a DFSP, an AFX, a spindled squamous carcinoma, or a sarcoma **i40.20**. Fortunately, close study of a desmoplastic melanoma will usually uncover 1 or more of the following features: focal areas of more conventional melanoma, areas of melanoma in situ, focal nuclear atypia, nerve invasion, an atypical lentiginous component, or collections of lymphocytes at the periphery of the tumor. About 1/2 of desmoplastic melanomas are associated with a conventional melanoma component, but pure desmoplastic melanomas often occur in the head and neck area and have a less aggressive course [PMID20564101]. Immunohistochemistry is of limited value in identifying pure desmoplastic melanomas because they are usually negative for Melan-A (also called MART-1) and HMB-45. An S100 stain is of somewhat greater value, but does not have the sensitivity that is seen in a conventional melanoma [PMID18399807].

Before making a diagnosis of either a desmoplastic melanoma or a spindle cell melanoma, a pigmented DFSP, an AFX, and a spindle cell squamous carcinoma should be excluded, and it is in these exclusions that immunohistochemistry has greater value. DFSPs generally stain for bcl-2 and CD34. AFX is usually positive for CD10. p63 expression favors a spindle cell squamous carcinoma [PMID20184665].

The spindle cell melanoma is also composed of spindled melanocytes and is also often HMB-45 negative, but the stroma is less desmoplastic. Some believe that the desmoplastic melanoma is a type of spindle cell melanoma.

Minimal deviation melanoma is a controversial lesion that some observers do not accept as a distinct entity. It is characterized by a dermal melanocytic nodule having an expansile growth pattern. The cells are individually unremarkable but form a nodule. There may be occasional mitoses and deep infiltration, but neither the nuclear atypia nor mitotic activity is striking. The lesion is less aggressive than the depth would suggest, and the clinical course is relatively benign [PMID16446716].

Melan-A may be more sensitive and specific for melanoma than S-100 or HMB-45, and its use has been recommended in sentinel nodes for ordinary melanomas [PMID11474288]. On the other hand, lymph nodes may rarely contain benign neval cells that will be usually stain with Melan-A or S-100, but not with HMB-45. If immunohistochemical stains are used in sentinel lymph node evaluation for melanoma, S100 and Melan-A positivity without HMB-45 positivity should alert one that the putative metastasis may be a deposit of benign neval cells. In problem situations involving a known melanoma (such as sentinel node), one may need to compare the immunohistochemical profile with that of the melanoma [PMID12717252].

Re-excising melanomas that are <2 mm in thickness with initially negative margins may not be necessary, but patients with thicker melanomas may still benefit from a wider excision [PMID12361412]. There are fewer local and regional recurrences for melanomas which are 2 mm or thicker if there is a 3 cm margin instead of 1 cm, but this does not translate into a significant overall difference in survival [PMID14973217].

Dysplastic nevi are atypical melanocytic proliferations, characterized by architectural and/or cytologic atypia, that are precursors of melanoma in at least some cases [PMID20055909]. The precise relationship between melanomas and dysplastic nevi remains disputed, but there is agreement that melanomas pass through some stage of intermediate histologic appearance in their evolution. Dysplastic nevi may be junctional or compound, but not purely intradermal, and the key histologic features are in the junctional component. Dysplastic nevi have asymmetry of the junctional component, bridging from one melanocytic nest to an adjacent nest, fibrosis of the papillary dermis, and if the nevus is compound, the junctional component usually extends beyond the dermal component **i40.21a**, **i40.21b**. In dysplastic nevi, a rare melanocyte may be found in the epidermis, but significant pagetoid invasion is not generally seen.

Some degree of interobserver variation in the precise observations and descriptions is to be expected in dysplastic nevi. The presence or absence of nuclear atypia should be specifically noted, and is the basis for a 2-tiered reporting system of low-grade and high-grade dysplasia that some employ for these nevi. The important points are to ensure complete removal and a surveillance of the site.

To my mind, melanoma in situ is overdiagnosed because too much reliance is placed on melanocytic hyperplasia at the dermal-epidermal junction, and not enough emphasis is given to nuclear atypia. Normal sun-damaged skin may have up to 15 to 20 melanocytes at the dermal-epidermal junction per high-power field (0.5 mm in diameter), vs 5 to 7 melanocytes in skin that has not been chronically exposed to sun. Benign sun-damaged skin may also have confluence of melanocytes. Up to 9 melanocytes may be adjacent, and there may also be extension along hair follicles [PMID16847203]. Nuclear atypia and pagetoid epidermal invasion remain essential features of conventional melanoma in situ **i40.22a**, **i40.22b**.

A similar situation exists for lentigo maligna, a form of melanoma in situ that is found in sun-damaged skin. Lentigo maligna differs from conventional melanoma in situ primarily in having a confluent row of atypical melanocytes at the dermal-epidermal junction without significant epidermal invasion. To my mind, this form of melanoma in situ is also often overdiagnosed because the extent of melanocytic hyperplasia and confluence in benign, sun-exposed skin is often not appreciated. For the diagnosis of lentigo maligna, the melanocytes must be clearly and significantly increased in number, they must be confluent to a greater extent than is seen in normal sun-damaged skin, and most of all, they must have nuclear atypia **i40.23**.

The pathologist should remember that a diagnosis of melanoma in situ or lentigo maligna will be perceived by the patient and his or her insurance company as a cancer diagnosis. This is highly likely to cause unnecessary anxiety for a patient who does not understand the difference between in situ and invasive processes, and who is not at risk for metastatic disease. Moreover, insurance companies have no understanding of the biologic potential of an in situ lesion, and once a patient is labeled with a "cancer" diagnosis, he or she will likely have great difficulty obtaining health or life insurance. Any malignant diagnosis, including that of an in situ lesion, should be made only if it is clear that the lesion has the potential to metastasize. For cases in which metastasis will not occur, such as in situ lesions, a diagnosis of atypical melanocytic hyperplasia or a dysplastic nevus, followed by a recommendation for complete excision and surveillance, accomplishes every legitimate objective of the examination and frees the patient from these added difficulties. The proper role of the pathologist in these situations is to verify the absence of invasion and comment on the status of the margins. It is also prudent to add a comment that if this is a biopsy of a larger lesion, invasive melanoma cannot be excluded in a location in the lesion that was not biopsied, and excision is recommended.

Any practicing pathologist would be hard-pressed to find any differential diagnosis that is more difficult than that between a Spitz nevus and a melanoma. There are a number of types of Spitz nevus [PMID17388217, PMID21549244], of which the most common is the epithelioid form. Other forms include the pigmented spindle cell nevus, the plexiform spindle cell nevus, the hyalinizing Spitz nevus, and the desmoplastic Spitz nevus. Different types may occur together in the same lesion.

The cells in the epithelioid variety of Spitz nevus are generally large, with large nuclei and often, prominent nucleoli. However, they are relatively uniform **i40.24a**, **i40.24b**, and if the observer subtracts the nucleoli in the mind's eye, the cells are not truly pleomorphic in the way that those of a melanoma are. There may be mitotic activity but usually only in the upper portion. Epidermal invasion, if any, is usually in the form of small clusters and rarely as single cells (ie, true pagetoid invasion is rare). Spitz nevi are generally symmetric and have some degree of maturation, meaning there is less melanocyte atypia in the deeper portion, whereas maturation is usually lacking in melanomas. Multinucleated cells may be seen in benign or malignant melanocytic processes, but are more common in Spitz nevi than in melanomas. An eosinophilic or ground glass appearance in the cytoplasm, and polygonal cells are features that are seen more often in Spitz nevi than in melanomas. In addition, almost 90% of melanomas have marked thinning of the epidermis at some point, whereas only 10% of Spitz nevi have this feature [PMID15577682]. A Spitz nevus may have eosinophilic globules (Kamino bodies) and artifactual separation of nests of melanocytes in the papillary dermis from the overlying epidermis **i40.24c**, though I have not found these features useful in my practice.

All of this having been said, however, it is important to note that there are cases in which the distinction of a Spitz nevus from a melanoma is simply not possible. For this reason, it has been my policy to recommend a complete excision and surveillance of the area in any lesion considered to be a Spitz nevus. Indeed, 2 of the patients in the original study by Sophie Spitz [PMID18859360] died of metastatic melanoma. Likewise, if there is any atypia in a Spitz nevus or any possibility of a melanoma, sentinel lymph node examination should be strongly considered. The morbidity of reexcision and sentinel node study pales beside the consequences of an untreated melanoma. Patients are often best served by a willingness to admit imperfect knowledge. Good pathologists become confident that they can reliably distinguish between a melanoma and a Spitz nevus. Great pathologists know this is often impossible.

The presence of melanocytes in a sentinel node removed for a presumed Spitz nevus does not necessarily change the diagnosis to melanoma, as cells from a Spitz nevus (and rarely, other melanocytic processes) may travel to a regional node without ill effects [PMID19123453].

The blue nevus is characterized by spindled, deeply pigmented melanocytes in the dermis. The cellular blue nevus is a different entity that is often found on the lower back. Cellular blue nevi have fascicles of nonpigmented spindle cells intermingled with isolated pigmented spindle cells **i40.25**. If cross-sectioned, these nonpigmented cells will appear as

ISBN 978-089189-5886

nodules. Cellular blue nevi may extend into the subcutaneous tissue. The atypical blue nevus overlaps with the cellular blue nevus, without universally accepted criteria for differentiation between the 2, though nuclear pleomorphism and mitotic activity are likely to engender a diagnosis of atypical blue nevus among most experienced pathologists [PMID21366456]. The cellularity, mild atypia, apparent lack of maturation, and extension into the subcutaneous tissue are alarming features.

The deep-penetrating nevus, described in 1989 [PMID2909196], may extend from the dermal-epidermal junction to, and into, the subcutaneous tissue. It may have spindled or epithelioid cells. While moderate nuclear atypia with small nucleoli may occasionally be seen, minimal nuclear atypia is the rule. There will generally be few mitoses and no epidermal invasion. The deep-penetrating nevus is well demarcated and circumscribed, and is often symmetrical. An important clue is that the cells often extend along adnexa [PMID21366455].

Compared to benign melanocytic proliferations, melanomas may have chromosomal abnormalities such as losses of 6q, 8p, 9p, and 10q, and they may also have copy number increases in 1q, 6p, 7, 8q, 17q, and 20q. Abnormalities of 6q23 and 11q13 appear most specific [PMID19561450]. There is hope that assistance in difficult cases may be forthcoming from FISH probes, but at this writing, FISH testing for chromosomal aberrations either has not added significantly to H&E interpretation [PMID20081813] or has only provided support for a malignant diagnosis if the H&E was suggestive [PMID21151100]. The Val600Glu in the *BRAF* oncogene (V600E) is found in a minority of cases of melanoma, as it is in some cases of papillary thyroid carcinoma and colon carcinoma. It may be important to identify this subgroup since there is now an inhibitor of the Braf enzyme (vemurafenib) [PMID21802280].

The definitive distinction of Spitz nevi, cellular or atypical blue nevi, and deep-penetrating nevi from melanoma is often impossible, even among the most experienced observers. Indeed, there is only moderate agreement in this area among so-called "experts" [PMID8666360], as is the case for numerous other diagnostically difficult situations, such as intraductal breast proliferations, follicular lesions of the thyroid, and the distinction of small cell from non-small cell carcinomas of the lung. Because of the great difficulty and interobserver variation in the distinction of Spitz nevi, atypical or cellular blue nevi, and deep-penetrating nevi from melanoma, and because there are examples of these tumors that are indolent even in the face of regional lymph node metastases, the proposal has been made that these entities be grouped under the label of melanocytic tumors of uncertain malignant potential [PMID20118771]. To my mind, this conception has appreciable merit and should be adopted until the situation is clarified by molecular techniques. There is ample precedent in many other body sites for a category of tumors of indeterminate potential, and it is time to acknowledge that there is a group of melanocytic lesions for which perfect prognostication is simply not possible.

A final comment on the difficult and evolving area of pigmented lesions is that frozen section en face evaluation (Mohs) is problematic for any melanocytic lesion and is not good for margins of melanocytic processes [PMID12931550].

Inflammatory Skin Lesions (Dermatoses)

No attempt is made here to provide a thorough discussion of inflammatory skin lesions, only to provide a brief overview of those dermatoses that are commonly encountered in general practice. For a thorough discussion, the reader is referred to the time-honored Lever textbook [Elder ISBN978-0781773638]. The convenient and useful listing of the major features and the corresponding differential diagnoses that Dr Ackerman compiled in his large textbook [Ackerman ISBN978-1893357259] is also recommended, and more recently, a similar approach based on the type and location of the inflammation has been offered [PMID18418089, PMID18948765]. The goal here is simply to introduce the basic patterns of inflammation and to offer a simple approach to the biopsy of an inflammatory skin condition.

It is rarely possible in a biopsy from an inflammatory skin condition to render a definitive diagnosis, as many dermatoses have similar histologic appearances and a precise diagnosis requires clinical correlation. The pathologist should strive to render a good differential diagnosis from which the dermatologist can select the entity that most closely matches the clinical situation. More than for any other tissue type, a back-and-forth dialogue between the pathologist and the dermatologist may be needed to reach the best diagnosis, as the correct diagnosis—the best match between the clinical and histologic appearances—may be the second choice for both the pathologist and dermatologist, or the pathologist's third choice and the dermatologist's first choice.

More than other processes in other body sites, inflammatory cutaneous lesions evolve with time and may have different histologic appearances depending on when in their course the biopsy was taken, a concept developed by Dr Ackerman [Ackerman ISBN978-0893520953]. If the clinician biopsies an older lesion, the characteristic histologic findings may no longer be specific. If a traumatized lesion is biopsied, the superimposed changes of the trauma will obscure the basic process. Clinicians should be encouraged to biopsy the newest, most pristine, and undisturbed lesions, because these afford the greatest chance for specific histologic findings.

The most important clinical point is whether the lesion is single or one of a small number on the one hand, vs a generalized eruption on the other. Inflammatory skin lesions that are clinically significant usually present with a multiple lesions. The pathologist should have a passing familiarity with dermatologic terms to allow him or her to understand the extent of the process on the patient. For example, patches and macules refer to flat areas; a patch is large macule.

An extremely important technique in assessing inflammatory skin lesions is to get multiple levels. Multiple levels often expose the point of origin of the inflammation or reveal a key diagnostic finding that is not present on other levels. More than any other situation in surgical pathology, numerous levels are important in the evaluation of inflammatory skin disorders.

The key questions to ask when approaching a cutaneous inflammatory biopsy are "What?" and "Where?" What are the cell types involved in the inflammatory reaction, and where are they located? Unlike other sites, the skin usually does not react to acute inflammation with neutrophils. Rather, lymphocytes are most commonly seen from the beginning. Neutrophils and eosinophils are seen in special situations, and their presence immediately calls into play specific diagnostic possibilities, including fungi, superimposed scratching, and the psoriasiform disorders.

Locations include the keratin layer, the epidermis, the junction of the epidermis and the dermis, around the blood vessels of the superficial dermis, around the vessels of both the superficial and deep dermis, interstitial (between rather than around blood vessels), around adnexal structures, and in the subcutaneous adipose tissue. The differential diagnosis is constructed from a stepwise assessment of the number and type of each inflammatory cell in each of these locations.

A shave biopsy for an inflammatory skin condition is almost sure to be futile because it does not have the depth necessary to show the distribution of inflammation. A punch biopsy is required. A 2 mm punch biopsy is unlikely to demonstrate all of the structures (hair follicles, sweat glands, etc) that may be involved in the process, and is also unlikely to permit the recognition of a recognizable pattern. A 4 mm punch biopsy is better and usually adequate, but a larger punch or even an incisional biopsy may be needed in a panniculitis or a lymphoproliferative disorder.

Acute and Chronic Dermatitis

Acute and Chronic Dermatitis with Epidermal Changes

Acute contact dermatitis is characterized by edema of the epidermis (spongiosis) i40.26. While edema is a hallmark of acute inflammation anywhere, another important hallmark of acute inflammation, neutrophils, are usually absent in acute dermatitis. If the acute contact dermatitis is of allergic origin, eosinophils may be identified, both in the epidermis and in the dermis. In acute contact dermatitis caused by irritation or direct toxicity rather than via an immune-mediated process, dyskeratotic or damaged keratinocytes may be found in the epidermis.

Photoallergic dermatitis, also called photocontact dermatitis, is a type of contact dermatitis caused by a hypersensitivity response to UV light, usually in conjunction with a sensitizing agent (often a drug). Extreme cases, in which there is epidermal damage, are called phototoxic reactions.

With increasing chronicity in a dermatitis, the rete pegs elongate and parakeratosis develops. Elongation of rete pegs is a much more reliable indicator of chronicity, as parakeratosis may develop a day or 2 after exposure because of the rapid turnover of the epidermis. The classic example of a well developed chronic dermatitis is psoriasis, which has extensive and relatively uniform elongation of the rete pegs, with fusion at their lower borders i40.27a. Psoriasis and related disorders typically have neutrophils both in the epidermis and in the parakeratotic layers (Munro abscesses) i40.27b, an exception to the general rule that neutrophils are rare in cutaneous inflammation (paradoxically, these chronic cutaneous inflammations are one of the few occasions in which large numbers of neutrophils may be found in the skin).

Lichen simplex chronicus is a chronic dermatitis that is usually caused by trauma or irritation of a preexisting condition. It has irregular elongation of the rete pegs, in contrast to the uniform elongation seen in psoriasis, and also demonstrates an unusual kind of fibrosis of the papillary dermis wherein the collagen fibers are perpendicular to the epidermis, running parallel between the elongated rete pegs i40.28.

There are numerous examples of so-called subacute dermatitis, with a histologic picture intermediate between acute and chronic dermatitis. Most cases of seborrheic dermatitis and the confusing group of disorders called "eczema" fall into the category of subacute dermatitis. In subacute dermatitis, there is a mild or uneven elongation of the rete pegs and inconstant fusion of the rete pegs in their basal portions. Neutrophils are rare and spongiosis is minimal i40.29. Pityriasis rosea is a subacute dermatitis that often has dermal microhemorrhage and discrete mounds of parakeratosis.

Acute and Chronic Dermatitis without Epidermal Changes

In cases where the epidermal changes do not provide a diagnosis, as they often do in acute contact dermatitis or in psoriasis, the type and distribution of dermal inflammatory cells is the primary mechanism for the construction of a differential diagnosis. Major patterns include a lymphocytic infiltrate around the vessels of the superficial dermis, a lymphocytic infiltrate around vessels of both the superficial and deep dermis, a mixed infiltrate that may include eosinophils or neutrophils, and a predominance of lymphocytes at the dermal-epidermal junction rather than around dermal vessels. The following synopses are based on commonly accepted patterns [Ackerman ISBN978-1893357259, PMID18418089, PMID18948765, PMID16311340].

A common pattern is perivascular lymphoid inflammation around the superficial blood vessels i40.30. This pattern is seen in conditions such as:

Superficial perivascular lymphoid inflammation

- Viral exanthems
- Pigmented purpuras
- Erythema annulare centrifugum (a poorly understood entity that is also called gyrate or figurate erythema)
- Drug eruption
- Urticarial reactions
- Arthropod bites/stings.
- Subacute dermatitis without diagnostic epidermal changes

If there are also eosinophils, then drug eruptions, urticarial reactions, and arthropod assault become more likely, and several other possibilities should also be considered:

Superficial perivascular lymphoid inflammation with eosinophils

- Drug eruption
- Urticarial reactions
- Arthropod assault
- Bullous pemphigoid that is not yet vesicular
- Pruritic urticarial papules and plaques of pregnancy if the patient is pregnant
- Allergic contact dermatitis without epidermal changes

If there is superficial perivascular lymphoid inflammation with plasma cells, additional considerations include:

ISBN 978-089189-5886

Superficial perivascular inflammation with plasma cells

- Rosacea
- Secondary syphilis
- Patch stage of Kaposi sarcoma
- Erythema chronicum migrans, a cutaneous manifestation of Lyme disease

Dermatoses that have perivascular lymphoid infiltrates around both the superficial and deep vascular dermal vessels are often clinically more serious. Dermatoses in this group include:

Superficial and deep perivascular inflammation

- Polymorphous light eruption
- The inflammatory stage of scleroderma
- So-called Jessner infiltration (an enigmatic entity that some believe to be related to lupus)
- So-called deep form of erythema annulare centrifugum

A distribution of inflammatory cells that is typically seen in dermatoses is a lichenoid (also called interface) distribution, in which large numbers of lymphocytes are found at the dermal-epidermal junction, forming a linear band in this location. Lichen planus is the prototype entity in this group of disorders **i40.31a**. The lichenoid inflammation is almost always associated with some degree of perivascular lymphoid infiltrate below this band, and often with vacuolar change or loss of the basal layer of the epidermis **i40.31b**, but the dense lymphoid infiltrate at the dermal-epidermal junction is characteristic of this group of disorders, which include:

Lichenoid inflammation

- Lichen planus
- Autoimmune disorders such as lupus and dermatomyositis
- Acute radiation dermatitis
- Erythema multiforme
- Drug eruption
- Lichen sclerosis et atrophicus
- Graft vs host disease

Bullous/Vesicular Disorders

The observational imperatives in addressing bullous disorders are the location of the vesicle and the nature of any associated inflammatory cells.

Autoimmune Subepidermal Bullous Disorders

In the autoimmune-mediated group, direct immunofluorescent studies are often very helpful, as these reveal the type and location of immunoglobulin and complement proteins that have been deposited.

The lesions of fully developed bullous pemphigoid have subepidermal blisters that contain large numbers of eosinophils **i40.32**, but in its early stages, prior to the blister, there may be an intact epidermis with an eosinophilic infiltrate at the dermal-epidermal junction. In direct immunofluorescent studies, there is linear deposition of C3 at the basement membrane in essentially all cases and also of IgG in most cases. Linear deposition of C3d is almost always seen and is very helpful in the exclusion of other bullous disorders [PMID19863700]. Pemphigoid gestationis (formerly called herpes gestationalis) is a rare autoimmune disorder of pregnancy characterized by pruritic blisters [PMID21163161]. Histologically, it is indistinguishable from bullous pemphigoid and requires the proper clinical setting for the diagnosis.

Subepidermal bullae associated with large numbers of neutrophils are seen in dermatitis herpetiformis **i40.33a**, **i40.33b**, an autoimmune disorder that is associated with celiac disease. Direct immunofluorescence usually reveals granular IgA deposition at the tips of the dermal papillae. Subepidermal bullae are also seen in epidermolysis bullosa.

The pemphigus group demonstrates acantholysis—breakup of the epidermis from disruption of the normal intercellular connections—rather than a distinct vesicle **i40.34**. These disorders are characterized by IgG autoantibodies against proteins that are important in intercellular connections in the epidermis, and direct immunofluorescence will usually demonstrate IgG deposition between cells. Pemphigus foliaceus and pemphigus erythematosus have acantholysis in the high epidermis, usually in the granular layer. Pemphigus vulgaris, pemphigus vegetans, and paraneoplastic pemphigus have a greater degree of acantholysis, involving the lower portion of the epidermis. Extension of acantholysis into follicular infundibula is virtually diagnostic of pemphigus vulgaris.

Nonautoimmune Bullous Disorders

In addition to these immune-mediated bullous disorders, there are a variety of skin lesions that may have vesicles. Keratosis follicularis (Darier disease) is a generalized eruption, characterized by an unusual manifestation of dyskeratosis. There are corps ronds, dyskeratotic cells in the granular layer (they are basophilic and have a halo) and grains, large parakeratotic cells in the keratin layer **i40.35a**, **i40.35b**. Darier disease is caused by a mutation in the *ATP2A2* gene, which codes for a calcium pump that is associated with an ATPase. This calcium pump is apparently necessary for the cell signaling and differentiation needed to create effective cell-to-cell adhesion. Warty dyskeratoma is a single lesion with an appearance that is very similar to one of the lesions in Darier disease.

Transient acantholytic dermatosis (Grover disease) is a multifocal acantholytic process characterized by suprabasal clefts and acantholysis. The disorder is usually self-limiting, and individual lesions come and go. There are several patterns, one of which resembles Darier disease, with corp ronds and grains. Other patterns resemble pemphigus or spongiotic dermatitis. A clue to the diagnosis of Grover disease is that different lesions may show different subtypes. For example, one lesion may resemble Darier and another pemphigus.

Focal acantholytic dyskeratosis (FAD) is a single lesion or a small number of lesions with simple histologic findings to Grover disease. There is acantholysis without corp ronds or grains, significant numbers of inflammatory cells, or deposition of immunoglobulin or complement. FAD is sometimes idiopathic, but many cases are simply an acantholytic actinic keratosis.

Stasis Dermatitis

Stasis changes may be the primary reason for the biopsy but are also commonly encountered as a secondary finding in biopsies that demonstrate another process, such as a neoplasm. Stasis dermatitis is seen mostly on the legs of older patients or those with peripheral vascular disease. It is characterized by mild epidermal hyperplasia, increased dermal capillaries, dermal fibrosis, and a perivascular lymphoid infiltrate i40.36. Extravasated erythrocytes are common and hemosiderin macrophages may be seen.

Other Autoimmune Disorders of the Skin

The 3 most common autoimmune disorders that are likely to receive skin biopsies are scleroderma (progressive systemic sclerosis; called morphea in its localized form), lupus, and dermatomyositis [PMID11094633]. In the acute phase of scleroderma/morphea, there is a dermal lymphoplasmacytic infiltrate that is perivascular and interstitial in the dermis i40.37a. In its chronic phase, inflammation is less pronounced, and there is dermal fibrosis i40.37b. This fibrosis blurs the normal distinction between the looser papillary dermis and the denser reticular dermis, and also encroaches on the adventitial dermis, resulting in adnexal structures that are closely surrounded by dense collagen instead of the looser adventitial dermis and adipose tissue that is normally seen [PMID18460891].

There are many morphologic manifestations of lupus, but one of the most common is a lichenoid infiltrate at the dermal-epidermal junction, with extension around adnexal structures and keratin plugging of hair follicles i40.38. The epidermis may be atrophic, with vacuolar change at in the basal layer. A thickened basement membrane is commonly seen. The histologic changes of dermatomyositis are nearly identical to those seen in lupus, requiring clinical correlation for their distinction [PMID19155727].

Infectious and Granulomatous Conditions of the Skin

A number of viruses, especially herpes, are found in the skin, but the most common infectious cutaneous disorders involve bacteria and fungi (dermatophytes). In both of these conditions, neutrophils are common, and the finding of neutrophils in either the epidermis or in the keratin layer should elicit a search for infectious organisms. A fungal stain is prudent in any dermatitis with neutrophils that is not clearly a member of the psoriasis family or in any apparent psoriasiform disorder that does not respond to treatment.

A number of infectious and noninfectious disorders are manifest as granulomatous dermatitis. Granuloma annulare is characterized by lymphocytes and macrophages insinuated between dermal collagen fibers, with punctate foci of damage to the fibers i40.39a. Overt granulomas are often absent. An important diagnostic feature is the presence of acidic mucopolysaccharides, detectable with colloidal iron or alcian blue stain at pH 2.5 i40.39b. The process is usually centered in the dermis, but the deep (subcutaneous) form of granuloma annulare is diagnostically challenging. Dermatofibromas that have an appreciable histiocytic component may also simulate granuloma annulare, but will be more discrete, with a mass effect, and without acidic mucopolysaccarides.

Granulomatous conditions in any body site are among the most frustrating entities in pathology because the etiology can rarely be established with certainty. Special stains are almost always negative and cultures are rarely informative. It is wise to obtain multiple levels of the process to exclude obvious etiologies such as ruptured inclusion cysts. Once this is done, examination with polarized light may reveal birefringent material, likely of foreign origin, that may provide an explanation. If these measures, and special stains for acid fast bacilli and fungi, have been performed and found to be negative, it may be beneficial to extend testing to the DNA level, as there are now nucleic acid tests that are more sensitive than the older cytochemical stains.

If these tests are all negative, an infectious etiology is not completely excluded, but additional diagnostic considerations include cutaneous sarcoid, necrobiosis lipoidica diabeticorum, and rheumatoid nodules. Sarcoid is a diagnosis of exclusion made after all of the above measures have failed to render a specific etiology, but this diagnosis simply pushes the problem back a step since the pathogenesis of sarcoid is unknown. The diagnosis of necrobiosis lipoidica diabeticorum should be restricted to those patients known to have, or who can be subsequently shown to have, diabetes mellitus. Likewise, the diagnosis of rheumatoid nodule is best made in patients with either seropositive rheumatoid disease or compelling clinical or radiographic evidence of rheumatoid arthritis. In most cases of granulomatous dermatitis, even the most thorough workup usually leaves both the pathologist and the clinician tired, uninformed, and frustrated.

The Panniculitis Conditions

Probably the most confusing group of cutaneous inflammatory disorders are the so-called panniculitis conditions, inflammations that are primarily centered the subcutaneous adipose tissue.

The first step in addressing a panniculitis is to determine the precise site or sites of inflammation. Only those cases that are primary in the subcutaneous tissue should be included in the group of panniculitis. Cases that have "downward spillover" of inflammation from the dermis or an "upward spillover" from the fascia are not a true panniculitis and should not be included this group. Primary panniculitis is divided into septal and lobular forms, the former centered on the fibrous septae that divide the adipose tissue into lobules, and latter centered on the adipose tissue.

The simplest of the panniculitis conditions, and the only one that is not usually a diagnostic conundrum, is erythema nodosum. The histologic findings in well developed cases of erythema nodosum consist of thickened fibrous septae, with chronic inflammation, in the subcutaneous tissue i40.40, with relative sparing of the fat itself. There may be acute inflammatory cells in the early stages [PMID18793974]. While erythema nodosum has been associated with infections, malignancy, and even pregnancy, it appears to be fundamentally autoimmune.

ISBN 978-089189-5886

Panniculitis involving the adipose tissue in the lobule is more difficult to classify. Most lobular panniculitis in adults is secondary to autoimmune disorders, vasculitis, or ischemia. Excluding these entities histologically and working with the clinician to do the same are usually more important than a precise diagnosis. Weber-Christian panniculitis has long been the archetype of subcutaneous inflammation that is centered on the adipose tissue, but this disorder appears to encompass multiple entities, and this term is rarely used now. Nodular vasculitis (formerly called erythema induratum) classically involves both the septae and the adipose tissue, but the inflammation is primarily lobular and this process is now understood to be a vasculitis.

The important points in addressing a panniculitis are to ensure that the process is truly centered in the subcutaneous tissue, to exclude erythema nodosum, and to exclude vasculitis, autoimmune disorders, and ischemia.

Core Points for the Skin

- Benign epidermal hyperplasia: general term for nonspecific epidermal hyperplasia without dysplasia.
  - Usually exophytic, but may be endophytic (acanthoma).
- Epithelial neoplasms: separate those that with local recurrence potential (eg, basal cell carcinoma and most neoplasms of adnexal origin) from those with metastatic potential.
- Mesenchymal processes: dermal, cutaneous counterparts to low-grade soft tissue lesions.
  - Atypical fibroxanthoma, the juvenile xanthogranuloma, the dermatofibroma (DF), and the dermatofibrosarcoma protuberans (DFSP).
- Distinction of dermatofibroma from DFSP: immunohistochemistry may help, but DFSP infiltrates fat and DF does not.
- Vascular neoplasms: malignancy indicated by atypia or mitotic activity of the endothelial cells, infiltration, or poor formation of vascular channels.
  - Vascular processes on breast may be secondary to unknown history of radiation therapy.
- Lymphoproliferative disorders: mycosis fungoides (MF) is low grade.
  - Early stages of MF closely resemble inflammatory processes.
  - Anaplastic lymphoma and lymphomatoid papulosis are primary cutaneous CD30+ lymphoproliferative disorders and have overlapping features.
  - Isolated cutaneous anaplastic lymphoma is often ALK– and indolent.
- Dysplastic nevi: architectural asymmetry and/or cytologic atypia
- Melanomas:
  - Nuclear atypia
  - Pagetoid invasion
  - Increased mitotic activity
  - Persistence of atypia into the deeper portion of the proliferation.
  - Immunohistochemistry is helpful, but not diagnostic.
- 0.75 mm is a relatively accepted prognostic "breakpoint" in melanomas.
- Unusual varieties of melanoma include desmoplastic and spindle cell types.
- Spitz nevus, the cellular blue nevus, and the deep penetrating nevus have some features of melanoma. Consensus opinion often impossible, even among "experts."
  - Proposal to place these problematic entities into a category of melanocytic tumors of uncertain malignant potential.
- Inflammatory skin disorders: often have similar histologic appearances, requiring a "best fit" between the clinical and histologic appearances.
  - Appearance changes with time and subject to superimposed trauma, so that the "classic" appearance may not be seen in a particular situation.
  - 4 mm punch biopsy of newest lesions is best for diagnosis.
  - Diagnosis centers on epidermal changes (spongiosis in acute dermatitis and rete peg elongation in chronic dermatitis) and type and distribution of inflammatory cells in the dermis.
- Bullous (blistering) disorders: often of autoimmune etiology.
  - May require direct immunofluorescence
- Vasculitis is often secondary
- Primary vasculitis:
  - Acute inflammation in the wall of the vessel that exceeds that of surrounding areas
  - Necrosis of the wall of the vessel
  - Fibrin microthrombi
  - Endothelial damage
  - Neutrophilic debris
  - Most common group of primary cutaneous vasculitis is small vessel type
  - Like all cutaneous inflammatory conditions, vasculitis evolves, and no single histologic picture is to be expected at all times.

i40.1 Normal skin illustrating the extension of the epidermis downward into the dermis (rete pegs), the more delicate collagen of the papillary dermis between the rete pegs, and the denser collagen of the reticular dermis, in the lower right.

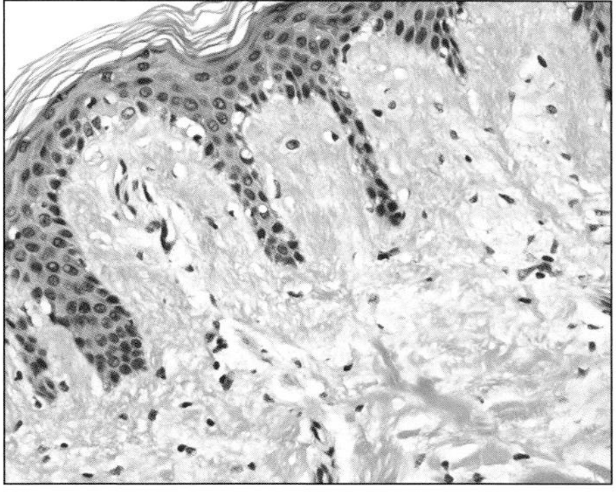

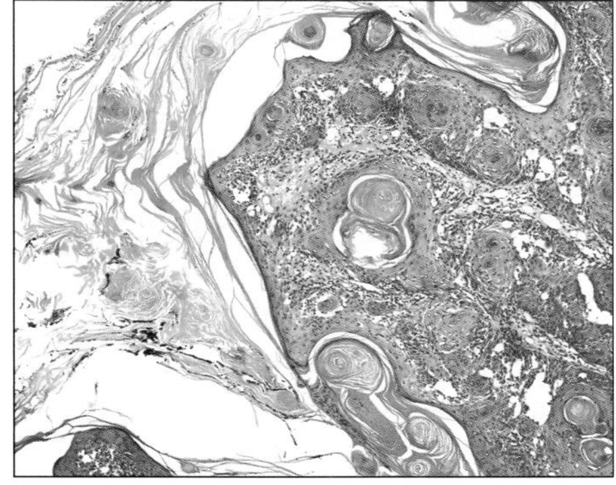

i40.2 A seborrheic keratosis. This common form of epidermal hyperplasia is characterized in most cases by an exophytic growth pattern and often by keratin cysts which are enclosed by squamous epithelium, as seen here.

i40.3 A verruca vulgaris. This form of benign epidermal hyperplasia usually has papillomatosis and can resemble a seborrheic keratosis. Not all verrucae have viral cytopathic effect, but in this example, there is prominent perinuclear clearing, characteristic of viral effect. There is a prominent granular layer except in foci where there is parakeratosis.

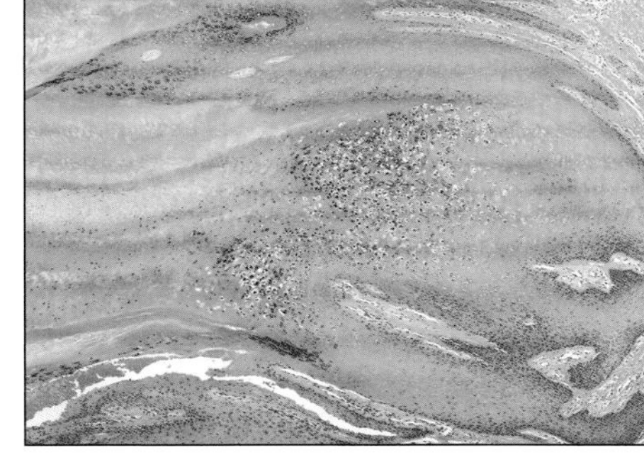

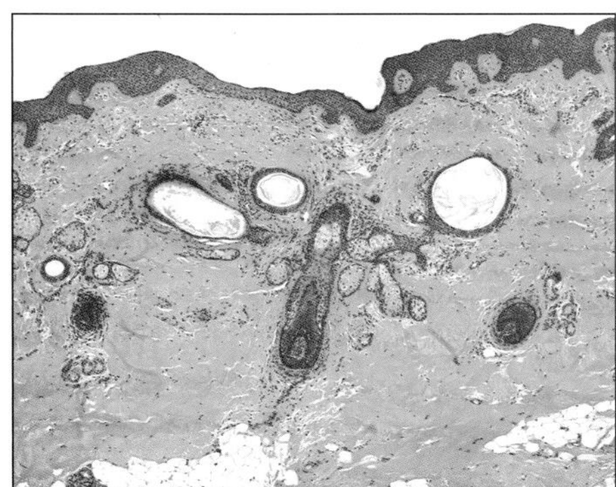

i40.4 A nevus sebaceous in a young child. Note the poorly developed pilosebaceous unit.

i40.5 An acanthoma, a group of epidermal hyperplasias with an endophytic growth pattern

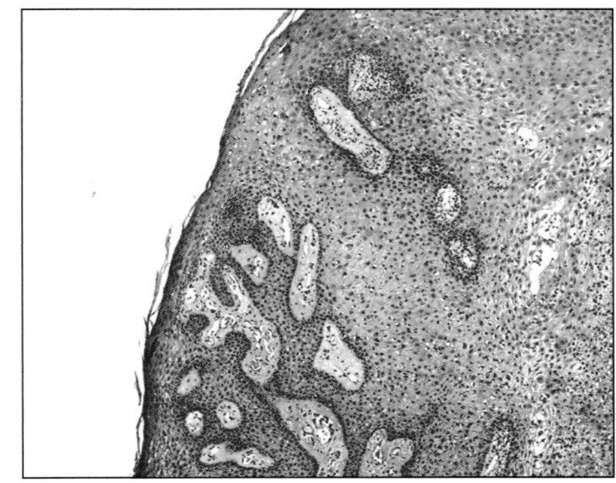

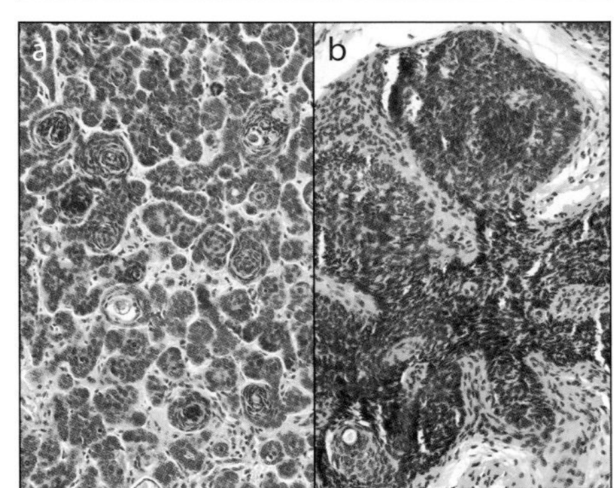

i40.6 a A trichoepithelioma. Although the neoplasm resembles a basal cell carcinoma, immature or incompletely formed hair follicles are evident. **b** A trichoepithelioma demonstrating an obvious attempt to form a hair follicle

i40.7 A Merkel cell carcinoma (primary cutaneous high-grade neuroendocrine carcinoma). Note the striking similarity to a small cell carcinoma of the lung, but the 2 neoplasms have different immunohistochemical and molecular characteristics. This neoplasm was positive for cytokeratin 20 and negative for thyroid transcription factor-1.

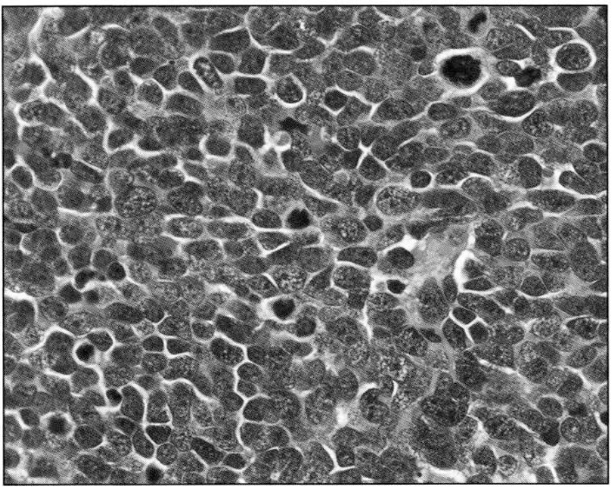

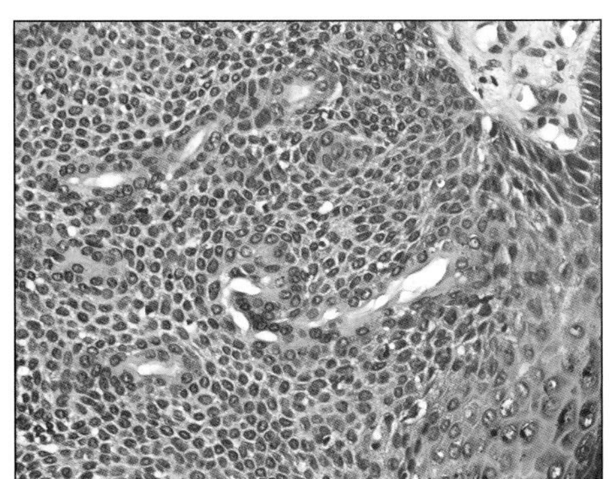

i40.8 A benign neoplasm arising from eccrine sweat ducts. Note the small gland-like structures lined by cells with distinctly eosinophilic apical cytoplasm (eccrine cuticles).

i40.9 A cylindroma with irregularly shaped clusters of tumor cells fitting together like pieces of a jigsaw puzzle

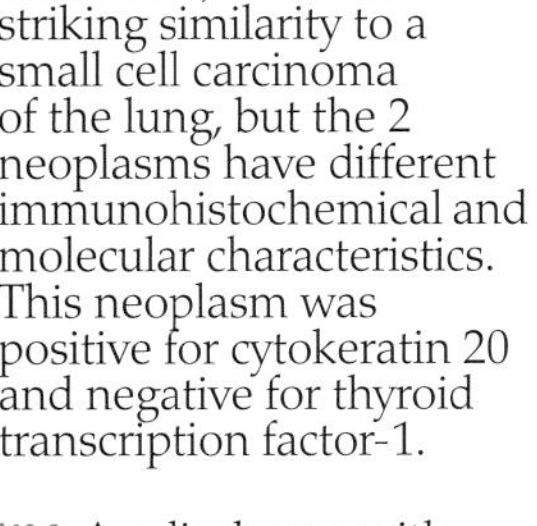

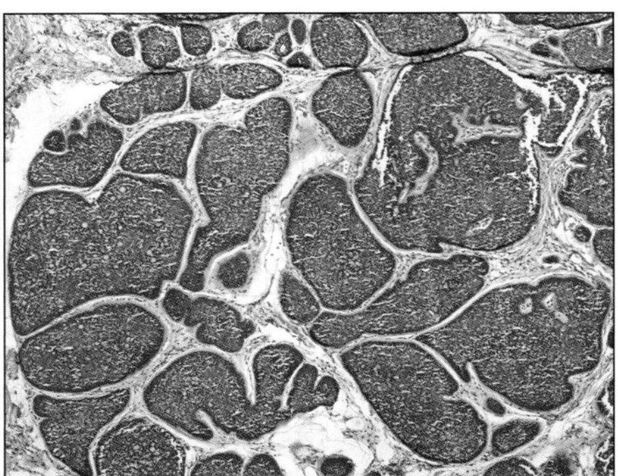

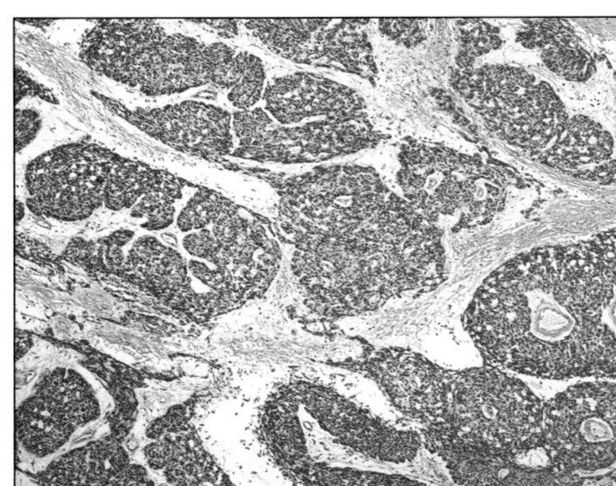

i40.10 An eccrine spiradenoma with more rounded clusters that are not as contiguous as the clusters in a cylindroma

ISBN 978-089189-5886

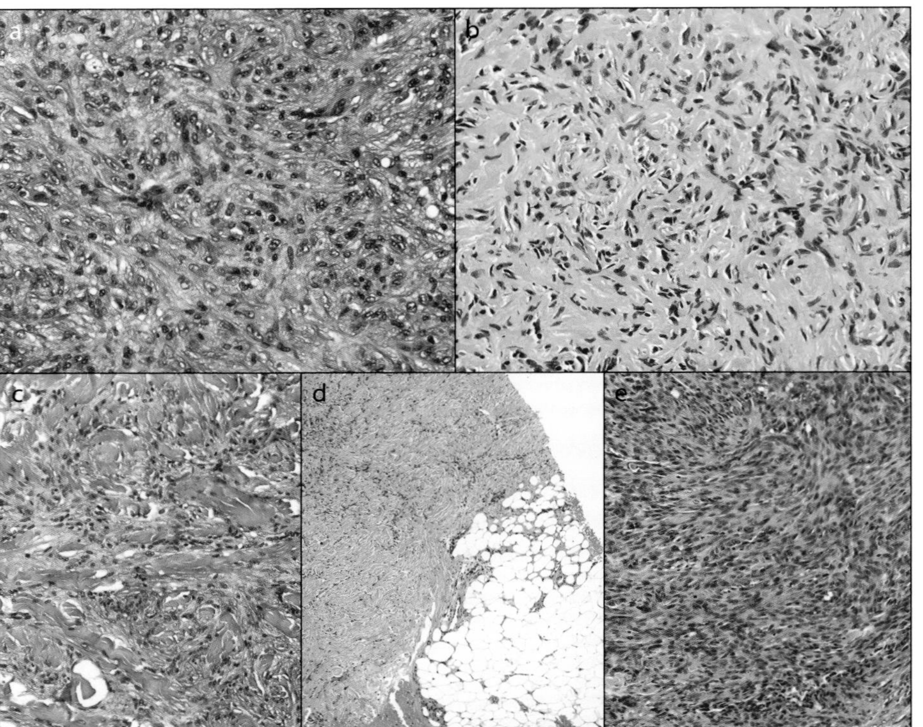

i40.11 a A dermatofibroma with plump fibroblasts

b A dermatofibroma with thin, spindled fibroblasts

c A dermatofibroma in which histiocytes intermingle with and damage dermal collagen

d Dermatofibromas do not significantly infiltrate the subcutaneous adipose tissue.

e A cellular dermatofibroma. Note the lack of significant mitotic activity or nuclear atypia. Like other forms of dermatofibroma, the cellular dermatofibroma does not infiltrate the subcutaneous adipose tissue to any extent.

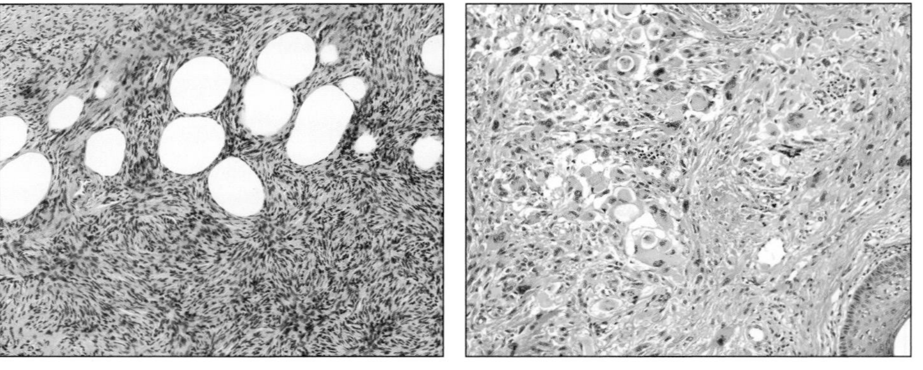

i40.12 A dermatofibrosarcoma protuberans (DFSP) infiltrating the subcutaneous adipose tissue

i40.13 An atypical fibroxanthoma (AFX) with very extensive generalized nuclear pleomorphism. Despite the pleomorphism, this dermal neoplasm does not have significant metastatic potential.

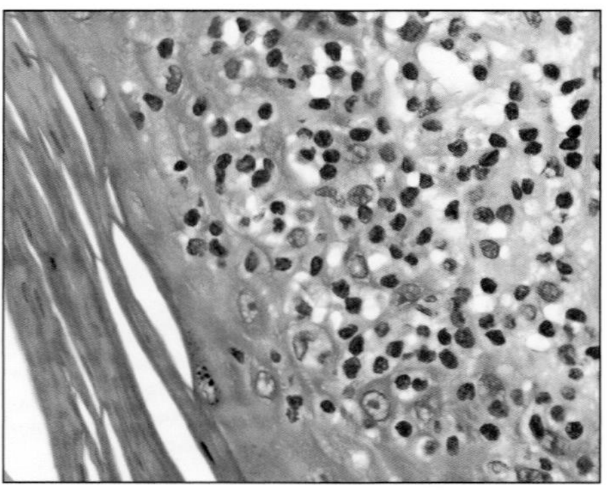

i40.14 A Pautrier abscess in mycosis fungoides

i40.15 a The very dense dermal infiltrate of cutaneous anaplastic lymphoma. This infiltrate often extends into subcutaneous tissue.

b A higher-power view of the same case as in i40.15a, illustrating the nuclear pleomorphism of the lymphocytes in anaplastic lymphoma

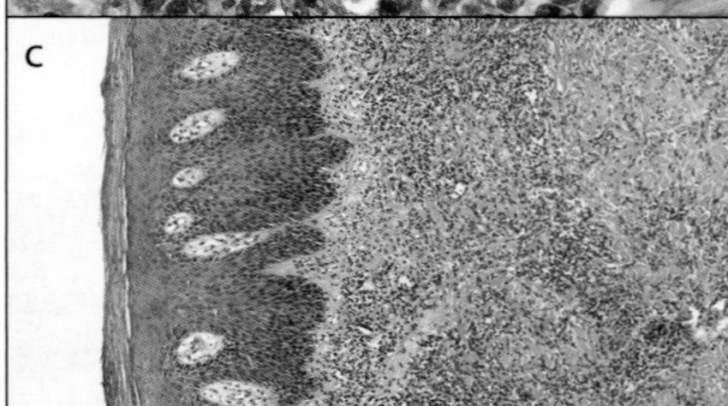

c Lymphomatoid papulosis with a significant dermal lymphoid infiltrate, but to the extent that these CD30+ cutaneous lymphoproliferative disorders can be separated, one that is less intense than in anaplastic lymphoma

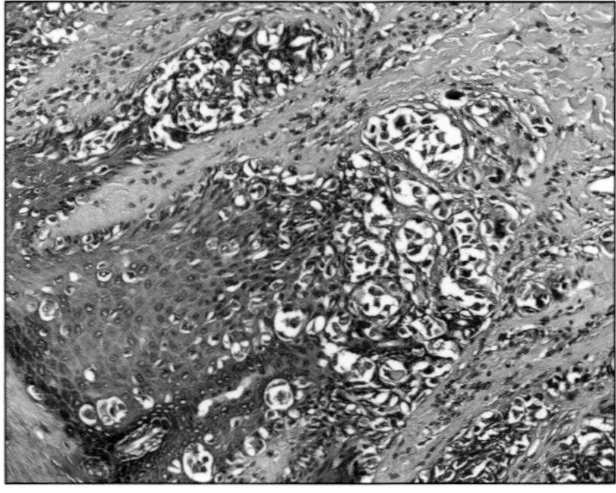

i40.16 A melanoma illustrating the pagetoid invasion of the epidermis (in a disorganized manner, predominantly as single cells), nuclear atypia, and invasion into the dermis

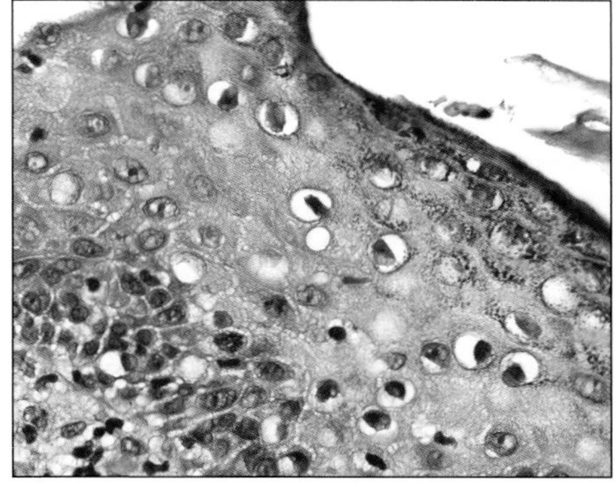

i40.17 Benign skin in which formalin fixation and paraffin processing has caused perinuclear clearing in the epithelial cells, resulting in an appearance that can simulate pagetoid invasion in the melanoma

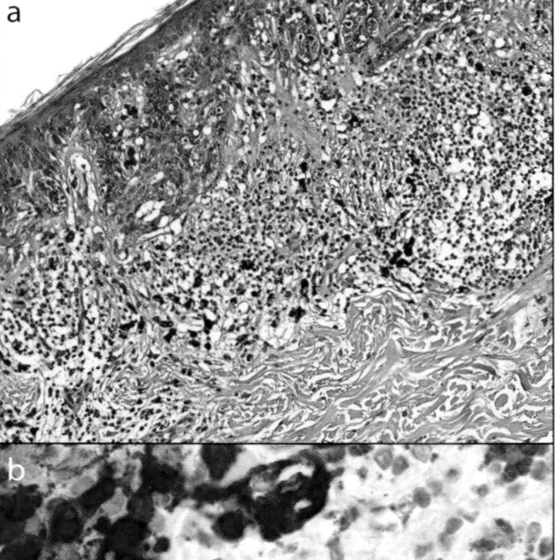

i40.18 **a** The use of immunohistochemical stains in melanoma. Melanoma in situ is readily apparent, primarily in the lentigo maligna form, at the dermal-epidermal junction, but it is not clear if the pigmented cells in the dermis are invasive melanocytes or melanophages.

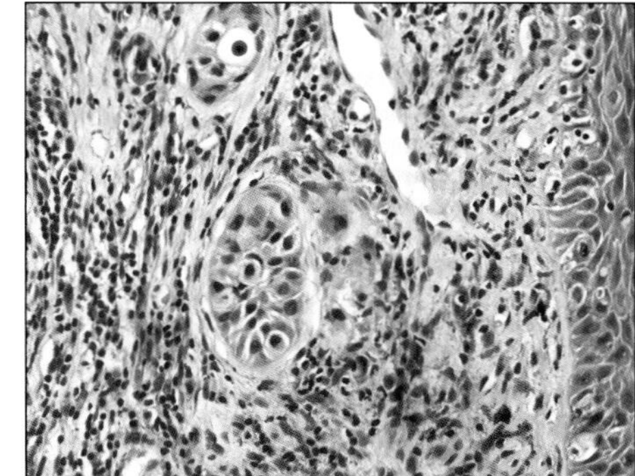

i40.19 An invasive melanoma with regression, evident as both an accompanying lymphoid infiltrate and by fibrosis

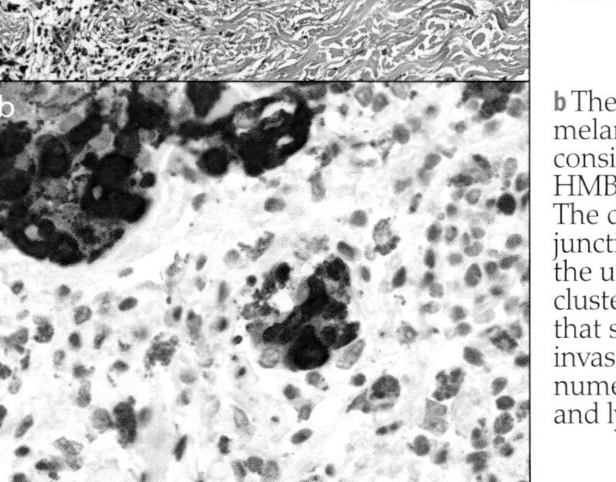

b The use of a pan-melanoma cocktail, consisting of S100, HMB-45, and Melan-A. The dermal-epidermal junction is evident in the upper left but the cluster in the center that stains positively is invasive melanoma amidst numerous melanophages and lymphocytes.

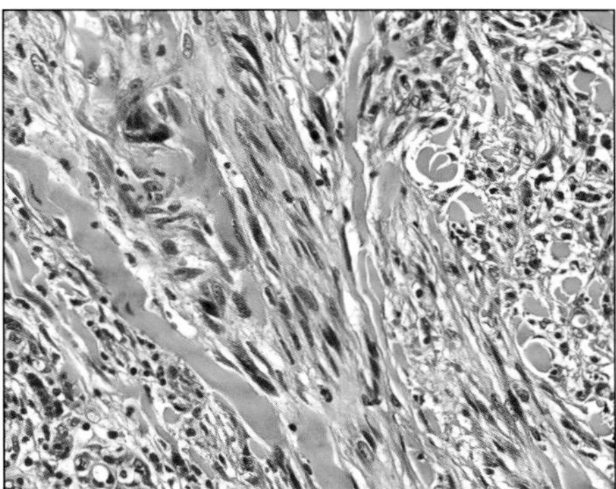

i40.20 A desmoplastic melanoma with spindled, atypical nuclei infiltrating between dermal collagen fibers, simulating a sarcoma

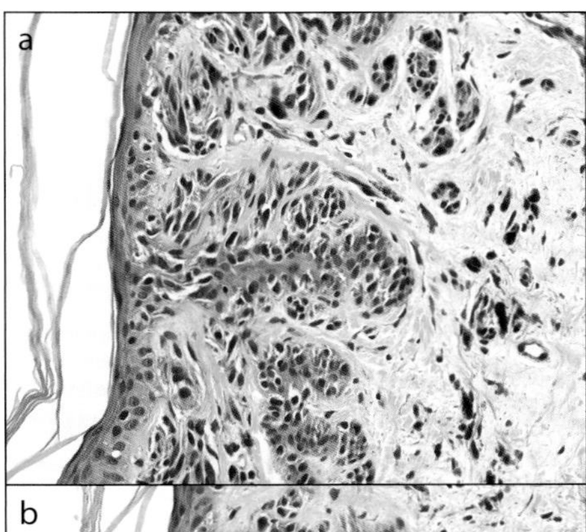

i40.21 **a** A dysplastic nevus illustrating the asymmetry of the junctional component and the fibrosis that surrounds the clusters of melanocytes at the junction

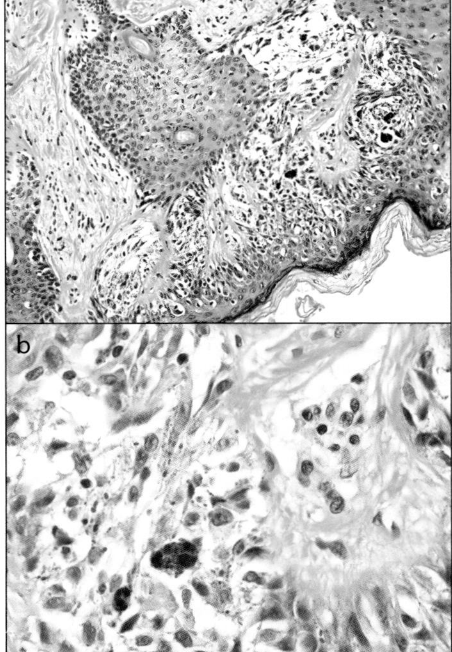

i40.22 **a** Melanoma in situ with pagetoid invasion of the epidermis. The process surrounds a hair follicle but because adnexal structures are part of the adventitial dermis, this does not constitute true invasion.

b A higher-power view of the same case as in i40.22a, highlighting the nuclear atypia of melanoma in situ

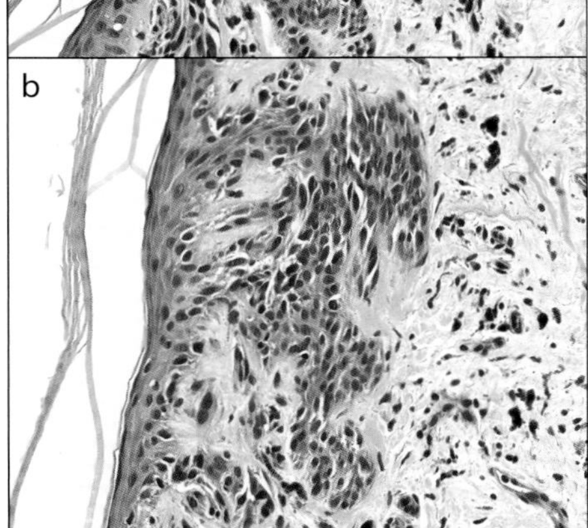

b A dysplastic nevus in which adjacent clusters of melanocytes merge with each other

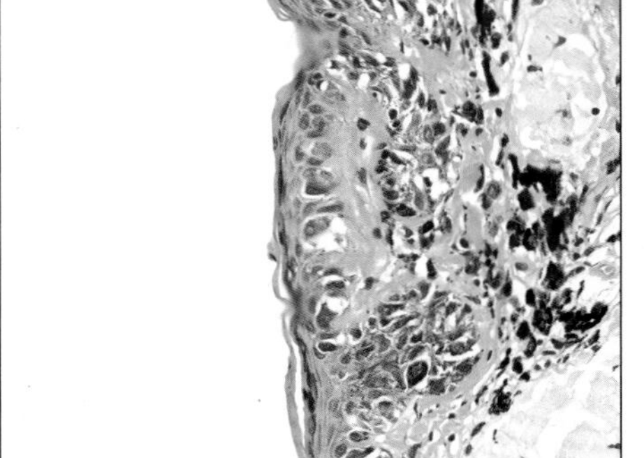

i40.23 Lentigo maligna, a form of melanoma in situ that is characteristic of sun-damaged skin. Note the nearly confluent array of atypical melanocytes at the dermal-epidermal junction, with an atrophic epidermis, but without pagetoid invasion of the epidermis. Note also that clusters of neoplastic melanocytes bulge into the dermis, but this does not constitute true invasion.

i40.24 **a** A Spitz nevus with extensive melanocytic cellularity. However, there is no pagetoid invasion of the epidermis and in the lower left some maturation can be identified.

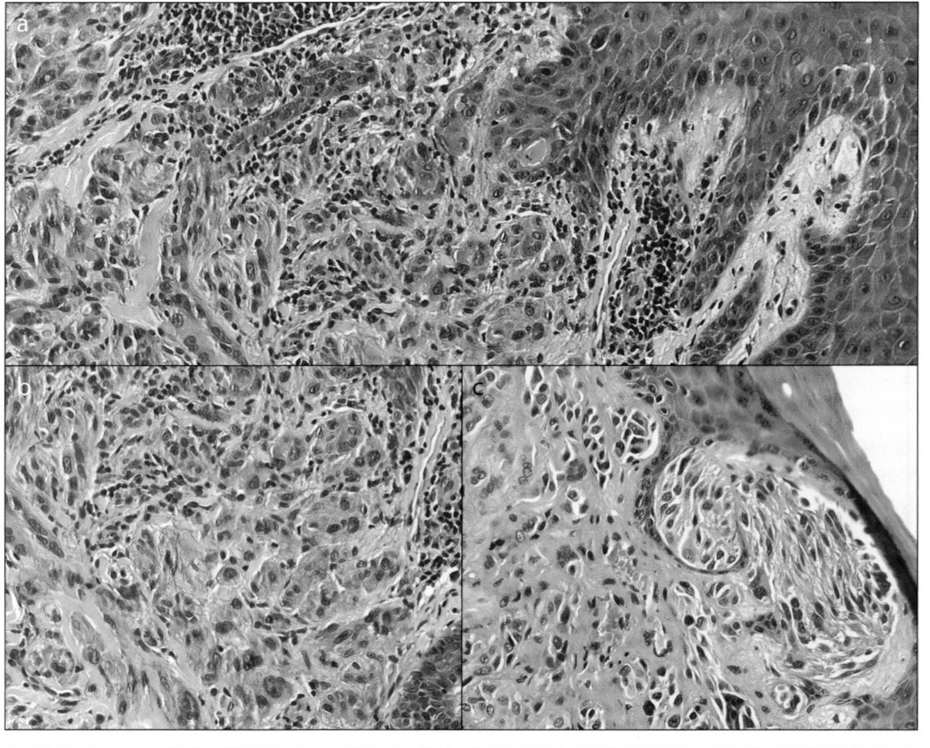

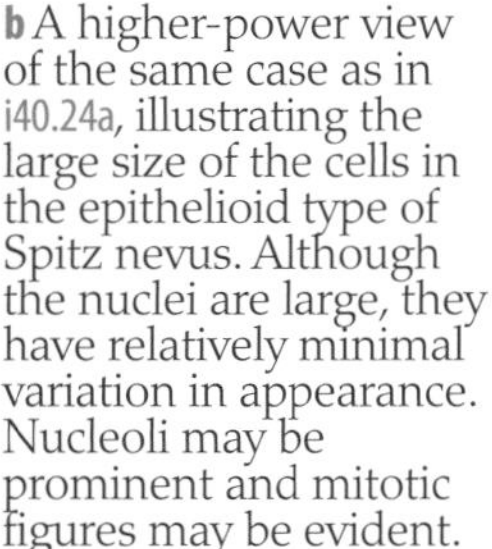

b A higher-power view of the same case as in i40.24a, illustrating the large size of the cells in the epithelioid type of Spitz nevus. Although the nuclei are large, they have relatively minimal variation in appearance. Nucleoli may be prominent and mitotic figures may be evident.

c A spindle cell variant of Spitz nevus with artifactual separation of the melanocytes at the dermal-epidermal junction from the overlying epidermis. Again, the process is quite cellular and worrisome, but the nuclei are not as pleomorphic as in an invasive melanoma, and pagetoid invasion is minimal.

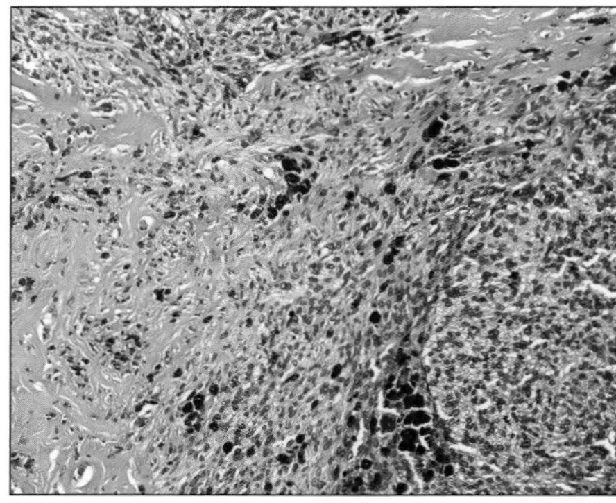

i40.25 A cellular blue nevus, illustrating nonpigmented spindle cells intermingled with pigmented spindle cells. The extensive cellularity makes this process difficult to separate from an invasive melanoma.

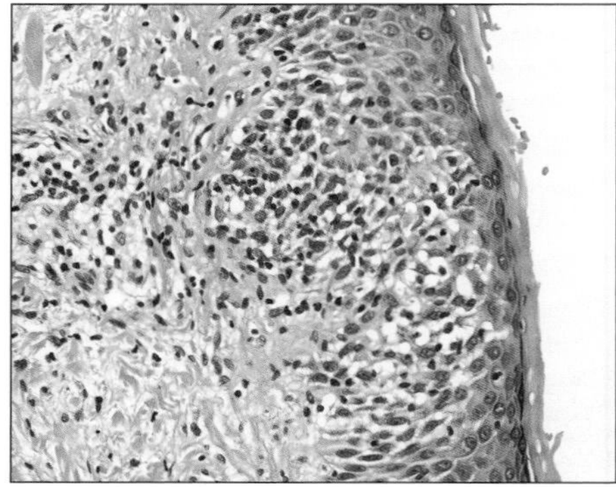

i40.26 Acute dermatitis characterized by spongiosis (epidermal edema)

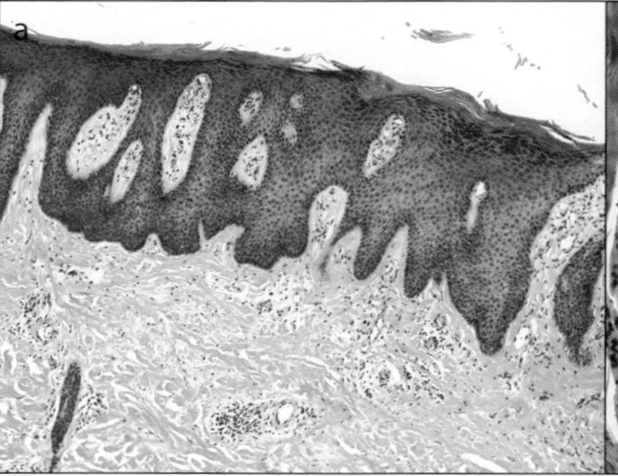

i40.27 **a** A chronic dermatitis characterized by elongation of the rete pegs, with fusion at their lower borders. At the left there is thinning of the epidermis. This histologic appearance is characteristic of psoriasis and chronic dermatitis conditions of the psoriasis family.

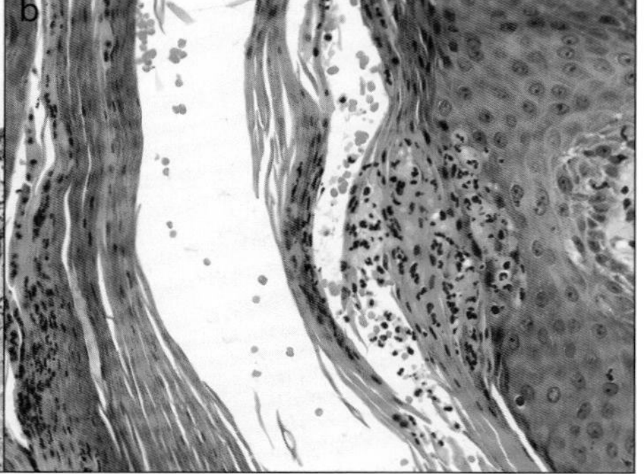

b Munro abscesses in psoriasis

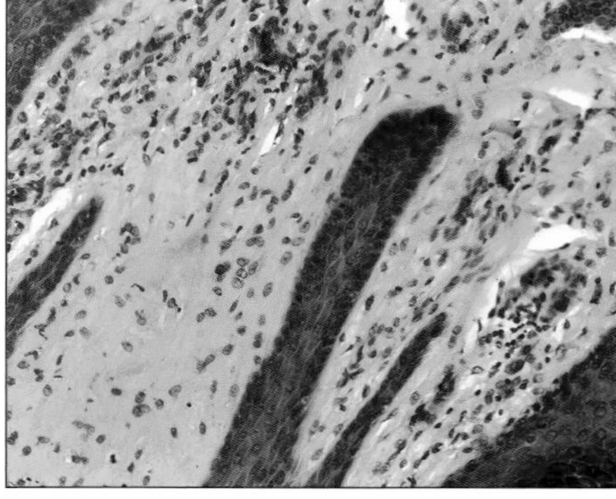

i40.28 Lichen simplex chronicus, characterized by irregular elongation of the rete pegs, without fusion at their lower border, and fibrosis of the papillary dermis that surrounds elongated rete pegs. Lichen simplex chronicus is usually a complication of another chronic dermatitis.

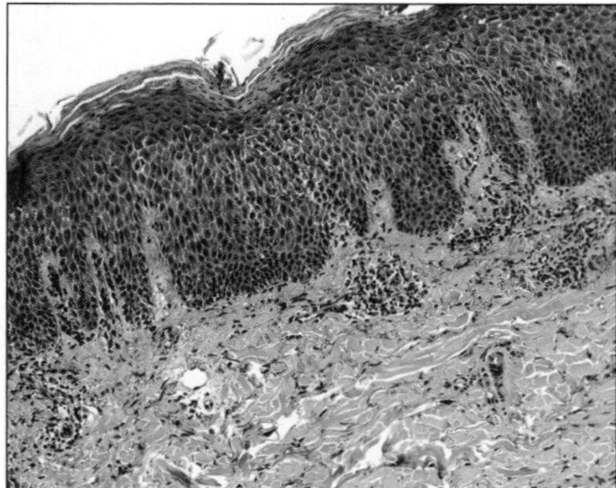

i40.29 A subacute dermatitis in which there is uneven elongation of the rete pegs, with minimal fusion of their lower portion. There is parakeratosis, but there is also spongiosis.

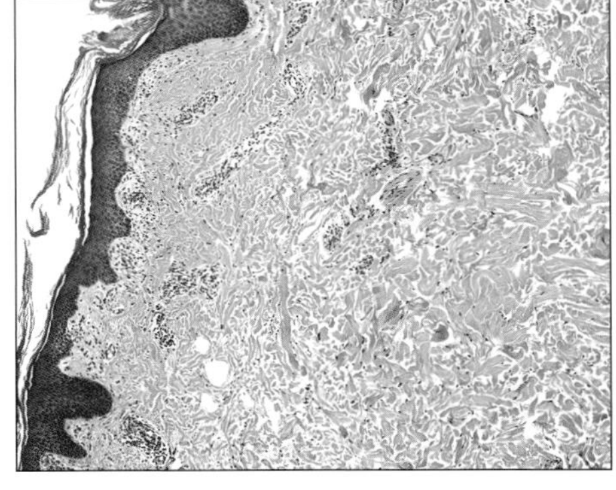

i40.30 A pattern of inflammation in dermatitis in which lymphocytes surround blood vessels in the superficial dermis.

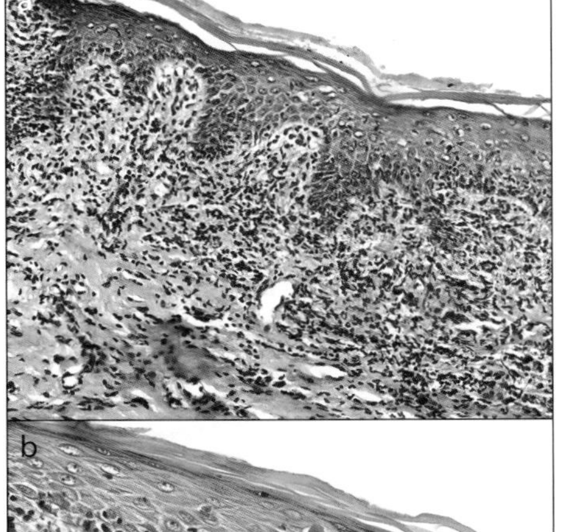

i40.31 **a** Lichen planus, illustrating another pattern of distribution of inflammatory cells in chronic dermatitis. In lichen planus and related disorders, lymphocytes are disproportionately found at the junction of the epidermis and the dermis. Rete pegs are elongated, but in a wedge-shaped manner, in contrast to the elongation that is seen in psoriasis.

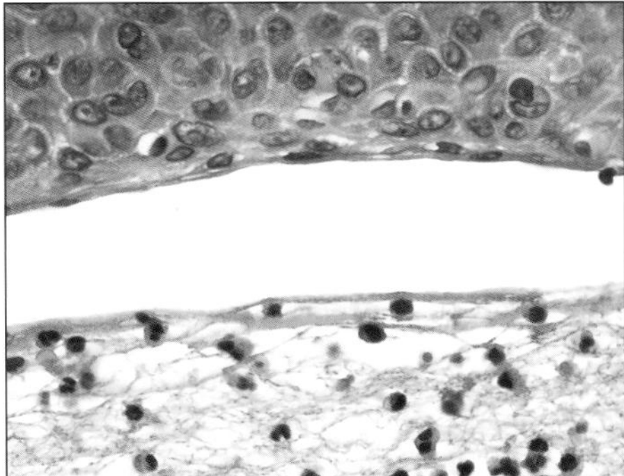

i40.32 Bullous pemphigoid in which there is a subepidermal blister containing eosinophils

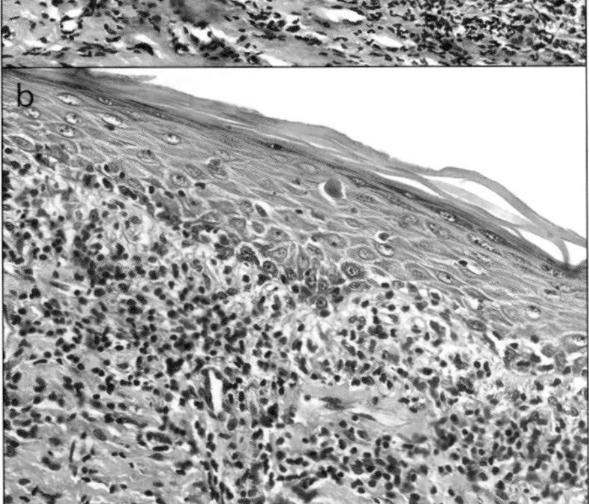

b In lichen planus and lichenoid keratosis, there is often attenuation of the basal layer of the epidermis and vacuolar change. Note the eosinophilic colloid bodies in the upper portion of the epidermis at the lower central portion of the photograph.

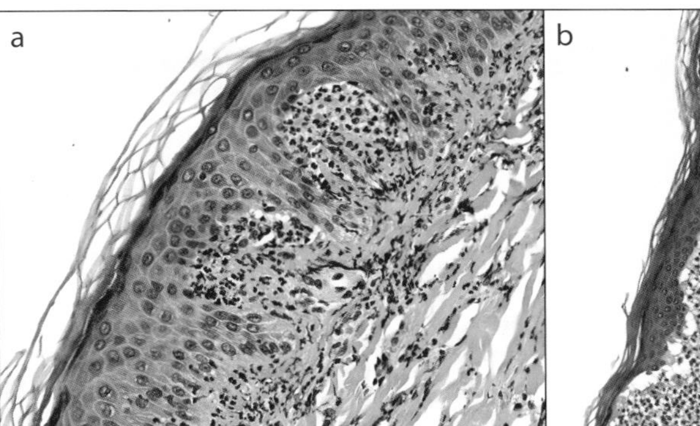

i40.33 **a** A case of dermatitis herpetiformis in the early stages, prior to formation of an overt vesicle. Neutrophils congregate at the dermal-epidermal junction.

b A well developed case of dermatitis herpetiformis in which neutrophils are found within a subepidermal blister

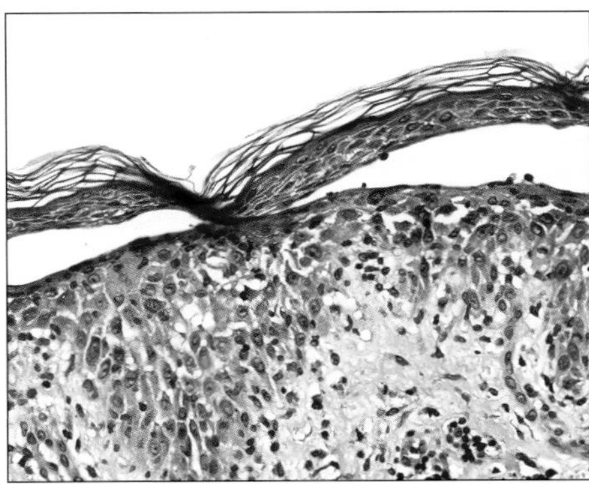

i40.34 An example of the pemphigus group of disorders in which there is loss of adhesion between adjacent cells of the epidermis

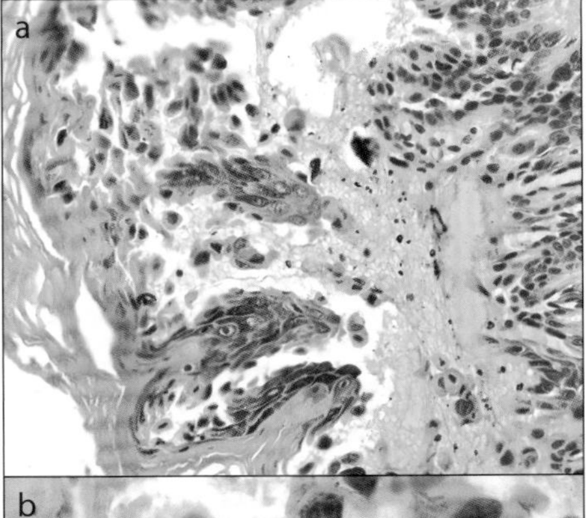

i40.35 **a** Darier disease, in which there is acantholysis and dyskeratosis

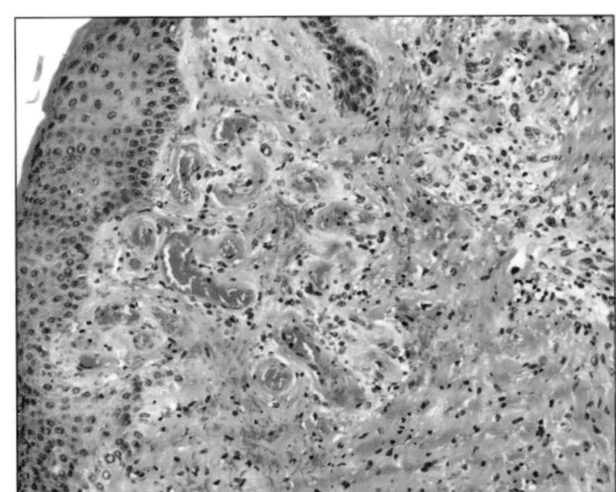

i40.36 Stasis dermatitis, illustrating the sharply increased number of capillaries in the upper portion of the dermis, fibrosis between the capillaries, and acute and chronic dermal inflammation. These changes are a reaction to ischemia.

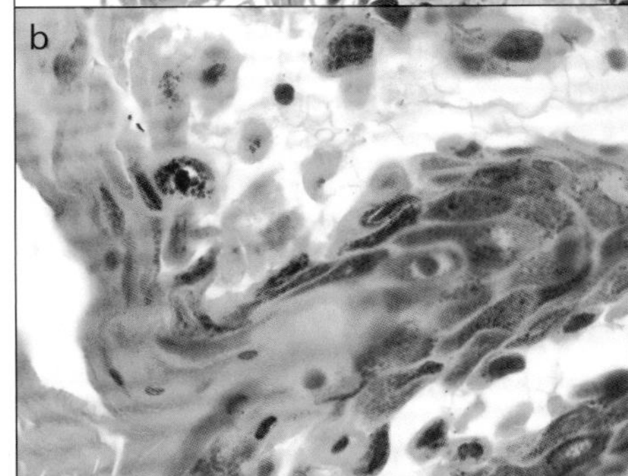

b The same case as in i40.35a, illustrating a corps rond, a dyskeratotic cell in the granular layer, with basophilic cytoplasm and a perinuclear halo

ISBN 978-089189-5886

i40.37 **a** An early stage of morphea in which chronic inflammation is still evident in the upper dermis but the lower dermis is fibrotic

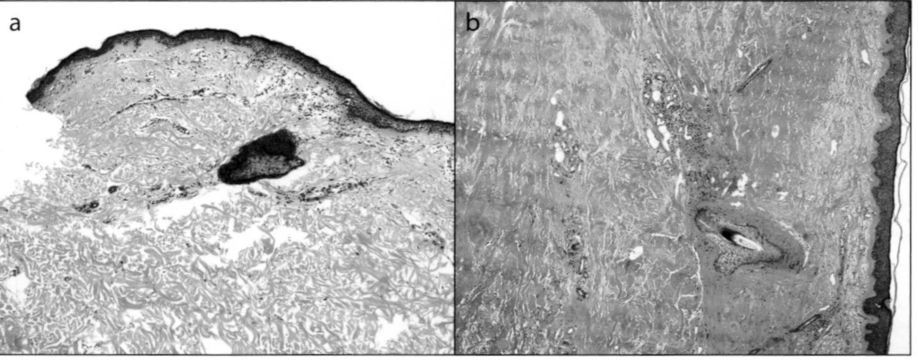

b A later stage of morphea in which the inflammatory cells are generally absent but there is dense fibrosis throughout the dermis, most evident around adnexal structures, which are no longer surrounded by a small portion of adipose tissue.

i40.38 Discoid lupus, illustrating chronic inflammation at the dermal-epidermal junction and surrounding a fair follicle, which is dilated and filled with keratin rather than containing a well formed hair

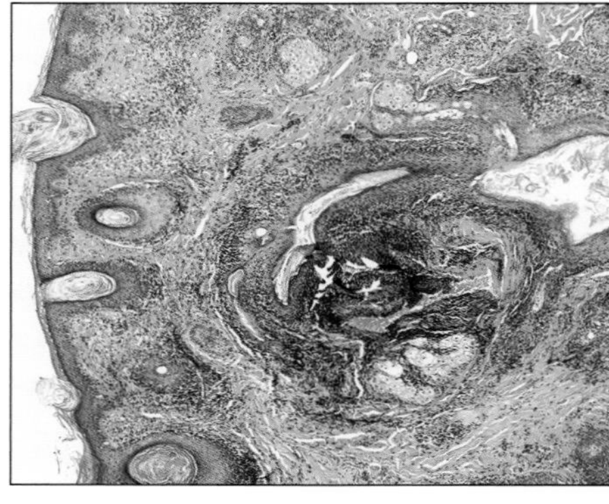

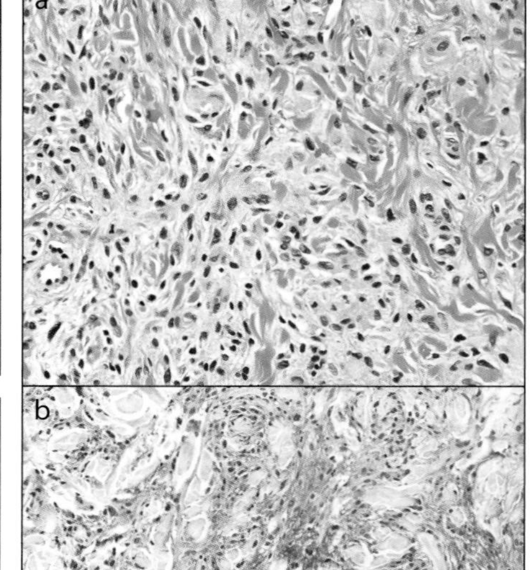

i40.39 Granuloma annulare. **a** illustrates histiocytes intermingling with dermal collagen. This appearance suggests a possible dermatofibroma but in **b**, acidic mucopolysaccharides are demonstrable by colloidal iron or Alcian blue stain.

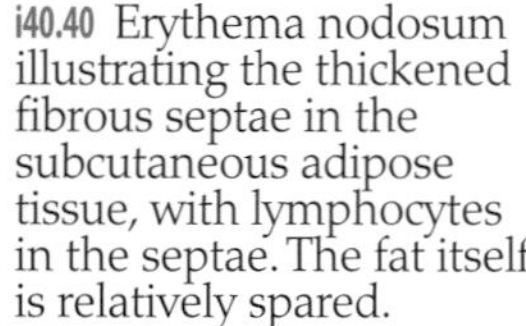

i40.40 Erythema nodosum illustrating the thickened fibrous septae in the subcutaneous adipose tissue, with lymphocytes in the septae. The fat itself is relatively spared.

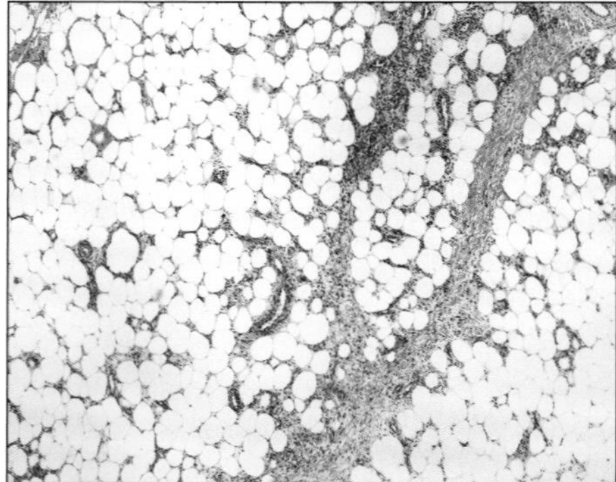

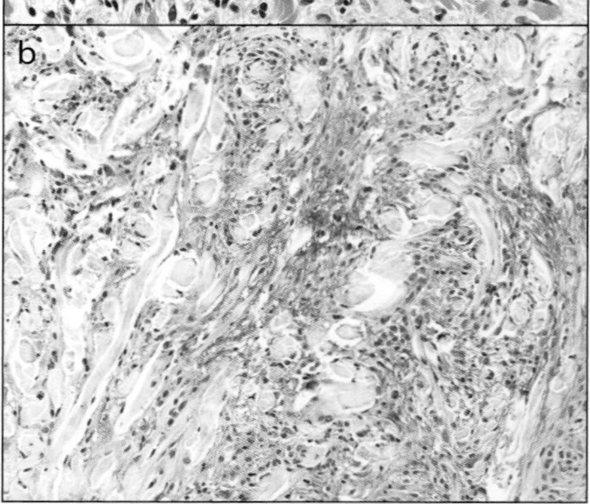

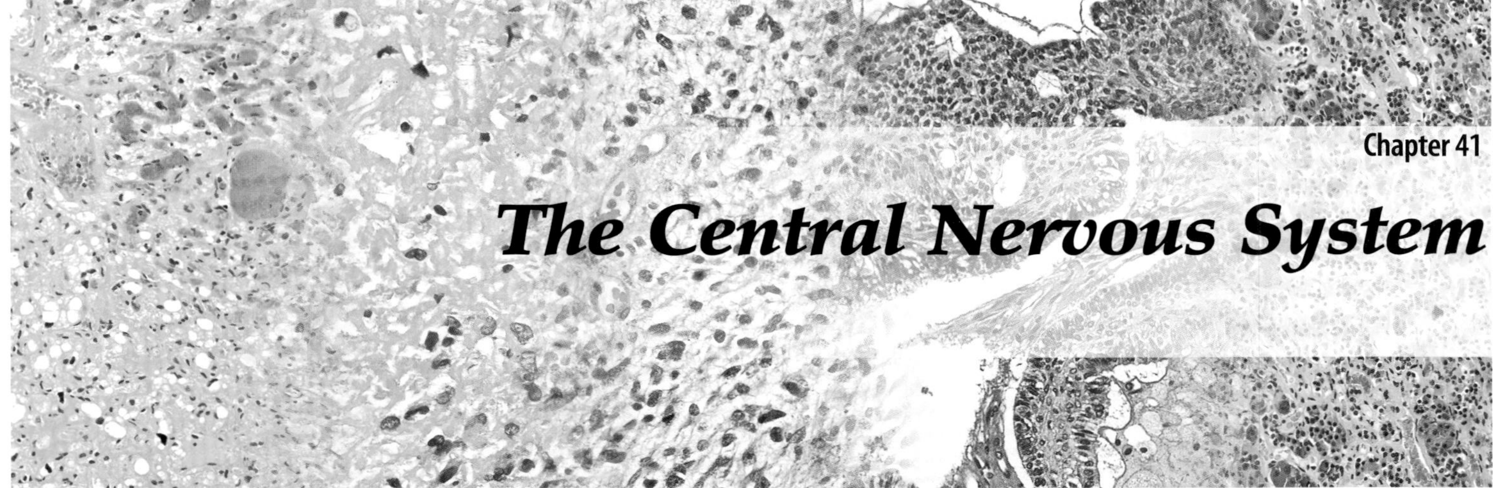

Chapter 41

The Central Nervous System

No attempt will be made to comprehensively discuss the pathology of the central nervous system (CNS), but only to introduce a few common problems and new developments that the general pathologist is likely to encounter.

Nonneoplastic Disorders of the CNS

Nonneoplastic neuropathology is not part of the typical practice of pathology, but a few comments are made here because this area is benefitting from developments in molecular pathology, a major focus of this work.

The terms "leukoencephalopathy" and "leukodystrophy" both refer to neurological disorders that primarily affect myelin or white matter. In general, the term "leukoencephalopathy" refers to an acquired condition, of many etiologies, usually inflammatory/autoimmune, toxic, or vascular. Leukeoencephalopathies are usually manifested in adulthood. The term "leukodystrophy" refers to a genetically determined, progressive disorder of myelination, with many etiologies and usually presenting in childhood.

Multiple sclerosis is an autoimmune disorder in which autoantibodies are directed against components of myelin [PMID11818475], though with progression, alterations in neurofilament proteins within axons and loss of axons themselves are also demonstrable [PMID21114565]. While the precise gene or genes involved have not yet been isolated, it is known that there is a susceptibility locus at 17q24 [PMID15256512]. The diagnosis is established by the clinical findings in conjunction with MRI. MRI is also used to monitor the effectiveness of therapy [PMID20182573]. Biopsies are rarely needed, but when done, the principal differential diagnosis is a low-grade glioma because of the gliosis that accompanies multiple sclerosis. This differential is discussed in the next section, but the triad of perivascular lymphocytes, macrophages and gliosis point to multiple sclerosis over a neoplasm i41.1 [PMID11304039], and the demonstration of demyelination with a myelin stain is confirmatory.

The CNS in dementia is discussed in Chapter 46 because developments in molecular pathology have greatly facilitated our understanding of this area.

Neoplasms of the Sella and Suprasellar Region

The pituitary gland is located in or near the sella turcica, a depression in the sphenoid bone. Resection of pituitary tumors often involves collaboration between an ENT surgeon and a neurosurgeon. Whereas the normal gland has a variety of cell types i41.2a, pituitary tumors are almost always adenomas with a single cell type i41.2b. Clinical manifestations of pituitary adenomas relate to the hormones produced or to visual compromise, since they often impinge on the optic chiasm. Approximately 20% of pituitary adenomas make no identifiable hormone (so-called null cell adenoma) and can only come to clinical attention via visual field defects. Of the approximately 80% of adenomas that are secretory, many secrete >1 hormone. Most functioning adenomas secrete prolactin, and prolactinomas are the most common form of pituitary adenoma that secretes only 1 product. Excess prolactin can cause amenorrhea or galactorrhea (Forbes-Albright syndrome).

The second most common product of pituitary adenomas is ACTH. Excess ACTH stimulates the adrenal cortex and causes Cushing disease, a subset of Cushing syndrome (increased adrenal cortical hormones from any etiology, including adrenal tumors). The third most common product is growth hormone, causing gigantism in children, whose epiphyseal plates have not yet closed, and acromegaly in adults. The product, if any, can usually be identified by immunohistochemistry, though there is an increasing role for the detection of mRNA by in situ hybridization, particularly in cases for which immunohistochemistry is negative [PMID10727285].

The craniopharyngioma is usually a tumor of childhood and is generally suprasellar rather than in the sella turcica. Its histology is similar to the ameloblastoma of the oral cavity, and like the latter tumor, the craniopharyngioma may have a number of appearances. Commonly, at least part of the tumor has a fibrous stroma lined by basaloid epithelium i41.3a. There is often peripheral palisading and cyst formation i41.3b. Focal calcification is common. Craniopharyngiomas are benign but may be locally recurrent and destructive, and there may be consequences of the surgery and radiation therapy used to treat them [PMID18226736].

ISBN 978-089189-5886

Neoplasms of the CNS

There are numerous classifications of CNS tumors, but the World Health Organization (WHO) classification of tumors of the nervous system [Louis ISBN978-9283224303] is becoming the standard and is the basis for these comments.

The first comment is that the specific location of the neoplasm and the age of the patient are critical in the diagnosis. For example, medulloblastomas tend to be found in the cerebellum or the roof of the fourth ventricle in children, while pineoblastomas are typically a cerebellar tumor in children. These 2 tumors share many properties with primitive neuroectodermal tumors and morphologically are small blue cell tumors i41.4, though their cytogenetic abnormalities are different from similar tumors in the periphery [PMID15018124]. Medulloblastomas often have abnormalities of chromosomes 1 or 17 [PMID9293446]. The desmoplastic medulloblastoma has micronodules of stromal desmoplasia and reduced tumor cellularity.

The diagnosis of meningioma is heavily dependent on the reliable radiographic demonstration of connection of the neoplasm to the meninges. Most meningiomas are of grade 1. These are benign, with the qualification that the CNS has very limited capacity to cope with mass effect, so even a tumor that would have a completely benign behavior elsewhere may result in a malignant course in the brain if there is a significant mass or pressure effect. Grade 1 meningiomas are usually well circumscribed. A few grade 1 meningiomas are invasive, but are still relatively indolent except for an increased incidence of local recurrence. There are a number of subtypes of grade 1 meningiomas, but most will be meningothelial (clusters of epithelioid cells with minimal pleomorphism and a syncytial appearance, separated by thin fibrovascular septae), fibroblastic, or a combination of these 2 patterns (transitional) i41.5a.

Any meningioma with mitotic activity of 4-19 mitoses per 10 high-power fields (HPF) is considered to be WHO grade 2 (atypical meningioma). Alternatively, 3 or more of the following features place a meningioma into grade 2: increased cellularity, small tumor cells with diminished cytoplasm, prominent nucleoli, a disorganized or sheet-like growth pattern, or significant necrosis i41.5b. There are also specific types of meningioma, such as clear cell and chordoid types, that are automatically of grade 2. Grade 3 meningiomas (anaplastic meningiomas) are aggressive and have >19 mitoses per 10 HPF or obvious and generalized pleomorphism that results in a frankly sarcomatous or carcinomatous appearance.

The hemangiopericytoma at one time was considered a type of meningioma, but is now recognized as a distinct tumor type in the CNS. True meningiomas lack the CD34 positivity that is usually seen in hemangiopericytomas.

Although the term "glioma" also encompasses ependymoma and medulloblastoma, in practice, it usually indicates an astrocytoma/glioblastoma multiforme, or an oligodendroglioma. In the WHO classification of astrocytomas, those of grade 1, also called pilocytic, are reasonably circumscribed and display only a minimal increase in cellularity and only mild nuclear pleomorphism. The very difficult differential diagnosis is reactive gliosis. Cases of low-grade astrocytoma vs reactive gliosis are exceptionally challenging and can cause angst among even experienced neuropathologists. As is the case for neoplasms in other body sites, most brain tumors, excepting gliomatosis cerebri, form at least a vague mass, in contrast to gliosis, but this may be difficult to appreciate radiographically and a biopsy may be too scant to identify a mass effect. Both gliosis and glioma are hypercellular, but a low-grade astrocytoma has a greater density of glial cells than a reactive gliosis, with more nuclear atypia. i41.6a, i41.6b, i41.6c, and i41.6d illustrate normal brain, reactive gliosis, and a low-grade astrocytoma.

Some assistance is available from immunohistochemistry and molecular methods. Immunohistochemical staining for glial fibrillary acidic protein (GFAP) will not distinguish between reactive and neoplastic astrocytes, but p53 expression favors a neoplasm [PMID8764745]. 80% of astrocytomas have chromosomal abnormalities, some of which can be identified by in situ hybridization, effectively excluding reactive gliosis [PMID11342694]. Macrophages are rare in gliomas unless there has been treatment for a previously diagnosed neoplasm. In the absence of a history of treatment, good numbers of macrophages suggest gliosis secondary to an infarct or a demyelinating disorder. Immunohistochemistry for CD68 and HAM-56, both markers of macrophages, may make the identification of macrophages easier. Ki-67 (MIB-1), a marker of proliferation, suggests neoplasia if significantly elevated but does not necessarily indicate gliosis if low, as some low-grade astrocytomas may have a low proliferation index [PMID15900115]. Perivascular lymphocytes are more suggestive of multiple sclerosis and are part of the traditional triad (with gliosis and macrophages) of that disorder.

If there is a history of a tumor treated with radiation i41.7, macrophages are to be expected [PMID17318000], and in such a situation, a paucity of this cell type (less than about 10% of total cells), confirmed by immunohistochemistry, suggests that a cellular area is likely to be residual/recurrent neoplasia. Ki-67 may help in previously diagnosed cases that have been irradiated, as the percentage of positive cells in cases where there is no residual/recurrent tumor rarely exceeds 1%, but typically is 3% or more in cases of residual/recurrent tumor [PMID10222423].

WHO grade 2 is the diffuse astrocytoma. It is more cellular, with more pleomorphism, and it is less circumscribed. Protoplasmic, fibrillary, and gemistocytic astrocytomas are all types of grade 2. The most pronounced example of a diffuse astrocytoma is gliomatosis cerebri, in which the tumor involves 2 of more lobes. A grade 3 astrocytoma is anaplastic, with obvious pleomorphism and mitotic activity i41.8, and a grade 4 astrocytoma is a glioblastoma multiforme, with profound pleomorphism, intense mitotic activity, and necrosis i41.9. Often, viable tumor cells surround a necrotic focus.

Glioblastomas are associated with abnormalities in copy number of chromosomes 7, 9, and 10, especially gains of chromosome 7 and losses of 9p [PMID21884817].

Oligodendrogliomas have relatively round and uniform nuclei, usually with prominent perinuclear clearing, resulting in the classic "fried egg" appearance i41.10. The WHO considers the classic oligodendroglioma to be grade 2 and recognizes a grade 3, with greater cellularity, atypia, and mitotic activity. Many oligodendrogliomas are associated with deletions of 1p and 19q, and tumors with these deletions are less aggressive [PMID21233669]. Other brain tumors may have deletions in portions of these arms, but loss of the entire arm,

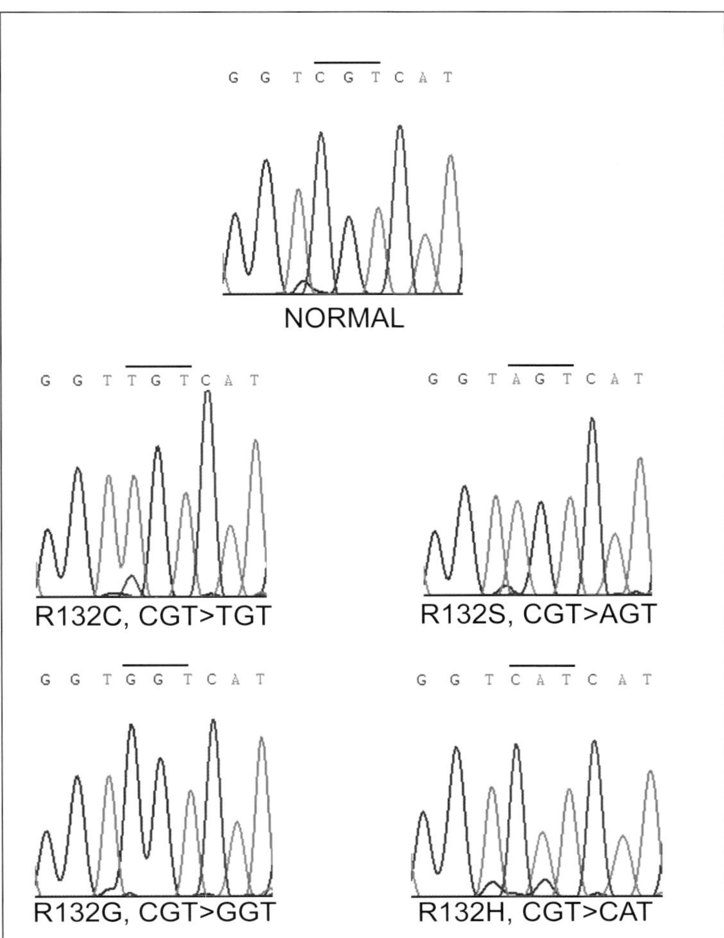

f41.1 The 132 codon is at top center. Normally, CGT codes for arginine. The most common abnormality is shown at bottom right. It is CAT in that codon and codes for histidine.

though not found in all oligodendrogliomas, is specific for that tumor when found.

Mutations in 1 of the 2 isozymes of isocitrate dehydrogenase (IDH) occur in 40% of astrocytomas and oligodendrogliomas but are not seen in nonneoplastic glial tissue. The mutation is generally in IDH1 and is usually a point mutation in exon 4 resulting in a substitution of histidine for arginine (R132H). Sequencing can be done in formalin-fixed, paraffin-embedded tissue **f41.1** [PMID19915484], and there is an immunohistochemical stain for the R132H form of the protein, which, if positive, can substitute for sequencing [PMID21643842].

The rosettes in an ependymoma are usually pseudorosettes around blood vessels **i41.11** rather than true rosettes, which occur around a lumen formed by the tumor cells. Occasionally, there will be true rosettes, like those in retinoblastoma, with a well defined central lumen and a basement membrane, but in the right location (adjacent to a ventricle), tumor cells surrounding a blood vessel suggest an ependymoma.

Hemangioblastoma is a very vascular tumor, but its vessels are not neoplastic. Only the fat-laden cells between the capillaries are neoplastic. Because of this combination of clear cells in a background of arborizing vessels **i41.12**, a hemangioblastoma may greatly resemble a metastatic clear cell renal cell carcinoma. The stromal cells of hemangioblastoma are positive for aquaporin1 and α inhibin (also called inhibin A), while those of metastatic renal cell carcinoma are negative [PMID20179436]. Metastatic renal cell carcinomas are positive for keratin, RCC, and CD10, while hemangioblastomas are negative for these markers [PMID18496143].

There are 3 final groups of tumor in the CNS—metastatic carcinoma, germ cell tumors, and lymphomas. Germ cell tumors may rarely occur in the CNS, and when they do, they occur in the midline, especially near the pineal. The properties of these tumors are identical to those in their more common sites, as discussed in Chapters 33 and 38. Likewise, the diagnostic evaluation of lymphomas and metastatic carcinomas is as described in other sites.

Inflammatory and Degenerative Conditions of Muscles

While nerves and muscles are not part of the CNS, discussions of biopsies of these tissues are traditionally included in neuropathology texts. The 3 most common idiopathic inflammatory myopathies are polymyositis, dermatomyositis, and inclusion body myositis [PMID19349710].

The muscle weakness in both polymyositis and dermatomyositis is proximal and symmetrical. Biopsies of polymyositis reveal muscle tissue with unevenly distributed degeneration and inflammation. Some areas will appear nearly normal, but other areas will show degeneration with necrosis, chronic inflammation with lymphocytes and macrophages, and central nuclei. The changes are most pronounced in the endomysium, the connective tissue that surrounds individual muscle fibers. There will be evidence of regeneration in the form of amphophilic or basophilic cytoplasm and large nuclei with vesicular chromatin [PMID19282137].

In addition to the skin involvement in dermatomyositis, there are subtle histologic differences between polymyositis and dermatomyositis. The inflammation in both is focal and chronic, but is predominantly perivascular or perimysial (the perimysium surrounds groups of muscle fibers) in dermatomyositis, rather than endomysial, as in polymyositis [PMID19282137]. Atrophy in dermatomyositis is most pronounced at the periphery of fascicles **i41.13**. Fortunately, though the symptoms of polymyositis and dermatomyositis overlap, there are differences, as well as differences in the precise autoantibodies that are found [PMID20146695], so the pathologist is relieved of the sole responsibility of distinguishing between them.

In contrast to polymyositis and dermatomyositis, the pattern of weakness in inclusion body myositis is often asymmetrical, and patients tend to be middle-aged or older adults. Like polymyositis, inclusion body myositis has patchy inflammation that is centered on the endomysium. The characteristic feature is tubulofilamentous bodies that range in size from 15 to 18 nm, thus requiring electron microscopy for definitive diagnosis. Inclusion body myositis is more refractory to therapy than polymyositis or dermatomyositis [PMID19864656].

Muscle biopsies are usually divided into 3 parts, 1 each for H&E, electron microscopy, and histochemical stains for important mitochondrial enzymes, such as ATPase. Immunohistochemical, molecular, or immunofluorescent studies may also be performed. Muscle biopsies may be clamped upon procurement and are often performed in

ISBN 978-089189-5886

academic centers to ensure that the 3 components are properly processed. In particular, histochemical stains for mitochondrial enzymes cannot be done in a community hospital and usually require snap freezing in liquid nitrogen. Likewise, few community hospitals have an electron microscope. However, travel to a tertiary medical center is often a substantial inconvenience to patients and may not be necessary. Clamping is rarely essential, and the general pathologist can make very important contributions in nerve and muscle biopsies by excluding vasculitis, infectious agents, granulomas, etc, and noting the patterns of degeneration and inflammation alluded to above. Moreover, improved clinical modalities, such as nerve conduction studies and electromyography, adequately complement routine histologic study and permit a diagnosis in many cases. In most cases, collaboration between a neurologist and a pathologist can achieve a diagnosis in a community hospital, and most of the remaining cases can be resolved by sending tissue for special studies to an academic center. Even electron microscopy and histochemical staining of mitochondrial enzymes, if required, can usually be performed if a portion of the specimen is frozen with dry ice and a second portion is placed in gluteraldehyde and sent to a neuromuscular laboratory.

Core Points for the Central Nervous System

- Multiple sclerosis: biopsies rare but if done, perivascular lymphocytes, macrophages, and gliosis.
- Low-grade astrocytoma: greater cellularity and more nuclear atypia than reactive gliosis.
  - Macrophages favor gliosis.
    - CD68 and HAM-56 stains highlight macrophages.
  - Low proliferation index not helpful, but increased proliferation favors an astrocytoma.
  - Many astrocytomas have chromosomal abnormalities, whose identification secures a diagnosis of neoplasia.
- Radiation treatment: macrophages are common.
  - If they are rare, recurrent/residual neoplasia is suggested.
- Pituitary tumors: adenomas in the sella turcica
  - Usually secrete one or more hormones.
    - The most common hormones are prolactin, ACTH, and growth hormone.
  - Symptoms in nonsecreting secondary to visual symptoms.
- Craniopharyngioma is a suprasellar tumor of childhood.
- Patient age and location essential in the diagnosis of CNS neoplasms.
- Meningioma: 90% benign.
  - But in the confines of the skull, even benign neoplasms can be problematic.
- Astrocytomas: 4 grades, from grade 1, which is easily confused with reactive gliosis, to grade 4, glioblastoma multiforme.
- Oligodendrogliomas: distinct perinuclear haloes
  - Grade 2.
  - Some have deletions of 1p and 19q.
- Ependymomas: often arise in the fourth ventricle.
  - Pseudorosettes consisting of tumor cells surrounding a blood vessel.
- Hemangioblastomas: may resemble a metastatic renal cell carcinoma, often requiring IHC.
- Lymphomas: usually of diffuse large B cell type.
- Metastatic carcinomas are common in the CNS.
- Muscle biopsies: examined by traditional H&E, electron microscopy, and stains for important mitochondrial enzymes, especially for ATPase.
  - After exclusion of vasculitis, infectious agents, and granulomas, diagnosis of polymyositis or dermatomyositis made in conjunction with additional information from other modalities.

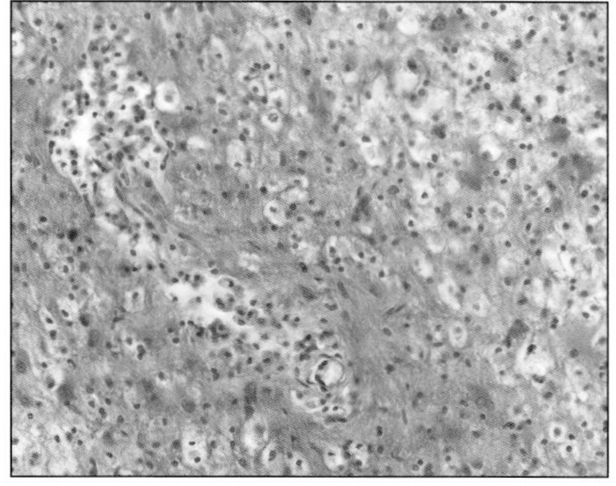

i41.1 Multiple sclerosis. Macrophages are seen at upper right. There is sclerosis in the central portion. The sclerotic tissue surrounds a blood vessel with a perivascular lymphoid infiltrate.

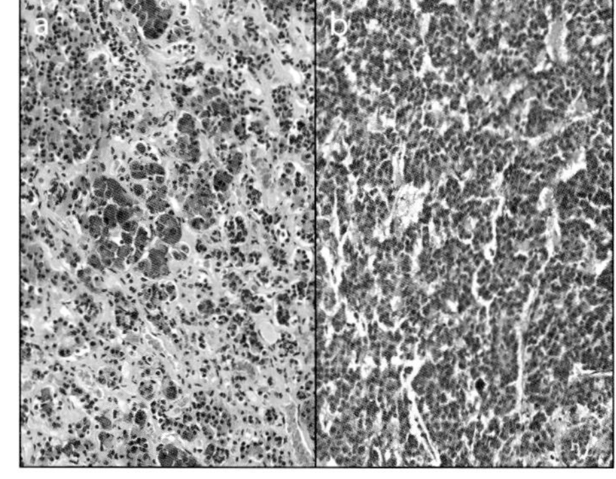

i41.2 **a** Normal pituitary gland with multiple cell types **b** A pituitary adenoma with only 1 cell type

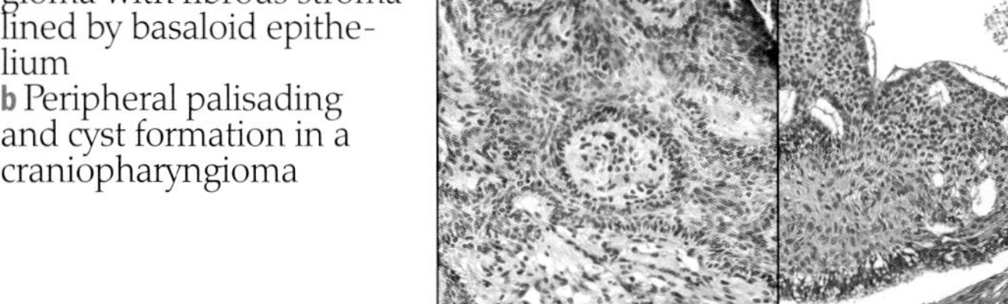

i41.3 **a** A craniopharyngioma with fibrous stroma lined by basaloid epithelium
b Peripheral palisading and cyst formation in a craniopharyngioma

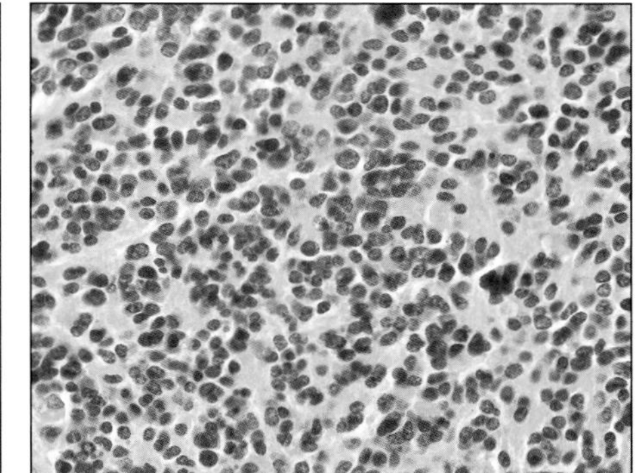

i41.4 A medulloblastoma. Note the resemblance to the primitive neuroectodermal tumor.

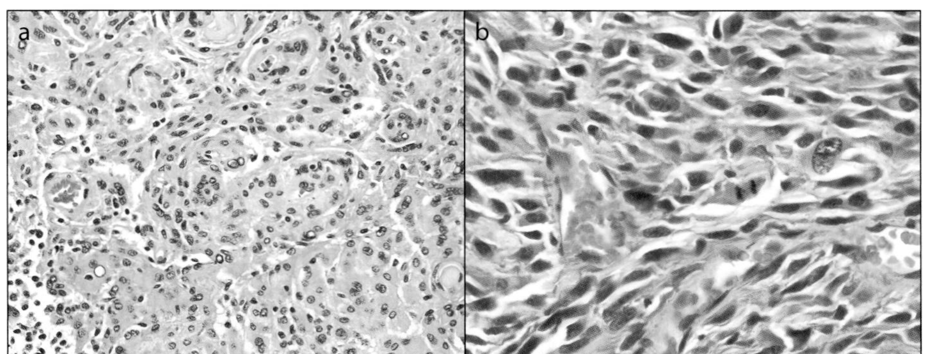

i41.5 **a** A transitional meningioma. Epithelioid cells are seen at the bottom while spindled, fibroblastic tumor cells are seen at the top.

b A grade 2 meningioma with nuclear pleomorphism, a mitotic figure, and several cells with prominent nucleoli

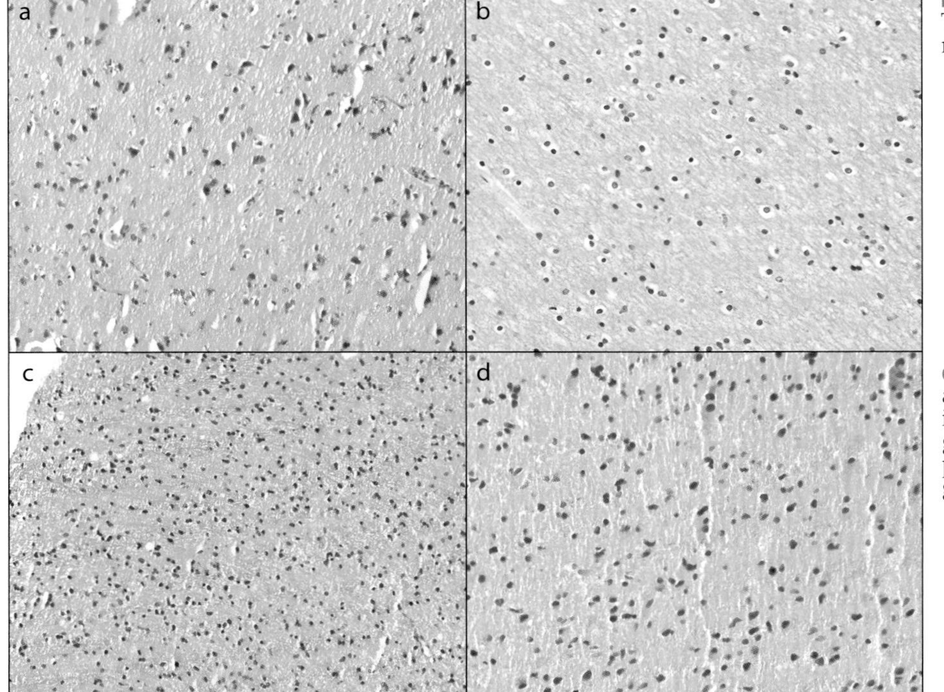

i41.6 **a** Normal brain tissue, illustrating a normal density of glial cells

b Benign reactive gliosis. This biopsy came from near a shunt site.

c A low-grade astrocytoma illustrating the higher cellularity relative to reactive gliosis

d A higher-power view of a low-grade astrocytoma illustrating the slightly greater nuclear pleomorphism relative to reactive gliosis

ISBN 978-089189-5886

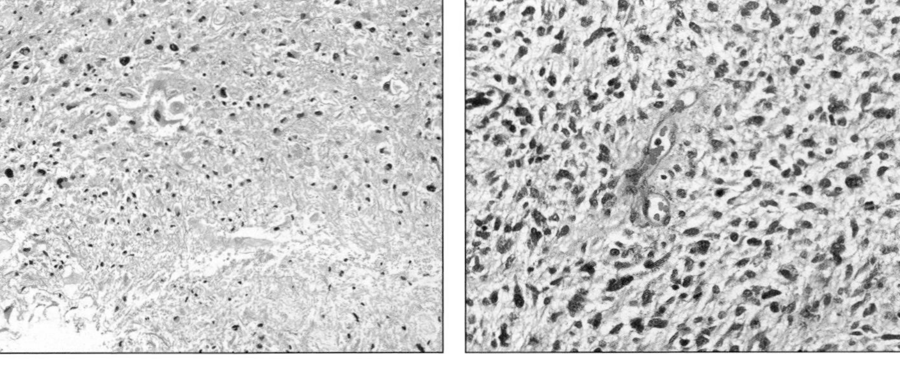

i41.7 An astrocytoma that has been treated with radiation therapy. Tumor necrosis is evident at the bottom, but viable tumor cells remain at the top.

i41.8 A grade 3 astrocytoma with nuclear pleomorphism

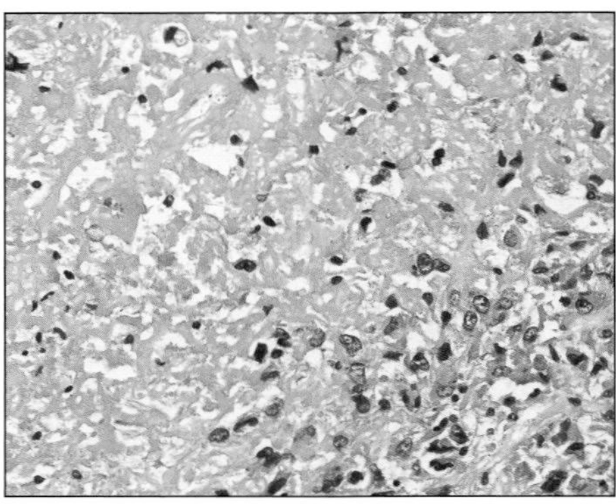

i41.9 A glioblastoma multiforme. There is tumor necrosis, not secondary to treatment, in the upper left and very pleomorphic tumor cells in the lower right.

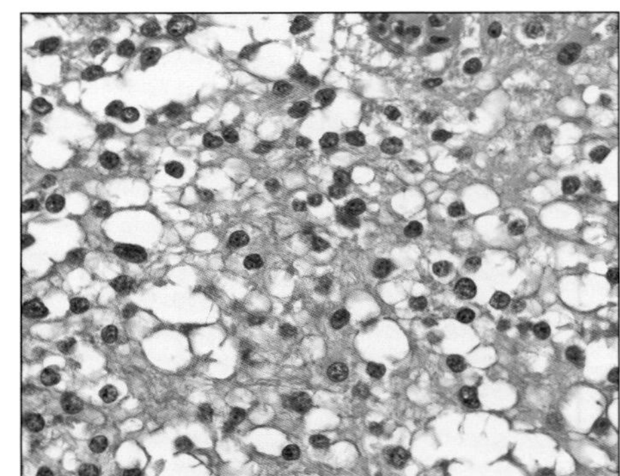

i41.10 An oligodendroglioma with relatively uniform, round nuclei, and appreciable cytoplasmic clearing

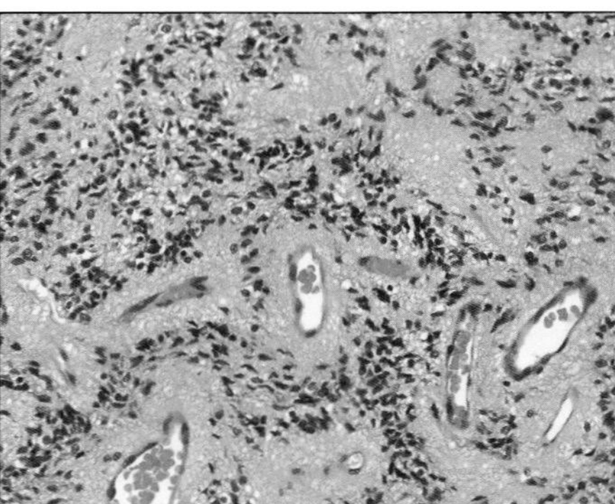

i41.11 An ependymoma with pseudorosettes around blood vessels

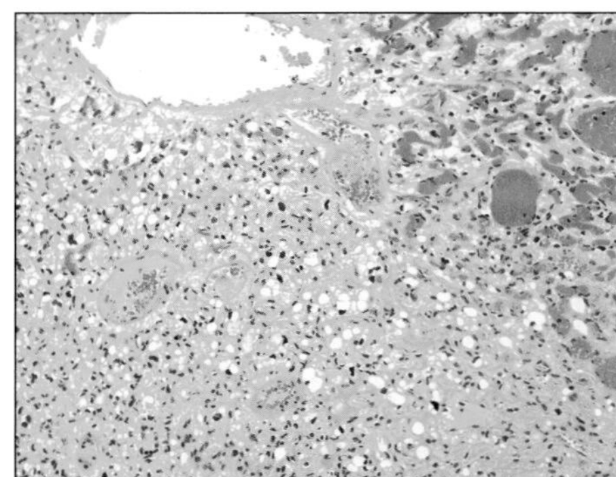

i41.12 A hemangioblastoma. The neoplastic cells are in the center and have clear cytoplasm. A large number of capillaries, characteristic of this tumor, are evident on the right. Note the similarity to a renal cell carcinoma.

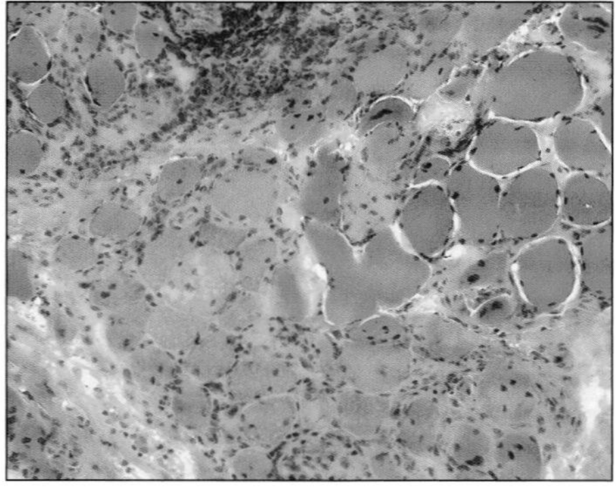

i41.13 A muscle biopsy in a patient with dermatomyositis. Relatively normal muscle fibers are seen in the upper right, while atrophic fibers are seen in the central and lower portions of the photograph. A lymphoid infiltrate is evident, particularly in the upper left.

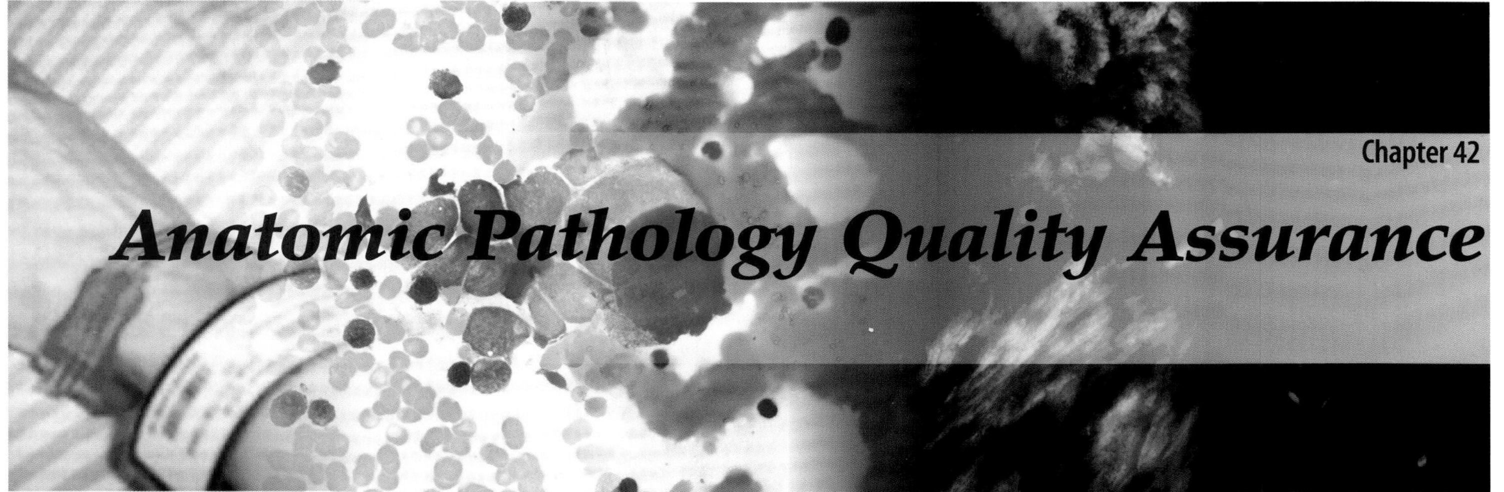

Anatomic Pathology Quality Assurance

In every field of medicine, optimal patient care involves a triad of good performance, good communication, and thorough documentation. As is the case for the clinical laboratory, testing in anatomic pathology can be divided into 3 stages. The preanalytic stage encompasses the time and activities from the initial patient-physician interaction to the receipt of the specimen in the laboratory, including specimen acquisition and transport. The analytic phase encompasses the time and activities while the specimen is actually in the laboratory, and includes the processing and examination of the specimen and the generation of the report. The postanalytic phase encompasses the time and activities after the report is generated, such as the conveyance of the report to the proper people in a timely manner.

The inherent subjectivity of anatomic pathology makes perfection unattainable, but mistakes in pathology fall roughly into 4 categories: mistakes of identification, mistakes of omission, mistakes of interpretation, and mistakes of documentation.

Mistakes of Identification

In mistakes of identification, the pathologist is dictating or signing a report on a different patient from the one he or she thinks is being served. Mistakes of identification occur when there is mislabeling of a specimen at the time of acquisition or anytime thereafter, including accessioning, the gross description, the microscopic examination, and the dictation of the final report.

Because of the generally manual methods employed in anatomic pathology, a higher percentage of errors are likely to be in the analytical phase than is the case for clinical laboratory specimens. In an 18-month study involving almost 30,000 cases, Layfield and Anderson found that 2/3 of labeling mistakes occur at the time of grossing [PMID20716804].

The key to prevention of errors of identification is double identification of the patient and the specimen at every stage in the process, from specimen acquisition to the signing of the report. In my experience, the laboratory should have a process for following each specimen from receipt to the final pathology report and should be able to demonstrate that there has been double identification at every stage. If 2 identical identifiers, such as a name and either a social security number or a date of birth, are found on both the specimen container and the accompanying requisition before the assignment of an accession number, and then all subsequent actions verify both the name and the accession number, double identification is achieved at every stage. This process must involve everyone who participates in patient care, including pathologists, assistants, and clerical and technical personnel, and comprises the following steps:

1. Ensuring a perfect match between the labeling on the specimen container and that on the accompanying requisition. Only after this verification is an accession number assigned to the specimen and the requisition.
2. During the gross dictation, the patient's name should be dictated with the accession number and the transcriptionist should be instructed that anything less than a perfect match must not be transcribed.
3. Assurance that the accession number on the cassette matches that on the specimen container and the requisition. When the cassette becomes the paraffin block, it will still carry that number.
4. Assurance that the slide carries the same accession number as the paraffin block from which it was cut. Patient names on slides, verified by the information system as matching that accession number, are highly recommended.
5. Even after there has been double identification of the patient at all stages, there are 2 causes of mistaken identification. The first occurs when the wrong slide is picked up from the tray. When dictating, the pathologist must be certain that the name and accession number on the slide being examined match those on the gross description. There is a natural tendency to examine slides in the order in which they are found on the tray, to turn the accompanying paperwork in the order in which it is present, and to assume that there is always a perfect correspondence between the paper and the slide.

Even when there is perfect correspondence between the paperwork and the slides, errors can occur when a slide is inadvertently skipped and the pathologist grasps a slide that is adjacent to the intended one. It is helpful to place slides that have been read back on the tray with the label facing the opposite direction from those that have not yet been examined. An added measure of confidence that the correct slide has been grasped is obtained placing the slide next to the gross description paperwork prior to being placed on the microscope, and ensuring that there is perfect correspondence of the accession number and name on the paper with those on the slide.

The second way in which a pathologist can unknowingly examine tissue from an unintended patient, even after double identification, is when there are transfer artifacts (colloquially called floaters). Almost all transfer artifacts arise from the cutting board at the time of gross examination or the water bath that is used by the histotechnologist during the cutting of the paraffin blocks [PMID12049100, PMID22031316]. Many of these are simply ignored, but the incidence is about 1-3% if specifically and prospectively looked for. A clue to the presence of transfer artifact from either source is fragments that differ from the other fragments, and an additional clue to extraneous tissue arising from the water bath is that it is not present in the paraffin block or is present in only 1 level.

The above suggestions will indicate to any future auditors that the pathologist took every reasonable step to avoid errors of identification.

Mistakes of Omission

Mistakes of omission occur when not every part of every fragment is examined. These mistakes may occur when there are numerous fragments on the slide, 1 of which was not examined. After examining 5 or 6 biopsies and finding them all to be normal, it is easy to conclude that the set of biopsies is normal and to complete the case without seeing another biopsy that might tell a different story.

The keys to preventing this type of error are to note the number of fragments mentioned in the gross description and be sure the same number is present on the slide. The paraffin block can be examined if there is any discrepancy. Each slide can be examined with the naked eye on a white background to determine the number and location of all fragments on the slide before placing it under the microscope, so that all fragments are accounted for during the microscopic examination. A 2× objective is worth its weight in gold because it allows one to locate every fragment on the slide. Another helpful activity is to examine the slide in a "grid-like" manner, such as the one employs in a cytology smear, so that every field is seen.

Mistakes of Interpretation

There are fewer interpretive mistakes than those involving identification or omission. There may be a disagreement about the precise type of tumor or its degree of differentiation, and there will be problematic cases that will inevitably have interobserver variation, but if correct patient identification is assured and every portion of the specimen is examined, only rarely will a qualified, experienced pathologist examine a given field and reach a conclusion that fundamentally cannot be justified. Aside from interpetive issues, there are a number of practices that pathologists may find helpful.

Be wary of cases in which an inadequate clinical history or clinical diagnosis is provided

The history and clinical findings are the context within which the tissue is interpreted, and if these are absent, they should either be obtained or it should be documented in the report that they were not given and an attempt to obtain them was not successful. At a minimum, there should be a limited history on the accompanying requisition, and it may be possible to obtain a more detailed history from the laboratory or hospital information system.

Both the pathologist and the clinician are busy, but it is precisely because they are busy that a history and clinical impression should be furnished on the requisition, so that no time is lost chasing these down later. Even if they are not provided on the requisition, the effort and time required from both physicians to obtain them before the pathologic diagnosis is rendered will be much less than that required for a cleanup campaign afterward if the case is misdiagnosed because of insufficient history.

One word of caution, however, in obtaining and using clinical history. It is remarkable and distressing how often major changes occur as information is anecdotally passed from one physician to another or is reiterated multiple times in the medical record. Remarkable transformations in the types and locations of tumors occur as physicians obtain information from other physicians. Situations in which information is conveyed verbally, as opposed to an examination of the record, are prone to errors. For this reason, I recommend getting primary source verification of all pertinent medical history. For example, instead of relying on a progress note or a telephone call that the patient has a history of chronic lymphoid leukemia, if one goes back to the original diagnostic tissue, or at least the pathology report on it, one may find that the actual history is that of a lymphoma of another type with a circulating component.

Even if the correct diagnosis for the correct patient is rendered, harm can occur if incorrect information on the requisition or from the record is transferred to the pathology report. For this reason, it is wise to indicate the source of any additional information, such as site, that appears on the pathology report. For example, if there is a biopsy from the right breast and the requisition erroneously indicates left breast, the pathologist increases the risk of wrong-sided surgery if he or she blindly dictates: "Biopsy of left breast: invasive adenocarcinoma." If there has been an error on the requisition or in the record, the pathologist minimizes the risk of its perpetuation and augmentation by dictating, "Breast biopsy (clinically left from the requisition): invasive adenocarcinoma," or "Breast biopsy (clinically left from the progress notes): invasive adenocarcinoma."

Do not read the history or clinical impression initially

As critical as the clinical history and a clinical diagnosis are in the formation of the final opinion, it is beneficial to form an initial impression without knowing them, as this minimizes the potential for prejudice. Many errors in diagnosis are caused by what I call "bandwagonning," whereby successive physicians assume that previous impressions must be accurate and do not need independent verification. For example, one might believe that because Dr X is a good clinician, if he or she thinks the lesion is malignant, it must be. If the case has been previously examined by another pathologist, there is a tendency to believe that because Dr Y is a good pathologist, his or her diagnosis is almost certainly correct, and the case therefore needs little attention. After an initial impression has been independently formed, the case can be reexamined with knowledge of the clinical history or previous opinions.

Examine the slide in a systematic manner, not in a haphazard or desultory fashion

As mentioned, a "grid-like" examination minimizes the risk that a fragment will be overlooked. Avoid a quick opinion on the principal process, as such an opinion that may be premature. The prototype example of this is the premature opinion that a malignancy is present when atypical cells are found, without appreciating a milieu that may cause severe reactive atypia. We tend to focus quickly and exclusively on the first apparent process that we see, believing that we have the case well in hand, without fully understanding the entire situation. Consider alternative processes that may cause a similar histologic picture.

Be watchful for unusual tumors or tumors that may have an unusual appearance, and begin with a wide differential diagnosis

The final opinion will be selected from the list of possibilities that the observer constructs. If the correct diagnosis is not on that initial list, there is no chance of a proper interpretation. For example, could this case be an angiosarcoma? Could it be an unusual type of melanoma? Could it be a thyroid medullary carcinoma? Could it be a reactive process despite its great cellularity and nuclear atypia?

Minimize distraction

Many errors are due to distractions during the interpretation process. I recommend making every effort to minimize telephone calls, knocks on the door, etc. This practice not only ensures more efficient workflow, it also makes it less likely that a mistake will be made. An "open door" policy is critical to good communication and an optimal work environment, and I wholeheartedly endorse such a policy in principle. But if this is interpreted literally, and everyone in the hospital is free to interrupt at any time, it is only a matter of time before a distraction causes an error. To my mind, "open door" means a very rapid, courteous, and complete response to an email inquiry. Moreover, receipt of questions via email permits a more reasoned response rather than an "off the cuff" answer that is likely to result from a knock on the door during a busy time or a difficult case. A better "open door" policy is an atmosphere where all feel free to express a concern via email or at specified times, with the knowledge that their concerns will be respected and promptly addressed.

The above steps, if followed assiduously, will convey the impression that the pathologist is meticulous, careful, and complete.

Errors of interpretation can often be prevented if the examiner requires that if anything is out of the ordinary, or if there is less than complete confidence, he or she performs additional examinations

Additional measures that can be taken and documented in the report may include:

1. Communication with clinicians.
2. Additional levels.
3. Immunohistochemical stains and molecular procedures.
4. A second opinion, either in-house or outside. There is a tendency not to document in-house second opinions. This can be done in the report or in a separate file. The former is generally preferred because the clinician can see from the report that a second opinion has been obtained.
5. A literature search. The literature in problematic cases can often be reasonably well and quickly searched through Pubmed at www.pubmed.com. Specifically citing these publications in the report conveys thoroughness and scholarship.

These steps, if followed assiduously, will show that the examining pathologist used every resource that was reasonably available to him or her.

Caution is indicated whenever the pathologist is in an area that has historically been difficult

In my experience, some of the situations that are more likely to lead to serious errors and/or litigation are as follows:

1. A frozen section diagnosis of thyroid carcinoma. As discussed in Chapter 6, this is an extremely treacherous area. Many benign processes may have some form of papillary structures. Frozen section compromises nuclear morphology and the peripheralization of chromatin—critical in the diagnosis of any form of papillary carcinoma, but especially in the follicular variant form—is an artifact of paraffin processing and cannot be appreciated at all on frozen section [PMID7536449, PMID10792769]. While such frozen sections may occasionally be diagnostic, there will be other cases in which even the most confident frozen section diagnosis is found to be in error.
2. Frozen sections of breast masses. In particular, florid adenosis and a well differentiated, small carcinoma cannot be reliably distinguished on frozen section. Frozen section interpretation of papillary and hyperplastic processes of the breast are also treacherous. Indeed, as discussed in Chapter 4, these situations are difficult on paraffin-processed tissue and often require immunohistochemistry.
3. The interpretation of these breast processes (florid adenosis vs carcinoma and papillary and hyperplastic lesions) even on paraffin-processed biopsies or resections. While the poor morphology of frozen section is eliminated, these remain difficult situations, responsible for a disproportionate share of errors, and there should be no hesitation in getting additional studies in either a biopsy or a resection of a cellular breast lesion.

ISBN 978-089189-5886

4. Fine needle aspirations of breast masses. It is often not appreciated that benign masses, such as fibroadenomas, may have substantial atypia on an aspirate and may also exfoliate single cells. Unlike frozen sections, there is a place for fine needle aspirations of breast masses, but only if they are conservatively interpreted.
5. A Pap smear diagnosis of negative, when there is actually high-grade dysplasia. This is especially frustrating because a Pap smear felt by the cytotechnologist to be negative is unlikely to even come to the attention of the pathologist. Hopefully, newer immunohistochemical stains, such as p16, increasing use of image-guided Pap smear interpretation, HPV assessment, and an evolving understanding of the molecular biology of cervical carcinoma will diminish these situations.
6. The Pap smear diagnosis of cervical dysplasia in middle-aged and older patients with no history of dysplasia. False positives can occur in patients of any age, but in older patients, mimics of dysplasia, such as squamous metaplasia and atrophy, are very likely to simulate dysplasia on a Pap smear or even on a biopsy. A typical scenario is an older patient with an unexpected ASCUS or low-grade Pap smear interpretation, followed by a biopsy that demonstrates epithelial cells with an increased nucleus to cytoplasmic ratio, diminished maturation (seen in atrophy), or perinuclear haloes (a nonspecific finding). The biopsy appears to corroborate the Pap smear findings, but studies for HPV , p16, and Ki-67 will show that the molecular accompaniments of dysplasia and proliferative activity above the basal layer are absent. The patient does not have dysplasia.
7. Melanoma vs benign mimics. The difficult differential diagnosis between a melanoma and a Spitz nevus is legendary, as discussed in Chapter 40. Many of these cases, and many examples of the deep-penetrating nevus and the cellular or atypical blue nevus are best regarded as melanocytic tumors of uncertain malignant potential [PMID20118771]. In these cases, there should be no hesitation in recommending verification of complete removal and close followup if the margins are negative, or re-excision if the margins are involved. A conservative interpretation of problematic or borderline melanocytic lesions, followed by a recommendation for complete excision if not already achieved, close followup, and possibly a sentinel lymph node study serves the patient well, often without an unnecessary cancer diagnosis.
8. Metastatic squamous carcinoma vs branchial cleft cyst in neck masses. Squamous cells should not be found in aspirates or biopsies of cervical lymph nodes, and their presence is disturbing. However, a branchial cleft cyst may have atypical cells and can be worrisome in limited material. A comment on the diagnostic possibilities, without a commitment, is prudent.
9. Small foci of atypia on prostate biopsies are responsible for both false-positive and false-negative diagnoses. As discussed in Chapter 37, immunohistochemistry is invaluable in elucidating the nature of small foci of atypia and is recommended in any situation where the diagnosis of prostate carcinoma is considered but not assured. Even after such stains have been performed, however, a small subset of patients is best served by the diagnosis of atypical small acinar proliferation (ASAP).
10. Failure to realize that urothelial carcinoma in situ (CIS) can have several morphologies [PMID11224606] and may still have umbrella cells. Both high-grade flat urothelial dysplasia/CIS and papillary lesions are associated with invasive carcinoma and difficult to detect in voided urine preparations because of low sensitivity, but it is prudent to suggest a cystoscopy with washings or biopsies for any urothelial atypia in a voided specimen.
11. Failure to take into account the milieu of atypical cells. Necrotic tissue, and the granulation tissue that often accompanies it, are likely to contain cells that are atypical, and may simulate malignancy. In a background of necrosis or severe inflammation, a conservative interpretation of atypia is warranted and a definitive diagnosis of malignancy in such material is usually unwise.

Unusual diagnoses demand convincing evidence

For example, the diagnosis of sarcoma in an organ is much more likely to be a carcinoma with sarcomatous metaplasia. Unless unusual entities are verified by additional evidence, the risk of an error is high.

Mistakes of Documentation

The pathology report should indicate that the clinical question was understood and addressed with all reasonable means available to the examiner. The report should indicate any communication with or attempt to communicate with clinicians concerning the acquisition of more clinical information or the conveyance of the pathologist's findings. Whatever is done on behalf of the patient should be documented, be these extra sections, special stains, another opinion, or a discussion. This ensures that all understand that every effort was made to do the best job.

The Anatomic Pathology Quality Assurance Program

A good analysis of error reduction in anatomic pathology has been published by D'Angelo and Zarbo [PMID17709316], whose experience has closely matched my own, and by Nakhleh and Fitzgibbons [Nakhleh ISBN978-0930304867]. The College of American Pathologists also publishes a comprehensive manual on Anatomic Pathology Quality Improvement [Nakhleh ISBN978-0930304751]. These publications, in conjunction with the triad of good practice, good communication, and good documentation, are the foundation of an anatomic pathology quality assurance program.

On a more specific level, a surgical pathology quality assurance program monitors the following areas:

- Correlation of the frozen section diagnosis and the final diagnosis, with discussion of discrepancies
- Correlation of the diagnosis rendered on cytology (both gynecologic and nongynecologic) with the biopsy or resection diagnosis, with discussion of discrepancies
- Documentation of in-house peer review, which should be about 5-6% [PMID20441505], and documentation of the resolution of any differences of opinion
- Documentation of reviews by other institutions, with discussion of discrepancies
- Discussion of any lost or compromised specimens, and documentation of a plan to minimize such losses in the future
- Amendments issued to provide new information (such as estrogen receptor status of a breast tumor) need only be noted, but a diagnosis that was fundamentally changed must be discussed, with a plan to prevent any recurrence of the error

Surgical Pathology "Critical" Values—What To Do?

The immediate communication of critical values is a well-accepted and long-established practice in laboratory medicine but has not traditionally been a part of anatomic pathology practice. However, because even the most conscientious clinician may not see a pathology report until 24 hours or more after it is generated, the suggestion has been made that in a few situations, the pathologist should contact the clinician to convey critical information immediately before or after the final report is generated.

Although there are no universally accepted "critical values" in surgical pathology, as there are in the clinical laboratory, the Association of Directors of Anatomic Pathology approved the concept in 2006 [PMID16867859], and suggested the following situations that might merit a telephone call to a clinician:

- Crescents in renal biopsies
- Primary vasculitis
- Bacteria within circulating leukocytes or bone marrow
- Evidence of any opportunistic infection
- Uterine contents though to be products of conception, but without villi or trophoblasts (possibly indicating an ectopic pregnancy)
- Evidence of transplant rejection
- Malignancy in a patient with superior vena cava syndrome
- Large vessels in a core biopsy
- Any tissue that suggests perforation, such as bowel tissue, fat, mesothelial cells, etc.

While the concept of rapid communication of surgical pathology critical values is sound, any such practice must balance the probability that rapid communication will improve patient care against several other considerations as follows:

- The ability to reach the clinician
- The possibility of misunderstanding in verbal communication
- The probability that the information, if successfully and accurately conveyed, will impact immediate patient care before the reading of the final report

It is often very difficult for even other physicians to reach their colleagues or their designees. Clinicians often leave cell phone numbers, but caution is needed to ensure compliance with HIAPA privacy regulations, as many cell phone conversations can be overheard, either via electronic eavesdropping or simply because the recipient may be in a public place at the time the call is made. In unsuccessful attempts to reach a responsible clinical party, the report should indicate that an attempt was made to contact the physician and that no one could be reached.

A major potential problem with telephonic communication of possible surgical pathology critical values is the possibility of a misunderstanding, especially since the information is likely to be conveyed to an assistant, followed by a second telephone call between the assistant and the physician. In contrast to laboratory values, which are typically simple numbers, the conveyance of a potentially critical finding in surgical pathology involves more complicated terminology that is more likely to be misunderstood on the telephone even by a physician, and often not understood at all by a secretary or nurse receiving the call who then relays the message to the physician. This means that a well-meaning attempt to telephone the contents of a report can cause more harm than good. For example, I am aware of a situation in which a telephone report was made to a physician's office that a patient "has an adenocarcinoma." This was repeated to the clinical physician as the patient "had no carcinoma."

The potential for confusion of patients is also much easier in a verbal communication because 2 physicians must both be certain of identity and neither is likely to use the normal double-identifier system in a hurried telephone conversation. A telephone call to a clinical colleague that "Mr. Johnston has such and such" could easily be heard and remembered as "Mr. Johnson has such and such."

Moreover, in most anatomic pathology critical value situations, the clinical circumstances dictate what action will be taken. In laboratory medicine, there are often situations in which patients with critical values, potentially on the verge of a significant event, may be relatively asymptomatic, and a rapid communication may be critical in preventing critical clinical symptoms (eg, patients with significant electrolyte abnormalities). Laboratory values can be communicated clearly and are often acted on even though significant clinical findings have not yet developed. In contrast, in anatomic pathology, even if there are significant unexpected findings, in most situations, no action will be taken unless clinical findings are evident. While the pathology findings are often indispensable in the long-term care of the patient, the clinical situation is much more sensitive in identifying patients who need immediate intervention. In most cases, the clinical situation alone, with or without a rapid communication from the pathologist, determines the immediate course of action. For example, a surgeon will usually know of a bowel perforation or significant bleeding after a biopsy based on the clinical examination even without telephone confirmation that bowel tissue or a large blood vessel were found. Likewise, if the patient is stable, it is very unlikely that the clinician will intervene based on a telephone call declaring the presence of bowel or vascular tissue.

In those rare cases where a hastened report appears truly necessary, I recommend direct telephone communication with the physician rather than with any assistant or employee. If this is not possible, an accelerated written report, even if only a preliminary report, can be conveyed to the office via fax or electronic means. This can be followed by a telephone call whose purpose is only to indicate that the physician should expeditiously review the faxed or electronic report, not to convey the information contained therein. An accelerated or preliminary written report mitigates the risk of a communication error, but still does not ensure that the information will make its way to the physician or modify the immediate care of the patient.

Core Points for Quality Assurance

- Preanalytic, analytic, and postanalytic phases in anatomic pathology, as in clinical laboratory testing.
- Mistakes of identification, especially during grossing, are common.
  - Can be reduced by a double identification system at all stages of the process.
- Mistakes of omission: may occur when one of many fragments on a slide is missed.
- Mistakes of interpretation: occur more often from an inadequate history, distractions, or an examination of a slide that is not systematic than from a fundamental lack of knowledge.
  - Probability increased in certain situations, such as frozen sections, fine needle aspirations, breast biopsies, and melanocytic lesions.
- Mistakes of documentation: when actions performed in service to the patient are not indicated in the report.
  - Communication with other physicians, additional sections, special stains, the acquisition of additional opinions, or the performance of a literature search.
- Surgical pathology quality assurance program: correlations of frozen section and final diagnoses, correlation of cytologic and biopsy/resection diagnoses, discussion of peer reviews and any discrepancies therein, and discussion of amended reports.
- Anatomic pathology critical values: meritorious concept with potential benefit.
  - But implementation must also consider:
    - Probability of reaching an appropriate person.
    - Possibility that the information will be distorted during its transmission.
    - Probability that it will change immediate patient care.

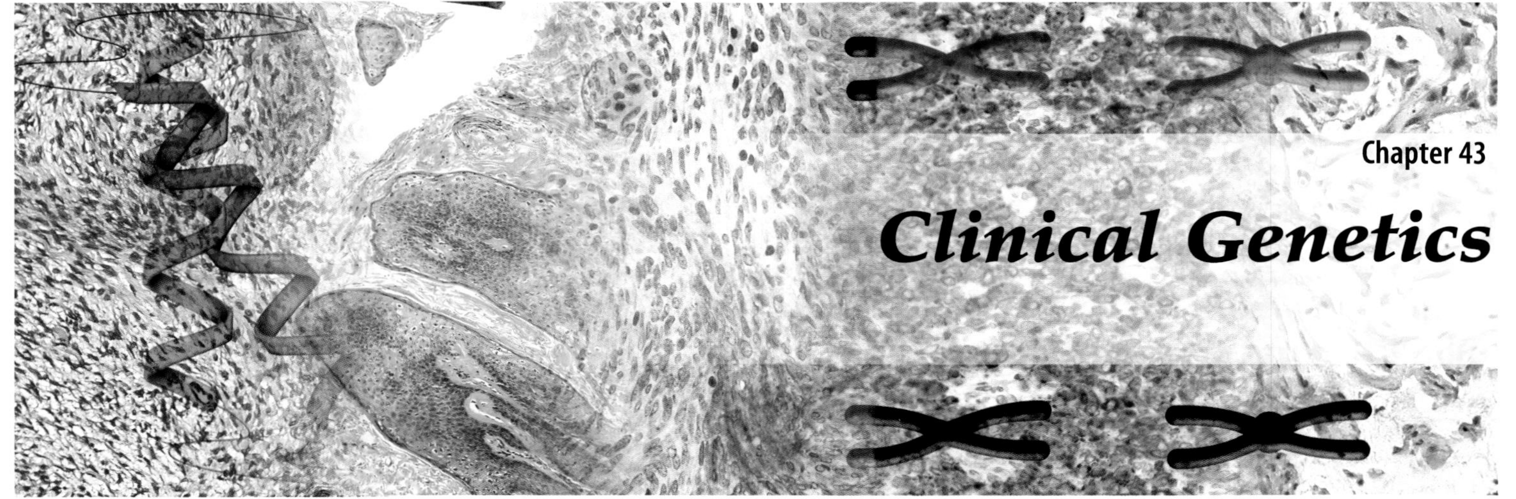

Chapter 43
Clinical Genetics

Because molecular biology and genetics are inextricably linked, we must review basic concepts in genetics before considering the wonderful field of molecular pathology in the second part of this work. For a comprehensive treatment of genetics, the Thompson and Thompson text is recommended [Nussbaum ISBN978-1416030805].

Humans have 46 chromosomes, which exist in sets of 2. A cell with 1 full set of chromosomes is haploid and a cell with 2, the normal state, is diploid. There are 22 autosomes and 2 sex chromosomes (the X and the Y). One set of chromosomes is inherited from the father and the other set is inherited from the mother. Males have 1 X chromosome and 1 Y chromosome and females have 2 X chromosomes.

In meiosis, there is 1 replication of the DNA in a diploid cell, followed by 2 cell divisions, resulting in 4 cells, each of which is haploid, containing 22 autosomes and 1 sex chromosome. Meiosis is illustrated in f43.1. Before DNA replication in meiosis, the chromosomes are organized into 23 pairs, with 1 member of each pair derived from the father and 1 member from the mother. After each of the 46 chromosomes is replicated, the DNA is still organized into 23 sets, but each set consists of 4, not 2, chromosomes. Each individual chromosome is now called a chromatid. This terminology came about because those who initially elucidated this process felt that the number of chromosomes should correspond to the number of centromeres, and each set of 4 chromosomes still has only the 2 original centromeres. Within each set, 2 of the 4 chromatids are from the father, representing the replication of his contribution to the original pair, and 2 are from the mother. Each of these homologous pairs of chromatids, sharing a common origin from 1 chromosome, is called a dyad. 2 of the 4 chromatids in each set—1 dyad—are sister chromatids from the paternal chromosome and 2 of the 4 chromatids in each set—the other dyad—are sister chromatids from the maternal chromosome.

All 4 chromatids within the set are precisely aligned so that corresponding genes are directly across from each other. In male mammals, even the X and Y chromosomes align, but

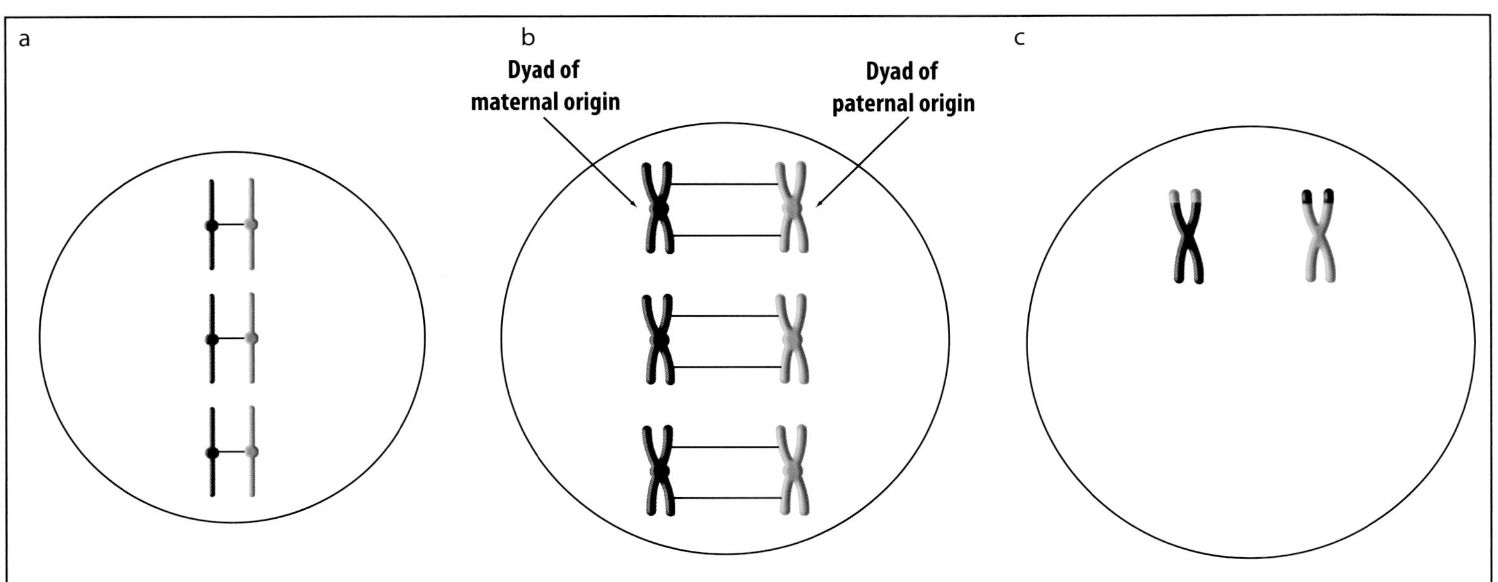

f43.1 Meiosis. This simplified diagram omits the individual stages, but emphasizes the mechanism whereby DNA from an individual's mother and father are combined.
a The black chromosomes are of maternal origin and the red are of paternal origin. At the beginning of meiosis, the 2 chromosomes in each pair line up in such a way that the corresponding genes are adjacent.
b The chromosomes then replicate, doubling the DNA content of each cell. Each chromosome replicates into 2 identical chromatids. The 2 chromatids from the chromosome of maternal origin form 1 dyad and the 2 chromatids from the chromosome of paternal origin form another dyad. The 4 chromatids within each set precisely align so that corresponding genes are adjacent.
c Recombination (crossing over) then occurs.

ISBN 978-089189-5886

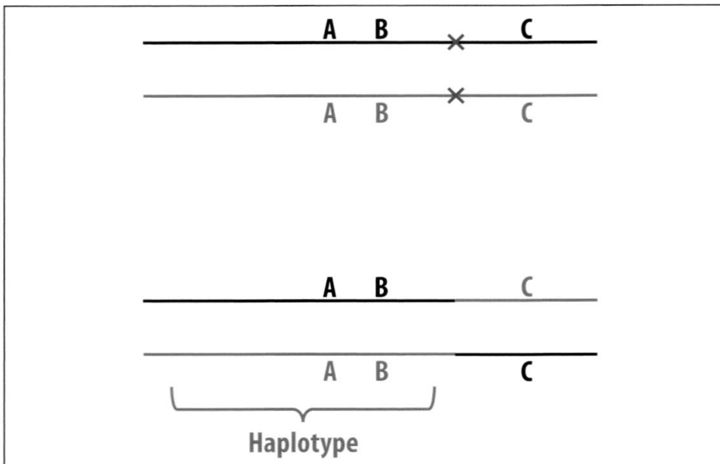

f43.2 The black chromosome is of maternal origin and the red are of paternal origin. The blue "x" indicates a breakage-prone point. Because genes A and B are on the same side of the breakage-prone point, they tend to stay together during recombination. Because gene C lies on the other side of the breakage-prone point, it is often separated from genes A and B during recombination. Genes A and B, and other genes that are within the same region, between 2 breakage-prone points, tend to be inherited as a unit called a haplotype.

because the small areas of homology are largely at the ends, the result is a nearly end-to-end alignment. This alignment brings paternally derived and maternally derived DNA into close proximity—something that never happens in mitosis, and something that could not happen if 1/2 of the 46 chromosomes in the original cell simply segregated to each pole of the cell.

This precise alignment of the chromatids permits recombination (also called crossing over)—the reciprocal sharing of DNA—between *nonsister* chromatids, ie, between chromatids from your mother and your father. Recombination is the actual physical cutting of the DNA in a chromosome and its reattachment at another location. We have seen the "cutting and pasting" of DNA in immunoglobulin synthesis, but it also happens in every meiosis. The enormous implication of this is that, instead of simply having 1 member of each pair of chromosomes migrate to a pole, there is recombination of *maternally derived* and *paternally derived DNA*. If 1 member of each of the 23 pairs of chromosomes simply migrated to a pole, there would be no such recombination.

The farther apart regions on a chromosome are, the more likely they are to undergo recombination. The reason for this is that there are regions of the chromosome that are prone to breakage and regions that are resistant to breakage [PMID15880103]. The farther apart 2 loci are, the more breakage-prone regions will lie between them, and the more likely it is that at least 1 of those regions will break and reattach to another region f43.2. Because recombination occurs less readily if the 2 loci are physically close and more readily if they are physically separated, 2 loci that rarely recombine are likely to be physically close, while 2 loci that are far apart will be much more likely to recombine. The maximal recombination rate is 50%. A recombination rate of 50% suggests that the loci are far apart or are on different chromosomes and exhibit independent segregation. The recombination frequency for 2 loci on the same chromosome is given by the Greek letter θ. θ varies from 0 (no recombination) to 0.5 (completely independent assortment, as if they were on different chromosomes). A smaller θ indicates that the 2 loci are closer and more tightly linked, while a θ of 0.5 indicates that the loci are completely unlinked, either by being on different chromosomes or by being so far apart on one chromosome that there will almost always be recombination. A θ of 0.01 means that there is roughly a 1% recombination rate between the 2 alleles. In honor of the great geneticist Thomas Hunt Morgan, this is referred to as 1 centimorgan. Genetic distances are roughly additive, so if genes A, B, and C are on the same chromosome and A and B are 1 centimorgan apart, and B and C are 1 centimorgan apart, then A and C will be roughly 2 centimorgans apart and will recombine in about 2% of meiosis. However, there is only rough correspondence between genetic distance—the probability of recombination—and physical distance. For long distances (high recombination rates) the observed frequencies underestimate the actual rate of recombination because there are situations in which a recombination is followed by a second recombination that returns the chromatids to their original state.

Because crossing over is partially related to whether a region of DNA is recombination-rich or recombination-poor, some regions are not typically exchanged and other areas are exchanged with great frequency. Recombination results in stretches of DNA that stay together during the process. Such stretches, which are passed to offspring as a unit, are called a haplotype. While DNA cannot be studied in light microscopy, new technologies allow us to identify where these breakpoints have occurred. A region that has undergone recombination is called a chiasma (plural "chiasmata").

After meiosis is completed, the final result is not only that the gametes have only 23 chromosomes, but also that those chromosomes that have undergone recombination have genetic material from both of the individual's parents. This is a new combination of DNA, never before present in the individual. When the gamete (egg or sperm) combines with a gamete from another person, its 23 chromosomes—each a genetic combination of that person's maternal and paternal DNA—will combine with the 23 from the other gamete—also a combination of maternal and paternal DNA—to reconstitute the full complement of DNA in the zygote with maximal mixing of genetic material. We have 2 parents, but we are the genetic result of 4 grandparents. Crossing over in meiosis, with subsequent merging of 2 sets of parental chromosomes, is the principal source of genetic variability, far outweighing random mutations.

Punnett squares are the simple 2×2 arrays of genetic probability, as we learned in high school. Punnett squares have the mother's gametes on the left and the father's gametes on the top, with the interior boxes containing the 4 possible combinations. For example:

	A	a
A	AA	Aa
a	aA	aa

A genetic family history is called a pedigree and is depicted by vertical lines representing different generations and horizontal lines representing one generation. A typical pedigree is depicted in f43.3. In pedigrees, squares represent males, circles represent females and diamonds indicate individuals of unknown or disguised gender. A diagonal line from the lower left to the upper right across a symbol

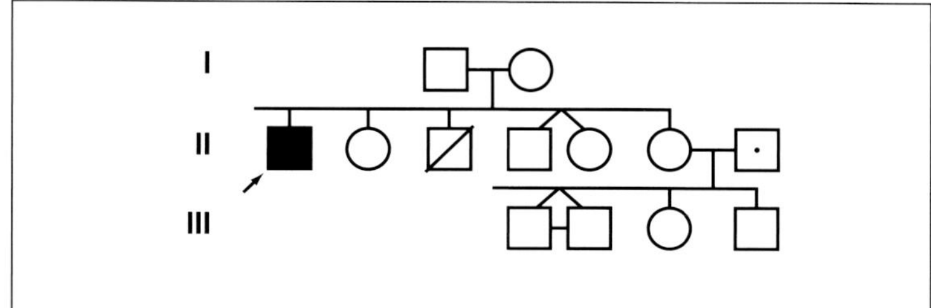

f43.3 Pedigree basics. In generation I, 2 phenotypically normal people mate. In generation II, their first child, a son, is the proband (the patient of principal interest), and is affected. His younger brother is deceased. He has fraternal twin siblings of different genders. His youngest sibling, a sister, has mated with a phenotypically normal man known to be a carrier. In generation III, there is a set of monozygotic twins, followed by a phenotypically normal girl and boy.

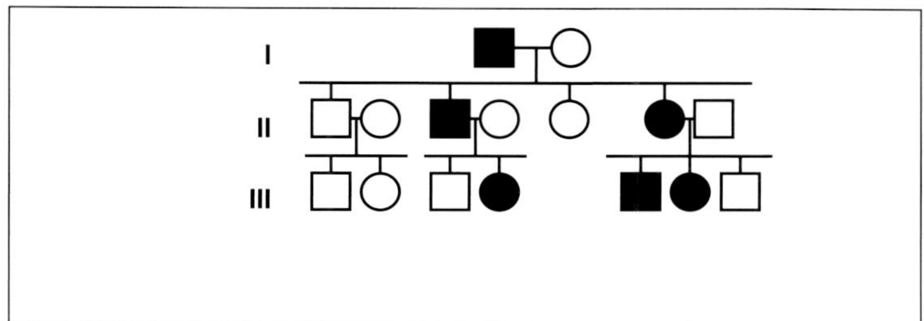

f43.4 A pedigree of an autosomal dominant trait. Even allowing for incomplete penetrance, variable expressivity, and de novo mutations, most complete pedigrees of autosomal dominant transmission will show an affected person in every generation and that males and females are affected equally.

indicates a deceased person. Offspring and their mates are denoted by a horizontal line (a sibship line) beneath a vertical line. In a sibship line, older children are depicted to the left of younger siblings.

Twins are indicated by diagonal lines connecting children to parents instead of a vertical line and a horizontal sibship line. A short horizontal connection between the diagonal twin line indicates that they are identical. Successive generations are numbered by Roman numerals, while individuals within a generation are designated by Arabic numerals, starting on the left (eg, II-3 refers to the third child in the second generation). Pedigrees typically depict phenotypes, not genotypes, with a few exceptions. A filled symbol indicates an affected person, while an open symbol indicates phenotypic normality, though complete openness of the symbol must not be construed as homozygosity for the wild-type gene or genes because often, a heterozygous state will also be phenotypically normal. An open symbol containing a dot indicates known heterozygosity. A circle with a dot in the center often indicates a female carrier of an X-linked trait. For a dominant trait, a partially shaded individual is affected but is known to be heterozygous. An arrow pointing to a symbol indicates the proband (the person of principal study).

Mendelian Inheritance

Disorders or characteristics caused by a mutation in a single gene are called Mendelian traits and are inherited in 1 of 4 ways—autosomal dominant, autosomal recessive, X-linked recessive, and X-linked dominant. X-linked dominant inheritance is rare, so in practice, there are 3 common modes of Mendelian inheritance—autosomal dominant, autosomal recessive, and X-linked recessive. Described disorders that are Mendelian or have a Mendelian component are given a specific number, the MIM (Mendelian inheritance in man). For example, the MIM number for cystic fibrosis is 219700. This classification permits an evaluation of possible relationships between phenotype and genotype, and is available at the Online Mendelian Inheritance in Man (OMIM) website at http://www.ncbi.nlm.nih.gov/omim.

There are 2 terms that are often used in describing autosomal dominant inheritance—"penetrance" and "variable expressivity." While these terms are occasionally used in other forms of inheritance, they are primarily used in autosomal dominant conditions. The term "penetrance" refers to whether or not there are sufficient clinical manifestations to make a diagnosis of the disorder in the presence of a genotype that generally causes disease. In incomplete penetrance, an individual inherits a copy of the defective gene and is expected to have the trait, but for multiple and as yet unknown reasons, the defective gene does not manifest in the disease. In clinical situations this means that most physicians would not diagnose the disorder. "Expressivity" refers to features of expression. Variable expression indicates different degrees of manifestation among different individuals, all of whom have a secure diagnosis of the disorder. Some diseases have many characteristic features any combination that could result in a diagnosis of the disorder. As an example, type I neurofibromatosis is autosomal dominant and has 100% penetrance, but has strikingly variable expression in which some individuals may have neurofibromas, but others may only have café au lait spots. The term "incomplete penetrance" means that only a subset of individuals with the disease-related genotype will have features of the disease.

In addition to penetrance and expressivity, another characteristic of autosomal dominant inheritance is that, unlike other modes of inheritance, these conditions may relatively frequently arise as de novo mutations, with neither parent affected.

In autosomal dominant inheritance, all affected individuals should have an affected parent unless there has been either a de novo mutation or incomplete penetrance. Even allowing for incomplete penetrance or a de novo mutation, there is usually a family history of the autosomal transmission of the trait, without skipping of generations. The trait occurs in parents as well as in siblings. There is generally a 50-50 gender distribution unless there are gender differences in penetrance or expressivity f43.4. About 50% of an affected individual's children should be affected. If an individual does not inherit the mutation causing the trait, all of their children will be normal. (If you don't get the genotype, it cannot be passed on). If a trait has incomplete penetrance, a seemingly normal carrier could pass on the genotype to their offspring. In autosomal dominant conditions, all children will be affected if either parent is homozygous, and 3 in 4 children will be affected if both parents are affected and heterozygous. 1 in 2 will be affected if there is 1 affected and 1 normal parent.

We may think that eventually, alleles conferring a severe disease would be removed, but failure to penetrate, variable expressivity, frequent late onset (after reproduction), lethality of the homozygous state, and the fact that some autosomal dominant conditions arise as de novo mutations maintain

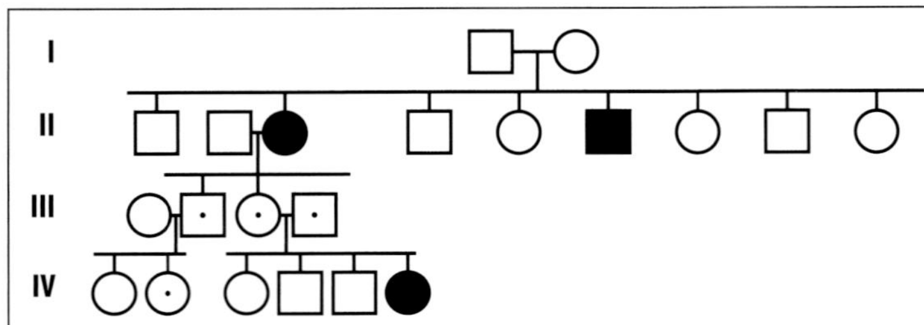

f43.5 A pedigree of an autosomal recessive trait. Note that the parents are phenotypically normal, that the 2 genders are equally affected, and that the trait appears to skip generations. The dots within the squares or circles indicate carrier status, but this can only be determined by testing, as carriers are phenotypically normal.

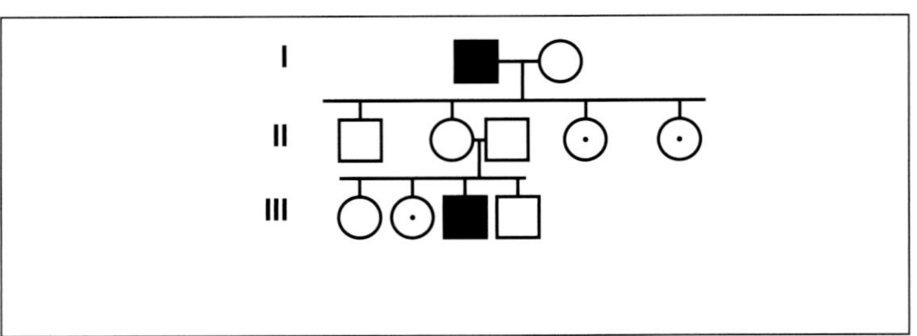

f43.6 A pedigree of an X-linked recessive trait. This mode of transmission is recognized by the skipping of generations and the invariable phenotypic normality of females.

these alleles in the population. The Hardy-Weinberg law in population genetics holds that in a large, stable, unperturbed population, with random mating and for which mutations do not affect reproductive fitness, allele frequencies do not change. For a single locus with 2 alleles, consisting of a dominant allele of frequency p and a recessive allele of frequency q, $p^2 + 2pq + q^2 = 1$. Major exceptions to the Hardy-Weinberg law occur when there are small, separated populations (founder effect) or when the randomness of mating is disturbed by stratification (preference for a particular subgroup, such as ethnicity), assortative mating (preference for certain traits, such as height), or consanguinity.

Though the Hardy-Weinberg law is used more for populations, it can occasionally be used in individual situations. For example, if a very rare autosomal recessive condition affects 1 in 1,000,000 people, the frequency for the responsible allele, q, in the population is 1/1,000. The dominant allele, p, must then have a frequency of 999/1,000. p^2 is the frequency of homozygous normal individuals who are not carriers, while q^2 is the frequency of an affected homozygous recessive. The central term of the Hardy-Weinberg law, "2pq," represents the carrier state. In this example, this probability of being a carrier is 2 × (999/1,000) × (1/1,000), or 1,998/1,000,000. This is equal to 0.002, indicating a 1 in 500 chance of being a carrier.

In autosomal recessive inheritance, there is often no family history of a disease because both parents are unaffected carriers. In contrast to autosomal dominant inheritance, the parents of a person with an autosomal recessive disease are usually phenotypically normal **f43.5**. In traits showing autosomal recessive inheritance, a second affected individual in a family is more likely to be a sibling of an already affected individual than a parent (ie, the trait runs more in siblings than in parents). Unless the recessive trait is very common in the population (such as blood group O), "skip" generations are the rule.

Both genders are equally affected in autosomal recessive inheritance. Whereas in autosomal dominant conditions, 3 in 4 children will be affected if both parents are affected and heterozygous, in autosomal recessive conditions, only 1 in 4 children will be affected if both parents are heterozygous (carriers). However, in a mating of 2 carriers of an autosomal recessive trait, of the 75% of offspring who are not affected, 2/3 will be carriers, and only 1/3 of the phenotypically normal children (1/4 of all children) will be homozygous normal and therefore incapable of transmitting the disease allele. If there has been any consanguinity or relatedness between family members, there can be a sharp increase in affected offspring.

X-linked inheritance can be dominant or recessive, as is the case for autosomal inheritance, though the former is very rare. The few described X-linked dominant inherited conditions, like Rett syndrome, are lethal in males. In any X-linked inheritance, the trait is never passed from father to son. Father-to-son transmission excludes an X-linked mechanism. In X-linked conditions, males are not spoken of as being either heterozygous or homozygous for the abnormality, as these terms are used only in reference to patients with 2 copies of a gene. Instead, the word "hemizygous" is used in X-linked conditions for males whose sole X chromosome carries the abnormality. Males are either both genotypically and phenotypically normal, or they are affected. They cannot be phenotypically normal carriers.

In X-linked recessive conditions, daughters of an affected male and a normal female are normal, but they will be carriers. Sons from such a relationship will be normal because they have not inherited any X chromosomes from their fathers (the trait is never passed father to son in any X-linked condition). In X-linked recessive conditions, females may be affected by 1 of 2 mechanisms. The first mechanism is a carrier with skewed lyonization of the normal X chromosome in embryogenesis (one X chromosome is largely inactivated in early embryogenesis in women in a random process called lyonization, after its discoverer, Mary Lyon; if by chance, a disproportionate number of normal X chromosomes are inactivated, the abnormal X chromosome may not be clinically silent). The second mechanism is that 1/2 of females who are children of a carrier female and an affected male will be fully homozygous.

In X-linked recessive conditions, males are much more likely to be affected than females. A typical pedigree for an X-linked recessive trait is an affected grandfather, phenotypically normal daughters, and about 1/2 of grandsons affected **f43.6**. Every affected male is linked to a female who is a carrier. A sufficiently well developed pedigree that has only males as affected individuals is highly likely to be X-linked recessive.

X-linked conditions may occasionally arise de novo, with neither parent affected. A final comment about X-linked recessive disorders is that while they generally require a female carrier, spontaneous mutations in the patient can account for occasional cases, in some instances up to 1/3 of cases.

X-linked dominant conditions are very rare, and unless otherwise specified, the term "X-linked" refers to "X-linked recessive." In X-linked dominant conditions, females are commonly affected. Indeed, all daughters of an affected male are affected because they will always inherit a defective X chromosome from their father. When males are affected, they have received an abnormal X chromosome from the mother, and they are usually more affected than females because they lack a normal X chromosome. Indeed, X-linked dominant conditions are often lethal in males. In situations where there is no lethality in males, the condition is twice as common in females because they have inherited an X chromosome from both parents and therefore have twice as many chances to have one that is abnormal. Because males inherit a Y chromosome from their father, their mother is the only possible source of an abnormal X chromosome. In contrast, females can inherit an abnormal X chromosome from either parent. X-linked dominant is the only pedigree that has more affected females than males, and it is the only pedigree in which all daughters of an affected male are affected.

A final comment about Mendelian inheritance concerns locus heterogeneity. *Allelic* heterogeneity refers to variations in the same gene, but *locus* heterogeneity occurs when the same clinical disease can be caused by defects in >1 gene at different loci. This can lead to multiple modes of transmission for the same clinical disorder. For example, there are >40 loci that can give rise to retinitis pigmentosa, some of which cause X-linked transmission, some of which cause autosomal dominant transmission, and some of which result in autosomal recessive transmission. *Allelic* heterogeneity leads to simpler situations than *locus* heterogeneity, but we must still keep in mind the possibility of a compound heterozygote, whereby an individual has 2 mutations in the same gene but different mutations on each of its 2 copies.

Y-linked Inheritance

A final mode of single-gene, Mendelian inheritance, extremely rare, is Y-linked. In Y-linked inheritance, a gene is passed down from father to son in every generation. Every man in a pedigree is affected if his father was affected, and all sons of an affected man are affected. Women are never affected. Like mitochondrial inheritance, Y chromosome genetics is non-Mendelian because of uniparental transmission but, like Mendelian or mitochondrial inheritance, is usually based on single genes.

The most important part of the Y chromosome is the *SRY* gene, which is the area that contains the genetic information to convert the embryo from its default female gender to male. One example of a Y-linked trait is male infertility as a result of *SRY* deletion or mutation. However, this disease has a low likelihood of being passed on unless assisted reproductive technologies are used. A major importance of the Y chromosome is that it has been used in tracing evolution and population migrations in a manner similar to that used for mitochondrial DNA.

Bayesian Analysis in Mendelian Inheritance

Probability calculations in Mendelian inheritance are generally quite simple but can be much more complicated if new information, such as knowledge of affected siblings or children, or results of screening tests are available. Accurate calculations of probability in Mendelian inheritance need to take such new information into account, and for this reason, they can be quite complex. Bayesian analysis is a statistical method in which new evidence is used to update an existing probability. As an analogy, the probability of pulling an ace from a deck of cards is 4 in 52, but if it is known that an ace has already been removed from an otherwise pristine deck, the probability of removing a second ace is not 4 in 52, but 3 in 51.

Bayesian methods are particularly important in genetic counseling because the probability of a particular person's being a carrier will change depending on what has already transpired. Using Bayesian inference, a baseline risk for having a disease or being a carrier that is inherent to a population is modified, depending on family history or the results of screening tests, to yield a much more accurate assessment of risk.

A brief summary of the technique will be followed by 5 examples. A typical Bayesian analysis consists of 2 columns and 4 rows. The 2 columns reflect mutually exclusive occurrences, usually being a carrier for a disorder in the left column and not being a carrier in the right column. In the first row, the probabilities are simply those of the patient's population or ethnic group, as if we knew nothing of the individual patient and had no additional information, such as the status of family members or the results of screening tests. This row is called the prior probability. It is the "starting probability" before any particular knowledge of that individual is considered. It is simply the probability of a comparable group.

In a simple example, if the probability of a woman's being a carrier of an X-linked recessive disorder is under investigation, and it is known that she had a normal father and a mother who was a carrier, this first row will be 1/2 | 1/2, reflecting the fact that until additional information is forthcoming, she has a 50% chance of being a carrier. For this patient, we would begin with:

	Probability of being a carrier	Probability of not being a carrier
Prior probability	1/2	1/2

The prior probability for any condition will vary among ethnic groups, and there are data available on the carrier frequencies for various diseases among different ethnic groups. For example, the carrier frequency of cystic fibrosis in Ashkenazi Jews is usually taken as 1 in 29 [PMID20494256], though 1 in 23 has recently been reported [PMID18264947]. For an Ashkenazi Jew undergoing testing for carrier state in cystic fibrosis, the prior probability (first row) would be:

	Probability of being a carrier	Probability of not being a carrier
Prior probability	1/29	28/29

For an individual patient, the actual probability will depend heavily on his or her family history, and a family history, if available, may modify published ethnically based prior probabilities. For this reason, a pedigree should be obtained before a Bayesian analysis is determined.

ISBN 978-089189-5886

The second row is called the conditional probability and is the probability of carrier or noncarrier, based *only* on the additional information that we have that is specific to the patient, such as the patient's relatives or the results of screening tests. Just as we ignored any information specific to the patient in the first row, so we ignore any general information about the patient's ethnic group in the second row. This new information is expressed in the first column (ie, the probability of being a carrier) of the second row. The entry in the second column of the second row will be 1, since this column is defined as noncarrier. This is perhaps the most confusing entry in a Bayesian table, as we might initially think that the conditional probability of not being a carrier is 1– the conditional probability of being a carrier. After all, in the prior probability row, the probability of noncarrier status was 1– the probability of carrier status, such that the sum of the 2 columns equaled 1. But in the conditional (second) probability row, the second column (noncarrier) is 1 by definition.

The third row is called the joint probability and is the product of the first 2 rows. This product takes into account both the general information concerning the patient's ethnicity and specific information concerning the individual patient. We need to convert any fractions in the joint probability row to achieve a common denominator.

The fourth and final row is called the posterior probability (also called or relative probability or residual risk; meaning after all knowledge is taken into account). Because the sum of all probabilities must equal 1, the probability for each outcome is calculated in the fourth row by dividing the joint probability for that outcome by the sum of the joint probabilities. In the posterior probabilities, the numerators are obtained by retaining the numerators of the joint probabilities, while the denominators are obtained by adding the numerators in the joint probability row (ie, the numerators in the fourth row are the same as the numerators in the third row, and the common denominator is the sum of the numerators in the third row).

Our first example concerns an X-linked recessive disorder. Consider a patient whose maternal grandfather was a hemophiliac. Both of her parents are normal, but her mother must be a carrier because she must have received a defective X chromosome from her father, the patient's grandfather, so the patient has a 50% chance of being a carrier. Her prior probabilities of being and not being a carrier are 1/2 and 1/2:

	Probability of being a carrier	Probability of not being a carrier
Prior probability	1/2	1/2

If the patient gives birth to an affected son, we know she must be a carrier. No further analysis is needed, and we need not proceed to a second row. But what if she gives birth to a normal son? She might still be a carrier, but her chances of being a carrier drop to somewhat <50%. How much less? In a Bayesian analysis of this situation, in the first row, the probabilities of carrier (first column) and noncarrier (second column) are 1/2 and 1/2 because we have not yet taken into account the additional information of a normal son. In the second row, the conditional probability, we do take into account the additional information for that specific patient, and we will express this in the first column. In this case, the first column of the second row is also 1/2. Half of the time, a carrier will give birth to a normal son. By definition, the second column of the second row is 1 because that column is defined as noncarrier:

	Probability of being a carrier	Probability of not being a carrier
Prior probability	1/2	1/2
Conditional probability	1/2	1

In the third row—the joint probability obtained by multiplying the first 2 rows—the first column is 1/2 × 1/2, or 1/4. The second column is 1/2 × 1, or 1/2. We convert this to 2/4 to get the same denominator as the first column, so that the third row reads 1/4 | 2/4:

	Probability of being a carrier	Probability of not being a carrier
Prior probability	1/2	1/2
Conditional probability	1/2	1
Joint Probability	1/4	1/2 (2/4)

Then we apply the rule that the numerators of the fourth row (posterior probabilities) are the same as the numerators of the third row (joint probabilities) and the denominator for the fourth row is the sum of the numerators of the third row, we have 1/3 and 2/3 as the first and second column of the fourth row:

	Probability of being a carrier	Probability of not being a carrier
Prior probability	1/2	1/2
Conditional probability	1/2	1
Joint probability	1/4	2/4
Posterior probability	1/3	2/3

The overall chance of her being a carrier is 1/3, and the chance of her being a noncarrier is 2/3. Because she has a normal son, her odds of being a carrier dropped from 1/2 to 1/3.

For our second example, consider the same woman who has had 2 normal sons. The first column is the probability that she is a carrier, and the second column is the probability that she is not. In the first row, the prior probability row, as if she had never had children, both of these numbers are 0.5:

	Probability of being a carrier	Probability of not being a carrier
Prior probability	1/2	1/2

In the second row, the conditional probability row, we take into account the additional information that she has 2 normal sons. In this row, the first column, representing the carrier state, is 0.5 × 2, or 0.25 . Only 1/4 of the time would we expect a carrier to have 2 normal sons. In the conditional probability row, the second column—noncarrier status—the probability is one by definition:

	Probability of being a carrier	Probability of not being a carrier
Prior probability	1/2	1/2
Conditional probability	1/4	1

In the third row—joint probability—we simply multiply the results of the prior and conditional probabilities. In the third row, the probability of being a carrier is 0.5 times 0.25, or 1/8. The joint probability of being a noncarrier is 0.5 times 1, or 1/2, which is written as 4/8, since we want the denominators of the 2 columns in the joint probability row to be the same:

	Probability of being a carrier	Probability of not being a carrier
Prior probability	1/2	1/2
Conditional probability	1/4	1
Joint probability	1/8	1/2 (4/8)

To calculate the final row—the posterior probability—the numerators for the 2 columns are the same as the corresponding numerators for the joint probabilities, and the denominator is the sum of the numerators in the joint probabilities. In this example, the denominator is 1 + 4, or 5. Thus, the posterior probability of being a carrier is 1/5 and the posterior probability of being a noncarrier is 4/5:

	Probability of being a carrier	Probability of not being a carrier
Prior probability	1/2	1/2
Conditional probability	1/4	1
Joint probability	1/8	1/2
Posterior probability	1/5	4/5

Given the totality of evidence available, her mother's carrier status and her own 2 normal sons, her final probability of being a carrier is 1 in 5, or 20%.

Similar analyses are conducted using the results of screening tests instead of, or in addition to, family history. To illustrate the incorporation of a screening test into Bayesian analysis, consider a third example concerning a screening test for cystic fibrosis, an autosomal recessive disorder. The chance of being a carrier for cystic fibrosis varies with the patient's ethnicity/race, and the sensitivity of screening tests also varies between patient populations. The 2 groups with the highest carrier risks are Caucasians and Ashkenazi Jews, being about 1 in 29 for both populations. At this writing, screening tests for cystic fibrosis are about 80% sensitive in Caucasians and about 97% sensitive in Ashkenazi Jews. What does a negative screening test mean for the carrier risk for an Ashkenazi Jew? Approaching this question from a Bayesian analysis, and again using the first column to indicate carrier state and the second column to indicate noncarrier state, the prior probability—the first row—is 1/29 in the first column and 28/29 in the second column. We *do not* take into account the results of the screening test:

	Probability of being a carrier	Probability of not being a carrier
Prior probability	1/29	28/29

In the second row, the conditional probability row, a negative test means there is a 3/100 chance of being a carrier, so this is the number used in the second row of the first (carrier state) column. Here, we take into account *only* the results of the test, and ignore her ethnicity. By definition, in the second column—the noncarrier state—we employ 1 (100/100) as the probability:

	Probability of being a carrier	Probability of not being a carrier
Prior probability	1/29	28/29
Conditional probability	3/100	1 (100/100)

In the third row, the joint probabilities are the products of the numbers in the corresponding columns in the first 2 rows. The joint probability of being a carrier with a negative test is 1/29 times 3/100, or 3/2,900. The joint probability of not being a carrier is 28/29 times 100/100, or 2,800/2,900:

	Probability of being a carrier	Probability of not being a carrier
Prior probability	1/29	28/29
Conditional probability	3/100	1 (100/100)
Joint probability	3/2,900	2,800/2,900

The posterior probability—the final number we seek—is then calculated in the fourth row. The numerators of the posterior probabilities are the same as the numerators of the joint probabilities, while the denominators are obtained by adding the numerators in the joint probability row. Thus, final probability of an Ashkenazi Jew with a negative screening test being a carrier is 3/2,803 and the probability of not being a carrier is 2,800/2,803:

	Probability of being a carrier	Probability of not being a carrier
Prior probability	1/29	28/29
Conditional probability	3/100	1 (100/100)
Joint probability	3/2,900	2,800/2,900
Posterior probability	3/2,803	2,800/2,803

It is conventional to express probabilities as "1 in ___," so in this case, 3/2,803=0.00107, the reciprocal of which is 934, so this patient has a 1 in 934 chance of being a carrier (this number can be more quickly reached by simply dividing 2,803 by 3). Because of the negative test result and the high sensitivity of screening in this population, this patient's chances of being a carrier fell from 1/29 to almost 1/1,000.

As a fourth example, we will consider a negative cystic fibrosis screening test in a Caucasian patient, where the typical screening test is only 80% sensitive. Intuitively, we know that a negative test will drop the odds of carrier status to less than the 1/29 that we started with, but not as much as in the Jewish patient. In the first row, we have 1/29 and 28/29, simply the odds for any Caucasian patient, and the same first row as for the Ashkenazi Jewish patient:

	Probability of being a carrier	Probability of not being a carrier
Prior probability	1/29	28/29

In the first column of the second row, we consider only the new information that is specific to this particular patient. Since the test was negative and is 80% effective in Caucasian patients, this entry is 20/100 (the results of the screening test alone, without taking into account the patient's ethnic group, suggest that she has a 20% chance of being a carrier). The entry in the second column of the second row is 1:

	Probability of being a carrier	Probability of not being a carrier
Prior probability	1/29	28/29
Conditional probability	20/100	1 (100/100)

In the third row, where we combine both the general ethnicity of the patient and her particular test results, the entries are 20/2,900 in the carrier column and 2,800/2,900 in the noncarrier column:

	Probability of being a carrier	Probability of not being a carrier
Prior probability	1/29	28/29
Conditional probability	20/100	1 (100/100)
Joint probability	20/2,900	2,800/2,900

ISBN 978-089189-5886

In the fourth row, the entries are 20/2,820 and 2,800/2,820:

	Probability of being a carrier	Probability of not being a carrier
Prior probability	1/29	28/29
Conditional probability	20/100	1 (100/100)
Joint probability	20/2,900	2,800/2,900
Posterior probability	20/2,820	2,800/2,820

The final probability of the patient's being a carrier, based on all of the available evidence, is 20/2,820=0.007092, the reciprocal of which is 141, so this patient has a risk of 1 in 141 of being a carrier, a smaller drop than for the Ashkenazi Jewish patient because of the reduced sensitivity of the test in Caucasians.

For our fifth example, consider a Caucasian man who is phenotypically normal and has a negative screening test for cystic fibrosis, but who has a brother with the disease. The analysis will unfold as in the fourth example except that his prior probability will not be 1/29. Since he has an affected brother, both of his parents must be carriers, and the patient's prior probability of being a carrier must be higher than 1/29. To understand the patient's prior probability, we need to consider Punnett squares. If each of his parents has 1 normal and 1 abnormal gene, the Punnett squares will be as follows, for "a" being an abnormal gene and "A" being a normal gene:

	A	a
A	AA	Aa
a	aA	aa

Since the patient is normal, his genotype cannot be aa. It must be 1 of the other 3, any of which will be phenotypically normal, but 2 of which will convey a carrier status. Thus, his prior probability of being a carrier is not 1/29, but a much higher 2/3. In the first row, we have 2/3 and 1/3:

	Probability of being a carrier	Probability of not being a carrier
Prior probability	2/3	1/3

The numbers for the second row, based on the screening test, are the same as in our previous example: 20/100 and 1:

	Probability of being a carrier	Probability of not being a carrier
Prior probability	2/3	1/3
Conditional probability	20/100	100/100

In the third row, where we multiply the results of the first 2 rows, we get:

	Probability of being a carrier	Probability of not being a carrier
Prior probability	2/3	1/3
Conditional probability	20/100	100/100
Joint probability	40/300	100/300

The fourth row, first column is the posterior probability of being a carrier. Finding the number for the fourth row, first column is the essence of Bayesian analysis. In this case, this number is 40/140, while his chances of not being a carrier are 100/140:

	Probability of being a carrier	Probability of not being a carrier
Prior probability	2/3	1/3
Conditional probability	20/100	100/100
Joint probability	40/300	100/300
Posterior probability	40/140	100/140

40/140 = 0.28, and 100/140 = 0.72, so he has a 28% chance of being a carrier and a 72% chance of not being a carrier. Stated another way, the reciprocal of 0.28 is 3.5, so he has a 1 in 3.5 chance of being a carrier. His affected brother greatly increased his prior probability, and the negative screening test dropped his chances from 2/3 to just <1/3.

Mercifully, there are computer programs for calculating Bayesian probabilities and Bayesian calculators are available online.

Mitochondrial Inheritance

Mendelian genetics pertains only to nuclear DNA, which is equally contributed to by both parents. Mitochondrial inheritance is an additional means of inheritance that involves the DNA in mitochondria passed on through the egg. Sperm have many mitochondria, but because they do not transmit them to the zygote, all of our mitochondria come from our mother, and the mode of transmission of mitochondrial genes is from an affected mother to all of her children. Males and females are equally affected, but they must be linked to an affected mother. Because of maternal inheritance, mitochondrial genetics is not considered Mendelian, though it shares with Mendelian inheritance the characteristic that it tends to be based on single genes.

In addition to maternal inheritance, mitochondrial inheritance has several unique features, and to understand them, we need to review mitochondrial DNA. Reflecting its prokaryotic origin, the mitochondrial genome is circular and very small (16,569 base pairs). Moreover, it consists of 44% G-C base pairs, an unusually high number. This makes one strand, containing many guanine bases, a heavy strand, and the other strand, with many cytosines, a light strand. 93% of mitochondrial DNA is coding vs only 1.6% for nuclear DNA. Moreover, mitochondrial DNA does not have introns, where mutations are less likely to cause disease. These 2 factors make mutations in mitochondrial DNA more likely to be symptomatic than those in nuclear DNA because there is precious little room for mistakes.

Because the 37 genes that are found in mitochondrial DNA primarily are important for oxidative phosphorylation and ATP production [PMID20544879], mitochondrial DNA-linked disorders are often encephalopathies or myopathies, since nerve and muscle tissue have a greater dependence on aerobic metabolism and oxidative phosphorylation.

Again reflecting its prokaryotic origin, mitochondrial DNA is transcribed in a polycistronic manner (ie, multiple genes are transcribed together from contiguous DNA and are cleaved afterward to generate individual functional genes). However, DNA replication in these organelles is dependent on many proteins encoded by nuclear DNA. Also, their DNA is not replicated like that of free-living prokaryotes, but rather is copied in a form of DNA replication called displacement loop (D-loop) replication.

Like the prokaryotes from which they are derived, DNA replication in mitochondria and chloroplasts begins from a single point of origin, but the heavy and light chains have different origins for replication, and they are replicated in opposite directions. The D-loop region of mitochondrial DNA is the small area that is noncoding and is important for 3 reasons. First, it is important in the regulation of

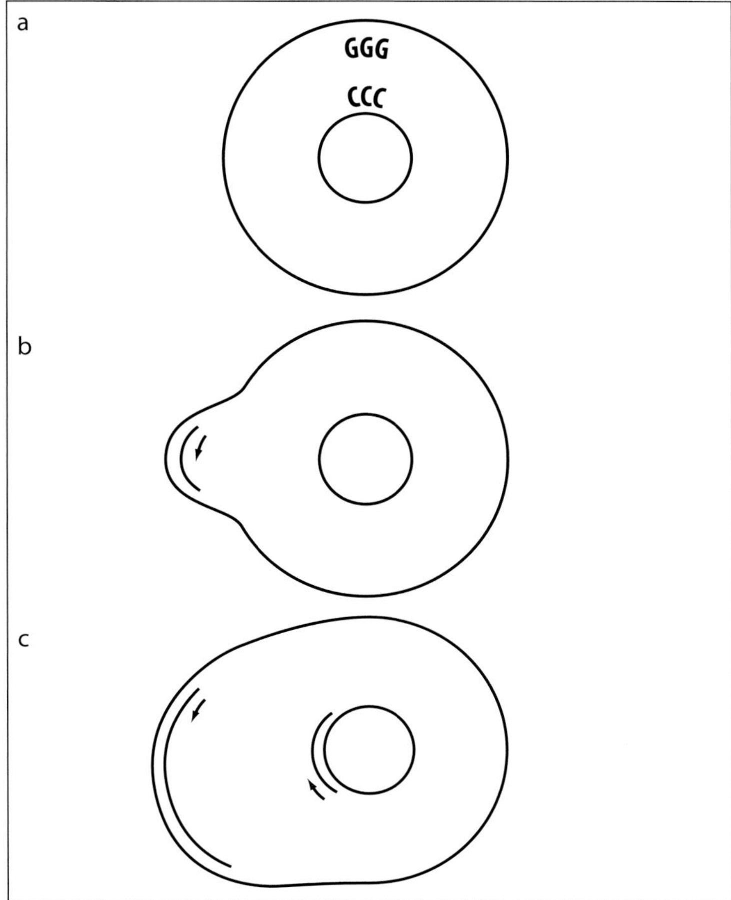

f43.7 **a** A diagram of mitochondrial DNA. It is circular, and one strand, the outer strand in this diagram, has a high guanine content and therefore is heavier than the other strand, which has a high percentage of the lighter base cytosine.
b The D-loop. Replication of mitochondrial DNA begins with the heavy strand. During the time before replication of the light strand commences, there are 3 strands of DNA—the original heavy strand, its complementary strand arising from replication, and the original light strand. This results in a configuration similar to the letter "D." The arrow indicates the direction of replication.
c When the origin point for light strand replication is reached, that strand is replicated in the other direction.

mitochondrial DNA replication. Second, it is the site of origin of replication for the heavy chain. Only after some heavy chain has been replicated without concomitant replication of the light chain, is the origin for the light chain reached and its replication begun **f43.7** [PMID9182553]. During replication of the D-loop area, before the origin of replication for the light chain is reached and parent-daughter strands are established, there may be a small triple-stranded region (2 heavy chains and 1 light chain that has not yet begun replication). The name of this form of replication comes from the fact that a diagram of it at this stage resembles the letter D.

The third reason the D-loop region is important is that because it is noncoding, mutations in this region are more likely to be clinically silent than a mutation in a coding region and therefore likely to accumulate over a very long time period without consequences to the individual, in sharp contrast to mitochondrial DNA in general. A woman passes down the set of mutations at the D-loop that she inherited from her mother, as well as mutations that occurred over the course of her lifetime, to her offspring. Mutations in this region accumulate over each generation, resulting in a rapid and predictable mutation rate in the D-region, with significant differences in this region from one individual to another, provided they are not maternally related. This high mutation rate is a characteristic of mitochondrial inheritance. In particular, the D-loop contains 2 hypervariable regions, HVR1 and HVR2, that have been especially useful in studies of evolution [PMID20230407].

Mutations in the D-loop are therefore very useful in phylogenetic and evolution studies. Studies of D-loop mutations in mitochondria have been invaluable in many aspects of the study of eukaryotic evolution. Also, direct sequencing of this tiny genome is far easier than the primary genome, and sequencing of the mitochondrial genome has been beneficial in identification of human remains. The Mitomap database (http://www.mitomap.org) has recorded known mutations in human mitochondrial DNA.

One unique feature of mitochondrial inheritance is that whereas there are normally only 2 copies of nuclear DNA, mitochondria routinely contain multiple copies of their DNA, and a cell can contain multiple mitochondria. During mitochondrial replication, these multiple copies replicate and sort independently and randomly among the newly synthesized mitochondria, so the DNA of daughter mitochondria may not be identical to that of the parent organelles. If there is a mutation in mitochondrial DNA, some daughter mitochondria will have more of the mutated DNA than others. This feature is called heteroplasmy and can result in incomplete penetrance or variable expressivity in mitochondrial disorders. Children who inherit more of their mother's mutated mitochondrial DNA will be more severely affected, and children who receive less of the mutated mitochondrial DNA may be less affected or appear unaffected.

Another unique feature of mitochondrial inheritance is that whereas nuclear DNA is meticulously divided evenly between the 2 daughter cells, mitochondria, like other organelles, are unevenly divided among the progeny cells. For example, if a cell contains 1,000 mitochondria before division, the 2 daughter cells may have 400 and 600 mitochondria. This is called replicative segregation. Because the multiple copies of mitochondrial DNA replicate and sort independently within individual daughter mitochondria and because the daughter mitochondria are unevenly divided between the daughter cells, if there is a mutation in mitochondrial DNA, some cells are likely to receive, for all practical purposes, a uniform population of either normal or abnormal mitochondria (called homoplasmy), or a mixture of mitochondria with normal and abnormal DNA (heteroplasmy).

Non-Mendelian Inheritance Secondary to Multifactorial Inheritance

The well-studied and time-honored Mendelian mechanisms actually account for only a small portion of human genetic abnormalities. Indeed, Mendel was fortunate in his studies to have selected traits in peas that conform to these simple laws. Most diseases and traits result from other forms of inheritance. The 2 most common modes of inheritance are multifactorial or complex inheritance and de novo chromosomal aberrations, both of which defy the simple Mendelian mechanisms described above.

Multifactorial or complex inheritance is a leading manner in which traits or diseases are passed from parent to offspring. In complex inheritance, 2 or more gene loci are involved, often in a nonequal manner. Multifactorial inheritance is further complicated by the influence of environmental or cultural factors.

Some cases of multifactorial inheritance are polygenic, while others result from additional nongenetic influences. The simplest form of multifactorial inheritance, pure digenic inheritance, results from the interaction of 2 genes at 2 loci. In uncomplicated polygenic inheritance, without a nongenetic component, in which all genes make an equal contribution, a cumulative effect that is essentially a Gaussian distribution of genotypic possibilities can be expected.

A number of techniques have been devised to determine the genetic and nongenetic contributions to the disorder in such cases, many of which involve twin studies. One of these methods is the comparison of the concordance of a trait in monozygotic (identical) twins relative to the concordance of the trait in dizygotic (fraternal) twins. There is often discordance between identical and fraternal twins (ie, one twin has the disorder and the other does not), indicating some nongenetic contributing factor(s). The higher the rate of discordance, the greater is the nongenetic component. Calculations for heritability (the percentage of a trait that is genetic) can be further confounded by in utero environmental factors, which are more likely to be shared by monozygotic than dizygotic twins.

A characteristic of multifactorial inheritance is familial aggregation, wherein the disease or characteristic clusters in families in a way that cannot be explained by genetics alone. Other characteristics are that the disorder can appear at what appears to be random, with affected patients often having unaffected parents. There is often an uneven gender distribution, and unlike Mendelian situations, there is a greater likelihood of the presence of the abnormality in a given individual if multiple siblings are affected. In many diseases with complex inheritance, a threshold of liability needs to be reached in order for the disease or trait to manifest. This means that an individual needs to inherit enough genetic factors or be exposed to enough of the environmental factors for the disease to be present. Thus, as families share many genetic factors and environmental risk factors, multifactorial diseases are more likely to cluster in families.

Chromosome Banding and Cytogenetics

In addition to multifactorial or complex inheritance, de novo chromosomal aberrations are a major cause of non-Mendelian inheritance. Abnormalities of chromosome structure may be inherited or may occur from chromosomal instability (causing abnormal breakages) or defects in repair. Chromosomal aberrations include translocations, deletions, duplications, inversions, trisomies, and monosomies. Among the many examples of conditions caused by chromosomal aberrations are Down syndrome, also known as trisomy 21, and Turner syndrome, in which, in most cases, the paternal X chromosome is lost, resulting in a karyotype of 45,X. These aberrations have been defined by traditional cytogenetics and chromosome banding, but as described later, they have been and are being substantially redefined by techniques in molecular biology.

Prior to banding, chromosomes were often divided into the following groups:

- Group A: chromosomes 1-3, metacentric
- Group B: chromosomes 4 and 5, submetacentric
- Group C: chromosomes 6-12 and the X chromosome, metacentric
- Group D: chromosomes 13-15, acrocentric
- Group E: chromosomes 16-18
- Group F: chromosomes 19 and 20
- Group G: chromosomes 21, 22, and the Y chromosome, acrocentric

The technique of chromosome banding was pioneered by Caspersson [PMID5422961]. One of the first banding methods was called Q-banding because it involved treating chromosomes with the fluorescent compound quinacrine, after which visualization with a fluorescent microscope revealed alternating bright (said to be Q bright) and darker (Q dull) bands. Later methods used primarily Giemsa, which produced a series of alternating light and dark bands that could be visualized in an ordinary microscope. The primary Giemsa method is G-banding. In G-banding, homologous chromosomes can be paired because of their identical patterns of light and dark bands. Changes in banding patterns indicate structural anomalies, such as translocations and inversions. G-banding has proven invaluable in medicine. It has low sensitivity (since the bands that are visualized and followed consists of large segments of DNA) and an inability to sort out complex or multiple abnormalities. Using techniques that either stop mitosis just after DNA replication or prevent chromosome condensation, it has been possible over the years to visualize more "stretched out" chromosomes, allowing for greater resolution. At this writing, such high resolution banding techniques have allowed many chromosomes to be resolved into about 1200 bands.

G-banding parallels Q-banding. A G positive band would be fluorescent in a Q stain. But unlike the earlier Q-banding, G-banding does not require a fluorescent microscope for interpretation, and the stain will not fade with time. G-banding, like Q-banding, stains AT-rich areas of the chromosome more than CG areas. G-positive bands contain few transcribed genes and are rich in long interspersed nuclear elements (discussed in Chapter 45). G-positive bands tend to replicate later in DNA replication than G-negative regions. In contrast, G-negative bands are rich in CG and contain many genes. They tend to have large numbers of short, interspersed nuclear elements, and they tend to be early replicating [Shaffer ISBN978-3-8055-8985-7]. The image of the G-banded, paired chromosomes is called a karyogram (the word "karyotype" refers to the written representation of a karyogram).

Conventional G-banding was a huge advance in medicine and forms the foundation for the more sophisticated and sensitive karyotyping techniques that are discussed in Chapter 45. It continues to be the most commonly used traditional banding technique, but it has 4 major disadvantages. The first of these is low resolution. Abnormalities must be about 4-5 Mb (4-5 million base pairs) to be detectable. The second disadvantage is that the cells to be studied must be cultured, so that metaphases can be obtained. Often, attempts to culture fail, either from lack of growth or from contamination, and obtaining sufficient metaphases from cells that have a very low rate of division, such as nerve and muscle, is nearly impossible. Third, even when culture is successful, it introduces at least a 10-day delay, often a critical time in prenatal studies. A fourth disadvantage is that interpretation is subjective.

There are other staining techniques based on Giemsa, though these have many of the same limitations of G-banding and have largely been supplanted by newer methods. R (for "reverse") banding yields bands that are the reverse of those obtained by G-banding (ie, bands that are light in G-banding are dark in R-banding and vice versa). Though rarely employed in the United States, R-banding is common in some places in Europe. An advantage of R-banding, prior to the more specific telomere banding that is now available, was that the telomeres are G negative and therefore much easier to study in R-banding. Giemsa techniques that stain constitutive heterochromatin (ie, chromatin that is always densely packed and rarely transcribed) are called C-banding methods (since most constitutive heterochromatin is in or near the centromere, C-banding is also called centromeric staining or centromeric banding). C-banding is good for identifying dicentric chromosomes and those with an excessive amount of satellite DNA, which tends to be preferentially located near centromeres. Telomere banding (T-banding) stains telomeres.

Nomenclature for chromosome banding has been standardized by the International System for Human Cytogenetic Nomenclature (ISCN) [Shaffer ISBN978-3-8055-8985-7].

In the technique of replication banding, the thymidine analogue BrdU is introduced at various times during the replication cycle. After all replication is complete, BrdU is visualized in the completed DNA by fluorescein isothiocyanate-labeled antibodies to BrdU. This work has shown that DNA in each band replicates independently of that in other bands and that there is a precise sequence of replication waves in a chromosome.

Classic examples of gene amplification include *MYC* and *HER2*. The demonstration of gene amplification may require fluorescent in situ hybridization (FISH), as in the case of *HER2*, but in conventional cytogenetics, the gene amplification may occur by other means which are detected cytogenetically in different ways. First, there may be small extrachromosomal fragments called double minutes (DM), which are very small, paired structures without centromeres. *MYC* amplification is usually in the form of double minutes. Second, there may be long homogeneously staining regions (HSRs) in the chromosomes, which are neither light nor dark (additional studies, such as FISH, may be needed to exclude an insertion). The amplification of the *RUNX1* gene on chromosome 21 in some cases of acute lymphoid leukemia is detected as HSRs. Episomes may be a rare cause of gene amplification, but these are never seen on G-banding and require FISH for demonstration. However gene amplification is initially detected, it is often confirmed by FISH.

Abnormalities of chromosome number may stem from nondisjunction, which is failure of the chromosomes to sort properly, resulting in an abnormal number in the daughter cell. Nondisjunction can occur in mitosis, resulting in an abnormality in chromosome number in only some cells, or in meiosis, resulting in abnormal chromosome number in gametes only. If nondisjunction occurs in meiosis I, only abnormal gametes can occur, but if it occurs in meiosis II, some gametes may be normal, while others will have trisomy or monosomy. Other causes of abnormal chromosome number include anaphase lag (whereby one chromosome does not migrate normally to a daughter cell and is lost), abnormalities of the mitotic spindle, some malignancies, and some inherited abnormalities.

Aneuploidy refers to a particular type of abnormal chromosome number in which the total number of chromosomes is not a multiple of 23. When aneuploidy occurs, more genes are affected than when point mutations or other more subtle mutations occur. "Polyploidy" refers to a number of chromosomes that is a multiple of 23. The most common cause of triploidy, a form of polyploidy in which there are 3 sets of chromosomes, is a normal egg that is fertilized by 2 sperm (dispermy). In contrast, the most common cause of tetraploidy, when there are 4 sets of chromosomes, is an error in early cleavage division.

In ISCN nomenclature of individual G-banded chromosomes, chromosomes are divided into regions, and each region is divided into bands. The centromere is first identified. Chromosomes have 2 arms, except for those which are acrocentric. The short arm of a chromosome is designated as the p arm (French for "petit"). The long arm is the q arm. Moving from the centromere toward the end, each arm is first divided into regions (eg, p1, p2, q1, q2). Each region is divided into bands, with higher numbers of bands moving distally from the centromere toward the next region (eg, p12 is the second band in the first region of the short arm and is further from the centromere than p11; q34 is the fourth band in the third region of the long arm and is further from the centromere than q33). Sub band and sub-subbands are recognized by additional numbers following a decimal point (eg, p21.23 refers to the second region, first band, second subband, third sub-subband of the short arm).

In ISCN nomenclature of karyotypes of G-banded chromosomes, the number of total chromosomes, called the model number, is specified first. Then, the nature of the sex chromosomes is given after a comma but without a space (ie, 46,XX or 46,XY). If there is a constitutional abnormality in the model number, the model number is followed by a comma, then a statement that clarifies the nature of the missing or excess chromosome (ie, 45,X designates Turner syndrome and 47,XXY designates Klinefelter syndrome).

If there are 1 or more abnormalities that involve portions of a chromosome, the model number is followed by a comma, after which the sex chromosomes are given, followed by a comma. Then the major process or processes are designated by an abbreviation, again without a space. Then, without a space or comma, the chromosome involved is given in parentheses. Without a space or comma, the region or regions of the chromosome are given in another set of parentheses. For example, 46,XX,inv(2)(p22q34) is a female karyotype that has an inversion on chromosome 2, the breakpoints of which can be shown to be region 2, band 2, of the short arm and region 3, band 4, of the long arm.

ISBN 978-089189-5886

A paracentric inversion is one in which the breakpoints are both in the same arm and the centromere is not involved (ie, it is not present in the inverted segment). Because there is minimal loss of DNA, paracentric inversions tend to be relatively asymptomatic in somatic cells unless the breakpoints are within a gene. However, if they occur in cells that will become gametes, there are more likely to be abnormalities produced in the gametes during meiosis. A pericentric inversion is one in which there is a breakpoint in each arm and the centromere is present in the segment that is inverted.

A reciprocal translocation is when pieces from 2 chromosomes are swapped equally and no chromosomal material is lost. In reciprocal translocations, after the total number of chromosomes and indication of the sex chromosomes, the translocation is designated by a "t," after which the 2 chromosomes involved in the translocation are given in parentheses, separated by a semicolon, followed by another set of parentheses indicating the precise breakpoints, with the first region in the second parentheses indicating the breakpoint on the first chromosome and the second region in the second parentheses giving the breakpoint on the second chromosome. For example, 46,XX,t(11;15)(q23;p34) indicates that in this female, everything distal to region 2, band 3, on the long arm of chromosome 11, and everything distal to region 3, band, 4 on the short arm of chromosome 15 have been exchanged. A semicolon indicates that >1 chromosome is involved. In this example, in the 2 parentheses, there is correspondence between what is on the left side of the semicolon in the first and second parentheses, and what is on the right side of the semicolon in the 2 parentheses (ie, q23 refers to chromosome 11 and p34 to chromosome 15). Within the first parentheses, the lowest numbered chromosome is listed first.

If translocations occur in gametes, there may be no consequences if they are balanced and reciprocal, or there may be trisomy for a portion of a chromosome, depending on what happens during meiosis.

A Robertsonian translocation occurs between acrocentric chromosomes (the 6 acrocentric chromosomes are numbers 13, 14, 15, 21, and 22, and the Y chromosome) and involves the loss of the 2 p arms, resulting in the fusion of the 2 q arms to 1 centromere. In a Robertsonian translocation, 1 centromere and the 2 p arms are lost. The resulting chromosome is often designated a "der," meaning that 1 chromosome is derived from 2 others. The number in parentheses refers to the chromosome with an intact centromere. For example, if chromosomes 14 and 15 engaged in a Robertsonian translocation, and the resultant single chromosome retained the centromere of chromosome 15, it would be designated "der(15)." A derivative chromosome is a rearranged, but stable and transmissible chromosome that is generated either by a translocation or by other abnormalities such as inversions and deletions.

In a Robertsonian translocation, there is usually no significant loss of genetic material and there are usually minimal clinical consequences in the immediate term because the p arm of acrocentric chromosomes is very small (it is often called a satellite) and usually codes only for ribosomal RNA. For this reason, Robertsonian translocations are often clinically equivalent to a balanced reciprocal translocation, but if the process occurs in a germ cell, a trisomy can result in the offspring.

An isochromosome is one that has experienced a translocation near the centromere between 2 sister arms, resulting in chromosomes that either have 2 short arms or 2 long arms. Isochromosomes are denoted by an "i." For example, i(18q) refers to a chromosome that consists of the 2 long arms of chromosome 18. A Robertsonian translocation is one cause of isochromosome.

A ring chromosome usually results from loss of telomeric material from both arms. This typically causes the 2 arms of the chromosome to loop around and bind to each other, although there may be fusion with another chromosome that has also lost telomeric material, in which case a dicentric (ie, having 2 centromeres) chromosome results. Because telomeric DNA is generally not critical to the functioning of somatic cells, ring chromosomes are often asymptomatic (though with important exceptions). In most cases, the larger problem is that during meiosis, crossing over will result in unstable structures. For example, crossing over during meiosis of a ring chromosome often leads to a dicentric chromosome that cannot participate further in normal meiosis. Even somatic cells may undergo a small amount of crossing over during mitosis, and here again, the presence of a ring chromosome may result in daughter cells with an abnormal amount of DNA. Also, ring chromosomes tend to be unstable, even without meiosis or mitosis, and to be lost, leading to monosomy. In cytogenetic nomenclature, a ring chromosome is designated by an "r," as in r(15).

Macrodeletion syndromes, or syndromes in which missing chromosomal material can be detected by G-banding, include Cri-du-Chat (del5p) and Wolf-Hirschhorn (del4p). Microdeletion syndromes are more common and include Smith-Magenis syndrome (del17p11.2), most cases of Prader-Willi, most cases of Angelman syndrome (both del15q11.2-q13), Williams syndrome (7p11.23), DiGeorge syndrome (22q11.2), and Miller-Dieker syndrome (17p13.3). Most microdeletions can be detected by FISH or by microarrays. Microarrays will be described in more detail in Chapter 45.

Whereas deletions typically involve 2 breakpoints, insertions require 3, 2 in the donor chromosome and 1 in the recipient, and may be rarer.

If there is an abnormality involving either sex chromosome, the normal sex chromosome is written first, before the abnormality is described. For example, a male who has lost his Y chromosome is denoted by 45, X,–Y, not as 45,–Y,X.

A marker chromosome is one that is of unknown origin. A marker chromosome is denoted by "mar" at the end of a designation, such as 47,XY, +mar.

Whereas constitutional chromosomal abnormalities occur in all cells because they arise early during meiosis or are passed down from a parent, somatic chromosomal abnormalities are those that occur late in development. As a result, somatic abnormalities occur in only some cells, making individuals with these events mosaics. A mosaic is an individual who has 2 or more genetically different cell lineages, each capable of replication. The term "mosaic" is usually understood to mean that all genetic material from all lineages is derived from the same zygote, as opposed to a chimera, in which there is DNA that is not from the zygote. However, as we will see in our discussion of gene modification, the term "mosaic" is occasionally applied to an organism with >1 distinct lineage that is capable of replication, even if 1 of the lineages contains foreign DNA that is not from the zygote.

"Mosaicism" refers to distinct lineages of cells that are capable of replication. The term is not used in connection with a rare, isolated cell with a different DNA content (indeed, no 2 cells have exactly the same DNA content down to the last base). A common cause of somatic mosaicism is chromosomal nondisjunction. Any patient who has a genetic abnormality that is expressed in only a subset of cells that can proliferate (eg, blood cells in leukemia) is a mosaic.

In contrast to somatic mosaicism, germline mosaicism is a spontaneous mutation in some of an individual's germ cells, such that some of his or her children are affected and others are not, in a way that does not conform to any known Mendelian pattern. Some autosomal dominant conditions that show up in multiple offspring of an unaffected individual may be due to germline mosaicism.

A clone is population of cells that is derived from a single progenitor cell. A clone is defined on the basis of cells that have similar gains or losses of genetic material, or similar structural abnormalities. If the definition is based on a gain of genetic material or the same structural anomaly, then there must be 2 or more cells with identical abnormalities. A clone can also be defined as a loss of a chromosome, but if it is defined in this manner, 3 or more cells that lack the same chromosome are required. The reason for this difference is that chromosomes are artifactually lost more easily than any material is artifactually gained, so if a clone is defined by loss of a chromosome, an extra cell is needed to exclude artifactual loss. The stem line is the primary abnormality associated with a given disorder (eg, the *BCR/ABL* translocation in chronic myelogenous leukemia). Secondary abnormalities (side lines) are additional aberrations that may be present in addition to the primary stem line. Side lines often occur later in the course of the disorder and are often indicative of a more aggressive clinical course.

Linkage and Association: Tracing a Gene

Determining the location of a gene, called gene mapping, is critical because only after its precise location is known can it be studied and the nature of the disease it causes be elucidated. Before the sequencing of the genome, there were 2 basic approaches to mapping a gene that is associated with a disease or trait: linkage analysis and association studies.

In linkage analysis, *families* are studied and the inheritance of the disease or trait is followed through pedigrees of successive generations. Linkage analysis is primarily suited to Mendelian (ie, monoallelic) inheritance. In association studies, *populations* are studied, and changes in the frequency of an allele or a set of alleles are identified in a group of affected people and compared to the corresponding frequency of unaffected people in the population. Association studies have been more useful in non-Mendelian situations.

Linkage analysis is largely of historical value and was based on the fact that in meiosis, there is recombination in the stage in which there are 4 chromatids, and that the closer 2 genes are, the less likely they are to recombine and the more likely they are to remain together. Genetic linkage is the phenomenon whereby 2 loci tend to be inherited together because they are close together on the chromosome and therefore tend not to recombine during meiosis. In linkage studies, one locus is the gene to be mapped, and the other is a marker that is close to it and that tends to be inherited with the gene. A marker is a DNA polymorphism, ie, a sequence of DNA that varies from one individual to another. A marker can be an allele, a haplotype, a variation in response to restriction endonucleases, a variation in the number of repeating units in a repetitive sequence, or a single nucleotide polymorphism (SNP) that is close enough to a gene or sequence of interest to be useful in tracking it across generations. Markers have been pivotal in identifying genes that are associated with diseases, and until recently, most of what we knew about the location of genes that lead to disease came largely through markers.

When geneticists studied linkage analysis through pedigrees, they were studying the probability that the allele of interest and the marker will or will not undergo recombination together during meiosis, depending on the distance between them on the chromosome. During recombination, 2 genes are likely to be separated if they are far apart, but likely to stay together in a haplotype if they are close together. If a parent is heterozygous for both the gene of interest and the marker gene, and a high percentage of his or her children have both the gene being traced and the marker, then it is likely that the gene and the marker are close together on the chromosome because they have stayed together during recombination. On the other hand, if a small percentage of the parent's children have both the gene of interest and the marker, then they have been subjected to separate recombination events and must be further apart. The goal in linkage studies was to identify a genetic marker that is always or nearly always present when the disease is present, but never or nearly never present in unaffected individuals. Once initial success was achieved, the process was continued, homing in on a progressively smaller area of the genome.

Now that the genome has been sequenced, traditional linkage analysis has largely been replaced by DNA sequencing of candidate genes from affected and unaffected individuals using the next generation DNA sequencing methods that we will examine in Chapter 45.

Association Studies

In contrast to linkage analysis, association studies are still very much in use. Linkage studies focus on families and have been very effective in monoallelic (Mendelian) inheritance, but even if nonparametric methods are used, they are very difficult to apply to multifactorial inheritance. Family studies, including those involving twins, have shed some light on multifactorial inheritance, but even those involving identical twins raised in different settings are complicated and often yield data that are difficult to interpret.

Association analysis, which has been recently well reviewed [PMID18522673], takes a different approach and studies gene frequencies in affected patients vs those in the population as a whole. For all practical purposes, association studies are the only means of investigating multifactorial inheritance. While association analysis is by no means new, it has been rejuvenated by the use of SNPs (discussed in detail subsequently). In particular, the combination of SNPs and microarrays has breathed new life into association studies.

Association studies depend on alleles at different loci being inherited together with a greater frequency than would be expected on a purely random basis. This is called linkage disequilibrium (LD), and to understand this, we must first understand linkage equilibrium. Linkage equilibrium indicates that genes at different loci on the same chromosome sort independently in a random manner relative to each other (ie, there is a very high θ).

For example, consider 2 loci, A and B, on the same chromosome, each of which has 2 alleles—"A" and "a" at one locus and "B" and "b" at the other. Let us assume that at both loci, the 2 alleles are equal in frequency (gene frequency of 0.5). If the 2 loci are in linkage equilibrium, we would expect that whenever we find an "A" allele at one locus, we would find a "B" allele at the other locus half of the time and a "b" allele half of the time. Similarly, when we find an "a" allele at one locus, we would expect to find a "B" allele at the other locus half of the time and a "b" allele the other half.

In the above example, the alleles "A" and "B" are in linkage equilibrium, so that A and B are found together only by chance. The probability of a haplotype—a collection of genes that tend to be inherited together on a single chromosome — containing both "A" and "B," P(AB), is the probability of "A" times the probability of "B": P(AB) = P(A) × P(B). In this case, P(A) = 0.5 and P(B) = 0.5, so P(AB) = 0.25.

But what if we find that if a chromosome has an "A" allele at the first locus, in 90% of cases, it has a "B" allele at the second locus? This is a nonrandom association of the alleles "A" and "B" at the loci A and B, and these 2 alleles, from different loci, are in linkage *disequilibrium* (LD [abbreviated D]), which is the nonrandom association of alleles at different loci. LD occurs when the haplotype frequencies depart from the values they would have if the alleles at each locus combined completely at random. When an allele at one locus and a second allele at another locus are found together on the same chromosome with a frequency that is greater than would be expected if the 2 loci were segregating independently, then those loci are said to be in LD. If alleles at 2 loci sort independently and randomly, they are in linkage equilibrium. If they do not, they are associated and are in LD. Strachan and Read [Strachan ISBN978-0815341499] point out with perfect fidelity that "allelic association" is a simpler, more intuitive, and less confusing term than "linkage disequilibrium," but old terms die hard.

The LD between A and B is defined by

$$D = P(AB) - [P(A) \times P(B)]$$

The first term of this equation, "P(AB)," is the actual percentage of the time we find the 2 alleles together, and P(A) × P(B) is what we would expect in random association. A positive value for D indicates that the alleles are associated with each other more often than would be expected from chance. In our example, where a chromosome has an "A" allele at the first locus and a "B" allele at a second locus in 90% of cases, then

$$D = 0.9 - [0.5 \times 0.5]$$

or 0.9 – 0.25, which is 0.65, and there is an association. If D = 0, then P(AB) = P(A) × P(B) and there is no LD and any association of the 2 alleles is purely by chance. D can be negative, indicating that alleles are associated less frequently than would be expected from chance.

LD of 2 alleles implies a physical proximity between them. However, there is a second, less remembered variable that affects LD. The degree of association between alleles tends to fall with time, as more meioses occur. As time passes and more meiotic recombination events occur, LD will fall unless the alleles are very close together. The longer the time since the origin of the LD, the greater must be their proximity for LD to be evident. LD may be lost altogether if sufficient time has passed. Since the LD between any 2 alleles is a function not only of distance between their loci on the chromosome, but also of the amount of time between the divergence of populations, different populations will have different values of LD for the same 2 alleles. In addition, it is possible for 2 SNPs to arise at the same location in different populations at different times. These alleles, although identical by sequencing, would fall on different haplotypes and thus have different LD with neighboring alleles.

Association studies are applied to populations, not to individuals or families, and seek to statistically identify polymorphisms that are associated with a disease. The most common polymorphic markers that are currently used in association studies are SNPs because they are easy to genotype and have a low rate of spontaneous mutation. Ironically, there is no assurance that the polymorphisms that are targeted in association studies are necessarily directly related to the disease at all. In all probability, many of them are simply close to and in LD with the true factor, which may not even be known.

Like linkage studies, association studies are heavily dependent on statistical analysis, but different kinds of statistics are used. Both forms of study use odds ratios, but instead of LOD scores, association studies are based on the disease odds ratio and the relative risk ratio (RR or RRR).

To understand these terms, we first consider a group of people who carry an allele that is suspected of playing an etiologic role and divide them into 2 groups—those who have the disease and those who do not. The odds ratio for this group is a/b, where a is the number of people who have the allele and the disease and b is the number of people who have the allele but not the disease. We then construct a similar ratio of people who do not have the allele of interest. Let group c be people without the allele who have the disease and group d be people without the allele who do not have disease. The odds ratio for this second group is c/d. The disease odds ratio is the ratio of the 2 ratios, ie, a/b divided by c/d, which equals ad/bc. A disease odds ratio of 1 indicates that the factor in question (in this case an allele) does not confer any additional risk, while a disease odds ratio that is >1 indicates that the allele confers risk.

For example, if there are 100 people with both the allele and the disease (group a), 10 people with the allele but without the disease (group b), 10 people without the allele who have the disease (group c), and 100 people without either the allele or the disease, then a/b = 100/10 =10. c/d = 10/100 = 0.1. The disease odds ratio is then 10/0.1, or 100. The disease odds ratio can also be written as ad/bc. ad = 100 × 100 = 10,000, while bc = 10 × 10 = 100, so ad/bc = 10,000/100, or 100. This high number suggests that the allele is strongly associated with the disease.

The disease odds ratio is commonly used in retrospective (case-control) studies, which begin with 2 groups of patients, 1 with and 1 without the condition of interest, then retrospectively determines how many people in each of these 2 groups were exposed to the risk factor or have the allele under investigation.

In cohort (prospective) studies, which begin with 2 groups of healthy patients—a group with the risk factor or allele and a control group without—and follows them over time, a related ratio called the relative risk ratio (RR or RRR) is used. The RR is the risk of the condition of interest subsequently developing as a result of exposure to the factor or the presence of the allele of interest.

Let us again consider 4 groups of people. Patients in group A have both the allele and the disease. Group B has the allele but not the disease. Group C does not have the allele, but does have the disease. Group D has neither the allele nor the disease. Like the disease odds ratio, the RR is a ratio of ratios. The numerator is the ratio of those who have the allele *and* the disease to all those who have the allele, *with or without the disease*, A/(A + B). The denominator is the ratio of those who do not have the allele, but who do have the disease to all those who do not have the allele, with or without the disease, C/(C + D). The RR is then written as:

$$RR = \frac{A/(A+B)}{C/(C+D)}$$

Using the same numbers as for our example of the disease odds ratio (A = 100, B = 10, C = 10, and D = 100), the numerator for the RR is 100/110, or 0.91. The denominator is 10/110, or 0.09. The RR is 0.91/0.09, or 10. As is the case for the disease odds ratio, a RR of one indicates that the allele or risk factor is not influential, while the higher the RR, the greater is the role of the risk factor or allele in the development of the disease. Statistical testing, such as the χ^2 test, determines if the ratios are significant.

Association studies are free of many of the restraints of linkage studies. They do not require large pedigrees collected over generations, nor do they require heterozygosity for the allele of interest or knowledge of the specific genotype of individuals. Association studies also offer the additional advantage that data is much easier to collect, especially now that the genome has been sequenced. Indeed, using SNPs, a genome-wide association study can be carried out on very large numbers of people, and SNPs that are associated with the disease can be rapidly determined by commercially available methods.

It is usually easier to obtain blood and perform a partial DNA sequence than to perform meticulous multigenerational family studies. In association analyses, one can obtain data from much larger samples than in linkage studies, increasing the chances of making a statistically valid conclusion. Because of larger samples, the effect of a gene that is only a minor contributor can often be detected, whereas linkage studies are sensitive only to genes that are strongly etiologic and do not detect genes that convey only a susceptibility.

On the other hand, in association studies there are potential difficulties with population stratification and incidental associations. Population stratification arises from subgroups that have different prevalences of the disease and also, by coincidence, different prevalences of an unrelated trait or allele. If people in such a subgroup preferentially mate with others in the same subgroup, the disease will artifactually appear to be associated with the unrelated allele. Imagine, for example, trying to identify "the" gene for prostate cancer by association studies without knowing that this condition is more common in African-Americans. Any other genes that are more common in African-Americans may appear to be linked to prostate cancer. One might conclude, for example, that the gene for hemoglobin S plays a role in prostate cancer. Of course, cohort studies are controlled for race and gender, but there may be unknown subgroups. This problem does not arise in linkage studies because there is no external control group—comparisons are made between members of a family.

Population stratification is particularly challenging because subgroups may not even be known when the study is commenced. Several methods have been developed to mitigate the effects of population stratification in association studies, often centering on using unassociated alleles whose frequency is known among different racial and ethnic groups to ensure essential comparability between the control and experimental groups.

Another potential problem with association studies is that the same mutation may arise more than once in different populations or even in the same population. Even if the mutation is the same in all cases (ie, we are not dealing with locus heterogeneity, where the same clinical disease is caused by defects in >1 gene), each time the mutation arises, the alleles surrounding it will be different because recombination constantly makes subtle changes in the position of genes. Each occurrence of the mutation has its own set of alleles with which it is in LD. No single occurrence of the mutation stands out, so no specific set of alleles that are in LD with it stands out. In these situations, we are trying to hit a moving target. Because there may be variation in the frequency of the mutation, or the number of times it arose, among ethnic groups, ethnicity plays a role in this difficulty, as it does in population stratification. In linkage studies, confined to one or a small number of families, this problem does not occur.

A particularly troubling concern with association studies is that they are based on the premise that factors that convey susceptibility to diseases derive from ancient, conserved blocks of DNA that have been passed down intact. This is called the common disease-common variant hypothesis. Is this a valid assumption? With rare exceptions, such as sickle trait conferring partial protection against falciparum malaria, would not natural selection operate against any such conservation of deleterious segments of DNA? For this reason, any individual susceptibility factors that are uncovered by association studies are likely to be small contributors to the disease. Were they large contributors, they would either have been removed by natural selection if they were early onset enough to affect reproductive health, or they must play an as yet unknown protective role in another context.

What if susceptibility factors arose from more recent mutations? In fact, there is considerable feeling that recent mutations, not conserved sequences, account for the presence of most susceptibility factors. This is called the mutation-selection hypothesis, and if it is verified, it would require a redirection of association studies away from the statistical

ISBN 978-089189-5886

techniques discussed above and towards the sequencing of candidate genes in large numbers of both patients and unaffected people because the responsible mutations are likely to be new alleles in the same gene (allelic heterogeneity) rather than locus heterogeneity. Only direct sequencing can identify recent new alleles at the same locus. It is likely that both of these hypotheses are true and that some susceptibility factors arise from conserved sequences and some from new mutations, but at this writing, this pivotal question has not been answered.

There is also the difficulty that most diseases have susceptibility factors that vary in the degree of influence, with some being more important than others. Consider a disease that is caused by 5 different susceptibility factors working in concert, one of which makes a much greater contribution than the other 4 combined. Such a disease, while multifactorial, is close to Mendelian. The line between Mendelian and non-Mendelian inheritance is blurred. Undoubtedly, many diseases fall into this category without our knowledge. Are such processes best studied by linkage/sequencing or association?

Like linkage studies, association studies association studies can be derailed at the beginning by either a poor definition or recognition of the target phenotype and are vulnerable to confusing results because of locus heterogeneity.

Genome-wide association studies (GWAS) are those that examine variations across the genome and their association with any trait, characteristic, or disease. There are many ongoing GWAS, described at http://gwas.nih.gov.

Linkage studies are effective in mapping a gene that is solely responsible for a disease (Mendelian inheritance), and association studies are generally superior to linkage studies in examining multifactorial inheritance. But both of these techniques require difficult statistics, are prone to errors, and involve working with fundamental gaps in knowledge. Our knowledge of diseases that have multifactorial inheritance lags far behind our understanding of Mendelian disorders, and it is likely that we will need to wait for a greater understanding of the genome than simply its sequence, such as the stop and start boundaries of introns and exons, the nature and interaction of gene products, and the regulation of DNA expression. Tracing a gene is an ongoing adventure without an end.

The Evolution of the X and Y Chromosomes

Before we leave the field of genetics, we need to review the origin of the X and Y chromosomes because many diseases involve sex chromosomes, particularly the X chromosome. The males of all vertebrate species have testes, but there is variation as to how those testes arise. While some reptiles use temperature-dependent gender determination, most vertebrates employ a genetic basis. When inheritance of a particular chromosome leads to the formation of a female, that chromosome is called a W, and its counterpart is called a Z chromosome. The W-Z system is used by birds and some reptiles. When a specific chromosome leads to male gender, that chromosome is called a Y, and its counterpart is an X. The X-Y system of sex determination is used by mammals [PMID18391511].

The X and the Y chromosomes are thought to have arisen from autosomes and to have been a matched pair of roughly equal size shortly after their evolution. These chromosomes were originally capable of considerable recombination, but are thought to have begun to diverge about 300 million years ago [PMID19609352]. Mammals arose about this time, and it may be that an important part of mammalian evolution was the divergence of the X and the Y chromosomes.

The Y chromosome contains essentially all of the genes needed for male fertility. Some of these genes appear to have relocated to the Y chromosome from other chromosomes [PMID18729722]. The advantage of this relocation is unclear, but it is likely that there was an evolutionary advantage to having all of these genes in one place so that they can be passed down from male to male without dilution by maternal DNA.

Clustering of male-related genes on the Y caused it to lose its essential homology with the X chromosome and to no longer be able to recombine with it. Only 54 of the X chromosome's 1,098 genes—about 5%—have a Y counterpart. These genes map to 2 very small regions where limited recombination still exists between the X and Y chromosomes, one at each end of the chromosomes. These are called pseudoautosomal regions [PMID18398439].

Recombination is essential to the long-term integrity of the chromosome, and the sharply reduced recombination that the Y chromosome has undergone over the course of evolution has greatly diminished its size, while the X chromosome, which has a partner in women, has not suffered this fate. One might therefore expect hard times for the Y chromosome, and in fact, its future is uncertain. At some time in the future, male gender may be determined by a simple XO status (ie, simple loss of the second X chromosome). Indeed, in some older men, the Y chromosome has been lost. But for now, the Y chromosome seems stable in the human population as a whole, in part because many important genes on the Y chromosome are present in multiple copies [PMID1998119].

Because both copies of a gene are normally expressed, and both copies of a chromosome are generally needed, the loss of an X chromosome in males would ordinarily lead to a critical shortage. Different species use different adaptations, but in general, this problem is avoided because one copy of the X is sufficient. But this raises another problem—why don't females experience excessive doses of the X? In females, inactivation of one X chromosome (lyonization; described earlier) occurs everywhere on one X except for the pseudoautosomal region that is homologous to the Y chromosome [PMID18729722]. There are a few genes on the inactivated X chromosome, in the pseudoautosomal regions, that have a working counterpart in the Y chromosome and that remain active, so that there is equal expression of this DNA [PMID8225310]. The loss of one copy of these genes in Turner syndrome (45,X) apparently accounts for the symptoms of that disorder [PMID18660847].

In summary, the X and Y chromosomes are incompletely understood, but appear to have resulted from the relocation of most of the genes related to male gender to the Y chromosome, followed by the degeneration of most of the rest of the Y chromosome, and the inactivation of most of the genes in 1 of the 2 X chromosomes in females.

Core Points for Clinical Genetics

- 46 chromosomes, 23 pairs, 22 pairs of autosomes and one pair of sex chromosomes.
  - o Males have 1 X and 1 Y chromosome, while females have 2 X chromosomes.
- All of the genes needed for male fertility have relocated to the Y-chromosome.
  - o Causing the male to lose 1 X chromosome.
  - o Because both copies of a chromosome are generally needed, this loss would normally be intolerable.
  - o But evolution has permitted one copy of the X chromosome to suffice.
  - o No excessive X chromosome effect in females because of inactivation of 1 of the 2 X chromosomes.
- Meiosis: 1 replication of DNA followed by 2 cell divisions, resulting in 4 haploid cells.
  - o After the DNA replication, chromosomes paired, permitting crossing over between paternally derived and maternally derived DNA
  - o A major cause of genetic recombination.
  - o DNA of the embryo is thus derived from the 4 grandparents.
- 2 fundamental modes of inheritance: Mendelian and non-Mendelian.
- Mendelian disorders: based on one or a very small number of genes.
  - o Governed by the Hardy-Weinberg law.
    - ▪ Allele frequencies do not change in populations that are large, stable, and demonstrate random mating.
  - o Have been assigned an MIM number (Mendelian inheritance in man)
  - o Inherited as autosomal dominant, autosomal recessive, X-linked, or rarely, Y-linked.
- Autosomal dominant inheritance: most patients have an affected parent, but de novo mutations are relatively common.
  - o Incomplete penetrance: gene is present, but clinical manifestations may be insufficient to make a diagnosis.
  - o Variable expressivity: the clinical diagnosis is established, but symptoms vary from one patient to another.
  - o Equal gender distribution and about 50% of an affected individual's children will be affected.
- Autosomal recessive inheritance: both genders equally affected.
  - o Both parents are unaffected carriers, and the disorder often skips generations, so family history often absent.
  - o Mating of 2 unaffected carriers will produce the disorder in 1/4 of children. 1/2 of children phenotypically normal carriers and 1/4 homozygous normal.
- X-linked recessive conditions: males much more likely to be affected.
  - o Generally require a female carrier, but spontaneous mutations can account for some cases.
  - o Daughters of an affected male and a normal female are phenotypically normal but are carriers.
  - o Sons of an affected father and a normal woman will be phenotypically and genotypically normal because they have inherited their X chromosome from their mother.
  - o Half of sons of a normal male and a carrier woman will be affected.
- Bayesian analysis: probability calculations in Mendelian inheritance if additional information, such as the status of siblings or children, or results of screening tests, are known.
- Mitochondrial inheritance is an additional means of single-gene inheritance, but not Mendelian because it does not involve nuclear DNA.
  - o Mitochondria are inherited only through the mother.
  - o Mitochondrial inheritance involves only a small number of genes in the mitochondrial genome, with disproportionate impact on neuromuscular diseases.
  - o 2 unusual features of mitochondrial inheritance: heteroplasmy and replicative segregation.
- Multifactorial (or complex) inheritance: more common than Mendelian inheritance.
  - o 2 or more gene loci are involved, often with substantial influence of environmental or cultural factors.
  - o Twin studies can be used to estimate the genetic and nongenetic components in multifactorial inheritance.
- Chromosomal aberrations: another means of non-Mendelian inheritance
  - o Became amenable to study with the advent of banding techniques.
  - o Giemsa banding is still used, but has been supplemented with newer techniques based on FISH and microarrays.
  - o Translocations, deletions, duplications, inversions, trisomies, and monosomies.
  - o May be inherited or occur de novo.
- Linkage analysis and association studies: ways to map genes.
  - o Linkage analysis: rare now, but were helpful in studying Mendelian inheritance.
  - o Genes or regions that are farther apart on a chromosome are more likely they are to undergo recombination because there are a larger number of breakage-prone regions between them.
  - o 2 loci that stay together over the generations are likely to be close to each other on the same chromosome.
- Association studies: particularly helpful in non-Mendelian situations
  - o Focus on populations, comparing the frequency of one or more alleles in a group of affected people with that of unaffected people.
  - o Association studies continue and have been applied to the entire genome.

ISBN 978-089189-5886

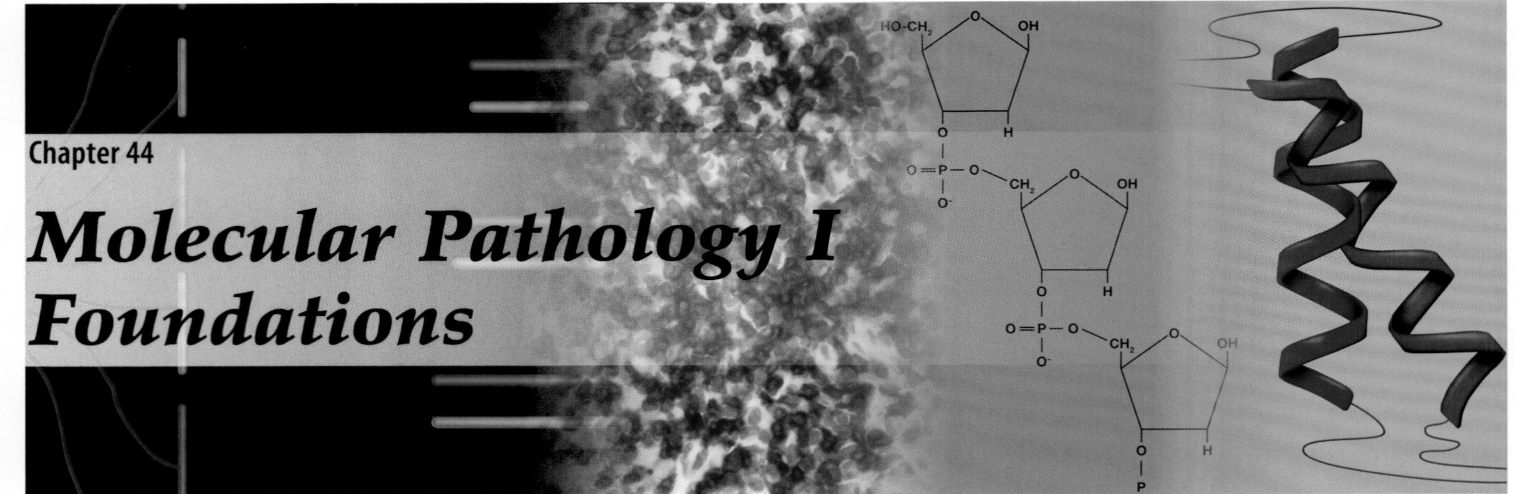

Chapter 44

Molecular Pathology I Foundations

In molecular pathology, we enter a world that is very different from that of the previous chapters. We no longer enumerate and describe the conditions that might be encountered in each organ or system, but rather navigate through different and less familiar concepts. To ease the journey, this section is divided into 4 chapters—foundations, techniques, applications and diagnoses, and frontiers. Most of us have a basic concept of DNA, how it is structured, and how it controls the actions of a cell. In this chapter, we will expand on and sharpen those concepts and strive for a more complete understanding of the workings of the cell.

Historical Background

There are in science a small number of triumphs that stand above all others. The elucidation of the structure of DNA, with relativity and quantum mechanics, was one of the great triumphs of the 20th century, and its entry into clinical use is a defining moment in the history of medicine.

DNA was actually discovered in 1869 by Johann Friedrich Miescher (1844-1895), who is curiously forgotten in this chapter of medical history [PMID15680349]. For decades after its discovery, no one had a clue what the function of DNA might be. It had long been assumed that large molecules must somehow store and convey genetic traits. The central role of chromosomes in the transmission of genetic traits was understood, and it was known that the cell's DNA was in chromosomes. Indeed, in the 1920s, Thomas Hunt Morgan showed that linkage—the tendency for some genes to be inherited together—was caused by physical proximity of those genes on a chromosome. But chromosomes also contain as much or more protein than DNA, and chromosomal protein was believed to be the genetic messenger.

In 1941—before the discovery of the structure of DNA—George Beadle and Edward Tatum proposed the famous "1 gene-1 enzyme" hypothesis. As we will see, only a small minority of DNA (<2%!) actually codes for a polypeptide, and indeed, the very definition of a gene is unclear, but the 1 gene-1 enzyme hypothesis was a great leap because all proteins are derived from the small portion of DNA that goes the classic transcription-translation route. Even today, the concept that a gene is a portion of DNA that eventuates in a distinct protein molecule has appreciable validity.

The first step in understanding DNA was to prove that it, not proteins, carried genetic information. In 1944, Avery, Macleod, and McCarty, in an ingenious series of experiments, showed that DNA carried genetic information. There are few statements in all of medical history that carry more power than this single sentence from their seminal paper [PMID19871359]:

"The fact that transforming activity is destroyed only by those preparations containing depolymerase for desoxyribonucleic acid and the further fact that in both instances the enzymes concerned are inactivated at the same temperature and inhibited by fluoride provide additional evidence for the belief that the active principle is a nucleic acid of the desoxyribose type."

In 1952, Hershey and Chase confirmed this by labeling viruses that target bacteria (phages) with 2 radioactive labels: 1 for the nucleic acid and 1 for the proteins [PMID12981234]. They allowed the phages to adhere to the bacteria, permitting them to initiate their attack. But before they could complete their attack on the bacteria, Hershey and Chase separated them and centrifuged the mixture. The lighter phages and any free proteins were in the supernatant, while the heavier bacteria were in the pellet. They found that the nucleic acid label was with the bacteria in the pellet, while the protein label was in the supernatant. Their correct interpretation was that the phage attack, which clearly commandeered the machinery of the bacteria to make new phage particles, used nucleic acid to do this, not proteins.

This was the background for the elucidation of the structure of DNA. Like any great idea, the discovery of the structure and function of DNA was the work of many people over a long time. The basic components of DNA were known, and Erwin Chargaff (1905-2002) made the indispensable observation that the number of adenine molecules equaled the number of thymine molecules and the number of guanine molecules equaled the number of cytosine molecules. Linus Pauling (1901-1994) showed that some proteins—macromolecules presumably comparable in structure to DNA—had helical structures.

Earlier, many workers, especially Max von Laue (1879-1960), had shown that x-rays could not only see through objects but could also elucidate their structure in many cases. Advances in x-ray crystallography then allowed 4 people—Maurice Wilkins (1916-2004), Rosalind Franklin (1920-1958),

Francis Crick (1916-2004), and James Watson (b 1928)—to come to the fore. Wilkins and Crick were trained as physicists, and Franklin had studied chemistry and become an expert on crystallography. Only Watson was classically trained in biology. Wilkins was the first to realize that x-ray crystallography could make an invaluable contribution toward elucidating the structure of DNA, and he obtained early crystallographs. Franklin soon improved these, and Watson and Crick synthesized all available information to make a bold hypothesis of the structure of the molecule.

In 1958, 5 years after the work of Crick and Watson, the central dogma of molecular biology was developed. The central dogma holds that DNA is transcribed to RNA, which is then translated into protein. Like the 1 gene-1 enzyme hypothesis of Beadle and Tatum, the central dogma has stood the test of time well, but as we will see, both of these pioneering hypotheses need modification and extension.

The Structure of DNA

The definitive text on molecular biology is by Alberts et al [Alberts ISBN978-0-8153-4111-6], to which the reader is referred for a comprehensive discussion of all aspects of nucleic acids and cell biology. Another excellent discussion of cell biology, basic DNA function in genetics, and molecular pathology can be found in the text by Strachan and Read [Strachan ISBN978-0815341499].

Distinction between Prokaryotes and Eukaryotes

The distinction between prokaryotes and eukaryotes is much more important than that between animals and plants, and is key to understanding nucleic acids and molecular pathology. To understand DNA, we must first review the newer classification of life. The old animal kingdom/plant kingdom system was replaced by a eukaryote/prokaryote classification, beginning in the 1960s [PMID13916221], because it was recognized that eukaryotes of all types—be they humans, insects, or trees—have far more in common with each other than they do with prokaryotes. Like it or not, we are much more like an insect than an insect is like a bacterium. Prokaryotes are essentially synonymous with bacteria, while eukaryotes include virtually all other living creatures, except viruses. Eukaryotes have a more complex cellular structure than prokaryotes, with organelles (often enclosed by a membrane), sterols in the cell membrane, and a more complex cytoskeleton than is found in prokaryotes. Chief among the membrane-enclosed organelles of eukaryotes is the nucleus. Remarkably, the nucleus, a small portion of the eukaryotic cell, is divided into many zones, each specialized for a particular purpose. For example, ribosomal RNA is transcribed only in a portion of the nucleus called the nucleolus. Many other zones of the nucleus, and their specialized functions, are just now beginning to be understood. Eukaryotes have a wide array of genes that have been remarkably conserved during hundreds of millions of years of evolution.

Archaea are a recently discovered group of organisms that resemble bacteria and are occasionally classified with them as prokaryotes. However, pioneering work begun by Carl Woese [PMID2112744] has shown that archaea differ from bacteria in being heat or salt loving; in making methane; in the structures of their transfer RNA, ribosomes, and RNA polymerase; in the chemical composition of their cell walls and cell membranes; and in the lack of a well defined cytoskeleton (though cytoskeletal proteins are found in archaea [PMID17189356]). Nucleic acid studies, especially comparison of sequences of ribosomal RNA, have also shown significant differences between bacteria and archaea [PMID19946133].

Because differences between bacteria and archaea make it difficult to combine them, it has been proposed that life be considered to have 3 domains—eukaryotes, prokaryotes (bacteria), and archaea—rather than kingdoms [PMID2112744]. The rationale for the term "domain" is that it leaves intact the older classification system that begins with kingdom and extends down to species. For example, under the eukaryote domain, one can still talk about the plant and animal kingdoms, and the phyla, classes, etc, that extend downward from these kingdoms.

Increasing understanding of DNA has confirmed this tripartite tree of life—eukaryote, bacteria, and archaea domains—and the concept has generally been accepted, though one still occasionally sees bacteria and archaea conflated into the prokaryote domain.

Life Is Based On 2 Sugars, 5 Bases, and a Phosphate Group

Now we consider the structure of DNA and RNA. Both of these nucleic acids are built in the same way, with only minor differences. The first difference between DNA and RNA is the sugar moiety. Both DNA and RNA use a pentose (5 carbon sugar), but in RNA, the sugar is ribose, in which hydroxyl groups are bound to the carbon atoms at positions 1, 2, 3, and 5. In DNA, the sugar is deoxyribose, in which a hydroxyl group is bound to carbon atoms 1, 3, and 5 only—not to carbon atom number 2 **f44.1**. In nucleic acids, 1 of these 2 sugars in bonded to 1 of 5 bases—adenine, guanine, cytosine, thymine, or uracil **f44.1**. Uracil is used in RNA instead of thymine; otherwise the bases are shared between the 2 nucleic acids.

A *nucleoside* is a base and a pentose **f44.2**. When combined with a pentose, the resulting nucleosides are called cytidine, thymidine, uridine, adenosine, and guanosine. A *nucleotide* is a nucleoside bound to a phosphate group **f44.3**. Nucleotides are named as for the nucleoside, plus the phrase "monophosphate." The nucleotides are cytidine monophosphate (CMP), thymidine monophosphate (TMP), uridine monophosphate (UMP), adenosine monophosphate (AMP), and guanosine monophosphate (GMP). A nucleoside may also combine with >1 phosphate group, in which case the product is not a nucleotide (which by definition has only 1 phosphate group), but a nucleoside diphosphate or triphosphate. These include cytidine triphosphate (CTP), thymidine triphosphate (TTP), uridine triphosphate (UTP), adenosine triphosphate (ATP), and guanosine triphosphate (GTP). These compounds are required for the synthesis of DNA because bases are added to DNA in their nucleoside triphosphate form.

When pentoses are part of a nucleotide, the numbers of their carbon atoms are followed by a prime mark (') and the carbon is referred to as "5 prime," "3 prime," etc. In the synthesis of each strand of DNA, bonding occurs between

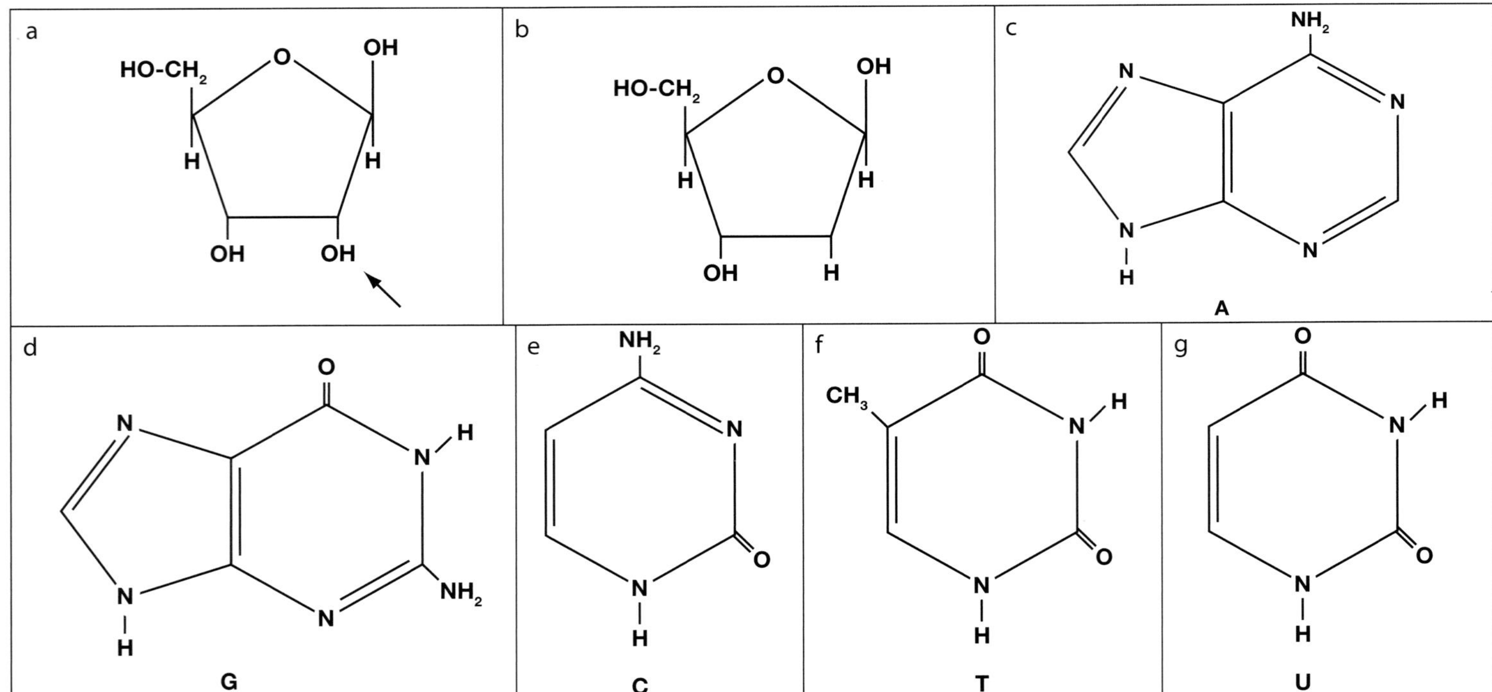

f44.1 The 7 molecules of life **a** The pentose ribose. Note that carbon number 2 (denoted by the arrow) and carbon atom number 3 both have hydroxyl groups. **b** The pentose deoxyribose. Note that carbon atom number 2 does not have a hydroxyl group. This does not affect its ability to participate in polymerization, as polymerization requires a hydroxyl group on carbon atom number 3. **c** The base adenine (A) **d** The base guanine (G) **e** The base cytosine (C) **f** The base thymine (T) **g** The base uracil (U)

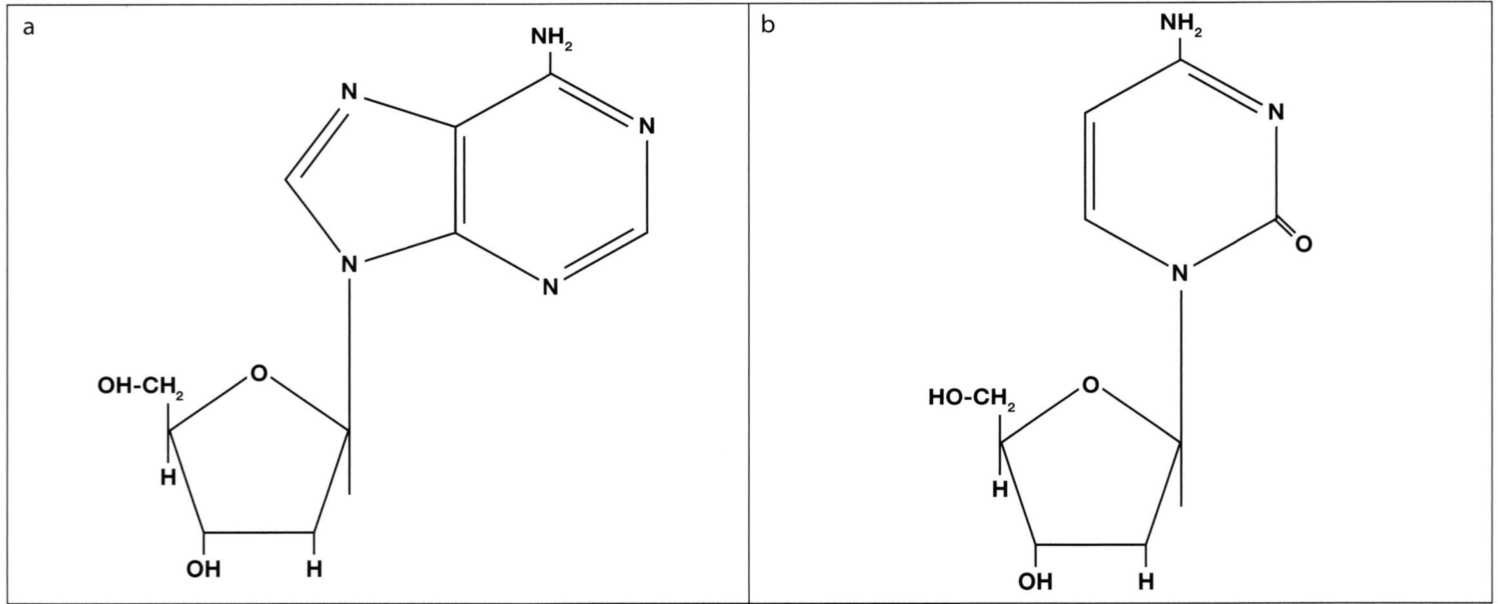

f44.2 **a** A nucleoside based on adenine (adenosine) **b** A nucleoside based on cytosine (cytidine)

the phosphate group of the 5' pentose of one nucleotide and the hydroxyl group of the 3' carbon from the pentose of the adjacent nucleotide f44.4. This creates a sugar-phosphate backbone from which the bases protrude into the center, to be met in the middle by a base attached to the other backbone, so that a double-stranded nucleic molecule is composed of 2 complementary strands of nucleotides, each strand being anchored by a sugar-phosphate backbone. This bonding requires the hydrolysis of the triphosphate molecule (ATP, GTP, CTP, or TTP, depending on which base is to be added) and results in the release of a water molecule and a pyrophosphate molecule (containing 2 phosphate groups), so that only 1 of the 3 phosphate groups is actually incorporated into the DNA molecule. The triphosphate forms of nucleosides are essential to DNA synthesis because they are the forms that are used in elongation. Moreover, nucleoside triphosphates, especially ATP and GTP, are of immense importance in other areas of biology, particularly in cell signaling.

For each strand, the 5' end of the DNA molecule has a terminal pentose that contains a phosphate group, while the pentose at the 3' end has an intact hydroxyl group. A single strand of nucleic acid can be denoted from the 5' end by using a single capital letter for each base, and a lowercase "p" to denote the intervening phosphate groups, for example 5'pGpApC3'. Since it is understood that a phosphate group must be between each base, this can be shortened to 5'GAC3'. By convention, a single

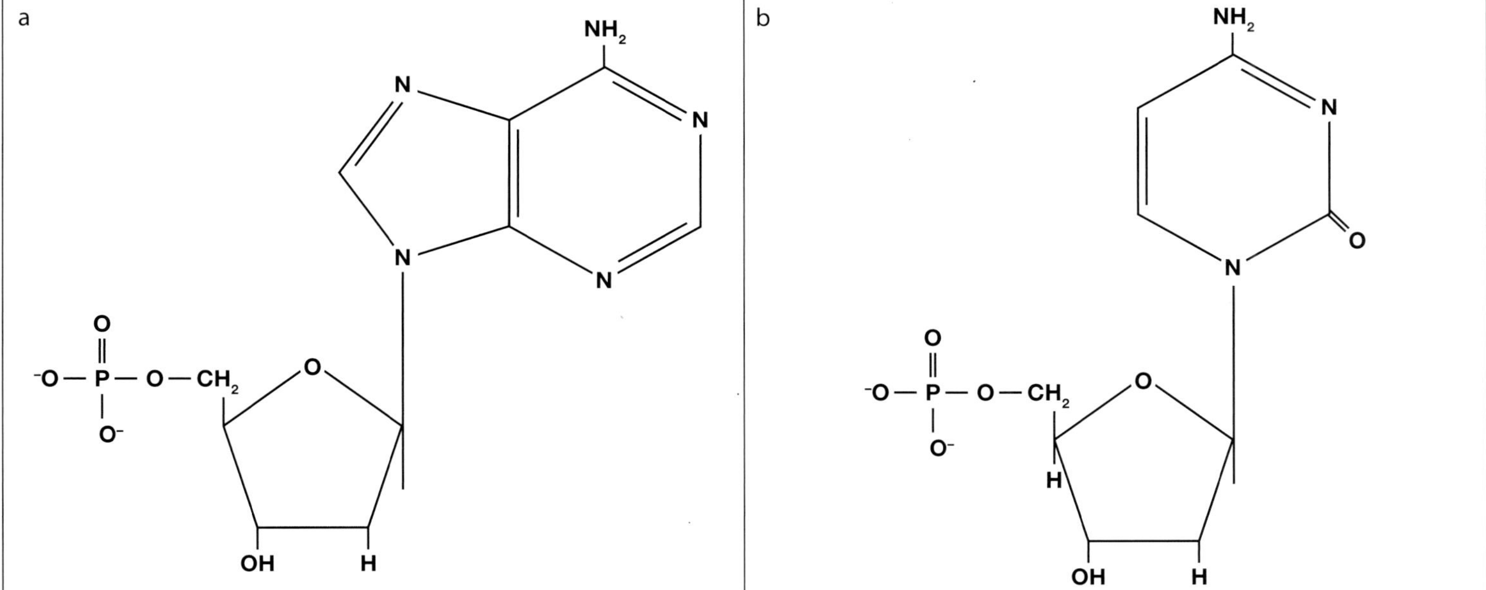

f44.3 **a** A nucleotide based on adenine (adenosine monophosphate) **b** A nucleotide based on cytosine (cytidine monophosphate)

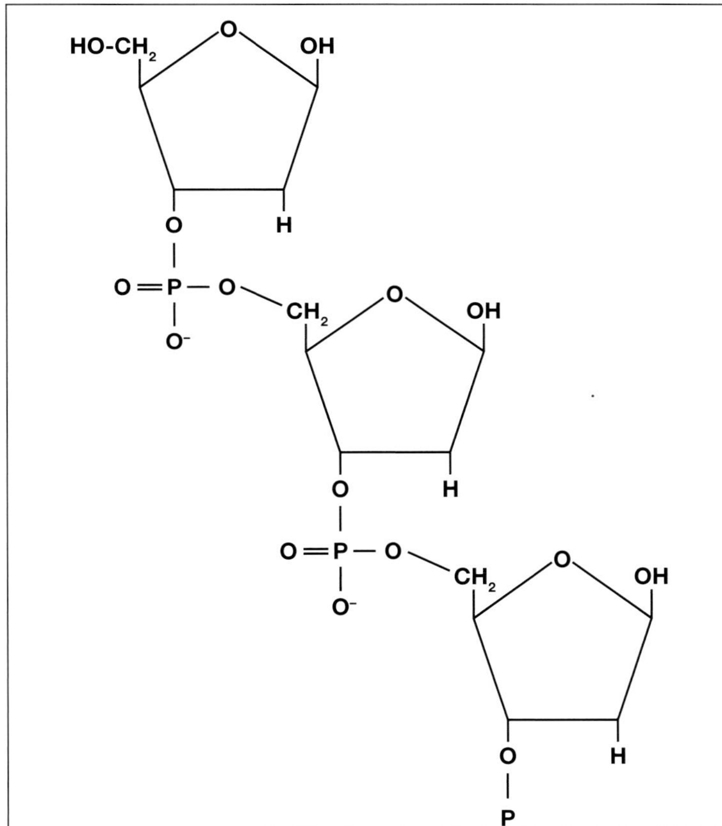

f44.4 The pentose-phosphate backbone of DNA. The 2 backbones are each composed of polymers of a pentose (ribose or deoxyribose) linked by phosphate groups. There are no bases in the backbone. The bases project from the backbone towards the center, to be met in the middle by a base projecting from the other backbone.

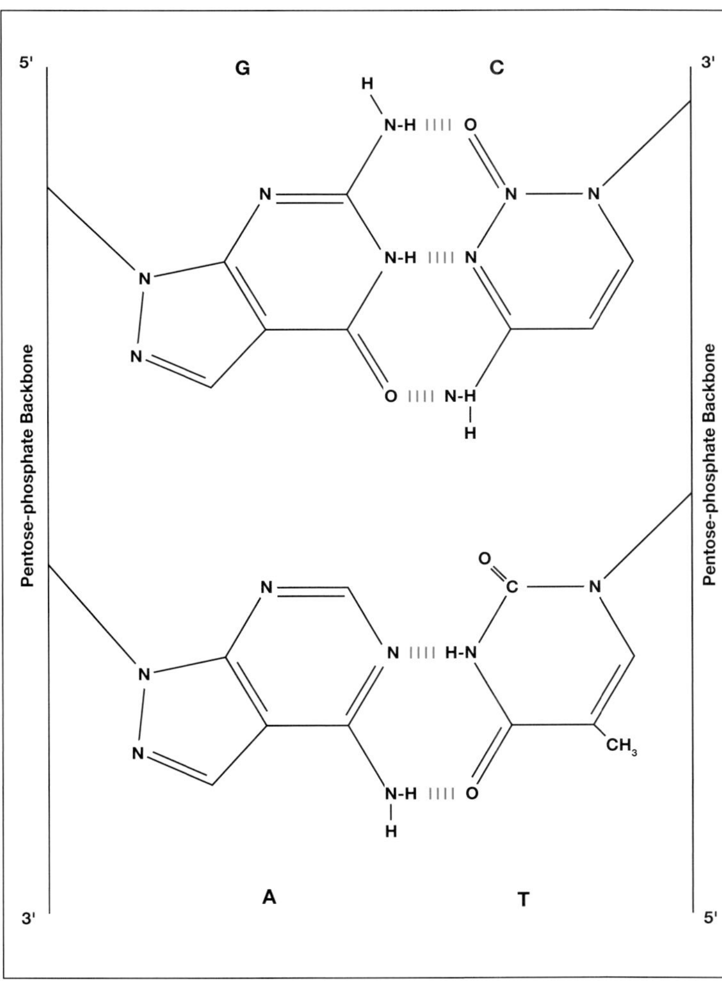

f44.5 The pentose-phosphate backbone depicted in f44.4 is depicted here as a simple line on either side. In the center, there is base pairing. At the top, the base guanine, attached to the pentose-phosphate backbone on the left, pairs with the base cytosine, attached to the backbone on the right. On the bottom, the base adenine, attached to the backbone on the left, pairs with the base thymine, attached to the backbone on the right. The red vertical lines indicate hydrogen bonds. Note that there are 3 of them between the bases guanine and cytosine, but only 2 between the bases adenine and thymine, making G-C bonds slightly stronger than A-T bonds.

strand of nucleic acid is written with the 5' end on the left side and the 3' end on the right side, so that the above sequence can be further abbreviated as simply GAC.

DNA exists as a double-stranded helix in which the adenine bases of one strand pair with the thymine bases of the other strand, and the cytosine bases of one strand pair with the guanine bases of the other f44.5. The 2 strands of DNA

ISBN 978-089189-5886

are aligned in what is said to be an antiparallel configuration. This means that they face each other in a mirror image manner such that the 5' to 3' direction on one strand is 3' to 5' on the opposing strand. Here is a simplified example of an antiparallel sequence of DNA:

5' GTAGCTACCATG 3'

3' CATCGATGGTAC 5'

The sugar-phosphate backbone, on the outside of the molecule, is negatively charged and is therefore relatively hydrophilic, since water is a polar molecule. The bases, on the other hand, are hydrophobic and are shielded from water in the interior.

There are no covalent bonds between the 2 strands of DNA. They are instead held together largely by the hydrogen bonding of the complementary bases in the center. An ionic bond is a *transfer* of electrons from one atom to another, while a covalent bond is a *sharing* of electrons between atoms. A hydrogen bond is an incomplete sharing of electrons, in which one atom has "custody" of the electron much more than the other and, roughly speaking, is a partial or incomplete covalent bond that is about 5% as strong as a covalent bond. There are 3 hydrogen bonds between the cytosine-guanine bases, but only 2 between the thymine and adenine bases, so DNA that is rich in G-C pairings is more strongly bound into a double-helix form.

In addition to the hydrogen bonds between bases, hydrophobic interaction of the bases provides a stabilizing force and helps maintains DNA structure. Counterbalancing both of these attractive forces is the mutual electrostatic repulsion of the phosphate groups. This repulsive force is neutralized by salt. Higher salt concentrations neutralize the repulsive force of the phosphate groups and lead to a more stable double-stranded structural formation of DNA. Low salt concentrations are usually used in situations where separation of the 2 strands is desired, so that maximal advantage can be taken of the mutually repulsive force between the phosphate groups. If highly specific binding is desired for in vitro work, lower salt concentration is utilized as only specific and very well matched base-pair binding can overcome the powerful repulsion of the phosphate groups in low salt conditions.

Each Cell Contains As Much As a Meter of DNA, Packed in an Intricate Series of Structures

Each chromosome consists of 1 linear DNA molecule and the proteins that are associated with it. Because there are 2 chromosomes per cell, there are 23 different pairs of DNA molecules per cell, not counting the mitochondrial genome, which is tiny, but very important in a number of neuromuscular diseases. Of the 23 pairs of chromosomes, there are 22 autosomes which all males and females possess. The 23rd pair of chromosomes is called the sex chromosomes since they vary by gender. Females have 2 Xs, which are large chromosomes. Males have 1 X, inherited from the mother, and 1 Y chromosome, which is very small and is inherited from the father.

In its normal state, all DNA molecules are coiled and tightly packed. The nucleosome is the basic unit and first order of DNA packing. It consists of a collection of 8 protein molecules called histones, 2 each of H2A, H2B, H3, and H4

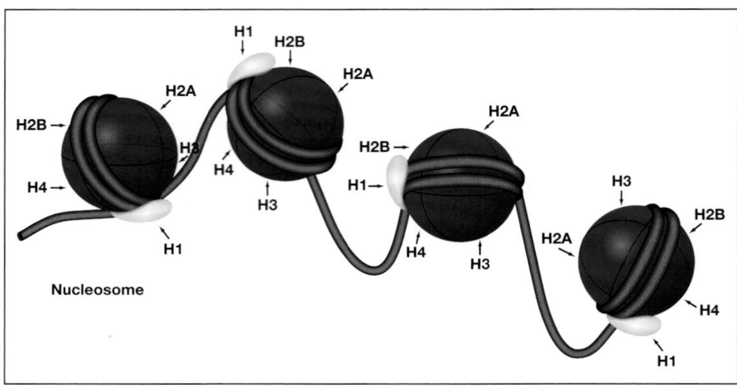

f44.6 The first order of DNA packing. The nucleosome is a spherical structure composed of 8 protein molecules (only 4 of the histones [H] are shown, but each of these is repeated behind the proteins shown). The nucleosome is stabilized by a ninth protein molecule (H1). DNA is wound around the nucleosome and then passes to the next nucleosome and wraps around it.

(sperm use a group of proteins called protamines instead of histones). A 147 base pair length of DNA is wound around the histone complex. A short spacer (or linker) sequence of DNA connects each nucleosome, resulting in an electron microscopic appearance that resembles a "string of beads" and that has a diameter of about 10 nm **f44.6**. The histone H1 is not part of the nucleosome but is immediately adjacent to it, contacting the DNA as it enters and exits the nucleosome [PMID19794910]. H1 stabilizes the nucleosome and is necessary for orderly packing.

The structure of nucleosomes is reasonably well agreed upon, but the details of higher degrees of DNA organization are less clear. When interphase nuclei are gently lysed, the chromosomes are usually in the form of 30 nm fibers, which appear to be a higher order of packing of nucleosomes and the "string of beads," but also 1 or more orders less packed than an interphase structure. The true structure of interphase chromosomes is unknown, and chromosomes in mitosis are even more tightly packed.

In general, the less tightly packed DNA is, the more likely the genes on it are to be transcribed. If DNA is "unwound" by a cellular signal, a gene or genes in the exposed region can be transcribed. In the interphase chromatin fiber, "euchromatin" is a term used to designate more relaxed areas of DNA organization. Genes in euchromatin may or may not be expressed, while those in the more tightly packed DNA, heterochromatin, are typically not accessible to DNA polymerase. Constitutive heterochromatin is always tightly packed and therefore, almost never transcribed. Indeed, it consists largely of repetitive DNA and has very few functional genes. Constitutive heterochromatin constitutes approximately 10% of the total DNA. Facultative heterochromatin may occasionally be "unwound" sufficiently for some degree of transcription.

The degree of chromosome packing is largely dependent on the conformation and activity of histones. Chromosome remodeling complexes are ATP-dependent enzyme complexes that can modify histones and change the structure of nucleosomes to allow enzymes to access the DNA, permitting transcription. In addition to the "accessibility" of the DNA, methylation of DNA affects transcription (methylation and its effects are considered in more detail in Chapter 47).

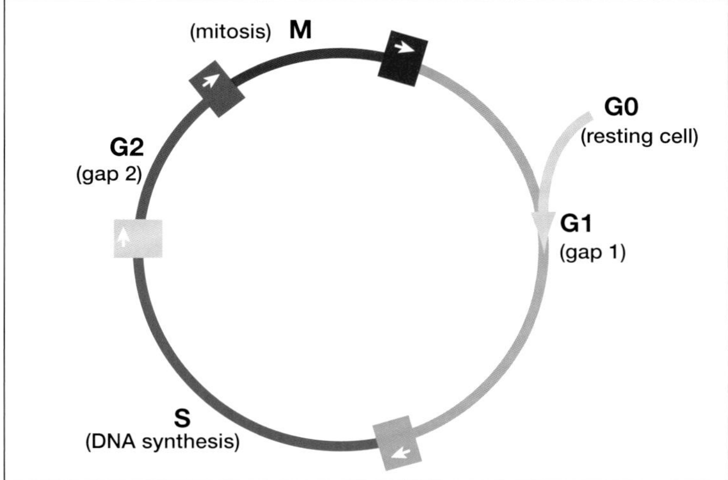

f44.7 The cell cycle. This diagram is read in a clockwise manner. A resting cell (G0) may enter the cell cycle at G1. DNA is duplicated during the S phase after which the cell has twice the normal DNA content (G2). The duplicated DNA, in the form of chromatids, is segregated to opposite ends of the cell during mitosis (M). The 4 shaded boxes indicate the checkpoints, which, if not successfully navigated, will arrest the cycle or destroy the cell.

The Cell Cycle Consists of Phases and Has Specific Regulatory Checkpoints

Before we consider DNA replication, we must consider the cell cycle and mitosis. The terms "mitosis" and "cell division" are sometimes used interchangeably, but mitosis refers only to the segregation of the previously replicated DNA to the ends of the cell in preparation for the division of the cell and is distinct from both the actual replication of DNA, which precedes it, and the division of the cell, which follows it.

The cell cycle consists of a G1 phase, in which the cell intends to divide but has not yet undergone DNA replication. The S phase is the period of DNA replication. After the S phase, the DNA content is briefly twice normal. This phase is called G2. G2 is followed by the M phase, which is the mitosis during which a normal complement of DNA is moved to each end of the cell f44.7. With only very rare exceptions, mitosis is followed by cytokinesis, the cell division that results in 2 daughter cells, each with a normal DNA content and each in the G1 state. Sometimes, the term "G0" is used for cells that do not divide to any extent, such as neurons and muscle cells. Cytokinesis is said to be symmetric if the daughter cells are identical and asymmetric if they are not (an example of asymmetric cell division is the division of a basal cell, with 1 daughter cell differentiating and the other remaining as a replacement basal cell).

There are 3 stages at which the cell cycle is subject to extensive regulation. These are the entry into the S phase (the G1-S checkpoint), a checkpoint entry into mitosis (the G2-M checkpoint), and a checkpoint in mitosis (also shown in f44.7) [PMID11063129]. A checkpoint in the S phase is also currently recognized [PMID21610326]. A simple way to remember this is that the 2 most critical stages—the replication of DNA and the movement of the DNA to each end of the cell—are regulated both before and during the process. Each of these stages is regulated by a specific protein or group of proteins, and the precise packing of DNA changes during the cell cycle. We will consider regulation of the cell cycle in more detail in our discussion of infection by the human papillomavirus, because the effect of viral proteins on cell cycle regulation has been most extensively studied in this situation.

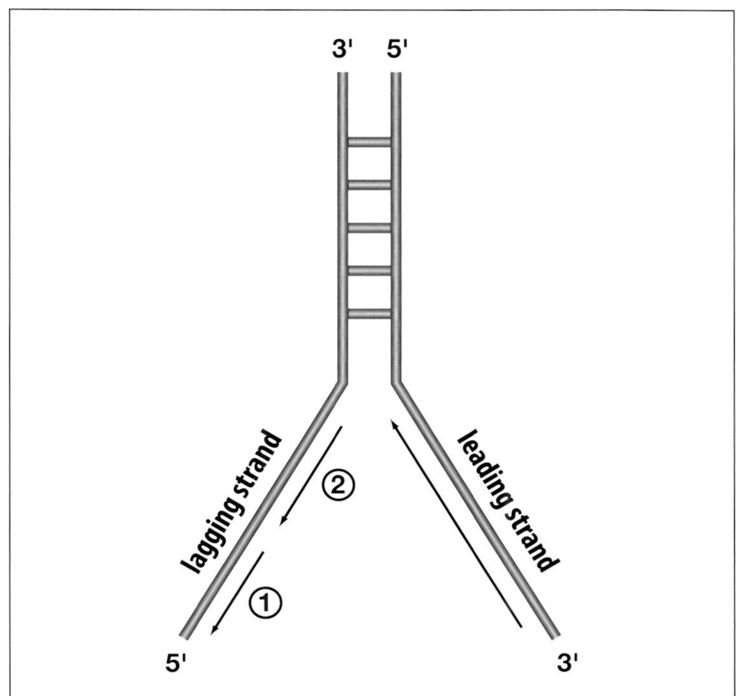

f44.8 DNA duplication. This diagram depicts the process after unwinding of the helix, separation of the strands, and binding of the RNA primers. The leading strand is replicated in a continuous manner, while the lagging strand is replicated in fragments that must be joined by a ligase.

DNA Replication

In both prokaryotes and eukaryotes, DNA is replicated by the enzyme DNA polymerase and must be released from its higher order packing so that a single strand can be presented to the DNA polymerase complex. Because higher order packing of DNA is not well understood, the details of how it is released are not clear, but it is known that 2 classes of enzymes, helicases and topoisomerases, are involved in permitting enzymatic access.

Helicases initiate the necessary unwinding and strand separation, after which topoisomerases complete the process of releasing supercoiling. Topoisomerases must break 1 or both strands of the double-stranded DNA. Type I topoisomerases break 1 strand at a time, while type II topoisomerases can break both strands simultaneously [PMID14993926]. These enzymes are occasional therapeutic targets. For example, the antibiotic ciprofloxacin works by inhibiting gyrase, a bacterial topoisomerase.

In both prokaryotes and eukaryotes, after separation and unwinding, DNA polymerase requires a double-stranded starting point, which is achieved by the addition of a short RNA primer at the beginning of replication. This primer is quickly removed after the enzyme commences its action. During DNA replication, both strands are copied in a 5' to 3' direction (relative to the template strand; replication is 3' to 5' relative to the newly-synthesized strands). Because the strands are antiparallel, 5' to 3' replication means that 1 parent strand, called the leading strand, is copied in 1 continuous fragment. The other strand, the lagging strand, must be copied in short pieces (Okazaki fragments), which are then joined by the enzyme DNA ligase f44.8.

ISBN 978-089189-5886

In prokaryotes, where the DNA is generally in the form of a single, circular chromosome, DNA has 2 primary forms of replication, θ-mode and rolling circle. In both of these forms, replication begins at a single point. In θ-mode, neither strand of DNA is broken. The 2 strands are separated, and there is bidirectional replication from one point. This results in a resemblance to the Greek letter θ. In the rolling circle mode, there is a nick in 1 of the 2 strands, after which replication proceeds in only 1 direction, using the strand that has not been nicked as the template. As replication proceeds, the strand that was nicked is displaced and becomes a long single strand that moves away from the chromosome. That displaced single strand then serves as the template for its complement, completing the process. The rolling circle mode is also called the σ-mode because it resembles that Greek letter.

In contrast to the circular DNA of prokaryotes, eukaryotic DNA is linear, and when it is replicated, there are usually many points of origin.

There Are Many Forms of DNA Polymerase, in Both Prokaryotes and Eukaryotes

The primary forms of DNA polymerase in prokaryotes are designated I and III [PMID11459973]. The function of DNA polymerase I is to excise the RNA primer and replace those bases with DNA. DNA polymerase I has "built-in" exonuclease activity in both a 5' to 3' and a 3' to 5' direction. However, the primary DNA replication enzyme in prokaryotes is DNA polymerase III, which also has exonuclease activity, but more in the 3' to 5' direction than in the 5' to 3' direction.

Eukaryotes have over a dozen DNA polymerases. The most well understood are the α, β, γ, δ, and ε polymerases, and of these, the primary enzymes are DNA polymerases α, δ, and ε. The α polymerase starts the process and is active in proofreading and repair. The distribution of labor between the δ and ε forms of the enzyme is unclear, but the δ form seems to do most of the work on the lagging strand, while the ε form is the primary form in the synthesis of the leading strand [PMID18824354, PMID18835809]. Whereas the other DNA polymerases are found in the nucleus, the γ polymerase is restricted to mitochondria and functions in replication of mitochondrial DNA. The β enzyme appears to function primarily in meiosis. The γ, δ, and ε forms have exonuclease activity, with correction potential. In addition to these 5 forms of the polymerase, a number of low-fidelity DNA polymerases have been found in mammalian cells, the function of which is not yet clear.

There Are Many Enzymes That Repair Damaged or Mismatched DNA

Although DNA is replicated with magnificent fidelity, no process is foolproof, and very rarely, the wrong base is inserted into the replicating double helix. A "transition" is a base pair substitution between 2 pyrimidines or 2 purines. Examples include a cytosine being substituted for a thymine or an adenine for a guanine. A "transversion" is between a pyrimidine and a purine, such as a cytosine for an adenine.

The most commonly used eukaryotic DNA polymerases, δ and ε, have "proofreading" and repair capability, and with their use, the mistake rate is perhaps 1 in every 10 million base pairs. But this is still not good enough, and behind the DNA polymerases are a variety of dedicated mismatch repair enzymes, which detect mismatched base pairs and cut out the incorrect base [PMID20951805]. In bacteria, MutS and MutL recognize mismatched bases and "call" MMR enzymes into action. Eukaryotes have a number of proteins that serve a similar function to MutS and MutL [PMID18157157].

Mismatch repair enzymes are a subset of repair enzymes that specialize in correcting base pairs that are incorrectly placed during replication. Consider a mistaken pairing of A-C. Because the correct pairing must be either A-T or G-C, one of these bases must be removed. But which one? Does the mistake lie in the placement of the adenine or the cytosine? Since DNA tends to methylate with time, the old strand of DNA, carrying the correct base, will be relatively more methylated than the new strand. So the mismatch repair enzymes remove the base from the less methylated strand. If these mismatch repair enzymes work properly, they reduce the error rate in DNA replication to about 1 in a billion.

Excision repair enzymes repair damage that occurs after replication from environmental damage (ionizing radiation, ultraviolet light, and various chemicals, especially alkylating agents). Excision repair enzymes may remove only a base or an entire nucleotide [PMID21414892, PMID19659577]. Enzymes that remove incorrect bases often act through a remarkable process called base flipping (or nucleotide flipping), in which the local structure of the DNA double helix is relaxed enough to permit a single base to leave the interior and flip outwards, coming to rest on the exterior, in the active site of the enzyme, so that the enzyme can work on it [PMID18000994]. Excision repair enzymes are deficient in xeroderma pigmentosum, resulting in patient's inability to repair ordinary environmental damage to DNA.

Other repair enzymes either arrest the cell cycle or initiate apoptosis, killing the cell [PMID19953589]. With these many repair enzymes, mistakes are extraordinarily rare, but the clinical consequences may still be great.

Mitosis Is the Separation of the Duplicated Chromosomes to Opposite Poles of the Cell

The mitosis portion of the cell cycle has been particularly well studied. After DNA replication, each chromosome is said to consist of 2 sister chromatids, each of which has the full complement of DNA of its parent chromosome. This terminology can be confusing because after DNA replication, the word "chromosome" now applies to a structure that has twice the DNA content that is normally associated with the term. As we saw in our discussion of meiosis, in the early days of cell biology, a chromosome was defined as having 1 centromere, and the 2 sister chromatids, while each having the same DNA content as the original chromosome, still have only 1 centromere between them. The DNA in sister chromatids is derived from either the mother or the father because a pair of sister chromatids represents the division of 1 chromosome. Although there may be occasional exchange of DNA between sister chromatids, there is no crossing over of maternally and paternally derived DNA (in contrast, during meiosis, pairing occurs in such a way that there can be crossing over and exchange of material between chromosomes from the mother and the father).

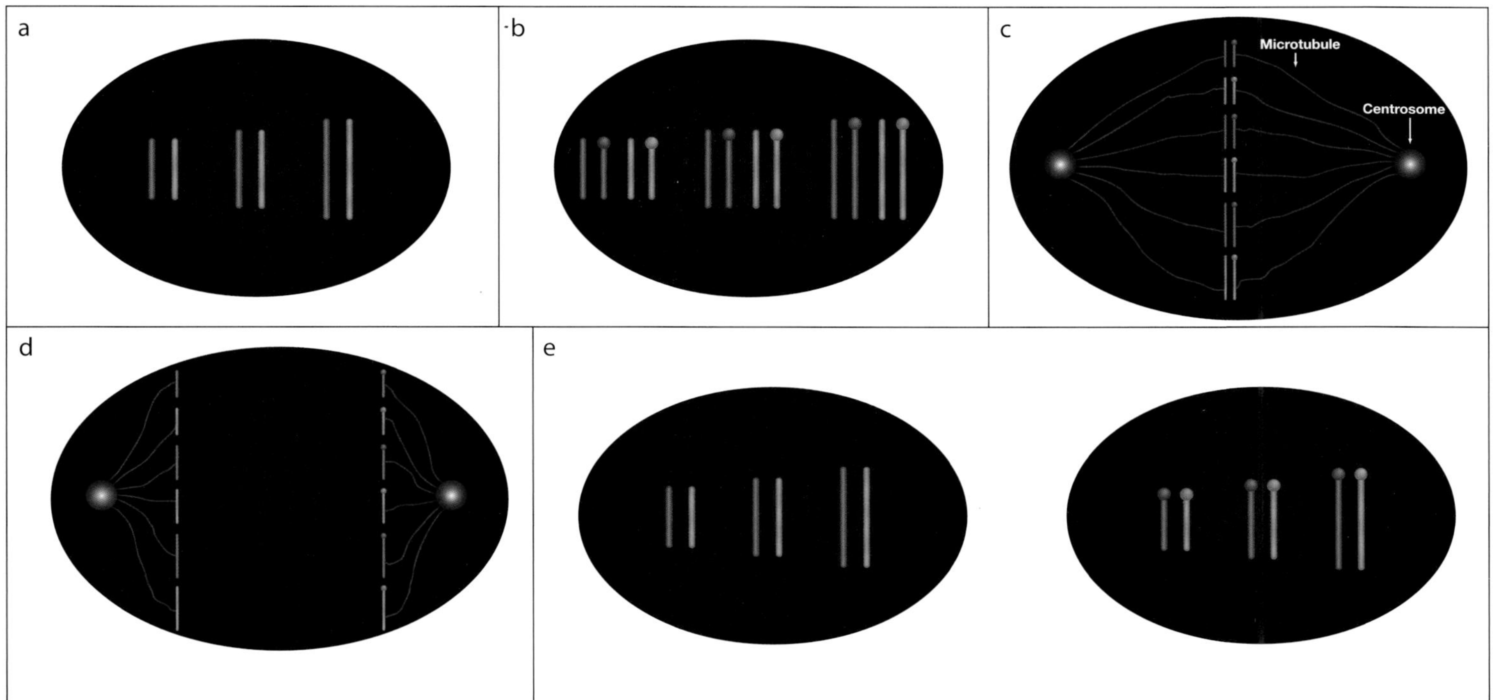

f44.9 The 5 images depict some of the stages of mitosis. a The normal state of the cell (G0 or G1) in which there are 2 copies of each chromosome. In this diagram, the black copy is derived from the mother and the red copy from the father. b The cell after DNA duplication (ie, during G2). The cell has twice the normal DNA content. In this diagram, the chromatids with dots on the top are newly synthesized. c The cell during the metaphase portion of mitosis, in which the chromosomes are aligned in the center and attached to microtubules, which in turn are attached to the 2 centrosomes at either end of the cell. d The cell during the telophase portion of mitosis, in which the chromatids have been pulled to either pole. Note that on the left, the original chromosomes are present. On the right, there are identical copies. e After cell division, there are 2 cells with identical DNA content.

After DNA replication, the chromatids are in groups of 4—2 sister chromatids from the mother and 2 sister chromatids from the father. Eventually, 1 of each sister chromatid will be partitioned into a daughter cell, guided by microtubules f44.9. The centrosome is normally located adjacent to the nucleus and is the major microtubule organizing center of the animal cell. It duplicates just before mitosis and the 2 centrosomes migrate to opposite ends of the cytoplasm and form the 2 spindle poles. Several types of microtubules emanate from the spindle pole, chief of which is the kinetochore microtubules, which extend from the spindle pole to the kinetochore, a protein structure that attaches to the centromere of the chromosome. The complex of the spindle poles and the different types of microtubules that arise from them is called the mitotic spindle (or spindle apparatus). The mitotic spindle forms in early mitosis and in conjunction with motor proteins called kinesins and dyneins, guides the chromosomes throughout the familiar phases of prophase, metaphase, anaphase, and telophase, until a complete set of chromosomes comes to rest at opposite poles of the cell. Cell division then ensues, resulting in 2 daughter cells with normal DNA content.

DNA Transcription and Translation

In 1958, Francis Crick correctly surmised that the connection between DNA, RNA, and proteins was that RNA was made from a DNA template and then served as the template for protein synthesis. This "central dogma" of molecular biology, whereby DNA is *transcribed* to RNA, which is then *translated* to protein, has undergone appreciable modification and elaboration over the years, but it has remarkably stood the test of time.

The structure of RNA is nearly identical to that of DNA except that it is uses the sugar ribose instead of deoxyribose, it is usually (but not always) single-stranded and uses the base uracil instead of thymine. The majority of DNA is transcribed into RNA, though only a small minority of the RNA is then translated into proteins. It has long been known that in most situations, both chromosomes are transcribed, but until recently, it was thought that only 1 strand of each chromosome was transcribed. While it has recently been learned that transcription may occur on both strands of both chromosomes, it occurs on only 1 strand at a time, and for our purposes, we will assume that transcription occurs on only 1 strand of each chromosome. The nomenclature of transcription is relative to the RNA and can be confusing. The strand of DNA that is transcribed may be called the template, complementary, or antisense strand. The strand that is not transcribed is usually called the sense strand but paradoxically may be called the coding strand. To avoid confusing terminology, I recommend the simple terms "transcribed strands" and "untranscribed strands."

Transcription Requires 1 of Several Forms of RNA Polymerase, a Promoter Site on the DNA, and a Number of Transcription Factors

Initiation of transcription is the major control point in protein synthesis. Transcription was initially studied in prokaryotes, where it was learned that unlike DNA replication, transcription requires a separate region on the DNA called a promoter, which is usually upstream (ie, toward the 5' end) from the actual gene to be transcribed. Eukaryotes also use

ISBN 978-089189-5886

promoters, but every aspect of transcription in eukaryotes is much more complicated than in prokaryotes.

There are 3 major RNA polymerases in eukaryotes. RNA polymerases I and III are primarily involved in the transcription of genes for ribosomal and transfer RNA, respectively, while RNA polymerase II is the primary enzyme in transcription that will ultimately result in translation into proteins. Although only 1 strand of the DNA can be transcribed at any one time, the RNA polymerase must recognize a double-stranded promoter, and it must work in conjunction with protein transcription factors (TFs). Prokaryotes may have both promoters and TFs [PMID20491932], but these are more common and more complex in eukaryotes. This discussion on promoters and TFs is restricted to eukaryotes.

Transcription often begins when RNA polymerase binds to a specific region of DNA called a promoter (although for reasons not understood, many genes apparently do not have promoters; the transcription trigger in these cases is not known). The most common promoter sequence in eukaryotes is called the TATA box. It consists of 7 or 8 base pairs, often TATAAAAA, on 1 strand of the DNA, but 1 or 2 of bases 5 through 8 may be T. The TATA box is generally located about 25 base pairs upstream (often written –25 since it is before the start site).

Many promoters contain essential elements that are upstream of the TATA box, and frequently, eukaryotes have a second promoter upstream called a CAAT box (usually GGCCAATCT), which binds a number of regulatory proteins. Occasionally, even a third promoter, called a GC box (usually consisting of the sequence GGGCGG), is found in eukaryote genes. The GC box is a binding site for a TF called SP1. More complex promoters, the use of alternate promoters, or other means of initiating and regulating transcription are thought to be one mechanism for the phenotypic complexity of humans, whose genome contains little more DNA and only a few more genes than that of a mouse. The use of alternative promoters may also result in greater isoforms, tissue-specific forms of individual proteins. Interestingly, these promoter sequences are not uniformly essential to the initiation of transcription eukaryotes and many genes do not have any known promoter. In these cases, unknown factors, perhaps including the conformation of DNA or the activity of histones, may initiate transcription.

Because promoters are sequences of DNA that modulate transcription only on the chromosome upon which they reside, they are said to be cis-acting. In contrast, TFs are proteins that can move or be transported to other chromosomes, and are said to be trans-acting. TFs generally have 2 domains (a protein domain is a portion of the protein molecule that has its own 3-dimensional structure and a specific function), so they may bind to other TFs, to DNA, or to RNA polymerase. If they bind to DNA, it is often to the promoter. General TFs work with many types of promoters, while some TFs may only regulate only a few or even a single gene. The TFs discussed here are general factors, operative in all eukaryotic cells, but there are also tissue-specific TFs that can modify transcription in individual tissues.

The promoter is the actual binding site for RNA polymerase II, but the polymerase cannot bind to the promoter until a complex of TFs has first done so. In a simple situation,

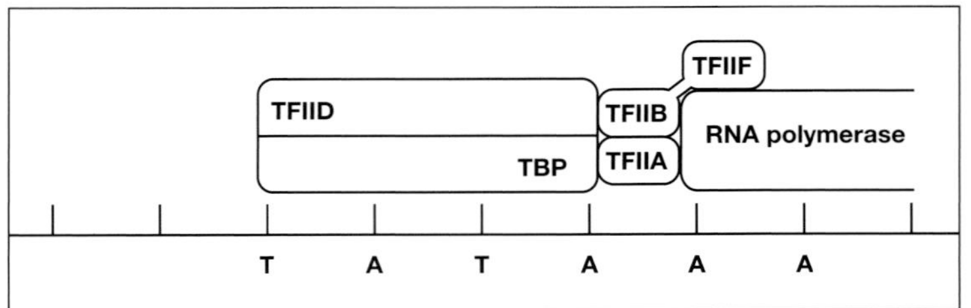

f44.10 The initiation of transcription. The TATA box binding protein (TBP), which is part of transcription factor IID, binds TFIIA and TFIIB. The latter transcription factor binds TFIIF, which binds RNA polymerase and allows it to bind to the promoter's site, initiating transcription.

the first step in DNA transcription is the recruitment of TFs to the promoter. This is done by a group of proteins called transcriptional activator proteins, which bind to the DNA, usually substantially upstream from the promoter. The next step in transcription is the sequential recruitment of TFs. The most important general TF is TFII, of which there are numerous components, some of which will begin transcription by creating the transcription-initiation complex.

The transcription-initiation complex begins with the binding of a portion of TF IID (TFIID) binds to the TATA site in the promoter. This portion of TFIID is called the TATA box binding protein (TBP). The binding of TBP to the TATA site changes the conformation of the DNA, permitting TF IIB (TFIIB) to bind to the complex of TBP and promoter DNA [PMID10884914]. The binding of TF IIB (TFIIB) and TBP to the promoter is stabilized by TF IIA. TFIIA and TFIIB bind to the TBP rather than to the actual DNA itself. This is sometimes called the DAB complex because the D, A, and B portions of TFII are bound to TATA). TF IIF then binds to TFIIB and mediates the binding of RNA polymerase to the DAB complex **f44.10** [PMID8621472].

TF IIE is then recruited. It serves as the anchoring protein for TF IIH. Preinitiation is completed when TF IIH binds to the complex. TF IIH is a helicase that unwinds the DNA helix and also activates RNA polymerase by phosphorylating it.

Additionally complicating the picture is that most eukaryotic genes contain areas of DNA called enhancers. Like promoters, enhancers are segments of DNA and are cis-acting and facilitate transcription by binding TFs. However, unlike promoters, enhancers may occur virtually anywhere, upstream from the promoter, far away from the gene in question, or even inside of it. Some TFs, called enhancer-binding proteins, bind to enhancers and cause conformational changes in the DNA. Yet another level of regulation is elongation factors, proteins that keep the RNA polymerase sufficiently close to the DNA until the transcription is completed.

Finally, environmental factors play a role in the transcription of many genes. An operon is a set of genes described in prokaryotes that are under the same control mechanisms. Well characterized operons include the lac (lactose) operon and the tryptophan repressor operon, which are sensitive to levels of lactose and tryptophan, respectively. Molecules from the environment can increase transcription by binding to and neutralizing repressor proteins, or they can decrease transcription by attaching to an activator so that it can no longer bind to DNA.

Gene expression is subject to 2 broad levels of control—transcriptional silencing and posttranscriptional silencing [PMID20569216], each of which has many facets and is incompletely

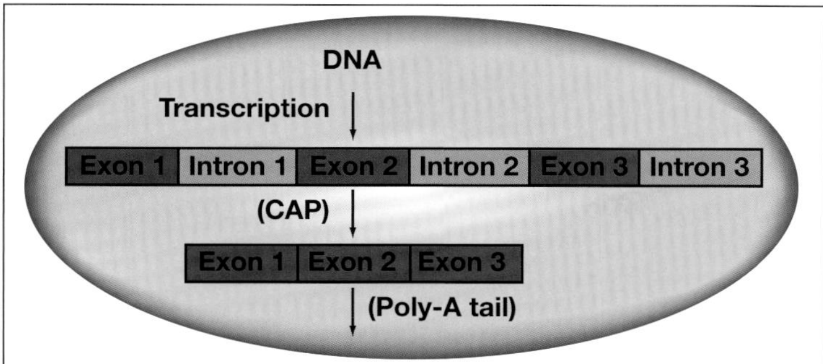

f44.11 RNA processing. After transcription of DNA, the primary RNA is in the nucleus (pink oval) and consists of areas that will eventually be translated (exons) and areas that will be sliced out (introns). After the addition of the cap, introns are removed and a poly-A tail is added, after which the mature RNA moves out of the nucleus into the cytoplasm and attaches to ribosomes.

understood, reflecting our general ignorance of the regulation of expression of DNA. We will consider posttranscriptional silencing momentarily. Transcriptional silencing of a gene in eukaryotes may involve negatively acting TFs that block the TATA box or the Inr region, fold DNA into an unfavorable conformation, or compete with positively acting factors. Silencers are proteins that dampen transcription by binding to TFs. A common situation is that positively acting factors are dimers, and inhibition is achieved when a monomeric unit of this dimer binds to a negative factor rather than to another monomeric positive factor.

Another means of transcriptional silencing of a gene involves antisense RNA, sequences of noncoding RNA that are complementary to the portion that is transcribed. Usually, there is an inverse relationship between the antisense RNA and the transcribed RNA. An increase in the transcription of the antisense RNA results in the recruitment of chromatin-modifying proteins to the promoter of the gene to be regulated, reducing its transcription [PMID20707673].

In bacteria, many related genes might be transcribed together in 1 long RNA molecule from 1 promoter. There are then multiple initiation sites for translation on the messenger RNA (mRNA) molecule. However, eukaryotic transcription and translation generally take place 1 gene at a time. Also, in prokaryotes, the RNA is often translated as it is being transcribed, whereas in eukaryotes, these processes are separated in both space and time.

Eukaryotic RNA Undergoes Modifications after Transcription, the Most Important of Which Is the Splicing of Introns

Another major difference between prokaryotic and eukaryotic transcription is that eukaryotic RNA undergoes several modifications after transcription. The initial messenger RNA molecule in eukaryotes is called primary RNA (it has a number of other names, including heterogeneous RNA, immature RNA, pre-RNA, or heteronuclear RNA). Primary RNA undergoes 3 major posttranscriptional modifications that result in mature messenger RNA, which is then transported to the cytoplasm for translation. The first of these posttranscriptional modifications is the addition of a 7-methyl guanosine residue at the 5' end. This is called a cap and assists in attachment of the messenger RNA to the ribosome.

Then, in a remarkable process called RNA splicing, some RNA is spliced out from the primary mRNA in eukaryotes before translation. The segments that are removed are called introns (short for intervening segment). Those that remain and are generally translated are called exons f44.11. Introns are rare (but not nonexistent) in prokaryotes.

There are several classes of introns, depending on the precise mechanism of their removal. The major class of introns in eukaryotes is spliceosomal introns, which are spliced out by special structures called spliceosomes, which consists of both protein and RNA. Spliceosomes are ribozymes, complexes of RNA and proteins that have enzymatic activity. The spliceosome consists of 5 types of small nuclear RNAs (snRNAs), called U1, U2, U4, U5, and U6. These are each complexed to proteins, forming small nuclear ribonucleoproteins (snRNPs).

The 5' end of U1 has a sequence UACUUAC that binds to GUAAGUA at the 5' end of the intron, a region called the splice donor. U2 binds the 3' end of the intron by a similar mechanism. Most introns have a GU dinucleotide at the 5' end (binding U1) and an AG at the 3' end (binding U2). After U1 and U2 bind to the intron, the other snRNAs bring them together, allowing excision of the intron through a lariat mechanism. In addition to their role in spliceosomes, snRNAs are involved in maintenance of telomeres and regulation of TFs.

While the spliceosome is a eukaryotic organelle and spliceosomal introns are found only in eukaryotes, self-splicing introns, of which there are 3 types, are ribozymes that do not require a spliceosome and may be found in bacteria and archaea as well as in some eukaryotic cells [PMID19443210, PMID12588294].

There may also be alternative splicing of introns in the primary RNA transcript. This can lead to different genes from the same sequence of DNA and is thought to be a major cause of the eukaryotic complexity and of human complexity relative to other eukaryotes.

In some cases, introns may occasionally be retained. While retained introns often result in poor transport of the primary RNA into the cytoplasm, preventing its translation, some of these mRNAs are functional and likely contribute to genetic diversity. Likewise, exons may rarely be discarded (exon skipping), which can also cause greater phenotypic complexity provided that a skipped exon is not essential and that its loss does not result in a frameshift mutation (ie, that the number of nucleotides skipped over is a multiple of 3).

There is also a theory that different proteins can be obtained from different combinations of exons in a process called exon shuffling, whereby exons are rearranged within a gene or even transferred between genes. The evidence for exon shuffling derives from the observation that some unrelated proteins share domains, suggesting that some exons have been swapped. For example, there are appreciable similarities in some regions of fibronectin, tissue plasminogen activator, and epidermal growth factor, all proteins from different families, with unrelated functions.

The final posttranscriptional modification of primary RNA is the addition of a poly-A tail, composed of about 200 adenine bases, at the 3' end. Like the 5' cap, the 3' poly-A tail is not translated. In addition, the regions immediately interior to the cap and the tail are untranslated. The poly-A tail is necessary for efficient translation and functions with the cap (at the other end of the mRNA molecule) to indicate an intact mRNA molecule.

The understanding of these differences between eukaryotes and prokaryotes has clarified that the fundamental divide in nature is not between plant and animal cells, or between the cells of "higher" and "lower" animals, but rather between eukaryotes and prokaryotes. In every way, we are far more like oak trees or squid or insects than we, or any of those species, are like bacteria.

Only a Minority of mRNA Is Ever Translated into Protein

In eukaryotes, the mature mRNA leaves the nucleus through the nuclear pore complex, which recognizes and passes only completed mRNA molecules, and the mature mRNA enters the cytoplasm. But not all of this mature mRNA will be translated into proteins. Many mRNA molecules instead function to regulate further transcription. Some mRNA will be subjected to posttranscriptional silencing, the second major form of transcription regulation, of which there are several forms, including the remarkable phenomenon called RNA interference (RNAi).

In RNAi, dsRNA is cleaved by an enzyme called dicer, resulting in short dsRNA fragments, with overhanging ends, called short interfering RNA (siRNA). siRNA are then separated into single-stranded fragments. One of these fragments is degraded, but the other, called the guide strand, is incorporated into a group of proteins, resulting in a riboprotein called RNA-induced silencing complex (RISC). The guide strand activates RNase in RISC. RISC captures any native single-stranded messenger RNA molecule in the cytoplasm whose sequence is complementary to the guide strand. If the captured RNA perfectly matches the sequences of the guide strand, it is degraded by an enzyme called splicer. If the match is good, but not perfect, the captured RNA may not be degraded, but its translation will be stopped. In either case, the result of RNAi is that the translation of certain single-stranded mRNA sequences is prevented.

In research, RNAi is often used to inactivate a gene to test its function or because its product is unwanted (but this technique is largely limited to cultured cells; to assess the function of a gene in multiple cell types or in an organism as a whole, another technique, called gene knockout, is used).

In nature, the dsRNA molecules that initiate RNA interference are often of viral origin (dsRNA is more common in viruses than in eukaryotes), and the process is a form of innate immunity. However, the primary natural function of RNAi seems to be in posttranscriptional gene silencing and in the regulation of gene expression. One pathway by which RNAi regulates gene expression is via microRNAs (miRNAs). miRNAs are short single-stranded fragments of RNA that are generated in the nucleus, then exported to the cytoplasm, where they are processed into a double-stranded form by the enzyme dicer (the same enzyme that processes siRNA and double-stranded viral RNA). As is the case for siRNA, the strands of miRNA are separated, one strand is degraded, and the other becomes part of RISC, after which RNAi acts on endogenous RNA whose sequence is complementary or partially complementary to the preserved strand of miRNA, resulting in its degradation or translational inhibition. The net result is that sequences of RNA that match those in miRNA are degraded or inhibited. RNAi is a form of epigenetic regulation of the genome (ie, a form of regulation of DNA expression that does not depend on the actual sequence of DNA, discussed in Chapter 47).

More than 1,000 human miRNAs have been identified, and it is thought that they are involved in regulating more than half of all human genes [PMID22642897]. miRNAs appear to play a role in modulating development [PMID14657504] and may function either as tumor suppressors [PMID20610624] or as oncogenes [PMID16024602]. miRNAs from different cells show considerable differences and are less conserved than other forms of RNA. In theory, this property makes miRNA a good candidate for specific cell identification, and indeed, a number of malignant tumors appear to have characteristic expression profiles of miRNA [PMID17060945] that can be detected by microarray studies (microarrays are discussed in Chapter 45). At this writing, miRNA studies are a promising means of identifying metastatic tumors of unknown primary site in cases where traditional histology and immunohistochemistry have failed [PMID17892365]. A reverse transcriptase-polymerase chain reaction (PCR) that targets 48 miRNAs, designed to identify up to 25 different possible primary sites, is available. miRNAs may be helpful in distinguishing specific types of neoplasms that resemble each other on H&E, such as different subtypes of renal tumors [PMID20595629] or the epithelioid type of malignant mesothelioma from pulmonary adenocarcinoma [PMID20864637]. A specific miRNA, miRNA-21, is associated with breast carcinoma, and serum levels of this miRNA show potential for both detection and staging [PMID21036945]. In addition, miRNA-499 has been reported to be cardiac-specific and therefore may be of benefit in the early diagnosis of myocardial infarct [PMID20395621]. miRNA can be studied in formalin-fixed, paraffin-embedded tissue [PMID18832457].

Both transcriptional and posttranscriptional regulation of gene expression offers theoretical therapeutic, as well as diagnostic, opportunities. Antisense drugs are oligonucleotides that are complementary to the mRNA made by tumors. By binding to this mRNA, antisense drugs make it double-stranded and subject to RNAi. An example of an antisense drug is Oblimersen (Genasense), which is complementary to the sequence of mRNA that codes for the product of the *BCL-2* gene (the bcl-2 protein inhibits apoptosis, thereby facilitating tumor growth). Oblimersen has been used in some cases of lymphoma [PMID21105187] and especially in chronic lymphoid leukemia [PMID20008230].

While a small portion of the RNA that is transcribed is conveyed to the ribosome for translation, most is sent elsewhere, often as combinations of protein and RNA called riboproteins (if these have enzymatic activity, the complex is called a ribozyme). "RNA trafficking" is the term used to describe the transport of RNA to different intracellular locations.

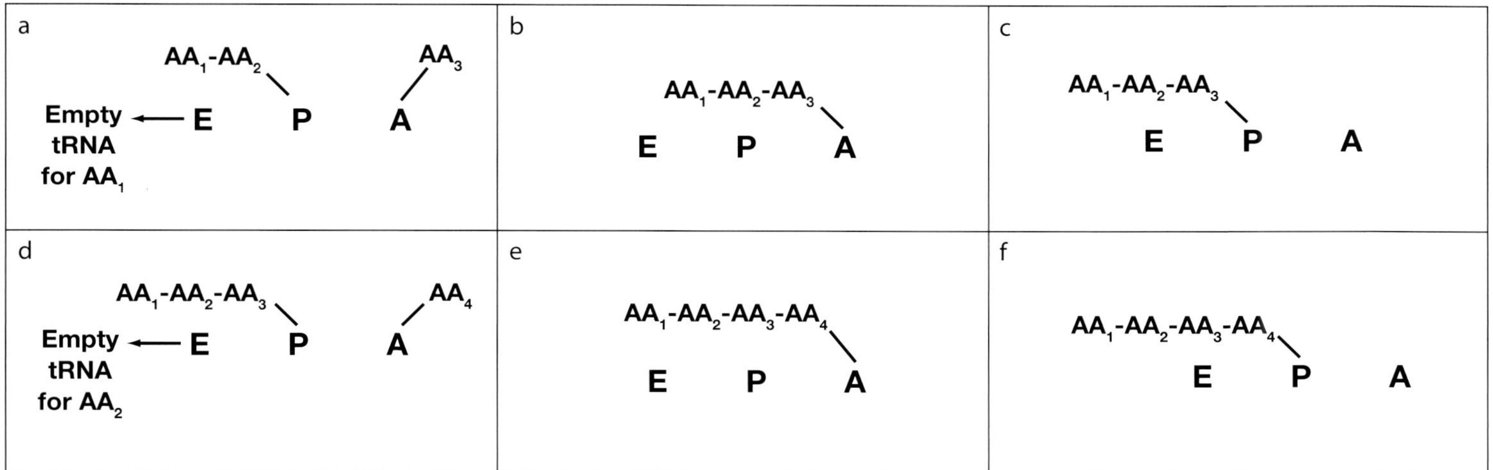

f44.12 **a** Translation. This diagram depicts the process of translation shortly after its initiation. 2 amino acids are attached to the P site of the ribosomes. A third amino acid arrives at the A site of the ribosome, at which time the transfer RNA that delivered the first amino acid, now empty, leaves the ribosome. **b** A peptide bond forms between the 2 amino acids on the P site and the third amino acid that has recently arrived on the A site. **c** The polypeptide, consisting of 3 amino acids, is transferred from the A site to the P site. **d** A fourth amino acid arrives at the A site, at which time the tRNA that brought the second amino acid, now empty, exits the ribosome. **e** A peptide bond forms between the 3 amino acids at the P site and the newly arrived amino acid at the A site. **f** The polypeptide, now consisting of 4 amino acids, is transferred to the P site so that a fifth amino acid can arrive at the A site.

Translation Involves Relative Motion between the Nascent Polypeptide Chain and 3 Critical Sites on the Ribosome

Translation, like replication and transcription, proceeds in a 5' to 3' direction. Amino acids are added according to a sequence of 3 base pairs called a codon. There are 64 triplet combinations of base pairs (4^3). The 3-base pair codons refer to base pairs in RNA, not DNA. Indeed, many of the bases in the genetic code for amino acids are uracil, which is not found in DNA. With the rise of genomics, however, there is some movement toward using 3 base codons based on DNA. There are 61 codons for the 20 amino acids, reflecting the redundancy whereby many amino acids have >1 codon. In addition, there are 3 stop codons (UAG, UGA, and UAA) and 1 start codon (AUG) to initiate translation. This totals 65 because the initiation codon also codes for the amino acid methionine. A stop codon does not necessarily follow every start codon. A sequence of DNA without a stop codon is called an open reading frame.

For each amino acid, there is a specific enzyme that recognizes the 3-base codon on the mRNA and binds that amino acid to a tRNA molecule for transport to the ribosome. Upon arrival at the ribosome, there is base pairing between the 3-base codon on the tRNA and the corresponding 3 base pairs on the mRNA.

Messenger RNA that will be translated attaches to the smaller 40S ribosomal subunit (the term "S" denotes size and is derived from the sedimentation characteristics after ultracentrifugation). Proteins called initiation factors facilitate this union and bring about the translation initiation complex. Translation starts when the 40S subunit binds to the mRNA and to an initiator transfer RNA that responds to the start codon AUG on the mRNA and attaches a methionine to the translation initiation complex. The first amino acid in all proteins is initially methionine, but this is often removed later, an example of posttranslational modification. After the start codon is found, the 60S ribosomal subunit is added to make the complete 80S ribosome.

To visualize translation, imagine 3 sites on the mRNA-ribosome complex, called, from left to right, E, P, and A. Initiation of translation begins when the start codon of the messenger RNA and the initiator tRNA, carrying a methionine amino acid, bind to the middle of these sites on the ribosome, the P site. This first amino acid is the only 1 that will directly attach to the P site of the ribosome. The mRNA at the next codon position then binds to the A site of the ribosome and receives another transfer (tRNA) molecule, carrying the second amino acid. The ribosome then attaches the 2 amino acids via a peptide bond, forming a dipeptide that is attached to the ribosome at the A site, freeing the first amino acid from its attachment to the P site. This dipeptide is transferred to the P site, freeing up the A site. At this time, the first tRNA is transferred from the P site to the E site, from which it will be released from the ribosome. A new tRNA binds to the now vacant A site. A peptide bond then forms again between this new amino acid and the peptide that is attached to the P site. This increases the length of the peptide by 1 amino acid and changes its site of attachment to the ribosome from the P site to the A site. The peptide is then transferred to the P site, again freeing up the A site. New amino acids arrive at the A site and the ensuing peptide bond releases the attachment of the peptide chain from the P site. Transfer to the P site then frees up the A site for the next amino acid. It is useful to think of the letters A, P, and E as standing for ***a***rrival of amino acid (AA), ***p***eptide chain, and final ***e***xit of tRNA, respectively f44.12.

There are no corresponding transfer RNA molecules for the 3 stop codons. When one of those stop codons comes into the A position, an enzyme called a release factor breaks off the peptide chain from the tRNA molecule that is attached to the P site.

We have seen that >1 codon can code for the same amino acid (the average is 3 codons per amino acid). Usually, the variation occurs in the third position. For example, both AGU and AGC code for serine, and if the first 2 bases are AU, then *any* third base will result in the amino acid isoleucine. This tendency for the redundancy of the genetic code to be manifest in the third base pair is called the wobble hypothesis. Because of the redundancy of the genetic code, a mutation in

ISBN 978-089189-5886

a single base pair may well be synonymous (ie, coding for the same amino acid), especially if the erroneous base pair is the third in the codon. In theory, all synonymous mutations are clinically silent, but a number of diseases are associated with supposedly silent mutations for unknown reasons.

The genetic code is nearly universal, but not completely. The primary example of lack of complete universality is slight differences between eukaryotes and prokaryotes. Also, the DNA in mitochondria and chloroplasts employ a genetic code that slightly differs from nuclear DNA and more closely resemble that used by prokaryotes. In fact, the great similarity between the DNA of free living bacteria and that of mitochondria or chloroplasts has made it a virtual certainty that these organelles are "captured" bacteria or archaea, an hypothesis put forth by Lynn Margulis [Margulis ISBN978-0300013535]. Although there is considerable redundancy in the genetic code, there is also codon bias for each species, especially for proteins that are highly expressed.

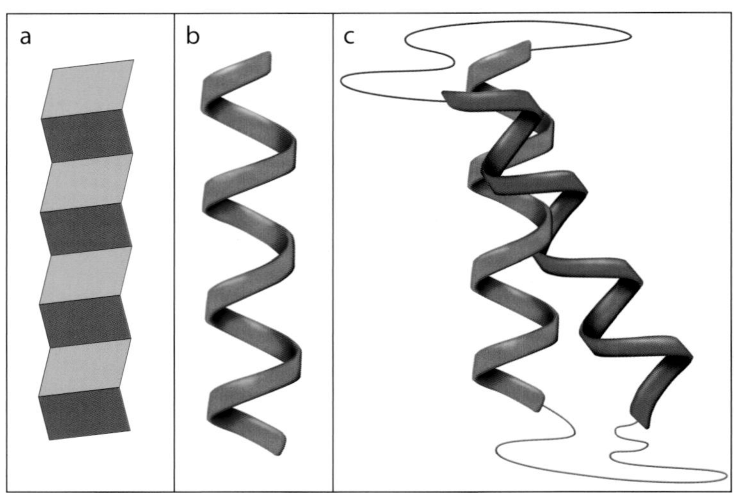

f44.13 **a** The β pleated sheet form of a polypeptide, one of the major forms of secondary structure
b The α helix form of a peptide, the other major form of secondary structure
c A simplified tertiary structure of polypeptide in which 2 helices are present, one of which folds over onto the other

Many Properties of Proteins Come from Posttranslational Modification

Posttranslational modifications provide critical properties such as assumption of the full 3-dimensional structure, attainment of enzymatic activity, and routing to the correct intracellular location with attachment to the correct intracellular structure. Posttranslational modifications are achieved by the action of specific enzymes and include cleavage of a precursor protein, phosphorylation, methylation, acetylation, carboxylation, and glycosylation. Glycoproteins, also called complex carbohydrates, are proteins to which oligosaccharides are covalently bonded to the side chains of some of the protein's amino acids. Glycosylation is largely restricted to those proteins that are to become part of the plasma membrane or are to be exported. By contrast, proteoglycans are proteins with repeating units of disaccharides, usually glucosamine or galactosamine. The repeating disaccharide units are called glycosaminoglycans (GAGs). Proteoglycans are usually destined for the extracellular matrix.

Once a protein has been completely synthesized and posttranslational modifications are made, it acquires its final 3-dimensional structure. Primary protein structure refers to the amino acid sequence, which determines a fundamental structure. Secondary structure refers to the basic structure of the protein's backbone and is determined by local interactions between different parts of the polypeptide chain. The 2 major secondary structures are the α helix and the β pleated sheet. In the α helix, there is hydrogen bonding between the carbonyl group of 1 amino acid and the amino nitrogen of an amino acid that is 4 amino acids away, resulting in a curved backbone. In a β pleated sheet, there is hydrogen bonding between adjacent polypeptide chains, resulting in a approximately planar surface in which side chains alternately point up and down. Tertiary structure refers to the overall 3-dimensional shape of one chain, not just the shape of the backbone, and is determined by interactions over a long distance **f44.13**. Quaternary structure refers to the structure of complex proteins that have >1 polypeptide chain.

Proteins that are not in the proper conformation may be nonfunctional, even if their amino acid sequence is correct. Chaperones are proteins that assist other proteins in attaining their proper folding and 3-dimensional conformation. The heat shock proteins (HSPs) are a major group of chaperones. Some HSPs are present at the time of translation and help newly-incorporated amino acids assimilate into the new protein in a proper 3-dimensional conformation. Other HSPs restore the proper 3-dimensional conformation to existing proteins that have lost it. Still other HSP guide the assembly of polypeptide chains into larger structures such as receptors. Chaperones—especially HSPs—are a potential target of pharmacologic therapy in some diseases. For example, the steroid receptor is bound to heat shock protein 90 (HSP90). Steroids, either endogenous or exogenous, bind to the steroid receptor and displace HSP90, after which the steroid/receptor complex crosses the nuclear membrane. After entering the nucleus, it is the receptor, not the actual steroid itself, that modulates transcription, though continued binding of the receptor to steroid is necessary.

Like RNA, the Fully Developed Proteins Must Be Transported to the Correct Intracellular Location

Routing of the protein to the correct intracellular location is achieved by localization signals, which are usually short amino acid sequences within the protein. These sequences are often removed once the protein has reached the desired destination, a final posttranslational modification. Abnormal proteins may not only have defective function, but also may not be properly routed within the cell.

All protein synthesis begins on free ribosomes in the cytoplasm, and many are completed in that location, after which they are routed to the correct portion of the cell by short amino acid sequences. However, the synthesis of proteins that are destined for the endoplasmic reticulum (ER) stops after 15-25 amino acids, after which a signal recognition particle attaches to the polypeptide chain. The signal recognition particle directs the entire ribosome to the ER, where it attaches to the external surface. The signal recognition

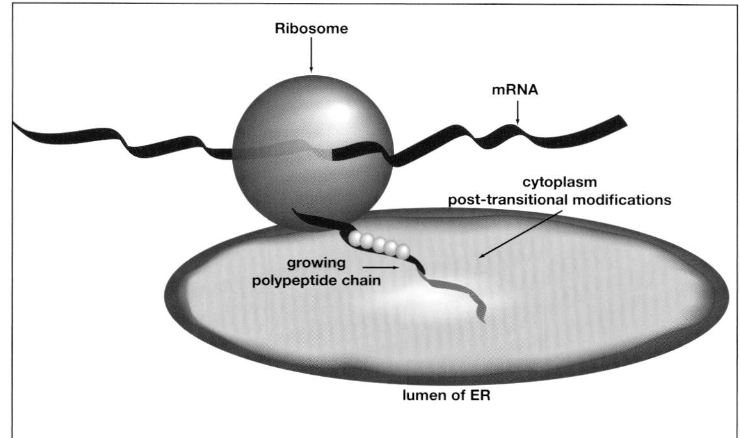

f44.14 Proteins that are synthesized in the endoplasmic reticulum (ER) reach that organelle because the entire ribosome attaches to the ER. As the polypeptide chain grows, it projects into the lumen of the ER, where it will undergo extensive posttranslational modifications.

particle is then released and the nascent polypeptide chain translocates through the membrane of the ER into its lumen. The growing polypeptide chain penetrates further into the lumen of the ER as it is synthesized, while the ribosome remains on the exterior of the ER f44.14.

The completed protein in the lumen of the endoplasmic reticulum often undergoes appreciable posttranslational modification before leaving the endoplasmic reticulum. In particular, the ER is also the place where the cell's lipids are synthesized and proteins and lipids made in the ER leave that organelle in membrane-coated vesicles and are transported to the Golgi apparatus, where they may be further modified and then either transported out of the cell or to a final destination within it. The ribosome remains bound to the ER throughout this process, transforming it from "smooth" ER to "rough" ER (these names are derived from early electron microscopy of the ER, where some ER appeared smooth and other appeared granular).

We have now followed a protein from DNA replication, through transcription, translation, posttranslational modification, assembly into a multimeric structure with a correct 3-dimensional conformation and properly interacting subunits, and proper intracellular localization. Because this complete sequence is necessary for proper protein function, a defect in any one of these steps can lead to phenotypic abnormality. The same clinical phenotype can result from mutations in different genes at different loci affecting different stages in the maturation and localization of a protein. This is called locus heterogeneity. By contrast, the term "polymorphism" refers to a difference in sequence at a specific locus in the DNA.

The total of all mRNA is called the transcriptome, and its study is referred to as transcriptomics. The collection of all of the proteins that are translated is called the proteome (not to be confused with the proteasome, an organelle involved in the destruction of senescent protein molecules), and the study of the full range of protein translation, structure, and interaction is called proteomics. With the sequencing of the human genome accomplished, the next frontiers are an understanding of the regulation of DNA expression, transcriptomics, proteomics, and the effect of individual genetic variations that govern the response to drugs (pharmacogenetics). Pharmacogenetics is discussed in Chapter 46. Proteomics and the personalized medicine that will emerge from our new understanding are discussed in Chapter 47.

In describing protein abnormalities, the expected (normal) amino acid precedes the position, and the actual amino acid that is present (the abnormal one) follows the number. For example, hemoglobin S (which causes sickle cell anemia if present in the homozygous state) is caused by Glu6Val, a substitution of valine for the normal glutamic acid at amino acid position 6 in the β globin chain. Amino acids also have single-letter abbreviations, so this can also be denoted as E6V (E denotes glutamic acid because "G" is used for glycine). Sometimes, a small "p" precedes the designation to indicate that a protein is being described, not nucleic acid. pR117H indicates that the normal arginine at amino acid position 117 has been replaced by histidine. Because there are no bases that are denoted by R or H, the preceding "p" is not necessary but may facilitate reading. F is the single-letter abbreviation for phenylalanine, and V617F is a substitution of phenylalanine for valine, seen in most polycythemia vera patients. Again, there are no bases that are abbreviated by a V or an F, so it is clear that a protein molecule is being discussed, but to ensure that there is no confusion as to whether a protein or nucleic acid abnormality is being described, this may be designated as pV617F. X denotes a stop codon and a Δ indicates a deletion, so G542X is a substitution of a stop codon for glycine at amino acid 542, resulting in a truncated protein, and ΔF508 is a deletion of the amino acid phenylalanine at position 508, seen in many cases of cystic fibrosis (see Chapter 45).

In describing DNA abnormalities, a similar nomenclature may be used, with the expected base, followed by the number, then the actual base (eg, A1000G indicates that a guanine has replaced the normal adenine at nucleotide position 1000). However, in nucleic acids, more often than not, the nucleotide position comes first, after which the expected base is given, followed by a ">," then the inappropriate substitution. For example, the replacement of adenine by guanine at nucleotide position 1000 is written as 1000A>G (a "→" sign may be used instead of an arrow, as in 1000A→G). For both proteins and DNA, the expected (normal) amino acid or base comes before the actual (abnormal) amino acid or base; the difference is in the placement of the number. In describing abnormalities in the DNA or RNA, more specific information is occasionally conveyed by preceding the designation with a "g." for genomic DNA, a "c." for complementary DNA, an "r." for RNA [PMID9450896, PMID18428344]. For example, g.1000A>G clarifies that the substitution is in genomic DNA. c.1444g>a is an adenine for guanine substitution in the cDNA, and r.100u>c is a substitution of cytosine for uracil at base position 100 in an RNA molecule (in describing genomic DNA, capital letters are used for the nucleotides, while lowercase letters are usually used in descriptions of cDNA and always in describing RNA). A nucleotide change preceded by an "m" denotes mitochondrial DNA. Additional nomenclature includes "del" and "ins" for deletions and insertion, respectively. For example, g.100_149del refers to a 50 base pair deletion in genomic DNA, beginning with the 100th nucleotide, while g.100_101insT indicates that a thymine has been inserted after nucleotide 100 in genomic DNA.

Mutations in introns may be symptomatic if they cause an exon to be deleted from the transcript. There are 3 ways to indicate a point mutation in an intron. In the first method, "IVS" (for intervening segment) is used. For example, IVS3+2T>A refers to the substitution of an adenine for a thymine at the second base of intron 3 of a gene. Sometimes a "+" sign indicates a splice donor site and a "–" sign indicates a splice acceptor site. Intronic mutations can also be denoted by reference to the nearest exon nucleotide in the complementary DNA sequence (cDNA does not contain intronic DNA). For example, one might write c.2000+2T>A for the same mutation, indicating that the full genomic sequence is not known or not indicated, but that it is known that the intronic mutation occurs at the second base after the 2000th coding nucleotide at the end of the adjacent exon. In either of these nomenclatures, the use of a "+" or a "–" sign and a number preceding the usual ">" sign is likely to denote an intronic mutation. A third method of denoting intronic mutations, if the full genomic sequence is known, is simply to indicate the nucleotide number of the entire, intact, genomic sequence. In this nomenclature, g.5000T>A means that the complete genomic sequence is indicated and the mutation is in the 5000th nucleotide of that sequence [PMID17251329].

In general, a single working copy of a gene product is sufficient for clinically normal function. While one non-functioning allele may have consequences for offspring if that allele is incorporated into a gamete, it is usually silent in an individual unless it is the X chromosome in males, and that individual has a normal phenotype. The exception to this is called haploinsufficiency, whereby 50% of a gene product is not sufficient for normal function. Conditions characterized by haploinsufficiency are, in effect, autosomal dominant because both copies of the gene must work to avoid manifestations.

The naming of genes is a problematic area because genes were often given whimsical names by their discoverers, and the same gene often had >1 name. The website http://www.genenames.org clarifies existing nomenclature, and policies have been put in place to regulate the naming of new genes.

So What Is a Gene?

Now that we have studied transcription and translation and seen that only a small minority of DNA actually experiences this pathway, we come to a central question in molecular biology today: What is a gene? Since <2% of DNA is eventually translated into protein, the original definition of a gene as a unit of DNA that codes for a polypeptide appears incomplete at best. Many experienced people have submitted new candidate definitions of a gene, but to my mind, the defining feature of a gene is that it is a subset of the genome that performs a specific function. Coding for a polypeptide is an example of a specific function, and until we know more about the genome, this function remains the best known and the most important in medicine, despite the fact that only a small amount of DNA is engaged in this capacity. Other functions include coding for ribosomal or transfer RNA, or coding for RNA that is regulatory. The sequence or sequences in a gene may or may not be contiguous, and any or all of the DNA in a gene may or may not be used for a similar or different function as part of a different gene.

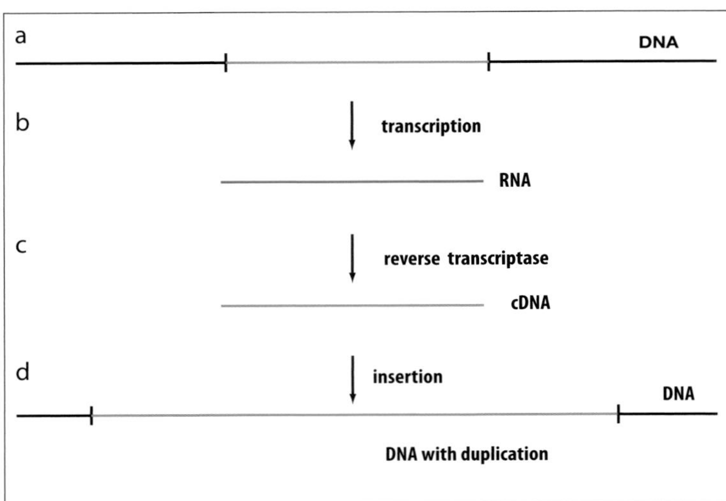

f44.15 How retrotransposons can expand the genome.
a In this sequence of DNA, the central blue area is a class 1 transposon (retrotransposon).
b After isolated transcription of the transposon, it exists as a detached RNA molecule.
c After the action of reverse transcriptase, there is a detached molecule of cDNA.
d The cDNA (retroelement) can then insert, resulting in duplication of that portion.

Mobile Genetic Elements

We are deeply indebted to Barbara McClintock for the discovery of transposons, then called "jumping genes," in 1948 [PMID15430309]. This was the entry point into the huge and fantastically important field of mobile (or transferrable) genetic elements (MGE).

There are many types of mobile genetic elements that can be transferred within a cell or between cells. Horizontal (or lateral) gene transfer has been an important driving force in the evolution of prokaryotes. Horizontal transfer and the rapid reproductive rate of prokaryotes are the 2 reasons that they evolve at a rate that is orders of magnitude greater than that of eukaryotic organisms.

Mobile genetic elements include transposons, insertion sequences (IS), genomic islands, plasmids, group II introns, and sequences of DNA that are transferred by bacteriophages. The term "mobilome" is occasionally used for the sum of all MGEs in a cell.

Transposons are genes that can move about within the genome of a single cell. There are 2 broad classes of transposons—those that use an RNA intermediate (class I transposons) and those that use a simpler "cut and paste" mechanism (class II transposons) [PMID20813032]. Class I transposons, also called retrotransposons, are the primary type in eukaryotes and work through an RNA intermediate. They can be transcribed alone, without concurrent transcription of the flanking DNA, after which reverse transcriptase (the DNA coding for which is often contained within the transposon itself) acts on the RNA, resulting in cDNA sequences called retroelements that can then insert back into the genome and furnish additional copies of the original DNA.

Because the original DNA is not removed or relocated, retrotransposition results in amplification and duplication of DNA, furnishing raw material for genetic variation. Retrotransposons result in repetitive DNA that has expanded

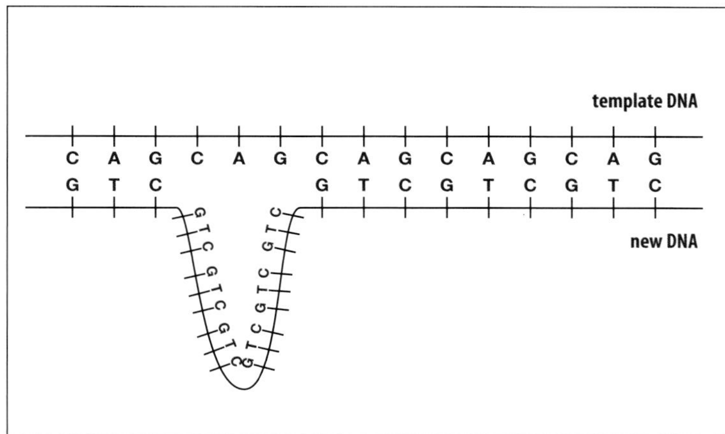

f44.16 Replication slippage. In this diagram, the sequence CAG repeats on the template DNA. If the growing DNA strand becomes dissociated from the template strand, because of the repeating sequence, it may not perfectly reanneal to the template, but rather may have an "outpouching." The result will be a newly synthesized strand of DNA that is longer than the original and contains duplications.

the eukaryotic genome f44.15. Indeed, almost 1/2 of the human genome appears to be derived from duplications of DNA, much of it from retrotransposons. Some retrotransposons result in long terminal repeats, sequences of DNA that are composed of many repeats of a smaller subunit, while other retrotransposons result in redundant sequences of DNA that are present in only 1 copy in each location in which they are found [PMID20885819]. Repetitive DNA is discussed in Chapter 45, but the important point here is that retrotransposition is one cause of pseudogenes, defective copies of functioning genes. There are almost as many pseudogenes known as there are genes. Pseudogenes have sequences that are very close to those of functional genes and can be formed in 2 ways: retrotransposition and duplication during replication [PMID21116863].

Pseudogenes formed by retrotransposition are called processed pseudogenes because they have been transcribed. Because the RNA that is reverse transcribed into DNA in retrotransposition does not include introns or promoters, a processed pseudogene lacks these areas and are not transcribed again except in rare cases where it integrates close enough to the promoter of another gene to use it, in which case it becomes a functional gene called a retrogene. Processed pseudogenes can inactivate a normal gene if they insert into or near it.

The second way in which pseudogenes can arise is from slippage during DNA replication. Replication slippage often occurs in areas of satellite DNA (ie, sequences that are repeated). During DNA replication, the 2 strands will occasionally be very slightly separated. They generally come back together perfectly and no harm is done. Rarely, in areas of satellites, the 2 strands will come back together imperfectly because the repeated sequences afford an opportunity for mistakes. If the new DNA strand bulges outward or loops back, there will be a duplication f44.16. Pseudogenes formed in this manner are called nonprocessed pseudogenes since the DNA they are derived from is not transcribed. Unlike processed pseudogenes, nonprocessed pseudogenes contain all of the introns and promoter sites of the original gene, but they are not transcribed, usually because the promoter is not functional.

Because processed pseudogenes are derived from retrotransposition, they are likely to be physically distant from their progenitor gene, while nonprocessed pseudogenes, because they are derived from adjacent satellite DNA, tend to be physically close to the ancestral gene from which they arose.

Because it is now known that DNA sequences do not have to be transcribed to have a function, pseudogenes may function in a regulatory capacity, possibly impacting how much the genes to which they are related are transcribed. In addition, pseudogenes of either type are important because they expand the genome and may serve as a source of genetic variation, leading to gene superfamilies, groups of genes with related structure and function that likely arose from slight variations on pseudogenes. Pseudogenes are important in molecular pathology testing because they may be inadvertently amplified in PCR.

In class II transposons, the DNA is simply cut from one place and reinserted in another place. This requires a transposase, which is often embedded in the transposon and which recognizes inverted repeats at each end of the transposon, but it does not require reverse transcriptase. In contrast to class I transposons, there is no duplication of DNA when class II transposons move, and therefore no expansion of the genome. Class II transposons are the primary type in bacteria, though they are also found in eukaryotes.

Some bacterial transposons are capable of conjugation, transfer between cells in a manner that is normally seen in plasmids [PMID12568331]. While transposons generally move *within* a single cell, conjugative transposons can excise themselves and form a separate, stable double-stranded circular structure. A single-stranded version of this can then be transferred to another bacterium via conjugation, after which it is reconstituted into a double-stranded DNA element that is inserted into the genome of the other organism.

Some class II transposons insert at random, while others recognize specific IS. IS are themselves mobile fragments of DNA. They are small, rarely exceeding 2.5 kilobases, are commonly found, and are widely dispersed throughout bacterial genomes. They are the smallest transposable elements in bacteria and in contrast to true transposons, IS have no accessory genes and carry only sufficient genetic information to govern their transposition and regulation, although they may also inactivate the genes into which they insert. Some consider IS to be the simplest type of transposon, while others believe they are too small and too simple to be included in the category of transposon. Because they do not convey antibiotic resistance, they are difficult to identify, and most known IS have been found by chance, based on their effects on genes they insert into.

Genomic islands (GIs) are another form of mobile genetic element. GIs share with transposons the ability to move within the genome, but the term "transposon" is usually used for elements that are transferred intracellularly, while GIs move between different bacteria (in fact, often between different bacterial species). GIs have characteristics that are different from the surrounding DNA, such as differences in G-C content or pattern of codon usage, that identify it as having originated in another species. GIs often have direct repeats on either side and are inserted into the genome by site-specific integrase enzymes. The integration sites are usually in genes for small RNA molecules such as tRNA. There are several types of GIs. Those that convey increased pathogenicity are called pathogenicity islands (PAIs). Most PAIs are on the chromosome, though they may be found on plasmids or in conjugative transposons. GIs that confer antibiotic resistance are called antibiotic resistance islands.

Conjugative plasmids can be transferred by conjugation, which is a mechanism of horizontal transfer. In conjugative plasmids, an enzyme called relaxase nicks one strand of the plasmid at the origin point for the transfer (oriT). Sometimes, the relaxase works with other enzymes in a complex called a relaxosome. After the nick, one strand is unwound from the plasmid in a rolling circle manner and transferred (this is called the T strand). After arrival into the recipient, the plasmid is reconstituted by the synthesis of a complementary strand.

Most introns in eukaryotes are removed by the spliceosome (spliceosomal introns), but a minority are self-splicing. The few introns in prokaryotes are all self-splicing and fall into 3 groups. Group II introns are MGEs because once spliced, they can undergo reverse transcription (they have their own reverse transcriptase) and reintegration into the genome. Group II introns have 6 domains which are stem-loop structures surrounding a central core. This structure brings its 5' and 3' breakpoints into proximity, and the intron excises itself through a lariat mechanism. This is very similar to the mechanism used by the spliceosome, and some believe that primary RNA splicing in eukaryotes via spliceosomes may have evolved from group II introns.

Conjugative transposons, genomic islands, conjugative plasmids, and group II introns are all mechanisms of horizontal transfer between bacteria. Other such mechanisms include transduction (involving a viral intermediary, such as a bacteriophage) and transformation (uptake of DNA from the environment by suitable environmental conditions). All forms of horizontal transfer have greatly augmented bacterial antibiotic resistance.

A Large Amount of DNA is Repetitive, and There Are Different Types of Repetitions

An unexpected characteristic of DNA is that much of it is repetitive, usually a consequence of either retrotransposition or an error in replication. These duplicated sequences are not necessarily useless, as they often furnish the material for genetic variation. In Chapter 45, we will discuss special kinds of repetitive DNA that are widely dispersed throughout the genome, and only 2 concepts are conveyed here. A tandem direct repeat, for example, GAAGAAGAA, may result in replication slippage, in which the DNA polymerase attaches to an incorrect site that is identical to, but adjacent to, the site to which it should have bound [PMID15165229]. Replication slippage is a cause of genetic variation.

An inverted repeat consists of 2 sequences on the same strand, usually with an intervening segment, that are complementary to each other and run in opposite directions towards each other. For example:

GGGAAA----------------------------TTTCCC

This results in sequences on the same strand that can bind to each other In the above case, for example, the G and the C bases may loop around and pair, and the A bases may bind with the T bases, resulting in an outpouching called a hairpin [PMID21119018]. Transfer RNA has hairpin structures. In addition, many inversions result from recombination between inverted repeats.

Core Points for Molecular Pathology I: Foundations

- Prokaryotes and eukaryotes are the 2 great categories of life.
  - All eukaryotes are more like each other than any are like prokaryotes.
- DNA consists of 2 strands, twisted into helices.
  - Each strand consists of a backbone of alternating sugar and phosphate groups, with bases projecting inward.
- Cell cycle, G1→S→G2→M→Cytokinesis, has specific regulatory checkpoints.
- DNA replication, transcription, and translation are all multistage and highly regulated processes
- Many enzymes repair damaged or mismatched DNA.
  - Deficiencies in many of these are responsible for some genetic syndromes.
- A large amount of DNA is repetitive, in large part because of mobile genetic elements.
- Transcription: requires an RNA polymerase, a promoter site on the DNA, and many transcription factors.
- After transcription, eukaryotic mRNA is modified, and introns are spliced out.
  - mRNA leaves the nucleus and is translated on 3 critical sites on a ribosome.
- Many proteins are not functional until they undergo post-translational modification.
- Once modified, proteins are transported to the correct intracellular location.
- Only a small fraction of DNA goes the route of transcription and translation (the classic "central dogma").
  - The definition of a gene has become a central question in biology.

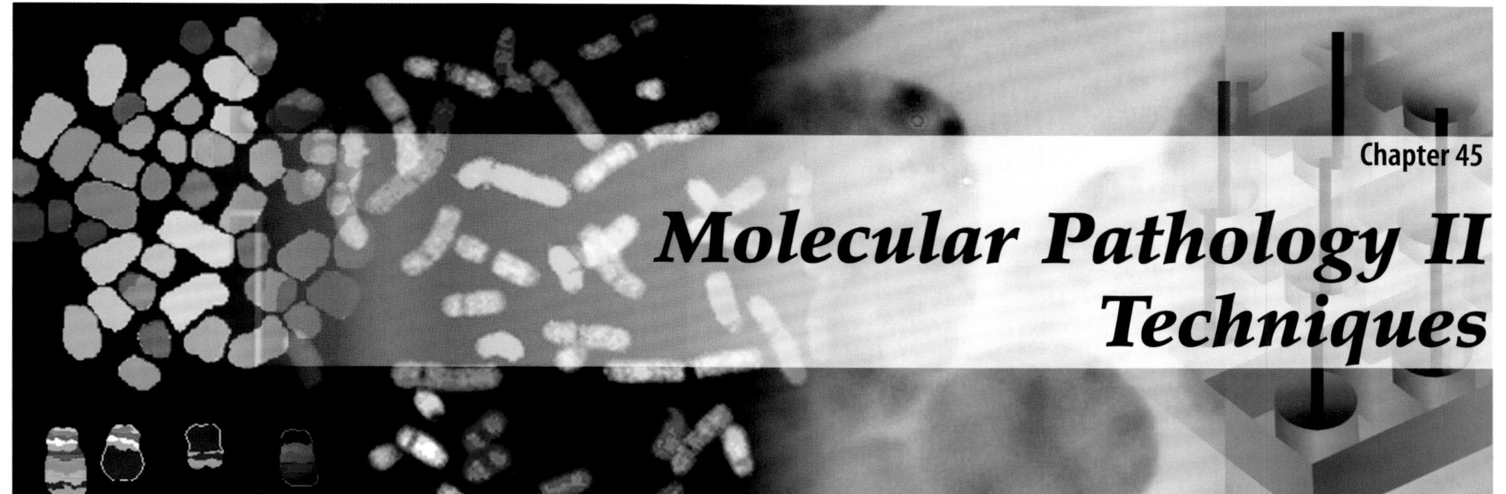

Molecular Pathology II Techniques

Now that we have examined some of the basics of molecular biology, we turn our attention to specific techniques used in diagnostic pathology. In addition to diagnosis, many molecular techniques hold promise as screening tests and in the assessment of residual disease or recurrence after treatment.

The principles of molecular testing are difficult for many people in pathology-related disciplines because they do not have a firm foundation in either molecular biology or in the techniques that are used. In Chapter 44, we addressed basic principles of molecular biology. The goal of this chapter is to understand molecular techniques and methods, based on nucleic acid analysis, which will enormously expand what we can tell patients and their caregivers. Many excellent works elaborate on the topics discussed here, but of particular merit is the text by Dale and von Schantz [ISBN978-0470017340].

Early Nucleic Acid Studies

Before the advent of nucleic acid amplification techniques, all nucleic acid studies began with extraction and purification of DNA or RNA.

Nucleic Acid Extraction and Measurement

Because many commercially available nucleic acid analyzers extract and purify the nucleic acid as part of the testing procedure, the pathologist is rarely concerned with nucleic acid purification, but should understand its principles because molecular techniques often begin with isolation of nucleic acid. Detergents are often used to solubilize membranes, after which enzymes degrade protein and inhibit nucleases. The DNA is then often purified by extraction steps, although the advent of polymerase chain reaction (PCR) and related amplification techniques make a rigorous purification of all DNA less important than previously since the sequence of interest can be amplified from less pure starting material. Many steps in the isolation process have been automated, and commercial extraction kits are available. Automated DNA extraction compares well with manual extraction in efficiency, though it is usually more expensive [PMID18556770].

Historically, after extraction, the purity, intactness, and amount of DNA was assessed. With the advent of nucleic acid amplification, these traditional verification procedures are less often employed because in most situations, the test of adequate extraction is whether or not it will generate a desired final product of sufficient quantity and purity. It is the final product, not the starting material, which is increasingly the target of verification assays, but some familiarity with these 3 assays remains important.

Purity is determined by spectrophotometry, taking advantage of the fact that nucleic acids absorb at 260 nm, while other molecules absorb at other wavelengths. In particular, the peptide bond of proteins, a leading contaminant, absorbs at 280 nm. Purity of the sample can be assessed by the absorbance at 260 nm divided by the absorbance at 280 nm [PMID18429085]. Because there is overlap in the spectrums of nucleic acids and proteins, a ratio of about 2.0 is generally accepted as an essentially "pure" sample of DNA. A ratio of 1.8 is usually considered acceptable, while a ratio <1.8 indicates a suboptimal sample that may contain a potentially problematic amount of protein [PMID19760105]. The absorbance at 230 nm is sometimes used to estimate carbohydrate contamination. Depending on the procedure used to extract DNA, other spectrophotometric measurements may be needed to determine if any chemicals that were used in the extraction process remain.

A determination of the intactness of the DNA is especially important when the source is poorly preserved tissue (ie, from a fossil or crime scene) or tissue from a paraffin block, and is often done by gel electrophoresis. Whereas proteins are usually examined by polyacrylamide electrophoresis (polyacrylamide is a type of plastic), DNA fragments longer than about 500 nucleotides are too large to pass through the pores of polyacrylamide, and agarose gels are necessary. Agarose is a polysaccharide obtained from agar and is prepared in lower concentrations than polyacrylamide (roughly 0.5-2% vs roughly 4-20% for polyacrylamide). The lower the concentration of agarose, the larger will be the pores and the larger are the fragments that can be effectively separated. Whereas polyacrylamide gels are typically run vertically, agarose gels are usually run horizontally.

Marker DNA fragments of known size are run on the gel to provide a comparison for the DNA that is being investigated. Visualization is by ethidium bromide, which binds to DNA and can be seen with ultraviolet light. The more intact the DNA is, the higher will be its molecular weight, the less it will migrate, and the closer to the point of origin it will be at the completion of electrophoresis. DNA that has been fragmented during extraction will appear as bands toward the bottom of the gel or, if degraded, as a smear without distinct bands, because it consists of smaller fragments that migrate more quickly and separate incompletely from each other.

If the sample is relatively pure, the quantity of DNA can be estimated by the amount of absorbance at 260 nm. However, contaminating protein or RNA will cause errors in the calculation of quantity.

Blotting

Blotting, the transfer of macromolecules that have been subjected to electrophoresis from a gel to a membrane, was the first clinically relevant method to be used in conjunction with electrophoresis.

The first nucleic acid studies to find clinical relevance were based on blotting. The term "blotting" refers to the transfer of protein or nucleic acid, after electrophoresis, from a gel to a membrane, so it can be fixed in position and detected. There are several types of blotting. "Southern blotting" refers to the transfer of electrophoresed DNA to a membrane. "Northern blotting" refers to the transfer of electrophoresed RNA. As we will see, PCR has reduced the need for Southern blotting and reverse transcriptase PCR (RT-PCR) has greatly limited the use of northern blotting. "Western blotting" refers to the transfer of electrophoresed proteins to a membrane, and unlike other forms of blotting, requires the use of an electric current to drive the proteins into the membrane. All forms of blotting are becoming increasingly rare in clinical medicine.

Types of Electrophoresis

There are many types of electrophoresis and many ways to detect the macromolecules after electrophoresis. Migration of nucleic acid fragments on an agarose gel depends on both size and conformation. For length determinations, double-stranded fragments are used. While double-stranded DNA is packed in a very complex manner in vivo, in vitro, double-stranded fragments, unless very large, tend to be linear, without complex folding. Therefore, double-stranded DNA generally separates on a gel only on the basis of size. Fragments of DNA of known size are run in an adjacent well in the electrophoretic gel to provide standards by which the size can be assessed.

Very large double-stranded nucleic acid fragments, once they are oriented in an electric field, may not be able to enter the gel, and if they can, they will not move through it in a purely size-dependent manner. Rather, the limiting factor in their migration is the time taken to achieve orientation with the electric field. Orientation eventually results in a linear configuration that can usually move slowly through the gel.

In pulsed field gel electrophoresis (PFGE), 24 electrodes surround the gel in a hexagonal arrangement and the polarity of the electric field is periodically reversed. With each reversal, large molecules must reorient themselves to again achieve a linear configuration that can move through the gel. Reorientation takes longer for larger molecules, so the net effect is to achieve a size-dependent migration that would not otherwise be possible for large molecules because they migrate poorly in a gel. In PFGE, the electric field drives the fragments toward the bottom of the gel, but the reversals cause the fragments to take a zigzag path to the bottom. Migration can take about 16 hours, depending on the switch interval (the time between changes in the direction of current flow). With large fragments, a longer switch interval is needed, since they require more time to reorient after switching of the direction of current. When the procedure is completed, the bands are visualized on the gel by ethidium bromide staining under ultraviolet light. PFGE is used in public health applications to type strains of bacteria.

Single-stranded DNA is less restrained than double-stranded and more able to adopt a variety of unusual conformations (such as looping back upon itself, etc) that will interfere with mobility. If it is desired to measure the length of a single-stranded fragment by electrophoresis, denaturing conditions, such as low salt concentrations (so that the mutual repulsion of the phosphate groups is not mitigated) or high temperature, are used to prevent these conformations. Single-strand conformation polymorphism (SSCP) runs single-stranded fragments under nondenaturing conditions (high salt or low temperature). This allows the single-stranded fragments to assume unusual conformations, so that they separate more on the basis of conformation than size. Because conformation is a reflection of sequence, this technique permits minimal base substitutions (sometimes even just 1 base pair) to be detected.

Heteroduplex assays (also called double-strand sequence specific conformation polymorphism assays [DSSCP]) is the double-stranded equivalent to SSCP and is based on the principle that 2 strands of DNA that are not a perfect match will have small areas of separation, called "bubbles," in the areas of mismatch. These bubbles will slow the electrophoretic migration of the fragment if nondenaturing conditions are used. PCR, followed by either SSCP or DSSCP, is one of the methods used to detect the presence of abnormal proteins.

Cleavase is an enzyme that cleaves at the junction of single-stranded and double-stranded DNA (such a junction is called a hairpin). Cleavase fragment length polymorphism (CFLP) is based on the principles that the sequence of a fragment of DNA determines where hairpin structures will be formed. By cleaving at a hairpin, CLFP is a way to determine sequence differences. An advantage of CLFP over SSCP or DSSCP is that the conformation need not be maintained during electrophoresis. Once cleavase has cut, separation is dependent on size, not conformation.

There are numerous ways to detect nucleic acid after it is has migrated in a gel. Ethidium bromide is an example of detection by fluorescence. In fluorescence, a compound absorbs electromagnetic radiation at one wavelength and emits at a longer wavelength. Ethidium bromide intercalates into the DNA double helix, after which exposure to ultraviolet light results in fluorescence in the orange spectrum. The difficulty with ethidium bromide is that it is carcinogenic and must be disposed of by a specific protocol.

Other fluorescent compounds are also used. SYBR green also intercalates into double-stranded DNA, after which it absorbs in the blue spectrum at 488 nm and emits green light at 522 nm. Although it also requires ultraviolet light, it is safer than ethidium bromide and does not require special disposal conditions. Fluorescein isothiocyanate (FITC) absorbs at 495 nm and emits at 521 nm, but is more often used in the construction of probes for in situ hybridization (ISH) studies than in the electrophoretic detection of DNA. Fluorescent methods are the usual basis of detection in capillary electrophoresis, in which DNA fragments in a liquid medium flow quickly past a laser that detects the labeled fluors that are integrated into the nucleic acid [PMID18428903].

The second method is direct detection, in which a compound that can be seen binds to the nucleic acid. An example of this is silver staining. The silver will deposit in the nucleic acid and render it visible in ordinary light. The difficulties here are that this cannot be done in agarose gels, in which most nucleic acids are run, and silver staining renders the nucleic acid unrecoverable from the gel for any further studies.

A third method of detecting DNA is isotopic labeling, in which a component of DNA is labeled with a radioactive molecule. The gel, or a membrane into which the migrated nucleic acid has been transferred from the gel, is exposed to x-ray film. The emission of a particle or γ ray from the label will precipitate silver particles on the film. There is now a digital photoimaging system, similar to charged-coupled devices, that affords a more convenient method of detecting the emission of radioactivity. An advantage of isotopic labeling is that the exposure times (and thus the sensitivity), can be varied. Another advantage of isotopic labeling is that intensifying membranes can be placed between the gel and the film. Atoms in the intensifying membrane receive the primary emitted particle from the isotopic label and then emit multiple secondary particles, causing amplification of the signal.

A fourth method of detecting nucleic acids in gels is chromogenic (color) detection, which uses an enzyme that is attached to a chromogen and which reacts with the DNA.

A fifth alternative is chemiluminescence, which is similar to fluorescent detection except that the light detected has not undergone fluorescence (ie, the light that is absorbed and emitted are of the same wavelengths). Like isotopic and fluorescent methods, variation of exposure times leads to varying sensitivity.

Proteins that are electrophoresed can be detected by methods similar to those used for DNA. Often staining the gel with coomassie blue, which allows proteins to be seen in visible light, is used. As we will see, there are a number of ways to detect protein and DNA sequences without electrophoresis.

Nucleases

Naturally occurring nucleases were one of the great discoveries of the 20th century. Nucleases were first isolated from bacteria. They can be exonucleases, which cleave bases from the end of a strand of nucleic acid, or endonucleases, which cleave in the interior of the DNA molecule. Most exonucleases serve to remove inappropriate bases from the ends of growing DNA chains, such as might occur in errors of DNA replication. In contrast, most endonucleases have a defensive function. Restriction endonucleases (the term "restriction" indicates that these enzymes restrict or attack foreign DNA) arose in bacteria and archaea as a protection against insertions of viral DNA. Bacteria methylate their DNA to protect it from their own restriction endonucleases, but the unmethylated viral DNA is vulnerable to these enzymes.

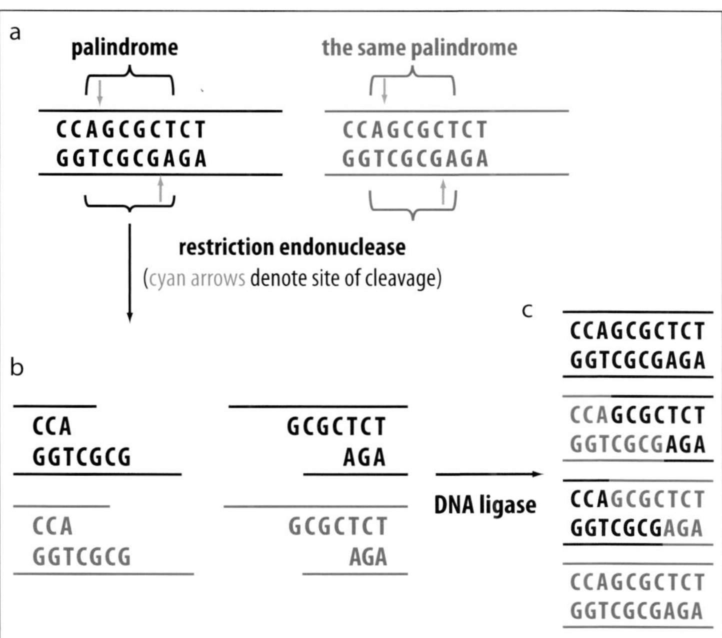

f45.1 The principle of restriction endonucleases. In a, the DNA sequence in black is derived from one species while that in red is derived from another species, but both sequences contain the same palindrome that is recognized by the restriction endonuclease. The cyan arrows denote the sites of cleavage. Note that the site of cleavage is identical on the 2 strands in the sense that the enzyme cleaves both strands between the same 2 bases, but because of the palindromic nature, these 2 cleavage sites do not cleanly cut the 2 chains but rather result in overhang. In b, the fragments of DNA in this case have 4-base overhangs. In c, at the completion of the process, 4 products will be obtained. 2 of these will simply be identical to the 2 sequences of starting DNA and are of no value, but the other 2 will be combinations of DNA from the 2 species, denoted here as sequences of both red and black bases.

Restriction endonucleases are divided into 4 broad classes—I, II, III, and IV—depending on their structure, cofactor requirements, the nature of their binding sites on the DNA, and the position of cleavage relative to the binding site. Type I restriction endonucleases cleave at a random site distant from their binding site. They are actually the most common in nature but are rarely used in research.

Type II endonucleases are the most diverse group and consists of a number of subsets. They are by far the most commonly used restriction endonucleases in research and medical work. Type II endonucleases generally bind to palindromes, sites whose sequence of base pairs reads the same both ways (eg, the sequence AGCCGA). Unlike the other types, type II endonucleases generally cleave at or close to the binding site [PMID15770420].

Type III restriction endonucleases cleave at a site a short distance from their recognition sequences and require 2 identical sequences in opposite directions in the same DNA molecule to become active. Type IV endonucleases are primarily important because they recognize DNA that has been modified, most often by methylation. As we will see, methylation is often used to silence transcription of DNA.

If a restriction endonuclease cleaves at a palindrome, the result will be 2 overlapping single-stranded ends of DNA that are complementary and will self-ligate without a ligase enzyme f45.1, though ligases are often needed to securely reseal the DNA backbone. Restriction endonucleases are identified by the first letter of the genus in which it was discovered, followed by the first 2 letters of the species, the first letter of the strain, and a Roman numeral indicating the order of discovery. For example, a commonly used endonuclease is EcoRI, referring to its origin from a bacterium of the *Escherichia* genus, *coli* species, strain RY13, and the first endonuclease isolated from this strain.

Variations in DNA may change the available cut sites, and hence the lengths of the DNA fragments after treatment with an endonuclease, by several mechanisms. In a minority of cases, the variation occurs in the DNA sequence in the actual site that the endonuclease recognizes, such that the enzyme no longer recognizes the site and does not cleave there. This causes a fragment of greater length compared to normal DNA. In most situations, the abnormality is not so fortuitously located, but variations in sequence cause variations in cleavage sites, resulting in fragments of differing lengths. One of the first methods of DNA analysis was based on variations in the sites of cleavage of endonucleases in DNA of different sequences, a technique called restriction fragment length polymorphism (RFLP). In RFLP, the application of a restriction endonuclease followed by gel electrophoresis resulted in fragments of differing length, whose varying sizes could be detected by Southern blotting to a membrane, followed by hybridization of a labeled probe. RFLP is rarely used today because it is labor-intensive, with its cumbersome sequence of electrophoresis, Southern blotting, and hybridization, and less sensitive than other techniques.

Cloning

The word "cloning" has 2 meanings, both referring to the making of copies that are identical to the original. The term may refer to the replication of a complete organism (in which case it is more properly called nuclear transplantation), but it is used here to refer to the amplification of a portion of DNA using genetic elements that have been modified. Like nucleic acid extraction, cloning is generally done by a manufacturer and is rarely a concern for a practicing pathologist, but a general knowledge of its principles will augment an understanding of nucleic acid testing.

Cloning has revolutionized biology in a myriad ways, but the major medical applications of cloning are sequencing and the production of large quantities of proteins that had previously been laborious to obtain. Cloning requires a portion of DNA that is capable of replication, called a vector, into which the DNA to be cloned can be inserted.

Vectors

There are many ways of cloning dna and many types of vectors are available. Plasmids are a commonly used vector for cloning DNA. A plasmid is a portion of bacterial DNA that is separate from the bacterium's single chromosome and self-replicating (a few plasmids, called episomes, can integrate into the bacterial chromosome). While plasmids from numerous bacteria have been used, most are derived from *E coli*. These plasmids, particularly one called ColE1, are the easiest and most commonly used bacterial vectors for DNA cloning.

The plasmid vector without its host bacterium and the DNA to be cloned are placed together in solution and exposed to endonuclease enzymes that cleave both samples of DNA in such a way that when the cleavages are repaired, the desired DNA is integrated into the vector. If the right endonucleases are chosen, they will not only cleave the DNA, but will also generate "sticky" ends on both the vector and the insert that will spontaneously reanneal in a way that inserts the new DNA into the desired location in the plasmid vector **f45.1**. If conditions are right, each plasmid molecule takes up 1 and only 1 insert fragment. A number of techniques are used to optimize the desired one-to-one relationship of vector and insert.

After integration is complete, some of the plasmids will have closed without incorporating any foreign DNA (called empty plasmids), while others will have incorporated foreign DNA that is not of interest. But a small percentage of the plasmids will contain the DNA that is to be amplified. At this time, all of the plasmids are placed in bacteria in a process called transformation. Bacteria are naturally (and understandably) resistant to taking in foreign DNA. Transformation is often achieved by raising the temperature or by using brief pulses of electricity that create minute holes in the cell wall (electroporation). Adjustment of ionic strength is often also a factor. One usually starts with a bacterial strain that has mutations that make it easier to transform with a plasmid.

Under conditions that have been worked out over the years, each cell takes in only 1 plasmid vector. The subsequent proliferation and plating of the transformed cells will produce many colonies on agar plates. In the ideal situation, each colony—the product of 1 cell—contains only 1 modified plasmid, and each plasmid in turn contains only 1 insert. Each cell in a colony contains the same modified plasmid, although many of these will not contain the desired fragment of DNA. The net effect is that a solution of myriad molecules of fragmented DNA, after reannealing, transformation, and plating, is converted into a series of colonies on an agar plate, each individual bacterium of which is transgenic (a term referring to any organism that has received DNA from another organism, of the same or a different species), containing a plasmid that contains the DNA to be cloned.

If it is desired to clone the entire DNA of a particular organism (this is called genomic cloning), the DNA is cleaved in multiple places by endonucleases, after which each fragment is inserted into a plasmid. After transformation into bacteria and plating onto agar, there will be colonies, each of which grows from one original transformed cell and carries a single vector that contains a portion of the organism's DNA. This collection of colonies is called a library. A genomic library is an organism's entire DNA, fragmented and inserted into the same vector. The collective inserts of the vector represent the entirety of an organism's DNA. Genomic libraries are invaluable in sequencing an organism's genome, and played a major role in the sequencing of the human genome. Because overlap among the inserts is unavoidable, genomic libraries contain more cloned DNA than the actual size of the genome of the organism they represent. The genomic equivalent is the ratio of the total DNA in the library to that of the organism.

Prokaryotic genomes are small enough that genomic libraries can be constructed. Genomic cloning has also been performed for eukaryotic organisms, but because of the greater size of their genomes, it is cumbersome and labor-intensive. The cloning and study of mRNA is more feasible and also allows the investigator to focus on which genes have been transcribed. mRNA is studied by its conversion into complementary DNA (cDNA) by the enzyme RNA-dependent DNA polymerase, discovered in 1970 and commonly called reverse transcriptase [PMID4316300]. Reverse transcriptase is an enzyme complex with 3 different enzymatic activities: generation of a single-stranded complementary DNA (cDNA) from the mRNA, lysis of the mRNA from the resulting DNA:RNA hybrid by an RNase that is part of the reverse transcriptase enzyme complex, and a DNA-dependent DNA polymerase which is also part of the complex and which is different from both the RNA-dependent DNA polymerase in reverse transcriptase and the separate, dedicated DNA polymerase that is used in DNA replication f45.2. These 3 activities of this one enzyme result in the production of a double-stranded DNA from a single-stranded mRNA. Both of the DNA polymerases of reverse transcriptase—using RNA and DNA as templates—require primers.

Reverse transcriptase requires primers to make cDNA. 3 types of primers may be used: those that are specific for a target sequence, random hexamers, or oligo-dT. Primers that are specific for a known target sequence are excellent if a particular gene is under investigation, but often either random hexamers, which bind indiscriminately, or oligo-dT, which binds to the 3' poly-A tail of mRNA, are used. The advantage of the latter 2 primers is that they are less specific and are therefore useful if a specific target sequence is not completely known. They can also amplify families of related RNAs and permit the study of the simultaneous expression of sets of genes. In a typical procedure, the making of a cDNA library commences with lysing of the cells, after which the mRNA is extracted and captured by column chromatography using oligo-dT to bind to the poly-A tail of mRNAs. The use of an oligo-dT primer will amplify only mRNA, not other kinds of RNA such as ribosomal or transfer RNA, because only mRNA has a poly-A tail. cDNA is then made from the captured mRNA by reverse transcriptase, after which any residual RNA is cleaved by RNase.

The DNA polymerase portion of the reverse transcriptase enzyme also requires a double-stranded primer, but whereas primers must be added to allow the synthesis of cDNA, the single-stranded cDNA that is formed often loops over on itself at the 3' end, forming a double-stranded template that can suffice for the DNA polymerase without the addition of a primer. Residual RNA may also bind to the cDNA and furnish the necessary double-stranded template for DNA polymerase.

mRNA cloning results in a smaller, more manageable library, composed only of those portions of DNA that are transcribed into mRNA, and is called a cDNA library or a gene expression library. Unlike a genomic library, a cDNA library may differ among different cell types in the same organism, or even among the same cell type at different times in its life, under different condition, or in disease vs health.

Libraries are often stored as a frozen suspension of pooled colonies. With the advent of microarray technology, many libraries exist on microtiter plates rather than on agar plates. These libraries, called arrayed or gridded, are the form in which most commercially available libraries are supplied.

Naturally occurring plasmids can only accommodate fragments of 5-10,000 base pairs. Plasmid libraries work reasonably well for most prokaryotes, but for eukaryotes, vectors are needed that can handle larger amount of DNA. Eukaryotes may also have plasmids, but these do not self-replicate as easily as their bacterial counterparts and are not often used in DNA cloning. Bacteriophage viruses, modified plasmids, cosmids, yeast artificial chromosome (YAC), and bacterial artificial chromosome (BAC), are all commonly used vectors for eukaryote work, and we will briefly look at each of these vectors.

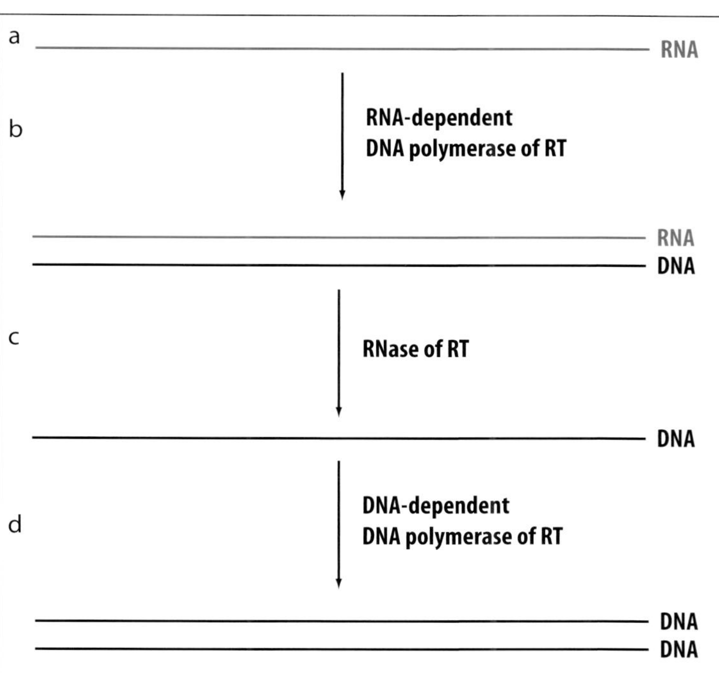

f45.2 The 3 sequential actions of the enzyme complex reverse transcriptase (RT).
In a, there is a single-stranded RNA molecule.
In b, the RNA-dependent DNA polymerase of RT uses a primer to form a complementary DNA molecule, resulting in a heteroduplex of RNA and DNA.
In c, the RNase of RT lyses the RNA, leaving a single DNA strand.
In d, the DNA-dependent DNA polymerase portion of RT forms a complementary strand, resulting in a double-stranded molecule of DNA.

A bacteriophage can accommodate larger amounts of DNA than most bacterial plasmids. The word "transfection" is used instead of "transformation" when referring to using a phage to introduce the desired DNA into a bacterium. Several bacteriophages are used, especially λ, P1, and M13. λ permits inserts of about 25,000 base pairs, more than twice the capacity of a plasmid. Another advantage of λ is that although transfection is inherently relatively inefficient, molecular biologists have several clever techniques that allow phage DNA to be introduced into bacteria with high efficiency.

Because it is larger than a plasmid, λ has more restriction sites but has usually been manipulated to remove most of these, and also to remove unnecessary DNA so that more can be inserted. The term "replacement vector" refers to a phage whose native DNA has been largely removed and replaced by DNA that facilitates its use as a vector. In nature, λ may replicate in a manner that destroys the bacterial cell (lysis), but it may also replicate without destroying the cell in a process called lysogeny. In using λ for cloning, the genes for lysogeny are removed, so lysis will result. Since the genes for lysogeny

ISBN 978-089189-5886

are removed, the lysis of a bacterial cell liberates more phages, which then lyse adjacent bacteria. The result is a clear area on the agar plate, called a plaque, not a bacterial colony, as was the case with plasmids. These plaques can then be removed and frozen as phage libraries, serving as a source of recombined genetic material, very much the same way that plasmid-based libraries can be frozen.

Some bacterial plasmids have been modified to accept a larger amount of DNA and combination vectors can be used. For example, the ends of the genome of λ contain cohesive end sites (COS) that have 12 unpaired and complementary base pairs, so that it easily forms a stable circle. A cosmid is any vector, usually a bacterial plasmid, that contains COS. A cosmid is a combination vector in which most of the λ DNA is removed, while preserving its beneficial sequences. At the same time, the plasmid features of a cosmid allow for easy detection on agar plates, as for simple pure plasmids. The result, in effect, is a plasmid with a larger capacity. A fosmid is a cosmid that is based on adding the λ COS sites to a particular plasmid from *E coli* called an F-plasmid.

While λ and cosmid vectors can handle larger amounts of DNA than a simple plasmid, cloning particularly large sequences (eg, genomic cloning in eukaryotes), requires even larger vectors. Molecular geneticists are very good at taking natural sources of replicating DNA, removing nonessential portion and creating vectors that will accommodate large inserts. One solution to the need to accommodate larger inserts was YACs, hybrids of a plasmid and a yeast chromosome. The YAC vector is maintained in bacteria, but after endonuclease digestion and recombination with the insert, the YAC replicates in yeast, usually *Saccharomomyces cerevesiae*. A YAC can handle up to 1,000,000 bp of foreign DNA and is used to construct a gene library for mammalian cells. YACs can accommodate very large inserts and were invaluable in the cloning of the human genome, but are difficult to work with because the insert is often unstable, resulting in a relatively low yield of cloned DNA.

At about the time that the difficulties of working with YACs were being realized, 2 new vectors became available. The first was an artificial chromosome based on the bacteriophage P1, which is larger than λ and can therefore accommodate larger inserts. These vectors are called PACs. The second was a modified bacterial systems based on the F-plasmid, called BACs. While BACs cannot accommodate as much foreign DNA as a YAC, the inserts are more stable and BACs are easier to work with than YACs. Moreover, BACs maintain many of the conveniences of bacterial systems since they do not use viral DNA (eg, screening and storage of BAC libraries is similar to ordinary plasmid libraries). More recently, artificial human and plant chromosomes have been developed to extend the advantages of YACs and BACs [PMID21750534, PMID21482517].

Libraries based on BACs were critical in the sequencing of the human genome. In the initial stages of the Human Genome Project, a technique called shotgun sequencing was employed, in which the genome was randomly fragmented into small segments that could be sequenced, the idea being that overlapping bases would permit the reconstruction of the genomic sequence. For example, the series of fragments AATCGG GTACCAA ACTGCGT can be reconstructed as ACTGCGTACCAATCGG.

While conceptually simple, there were 2 difficulties with this approach. First, the sheer volume of data tendered the approach untenable, even with the best of computer support. Second, repetitive DNA sequences negated the simplistic reconstruction illustrated above. For example, if the above sequence contains numerous areas of repeating G bases, and its in vivo sequence was:

GGGGACTGCGGGGGGTACGGGGCAATCGG

the fragments, when sequenced, might read:

GGGGACTGCGG GGGGGGTACGG GGCAATCGG

These sequenced fragments are far more difficult to assemble into a completed sequence.

To address these problems, partial endonuclease digestion was used to generate smaller fragments. Had the digestion been complete, identical copies of the same sequence would be fragmented into identical shorter segments, but because the digestion was only partial, identical copies were cleaved slightly differently, so that the initial sequence was converted into a series of short, slightly different fragments with overlapping ends. The slightly different fragments were then cloned, often in YACs or BACs.

After sequencing of an initial fragment, a labeled probe was prepared that hybridized to that fragment. Because of overlap, this probe also hybridized to fragments that were similar but not identical. Those very similar fragments were then sequenced and probes prepared for the second set of fragments. These probes, in turn, were hybridized to a third set of fragments that were similar to the second set. Sequential hybridizations, sequencing, and preparation of new probes in this manner yielded ever-larger fragments of known sequence. This technique is called chromosome walking and allows a genomic library to be ordered. Ordered libraries, consisting of clones whose inserts have overlapping sequences, were invaluable in sequencing the human genome.

If instead of sequencing, it is desired to retrieve a colony with a particular insert so that the insert can be amplified, then the library must be screened to identify the appropriate colony. The screening procedure depends on the type of vector and the details of how the library is set up. Historically, screening consisted of a primary phase intended to pinpoint a group of colonies (often based on antibiotic resistance), followed by a secondary phase intended to identify a specific relevant colony. Today, with advances in technology, screening can often be accomplished in a single step. A common procedure is that a membrane is placed on top of the colonies on a plate, touched lightly, then lifted, so that a few bacteria will come off each colony (or a few λ particles will come off each plaque) onto the membrane. The cells on the membrane are then lysed and their DNA is denatured to permit access to a labeled probe which is made so that it will only hybridize to the DNA sequence of interest. After hybridization, the location of the signal identifies the correct colony on the membrane. Because the orientation of the membrane and the original plate has been maintained, it is possible to identify the corresponding colony on the plate. Often, to increase purity of the product, 2 probes are used, or the candidate colony and adjacent colonies are harvested together, then resuspended, replated, and screened again.

If the desired fragment of DNA codes for an enzyme, an enzymatic assay may be used instead of hybridization (this method is called expression assay). Sequencing is the ultimate verification that the candidate colony is the correct one. Once the colony of interest is identified, portions of it can be transferred to other plates for amplification.

If large quantities of protein production are desired (eg, human insulin), expression cloning, using an expression vector, can be used. An expression vector is so named because its purpose is the expression of a protein, not the construction of a library of genomic or cDNA. An expression vector has a promoter and may also have translational signals.

In expression cloning, a eukaryotic host may be preferred because of the large amount of posttranslational modification that eukaryotic proteins have. For example, the hepatitis B surface antigen can be cloned in *E coli*, and the amino acid sequence is correct, but it is not immunogenic because it does not have the correct 3-dimensional conformation. Cloning in the yeast *Saccharomyces cerevisiae* solves this problem and permits the production of recombinant proteins that are effective for use as vaccines. Other proteins that are often expression cloned include the interferons, growth hormone, tissue plasminogen activator, granulocyte-macrophage stimulating hormone, factor VIII, and erythropoietin. Libraries constructed with an expression vector can be screened by nucleic acid hybridization, by enzymatic assay, or by the binding of antibodies to the desired protein.

Gene Modification

Vectors can be used for purposes other than amplification of DNA or increased protein synthesis. An important use of vectors is to modify the expression of genes, a technique called gene targeting. In gene targeting, the expression of a gene can be increased or decreased. In bacteria, a gene can be inactivated by inserting into it a fragment of DNA that will impede its transcription (eg, by disrupting the promoter or by introducing a premature stop codon). This is called gene knockout. In bacteria, gene knockout is often done by constructing a DNA sequence that will inactivate the gene, then inserting it into the host DNA by endonuclease treatment. Sometimes, gene knockout can be done without nucleases if the DNA sequences of the host and insert are similar. In this case, homologous sequences between the 2 portions of DNA may recognize each other and spontaneously form hybrids in a process called homologous recombination, as occurs in meiosis.

Gene knockout may also inactivate genes adjacent to the insertion site in addition to the target gene. This is called polar effects or polarity. Before a gene is implicated because knocking it out causes a particular phenotype, polarity must be excluded by showing a return to normal phenotype upon insertion of the purified target gene, without adjacent sequences, into the knocked-out animal, a procedure called complementation. Knockout and complementation is the acid test of a gene's direct involvement, the genetic equivalent of Koch's postulates.

The expression of a gene can be increased by inserting it next to the promoter of an active gene, so that the promoter can also activate the gene of interest (called gene knock*in*).

Gene knockout in eukaryotes is more difficult than in bacteria. RNA interference (RNAi) can be used to inactivate a eukaryotic gene because the presence of double-stranded RNA silences the expression of the corresponding gene. However, this method is largely limited to invertebrates or to vertebrate cells in culture, and gene knockout in eukaryotes usually requires inactivating the target gene by introducing DNA during embryogenesis.

A number of techniques have been used to introduce DNA into embryonic cells during development, and different techniques have been established for different animals and plants. In evaluating the method used to produce genetic modification in animals, it is important to understand that modification in different ways and at different times may result in the modification of all or only of some of the cells in the adult. For example, microinjection of DNA into a fertilized egg or into the sperm pronucleus results in modification of all cells if integration is immediate, but of only some cells if there is delayed integration because some cells will contain the new DNA and some will not. If all cells are modified in the embryo, all of the cells in the adult will have the same genotype and all will contain foreign DNA. The result is a true transgenic animal. Animals in which only some cells have been modified are referred to as mosaic because there are different lineages that do not have the same genotype, though others restrict the term "mosaic" to those situations in which there are multiple lineages that are all derived from the DNA of 1 zygote. Mosaic animals may suffice if the germ cells are modified and if the modification is transmitted to offspring.

In a typical example, embryonic stem cells (ie, of the inner cell mass) are injected with a DNA construct that contains 1 sequence that will inactivate the gene and another sequence that will permit integration. These cells, with the gene inactivated, are then injected into a blastocyst from another embryo, where they join the other cells of the inner cell mass. This means that some cells of the inner cell mass will have an inactivated gene, while other cells will be normal. After birth, the animal will be chimeric because some of its DNA is not from the zygote, and it will be heterozygous for the gene of interest. Subsequent breeding will produce animals that are homozygous for a nonfunctional gene. In these animals, the gene has been knocked out. Similar procedures can increase the expression of a gene in animals (knockin). These methods have proven invaluable in obtaining animal models for many diseases. Indeed, there is an International Mouse Knockout Consortium that seeks to knockout all mouse genes and to provide researchers with mice in which any desired gene has been inactivated [PMID17218247].

Gene transfer with retroviruses has been achieved, but is more likely to be effective in producing mosaics than truly transgenic animals. The hope for retroviruses is that they can deliver "corrected" gene copies to the specific tissues that are affected by a disease (eg, a working copy of the dystrophin gene to muscle cells in muscular dystrophy patients). Unfortunately, the introduction of new and functional genetic material into human or animal cells in the postembryonic state for therapeutic purposes (so-called gene therapy) has proven to be far more difficult than the techniques described above. The difficulties have been getting the desired genes into animal cells, getting them to integrate in the right location,

ISBN 978-089189-5886

and ensuring that they are properly expressed and controlled. Even after successful delivery of the gene into the cell, only a fraction of the DNA will integrate at all into the host DNA, and because the location of integration is largely a matter of chance, only a much smaller fraction of the integrated gene will be in the proper location, and assume normal function.

A number of techniques are currently used to introduce a gene into a eukaryotic cell. In bacteria, "transfection" is generally understood to refer to transfer by a phage virus and transformation implies nonviral means. In eukaryotes, however, because the term "transformation" was in previous use to indicate neoplastic growth, the term "transfection" refers to nonviral means of DNA transfer and corresponds to transformation in bacteria. Transduction refers to viral means of transferring DNA into eukaryotic cells. Examples of transfection techniques in eukaryotes include chemicals, liposomes, temperature elevation, direct injection, electroporation, receptor-mediated endocytosis, microinjection, and sperm-mediated DNA delivery (sperm heads bind DNA in vitro).

Despite its disappointing results, gene therapy remains one of the most exciting prospects in medicine, and some incipient progress has been made. There are even a few explicit bright spots. Severe combined immunodeficiency (SCID) secondary to deficiency of the enzyme adenine deaminase has been well treated with ex vivo retroviral transduction of the enzyme into T lymphocytes, with excellent results [PMID20966749]. Some success has also been achieved with the X-linked form of SCID. The X-linked form of SCID is caused by an abnormality in the γ chain of the Il-2 receptor, and bone marrow stem cells from patients have been transduced with a retroviral vector containing this gene, after which return of the stem cells to the patient has resulted in apparent cures, although some patients treated with retroviral vectors have experienced lymphoproliferative disorders [PMID20071242]. Excellent results have also been achieved by using a virus to deliver a missing gene into the retinas of patients suffering from the rare condition Leber Congenital Amaurosis [PMID20399883]. In theory, almost any disease, and certainly almost any cancer, is ultimately caused by an abnormality of DNA, and could be treated by replacing a dysfunctional enzyme, blocking the transcription of an oncogene, increasing the amount of DNA coding for a tumor suppressor gene, etc.

Gene knockout and knockin are examples of gene targeting. Larger modifications in the expression of DNA, involving regions of chromosomes rather than single genes, can be achieved by chromosome engineering [PMID16824018, PMID16839184]. In chromosome engineering, gene targeting is used to insert a site-specific recombinase enzyme into stem cells, resulting in translocations, deletions, inversions, etc. Like gene knockout, chromosome engineering is more difficult in animals and achieving animal models for human chromosomal disorders will be more challenging. Moreover, because so many human diseases do not conform to simple Mendelian inheritance, even a successful effort by the International Mouse Knockout Consortium will not leave us with effective models for many diseases [PMID17172731].

The ultimate in genetic modification will be DNA reprogramming, so that stem cells can be made into any desired cell type. Indeed, in theory, even a differentiated cell could be deprogrammed, then redirected along another pathway, so that, for example, pancreatic β cells, made by directing stem cells, or even by redirecting an already differentiated cell, can be given to patients with type I diabetes. Stem cell research is controversial, but it offers many potential advances in disease treatment.

Amplification Techniques

Nucleic acid amplification techniques, of which polymerase chain reaction was the first, are the basis of molecular medicine.

Polymerase Chain Reaction

Few advances have fundamentally changed DNA technology as profoundly and quickly as PCR [PMID3472723]. PCR begins with the use of an elevated temperature—about 94°C—to separate the 2 strands, a process called melting. In the presence of new bases and appropriate conditions of ionic strength, primers that bind to the regions of the DNA *adjacent* to the area to be amplified are then added. The temperature is then lowered to permit the primers to anneal to the single-stranded DNA molecules (the exact temperature employed during this step will influence the specificity of primer binding), and DNA polymerase is added. The primers then hybridize at both ends of the target sequence. The DNA polymerase then creates a short complementary strand whose length is determined by the distance between the primers. The temperature is then elevated to denature the new DNA molecules, and the process is repeated, using both the old and the new DNA molecules as templates. At the beginning of this second cycle, there are twice as many copies of the desired DNA sequence compared to the starting material **f45.3**. These

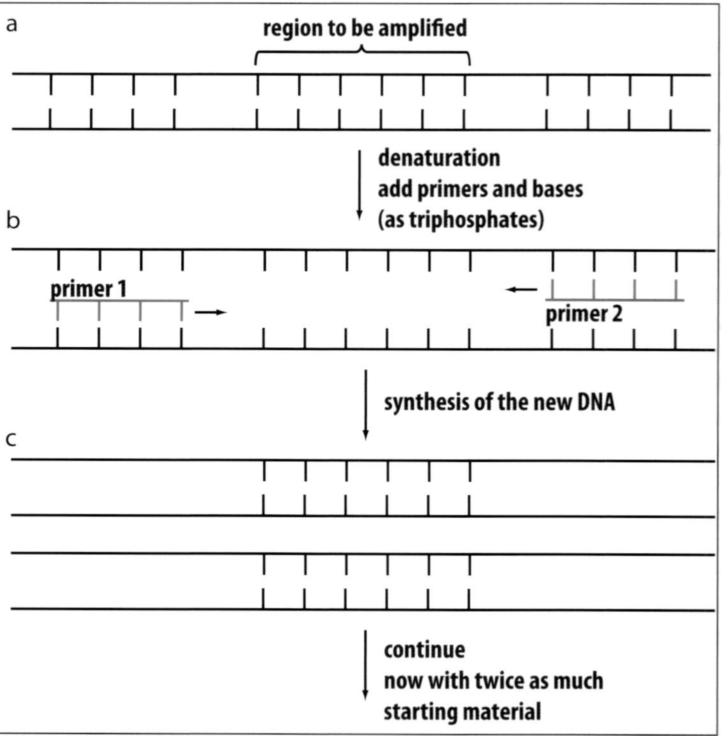

f45.3 Polymerase chain reaction. **a** depicts the native double stranded DNA with the region of interest that is to be amplified. In **b**, after denaturation and the addition of primers and bases, the primers bind to the portions of the DNA that are adjacent to the region to be amplified. In **c**, after the process goes to completion, there are 2 copies of the region of interest, 1 derived from each of the original strands. Not indicated in this figure is the need for thermocycling. The DNA must be heated to achieve denaturation, but then cooled to permit binding of the primer and the synthesis of new DNA strands.

continual cycles of raising the temperature to denature, lowering it to permit primer annealing, allowing synthesis of complementary strands between the primers, and raising it again doubles the amount of the desired DNA sequence with each cycle.

The DNA polymerase Taq (*Thermophilus aquaticus*), from a thermophilic archaebacterium, was initially used in PCR because it could withstand the melting temperature, obviating the need to add fresh polymerase with each cycle. The Taq enzyme made PCR practical, but it lacks a "proofreading" exonuclease, which could result in significant errors in the fidelity of the final products. In practice, this is usually not a big problem unless one is sequencing or unless Taq makes a mistake early in the process, such that the error is perpetuated in subsequent cycles. However, thermostable bacterial (as opposed to archaea) DNA polymerases are often used today. For example, Pfu and Pwo are thermostable DNA polymerases that do have proofreading ability and can also amplify longer stretches than Taq. The products of PCR are called amplicons.

This process has been automated and can be carried out by a variety of commercially available instruments. Many of these instruments perform nucleic acid extraction and purification as part of their procedure (many tests in molecular pathology are now available in kit form, as is the case for most testing in the general laboratory). For those situations in which a PCR assay must be developed de novo, the most important part of the development is the design and use of the primers. There are internet resources available to assist molecular biologists in the optimal design of primers and to ensure that they do not bind nonspecifically, form unwanted loop structures, or have difficult hybridization characteristics.

As the PCR reaction proceeds, the amount of primer that is needed will increase exponentially, so there must be an initial excess of primer to allow for this. On the other hand, primers will bind to a slight extent to nontarget DNA, and excess primer increases nonspecific amplification. In a well-executed balancing act, in many PCR reactions, even though exponential amplification is the rule, the process will eventually plateau. One reason for this is that there are insufficient primers for the larger numbers of binding sites made possible by the amplification. Another reason is that as the PCR process continues, the number of amplicons increases and the ratio of amplicons to primers increases, so amplicon-primer hybridization, which leads to DNA synthesis, becomes less common, and amplicon-amplicon hybridization, which does not lead to synthesis, become more common. The DNA polymerase must also be added in excess to allow for the much greater amounts that will be needed towards the end of the reactions, but again, a large excess of the enzyme opens the door to nonspecific reactions. It is important to add the DNA to be amplified last, as this minimizes unwanted amplification while one is preparing the final aspects of the reactions.

A huge advantage of PCR, even more than the actual amplification, is that one can start with less pure material and still obtain a pure product at the completion of the process. Historically, some degree of purification of DNA has been necessary to remove substances that inhibit the reactions, but PCR sharply reduces laborious purification steps and progress is being made in developing methods that will produce the desired product from crude starting material with no antecedent purification at all [PMID20075207].

A weakness of PCR is that if the defect is caused by a large deletion, especially if both the pertinent sequence and flanking sequences are deleted, there may be no place for the primers to bind, and one may not be able to get amplification. Fluorescence ISH (FISH) is generally better than PCR in the detection of deletions or inversions, and PCR should not be the sole means of searching for a mutation unless it is known that the mutation does not involve a large deletion, or it has been established that there is a PCR procedure that can amplify across such a deletion from an adjacent site.

Another weakness of PCR is that in general, only short sequences can be amplified, although newer protocols make longer sequences amenable to the process. This is called long PCR or long-range PCR and usually involves the use of 2 polymerases, 1 with and 1 without proofreading ability, so that one can simultaneously have polymerase activity over a long stretch of DNA (from the nonproofreading enzyme) and also have 3' to 5' exonuclease proofreading, from the other polymerase, for the specific sequence of interest.

Another difficulty with PCR is that not all areas of interest are necessarily amplified to the same extent. This is called amplification bias. Amplification bias can result from many technical considerations, such as number and accessibility of the target sequence, and random fluctuations in the efficiency of each cycle. While amplification bias is unlikely to affect qualitative PCR, it can cause a false copy number determination in quantitative PCR (qPCR).

A final potential weakness of PCR is that it requires that the DNA sequences flanking the region of interest be known, so that appropriate primers can be constructed, though with the sequencing of the genome, this is rarely a serious problem. Moreover, this apparent weakness can be utilized as a strength. Since any primer can be constructed, one can adjust the primers to allow for the selective amplification of a specific sequence. Any sequence of DNA for which a specific PCR test is available (ie, for which primers that will hybridize to the adjacent regions are available) is said to be a tagged sequence. For example, there are allele-specific primers that will hybridize only to a specific mutated DNA sequence, so that amplification occurs only in the presence of that particular abnormality (allele-specific primers are used in conjunction with conditions of high hybridization stringency, such as low salt or higher temperature). This is allele-specific PCR amplification, sometimes called sequence-specific PCR, PCR with sequence-specific primers (SSP), or amplification refractory mutation system (ARMS). These allele-specific primers are often used in parallel with primers that amplify only normal DNA, so that the ratio of normal to abnormal DNA can be assessed.

Allele-specific PCR is a leading method to detect abnormal proteins. A difficulty with this method, however, is that a primer need not hybridize perfectly for PCR to occur, so there may be inappropriate amplification of an allele that does not correspond to the primer [PMID2179874]. To address this problem, PCR clamping was developed. In PCR clamping, the primers for the normal DNA are constructed from peptide nucleic acids (PNAs). PNAs [PMID1962210] are nucleic acid analogues that contain a base, but have a peptide bond, as is found in proteins, in their backbones rather than the weaker sugar-phosphate bond of normal nucleic acids. PNAs have 2 important properties. First, because PNAs lack a charged phosphate group, they do not experience mutual repulsion with the phosphate groups of the nucleic acid sequence to which they have bound and therefore bind to a complementary strand with greater affinity compared to normal oligonucleotides. This allows PNA-based primers to effectively out-compete partially matched, allele-specific primers at binding sites on normal DNA and prevent inappropriate primer binding. Second, PNAs are not recognized by DNA polymerase, so there will be no amplification of any DNA to which PNA primers are bound. PNA oligonucleotides, therefore, bind to and "clamp" the DNA to which it has hybridized from any further amplification. If one constructs PNA primers that are specific for the normal sequence, while using normal nucleotide primers for the abnormal sequence of interest, only the latter sequence will be amplified [PMID11464917]. PNAs also have potential use in antisense therapy since they could theoretically be constructed to bind to and inactivate abnormal DNA in vivo.

Allele-specific PCR can also be performed with locked nucleic acids (LNAs), which are nucleotides that have been modified by using a methylene unit to link the 2'-oxygen and the 4'-carbon atoms of a ribose molecule in RNA [PMID9873516]. Unlike PNAs, LNAs are modified in the sugar moiety, not in the backbone, and they do contain phosphate groups. Oligonucleotides made from LNA bind more strongly than natural nucleotides because they are fixed into the ideal conformation for hybridization. Unlike primers made from PNA, primers constructed from LNA do not prevent PCR. Indeed, because their affinity is higher, allele-specific primers made from LNA not only support PCR, but can also be shorter and can detect mutations even if only 1 base pair is abnormal (ie, single nucleotide polymorphism [SNP]) [PMID16683135, PMID12528362]. In fact, LNAs are excellent for any hybridization application that benefits from high affinity. There is also hope that they might be used in antisense therapy.

COLD-PCR enriches for mutations that are present in very small numbers. In COLD-PCR, a number of cycles of regular PCR, at the usual denaturing temperature, are performed, after which additional cycles are performed at a lower denaturing temperature. Because mutant sequences are rare, most of them will be paired with wild-type sequences in heteroduplexes (molecules formed from a hybridization of a mutant strand with a wild-type strand) instead of being in homoduplexes with other mutant sequences, as would be the case if they were present in greater numbers. These heteroduplexes are not hydrogen bonded as strongly as duplexes formed between 2 wild-type strands. At the lower temperature, heteroduplexes containing the mutant DNA sequence tend to separate and are amenable to further PCR, while duplexes formed from 2 wild-type strands will remain hybridized, and are refractory to PCR, resulting in preferential amplification of mutant sequences. [PMID18408729]

It is occasionally necessary to extract DNA from a paraffin block for PCR amplification. Because formalin fixation fragments DNA into small sequences that will bind primers, but are incapable of complete amplification, only short sequences of DNA can be amplified from paraffin blocks, no more than about 400 base pairs [PMID21142742]. However, procedures are being developed that minimize these small fragments in DNA extracted from paraffin blocks.

A variety of other fixatives have been marketed with the claim that they provide for superior DNA amplification from paraffin blocks, but at this writing, these new fixatives are unproven in their ability to improve DNA recovery and, more importantly, are unproven in their ability to offer adequate morphologic detail on H&E examination, which continues to be the overwhelming priority of tissue fixation. Alcohol-based fixatives are no better than formalin in DNA studies [PMID21917676]. Fixatives containing mercury or picric acid, and the acid used in decalcification, render the DNA in a sample unsuitable for PCR [PMID1452690]. At this writing, good fixation with conventional neutral buffered formalin is difficult to improve upon in DNA studies in paraffin material. While formalin overall continues to be the fixative of choice, RNA is less well preserved in formalin than DNA [PMID20502189], underscoring the need to find a fixative that is optimal for morphologic assessment and studies of all nucleic acids.

DNA studies from actual histologic slides are even more difficult than those from paraffin blocks because a typical 6-μm section contains only fragments of the nucleus with less likelihood of obtaining quality DNA. This situation is to be avoided if at all possible. Cytology preparations are more amenable to DNA studies than tissue sections because the entire cell is present on the slide and paraffin processing is avoided. However, success is far from assured and discretion is needed, as the use of smears destroys irreplaceable morphologic evidence.

Amplicons arising from PCR are usually electrophoresed, after which they may be detected in several ways. In the traditional gel system, the simplest detection method is staining with ethidium bromide, which reveals the bands upon examination with ultraviolet light. If blotting is performed from a gel onto a membrane, hybridization with a labeled probe (do not confuse primers and probes; primers get the process started, while labeled probes identify the target sequence afterward) that is specific for the sequence of interest can be used. This is called a sequence-specific oligonucleotide probe, or SSOP. This provides 2 different means of establishing the identity of the amplicon: its migration pattern and its hybridization characteristics. The shorter the probe used in hybridization, the more precise must be the match, and therefore shorter probes are less likely to lead to errors. Longer probes are likely to be mismatched in a few areas but may still have sufficient overall complementarity to anneal and permit a signal, but the annealing may be to a sequence that is not the precise target. PCR with SSP is an invaluable technique, and although blotting is rarely used now, some form of hybridization with a specific labeled probe is also widely used.

A typical probe design is called a molecular beacon [PMID9630890]. In this design, a probe that is complementary to the target sequence bends back on itself in a loop structure such that the 2 ends of the probe are in very close proximity. One end contains a fluorescent compound and the other end contains a quencher molecule that absorbs the light emitted by the fluorescent compound. Before annealing, the fluorescent compound and the quencher are very close together and any fluorescence is quenched and not detected. After binding to the target, however, the fluorescent compound and the quencher are separated by a sufficiently large distance that the fluorescence is no longer quenched, and a signal can be detected.

Newer modalities of detection include capillary electrophoresis. Like conventional electrophoresis, capillary electrophoresis is based on the principle that the smallest fragments migrate faster. In capillary electrophoresis, the amplicons are tagged in some way—usually with a fluorescent dye—and passed through very thin tubes past a laser, which then interrogates the reporter molecule that is attached to the amplicons through a small section of the capillary tube that is transparent. Capillary electrophoresis is not only much faster than traditional gel electrophoresis, but is also more precise and can be interpreted in a much less subjective manner.

Microchip-based electrophoresis is a variant of capillary electrophoresis in which microchannels are etched in a glass plate. Minute amounts of sample are placed at one end and a current carries these samples past a point of interrogation (eg, a fluorescently tagged sample is carried past a fluorescence detection system) [PMID17094291].

As is the case with any procedure, PCR must balance sensitivity (the ability to amplify the desired sequence to a detectable level) with specificity (the ability to exclude undesired sequences from amplification). False positives can occur in PCR because the primers may bind to a sequence of DNA without perfect homology, leading to amplification of the wrong portion of DNA. Likewise, a larger number of cycles will increase the yield of the target DNA, but at the price of some amount of amplification of unwanted sequences. Stringent hybridization conditions, such as low salt or higher temperature, diminish imperfect or nonspecific binding and increase specificity. In addition, there is the concept of fidelity, which pertains to the *accuracy* of the amplified transcript, whereas specificity pertains to amplification of the correct sequence. Another potential problem with PCR is that the genome of many microorganisms changes.

There are a number of types of PCR that are used in specific situations. One of these is multiplex PCR, in which multiple sets of primers are employed to simultaneously generate multiple sets of amplicons in the same tube. Another variant of PCR is the 2-step nested PCR. In this technique, PCR is initially carried out with a set of primers that is not immediately adjacent to the sequence of interest, but rather separated from it, such that the amplicons contain the sequence of interest and the DNA adjacent to it. An aliquot of the amplicon is transferred to a new tube and the process is repeated with a different set of primers that binds adjacent to the target sequence. The second primers are called the inner or nested primer pair and will code for a shorter amplicon than the first set. The advantage of the 2-step nested PCR is that it permits the second amplification step to start with material that has already been enriched for the target sequence.

Forms of PCR

There are many forms of PCR, the 2 most important of which are reverse transcriptase (RT-PCR) and quantitative (qPCR).

Reverse Transcriptase PCR

Now we turn our attention to the 2 most common variants of PCR—RT-PCR and quantitative PCR (or qPCR; formerly called real-time PCR). RT-PCR is used to amplify mRNA, not DNA. Because mRNA is unstable and is quickly degraded by RNases (the reason for this is to prevent excessive translation), there are 3 options to work directly with RNA. One must either freeze the tissue quickly, inhibit RNases, or, more commonly, use RT-PCR. The abbreviation formerly indicated real-time PCR, a different process now called qPCR and discussed subsequently.

In RT-PCR, single-stranded cDNA is made from mRNA by the enzyme reverse transcriptase. Although the complete reverse transcriptase enzyme also lyses the mRNA and uses its own DNA polymerase to create a double-stranded DNA molecule, in RT-PCR, only the generation of the single-stranded cDNA is important because PCR begins after cDNA is made. In contrast to cloning applications and the construction of a cDNA library, where double-stranded DNA is required, the RNase and DNA polymerase portions of the enzyme are not needed in RT-PCR. Indeed, the RNase and DNA polymerase activities are often removed from the enzyme if it is used in RT-PCR.

RT-PCR, by amplifying only the DNA that is transcribed into mRNA, permits the study of gene expression, while simultaneously avoiding the inherent instability of mRNA. Many translocations are now studied by looking for the mRNA that results from the translocated DNA, not the actual DNA itself. For a given situation, the best test may be a FISH study performed on the DNA or an RT-PCR performed on amplified cDNA. In searching for translocations by RT-PCR, typically 1 primer binds to 1 of the chromosomes involved in the translocation, while the other binds to the second chromosome. If there has been no translocation, the primers will be on different chromosomes and there will be no amplification. But if the translocation is present, the 2 primers will be in proximity and amplification will result.

It is convenient to perform RT-PCR in 2 steps. The first step is the isolation of mRNA and the creation of the cDNA. The second step is the amplification of the cDNA. Isolation of mRNA is often done with a commercially available oligo-T sequence that binds to the 3' poly-A tail of RNA. cDNA is then made from this mRNA, using reverse transcriptase (usually from *E coli*) in the presence of bases and primers. The oligo-T sequence serves both to isolate mRNA and as a primer in the creation of cDNA. SSP can also be used if a specific sequence is targeted and well characterized, and random hexamers can also be used as primers.

Whereas DNA replication, transcription, and translation all proceed in a 5' to 3' direction, reverse transcription proceeds in a 3' to 5' direction because it begins by binding of the reverse transcriptase to the poly-A tail at the 3' end of the mRNA. A potential problem with RT-PCR is that the reverse transcriptase enzyme may not reach the 5' end of the mRNA because the template may become detached, the secondary structure of the mRNA may impede the enzyme, or proteins may bind to the RNA and inhibit the enzyme. An advantage of random hexamer primers is that with them, the enzyme is more likely to reach the 5' end (another advantage of random primers is that there are a few mRNA molecules that do not have a poly-A tail). There is also a special technique, called rapid amplification of cDNA ends (RACE), that is designed to address this problem, but in many cases, this is not necessary.

The second step, once cDNA has been obtained, is the actual amplification, via traditional PCR. One can generate the cDNAs from many samples at one time, and subsequently perform the amplifications simultaneously at another time.

ISBN 978-089189-5886

One problem with RT-PCR is that there is likely to be some contaminant DNA in the mRNA preparation that will also be amplified during the amplification stage. For this reason, in RT-PCR, either DNases must be used, or primers must be designed so that they anneal to different exons that become adjacent only after splicing. In the latter case, if there is contaminating DNA, there either is no amplification of the DNA because the intervening intron places the primers too far about, or if there is amplification, the amplified product is readily recognizable because of its large size. The major technical problems with RT-PCR are the need to isolate mRNA with minimal loss and the need to deal with potentially contaminating DNA by 1 of these 2 methods.

RT-PCR can be used to quantitate viral load for RNA viruses if an internal standard is used. In this use, the products of RT-PCR, derived from viral RNA, are hybridized to a well and detected colorimetrically. Quantitation is by reference to a quantitation standard optical density.

At this writing, gene expression as elucidated by RT-PCR has not yet replaced immunochemistry as a means of identifying tumors of unknown origin, but progress is being made and a 92 gene RT-PCR system has been described which can perform as well or better than immunohistochemistry in the identification of a primary site in metastatic deposits in paraffin processed tissue [PMID20427384].

RT-PCR can also be done in situ, meaning in the actual place that has been visualized on the H&E stained slide. In situ PCR is a RT-PCR method that permits correlation of traditional morphology and molecular pathology techniques.

Quantitative PCR

qPCR, formerly called real-time PCR, was developed to allow quantitation of the amount of product [PMID1368485]. qPCR relies on the use of a fluorescent marker that becomes evident when a cycle of PCR is completed. In qPCR, one can see the results of the assay as each cycle is completed. qPCR obviates the need for electrophoresis, either in gels or by capillaries.

There are a number of variants of qPCR, depending largely on the fluorescent marker that is used [PMID16460794]. The TaqMan assay (Applied Biosystems; also called the 5' exonuclease assay) is a form of qPCR in which results can be seen immediately by a change in fluorescence. The TaqMan assay is made possible by the 5' to 3' exonuclease activity of the Taq polymerase. The principle of the TaqMan assay is somewhat similar to the principle of the molecular beacon. It uses a probe that is attached to both a fluorescent molecule and a quencher. The quencher neutralizes the fluorescence. As the probe becomes incorporated into the new DNA during the PCR process, the exonuclease activity cleaves off the fluorescent probe, freeing it from the quencher so that its signal can be detected. Greater fluorescence indicates a greater amount of hybridization and therefore a greater amount of amplified target. A control included, so that the ability of the system to amplify and detect the amplicons can be verified.

Another variant of qPCR uses the dye SYBR green. SYBR green intercalates into double-stranded DNA and then undergoes fluorescence if exposed to its excitation wavelength. Whereas in the TaqMan assay, the signal is generated immediately after hybridization, when the exonuclease activity separates the fluorochrome from the quencher, in the use of SYBR, the signal is generated upon full intercalation into a complete double-stranded DNA, not upon hybridization. An increase in its fluorescence indicates greater product.

Another form of qPCR uses FRET (fluorescence resonance energy transfer) probes. FRET probes are a pair of probes that bind to the same strand of amplified DNA. The 2 probes carry fluorescent molecules that are excited by different wavelengths in such a way that the emission spectrum of the first probe, called the donor, overlaps with the absorption spectrum of the second probe, the acceptor. The wavelength of the light emitted from the first probe, even if not quenched, is too short to be detected by the detector; only if it is absorbed and reemitted at a longer wavelength by the second probe can it be detected. When the probes are not bound, the light that is emitted from the first probe simply leaves the system without detection. But when there has been amplification and hybridization, the 2 probes are close enough so that after the incident light excites the first probe, the light it emits will excite the second probe, which then emits light of a longer wavelength than that emitted by the first probe. This longer wavelength light is detected. Whereas the TaqMan probe is based on exonuclease activity and SYBR green is based on intercalation, FRET probes are based on molecular energy transfer without photon emission between 2 very closely spaced molecules [PMID5233469]. For FRET probes to be effective, the following conditions must be met:

- The amplified segment of DNA must be able to bind 2 probes.
- The detector must not be able to detect either the background light or light emitted by the first probe.
- The excitation wavelength of the first probe must be able to excite the second probe.
- The distance between the 2 bound probes must be short enough that energy transfer can take place. This is usually 2-5 base pairs.
- The detector must be able to detect light from the second probe.

Hybrid systems, using elements of both TaqMan and FRET, have been described [PMID19594451]. In any form of qPCR, the patient sample is mixed with a known amount of the DNA of interest, called the standard or calibrator. In addition to the standard, 2 controls are important in qPCR. The first is a different sequence of DNA, called a reference or specimen processing control, that is also amplified. The amplification characteristics of the reference are well known and reproducible, and its inclusion in the assay proves that the assay is capable of generating high-quality DNA with high efficiency. Failure of the reference to amplify indicates a defect in DNA extraction, if that is one of the instrument's functions, a defective reagent, or the presence of an inhibitor.

The second control has no nucleic acid at all (a so-called water control or probe check control). The purpose of this control is to ensure that there is no significant background fluorescence and that the fluidics of the system work properly.

TaqMan, SYBR green, and FRET probes are 3 ways of producing fluorescence as PCR proceeds. However fluorescence is produced, fluorescence intensity for the standard or the patient sample is plotted on the Y axis against the number of cycles of amplification on the X axis.

qPCR assays have 4 time periods. The first is when there is not yet any discernible amplification and the curve appears flat. The second is a discernible exponential phase of amplification. Although qPCR theoretically has exponential amplification at all times, in practice, a number of factors, such as limited primer availability and exhaustion of fluorescence capacity in the fluorochromes, limit the exponential phase to a brief portion of the total run. The third phase is a linear amplification and the fourth phase is a plateau.

The number of cycles required to obtain a discernible rise over background is called the cycle threshold or crossover threshold, C_T, because at this time, the signal crosses over background threshold and exponential amplification is apparent. The C_T is not the point where the fluorescent signals from the standard and patient samples cross, but the point where either exceeds background. The the number of cycles necessary to pass C_T is inversely proportional to the amount of starting nucleic acid in the sample. The C_T cannot be reliably visualized on a graph because the difference between the fluorescence of the sample and the background fluorescence is very small at this point. One must rely on the instrument's internal calculations to furnish the C_T values for the standard and the unknown.

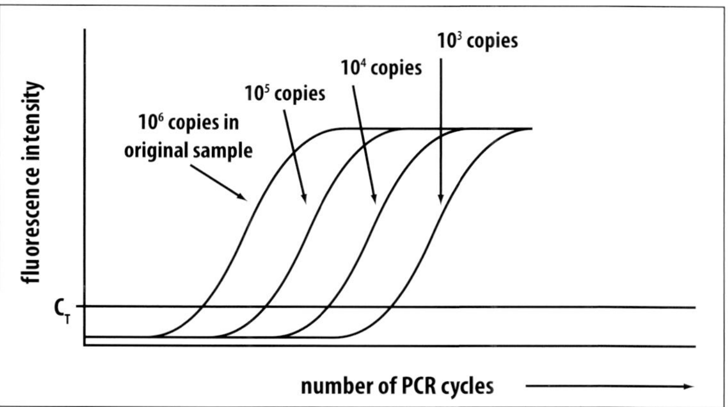

f45.4 Quantitative PCR. Increasing number of PCR cycles is depicted on the X axis and increasing fluorescence intensity on the Y axis. C_T, the point at which fluorescence becomes distinguishable from background, is depicted by a line that is parallel to the X axis. Regardless of the number of copies in the original sample, amplification occurs in 4 phases. First, there is no discernible amplification. Second, there is an exponential phase, the beginning of which is the most important part of the assay. Third, there is a linear phase, and fourth, a plateau phase. Quantitation is derived from the number of cycles required to pass C_T.

Comparisons between the unknown amount of patient nucleic acid and the known amount of standard nucleic acid are not made in the late, linear phase, but rather are made only in the exponential phase, just after there is sufficient amplification to commence the exponential phase f45.4. In most areas of laboratory medicine, we make comparisons in the linear phase, but in qPCR, comparisons are made only in the preceding exponential phase.

There are several ways to perform a quantitative analysis using qPCR. The simplest method, used by many laboratories, is called the comparative C_T method or the δ-δ C_T method. There are 2 C_T values, 1 for the standard sample and 1 for the patient sample. The δ-δ C_T method is the comparison of these 2 C_T values. For example, if the C_T of the standard is 30 (meaning it took 30 cycles of PCR for the fluorescent signal to be significantly above background) and the C_T of the patient is 25, we can say that it took the standard 5 more cycles to rise above background. This tells us that there had to be less standard nucleic acid than patient nucleic acid, since the standard had to undergo 5 more cycles of amplification to reach the same detectable level. Since each cycle is a doubling of nucleic acid, and $2^5 = 32$, there was 32 times as much patient nucleic acid as standard in the sample. The general equation in this method can be written several ways, but is of the form:

$$\text{target DNA in unknown} = [\text{target DNA in standard}] \times 2^{(C_T \text{ of standard} - C_T \text{ of unknown})}$$

In the example above, if there were 1000 copies in the standard, the patient sample would contain $1000 \times 2^{(30-25)}$, or 1000×2^5, which is 1000×32, or 32,000 copies. The comparative C_T method is an approximation that usually assumes there is 100% efficiency of replication with each cycle. In actual practice quantitation must take into account an estimate of efficiency.

A second method of quantitation uses a series of dilutions of a known standard. For example, an aliquot of patient plasma may be compared to 100, 1000, 5000, and 10,000 copies of the viral nucleic acid. For each known copy number of "spiked in" nucleic acid, there will be a given number of PCR cycles until the threshold, C_T, is triggered (the larger the number of added control copies, the lower will be the number of cycles needed to trigger threshold). After all of the runs of known amount are completed, the results are usually plotted as the number of cycles necessary for threshold on the Y axis vs the copy number on the X axis. The patient sample is then allowed to undergo PCR until it reaches threshold. The number of cycles needed for the patient sample to reach threshold is located on the Y axis of the standard curve, and the corresponding X value is obtained.

A third method is called the Pfaffl method, after its inventor, Michael Pfaffl [PMID11328886]. This method is similar to the δ-δ C_T but takes into account the fact that the efficiency of replication is <100% (ie, the number of copies of DNA does not quite double after each cycle) and that the efficiency of replication of the reference gene may differ from that of the gene of interest.

Many qPCR instruments can use multiple fluorochromes, each with a different combination of exciting and emission wavelengths. Each fluorochrome has its own channel, with a detector set to its particular emission wavelength, so that multiple segments of DNA can be tested simultaneously. For example, in searching for methicillin-resistant *Staphylococcus aureus* (MRSA), one channel may be devoted to a segment of DNA that is indicative of *Staphylococcus aureus* in general, while a second channel detects the MRSA gene.

There are 2 general caveats in viral load testing. First, it is important not to compare results obtained by different methods. Certainly, results obtained by any of the qPCR methods should not be compared to a non-PCR method, and even results obtained by different forms of qPCR should not be compared if possible. Second, even in the best of laboratories, the same specimen run by the same technique may generate a difference of up to 30%. A C_T difference of 1.0, while theoretically implying a 2-fold difference, is considered within experimental error and therefore clinically insignificant. Only C_T values that imply a 3-fold or greater difference (ie, C_T differences of about 1.7 or more) are considered significant, and major clinical decisions are generally not made unless there is a 10-fold increase in viral load, corresponding to a C_T difference of 3.3. If there is a 10-fold increase in viral load during therapy, it is wise to confirm with a second result demonstrating the same findings. If such confirmation is obtained, resistance to the antiviral regimen being employed is likely and should be confirmed by viral genotyping.

Viral load (quantitation) studies are usually done on plasma, not on tissue. In the case of the BK virus, there are large amounts in urine, but plasma is the preferred specimen. Hepatitis C and HIV are the 2 RNA viruses that are often quantitated. This is usually done by conversion to cDNA, followed by qPCR. In these 2 viruses, it is important to promptly separate the plasma. Otherwise, proviral DNA (cDNA that has been made from viral RNA but has not yet been incorporated into the host's genome) will leak out from the cell into the plasma and give spuriously high results.

As is the case for PCR in general, qPCR is excellent for the detection of known allelic variations or variations in the copy number of a repeating sequence, but it is not good for the detection of inversions, deletions, or translocations. FISH is often the technique of choice in these situations.

A final comment on PCR testing is that it requires rigorous technique to avoid contamination. The products of PCR may become aerosolized and travel to another part of the laboratory, where they may become inappropriate substrates for PCR activity in that area. Research PCR laboratories are rigorously designed to prevent amplicons from traveling. Work areas employ a unidirectional flow of work so that amplified DNA cannot return to the amplification area (for example, on a worker's clothing). PCR reactions are generally set up in a hood, both to minimize unwanted DNA from spreading throughout the laboratory and to minimize dust (which has DNA) from entering into the reaction. Close attention is given to air flow. Separate areas for preparation, processing, and detection are required, with unidirectional passage.

These requirements are substantially mitigated in PCR instruments that are designed for routine clinical use because these instruments are self-contained, multichambered, and closed, with the use of reagents that bind to and inactivate amplicons to prevent their being transferred from one chamber to another. These commercially available instruments have largely addressed the concerns of aerosolization and contamination, but these remain serious concerns in research use. In most cases, single, self-contained instruments can be obtained and placed without difficulty, but if the laboratory is considering performing large amounts of PCR testing with multiple instruments, it might be wise to visit several existing laboratories to learn how they perform QA and comply with the many regulations of such testing.

Other Methods of DNA Amplification

PCR is only 1 of a number of nucleic acid amplification methods. Another procedure is ligase chain reaction (LCR) [PMID2744765]. In contrast to PCR, in ligase chain reaction, the actual sequence to be amplified must be known, but not the flanking sequences. The DNA to be examined is first heated to create 2 separate strands. After cooling, 4 oligonucleotide probes, 2 for each strand, are allowed to hybridize on each strand. On each strand, both probes hybridize within the actual sequence to be amplified, not on its periphery, and they bind to immediately adjacent sites. These are large probes, so that together, the 2 adjacent probes on each stand hybridize to the entirety of the sequence to be amplified, but the 2 probes are not joined to each other. If—and only if—both probes are a perfect match for the original strand, DNA ligase will ligate them, in which case the resulting single probe hybridizes completely to the original target sequence and the original double-stranded DNA of the target sequence is perfectly reconstituted. The temperature is then raised to cause denaturation and the process is repeated, resulting in amplification. If there is even a single nucleotide mismatch in the hybridization of any probe to the target DNA, DNA ligase will not work, the original DNA is not reconstituted, and there is no amplification. Because the sequences of the probes correspond to the wild-type sequence, any mismatch means that the patient's sample contains a mutation. Therefore, absence of amplification implies the presence of a mutation.

The technique could also be used to search for a specific, known mutation by designing probes that would only anneal to that specific mutation and therefore would only be ligated if that mutation is present, in which case amplification implies the presence of that particular mutation. Because the target sequence must be known, LCR is not suitable for gene research but is excellent at identifying subtle mutations (even a single nucleotide) that have been characterized.

Ligation-dependent PCR (LD-PCR) is a variant of ligase chain reaction that also uses 2 hemiprobes that bind to immediately adjacent areas on one strand of target DNA. These hemiprobes are separated by only a tiny nick, as in ligase chain reaction. If and only if there is perfect hybridization of the probes to the target DNA, DNA ligase will ligate the 2 hemiprobes, resulting in a single strand of DNA, complementary to the original target, which is then amplified by traditional PCR. PCR occurs not on the original target sequence itself, but on the ligated, complementary hemiprobes. PCR cannot occur unless the 2 hemiprobes are ligated, and ligation cannot occur unless both probes have perfectly hybridized to the target. Because in LD-PCR, the hemiprobes are selected to match a specific abnormal allele, perfect hybridization—and hence PCR and the visualization of an amplicon on electrophoresis—can occur only if that specific abnormal allele is present on the original patient DNA.

Multiple pairs of hemiprobes, each designed to anneal to a particular known abnormality, can be employed in the same test, permitting the simultaneous testing of multiple possible abnormal foci. After PCR, all of the amplicons can be simultaneously taken and electrophoresed. The finding of any amplified band indicates an abnormality in the original DNA. Any amplicons that are present can be sequenced. The major clinical variant of LD-PCR is oligonucleotide ligation assay (OLA), which we will encounter in our consideration of cystic fibrosis.

LD-PCR can also be performed in a multiplex manner, wherein multiple sites are simultaneously investigated using a single set of primers. This is called multiplex ligation-dependent probe amplification (MLPA) **f45.5** [PMID12060695, PMID19557334]. MLPA is a form of multiplex PCR in which multiple

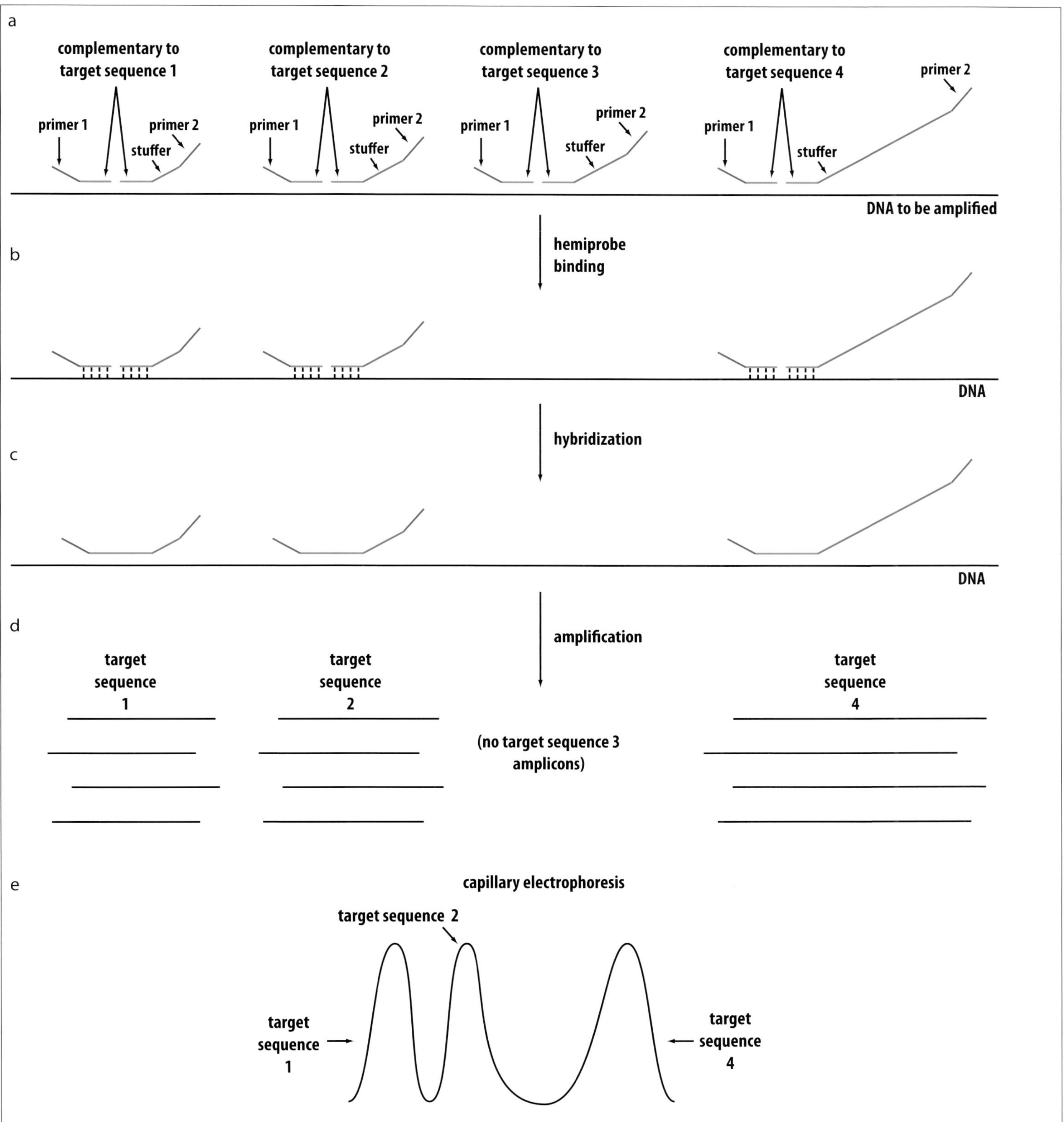

f45.5 Multiplex ligation-dependent probe amplification (MLPA). In MLPA, multiple different sequences can be simultaneously targeted and amplified. The same set of primers is used for all target sequences.
a The solid black line is the DNA with multiple sequences of interest. For each sequence of interest, the probe is divided into 2 hemiprobes. In this diagram, all hemiprobes are green, even though they each recognize a different target sequence. Each hemiprobe is attached to 1 of the 2 primers. A stuffer sequence of a variable length that corresponds to the specificity of the hemiprobe is inserted between one of the hemiprobes and the primer. The primers and the stuffers do not bind to the DNA.
b The hemiprobes bind to their target sequences, if present.
c After all hybridization has occurred, a ligase enzyme will join the 2 hemiprobes into a single probe if they have bound to the sample DNA.
d After ligation, PCR is simultaneously carried out, using the single set of primers, on all bound probes. Only hemiprobes that have been bound and ligated are amplified. Because target sequence 3 was not present in the sample, the hemiprobes specific for it did not bind and neither they, nor the stuffer sequence attached to them, were amplified. Because target sequences 1, 2, and 4 were present, the hemiprobes specific for them bound, were ligated, and amplified. Although the stuffers and primers did not bind to the sample DNA, they are included in the amplifications, resulting in amplicons of different lengths. Because the lengths of the stuffers correspond to the specificity of the attached hemiprobe, the final lengths of the amplicons correspond to a unique sequence of target DNA on the original sample.
e After capillary electrophoresis, the result is 3 amplicons of different lengths resulting from stuffer sequences whose lengths were chosen to correspond to hemiprobes specific for targets 1, 2, and 4.

targets—up to 50 at this writing—are simultaneously amplified using different probes for each target sequence, but only 1 pair of primers. Each of the probes consists of 2 hemiprobes, one of which has a stuffer sequence added to it. This stuffer sequence has no function except to make the length of that hemiprobe different from the length of any other hemiprobe for any other target. The length of the stuffer sequence is coordinated with the specificity of the hemiprobe. For example, if a hemiprobe hybridizes to gene A, it might have a stuffer sequence of 100 base pairs. If another hemiprobe hybridizes to gene B, the stuffer might be 200 base pairs, etc.

Each of the 2 hemiprobes contains a sequence that will specifically hybridize to the target DNA and also a sequence that will not. The portions of the 2 hemiprobes that are specific for any given target bind at adjacent sites so that they are separated by only 1 base pair. After the 2 hemiprobes hybridize to the target DNA, a ligase will concatenate them into a single probe. There is now 1 probe, with 2 sequences of unbound DNA, 1 at each end, derived from the portions of the hemiprobes that were not designed to be complementary to any target. At one end of the bound probe, the unbound DNA is the stuffer DNA, whose length uniquely corresponds to the target sequence.

The cleverness of MLPA lies in what happens at these unbound ends. The nonspecific portions of the hemiprobes—now the unbound ends of a single probe—contain the only sites that are recognized by the 2 primers. The same pair of primers is used for any number of targets. One of the primers is fluorescently labeled. After hybridization and ligation, what is actually amplified and measured is not the target DNA itself, but the probes, including the unbound portions of the probes that are not complementary to the target DNA, one of which contains a stuffer sequence. Because of the labeled primer and the different-sized stuffer sequences for each target, PCR results in fluorescently labeled amplicons that are of different length for each individual target. After amplification, the amplicons are separated by capillary electrophoresis. By comparing the fluorescence for that target—identified by its length—to a control, the amount of each target sequence can be determined. A technical concern with MLPA is that after ligation, the stuffer sequences result in long probes that can be difficult to work with.

MLPA is a leading method of detecting copy number variation (CNV), and in fact, was developed for that purpose. CNV refers to areas of the genome, 1,000 bases or larger, that are present in more or less than the expected 2 copies (eg, a copy number of 1 is loss of heterozygosity [LOH]). The affected area may or may not correspond to 1 or more distinct genes. CNVs are basically the same as deletions or duplications, but also include such entities as trisomies (which would not be considered a duplication) and abnormally large numbers of trinucleotide repeating units found in some diseases such as Huntington disease and fragile X. In contrast to deletions or duplications, which are unbalanced chromosomal abnormalities, inversions and reciprocal translocations, while of immense potential clinical significance, are balanced chromosomal abnormalities and therefore are not examples of CNV. CNVs have been associated with numerous diseases, including many cancers. CNVs can be detected by direct sequencing, though this is often impractical, and are increasingly identified by microarrays (discussed subsequently).

Isothermal Nucleic Acid Amplification Techniques

A variety of other techniques to amplify nucleic acids have been formulated that do not require the temperature cycling [PMID18260008, PMID16111667], though automated thermocycling has made temperature cycling more convenient.

Nucleic acid sequence-based amplification (NASBA) is an isothermal process that is used for RNA amplification and is especially used to study RNA viruses. The initial steps of NASBA are similar to those of RT-PCR, but its product is RNA, not DNA. NASBA uses 3 enzymes—reverse transcriptase, RNase, and RNA polymerase (an enzyme not used in RT-PCR) [PMID1706072]. The process starts when one primer binds to the RNA molecule that is of interest, permitting reverse transcriptase to make a single-stranded cDNA molecule, resulting in a hybrid DNA:RNA molecule. RNase then cleaves the RNA strand, after which a second primer binds to the DNA strand. DNA-dependent DNA polymerase activity of the reverse transcriptase then generates double-stranded DNA copies that have an intact RNA polymerase promoter. RNA polymerase then generates RNA copies from this DNA. In addition to being an isothermal process, the product is the actual RNA itself, making this a good technique for studying RNA. There is a quantitative variant of this technology that allows quantitation of target RNA.

A related technique is transcription-mediated amplification (also called self-sustained sequence replication) **f45.6**. Transcription-mediated amplification can begin with DNA or RNA, but usually starts with RNA, often ribosomal RNA. The RNA is converted into double-stranded DNA by reverse transcriptase, as in NASBA, after which RNA polymerase transcribes the DNA, generating amplified RNA. The RNA products are then acted on again by reverse transcriptase. There is amplification from the multiple copies of double-stranded DNA produced from RNA by reverse transcriptase and also from the multiple copies of RNA produced from the double-stranded DNA template by RNA polymerase. This process is particularly suited for amplification of ribosomal RNA because this is usually present in large quantities, providing ample starting material. The procedure is also technically simpler because only a single temperature is required, a single tube can be used, a nucleic acid purification step is not required, and there is less risk of contamination from unwanted RNA because it is less stable than DNA.

The usual means of detection in transcription-mediated amplification is the hybridization protection assay, wherein labeled commercial probes hybridize to the amplified RNA. After hybridization, any free label is hydrolyzed, but the label on those probes that has hybridized to the RNA is protected within the double helix and can be detected.

The APTIMA and PACE systems by Genprobe for *Chlamydia trachomatis* and *Neisseria gonorrhoea* do not use PCR amplification. Both target rRNA (specifically, the 23S rRNA that is found in the larger subunit of the ribosome). The PACE system is a direct hybridization of a labeled probe to the rRNA without amplification. The Aptima system amplifies the RNA target by transcription-mediated amplification. Genprobe also has a

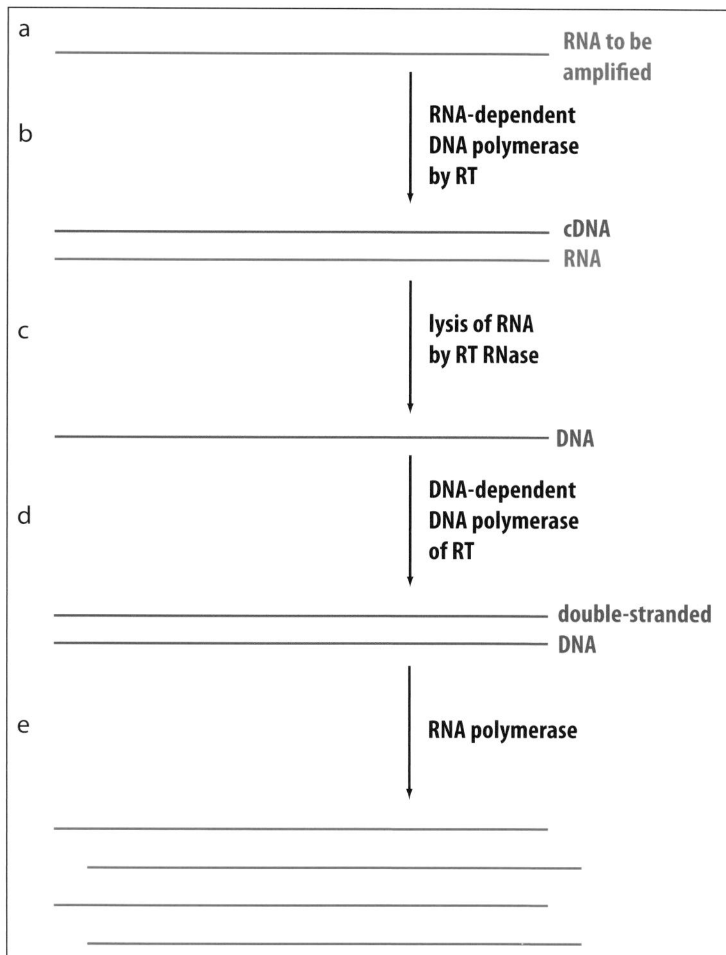

f45.6 Transcription-mediated amplification. **a** is the RNA to be amplified. In **b**, after action of RNA-dependent DNA polymerase of reverse transcriptase, there is a heteroduplex of RNA and cDNA. In **c**, there is only a single stranded DNA molecule after the action of the RNase portion of the RT. In **d**, the action of the DNA-dependent DNA polymerase of RT has resulted in a double-stranded DNA molecule. In **e**, the action of RNA polymerase, a different enzyme, has resulted in the transcription of the double-stranded DNA and multiple copies of RNA, which can be amplified in the same manner as the original starting RNA.

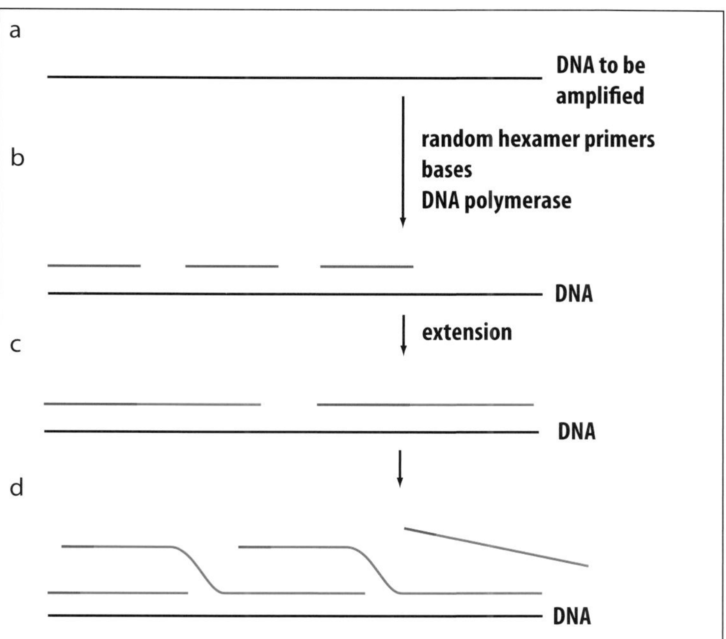

f45.7 Strand displacement amplification. **a** is the DNA to be amplified.
In **b** primers, usually random hexamers, are added along with bases and DNA polymerase, resulting in the extension that is seen in **c**.
In **d**, each newly synthesized DNA strand undermines and displaces the strand in front of it. The displaced strands, consisting of the 6-base pair primer and the extension, float away. In practice, polymerization begins on the new strands before they detach, forming hyperbranched structures.

variety of tests called Accuprobe that are nonamplified tests based on a chemiluminescent DNA probe that will hybridize to an rRNA of the target organism.

The strand displacement amplification (SDA) **f45.7** method of isothermal nucleic acid amplification relies on the synthesis of successive strands of DNA from the same site displacing previously synthesized strands [PMID1309614]. The DNA is denatured and mixed with an excess of 4 primers, 2 for each strand, in the presence of DNA polymerase. For each strand, both primers are on the same side of the target area, not on opposite sides as in PCR. Each of these 4 primers contains a recognition site for a restriction endonuclease because the DNA polymerase requires a nick in the double-stranded DNA. After denaturation, primer binding, and endonuclease nicking, DNA polymerase extends both strands from 2 locations, 1 at each primer. On each strand, the extension of the outermost primer displaces the product of the innermost primer. This produces 2 displaced fragments of DNA, arising from the inner primers of each strand. Extension of these displaced fragments in the opposite direction produces DNA that contains binding sites for the outer primers. After both sets of primers again bind to the newly-synthesized DNA, the process repeats. The result is exponential amplification of both strands of the original target DNA. In the most common use today, called multiple SDA, the same process occurs simultaneously at multiple sites.

Detection in SDA is by a fluorescent probe that hybridizes to the target DNA and is in real time, concomitant with amplification. SDA is available commercially for the detection of *Chlamydia trachomatis* and *Neisseria gonorrhoea* (the ProbeTec assay by Becton-Dickinson, an alternative to GenProbe).

Signal Amplification Techniques

Rather than amplifying the nucleic acid of interest (target amplification), some tests are designed to increase the sensitivity of detection by amplifying the signal (signal amplification). Branched chain nucleic acid technology is one such method. Branched chain technology increases the sensitivity of detection through a series of hybridizations. The process commences with a commercially available capture probe that is covalently bound to a well. The target nucleic acid hybridizes to this probe. Additional commercially available capture probe is then hybridized to the portion of the target protruding from the probe-target hybrid. Additional target nucleic acid then binds to the portion of the capture material that protrudes from the probe-target hybrid. This process is repeated and generates multiple sites for detection. Eventually, capture probe with a detection signal is used.

Branched nucleic acid detection permits quantitation of viral load in some cases, though PCR is replacing this technique.

Melting Curve Analysis

In melting curve analysis [PMID11901805] (MCA; also called melting point analysis or melting analysis), the primers are not allele specific. Rather, PCR is performed across the entire area to be studied, be it normal or abnormal. After amplification, a labeled probe that is specific to the wild-type sequence is used. This probe will bind an abnormal area less strongly. The probe's fluorescence is stronger when it is hybridized and weaker when it separates from the patient's DNA. The temperature is gradually increased, and the change in fluorescence is measured. Typically, the temperature is on the X axis and the fluorescence on the Y axis. Because in the mutant allele, the 2 strands are not as tightly bound, there will be a more rapid reduction of fluorescence in the abnormal sample as temperature increases, creating a peak to the left of that seen in the wild-type. A bimodal peak will be seen in a heterozygous patient. Usually, the fluorescent data is converted to a negative derivative curve (–dF/dT) by software, and this is plotted against temperature so that on the graph, the decrease in fluorescence appears as an upward peak **f45.8** [PMID18502416]. Standards of known sequence are generally run for comparison **f45.9**.

There is also a variant of MCA that uses a label (SYBR green) that is only fluorescent when bound to double-stranded DNA rather than a label that is attached to the actual probe itself. SYBR green is not fluorescent in the presence of single-stranded DNA. Fluorescence falls as temperature rises, and again falls faster for a mutant allele because the probe binds less strongly.

At this writing, high resolution MCA is being used in ever-greater number of assays because it obviates the need for allele-specific primers. In addition, high resolution MCA can often detect subtle sequence variations that might escape detection by PCR because the latter method may proceed normally in the presence of a minimal variation in sequence if the primers can hybridize to the abnormal area. In many cases, an SNP can be detected by high resolution MCA. While we may think of DNA sequencing as the "last word" in molecular pathology, the resolution of MCA can even surpass that of direct sequencing for some heterozygous mutations and in somatic mosaicism [PMID19418555]. LNAs are sometimes used in MCA because they result in higher melting temperatures and can better discrimination between normal and abnormal sequences [PMID12528362]. The Roche LightCycler is a commonly used instrument that combines qPCR with MCA [PMID19196999]. In addition to the detection of mutations, MCA is also used to detect CNVs and the presence of methylation.

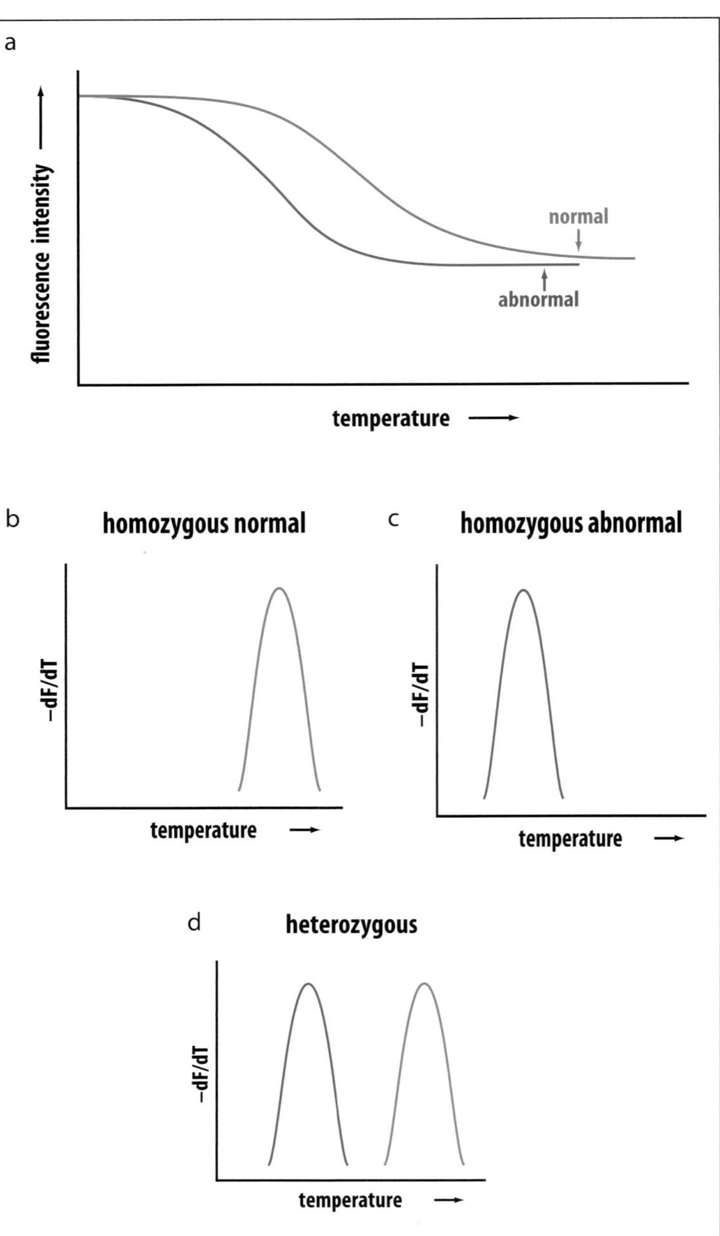

f45.8 Melting curve analysis. In **a**, a fluorochrome is used that fluoresces more intensely if it is part of a duplex and less brightly if it is not hybridized. Increasing temperature is shown on the X axis and increasing fluorescence intensity is on the Y axis (fluorescence change by temperatures, ie dF/dT). Because the normal DNA, with perfect base-pairing, is bound more tightly, the fluorescent probe tends to remain in a duplex and higher temperature is required to separate the strand and cause a decrease in fluorescence. For a given temperature, fluorochromes that are part of an abnormal DNA structure, with mismatched base pairs, are bound less tightly and therefore fluoresce less intensely than normal DNA. In **b**, homozygous normal, significant temperature is required to result in melting of the 2 DNA strands. In **c**, homozygous abnormal, separation of the strands, and reduction in fluorescence, is achieved at a lower temperature. In **d**, there is a heterozygous state. The 2 strands of DNA in the normal chromosome (red) separate at higher temperature, while the 2 strands of DNA in the abnormal chromosome (blue) separate at a lower temperature.

In Situ Hybridization and FISH

Hybridization—the binding of a probe to a target—can occur in solution, or on a number of commercially available substrates. Here, we consider ISH, in which hybridization of a sequence of nucleic acid which is bound to a reporter probe to a target occurs in the cell of interest **f45.10**. The advantage of ISH is that the results can be correlated with morphology because the precise location of the target nucleic acid within a cell can be determined. In the case of some viruses, it is possible to determine if the viral nucleic acid has integrated in to the host DNA or not.

ISH often uses a fluorescent-labeled probe that binds to a target. This is FISH. FISH grew out of the use of fluorescent compounds that adhere to individual proteins to identify

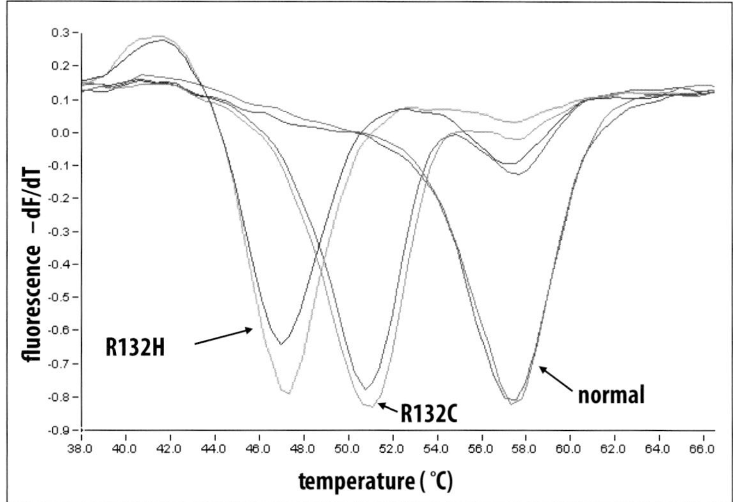

f45.9 Melting curve analysis for the gene *ICD1* (coding for the protein isocitrate dehydrogenase), which is important in some gliomas (see Chapter 41). Peaks usually rise (see f45.8), but in this particular version of the technique, they are inverted (and each peak records in duplicate). At the right is the pair of curves for the homozygous normal form of the gene, melting (ie, dissociating) at the highest temperature. At left is the pair of curves for a patient who is homozygous for an allele that codes for the R132H form or the protein. The decrease in fluorescence, indicating dissociation, occurs at a lower temperature. The center pair of curves represents a patient who is homozygous for an allele that codes for the R132C form of the protein.

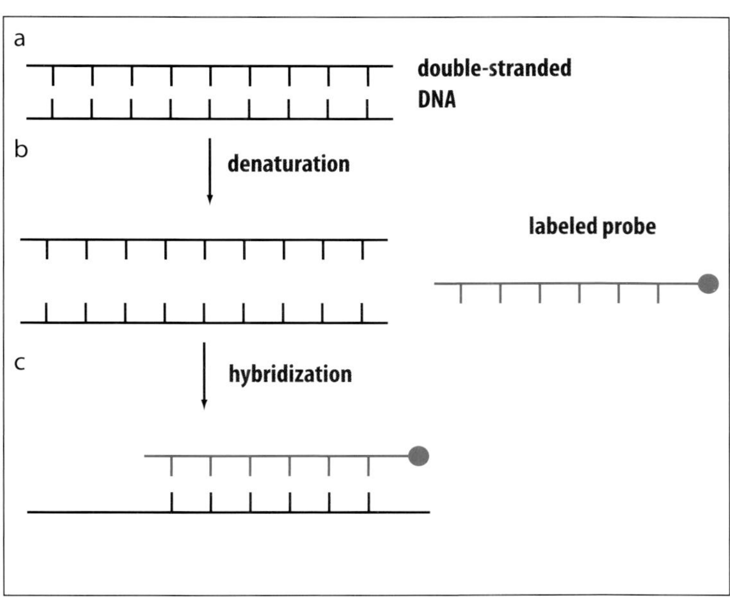

f45.10 The principle of hybridization and gene probes. In **a**, there is double-stranded DNA that contains the sequence of interest. In **b**, after denaturation, a portion of nucleic acid with a reporter molecule, called a probe, is added, after which the DNA is returned to conditions that favor hybridization. In **c**, if the target sequence is present, the probe will bind to it and this binding will be detectable by the reporter molecule, usually by fluorescence.

both the intracellular location of the protein and follow its movement in the cell. After this technology, involving only proteins, was mastered, fluorescent probes that bound to nucleic acids were developed. In FISH, the probe is a specifically designed sequence of nucleic acid—usually DNA—that is labeled with a fluorescent compound and the target is DNA or RNA from the patient to be tested. After exposure of the patient sample to the probe and a washing step, the presence of the fluorochrome in the sample indicates that the target sequence is present. Because fluorescence microscopy is required, the target may have a weak fluorescent counterstain to permit it to be seen, but the primary fluorescent material is the probe.

3 commonly used fluorochromes in FISH are FITC (also commonly called fluorescein), rhodamine, and Texas red. FITC absorbs light of about 495 nm and emits at about 525 nm, in the green part of the spectrum. Rhodamine absorbs at 540-560 nm and emits at 580 nm, in the orange/red portion of the spectrum. Texas red absorbs at 596 nm and emits at 615 nm, in the red portion of the spectrum.

FISH can also be done with PNAs, analogues of nucleic acids that contain a base, but also have a peptide bond. PNA-FISH is often used to identify organisms using a fluorescein-labeled PNA probe attached to a polyamine backbone that diffuses into the cell and binds its target, usually the gene coding for one of the RNA molecules in ribosomes.

Limitations of FISH

FISH is usually not as good as pcr for single nucleotide polymorphisms. FISH is rarely used to detect minimal abnormalities such as an SNP because the probe is sufficiently large (a typical size for a probe is 8-10 kilobases) that it will "forgive" a small mismatch and hybridize to the abnormal area as well it does to the normal nucleic acid. Allele-specific PCR is better for SNPs because PCR primers are much shorter than FISH probes and are much more likely to be significantly affected by small mutations (the corollary of this is that PCR is often poor at detecting larger inversions or deletions because the primers cannot amplify over a large gap). Other difficulties with FISH are that it requires a fluorescent microscope and that the signal fades with time. Fluorescent signals will last longer at cold temperatures, but will still fade after some months. For this reason, fluorescent images are either photographed or captured on a digital imaging system.

FISH works well on many types of preparations. The 2 major exceptions are that is does not work well in tissue that has been fixed in something other than formalin, and it does not work well in tissue that has been decalcified. It should also be restated that because of the large size of the probe used in FISH, it is "forgiving" in situations where only 1-2 base pairs are mismatched, so it is not as good as PCR in identifying single nucleotide polymorphisms.

There is a colorimetric (also called chromogenic) ISH (CISH) that works like FISH, except the detection is colorimetric rather than fluorescent. CISH is also called brightfield ISH because it uses an ordinary brightfield microscope. CISH assays potentially offer easier use, since a fluorescent microscope is not needed, and the signal is stable. CISH assays for the nucleic acid of HPV and EBV have been established, but at this writing it remains to be seen if CISH assays will provide sufficient sensitivity in all situations to completely replace FISH. Moreover, as we will see, fluorochromes can be used in combination to create a large number of colors. The colors available in colorimetric methods are much more limited and cannot be combined to offer the gradations that fluorochromes afford. Rarely, ISH is performed with a silver stain (SISH).

FISH Preparation

FISH probes must be labeled, and both the probe and the target must be prepared for hybridization. Most clinical laboratories purchase their FISH probes, but for the daring that wish to make them, the steps in the process involve producing the DNA that is to be used as the probe (using either cloning technologies or PCR), labeling it with a fluorochrome, and subjecting the probe to preannealing steps so that it will be able to anneal to the target sequence.

Labeling the probe consists of ensuring that some of its nucleotides will be labeled with a reporter molecule. There are 2 ways to include a reporter molecule. The first is an indirect method, in which reporter compounds that are not fluorescent, but which can subsequently be attached to fluorescent labels, are joined to the nucleotides of the probe. The 2 most commonly used nonfluorescent reporter compounds are biotin, a naturally occurring vitamin in the B-complex family, and digoxigenin, a plant compound that like digoxin, is obtained from *Digitalis*. Biotin has a natural affinity for avidin, and in a biotin-based system, avidin is attached to fluorochromes. In a biotin system, after probe-target hybridization, avidin-fluorochrome is added. If the probe has bound, the avidin-fluorochrome will bind to the biotin on the probe. In the other common indirect labeling method, digoxigenin is attached to the probe and after hybridization to the target, antibodies to digoxigenin, attached to fluorochromes, are added. If the probe has bound, the digoxigenin will bind the antibody-fluorochrome.

If the target sequence is short, or if interphase cells are used, it may be necessary to amplify the signal. If the original reporter molecule was biotin, additional layers of biotin that bind to the fluorochrome-conjugated avidin may be needed, so that there are more binding sites for additional fluorochrome-conjugated avidin. In the case of digoxigenin, one may elect not to conjugate the digoxigenin antibody to the fluorochrome, but rather to employ antibodies to the original digoxigenin antibodies and attach the fluorochrome to this second antibody, so that there will be a greater accumulation of fluorochrome around the digoxigenin. Such procedures of colloquially referred to as "stacking."

The second method of labeling is direct labeling, in which a fluorochrome is directly attached to the nucleotides that will be incorporated into the DNA probe. This leads to immediate fluorescence as soon as the probe binds the target. These probes are more expensive and typically generate a slightly weaker signal, but they are quicker and easier to use. "Stacking" is rarely used in direct labeling.

Whether indirect or direct labeling is employed, the nucleotides carrying the reporter molecules or the compounds that will react with the reporter must be introduced into the double-stranded cloned DNA that is to become the probe. One could simply use an enzyme to add a labeled nucleotide to one end of the probe, but this results in a probe that carries only 1 label and will therefore generate a weak signal. It is better to use a process that continually incorporates label during synthesis, so that the probe will carry many labeled nucleotides. This is often done by PCR, in which case, if the primers are correctly designed, labeled nucleotides will continuously be incorporated into the growing chain.

Another way to incorporate label throughout the probe is a process called nick translation. Nick translation uses 2 enzymes. The first is a eukaryotic DNase that nicks 1 of the 2 strands of DNA. The second enzyme is the prokaryotic enzyme DNA polymerase I, which in prokaryotes functions in DNA replication both to excise the RNA primer and to replace those bases with DNA. In nick translation, DNA polymerase I attaches to the site that has been nicked by the eukaryotic DNase, removes about 10 base pairs, then fills in the gap using the labeled nucleotides.

Less commonly, probe labeling occurs by random primer extension, in which the DNA to be labeled is denatured and labeled nucleotides are added in the presence of random primers. If this method is used, it is necessary to use a DNA polymerase that does not have exonuclease activity in the 5' to 3' direction, as this is the direction of synthesis and any such exonuclease activity will negate incorporation. Prokaryotic DNA polymerase I has exonuclease activity in both directions, but if it is treated with a protease, it is split into 2 fragments, the larger of which retains polymerase activity and an exonuclease activity in the 3' to 5' direction, but not in the 5' to 3' direction. This is called a Klenow fragment and will add labeled nucleotides to DNA in the presence of oligonucleotide primers (a Klenow fragment can also be produced from a gene that has been truncated).

Before the probe is ready for use, it must undergo a number of preparatory steps. Because repetitive sequences are found throughout the genome, both probe and target DNA may contain repetitive sequences. If both probe and target do contain repetitive sequences, when they are denatured and exposed to each other, hybridization of counterpart sequences in the repetitive regions will cause nonspecific hybridization that interferes with the specific hybridization signal that is sought. Signals from repetitive sequences can be substantially diminished by adding a mixture of commonly found repetitive DNA sequences to the probe prior to exposure to the target. Such DNA is called blocking DNA. By binding to repetitive DNA sequences in the probe, blocking DNA makes them unavailable for binding to the target. Cot-1 is a fragment of human DNA that is composed primarily of repeating sequences and is often used as blocking DNA. Most commercially available probes have already been "blocked."

The target must also be prepared. There are 2 requirements for the target. It must be fixed, so that its morphology is preserved and can be visualized, and its cell membranes must be rendered permeable, so that the probe can enter the cell and find its way to the chromosomes. Targets such as blood and bone marrow smears can generally be prepared with simple, time-honored techniques that are very similar to those used for the old G-banding procedures. Archival materials, such as formalin-fixed, paraffin-embedded tissue blocks require special techniques to remove the paraffin and permit access of the probe to the target. Considerable experience has been gained in this area and established, reasonably effective procedures are now well in hand for many commonly used probes.

The second phase of target preparation is a pretreatment that will facilitate hybridization with the probe. There are a number of protocols for specific situations. For example, in some situations, positive charges on the target must be neutralized to permit access of the probe. In other situations (especially when the target is derived from a paraffin block, where there has been precipitation or cross-linking of proteins), proteinases and detergents may be needed.

The target DNA must then be denatured to permit access of the probe. High salt favors duplex formation by neutralizing the negative charge of the phosphate groups. Low temperature also favors the double-stranded form. Consequently, before there can be hybridization, the target is typically exposed to a low salt and high temperature. In addition, a compound called formamide promotes dissociation of the DNA duplex into single strands by lowering the melting temperature (T_m is the temperature at which 50% of the duplexes have been separated into single strands) to a more convenient number.

Many protocols simultaneously denature both the probe and the target. Often, both the target and the probe are quickly chilled after denaturation, so that they cannot re-form duplexes until exposed to each other. Finally, additional blocking DNA must be added to diminish nonspecific binding that is unrelated to repetitive sites or even to base pairing. This second set of blocking DNA need not be of human origin, and in fact, DNA from herring or salmon sperm is often used for this purpose.

The probe is now ready to anneal to the target. In addition to salt concentration and the presence or absence of formamide, the percentage of G-C base pairs influences T_m because these pairs have 3 hydrogen bonds whereas adenine and thymine share only 2 such bonds. Finally, the length of the probe is important because longer probes bind with greater stability. All of these factors are expressed in the following equation:

$$T_m \text{ (in Celsius)} = 81.5 + 16.6(\log_{10}[\text{Na+}]) + 0.41(\%\text{G} + \text{C}) - 0.63(\%\text{formamide}) - (600/\text{L})$$

where T_m is the melting temperature that must be attained to denature the DNA and allow target-probe hybridization and L is the length of the probe.

Once the probe and the target are heated to T_m and combined, the actual hybridization usually takes from 3 to 12 hours. Longer times provide for greater hybridization, but also permit more nonspecific binding, and one must balance sensitivity and specificity.

After hybridization of probe and target, washing steps are needed to remove nonspecifically bound probe. As is the case for all steps in the FISH process, considerable experience is needed to determine the precise constituents and temperature of the washing solutions. For example, if the washing solution is too warm, it may remove some specific signal. On the other hand, if there is high background fluorescence, one may need to wash at a higher temperature, with a different washing solution, or for a longer time.

A weakly fluorescent background stain is used to allow the observer to see the chromosomes. Propidium iodide and DAPI (4,6 diamino-2-phenyl-indole) are often used for this purpose. The former fluoresces red-orange and is conveniently used when the signal of interest is green (such as in fluorescein-labeled probes). The latter fluoresces blue and is a good counterstain for green (fluorescein), red (rhodamine), or orange (orange spectrum) probes.

FISH Is Limited to Characterized Abnormalities

A major application of FISH is in cytogenetics, but it can only detect previously characterized abnormalities. In all of the many applications of FISH, because the probe must be specifically designed, it can only be used to detect the presence or absence of previously identified chromosomal aberrations. It cannot be used to identify new abnormalities.

Many of the uses of FISH pertain to cytogenetics, and FISH is in essence the next generation of cytogenetic techniques. In addition to the opportunity to correlate with morphology, FISH is also more sensitive than conventional metaphase cytogenetics and permits the detection of abnormalities that are beyond the sensitivity of the older technique. FISH can be done on paraffin section, on smears, or on disaggregated nuclei from a paraffin block, and may be used to assess DNA or mRNA. The major types of FISH probes in cytogenetics are locus-specific (looking for a particular abnormality, often translocations), centromeric (used for chromosome identification), subtelomeric, telomeric, and whole chromosome paints.

When FISH is used to detect monosomy or trisomy, metaphase spreads are used and a fluorescent probe that is complementary to the centromere of the chromosome to be tested for is applied. It is not simply a matter of counting signals in the test cells; normal controls are run concurrently and the cells of interest are compared to the control group. The mean number of signals for the control group should certainly be close to 2 but will rarely be exactly 2. For the control group, the mean and standard deviation is obtained. If a cell being tested has a number of signals that is above or below 2 standard deviations from the control group, it is considered to have an abnormality in the number of that chromosome. On the other hand, if the tested cell has a signal number that is within 2 standard deviations of the control mean, it is considered to have a normal number of that chromosome. Care must be taken to count only in areas in which the cells are not overlapping and in which the nuclei are intact and the chromosomes are well seen. 2 signals that are very close together or are separated by only a thin fluorescent strand are counted as a single signal.

In microdeletion analysis, metaphases are generally studied and a fluorescent DNA probe that is complementary to the DNA that may be deleted is used. After hybridization, a significant loss of fluorescent signal implies a microdeletion. Again, one cannot simply examine the test cells in isolation. A fluorescent DNA probe for part of the chromosome, typically the centromere, is labeled with a fluorochrome of a different color to distinguish it from the test DNA probe and used as a control to ensure that an apparent deletion is not caused by a diminished number of chromosomes.

Whereas metaphase chromosomes are used in determinations of chromosome number and in microdeletion studies, translocations are usually detected with interphase chromosomes. Using FISH for translocations is more problematic from an interpretational viewpoint because it is not just a matter of presence or absence of signal. A common procedure is to employ DNA probes that are specific for the portions of DNA that are on either side of the possible translocation, not for the abnormal DNA itself. In one form of testing, a different color conjugate is used for each side. In normal situations, where there is no translocation, the 2 colors are so close together that they merge into a single, intermediate color. In

ISBN 978-089189-5886

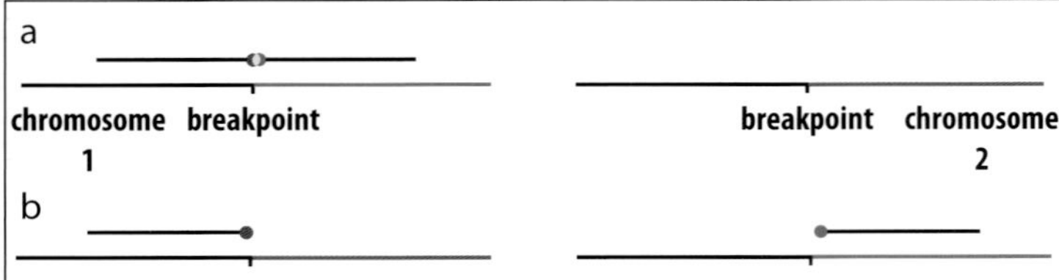

f145.11 Break apart FISH strategy. **a** depicts 2 normal chromosomes. In chromosome 1 the DNA to the left of the breakpoint is black, while the DNA to the right of the breakpoint is red. In chromosome 2, the DNA to the left of the breakpoint is black while the DNA to the right of the breakpoint is green. Sequences of DNA that are complementary to the sequences immediately on either side of the breakpoint, labeled with fluorescence probes of different colors, come to rest immediately on either side of the breakpoint. If there is no translocation, the 2 colors are too close together to resolve and appear as a single color (yellow). In **b**, there has been a reciprocal translocation. Both chromosomes have broken and the green portion of chromosome 2 and the red portion of chromosome 1 have changed places. In this case, the 2 probes bind to complementary sequences that are now on different chromosomes. Their separate colors, green and red, are readily apparent.

a ABL BCR

b BCR ABL

f45.13 Dual-fusion FISH strategy.
a a probe with a red fluorochrome is specific to the ABL locus on chromosome 9 and a probe with a green fluorochrome is specific to the BCR locus on chromosome 22. In the normal state, where there has not been a translocation, the colors are widely separated.
b If there has been a translocation, the 2 colors are brought together and are either seen as immediately juxtaposed or as a merged single color (yellow).

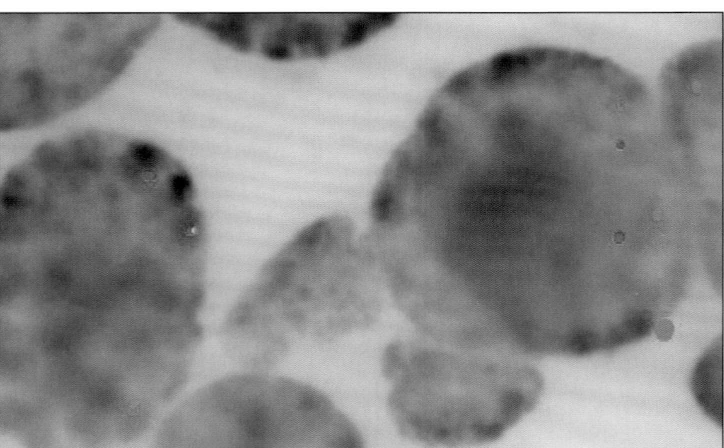

f45.12 Break apart FISH. Note the separation between the red and green signals.

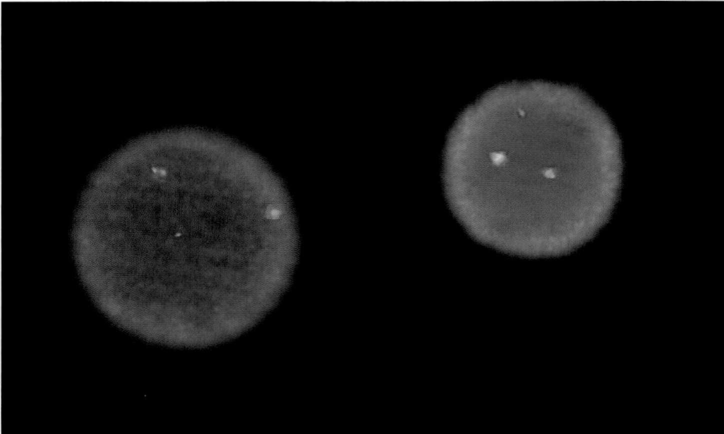

f45.14 Dual-fusion FISH study confirming the t(9;22) in a case of CML. In the normal case, the red and green signals remain separate, but in a translocation, they are fused, as is seen by the yellow signal.

situations where the translocation has occurred, the 2 colors are separated and will appear as 2 distinct colors (this is called break apart FISH) **f45.11a-b, f45.12**.

The process can also be reversed, so that in the normal situation, the probes are hybridized to areas that should be far apart, with 2 distinct colors. If there has been a translocation, it will bring the 2 colors together and merge them into a new color (this is called double fusion strategy) **f45.13a-b, f45.14**. A common example of this is that a red probe is used for the normal *ABL* gene on chromosome 9 and a green probe for the normal *BCR* gene on chromosome 22. If there has been a *BCR/ABL* translocation, the 2 probes are inappropriately fused, resulting in a yellow color.

One can also employ a probe that is specific for the post-translocation DNA. This is a single-color test, in which the probe, labeled with a color that is different from the background color, simply binds if the translocation is present and fails to bind if it is not (this is called single fusion strategy).

FISH can also be used to detect inversions. The detection of these abnormalities is based on the same principles as in the detection of translocations. In one approach, portions of DNA that should be adjacent are labeled with different color probes. As long as the relevant portions remain adjacent, these colors will merge into a single, intermediate color. An inversion causes the component colors to separate, resulting in 2 separate signals of different colors **f45.15**. Another approach to

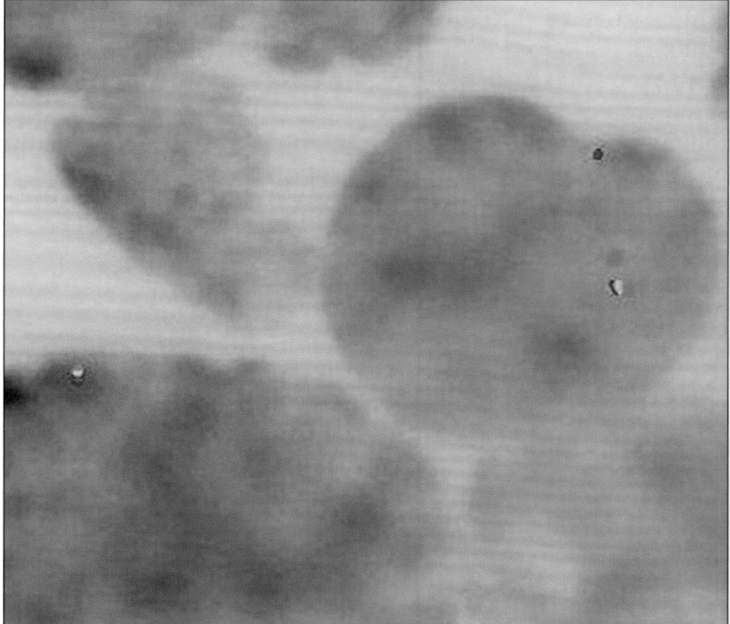

f45.15 Break apart FISH (ALK inversion in a case of NS-CLC, see Chapter 16). Fluorescent probes of different colors (in this case, red & green) are hybridized to either side of the breakpoint in the ALK inversion. If there is no inversion or translocation, the 2 colors are very close together, sometimes with a small area of intermediate color between them (yellow in this case), or merge into a single color. Where there has been an inversion or translocation, the 2 colors are separated. The cell at center contains an area in which the 2 colors remain adjacent and another area in which they are separated: this patient has an ALK inversion on 1 of the 2 chromosomes.

detecting inversions with FISH is to use a single color probe that spans the breakpoint for the inversion. If the inversion is present, the presence of the probe indicates that there has been an inversion.

As is always the case in FISH studies, overlapping nuclei should be avoided, though software is available to sort out signals in such situations. Interpretation is especially difficult when there has been previous treatment (for example, looking for *BCR/ABL* in a previously diagnosed CML who has been treated with imatinib). As is the case for immunohistochemistry, the interpretation of FISH is primarily manual, but automated methods, hopefully reducing interobserver variability in interpretation, are emerging [PMID19430291].

There are some terms that may be used only in cytogenetic studies of malignancies. "Hypodiploid" is usually used to indicate that there are 43 or fewer chromosomes, and "hyperdiploid" refers to 47 or greater, though some will say there must be 48 chromosomes to be truly hyperdiploid. Some cancers, such as some cases of childhood ALL may have >50 chromosomes per cell. These are called high hyperdiploid. Pseudodiploid refers to the normal number of 46 chromosomes, but with aberrations.

Rarely, the probe and target in FISH will be reversed and a probe will be prepared from a patient sample and applied to a commercial or constructed target, such as a metaphase spread. This is called reverse FISH. The principal example of reverse FISH is comparative genomic hybridization (CGH), discussed momentarily.

FISH results are usually reported in the International System for Human Cytogenetic Nomenclature (ISCN) nomenclature that is used in G-banding in clinical genetics. For FISH results performed on immobilized metaphase chromosomes, the traditional G-banding result, if available, is given first, followed by a period, followed by the letters "ish," followed by a more detailed description of the abnormality as elucidated by FISH. For normal findings, the FISH results that follow the G-band results are reported as the number of the chromosome followed by the band in which the tested locus resides, followed in parentheses by the name of the locus, with a multiplication sign and a number indicating the number of signals. For example, 46,XX.ish Xcen (DXZ1x2) is a normal female G-band karyotype (46,XX), followed by FISH results that indicate that the centromeric region of the X chromosome was specifically studied by FISH. This study revealed 2 copies of the locus DXZ1, which is found at the centromere. In normal findings, the chromosome is not in parentheses.

For abnormal findings, the G-banding pattern is again given first and followed by a period, after which the letters "ish" are again used. After "ish," the specific type of abnormality is given (eg, del for deletion, inv for inversion, t for translocation, dup for duplication, etc). The affected chromosome follows, but is in parentheses. The breakpoint or breakpoints follows the affected chromosome, again in parentheses. The specific locus is then given, followed immediately by a "–" sign if it is absent and a "+" sign if it is present, also in parentheses. For example, 46,XY.ish del(22)(q11.2q11.2)(D22S75–) refers to a male that was normal with G-banding, but upon FISH studies, was shown to have a deletion in the D22S75 locus in the 11.2 region of the long arm of chromosome 22 (this is the DiGeorge syndrome critical region).

Unless the nomenclature specifically indicates otherwise, it is conventional to assume that the other chromosome is normal. In the above example, the deletion of the D22S75 locus occurs on only 1 chromosome, while 46,XY.ish del(22)(q11.2q11.2)(D22S75–x2) indicates such a deletion on both chromosomes. Likewise, 46,XY.ish dup(17)(p11.2p11.2)(RAI1++) indicates a duplication of the RAI1 locus on only 1 copy in the 11.2 region of the short arm of chromosome 17 (a single plus sign indicates a single copy of the locus on that chromosome, which is normal). The other chromosome is not mentioned and is therefore presumed to be normal. On the other hand, 46,XY.ish dup(17)(p11.2p11.2)(RAI1++x2) indicates that the locus is duplicated on both chromosomes, for a total of 4 copies.

Unlike conventional G-banding, which requires metaphase spreads, FISH may also be done on intact nuclei, where the chromosomes will be in interphase. This is called nuclear ISH (nuc ish). Because this involves interphase chromosomes rather than metaphases, nuclear ISH is also called interphase ISH. FISH is the leading manner in which interphase cytogenetics is performed. There are 3 advantages to interphase cytogenetics.

- The chromatin in interphase chromosomes is more open and accessible to probes than those in metaphase. Investigations for translocations, for example, are more easily done in the relative openness of an interphase chromosome.
- There are many situations in which metaphase spreads cannot practically be obtained. For example, some tissues, such as muscle and nerve, have a very low mitotic rate and metaphases will be very rare at best. Even in some tissues that do undergo mitoses with reasonable frequency, metaphases may be difficult to obtain.
- Interphase cytogenetics can be done more quickly because one does not have to wait for a significant number of mitoses to develop or use a drug like colchicine to attempt to increase the number of metaphases. Rapid turnaround time is particularly important in many obstetrical settings, where decisions must be made quickly.

ISCN nomenclature also applies in nuc ish, but because G-banding is impossible in interphase chromosomes, G-banding nomenclature does not precede the nuc ish nomenclature unless it has been performed separately on metaphase spreads. Without separate G-banding, the nomenclature begins with nuc ish, after which the locus is designated, followed by a multiplication sign, after which the number of signals seen is given. For example, nuc ish(DXZ1x2) indicates that there were 2 fluorescent signals for this locus on interphase FISH testing. If the chromosome band at which the locus resides is known, it is included after the chromosome number and before the locus. For example, nuc ish 8cen(D8Z2x2) indicates that there were 2 signals from locus D8Z2 on the centromeric region of chromosome 8.

In the testing of neoplastic cells, the number of nuclei examined is indicated in brackets at the end. For example, nuc ish(NMYCx4)[50] means that 50 nuclei from a tumor were examined, and there was an average of 4 signals of the *NMYC* oncogene per nucleus. In reporting the nuc ish findings for translocation studies, the precise nomenclature depends slightly on the methodology and the number of probes used (ie, it will differ slightly if single fusion, double fusion, or break apart probes are used). But in a typical single fusion study for possible CML, nuc ish(ABL1,BCR)x2[200] means that 200 nuclei were examined, with the finding that they each had 2 *ABL1* loci and 2 *BCR* loci (normal finding, no translocation). But nuc ish(ABL1x2),(BCRx2),(ABL1 con BCRx1)[200] means that while the expected number of signals from *ABL1* and *BCR* were found, the examination revealed a juxtaposition of the *ABL1* and *BCR* signals (indicative of a translocation) on 1 chromosome in each of the 200 nuclei that were studied. In this case, the first 2 sets of parentheses indicate the total number of signals for *ABL1* and *BCR* (the normal 2 signals for both) and the third set of parentheses, (ABL1 con BCRx1), indicates the number of signals that are juxtaposed per nucleus (1). nuc ish(ABL1x2),(BCRx2),(ABL1 con BCRx2)[200] indicates that the cells have the expected number of *ABL1* and *BCR* signals (2), but that a translocation has occurred on both chromosomes in all 200 nuclei that were examined. nuc ish(ABL1x2),(BCRx2),(ABL1 con BCRx1)[50/200] describes a translocation in only 50 of the 200 nuclei that were examined.

An example of nuc ish is testing for *HER2*, which resides on 17q21. Because this procedure is often done on formalin-fixed, paraffin-embedded tissue that cannot be treated to increase the number of metaphases, nuc ish is necessary. In this procedure, a fluorescent probe specific for the *HER2* locus is used and the number of signals per neoplastic nucleus is tabulated. Because amplification of chromosome 17 is relatively frequent in breast cancer cells (reports range from about 10% to 50%), it is necessary to control for abnormal copy number of this chromosome. As subsequently discussed, α DNA is a form of repetitive found primarily at centromeres. Most chromosomes have a characteristic number of repeats of the basic unit in their α DNA and can be identified by fluorescent probes that hybridize to a known number of repeating units. These probes are called chromosome enumerator probes (CEP). By using a CEP for chromosome 17, which is stained with a fluorochrome of a different color from that used to detect *HER2*, one can determine if an increased *HER2* signal results from amplification on 1 or both chromosomes, or from an extra chromosome. A typical dual-probe testing procedure uses direct labeling of both the *HER2* locus and the chromosome 17 CEP, the former with rhodamine and the latter with FITC. The final results are then expressed as the ratio of the number of signals for *HER2* per neoplastic nucleus divided by the number of signals for CEP17 **f45.16, f45.17**. Ratios <1.8 are considered negative (ie, no amplification of *HER2* per chromosome). Ratios between 1.8 and 2.2 are considered equivocal, while ratios >2.2 indicate *HER2* amplification per chromosome [PMID17159189]. In addition to the use of a ratio of 2.2 as an indication of amplification, it is also important to determine the number of cells expressing this ratio, as breast cancers are often heterogeneous. A ratio of *HER2*/CEP 17 that equals or exceeds 2.2 in 30% of tumor cells appears to be a prognostic breakpoint [PMID21757600].

Difficulties with any FISH study performed on formalin fixed, paraffin-embedded tissue are nuclear truncation artifact, where copy number is underestimated because a particular section is thinner than an intact nucleus and may

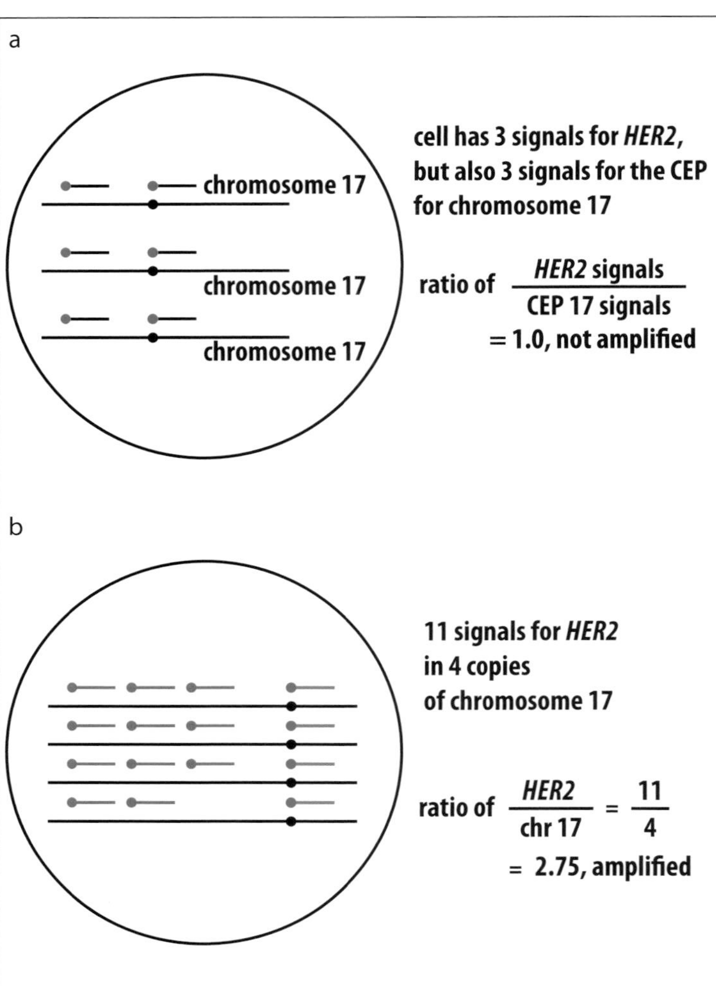

f45.16 *HER2* testing by FISH. The *HER2* gene is on chromosome 17, the centromere of which is indicated by the black dot. In **a**, the cell has 3 copies of chromosome 17 (increased copy number of this chromosome is relatively common in breast cancer). This is determined by a chromosome enumerator probe (CEP) that binds to the centromere and which is green in this illustration. A sequence complementary to the *HER2* focus carries a fluorescent probe of a different color from the CEP (red in this illustration). In **a**, there are 3 copies of the *HER2* gene in the cell instead of the expected 2 copies, but there are also 3 copies of chromosome 17, as determined by the CEP for that chromosome. The ratio of *HER2* signals to chromosome 17 is unchanged, and an increase in the number of *HER2* genes resulting from a copy number increase in chromosome 17 does not count as amplification. In **b**, there are 4 copies of chromosome 17 in the cell, but the number of *HER2* genes is increased even compensating for this. There are 11 signals from the *HER2* probe and 4 from the CEP for chromosome 17, resulting in a ratio of 2.75, which is amplification.

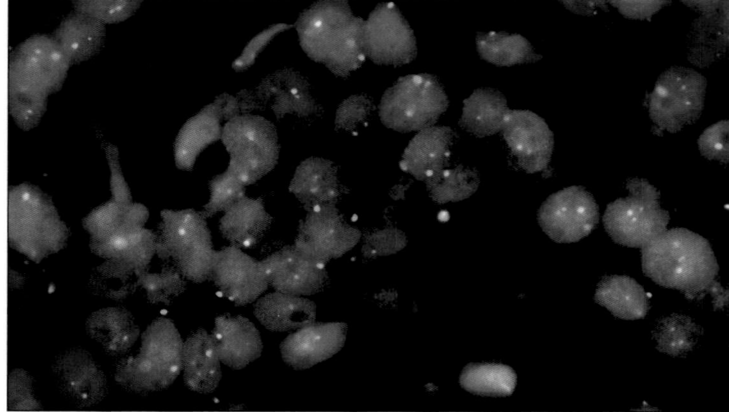

f45.17 A dual-color FISH study in breast cancer. The red signals indicate *HER2* DNA sequences and the green signals indicate a chromosome enumerator probe (CEP) for chromosome 17, the chromosome containing the *HER2* locus. The ratio of *HER2* signals to CEP signals is 2.33, indicating slight amplification. Modified from [PMID19019769] with permission.

not contain the necessary DNA for the probe to bind to [PMID12861068], and autofluorescence caused by the fixation of proteins [PMID9536283].

It may occasionally be advantageous to target a FISH study at mRNA rather than DNA because protein overexpression may result not only from increased copy number of the gene, but also from excess transcription of a normal amount of DNA. FISH studies for mRNA may identify tumors that have excess mRNA even without an increase in the number of *HER2* genes [PMID18985033]. If ISH is directed at mRNA, the probe is usually a specially constructed labeled single-stranded RNA, complementary to the target mRNA, called a riboprobe. A riboprobe that is not complementary may be employed as a control for nonspecific binding.

Multiple Probe FISH

FISH can be used with multiple probes of different colors and can be combined with other techniques. Instead of looking for specific abnormalities, one can also analyze the entirety of a chromosome with fluorescent probes of different colors. The collective hybridization of these probes, each labeled with its own color, permits individual chromosomes to be studied in greater detail than is possible with traditional FISH. Chromosome libraries are collections of FISH probes of different colors that collectively "paint" an entire chromosome (this is called whole chromosome painting). Many such libraries have been constructed by needletip dissection and removal of specific bands from a chromosome (called chromosome microdissection), followed by the construction of a FISH probe that specifically hybridizes to that band, whether or not it contains any known abnormalities. Because traditional FISH is useful only for known abnormalities, whole chromosome painting may occasionally disclose abnormalities that traditional banding or FISH techniques may not reveal.

In reverse chromosome painting, abnormal or marker DNA (a marker chromosome or fragment is one that is of unknown origin) is amplified and labeled, after which it is hybridized to normal metaphase spreads [PMID14984099]. The location of hybridization reveals the origin of the unknown sequence. In a related technique, if the sequence of a gene is known, but not its location, a FISH probe can be designed that is complementary to the gene and hybridized to metaphase spreads. More advanced techniques using hybridization of the probe to interphase nuclei might provide a more precise location of the gene.

FISH can be combined with immunohistochemistry, allowing a particular population of cells in a section to be studied. For example, if one wants to study T lymphocytes in a mixed population of cells, one can ignore all FISH signals except those emanating from cells that have previously immunohistochemically stained for CD3 [PMID20966547].

FISH can also be combined with flow cytometry. Metaphase chromosomes can be stained with a fluorescent probe that binds a known sequence of DNA and subjected to flow cytometry, which can measure the fluorescence intensity relative to normal metaphases and determine the amount of that particular DNA sequence in the sample relative to normal controls [PMID20687474]. This is a rapid, reproducible, and quantitative technique that in conjunction with the judicious choice of fluorescent probes, can provide excellent information, but it requires metaphase spreads, it is expensive, inversions and translocations will not be detected because they do not change the DNA content, and the instrument cannot determine where on the spreads the probe has bound.

Laser capture microdissection (also called laser-assisted microdissection) is used in FISH studies to separate cells of interest from surrounding cells in paraffin blocks (such as tumor cells from stromal cells). In this technique, an ethylene vinyl acetate film is placed over the area of interest in a paraffin block. A laser then melts the film, after which the molecules of the film diffuse into the block and surround the area of interest, permitting it to retain its integrity after removal from the block. This permits tiny areas of a biopsy or particular tissue types to be isolated and studied [PMID18989416]. For example, one could theoretically separate the epidermis from the dermis in a paraffin block of a skin biopsy and study it by FISH without interference from other tissues.

Another developing area is the use of FISH on extended chromatin fibers (fiber-FISH). DNA is packed in an extraordinarily complex manner, with a basic unit, called a nucleosome, consisting of a 147-base-pair unit of DNA wound around a collection of 8 histone proteins. A spacer sequence of DNA connects each nucleosome, resulting in a "string of beads" that can be seen in the electron microscope. Multiple levels of complex coiling of this string produce the normal interphase chromosome. In extended chromatin fibers, the chromosomes are physically stretched so that they are no longer in the coiled configuration that is characteristic of interphase [PMID8919917, PMID20809301]. This permits probes to have greater access to many portions of the DNA, but the trade-off is loss of recognizable chromosome morphology. Information obtained from fiber-FISH studies are designated with the prefix "fib ish."

Although there is a technique, called chromosome combing, that stretches DNA in solution, most extended chromatin fiber preparations are usually performed on a glass slide. The cells are typically fixed on a slide and lysed, after which they are placed vertically in an ethanol solution for a few minutes. Slow pulling of the slide out of the solution will pull the chromosomes into an extended fiber configuration.

Comparative Genomic Hybridization

CGH is an extension of FISH that has applications in both tumor pathology and cytogenetics. CGH provides an assessment of DNA gains or losses in populations of cells without cell cultures. In a typical situation, tumor (or other potentially abnormal) DNA and control DNA are extracted and labeled with fluorochromes. Often, the normal DNA is labeled with a red fluorochrome and the test DNA with a green fluorochrome. The normal and abnormal DNA populations are then mixed 1:1 in a buffered solution and applied to a substrate that contains normal metaphase spreads. These immobilized normal metaphase spreads are called the target. The 2 DNA populations will then compete for hybridization to the normal metaphase spreads. The ratio of green to red at a given

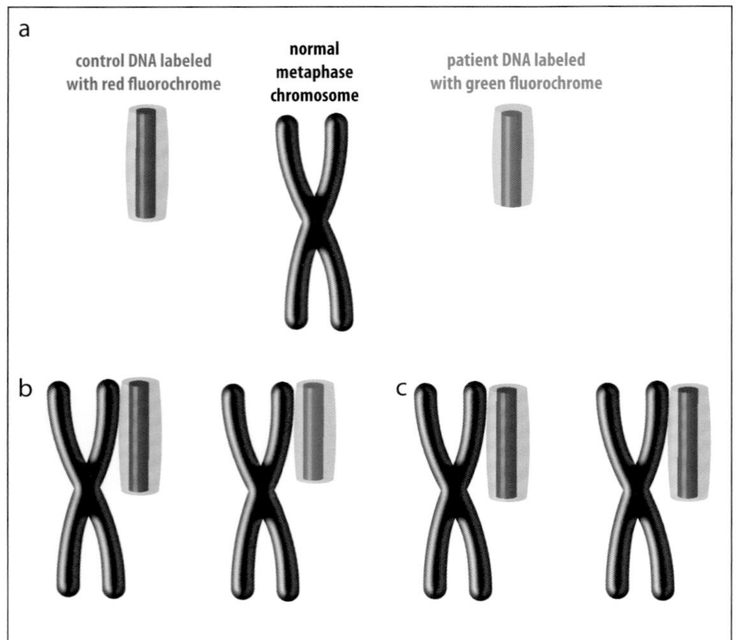

f45.18 Comparative genomic hybridization (CGH).
In **a**, control or reference DNA is labeled with a red fluorochrome while the patient's DNA is labeled with a green fluorochrome. These labeled sequences of DNA compete for hybridization on normal metaphase chromosomes.
In **b**, the control and patient DNA bind the normal metaphase chromosomes in equal amounts, indicating that the patient does not have significantly more or less of that DNA sequence than the control.
In **c**, only the control DNA has bound to the metaphase chromosomes, indicating that the patient has significantly reduced or absent amounts of that DNA sequence.

location on the metaphase spreads indicates if the tumor cells have more or less DNA than normal cells at that locus **f45.18**.

Repetitive sequences in either the control or test DNA can cause high background fluorescence in CGH, as is the case for ordinary FISH, and blocking DNA, such as cot-1, is used. The actual hybridization step lasts longer than in ordinary FISH, usually several days.

CGH requires a fluorescent microscope, but because 3 fluorochromes are used (1 each for the control and test DNA, and a third as a counterstain to allow visualization of the metaphase spreads), a more complex set of filters is needed than is the case for ordinary FISH. An important difference from ordinary FISH is that in CGH, it is not simply a matter of the presence or absence of a signal. Rather, results are in the form of a blending of color from the 2 fluorochromes as both normal and test DNA hybridize to some extent at virtually all locations along the metaphase spreads. The eye is not sensitive enough to detect the many gradations of color that occur as the 2 fluorochromes blend in myriad possible combinations. Therefore, digital imaging is needed to differentiate and quantitate the 2 colors of the control and test DNA. Because of signal fading, results must be preserved in some way, usually by digital imaging.

The first step in analyzing data from CGH studies is to digitally convert the counterstain fluorescence from the metaphase target spreads into a pseudo-Giemsa banding. This ensures that each chromosome in the target is properly labeled so that the control and test hybridizations can be properly assessed band by band.

Imaging software then measures the fluorescent signals from the test and control probes at intervals along a target metaphase spread. Multiple metaphase spreads are measured in this manner and for each interval, a mean and a standard deviation for fluorescence intensity are calculated for the normal sample. The software is generally set to flag any interval for which the fluorescence of the test DNA is more or <2 standard deviations from the mean fluorescence of the normal sample. That interval is then considered to have abnormally high or low expression of DNA.

CGH permits the study of a pathogenic organism's genome relative to the genome of a related, nonpathogenic organism. It also permits the investigation of changes in its gene expression during pathogenesis or as a response to antibiotics. However, there are limitations of CGH.

- It is difficult to obtain good data from intervals near a centromere, from regions of heterochromatin (condensed chromatin that is not often transcribed) or from the p arm of an acrocentric chromosome (numbers 13, 14, 15, 21, and 22) because the chromatin is condensed in all of these areas. Likewise, signals from telomeres are fainter than from other regions, making CGH less reliable in these areas. Suspected telomeric abnormalities should be confirmed by a FISH study specifically targeted at those areas.
- CGH cannot detect inversions or balanced translocations since, despite their potential clinical significance, they do not create an actual gain or loss of DNA and will hybridize to the same degree as normal DNA.
- Statistically significant differences in signal ratios generally require a gain or loss of 10 million base pairs or more of DNA. Smaller changes frequently escape detection, and SNPs will surely be missed.
- While CGH will certainly detect monosomies or trisomies (changes in the number of 1 chromosome in an otherwise normal number of chromosomes, such as 47,XXY), it will not detect generalized ploidy changes such as triploidy or tetraploidy, where all of the chromosomes are present in an abnormal number because the ratios of the 2 signals does not change (the term "-somy" refers to 1 chromosome, while the term "-ploidy" refers to the entire set).
- Even with the use of blocking DNA, it is difficult to use CGH to assess copy number in any area where repetitive DNA is common.
- CGH may indicate an abnormality without being able to provide specific information on the nature of the precise structural anomaly.
- Because the DNA from many cells within the 2 groups being tested is pooled (for example, one might pool the DNA from 1,000 normal cells to create the control group and from 1,000 tumor cells to create the test group), low-level mosaicism may be missed. For example, if 10% of the tumor cells have an abnormality at a particular location and the other 90% do not, the overall fluorescence emission from the tumor population may appear within 2 standard deviations of the normal DNA, and the minority population may be missed.

Most applications of CGH have been in solid tumors, though it is also used to supplement conventional cytogenetics if insufficient metaphases are recovered or if there is maternal DNA or bacterial contamination. Many applications of CGH are now carried out on microarrays (aCGH) because of its much higher resolution (see discussion of microarrays).

Nomenclature in CGH is also governed by the ISCN. In conventional FISH, a commercially available probe is used to hybridize to the patient's DNA. In contrast, in CGH, patient DNA is used, along with control DNA, to hybridize to reference metaphase spreads. For this reason, CGH is considered a type of reverse FISH. If a conventional karyotype has been performed, it is given first, followed by a period, followed by the phrase "rev ish" to indicate that the remainder of the nomenclature is from CGH. The designations "enh" and "dim" indicate that CGH has identified an enhanced or a diminished (respectively) number of copies of a chromosome or a part of a chromosome from the test DNA. For example, 47,XX,+mar is a conventional G-banding designation for a female with an extra chromosome and further indicates that the nature of that extra chromosome is unknown (marker chromosome). 47,XX, +mar.rev ish enh (11)(q) indicates that the extra chromosome is derived from the long arm of chromosome 11. In 46,XX,add(7)(q25).rev ish der(7)t(7;21)(q25;q22) enh(21)(q22), the notation in front of the period indicates that there is a female karyotype, but that there is additional material on chromosome 7, which has an expanded region 2, band 5, on the long arm. After the period, we see that there is a derivative chromosome, based on chromosome 7, that is derived from a translocation between chromosomes 7 and 21, causing extra material from region 2, band 2, of the long arm of chromosome 21 to be translocated to, and thus to enhance region 2, band 5, of the long arm of chromosome 7. The additional material on chromosome 7 that was identified on G-banding is shown by CGH to be derived from the long arm of chromosome 21. 46,XY.rev ish dim(18q23) indicates that a male whose conventional karyogram is normal, but who has reduced DNA in region 2, band 3 of the long arm of chromosome 18.

Multicolor FISH and Spectral Karyotyping

FISH probes of different colors can collectively "paint" an entire chromosome in a technique called whole chromosome painting. In 1996, 2 groups described slightly different methods of simultaneously painting all 24 different human chromosomes (the 22 autosomes and the 2 sex chromosomes). One technique is called multicolor (or multiplex) fluorescence ISH (M-FISH) [PMID8630489]. The second technique is called spectral karyotyping (SKY) [PMID8662537].

M-FISH and SKY are related techniques in which the target is the patient's metaphase chromosomes, denatured and immobilized on a substrate. Sets of probes that are specific for each chromosome are prepared by PCR and fluorescently labeled. All of the probes in each set have a unique color. For example, all the probes for chromosome 1 might be yellow, all those for chromosome 2 might be green, all those for chromosome 3 might be purple, etc. Because there are not enough separate fluorochromes to generate 24 unique hues, combinations of 5 fluorochromes are used. For a number of fluorochromes given by N, used in every possible combination, $2^N - 1$ different hues are possible. With 5 unique fluorochromes mixed in every possible combination, we can have 31 separate hues with combinatorial labeling because $2^5 - 1 = 31$. This is called combinatorial labeling. For example, all of the probes to chromosome one might be labeled with fluorescent dye number 1, which is yellow, and all of those that hybridize to chromosome 2 may have a combination of dyes 1 (yellow) and 2 (blue), making green. All of those specific to chromosome 3 may be tagged with dyes 2 (blue) and 3 (red), making purple, etc. The result is a set of probes for each chromosome, which collectively hybridize to most areas of the chromosome and give it a unique color **f45.19**.

M-FISH uses sets of excitation filters and corresponding dichroic mirrors (that reflect light of 1 color and transmit light of other colors). One set of filters and mirrors is used for each of the 6 wavelengths of the individual fluorochromes (the 5 fluorochromes used in the probes plus the DAPI counterstain used on the metaphase spreads). At some time in the analysis, each of the fluorochromes is exposed to the one wavelength that will make it fluoresce. Multiple images are taken, 1 for each wavelength, after which computer software digitally sums the images. At this writing, the 24 Xcyte system by MetaSystems is the leading method of M-FISH. A good review of M-FISH, including basic procedures and applications, has been published by Kearney [PMID16954655]. A detailed discussion of the procedures of M-FISH can be found in Geigl et al [PMID17406400].

SKY is a very similar technique that also uses combinatorial labeling, but that uses the splitting of light beams and mathematical analysis to allow a single imaging to suffice **f45.20**. Although mathematically more complicated than M-FISH, the end result is the same and SKY offers the convenience of a single exposure.

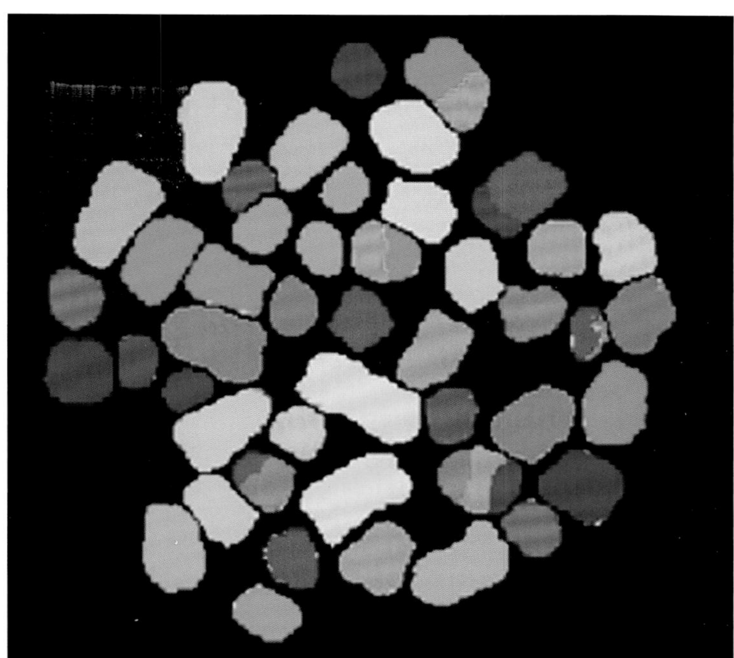

f45.19 Multicolor fluorescence in situ hybridization (M-FISH) in a child with ALL. Using combinatorial labeling, each chromosome has a unique color.

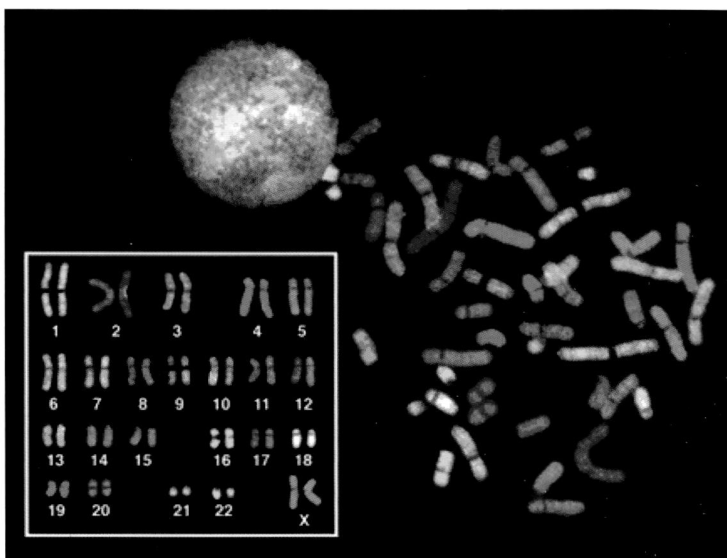

f45.20 Spectral karyotyping (SKY) is similar to M-FISH in that it also uses combinatorial labeling, but the splitting of light beams and mathematical analysis are used to allow a single imaging to suffice. Although mathematically more complicated than M-FISH, the end result is the similar, and SKY offers the convenience of a single exposure.

Also, new fluorochromes in M-FISH require the physical addition of a new filter, while the mathematics of SKY allows it to accommodate new fluorochromes without filters. On the other hand, M-FISH allows the operator to favor a particular fluorochrome that may be weak, thus "teasing" out a subtle fluorescence that might be missed with SKY.

As is the case for CGH, target and probe DNA must be denatured, and hybridization takes several days. After hybridization, the preparations are washed to remove nonspecific binding of fluorochromes and the target chromosomes are counterstained with DAPI. As is the case for CGH, the target chromosomes must be properly classified. After hybridization, washing, and DAPI counterstaining, software pseudokaryotypes the target metaphases by translating their DAPI counterstains into a rough G-banding pattern called reverse-DAPI. Any target spreads that the software cannot confidently classify must either be confidently classified by hand or discarded.

The individual chromosomes in the target metaphases are then scanned to detect the amount and color of each fluorochrome for each interval of each chromosome. This is called a fluorescence intensity profile. For each chromosome, the fluorescence intensity profile consists of a separate graph for each fluorochrome for each homologue. For example, if chromosome 1 is labeled only with 1 fluorochrome, then its fluorescence intensity profile will consist of only 2 graphs, 1 for each homologue of the pair, since the other 4 fluorochromes will be absent. On the other hand, some chromosomes are labeled with 4 fluorochromes, and their fluorescence intensity profiles consist of 8 graphs, 1 of each of the 4 colors for each of the 2 homologues. The summation of the fluorescence intensity of each fluorochrome at each interval along the fluorescence intensity profile results in a composite image for each chromosome. This composite image is then used to generate an artificial pseudocolor for that chromosome, making it possible to distinguish the different chromosomes.

As is always the case, most errors of interpretation in M-FISH and SKY stem from suboptimal material or preparation, such as poor fixation of the metaphase spreads, poor denaturation so that the probe and target cannot anneal properly, insufficient or excessive washing after hybridization, etc. One of the potential problems that may occur in even well-prepared material is called flaring (or sandwich effect). In flaring, a translocation between 2 chromosomes may result in a mixing of fluorochromes at the site of translocation that initially suggests the presence of DNA from a third chromosome. For example, if chromosome 1 is labeled with fluorochrome 1, and chromosome 3 is tagged with fluorochromes 3, 4, and 5, and there is a translocation between chromosomes 1 and 3, at the site of translocation, we may see fluorochromes 1, 3, 4, and 5. If this is the combination used to highlight chromosome 7, then we may believe that a portion of chromosome 7 has translocated to chromosome 1 or chromosome 3. While small translocations and insertions may unavoidably simulate the presence of a third chromosome, many cases of flaring can be resolved by realizing that if the colors are from a third chromosome, they will be intimately mixed, but if the mixture of colors results from flaring (ie, from a translocation), close study often reveals that they are juxtaposed but do not intermingle.

Because M-FISH and SKY can determine multiple parameters at one time, applications include analysis of multiple abnormalities, assistance in understanding complex karyotypes, identification of abnormalities for which there is no specific probe, and identifying marker chromosomes in cancers. M-FISH and SKY have been used effectively in elucidating chromosomal aberrations in many tumors.

A significant limitation of M-FISH and SKY is that they must be performed on patient metaphase chromosomes and are not yet suitable for interphase applications. The necessity for metaphase spreads from the patient requires that the patient's cells be cultured and that a sufficient number of metaphases be recovered.

A second limitation of M-FISH and SKY is that at this writing, they have relatively low resolution. Inversions, translocations, and duplications are likely to escape detection unless they are larger than about 2 million base pairs. While these techniques provide a "bird's eye" view of the genome and are excellent for situations where there are multiple abnormalities, they are not techniques of choice in looking for a specific, previously characterized abnormality.

M-FISH and SKY are also more effective in detecting abnormalities among different chromosomes than within a single chromosome, which makes them particularly useful for assessing tumors in which there are chromosomal aneuploidies or translocations between different chromosomes. However, the low efficiency in identification of intrachromosomal abnormalities has led to the development of higher-resolution techniques.

One approach to increasing the sensitivity of detecting abnormalities within individual chromosomes is multicolor banding (M-banding). M-banding is similar to M-FISH except that it uses a larger number of fluorochromes and shorter probes for each chromosome. These probes hybridize to smaller, sequences of DNA, the end result being the painting of shorter segments of chromosomes. For example, in M-FISH, a maximum of 4 fluorochromes are used for any one chromosome, but in M-banding, 8 or more fluorochromes may be combined to paint a single chromosome. The short labeled probes used in M-banding are called region-specific partial chromosome paints (RPCP). Each RPCP overlaps with the adjacent RPCP, so that the entire chromosome can be painted.

In M-banding, after hybridization with immobilized patient or test cell metaphases, the fluorescent signals of each fluorochrome are obtained, and they are summed as is the case for M-FISH. Again, artificial pseudocolors are assigned to the fluorescent pattern. Unlike M-FISH, in M-banding, individual chromosomes are not all painted in a single color. 20-30 different bands are obtained for each chromosome, and about 500 distinct bands can be obtained for the haploid genome in M-banding [PMID10393418]. The number of different colors that can be obtained from n different fluorochromes is $2^n - 1$, so achieving 500 different colors is not as daunting as might be thought. 9 fluorochromes will do the job ($2^9 = 512$).

M-banding is an ideal follow-up step once M-FISH has implicated a particular chromosome, since it permits the study of that chromosome in much greater detail **f45.21**. Processes such as deletions and inversions that involve a single band can often be identified on M-banding, whereas these are likely to be missed with M-FISH or SKY. Also, because M-banding focuses on an individual chromosome, it can identify specific breakpoints much

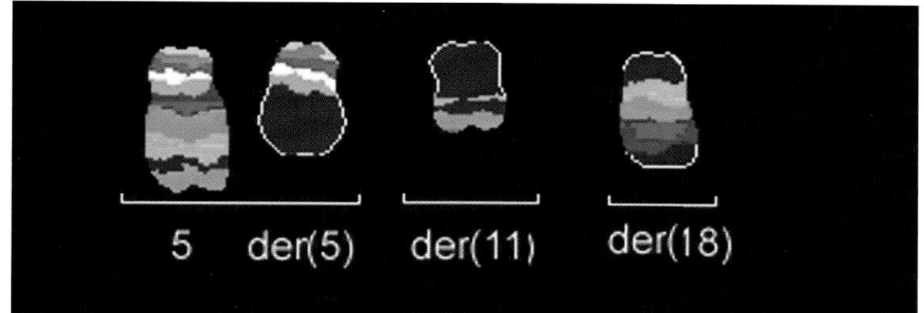

f45.21 M-banding focused on chromosome 5. Individual chromosomes are multicolored, unlike M-FISH (see f45.19), because a greater number of fluorochromes are used for each chromosome. The normal chromosome 5 is at the far left. Next to the normal chromosome 5 is its abnormal counterpart, der(5), which is missing several bands. Bands from chromosome 5 are seen in abnormal chromosomes 11 and 18, labeled der(11) and der(18).

more effectively than M-FISH. Many M-FISH studies suggest abnormalities that are either confirmed by ordinary FISH—if the suggested abnormality in known and a probe for it is either available or can be made—or are studied in greater detail by M-banding.

Another higher-resolution technique is ArmFISH, a 42-color application of multicolor FISH that has specific colors for the p arm and the q arm of each chromosome (excepting the y chromosome and the p arms of the acrocentric chromosomes) [PMID11107184].

DNA Sequencing

The most common mechanism for DNA sequencing has been the chain termination method, typically using dideoxy (dd) nucleotides, pioneered by Frederick Sanger [PMID271968]. In this procedure, the DNA to be sequenced is divided into 4 samples. Each of these samples is denatured and incubated in a solution of DNA polymerase, primers, and the 4 bases in nucleoside triphosphate (NTP) form, so that a complementary strand can be generated. But in each of the 4 reactions, a small amount of a modified NTP, a dideoxy NTP, is added. A dideoxy NTP contains the sugar dideoxyribose, which lacks hydroxyl groups at both the number 2 and the number 3 carbon atoms. Ribose, used in RNA, has hydroxyl groups at both of these positions, and deoxyribose, used in DNA, has an hydroxyl group only in the number 3 position. Extension of a nucleic acid requires the bonding from the 5' carbon of one sugar to the 3' carbon of the adjacent sugar via the binding of a phosphate group attached to the 5' carbon to an hydroxyl group attached to the 3' carbon. Hence, either ribose or deoxyribose can sustain elongation of the nucleic acid, but dideoxyribose cannot because it lacks a hydroxyl group at the 3′ position of the sugar.

Each of the 4 reactions uses copious amounts of all 4 normal bases and a small amount of 1 base in dideoxy form. Each of these dideoxy NTPs (ddNTPs)—ddATP, ddGTP, ddCTP, or ddTTP—is labeled. The original label was radioactive, but now the label is usually a fluorescent tag. Synthesis of the complementary strand terminates when a dd base is encountered because the dideoxy structure prevents any further addition. The double-stranded DNA so created is then denatured. The complementary strands in each of the 4 reactions will be a series of truncated fragments, each of which was terminated when a ddNTP of the one type that is present in that reaction mixture successfully competed with its normal analogue. For example, in the reaction containing ddATP, the shortest

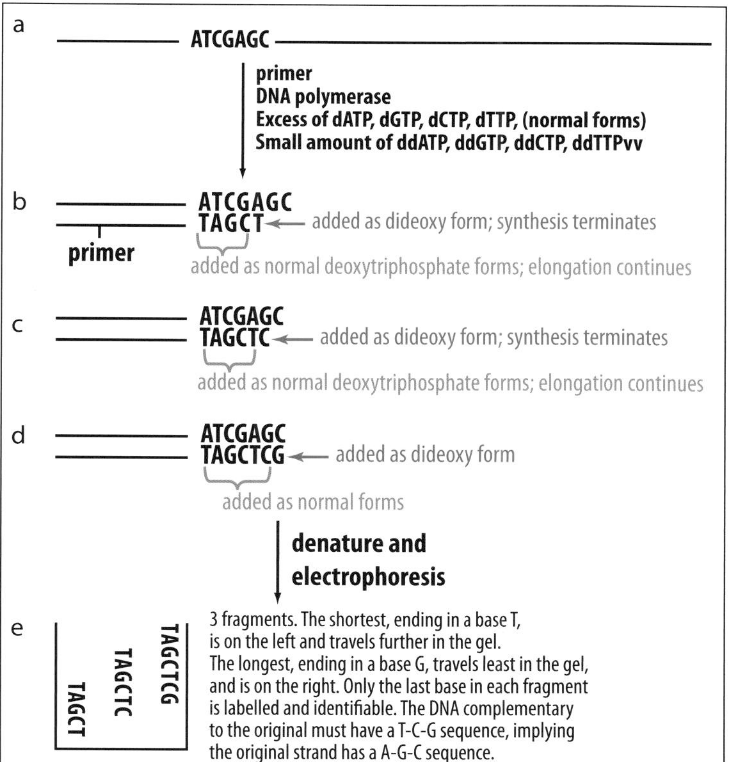

f45.22 Sanger DNA sequencing. a depicts the DNA sequence to be sequenced. It is incubated with DNA polymerase, primers, large amounts of the normal triphosphate forms of the bases and small amounts of the dideoxy forms of the bases in which the required hydroxyl group at carbon number 3 of deoxyribose is absent, so synthesis cannot continue because the pentose cannot bind a phosphate group. In b, the first 4 bases—T, A, G, and C—are added in their normal forms and synthesis continues. But then, base T is added in a dideoxy form and synthesis stops. In c, the first 5 bases of the growing DNA strand are added in their normal forms, but 6 base, C, is added in dideoxy form, terminating synthesis. In d, synthesis terminates after the seventh base, a G, is added because it is in dideoxy form. In e, the original DNA and the newly synthesized complementary strands of different lengths are denatured and subjected to electrophoresis. The shortest fragments travel further in the gel and are closer to the bottom. In this example, on the left, nearest the bottom, is the 5 base-pair sequence that resulted from the situation depicted in b when the fifth base was added in the dideoxy form. On the right, furthest from the bottom, is a 7 base-pair sequence depicted in d when synthesis proceeded until the seventh base was added. Because each of the dideoxy forms of the base carry their own specific fluorescent labels, the bases at the end of the sequences (T, C, and G) can be identified. The complementary DNA must have a sequence of T-C-G, meaning that the original strand must have a sequence of A-G-C.

fragment is a complementary strand that was terminated quickly when a ddATP replaced a normal ATP very soon after replication began. A slightly longer fragment results from a complementary strand that was terminated a little later by the incorporation of another ddATP. For each of the 4 reactions, the longest fragments are those in which the dd analogue did not compete successfully with its normal counterpart—and thus terminate synthesis—until the complementary strand was almost completed f45.22.

The products of all 4 reactions are then separately subjected to electrophoresis. In a gel system, for each of the 4 reactions, the smallest of these fragments, at the bottom of the gel, represents a complementary sequence that was terminated soon after replication began, close to the point of origin of the replication. The largest fragment, at the top of the gel, represents a complementary sequence in which the dideoxy nucleotide was not incorporated until near the end of the sequence. By comparing all 4 wells, one can read the sequence by walking up the ladder from the bottom of the gel. For example, in the reaction that contained ddATP, the fragments may have lengths of 4 base pairs, 8 base pairs, and 12 base pairs. Reading from the bottom of the gel to the top, in the reaction products from the ddCTP reaction, the fragments may be of lengths 5, 9, and 13 base pairs. For the products from the ddTTP reaction, the products may be of 6, 10, and 14 base pairs in length. The products emanating from the ddGTP may have bands at 7 and 11 base pairs in length. Putting all 4 of these results together, the sequence of DNA must be ACTGACTGACT (actually, this is the order of the tagged dd bases; the actual sequence of the original DNA would be the complement of this, or TGACTGACTGA).

One can combine these reactions in a single well by using a different fluorescent label for each terminating ddNTP. More recently, capillary electrophoresis is used, wherein each ddNTPs has its own unique fluorescent signature, and the products are fed through very thin tubes past a laser. The first products to pass the laser are the smallest, analogous to the bottom of the gel. The order in which the 4 unique fluorescent signals pass, read by a computer, gives the DNA sequence. An automated Sanger process using 4 separate fluorochromes and capillary electrophoresis was important in the Human Genome Project. Because fluorescent tags are used and the reading is done after synthesis stops, this is one of the so-called "dye-terminator" methods of sequencing.

In any sequencing of DNA, there are 2 potential pitfalls. The first is heterozygosity. If both strands of a patient's DNA are not sequenced, a potentially clinically important heterozygous state may be missed. If the patient whose DNA is being sequenced is heterozygous for the allele in question and both strands have been sequenced with a gel or capillary electrophoresis method, we will encounter 2 bands that have migrated to the same extent in the gel or have passed by the laser at the same time.

The second potential problem in DNA sequencing is that there are many areas in the human genome in which the same sequence of DNA tandemly repeats, and the number of repeating units often differs between the 2 chromosomes. If such a region is encountered, there will be a series of repeated bands that is likely to cause confusion as one attempts to read the sequence from the bottom of the gel upwards.

Newer Methods of DNA Sequencing Based on Synthesis, Not Termination

The Sanger method of DNA sequencing was a triumph of modern medicine, but it is expensive. A number of new technologies that can process multiple samples simultaneously, resulting in lower cost per sample, have come forward. In contrast to the methods based on the Sanger technique, in which information is obtained as synthesis stops (so-called terminator methods), information is derived in these newer methods as each new nucleotide is added. They are therefore sometimes called "sequencing by synthesis" [PMID15143316]. Unlike the Sanger method, DNA sequencing by synthesis can only read short sequences, but these methods are faster and less expensive, and work well for known, targeted mutations.

Although at this writing, alternative technologies are being developed that can sequence single DNA molecules, the currently available alternative sequencing by synthesis methods require very large numbers of identical DNA fragments, so that the summation of chemiluminescent or fluorescent signals has sufficient magnitude to be detectable. Therefore, the DNA of interest is amplified by PCR and each of the amplicons is simultaneously sequenced.

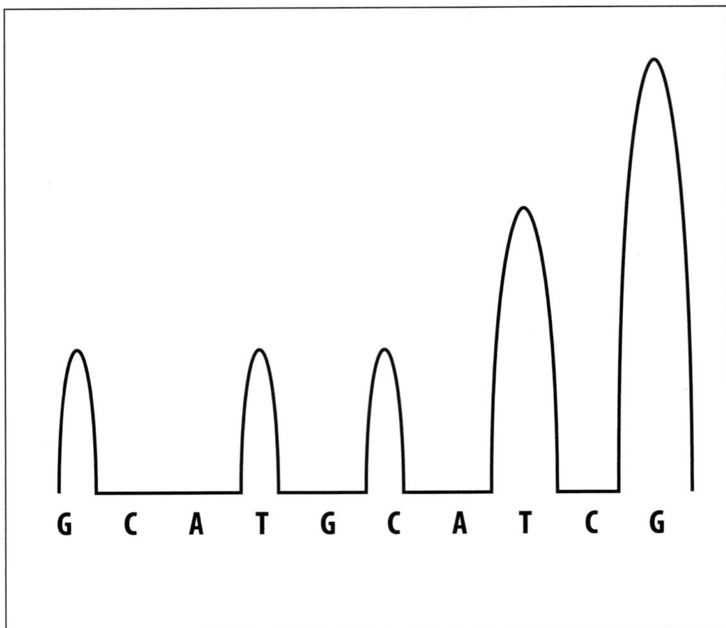

f45.23 A pyrogram. Reading from left to right, when the base guanine is added, light is generated, indicating that the base was accepted and was complementary to the next available base on the original sample. When the bases cytosine and adenine were added, no light was generated, indicating that neither of them was complementary to the next available base. The addition of thymine resulted in a generation of light, indicating that it was complementary. Guanine was not complementary to the next available base pair, but cytosine was. Adenine was not complementary to the next available base pair but the addition of thymine resulted in a double signal, indicating that on the original sample, the next 2 bases both paired with thymine. Cytosine was not complementary to the next base, but the addition of guanine resulted in a triple signal indicating that the next 3 bases were complementary to guanine. The sequence of the growing DNA strand therefore must be G-T-C-T-T-G-G-G, implying that the corresponding sequence of the original DNA must be C-A-G-A-A-C-C-C.

The first alternative to the Sanger method is pyrosequencing [PMID8923969]. In pyrosequencing, amplicons are converted into single strands and immobilized onto beads that are coated with streptavidin. Primers and DNA polymerase are added, but only 1 of the 4 bases, in its NTP form, is added. Luciferin, luciferase, adenosine 5' phosphosulfate, and the enzyme ATP sulfurylase are also added. When a base is added to a growing strand of DNA, pyrophosphate is released. If the added base is not complementary, there is no reaction and pyrophosphate is not released. If the base is complementary, pyrophosphate is released and ATP sulfurylase converts this pyrophosphate and adenosine 5' phosphosulfate into ATP. This ATP drives the luciferase, resulting in light emission if the base that was added complements the first unpaired base of the immobilized sequence. Since bases are added in their NTP form, adenine would normally be studied by adding ATP. Since this would trigger the enzyme luciferase even if adenine is not the appropriate base, a modified form of ATP (dATP-α-S) is added when adenine is tested.

Any unused ATP must be removed before the next nucleotide is tested. In the liquid variant of pyrosequencing, this is done by the enzyme apyrase, which degrades ATP. In the solid variant of the technique, there is a washing step before the next nucleotide is added.

Bases are added one at a time, making use of the fact that growth proceeds one base at a time and that only the first unpaired base can receive a complement (ie, bases cannot be skipped). As the sequential addition of bases proceeds, a record called a pyrogram **f45.23** is made of which bases were added and when. For example, if light is generated when GTP is added, then is not generated again until TTP is added, then is not generated again until dATP-α-S is added, the sequence of the complementary strand being synthesized is GTA. If the sequence is GTTTA, the amplitude of the light generated when TTP is added will be 3 times that of the other nucleotides and 3 times that of the amplitude from TTP in the sequence GTA.

As is the case for most techniques in molecular pathology, pyrosequencing has been automated, as one of the so-called next generation (or second generation) sequencing methods, in which the DNA to be sequenced is fragmented, amplified, and each cloned fragment is sequenced in parallel. Because innumerable fragments are simultaneously sequenced, with additive output, these methods are often said to use a massively parallel testing format. The term "deep sequencing" is used for targeted sequencing of a region of interest by a massively parallel format. Instruments using next generation sequencing in a massively parallel format have been reviewed by Natrajan and Reis-Filho [PMID21545259], by ten Bosch and Grody [PMID18832462], and by Voelkerding et al [PMID20805560, PMID19246620].

The Roche/454 FLX Pyrosequencer uses emulsion PCR, wherein genomic DNA is fragmented, often by nebulizing, after which it is attached to short sequences of nucleic acid called adaptors. One of the adaptors contains biotin f45.24a-c and will bind to beads that are coated with streptavidin, attaching the DNA to the bead. The double-stranded DNA is denatured and the strands that are not attached to the biotin are freed f45.24d-f. These strands are then mixed with beads that are coated with oligonucleotides that bind to the adaptors in such a way that each bead binds only 1 fragment. The beads are then placed in a water/oil medium and vortexed, after which they will occupy a small aqueous space encapsulated by oil. These aqueous micelles contain PCR reagents and PCR, with a primer directed to a sequence on the adaptor, takes place on the surface of the bead in the tiny aqueous space f45.24g,h. Because each bead contains only 1 fragment before amplification, each bead contains millions of copies of one of the original fragments after amplification. Because these copies are obtained from PCR, they are sometimes called polonies. The beads are then immobilized onto wells, after which pyrosequencing renders the sequence of the individual fragments, which are then assembled by software into the sequence of the original genomic DNA. Each individual bead is not particularly impressive in the length of the fragment it sequences, but the strength of the technique is that thousands of different fragments, each containing a different sequence and each on its own bead, can be simultaneously sequenced and assembled into a single sequence. The 454 FLX Pyrosequencer was used to sequence the genome of James Watson, which was then given to him as an expression of gratitude.

The SOLID (Sequencing by Oligo Ligation Detection) sequencer by Applied Biosystems uses a similar process of fragmentation, adaptor attachment, and emulsion PCR, but sequencing is by sequential ligation, with DNA ligase and with fluorescently labeled oligonucleotides rather than by pyrosequencing. The Illumina Solexa Genome Analyzer also fragments the DNA and attaches adaptor sequences to the fragments. However, the Solexa system then attaches the fragments to a glass surface. Amplification takes place on the surface, after which the double-stranded DNA is denatured and a sequencing primer is added. Sequencing occurs by the incorporation of uniquely fluorescent-labeled nucleotides, using a modified DNA polymerase. After each nucleotide is incorporated and identified by its unique fluorescence, the fluorescence is removed by washing so that the next nucleotide can be incorporated and identified (techniques based on this principle are sometimes called reversible dye-terminator techniques).

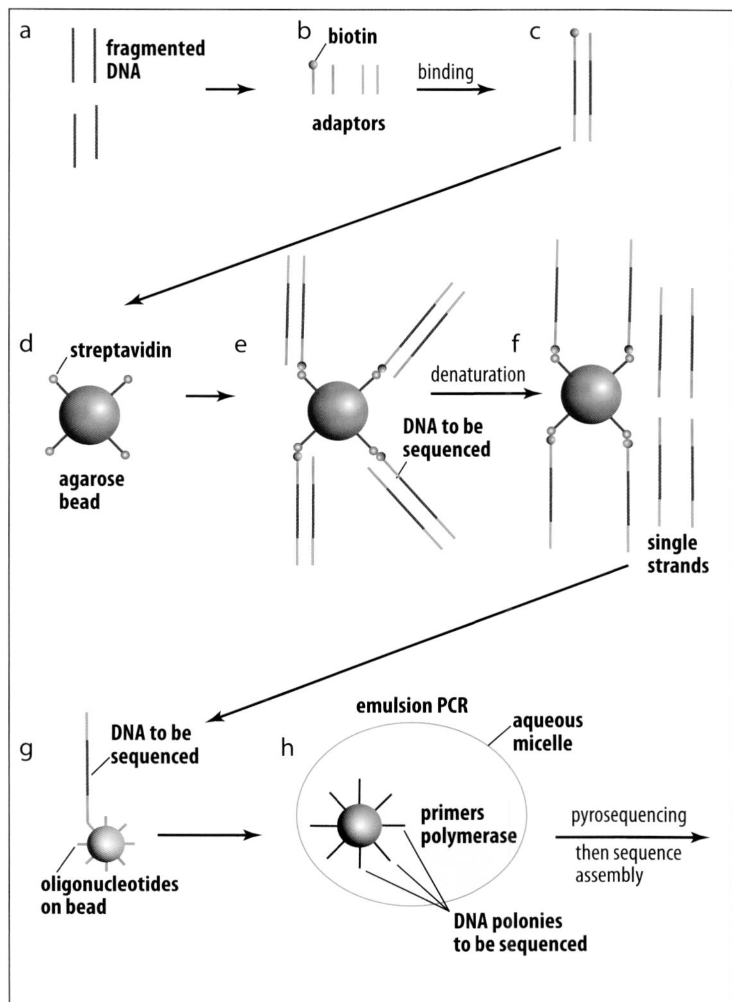

f45.24 Simplified diagram of massively parallel DNA sequencing
a Genomic double-stranded DNA is fragmented, usually by a nebulizer.
b The fragmented DNA is exposed to 2 short oligonucleotides called adaptors, one of which is attached to a biotin molecule (red ball).
c The adaptors bind to the ends of the double-stranded DNA fragments.
d The fragments, with adaptors, are exposed to beads that are coated with streptavidin.
e The streptavidin on the beads binds to the biotin molecules on the adaptors, attaching the DNA fragments to the beads.
f The DNA on the beads is denatured. The strands that are attached to the portion of the adaptor that contains the biotin molecule remain fixed to the bead, but the other strands are freed.
g The free strands are exposed to beads that are coated with an oligonucleotide that binds the adaptor sequence. The concentrations and conditions are chosen so that only 1 DNA fragment is bound to each bead.
h The beads are placed in aqueous micelles in an oil medium. Emulsion PCR takes place within the micelles, resulting in beads that are coated with large numbers of identical fragments (polonies). Within the aqueous micelle, each bead is bathed in PCR reagents, including primers and DNA polymerase. Other beads in separate micelles are coated with large numbers of different fragments (all fragments on each particular bead are identical).
After the emulsion PCR step, the sequence of the DNA fragments on each bead is determined by pyrosequencing, and an overall sequence is assembled by software.

Some next generation massively parallel DNA sequencing can sequence fragments of DNA without amplification. The first of these instruments, the HeliScope, by Helicos Bioscience, became available in 2008. Like the Illumina Solexa Genome Analyzer, the Helicos HeliScope immobilizes DNA fragments and sequences by iterative addition of labeled nucleotides, but differs in that there is no amplification. Despite the lack of amplification, this is still a massively parallel format since sequencing takes place simultaneously on millions of fragments.

Another next generation massively parallel sequencer that works without amplification is the Single Molecule Real Time sequencer (SMS or SMRT) by Pacific Biosciences, in which unique single fragments to be sequenced are deposited on an aluminum film punctuated by minute perforations. At each perforation, there is a DNA polymerase molecule that adds a fluorescently labeled nucleoside triphosphate (NTP) with loss of a pyrophosphate molecule. 4 different labels are used, 1 for each base, but the label is attached to one of the phosphate groups on the NTP that will be removed at the time of attachment (recall that bases are added in their triphosphate form, with loss of 2 phosphate groups). This would seem to be the wrong place to put the label, but the cleverness of this system is that the polymerase holds the NTP in place long enough for the label to be measured before lysis of the pyrophosphate group. In addition to its use as a sequencer, the SMRT system holds the promise of actually visualizing the synthesis of DNA.

Yet another alternative method of DNA sequencing, overlapping with the next generation methods, is the use of microarrays, discussed in the next section. Next generation DNA sequencing technologies hold the promise of permitting direct sequencing for virtually any clinical condition, even in small facilities. Indeed, at this writing, the 3 "hottest" technologies in molecular pathology are qPCR, high-resolution MCA, and next generation sequencing technologies.

Bioinformatics and Public DNA Databases

Bioinformatics and public databases of DNA sequence information are an essential and novel tool in research. Not long ago, data analysis consisted of basic statistics, such as mean, mode, standard deviation, the χ^2 test, etc. But now, data analysis in molecular biology involves computers to so great an extent that a new science, bioinformatics, has arisen from the union of computer science and molecular biology. Bioinformatics is the analytical branch of molecular biology and came to the fore in the sequencing of the human genome, which required enormous computer power to analyze the voluminous data. Bioinformatics continues to be important in the sequencing of the genomes of an increasing number of organisms, but in humans, it has shifted to play a central role in the creation and maintenance of databases to which newly acquired data can be compared. Major applications of bioinformatics include comparing DNA and protein sequences to identify evolutionary and functional relationships, identifying patterns in data that are not readily apparent (data mining), drug design, and developing 3-dimensional models of macromolecules to enable an understanding of their in vivo structure, function, and interactions. A number of works, both in print and online, are devoted to bioinformatics. Dale and von Schantz [Dale ISBN978-0470017340] cover the topic well, but for those of us who are less proud, a good starting point is *Bioinformatics for Dummies* [Claverie ISBN978-0-470-08985-9].

There are 3 major public databases of DNA sequence information, permitting further study of the genome and the comparison of any sequence of interest to the full genome. These databases are GenBank (http://www.ncbi.nlm.nih.gov), EMBL (http://www.ebi.ac.uk/embl), and DNA Database of Japan (http://www.ddbj.nig.ac.jp). These 3 databases routinely link information, so that an inquiry need not be posted to all 3 separately. These databases are typically queried through programs such as FASTA, which can compare nucleotide or amino acid sequences, or BLAST (Basic Local Alignment Search Tool), of which there are a number of variants, including one that compares nucleotide sequences (eg, BLASTN and BLASTX), one that compares amino acid sequences (eg, BLASTP), and one that allows the design of primers for PCR of a specified sequence. A newer querying program is BLAT (BLAST-Like Alignment Tool).

The sequencing of the normal human genome and the identification of some aberrations in this sequence in some cancers has resulted in the Cancer Sequence Genome Atlas (http://www.genome.gov/17516564), a project intended to catalog all of the DNA abnormalities identified in all forms of cancer [PMID20238077]. When this atlas is finally completed, and when our currently awkward and impractical ability to modify the DNA sequence matures, it will become possible to study and treat any cancer based on its specific aberration.

Need for Faster, Cheaper DNA Sequencing and Annotation of the Genome

Now that the human genome has been sequenced, the first challenge is to make sequencing much cheaper and faster, so that it can be used on a routine clinical basis. The second challenge is to annotate the genome. Annotation refers to understanding the biologic processes that are made possible by DNA. Sequencing is only the first step of this understanding. As an analogy, imagine being presented with a sequence of 3 billion letters without punctuation. One could read a few sentences here and there, but much of the text would be incomprehensible. Annotation is the process of better understanding the expression and regulation of DNA, and the function and interaction of its products.

Roughly, there are 2 types of annotation, structural and functional. Structural annotation attempts to identify promoters, start and stop codons, coding regions, intron-exon boundaries, probable products (RNA or protein), and regulatory areas. Functional annotation studies the functions of genes (remember, many genes do not code for a protein) and the structure, function, and interaction of their products, be they protein or RNA. Functional annotation overlaps with the fields of functional genomics and proteomics and seeks a complete understanding of the information that is contained in the DNA sequence. Full annotation is the combination of structural and functional annotation and searches for all information beyond the sequence, starting with promoters and start and stop codons, and ending with an understanding of the functions and interactions of DNA, RNA, and proteins. As was the case with the sequencing of the genome, full annotation will require huge computing power and a collaborative effort across many disciplines.

A difficulty in structural annotation is that many genes do not have any identifiable sequence that serves as a promoter, so one cannot simply look for TATA, CAAT, or GC sequences as initiators of transcription. Often, it is simply not known what triggers transcription. Without this knowledge, we do not know where new "sentences" begin.

Another difficulty in structural annotation is that genes are rarely simple, discrete entities. Rather, a segment of DNA can code multiple transcripts, depending on the specific start and stop codons, which introns are spliced out, which exons are transcribed, and what other transcriptional regulatory features come into play. In some cases, the DNA coding for one protein is completely contained within a sequence of DNA that codes for another, very different protein.

There are a number of approaches to functional annotation. One of these is sequence comparison (homology), which is based on the premise that similar sequences in DNA imply similar functions in the proteins they encode (eg, if an enigmatic DNA sequence is similar to that encoding for a protein in the immunoglobulin superfamily, a function in immunity is inferred). This technique has substantial potential but also 2 limitations. First, many sequences of DNA have been repeated in genes of diverse functions over the course of evolution. Nature has found that it is easier to employ existing DNA sequences in new genes, rather like the way one may use prefabricated building blocks in the construction of buildings of different purposes. Indeed, it is well known that genes with sequences similarities may encode very different proteins. A partial solution to this limitation is to compare large blocks of DNA, corresponding to multiple domains in proteins, as these are unlikely to represent merely "recycled" genetic material and are more likely to indicate genetic material that has a common purpose. A second limitation to functional annotation by homology is that the sequence of some genes simply does not match that of any known gene.

Repetitive DNA

If one were to pick the 5 most important advances in molecular biology in the last 35 years, good choices would be the discovery of restriction nucleases, the discovery of nucleic acid amplification techniques (of which PCR was the first), the discovery of sequencing techniques, the integration of computer technology (bioinformatics), and the discovery of hypervariable regions of the genome. Most hypervariable regions in clinical use involve repetitive DNA, sequences of DNA that are repeated throughout the genome, either as single units or as a variable number of repeating units. Along with single nucleotide polymorphisms SNPs and CNV, repetitive DNA is a major cause of the minor differences in DNA from one person to another.

To a great extent, repetitive DNA accounts for the appreciable similarity of DNA across many species. Duplication also furnishes another mechanism for genetic diversity because a duplicated area can undergo change while the original area continues the function of the sequence, very much as one would make a copy of a document before editing it. In particular, duplications are thought to give rise to families and superfamilies of related genes that share structural similarities.

Broadly speaking, repetitive portions of DNA may be divided into 2 groups. The first group is called interspersed (or dispersed) repetitive DNA and is comprised of those sequences which are *singly* repeated and which are dispersed throughout the genome. The second group consists of sequences that are repeated and dispersed as *tandem* duplications [PMID19052325].

There are several classes of interspersed repetitive DNA. The 2 best known are the short interspersed nuclear elements (SINEs) and the long interspersed nuclear elements (LINEs). Although there is no sharp dividing line, SINEs generally have <500 base pairs. An example of the SINE family is Alu, a sequence of approximately 280 base pairs, unique to primates, which is the single most abundant human DNA sequence, comprising about 10% of our total DNA. Recently, the Alu sequence has been found at several locations in the human genome where it is absent in other primates. Like many members of the SINE family (and possibly also some members of the LINE family), Alu appears to have arisen and propagated through retrotransposition (or retroposition) [PMID19621349].

The second group of repetitive DNA is comprised of those sequences that are repeated as *tandem* duplications, meaning that the repeated unit consists of multiple reiterations of a smaller sequence, one immediately following another. The terminology for this type of repetitive DNA can be confusing. Depending on the length of the repeating element and the number of repeats, these sequences of DNA are called satellites (the longest repeating unit), minisatellites, or microsatellites (the shortest repeating unit) [PMID18428214]. An alternative name for tandemly repeated DNA is "variable number of tandem repeats" (VNTRs), though the latter term often refers specifically to a type of minisatellite. Unlike interspersed repetitive DNA, tandemly repeated DNA is not randomly distributed throughout the genome, but rather concentrated in specific areas.

Tandemly repeated DNA apparently has a different origin from interspersed repetitive DNA and is not so clearly linked to retrotransposition. The basic unit of tandemly repeated DNA may be as small as a single base pair or as large as several hundred base pairs, but the important concept is that this building block is repeated many times, resulting in a final sequence that can be as long as several million base pairs in the case of satellites.

Satellite DNA is a type of tandemly repeating DNA that is composed of the longest repeated unit. Satellite DNA is not transcribed, and in fact, is often found in heterochromatin (the dense portion of DNA that is not transcribed), especially near centromeres. An example of satellite DNA is α (or alphoid) DNA, consisting of a basic unit of 171 base pairs. α sequences are found primarily at centromeres and seem important in the organization and maintenance of centromeres, although interestingly, they are not exclusively found in this location [PMID15289662]. Tandem arrays of this unit result in repeating structures called α subfamilies, defined by the number of repeating units of the 171 base pair monomer. At this writing, there are 33 α subfamilies. α subfamilies comprise 3-5% of all human DNA. Some of these subfamilies are specific to certain chromosomes and some are not. Some chromosomes have only 1 α subfamily at their centromeres, while others have >1. For example, the centromere on chromosome 7 contains an α subfamily consisting of 16 α monomers, resulting in a 2.7 kb structure that can be recognized, identifying the chromosome.

Most chromosomes can be identified in this manner, based on the number of repeating α subunits at their centromeres, usually determined by FISH (PCR is not good at determining the lengths of very long segments of DNA). Because some chromosomes have >1 α subfamily at their centromeres, chromosome identification often requires the use of blocking DNA (eg, cot-1) and special hybridization conditions that are usually proprietary. α probes are useful in identifying marker chromosomes (chromosomes of unknown nature). However, the acrocentric chromosomes (13, 14, 15, 21, and 22) are very difficult to distinguish in this manner, and chromosomes 13 and 21 have virtually identical repeat numbers of the α subunit and cannot be distinguished at all by this method.

Minisatellites are composed of repeating DNA units that are smaller than those in satellites. Microsatellites are composed of still smaller repeated units. There is some overlap in length between microsatellites and minisatellites, and the distinction is made on a combination of the length of the monomeric unit, the number of repeats, and tradition. In general, minisatellites consist of those tandemly repeated units whose monomer is about 15 to 50 base pairs, and whose total length is about 1,000-20,000 base pairs.

There are 2 types of minisatellites. The first type is telomeric. Telomeres, found at the ends of chromosomes, are minisatellites consisting of 6 base pairs (usually TTAGGG), repeated up to about 2,000 times. Although the monomeric unit is only 6 base pairs, the number of repetitions and the resulting overall length places the telomere in the category of minisatellite, not microsatellite. A number of proteins are associated with this repetitive DNA in telomeres. Telomeres appear to protect the chromosome from degradation and may have a function in orienting chromosomes during mitosis. Over time, some of these repeated units of TTAGGG are lost, and it has been suggested that this loss is a factor in aging. Some cells (germ cells, stem cells, lymphocytes, and most malignant cells) have telomerase, which is a ribonucleoprotein (combination of an enzyme and RNA) that restores the TTAGGG repeats (typically, the suffix "-ase" for an enzyme implies a cleavage function, but telomerase rebuilds telomeres rather than cleaves them). The protein portion of telomerase is a reverse transcriptase. In contrast, most normal cells do not have telomerase and cannot repair damage to telomeres. In somatic cells, telomere length provides an estimate of how many times that cell has divided and may soon be used to estimate cellular age.

The second type of minisatellite is the hypervariable type, discovered in 1985. Hypervariable minisatellite DNA is found in multiple locations in the human genome. In hypervariable minisatellite DNA, the basic unit is from 6 to >50 base pairs, and the overall numbers of repeats is highly variable between individuals, accounting for the name hypervariable. This type is often referred to as VNTRs, though this term is sometimes used for all forms of tandemly repeating DNA in general. Because of different numbers of the basic repeating unit in hypervariable minisatellites among different people, restriction endonuclease treatment gives rise to fragments of different lengths in different individuals. This was the basis of the first "DNA fingerprinting" (now called identity testing or DNA profiling), introduced by Jeffreys [PMID3856104, PMID2989708]. If there are 1,000 repeats of the basic unit in one person and only 500 in another, with an endonuclease site on either side of the entire repeated unit, the use of that endonuclease will result in a longer fragment in the first person than in the second. In the initial DNA profiling work, after endonuclease treatment of DNA, gel electrophoresis resulted in fragments with different migration positions. After blotting onto a membrane, labeled probes that bond to the core sequences that are repeated in these minisatellites were then hybridized to the fragments, so that their positions could be seen. In the first person, with the longer number of repeats, the fragments were larger, and the labeled probe showed that it had not migrated as far into the gel as the fragment from the second person. This procedure replaced RFLP, which was not suitable for profiling, but the cumbersome steps in Southern blotting were still necessary.

Today, microsatellites have replaced minisatellites in DNA profiling. The individual monomeric unit in a microsatellite is from 1 to about 13 base pairs, and the total length of the microsatellite is about 150 base pairs. Other names for microsatellites are short tandem repeat polymorphisms (STRP), simple sequence repeat polymorphisms (SSRP), and short tandem repeats (STR). Although class 1 transposons (retrotransposons) may occasionally give rise to long terminal repeats (LTRs) in eukaryotes, LTRs are primarily found in retroviruses, where they flank functional genes and serve to assist in their insertion into host DNA.

Unlike satellites and minisatellites, microsatellites are spread evenly throughout the genome. Bacteria use microsatellites to vary their antigenic profile, but they have no known function in humans.

In microsatellites, the number of repeated units is often not the same in the 2 corresponding chromosomes. The number of repeated units is variable because these repeated regions may form outpouchings during DNA replication. If these outpouchings are in the template strand, that DNA will be left out of the replication process and a deletion will result, diminishing the number of repeating units. If they are in the strand that is being synthesized, the number of repeated units will be increased and an insertion will occur, increasing the number of repeating units.

As is the case for minisatellite analysis, in microsatellite analysis the DNA abnormality need not be in an actual endonuclease site. A huge advantage of microsatellite analysis over minisatellite analysis is that the shorter length of the basic unit makes it highly amenable to PCR. Microsatellite analysis by PCR is based on the fact that the sequences flanking the microsatellite are conserved. Primers are designed that will hybridize to the adjacent conserved region, after which PCR will amplify the entire repeated region and generate amplicons whose length depends on the number of repeats. The amplicons are allowed to react with a fluorescently labeled probe, followed by capillary electrophoresis, thus obviating the laborious techniques of restriction endonuclease treatment and Southern blotting (Southern blotting is rarely used now in routine diagnostic molecular pathology). Microsatellite analysis is much faster than the restriction endonuclease-gel electrophoresis-Southern blotting procedure that was employed in minisatellite analysis.

Although the number of repeated units varies from person to person and even from one chromosome to its counterpart within a person, it is usually constant throughout different tissues on a given chromosome in a given person (eg, if a patient has 30 repeating units in one chromosome and 40 repeating units in the second chromosome in the skin, those same numbers are likely to be found in the bone marrow or the lung). But in certain tumors, it was noticed that the microsatellites from the malignant cells were either longer or shorter than the counterpart normal tissue. In some cases, the entire repeating focus is lost in one chromosome. This is called loss of heterozygosity (LOH), and is detected as the loss of a band or a set of bands after endonuclease digestion, electrophoresis, and hybridization with probes that are specific for a given microsatellite. LOH is actually a microdeletion and is often clinically important because the microsatellite repeats are often within tumor suppressor genes, or so close to them that they are functionally within them, so that loss of the microsatellite often means that a tumor suppressor gene is lost or inactivated as well. There will be loss of tumor suppression if there is also a mutation in the tumor suppressor gene of the chromosome which has not sustained LOH, and possibly even if the other chromosome is normal, because some heterozygotes appear to have an increased risk for some tumors [PMID17349581].

Although LOH in its broadest sense can refer to any situation where 1 of the 2 copies of an allele or a DNA sequence is lost, in most discussions of tumor biology, it refers to the physical loss of 1 of 2 tumor suppressor genes and is usually detected by the loss of a marker that is close to a tumor suppressor gene. The first such markers, still commonly used, were microsatellites because they are common and are spread throughout the genome, and it is likely that a microsatellite will be close to a tumor suppressor gene of interest. SNPs are increasingly used today as markers for tumor suppressor genes instead of microsatellites. As determining the DNA sequence of individual patients becomes more feasible, direct testing for a mutation will become the rule, precluding the need for testing for genetic abnormalities by association with markers.

In LOH/microsatellite analysis, one must compare the tumor to normal tissue. Because the number of microsatellite repeats normally varies between the 2 chromosomes but is constant between tissue types, there will usually be 2 bands of generally equal fluorescence intensity for each microsatellite in normal tissue, but only 1 in tumor tissue if there is LOH. In practice, the absent microsatellite is often present in the associated nonneoplastic tissue that is invariably present in samples of tumor (eg, stroma and blood vessels), and there will be a faint band that may cause LOH to be missed [PMID10580104]. For this reason, in searching for LOH, every effort should be made to test a sample in which at least 70-80% of the cells are actual tumor cells and LOH should be excluded if there are 2 bands of unequal fluorescence intensity in the tumor tissue. If LOH is detected, it might be desirable to sequence the suppressor gene on the other chromosome and to study family members of the patient.

It is also possible that the repeated region will not be deleted in a tumor, but that the number of repeated units in it changes relative to the patient's normal cells. This is called microsatellite instability (MSI) and is detected not as a loss of bands, but as a change in their migration pattern after PCR and gel electrophoresis or as a change in the time to pass the laser in capillary electrophoresis. Diminished *intensity* of a band suggests LOH, but different *positions* indicate MSI. Contaminating normal tissue is less likely to mislead in MSI studies than in LOH studies because the bands in MSI will occur in areas where there is no counterpart in the normal tissue.

Whereas LOH often indicates diminished tumor suppressor function, MSI frequently indicates poor DNA repair because normal DNA can usually repair an incorrect number of repetitions of the basic unit of the microsatellite. Although MSI does not appear to directly cause neoplasia, it is associated with some types of tumors, probably because the poor DNA repair that led to MSI also compromises DNA fidelity during replication. Because microsatellites are near to and a marker for a number of genes, MSI can be used in selected patients as a "screening" test to identify patients who have a higher risk of some types of tumors, especially hereditary nonpolyposis colon cancer syndrome (HNPCC; also called Lynch syndrome).

PCR/electrophoresis analysis of microsatellites, as in LOH/MSI analysis, is prone to a difficulty called "stutter" bands (or shadow bands). Stutter bands are false bands that are very slightly smaller (usually just 1 repeat unit) than the main band, and therefore, they are manifest on a gel as a faint band that runs just below (ie, is slightly smaller than) the main band. Stutter bands are thought to occur from "slippage" during DNA amplification by PCR. Stutter causes small, adjacent bands or peaks which should be disregarded.

Microarrays

Microarray technology developed from progress in 3 fields: the Human Genome Project, the fabrication of integrated circuits, and increased computer power. Most often, microarrays are small collections of DNA, in a checkerboard pattern, mounted onto a substrate. Microarrays (often called gene chips) can be constructed by 2 mechanisms [PMID19381969]. In the first method, DNA is cloned by such methods as BACs, PACs, etc, and amplified by PCR in solution. A drop of the solution is then transferred to a specific, minute area of the substrate (often called a well) by spotting or dropping with a fabricating instrument that ensures uniform size and even spacing.

The second method of fabricating microarrays is in situ synthesis of an oligonucleotide on the substrate, where one end of a DNA strand is extended while the other end is attached to the substrate. Synthetic oligonucleotide arrays are often more sensitive than arrays constructed from cloned sequences and can detect smaller deletions and duplications if the abnormality is represented by the oligonucleotide that has been designed and fabricated.

PNAs may substitute for oligonucleotides in the construction of synthetic microarrays. PNAs are nucleic acid analogues that contain a peptide bond rather than the weaker sugar-phosphate bond of normal nucleic acids in their backbone. The lack of phosphate groups in PNAs means that there is no mutual repulsion with the phosphate groups of the nucleic acid sequence to which they have bonded, resulting in increased affinity for a complementary strand compared to normal oligonucleotides.

In microarray use, the words "probe" and "target" often have reversed meanings from the other techniques we have discussed, and one must be sure of the writer's meaning. In most techniques (eg, FISH, CGH, M-FISH, M-banding), the word "probe" referred to a labeled oligonucleotide of known sequence, in *solution*, and hybridized to an *immobilized target* whose sequence is unknown and will be determined by whether or not it binds to the probe. However, in microarrays, the terminology is often reversed—the material immobilized on the slide or substrate is of known sequence and is frequently called the probe. The material in solution that is applied to the array (often a patient sample) is called the target. Care must be taken to ensure that the reader understands the writer's use of these 2 terms. The reason for the frequent reversal of terminology is that the word "probe" actually refers to a known sequence, be it immobilized or in solution, while the term "target" refers to an unknown sequence, either immobilized or in solution (ie, the correct term stems from whether or not the sequence is known, not whether or not it is immobilized or in solution). In conventional FISH and related techniques, the "unknown"—the patient sample—is generally immobilized and exposed to a known probe in solution, but in microarrays, the known sequence is immobilized and the unknown sample is in solution.

All uses of microarrays involve hybridization between the labeled target or targets and the unlabeled, immobilized probe, after which a washing procedure is performed to remove nonspecific binding. Digital imaging and software then provide information about the degree and location of binding of target to probe. Like M-FISH or SKY, microarrays address large portions of the genome in a single study, and whole genome arrays are becoming available. Some arrays are partially annotated, meaning that in addition to the known sequence of the DNA in the wells, the starting and stopping points for genes and regulators of gene expression for that DNA are also known.

Applications of Microarrays Legion and Growing

There are growing applications for microarrays [PMID19381982], but at this time, microarrays are used primarily to determine DNA sequence, to identify chromosomal abnormalities, study proteins that are associated with DNA, and to assess gene expression. When used to determine DNA sequence, microarrays consisting of thousands of short probes of known sequence, such that much of the genome is covered, are exposed to the target DNA whose sequence is sought. These chips are commercially available, and both the exact sequence and location on the chip of each oligonucleotide probe is known. The target fragment is amplified, and the many copies are tagged with a fluorescent dye, after which they are allowed to hybridize to the fixed sequences on the chip. One is not looking for the single perfect match that will immediately render the sequence. Rather, the pattern of numerous hybridizations of the target to many probes gives the sequence of the target. Most of the fragments will not hybridize at all; some will hybridize a little to some of the bound sequences to which they are partially complementary. A few fragments will hybridize more strongly because they are nearly complementary. After a washing step to remove nonspecific binding, computer quantitation will determine which probes on the chip the target hybridized to, and to what extent. The software determines the percentage of binding of the target to each of the thousands of probes. Knowing the sequence of each probe to which the target hybridized, the extent of the hybridizations, and the overlapping sequences of the probes, the sequence of the target can subsequently be calculated. A control target of known sequence is run concurrently. This method of sequencing is used for relatively short fragments of DNA. Repetitive sequences can be problematic.

A second use of microarrays is a variation on the sequencing strategy, called allele-specific oligonucleotide hybridization (ASO). This technique uses a series of synthetic oligonucleotide probes, differing in only a single base, encompassing all of the known polymorphisms, including SNPs, of a single gene. One of these oligonucleotides will hybridize to normal DNA, while others will hybridize only to DNA that has one specific mutation or polymorphism. Labeled fragments from a patient are applied to these immobilized synthetic oligonucleotides. After a washing step, only those patient fragments that perfectly match one of the oligonucleotide probes will remain bound and can be detected by its signal. Since this probe is of known sequence and location, the location of the signal discloses the sequence of DNA in the patient sample. Microarrays have merged as a leading method of detection of SNPs.

A third major use for microarrays is to replace conventional CGH. CGH is used to compare the DNA of a normal and an abnormal cell by tagging the cells' DNA with fluorochromes of different colors and allowing the 2 tagged DNA samples to compete for hybridization with normal metaphases. The ratio of the 2 colors provides information on the relative abundance of the DNA in the normal and abnormal cells and on CNV. A limitation of CGH is that normal metaphases are required, and chromosomes in metaphase have many areas in which the DNA is condensed and effectively inaccessible to the probe. Using metaphase spreads, one can only detect regions, or perhaps bands that are differentially expressed.

In the microarray modification of CGH (aCGH), introduced in 2001, patient DNA (often, but not always from a tumor) and control DNA are labeled with different fluorochromes, mixed, then applied to the arrays and allowed to compete for hybridization to the bound probes of the array **f45.25**. In aCGH, the probes are short oligonucleotides and the target is often portions of the patient or test genome that have been cloned by the use of BACs, PACs, or cosmids, or amplified by PCR. Because neither the probe nor the target is in metaphase, aCGH has greater sensitivity than CGH. In aCGH, microdeletions and microduplications that are beyond detection in conventional CGH can be identified [PMID17558419]. In addition to greater sensitivity, another advantage of aCGH is that data are obtained by a scanner rather than by a fluorescent microscope, permitting greater speed and decreasing subjectivity.

Using synthetic oligonucleotide sequences as probes, it is possible to construct arrays that collectively, encompass all of the genome (called whole genome arrays, though at this writing, they do not quite yet encompass the entire genome). A more typical use is to construct an array that encompasses a complete chromosome, so that specific regions of a chromosome can be studied in high resolution. For example, one might employ arrays that cover all of chromosome 3 in the study of renal cell carcinomas or chromosome 1 in the study of oligodendrogliomas, etc. These are called targeted arrays.

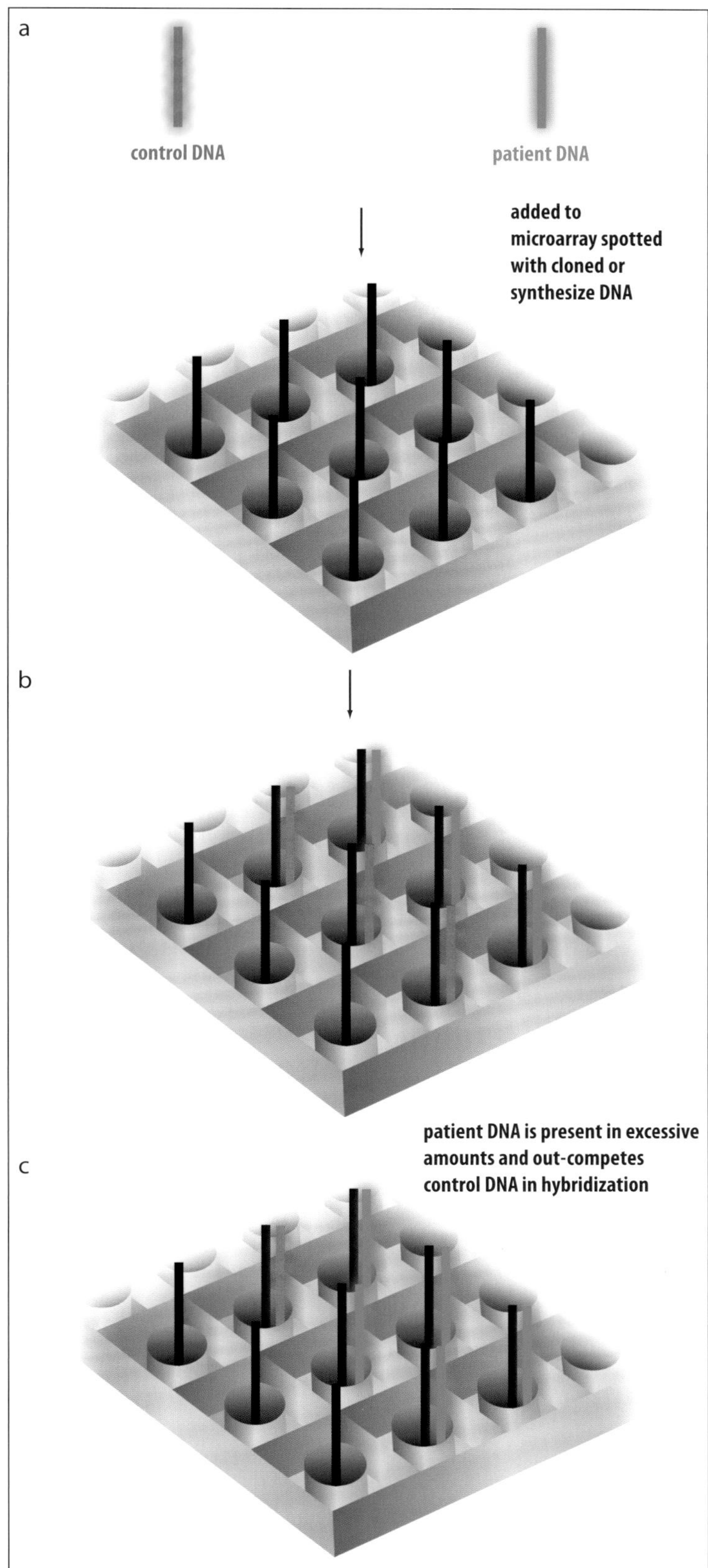

f45.25 Array comparative genomic hybridization (aCGH). Control DNA and patient DNA, labeled with fluorochromes of different colors, compete for hybridization, as in **f45.17**, but to cloned or synthesized DNA of known composition on microarrays, not to normal metaphase **a**. In **b**, the patient and control DNA samples bind to the array in equal amounts. In **c**, the patient DNA preferentially binds to the array indicating that the patient has an increased amount of DNA that is complementary to the sequences represented by that portion of the array. Because the sequences on the array are known, findings provide information about the patient's DNA sequence, chromosome copy number, or cytogenetic abnormalities.

Like conventional CGH, aCGH may miss a small minority population in a mosaic sample and like conventional CGH, aCGH will not generally detect balanced rearrangements, though a method to do this in aCGH has been developed [PMID21907824]. In this use, patient and control DNA are amplified and the amplicons are labeled with different dyes and applied to an array that contains normal DNA and known potential fusion products. The control amplicons bind only to normal areas on the array that correspond to one of the fusion partners, but an abnormal amplicon will bind to an area that spans the breakpoint of a translocation. The ratio of the 2 signals and the knowledge of the sequence they bind to provides information about balanced rearrangements.

A fourth application for microarrays, really a form of aCGH, is more sensitive cytogenetics [PMID18617013]. Conventional G-banding was a great advance, but is of low resolution and interpretation is subjective. Moreover, the requirement for metaphase chromosomes means that the cells must be cultured, so that even in the best of circumstances, there will be a delay, and often, culture is not possible because of a poor specimen, the nondividing nature of the cells, or contamination. Conventional FISH greatly improves turnaround time but can be used only when a specific, previously characterized abnormality is suspected.

Array CGH has transformed cytogenetics by permitting screening of a much higher percentage of the genome at high resolution. In this use of microarrays, called cytogenetic microarray analysis (CMA) or occasionally molecular karyotyping, patient DNA is labeled with one color and control DNA with another color, after which the two are mixed and then are hybridized to arrays that contain cloned and amplified normal genomic DNA or oligonucleotide sequences of known sequence. Chromosomal abnormalities in the patient will be evident by a ratio of the 2 colors that is significantly greater or less than 1. As is the case for other applications of microarrays, synthetic oligonucleotides are replacing cloned DNA as the probe on the substrate in CMA, especially if a specific abnormality is suspected, though cloned DNA is still used for the probes in wider screening.

Unlike the use of FISH without arrays, CMA offers the potential of identifying abnormalities that have not yet been characterized. With CMA, it is possible to show differences in the hybridization patterns of normal and abnormal DNA without testing for a specific, known abnormality. For example, if a patient sample exhibits diminished hybridization relative to a control sample in specific well of the microarray, because the DNA sequence of the probes in those wells is known, statements can be made about the nature of the abnormalities in the patient sample even if no such abnormalities have been previously described or sequenced.

CMA has shown that CNV is much more common than had been thought, involving approximately 12% of the total genome and thousands of genes [PMID17597776]. Some CNVs are seen in a sufficient number of patients (over 1%) that they are better regarded as variants of normal than as pathologic. These are called copy number polymorphisms. All CNVs are submitted to public databases, such as the Database of Genomic Variants (DGV) and the Database of Chromosomal Imbalance and Phenotype in Humans (DECIPHER). However, much of the information in these databases has been derived from surveys of phenotypically normal people. Consequently, as valuable as these publicly accessible databases unquestionably are, they suffer from 2 drawbacks. First, many of the reported "abnormalities" may not be germane to a clinical condition and may even be a variant of normal that has not yet been recognized. Second, because the field and the technology are young, many clinically significant abnormalities have not yet been characterized, and arrays that can detect any and all abnormalities of DNA sequence are not yet widely in use.

In theory, CMA can screen the entire genome at high resolution, with a rapid turnaround time, and does not require knowledge of a specific abnormality. In practice, although the human genome has been sequenced, microarrays do not yet carry the entire genome and therefore cannot screen for all abnormalities in the entire genome of a patient sample. Most CMAs are performed with arrays that have been constructed to identify all common abnormalities and to provide some degree of random coverage. However, whole genome arrays are nearly a reality at this writing. For example, tiling arrays cover many sequences, with some overlap, that together span a large region of the genome and are nearly whole genome. As true whole genome arrays become more common, all of the many advantages of microarrays will be greatly augmented.

At this writing, CMA is performed in conjunction with conventional karyotyping, but it is an evolving standard that is likely to replace conventional karyotyping because of its outstanding combination of high resolution and ability to screen for abnormalities that have not yet been characterized. For example, using array cytogenetics, abnormalities have been found in about 8% of patients with idiopathic dysmorphism, mental retardation, or developmental delay [PMID17389918], a significantly higher number than conventional G-banding.

A limitation of CMA is that it cannot detect balanced translocations and inversions (this is a major reason why conventional karyotyping is still needed). However, many apparently balanced rearrangements have small gains or losses at the breakpoints, and these might be detectable by array technology in the near future. A second potential limitation of CMA is that, as is the case for conventional CGH, low-level mosaicism can be missed (ie, the fluorescent signals of a small population of cells may not be detectable).

A fifth application of microarrays is in the study of the interactions of DNA and proteins such as transcription factors and regulatory proteins. This method is often called ChIP-chip because the DNA that is applied to the microarray chip is obtained by chromatin immunoprecipitation (ChIP). In ChIP, DNA is allowed to react with the protein of interest, after which it is fragmented and exposed to an antibody to the protein under investigation. Crosslinking of this antibody results in precipitation of the protein and the DNA that is bound to it. The DNA is then applied to the microarray chip, after which its hybridization characteristics are used to detect its location in the genome. It can then be seen where in the genome the protein is active.

A sixth major application of microarrays is to study messenger RNA (ie, gene expression analysis). mRNA is usually studied by conversion to cDNA with reverse transcriptase. In the simplest version of gene expression analysis, fragments of cDNA from 2 cell types (eg, a muscle cell and a skin cell) are bound to fluorescent tags of different colors. The tagged cDNA fragments are then hybridized to oligonucleotides in microarray wells. If both types of cells make that mRNA, then both colors will be seen. If one cell type makes the mRNA and the other does not, only 1 color will be seen. If both cell types make the mRNA, but in different amounts, gradations of color, as detected and analyzed by fluorescence microscopy and software, will permit statements regarding the relative amounts of mRNA made by cells in the 2 samples. Microarray studies of mRNA have been useful in studying gene expression in different types of cells, in one type of cell under different conditions, in neoplasia, during the cell cycle, in development, or in response to a drug.

Any step in this procedure, from extraction of RNA through hybridization of probes, may be more efficient for 1 of the 2 populations of cells, leading to spurious results and meaning that conclusions should be drawn only from significant differences in expression. One should be wary of a conclusion that one cell population transcribes 90% as much of a given DNA sequence as another population, but if the data are properly analyzed, quantitative statements can be made, such as abnormal cells transcribing 1/4 as much or 3 times as much of a particular DNA sequence as normal cells. This is called differential screening, and identifies those genes that are overexpressed or underexpressed in tumors. This approach has been useful in demonstrating that abnormal cells such as in tumors, transcribe DNA differently.

Once this technology is fully mature, the pattern of gene expression may replace morphology and immunohistochemistry in the diagnosis of neoplasia and in the assessment of prognostically important proteins. Initial forays into this area have come in attempts to determine the primary site when a metastasis has been sampled. Because RNA is degraded in formalin-fixed, paraffin-embedded (FFPE) tissue, much work in this area is done with fresh frozen tissue, though FFPE tissue has been adapted to the process [PMID20522636, PMID20688907]. 2 systems have been approved to assist in tumor identification by gene expression study in FFPE tissue. The first is the Pathwork Tissue of Origin Test (Pathwork Diagnostics, Redwood City, CA), using a microarray platform [PMID21602661]. The second is THEROS CancerTYPe ID (bioTheranostics, San Diego, CA), based on RT-PCR rather than microarrays [PMID16594740, PMID21708287]. While gene expression has not yet reached the point where it can substitute for traditional histology and immunohistochemistry, it can complement the traditional approach, and hybrid identification systems, employing both immunohistochemistry and gene expression, have been described [PMID20558571].

Once important genes in a disease have been identified, another possibility is to assess the response of those genes to drugs. In infectious disease, microarrays might allow the determination of how pathogenic genes respond to antibiotics. Gene expression profiling could potentially offer the opportunity to assess a patent's particular tumor at the molecular level and to design a drug regime specific for that tumor, overlapping with pharmacogenetics in the development of personalized medicine.

Expression vectors are changes in the expression of a gene over a set of different conditions (this use of the term "expression vector" is not to be confused with an expression vector that is used to generate quantities of protein in cloning, discussed earlier). A simplified expression vector in microarray studies for a gene over 3 different experimental conditions (exp con) might look something like this:

Exp con 1	Exp con 2	Exp con 3
0.5	1.0	1.3

where the numbers 0.5, 1.0, and 1.3 refer to the ratios of the fluorescence of the cDNA fragments from the gene under investigation to that of a control gene or a group of control genes (ie, under the first experimental condition, the gene is only half as transcribed as the control; under the second condition, it is equally transcribed, and under the third condition, it is transcribed at a slightly higher rate than the control).

Sets of expression vectors, encompassing multiple genes, constitute an expression matrix, a simplified example of which is the following:

	Exp con 1	Exp con 2	Exp con 3
Gene 1	0.5	1.0	1.3
Gene 2	0.5	0.4	0.2
Gene 3	2.1	0.3	2.3

An example of an expression matrix is seen in **f45.26**. There are a number of artifacts that must be compensated for prior to data acquisition and conclusions in microarray studies. First, not all wells are uniformly constructed or evenly placed on the substrate, and not all probes are uniformly constructed or placed within a well. Either of these difficulties will adversely affect results because the mathematical analysis assumes uniform construction and placement of wells and probes. For example, probes that are not perfectly round will result in aberrant signals. In addition, background fluorescence can be caused by nonspecific binding of target to probe or to the substrate itself. Minute particles of dust may obscure a signal. Different fluorochromes may not all have the same affinity for the probes. There are also variations between different substrates used in fabricating the same array.

Software is available to provide an estimate of background fluorescence, using fluorescence from negative controls, and an estimate of signal-to-noise ratio. Software is also available to identify signals that are suspicious because of their faintness, because the shape of the fluorescent area suggests a probe that is improperly made, shaped, or placed, or because the signal appears to have been modified by dust particles.

But even with the best software correction, the statistical analysis of microarray data can be immensely complex. Literally tens of thousands of simultaneous statistical analyses are necessary to analyze the signals emanating from the thousands of probes on the substrate. Computing plays such an integral role in microarray studies that databases exist solely to deal with this matter. One of the leading microarray databases is the Stanford Microarray Database (http://smd.stanford.edu) [PMID17182626]. To increase the standardization of data obtained from microarrays, the Microarray Gene Expression Database Group (MEGD), a consortium that includes investigators from the European Bioinformatics institute (EBI) and the National Institutes of Health (NIH), has created a standard format for the design of microarray experiments called the Minimum Information about a Microarray Experiment (MIAME). It is hoped that MIAME will standardize microarray data from different experiments and different institutions and permit free exchange of data [PMID11726920].

After partial software correction of the data, many of the remaining difficulties in the analysi THEROS CancerTYPe ID s of data from microarrays are addressed by statistical methods.

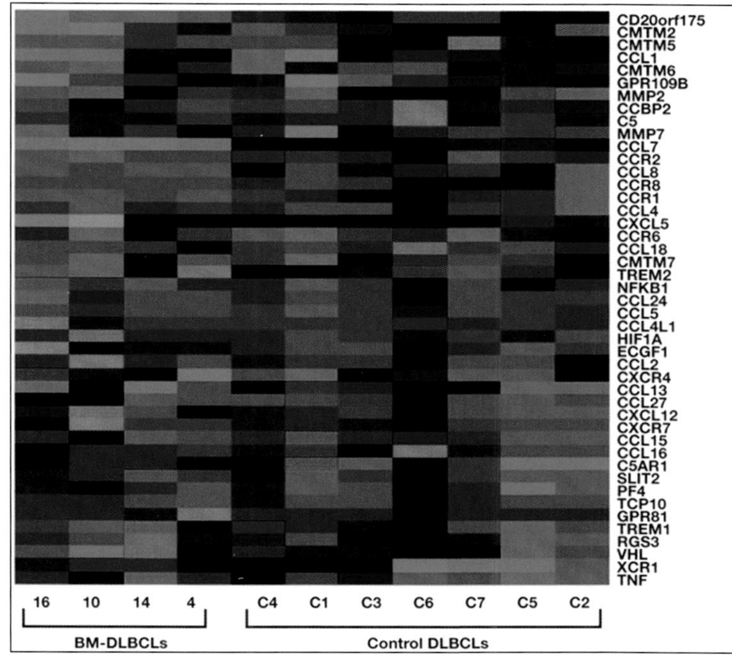

f45.26 A microarray-based study of gene expression in "ordinary" diffuse large B-cell lymphoma (DLBCL) at right vs DLBCL originating in the bone marrow at left. The expression of approximately 50 genes, enumerated on the right, is studied. Red indicates high levels of expression, and green indicates low levels. While the morphology and immunohistochemical features are essentially identical for the 2 types of DLBCL, there are clear differences in gene expression, suggesting that DLBCL may be a collection of neoplasms.

All of these methods involve a process of mathematical corrections called normalization [PMID18629271]. Normalization is based on the comparison of data signals to those obtained from reference points. It is, in effect, a calibration of the system. Using normalization, one first uses software to exclude obvious outlying data points, aberrant signals, and background fluorescence, then applies correction formulas to compensate for the imperfections of the system. Normalization works better for systematic errors (a general bias) than for individual errors affecting small regions of an array.

There are 3 sets of genes that can be used as internal controls in the normalization process: all genes, a subset of genes whose expression is thought to be relatively constant throughout a variety of conditions and circumstances, and genes that are extrinsic to the experiment (so-called "spiked in" control genes). Most often, normalization is based on all of the genes on the array. The rationale for this is that in most experiments, while the expression of 1 or a small number of genes may vary, the expression of most genes does not, and the expression of all genes as a whole is relatively constant.

Normalization is an attempt to compensate for errors and problems that are not fully understood, and, therefore, is destined to some degree of failure from the start. Indeed, normalization adds its own set of errors. The hope is that the user can exchange one set of errors, many from unknown causes, for a smaller set of errors of more predictable causes.

Common normalization programs include Bioconductor [PMID18563370, PMID16939789], TM4 software system, available from the Institute for Genomic Research (http://www.tigr.org/software), and BASE, a Web-based system developed at Lund University (http://base.thep.lu.se).

Data generated by molecular techniques, especially those involving microarrays, are often said to be "in silico," corresponding to the older terms "in vivo" and "in vitro." Thus, one may read in the literature that "... has been shown in silico."

Because of their relatively standardized construction, microarrays should permit easier and more reliable meta-analysis. In meta-analysis, results of different studies are combined, as if there had been one large study. Medical literature in all fields is increasingly using meta-analysis because statistical statements are more accurate when based on large numbers, and many studies cannot examine a sufficiently large number of patients to make statements with a high level of confidence, particularly for rare diseases. On the other hand, meta-analysis is heavily dependent on the component studies being similar with regard to patient populations and fundamental study designs, and on the studies being of comparable quality, so that combining their data is reasonable.

To my mind, improved meta-analysis is much needed. There are too many variables that cannot be well controlled in meta-analysis, such as selection of patient and control groups, and differences in protocols between different studies, but with the quantitative data from different microarray experiments, one can hope for more reliable, apples-to-apples meta-analysis studies.

Even the best of techniques are not perfect. Microarrays currently have 2 general limitations. First, current microarray technology may miss an abnormality because not every base pair of the genome is present on the chip, but it appears certain that this will be corrected in the near future with true whole genome arrays. A second general limitation with microarrays is that they often require relatively large amounts of DNA, necessitating amplification of the starting nucleic acid, generally by some form of PCR. Since microarrays are often used to investigate large areas of the genome, this means that whole genome amplification (WGA) may be necessary. WGA is technically difficult and prone to bias because not all areas are amplified to the same extent or to the same level of fidelity [PMID16928277].

When used in conjunction with bioinformatics, the myriad possibilities of microarrays have the potential to revolutionize every aspect of pathology, including the identification of tissue type and its benign or malignant nature. It is with a curious mixture of sadness and excitement that I confidently predict that the time-honored study of tissues under a microscope will come to an end as we move towards a "lab on a chip" technology.

Molecular Techniques: Closing Comments

2 comments are in order before concluding our discussion of molecular techniques. First, we must keep in mind whether we need to search for a mutation that is very rare or has not yet been characterized, or if we only need to determine if a well-known and previously characterized mutation is present. In the former case, we may need complete sequencing. But if the great majority of cases are secondary to known mutations, targeted tests such as commercially available FISH probes or PCR primers will suffice.

Second, a decision must be made to test DNA or RNA. Most molecular testing is done at the DNA level because it is more stable than RNA (indeed, RNA can usually only be studied by conversion to cDNA), and in clinical practice, the presence of abnormal DNA correlates well with the clinical phenotype even though only a tiny percentage of DNA actually codes for a protein. On the other hand, studying RNA, usually by conversion to cDNA, can be faster because we are rarely concerned with intronic DNA (with some exceptions that affect intron splicing, such as familial dysautonomia, mutations in introns are usually relatively silent clinically), we can recognize abnormal splicing of the RNA transcript, and we can study gene expression.

Core Points for Molecular Pathology II: Techniques

- DNA can be cloned in an organism from which it did not originate.
  - o Basis for the production of proteins such as insulin and those used in vaccines.
  - o Also the basis of gene modification.
  - o Using cloning, either an organism's entire genome can be copied (genomic library) or the portion that is transcribed can be studied (gene expression libraries).
- PCR: First and most common nucleic acid amplification method.
  - o Many forms, most important of which are reverse transcriptase, quantitative, and allele-specific.
- Also isothermal nucleic acid amplification techniques (strand displacement and transcription-mediated).
- In situ hybridization: allows the identification of specific mutations, often in paraffin-fixed tissue.
  - o But is limited to those mutations that have been characterized.
  - o Reporter molecule is usually fluorescent (FISH).
  - o Many uses, variations, and elaborations on FISH.
  - o Used for translocations, deletions, and inversions.
  - o Has been expanded into comparative genomic hybridization, multicolor FISH/spectral karyotyping, and microarrays.
- High resolution melting curve analysis: the binding force between the 2 strands of DNA is slightly lower in mutations than in the wild type
- DNA sequencing: Sanger method still used, but also a new generation using high throughput sequencing by synthesis, often in a massively parallel format.
- Bioinformatics and databases are now an integral part of medicine.
- The many repetitive sequences in DNA can be classified by the length of the subunit and the length of the entire repeated segment.
- Microarrays: based on the Human Genome Project, the fabrication of integrated circuits, and increased computer power.
  - o Becoming a platform of virtually every aspect of molecular medicine.
- Frontiers: easier and faster DNA sequencing, full annotation of the genome, and the ability to understand the response of each individual patient to a disease and treatment (personalized medicine).

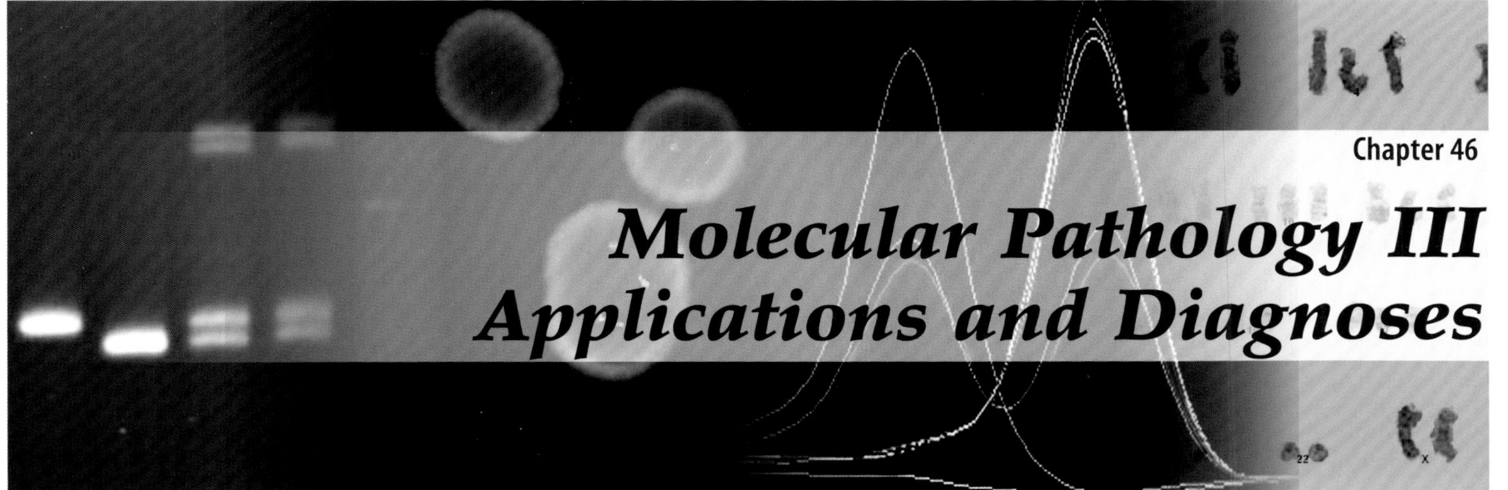

Molecular Pathology III Applications and Diagnoses

Having considered DNA structure and function, and the large range of techniques in molecular pathology, we are now ready to examine specific applications. In this chapter, we will see how testing at the molecular level enormously expands the repertoire of diagnostic medicine. First, we must realize that these new means of testing and diagnosis have legal and ethical implications because they can make broad statements about the patient *and about his or her relatives*. For this reason, molecular testing carries newer and more stringent regulations than general laboratory testing, and we must be aware of them before we consider the vast opportunities afforded by molecular diagnosis.

Regulatory, Ethical, and Legal Issues in Molecular Pathology

The terms "DNA testing" and "genetic testing" are not strictly synonymous, but there is substantial overlap. Most, but not all, genetic testing will be at the DNA level. Although there is no universal agreement on the definition of genetic testing, it can reasonably be defined as testing of a patient's nucleic acid or of proteins that are associated with nucleic acid, to confirm a suspected diagnosis, to influence or monitor treatment, to assess the probability of developing a disease, or to assess the probability of a family member developing a disease. The National Institutes of Health have released guidelines on the definition, scope, purpose, and regulation of genetic testing (Secretary's Advisory Committee on Genetics, Health, and Society [SACGHS]). Any testing that qualifies as genetic carries a large array of legal and regulatory requirements from many regulatory agencies, and the laboratory must be aware of possible ethical and social implications of its test results. The ethical, legal, and social issues of genetic testing are collectively called ELSI.

As is the case for any section of the laboratory, molecular pathology testing must be compliant with the Clinical Laboratory Improvement Act (CLIA), which is enforced by the Centers for Medicare and Medicaid Services (CMS), in conjunction with the Food and Drug Administration (FDA) and the Centers for Disease Control (CDC), and compliance with CMS guidelines is additionally required for Medicare or Medicaid reimbursement. Verification of CLIA compliance is often entrusted to other organizations, most commonly the College of American Pathologists (CAP). Even if the CLIA-conferring organization is not the CAP, a review of the CAP guidelines is very helpful.

The CDC, in conjunction with CMS and the Clinical Laboratory Improvement Advisory Committee (CLIAC), has promulgated recommendations for DNA-based molecular testing of inheritable diseases in the June 12, 2009, issue of *Morbidity and Mortality Weekly Report* [PMID19521335]. This is a comprehensive discussion of appropriate use of molecular testing, preanalytic, analytic, and postanalytic phases of testing, legal concerns, practice guidelines for laboratories, and qualifications of personnel.

Additional organizations may furnish guidelines or regulations, depending on the precise testing to be performed. The Department of Health and Human Services has established the Secretary's Advisory Committee on Genetic Testing (SACGT) to evaluate the implications of genetic testing and to safeguard the public's interest. The American Society for Histocompatibility and Immunogenetics also has guidelines on nucleic acid testing. Laboratories that perform genetic testing may also need to register with the FDA.

Particular attention must be paid to such matters as the following:

- Did an authorized person order the test?
- Are results being released only to authorized persons, and are safeguards in place to prevent unauthorized people or organizations from acquiring results?
- Are the results being released with necessary and appropriate additional information, such as disclosures, disclaimers, etc?

The Association for Molecular Pathology maintains a list of tests that have FDA approval. For those tests that do not, an analyte specific reagent (ASR) disclaimer must appear on the report. ASRs, and the disclaimers that should accompany their use, are discussed in FDA document 1590, issued September 14, 2007. The website http://www.genetests.org lists the laboratories that currently perform a given molecular test.

As is the case for any new test in any area of the laboratory, new molecular tests must be shown to have both analytical validity and clinical utility. For commercially obtained molecular testing kits, verification is done by the manufacturer prior to marketing, but the laboratory must conduct its own validation study, as is the case with any area of the

ISBN 978-089189-5886

laboratory. In general laboratory testing, reference material is critical, and a control is run with each test to ensure accuracy of results. In molecular testing, reference material is more difficult to find, but attempts are underway in every area to produce and disseminate reliable reference material. The laboratory should be aware of any generally accepted reference material that is available in the areas it offers testing in.

A laboratory-developed test (LDT) is one that does not come as a commercial kit, but has been developed by a specific laboratory. LDTs are permitted in clinical use by the laboratory that developed them, provided that they have been validated by that laboratory. LDTs are not FDA approved, but this approval is not required, and the report should indicate that such approval is not needed. However, if a laboratory wishes to market its in-house developed test, a significant series of requirements will follow.

CAP permits the use of research use only (RUO) kits if there is no commercially available FDA-approved or ASR alternative, and the lab has documented the absence of an acceptable alternative. Reimbursement problems should be anticipated in RUO tests.

Unlike most other areas of the laboratory, molecular pathology testing also carries unique social and ethical considerations that the laboratory must be prepared for. These include the potential stigmatizing of patients who are found to be carriers for a disease, patients' fears that their employers or insurance companies may learn of their status, resulting in their exclusion from further care, concerns that partners or potential partners may have if a patient is found to be a carrier for a disorder, concerns regarding racial and ethnic identity, and concerns regarding the ability of health care professionals who receive test results to properly use the information. Anyone involved in molecular testing should take a moment to place himself or herself in the position of a patient who has just learned that he or she has tested positive for an autosomal-dominant, late-onset disorder such as Huntington disease.

Additional ethical considerations arise when we realize that the testing of 1 family member for a genetic disease may provide unwanted information to another family member regarding their risk of the disease. Another sensitive issue is that in 5-20% of families in the United States, there is unknown nonpaternity (ie, the father is not the biological father and does not know it). Genetic testing is likely to reveal this fact, causing potentially shattering consequences to the family if they are not prepared. It is therefore essential that physicians and families be aware of this possibility prior to undergoing testing. Likewise, genetic testing has the potential to reveal incest, likely leading to incendiary consequences.

Particular care must be taken to ensure that the results of genetic tests are given only to appropriate individuals. This of course is true for any testing but is especially true for genetic testing because of its highly sensitive nature. In addition, some physicians may not fully understand the results and implications of a test and may not be equipped to appropriately counsel patients and family members. The laboratory and those involved in patient care must be especially skilled in dealing with and conveying the uncertainty that inevitably accompanies many molecular tests. Many of these issues were foreseen at the beginning of the Human Genome Project, and are considered in detail on the government website http://www.ornl.gov/sci/techresources/Human_Genome/elsi/elsi.shtml. While the laboratory cannot control all of these issues, it must be aware of them, and it must follow policies—especially those concerning release of information—that minimize potential ethical and social difficulties.

There are 2 additional legal caveats for laboratories performing molecular testing. First, unlike the general laboratory, some molecular tests may be patented and it may be necessary to license the technology from the owners of the patent. Polymerase chain reaction (PCR) testing, in particular, is likely to be patented (though the patent for purely qualitative PCR—is a fragment of DNA present or not?—has expired). Second, while no special patient consent is required in most molecular pathology testing beyond standard informed consent, any testing for *hereditary disease* often requires special consent beyond a general consent for testing and treatment. The molecular pathology laboratory is well advised to obtain full legal counsel regarding required permissions for all of its testing.

The Genetic Information Nondiscrimination Act (GINA) of 2008 prohibits employers from discriminating in employment hiring, promotions, wages, or termination on the basis of genetic information. It also prohibits insurance companies from using genetic information to discriminate in either the offering of coverage or in rates. However, GINA does not apply to life insurance.

Finally, it is generally wise to place a note on each report that the results are exquisitely sensitive to contamination and that the report is based on the assumption that there has been no contamination of the specimen prior to receipt in the lab.

Oncogenes and Tumor Suppressor Genes

In an individual, germline mutations are those that are present in every cell. This includes the gametes, so a germline mutation has a 50% chance of being passed on to that individual's children. In contrast, somatic mutations are acquired over one's lifetime and are present only in the cell in which they arose and in the daughters of that cell that arise from mitosis. Somatic mutations affect only a subpopulation of cells and cannot be passed on to offspring.

With some exceptions, most cancers arise from somatic mutations. While many cancers are facilitated by particular environments or activities (eg, cigarette smoking and lung cancer), almost invariably, the final cause of cancer lies in our chromosomes. One of the triumphs of 20th-century medicine, after looking for the cause of cancer anywhere and everywhere, was to learn that the cause lay within us all along.

The somatic mutations that cause cancer can arise from a variety of mechanisms. Some are point mutations, affecting a single base pair. A second class of somatic mutations is deletions and insertions, which are types of copy number variants (CNVs) within chromosomes. A third class is other types of CNVs, such as trisomies. A fourth class of somatic mutations in cancer cells is rearrangements, such as translocations. Less commonly, the mutation is derived from an exogenous source such as a virus (examples include the human papillomavirus and cervical cancer, Epstein-Barr virus (EBV) and Burkitt lymphoma, and human herpesvirus 8 and Kaposi sarcoma), but even in these cases, the virus usually modifies host DNA or its expression, or relies on a mutation in host DNA. Rarely, cancers arise from a mutation in mitochondrial DNA. Still less commonly, a cancer is associated with a change in the epigenetic regulation of DNA, discussed in Chapter 47.

The bewildering array of genes that are now part of medical practice is intimidating and confusing. There are numerous websites that can guide the practitioner it this area. One of the best—maintained by experts and peer-reviewed—is GeneTests (http://www.ncbi.nlm.nih.gov/sites/GeneTests/?db=GeneTests). This website can also guide pathologists to laboratories that perform esoteric testing for rare mutations.

While a number of mechanisms may cause a somatic mutation that leads to cancer, these mutations are fundamentally of 2 types. About 90% of them involve oncogenes, normal genes that have attained a gain of function that causes unrestrained cellular proliferation. These mutations act in a dominant manner (ie, a single copy leads to an increased risk of a cancer). About 10% of sporadic cancer-causing mutations are in tumor suppressor genes, genes that are necessary in their normal function because they restrain cellular proliferation. These mutations usually act in a recessive manner (ie, both copies must be defective) because in most cases 1 working copy of a tumor suppressor gene suffices to properly control the cell.

Oncogenes Are Normal and Necessary Genes That Have Undergone a Gain of Function Mutation That Facilitates Cancer

Oncogenes were originally found in transforming retroviruses and were subsequently found to be ultimately derived from host DNA. The term "proto-oncogene" is used for the normal gene, whereas the term "oncogene" refers to the abnormal tumor-causing form of the gene. Generally speaking, proto-oncogenes are normal and necessary genes that are involved with regulating cell growth and replication. A gain of function mutation of a proto-oncogene in either chromosome transforms it into an oncogene.

Oncogenes may cause transformation by altering the response to an extracellular signal (such as a growth factor), altering cell cycle regulation, altering DNA replication or repair, or inhibiting apoptosis (programmed cell death that is normal and necessary). For example, the steps in the cell cycle depend on progressive activation and inactivation of cyclins, a family of proteins that bind to and activate kinases (enzymes that transfer phosphate groups). Overexpression of cyclins has been demonstrated in some malignancies, and some oncogenes affect the cell cycle either by acting on the cyclins, their associated kinases, or proteins that regulate them.

Important proto-oncogenes include *MYC, HER2, ABL, FGFR3, BRAF, C-KIT, RET, BCL-1* (cyclin D1), *BCL-2*, and the *RAS* family. Geneticists use italicized capital letters for genes and nonitalicized capital letters for proteins, but for clarity, this work uses nonitalicized lowercase letters for proteins, except in rare cases where there is a strong convention for capital letters, in which case nonitalicized capital letters are used. The ret protein is transmembrane, and after binding

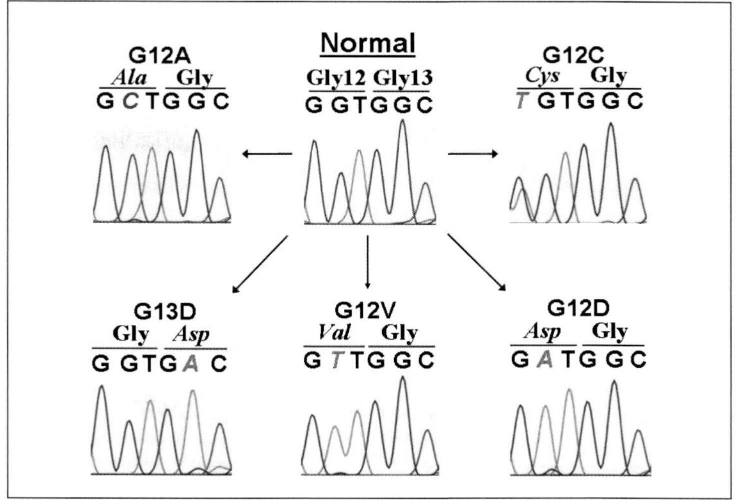

f46.1 Sanger sequence of the *K-RAS* gene. The normal sequence seen at codons 12 & 13 is seen at top center. The 5 most common mutations are shown in proximity. The colors represent different fluors used with the chain terminators (for more Sanger sequencing, see Chapter 45).

its ligand, dimerizes (binds to itself) and then transmits a signal internally via tyrosine kinase. Gain of function mutations in *RET* gene that enable the ret protein to bind its ligand more strongly causes familial thyroid medullary carcinomas, MEN type II, and some thyroid papillary carcinomas. Loss of function of the ret protein, generally caused by defective posttranslational modification of the protein rather than a mutation of the *RET* gene, causes Hirschsprung disease [PMID18365214].

There are several mechanisms by which a proto-oncogene may undergo a gain of function mutation, and the precise mechanism must be known before effective therapy can be instituted. The first way in which a proto-oncogene can become overactive is a point mutation, such as occurs with the *RAS* gene family. Ras proteins are normal and are required for an appropriate response to critical cell signaling pathways. They are monomeric GTPases that are activated upon binding GTP and transmit a mitogenic signal from the surface to the interior through a set of proteins called mitogen-activated protein kinases (MAP kinases), eventually resulting in the production of the transcription factor AP-1. A point mutation in a *RAS* gene encoding for a ras protein may result in an abnormal protein that acts autonomously and is not subject to normal regulation, thus enhancing tumor development and growth. In particular, a point mutation in the *K-RAS* gene is important in some cases of colon cancer f46.1. Other proto-oncogenes that can undergo point mutations to become oncogenes include *EGFR* and *BRAF*.

A second way in which a proto-oncogene may become an oncogene is a translocation that places the gene in an abnormal location that results in overexpression. Examples of this mechanism include the *EWS* gene translocation to the *FLI-1* gene in Ewing sarcoma/primitive neuroectodermal tumor, the t(8;14) in Burkitt lymphoma, which causes overexpression of the *C-MYC* gene by placing it next to the immunoglobulin heavy chain locus, the translocation of the *ABL* gene from chromosome 9 to chromosome 22 in CML, where it comes to rest next to the *BCR* gene, and the t(2;5) found in some cases of anaplastic lymphoma, which causes a fusion of the *ALK* gene and the *NPM1* gene. In some of these cases, the products of the proto-oncogene are found in normal cells in small amounts, but overexpression results when a translocation leads to physical proximity to another gene that increases its transcription. Examples of this include the *EWS/FLI-1* translocation. *FLI-1* is a transcription factor that becomes overactive when adjacent to the *EWS* gene. Another example is the t(8;14) that places the *C-MYC* proto-oncogene adjacent to the immunoglobulin heavy chain gene. A general rule in the transformations of proto-oncogenes into oncogenes is that a translocation for which one of the partners is an immunoglobulin gene will cause the overexpression of a normal protein. On the other hand, the *BCR/ABL* translocation in CML and the t(2;5) found in some cases of anaplastic lymphoma result in sequences of DNA that when transcribed and translated give rise to proteins that are novel and not normally present.

Reverse transcriptase PCR (RT-PCR) can be used to detect translocations, generally by designing primers that hybridize to the abnormal mRNA (ie, to the cDNA) that results from the translocation, such that there is amplification if there has been a translocation and none if there has not been. After the generation of cDNA, RT-PCR can be carried out in a quantitative manner like conventional quantitative PCR (qPCR). But there are 4 caveats in RT-PCR testing for translocations. First, care must be taken to ensure that native DNA is not amplified, either by using DNase enzymes or by using primers that hybridize to exons that become adjacent only after splicing, so that amplification of native (unspliced) DNA is aborted because the primers are too far apart or is evident as a very large product. Second, one must verify that the reverse transcriptase enzyme, which works in a 3' to 5' direction, has reached the 5' end of the mRNA. Third, it is difficult for RT-PCR to detect translocations that occur in introns because it is performed on cDNA derived from mRNA, from which introns have been removed during RNA processing. However, if primers are well designed, it may be possible to detect intronic translocations because one will find exonic regions that are abnormally adjacent because of the translocation. Fourth, PCR primers are short relative to the size of fluorescence in situ hybridization (FISH) probes, so PCR may miss a translocation if there is not a perfect match between the primer and the cDNA because the primers will not bind. On the other hand, because of their greater length, larger FISH probes are more tolerant of a short mismatched sequence and more likely to bind in cases of imperfect match.

So the precise manner in which a translocation is detected depends on the location of the partners and whether or not reliable primers can be obtained. If the study is directed at mRNA and 1 or both of the translocation partners is intronic, or if reliable primers cannot be obtained, FISH is usually employed. But if both partners are in exonic DNA and reliable primers can be obtained, RT-PCR is excellent for detecting translocation. But even if FISH is used for initial detection, qPCR is usually better for monitoring disease progression and response to therapy, as FISH is not sensitive to low levels of residual disease (in FISH, one can attain quantitation by counting the number of cells with the signal, but such quantitation will be manual and insensitive at low levels).

A third mechanism for the transformation of a proto-oncogene into an oncogene, in addition to point mutations and translocations, is an increase in the amount of the DNA. This occurs in *HER2* and *N-MYC*. The Her2 protein is a member of the epidermal growth factor family and is a growth factor itself. Like many growth factors, Her2 has both an extracellular and an intracellular portion, and it must dimerize (ie, bind to itself) before becoming active. If Her2 dimerizes, it facilitates cell division via an intracellular tyrosine kinase. The number of copies of the *HER2* gene is increased in some breast cancers. In these cases, Herceptin, which binds to the receptor and prevents its dimerization, may be used. In another therapeutic approach, Lapatinib (Tykerb) inhibits the intracellular tyrosine kinase that is activated by Her2 dimerization.

Tumor Suppressor Genes Undergo a Loss of Function Mutation to Facilitate Cancer

The discovery of tumor suppressor genes arose from the observation that some cancers were associated with deletions of DNA. Whereas proto-oncogenes code for proteins that permit normal functioning of the cell, tumor suppressor genes code for proteins that restrain proliferation or safeguard the integrity of the DNA. Whereas 1 copy of an oncogene, even in the presence of a second, normal copy is oncogenic, only if both copies of a tumor suppressor gene are defective is cancer likely because even 1/2 of the normal protein product can regulate proliferation and maintain DNA. This is the famous "2-hit" hypothesis put forth by Knudson [PMID11905807]. For this reason, oncogenes usually operate in a dominant manner while tumor suppressor genes operate in a recessive manner. However, as we will see, there are exceptions to this rule, and mutations in some tumor suppressor genes in hereditary cancer syndromes are effectively dominant.

Tumor suppressor genes include *P53* (also called *TP53*), retinoblastoma gene (*RB*), *P16* (also known as *CDKN2A* or *INK4A*, which codes for the p16 protein), *P21*, *APC* (adenomatous polyposis coli), *VHL* (von Hippel-Lindau), *P27*, *NF1*, *PTEN* (phosphatase and tensin homolog; involved in regulation of the cell cycle), *CDH1* (coding for the E-cadherin gene), *BCL-2*, *BRCA1/2*, and *MSH2*, *MLH1*, *MSH6* (coding for DNA mismatch repair (MMR) proteins), and *MGMT* (whose product repairs G to A transversions).

Tumor suppressor proteins usually work by 1 of 4 mechanisms [PMID16468415]. First is a suppression or regulation of DNA replication, often by modulation of transcription factors. The second mechanism is by promotion of apoptosis, such as the product of *BCL-2*. The third is by maintaining the integrity of the genome through DNA repair, such as the products of *MSH2* and *MLH1*. The fourth method is regulation of the cell cycle, such as the products of *RB* and *P53*.

Tumor suppressor genes can be inactivated by deletions or point mutations. In contrast to oncogenes, translocations rarely cause clinically significant mutations of tumor suppressor genes. Tumor suppressor genes can also be inactivated by hypermethylation of their promoters, which silences their transcription. Examples of tumor suppressor genes that are at least sometimes inactivated by hypermethylation of a promoter include *RB*, *MLH1*, *BRCA1*, *VHL*, *P16*, and *MGMT*. Promoter hypermethylation is epigenetic (outside the actual DNA sequence) and theoretically treatable with a hypomethylating agent such as 5-azacytidine. A tumor suppressor gene may be inactivated by >1 mechanism. Indeed, since both copies of a tumor suppressor gene must be inactivated, there may be different inactivating mechanisms on the 2 chromosomes.

Abnormalities in tumor suppressor genes are often associated with hereditary cancer syndromes. Examples of diminished tumor suppressor activity and their associated hereditary cancer syndromes include the *P16* gene in some cases of melanoma, *APC* in hereditary polyposis cancer, *MSH2*, *MLH1*, and *MSH6* in hereditary nonpolyposis colon cancer, *P53* in the Li-Fraumeni syndrome, *RB* in retinoblastoma and some cases of acute lymphoid leukemia, and *BRCA1*/*BRCA2* in hereditary breast and ovarian cancer.

2 of the most important tumor suppressor genes are *RB* and *P53*. *RB*, on chromosome 13, inhibits several transcription factors and is deleted in retinoblastoma. *RB* is also deleted in many cases of acute lymphoid and acute myeloid leukemia [PMID9517499].

P53 is an especially important tumor suppressor gene. It encodes a transcription factor that controls several important cellular functions, including apoptosis and entry into the S phase [PMID20494116], so abnormalities of the p53 protein lead to unchecked mitosis or to mitoses that are abnormal. P53 protein can be assessed by immunohistochemistry, but interpretation is difficult because it is a normal (indeed, necessary and important) protein, and at this writing, there are no immunohistochemical stains that target specific abnormal forms of the p53 protein. Wild-type p53 protein has a very short half-life (<30 minutes) and is normally not detected by immunohistochemistry. Positive immunohistochemical staining for p53 is seen in some malignancies and often portends a more aggressive course. Possible explanations for this are that its aberrant form is more stable but still binds the antibody raised against the wild-type protein or there is a defensive increase in the amount of normal p53, but this matter has not been settled [PMID15668707]. Even in those cancers where there is a mutation in the p53 pathway, it may be in any number of proteins that are downstream from the action of p53 rather than in p53 itself, so immunohistochemical staining for p53 may be of little or no value.

The terms "oncogene" and "tumor suppressor gene" are sometimes inappropriately used synonymously. One may occasionally hear, for example, that *P53* is an "oncogene" because it is perceived to be implicated in tumorigenesis, but in fact, the wild-type *P53* is protective against tumors. It is a tumor suppressor gene, not an oncogene. The terms "oncogene" and "tumor suppressor gene" should be used separately because of their different mechanisms of action, the different manners in which they were discovered (viruses for oncogenes and DNA deletions for tumor suppressor genes), and the different modes of inheritance (autosomal dominant for oncogenes and autosomal recessive for tumor suppressor genes).

The International Cancer Genome Consortium (ICGC), founded in 2008, has proposed that all pathogenic mutations be identified in 50 common types of cancers. The data for this study form the Cancer Genome Atlas (TCGA). This laudable and herculean task will face 2 challenges. First, the effort will require considerable DNA sequencing, still an expensive undertaking. Second, many—indeed, most—mutations in cancer cells are incidental, not causative (these are sometimes called passenger mutations, as opposed to driver mutations, which are causative). Even complete sequencing of cancer genomes and a thorough understanding of all mutation associated with any given type of cancer may still leave us without the knowledge of which mutations are truly causative and therefore appropriate targets of therapy [PMID19360079].

The understanding of oncogenes and tumor suppressor genes, and the molecular biology behind their actions has unfortunately not been matched by an equal understanding of why cancers metastasize. After all, it is the metastases, not the primary tumor, that lead to death in almost all cases of cancer.

A final point in oncogenes and tumor suppressor genes is that the proper specimen must be sent for testing for possible mutations. If the goal of the testing is therapy for the patient, then a sample *of the tumor* must be sent, because the goal is to understand the molecular biology of the tumor cells. On the other hand, if the goal is to determine the risk for the patient's relatives, then a nonneoplastic tissue is generally preferred, as this is more representative of the genome of the patient's gametes. The somatic mutation that occurred in the tumor cells cannot be passed to the patient's children. For example, Her2 or *HER2* testing must be done on a sample of the breast tumor, but *BRCA1* and *BRCA2* testing, which is done to determine the patient's risk of another type of malignancy or the risk to her relatives once she has been diagnosed with breast cancer, is done on blood. In some cases, such as testing for microsatellite instability (MSI) for hereditary nonpolyposis colon cancer syndrome, both tumor and normal tissue must be submitted, but this is for a different reason—one is comparing the number of microsatellite repeats in the normal and tumor tissue.

Hereditary Cancer Syndromes

Almost all hereditary cancer syndromes are secondary to a germline defect (ie, affecting all tissues, as opposed to a somatic mutation) in a tumor suppressor gene in 1 chromosome followed by a second, somatic mutation in the remaining tumor suppressor gene in the affected tissue (the "2-hit" hypothesis). Because both copies of the tumor suppressor gene must be inactivated, one would expect autosomal recessive inheritance in these syndromes. Autosomal recessive inheritance is indeed the case in *sporadic* cases of cancer caused by a defective tumor suppressor gene, but most hereditary cancer *syndromes* are inherited in an autosomal dominant manner. In these syndromes, a germline defect in one tumor suppressor gene is strongly associated with a second, somatic mutation in the other copy of the gene in certain tissues (eg, nerve sheath in neurofibromatosis or colonic epithelium in hereditary nonpolyposis colon cancer syndrome), making the syndrome effectively autosomal dominant.

ISBN 978-089189-5886

The reason for this is not fully elucidated. Rarely, a germline mutation inactivates both copies of a tumor suppressor gene, but this is unusual. If there were germline mutations in both chromosomes, one would expect an enormous array of malignancies throughout the body, and this is not seen. In some cases, it is probable that 1 working copy of the gene simply does not generate enough protective protein (haploinsufficiency) [PMID20307317]. It may be that a germline mutation somehow increases the probability of a second, somatic mutation in certain tissues. There are some hints that in some cases, a germline mutation causes the production of a protein product that interferes with, directly or indirectly, the functioning of the protein product of the normal allele (this is called a dominant negative effect). In some cases, inactivation of the second allele appears to result from hypermethylation of its promoter (silencing transcription) rather than from a mutation in the actual gene [PMID20951312].

It is wise to determine the precise mutation that a proband with a hereditary disorder may have because his or her family members are at increased risk only for that specific mutation. If a proband has been identified as having a specific mutation, testing in other family members can usually be limited to that particular mutation.

Clinical clues to the presence of a hereditary cancer syndrome include the following [PMID15322516]:

- Young age of onset
- Strong family history
- Synchronous or metachronous tumors (the terms "synchronous" and "metachronous" have different meanings to different people, but typically, the term "synchronous" refers to tumors that are detected within 6 months of the first tumor, while the term "metachronous" refers to tumors identified 6 months to 2 years after the initial neoplasm).
- Multiple primary tumors in different organs (eg, endometrium and colon)
- Bilateral tumors in the same organ type (eg, 2 separate breast cancers)
- Multifocal tumors in the same organ

If a hereditary cancer syndrome is suggested but no previously characterized mutation can be found, environmental factors or mutations specific to that family should be considered.

Major examples of familial cancer syndrome caused by insufficient tumor suppressor activity include neurofibromatosis type 1 (caused by a mutation in *NF1*), *BRCA1/2*-associated hereditary breast and ovarian cancer syndrome, familial adenomatous polyposis syndrome (FAP; caused by deficient function of the *APC* gene), and hereditary nonpolyposis colon cancer syndrome (HNPCC; also called Lynch syndrome).

A germline mutation in 1 copy of *NF1* is strongly associated with a subsequent somatic mutation in the second copy in certain tissues (ie, nerve sheath), and a germline mutation in *BRCA1* or *BRCA2* nearly guarantees a subsequent somatic mutation in certain organs (ie, breast, ovaries), making the inheritance of both of these tumor suppressor genes effectively autosomal dominant. Likewise, FAP is autosomal dominant and HNPCC is inherited as an autosomal-dominant condition with about 80% penetrance.

HNPCC Is One of the Best Understood Hereditary Cancer Syndromes

A minority of colon cancer cases are hereditary, but the precise number is unclear. Estimates range from as low as 2-4% [PMID18298004] to as high as 10%. Most hereditary colon cancer cases are HNPCC, which is caused by inherited mutations in or the transcriptional silencing of 1 or more of some 500 MMR genes. These MMR genes encode for enzymes that repair damaged DNA, and are all tumor suppressor genes. Fortunately, only a few are clinically important. Mutations in 6 MMR genes—*MLH1*, *MLH3*, *MSH2*, *MSH3*, *MSH6*, and *PMS2*—account for almost all cases, and of these, *MLH1* and *MSH2* together account for about 85-90% of cases [PMID19466295, PMID19659756].

MSI is an indication of a defect in one or more of these MMR enzymes, because these enzymes are required to keep the number of repeating units in microsatellites constant. MSI does not cause HNPCC, but it is a marker of ineffective MMR enzymes. In particular, the National Cancer Institute has recommended MSI analysis on 5 microsatellites as screens for MMR genes. These microsatellites are the mononucleotide repeats BAT25 and BAT26, and the dinucleotide repeats D2S123, D5S346, and D17S250. Some laboratories examine additional microsatellites, though it is not clear that this is helpful. Normal tissue from the same patient is studied as a control because the comparison is between the number of repeating units in the patient's normal tissue vs the number in his or her tumor tissue. In capillary electrophoresis, a smaller number of repeating units (ie, deletions) in the tumor results in smaller fragments that run ahead of the normal tissue. An increased number of repeats (ie, duplications) results in longer fragments that run more slowly than normal tissue. Because of tumor heterogeneity secondary to defects in MMR, one usually sees a series of peaks in MSI vs a relatively sharp peak in normal tissue.

If 30% or more of the microsatellite markers show instability relative to the patient's normal tissue, it is considered to be a high level of MSI and is designated MSI-H. If <30% of these markers show instability, it is considered a low level and is designated MSI-L. The clinical significance of MSI-L is unclear, and currently, only MSI-H is acted on.

HNPCC and MSI are associated entities that do not necessarily occur together. HNPCC is a *clinical diagnosis* that is usually, but not always, supported by MSI-H or a proven defect in an MMR enzyme. There are exceptions in both directions: 15% of sporadic colon carcinomas will have MSI-H, and about 80% of MSI-H colon carcinomas will *not* be HNPCC.

The revised Bethesda guidelines for the testing for MSI in colon carcinomas [PMID14970275] are as follows:

1. Colon carcinoma in a patient <50 years of age.
2. The presence of synchronous or metachronous colorectal tumors or tumors of other body sites involved in HNPCC syndrome, regardless of the age of the patient. These other tumor types include stomach (of the intestinal type, not the signet ring type), small bowel, endometrial and ovarian; urothelial carcinomas of the ureter or renal pelvis (but not bladder); biliary tract, pancreas, glioblastoma, sebaceous gland adenomas, and squamous cell carcinomas of the skin of the keratoacanthoma type.
3. The colorectal cancer has a morphology that is typical of MSI tumors (eg, lymphocytes within the tumor cells, poorly differentiated tumors with mucinous, signet-ring, or medullary features) in a patient <60 years of age.
4. The patient has 1 or more first-degree relatives with colorectal cancer or another cancer related to HNPCC syndrome, but 1 of the cancers in a relative must have been diagnosed before that patient was 50 years old.
5. The patient has 2 or more first-degree relatives with colorectal cancer or another cancer related to HNPCC syndrome, regardless of age at the time of diagnosis.

Although not specifically enumerated in the revised Bethesda criteria, 2/3 of HNPCC cases are right sided. A number of good reviews of HNPCC are available [PMID14964310, PMID17631130].

MLH1 (also called hMLH1) and MSH2 (also called hMSH2) are MMR proteins whose presence or absence can be detected by immunohistochemistry (in deference to convention, MMR proteins are denoted in this work by nonitalicized capital letters rather than lowercase letters). Loss of nuclear staining for either of these proteins—implying diminished ability to repair DNA—is highly predictive of MSI and is a good surrogate test for MSI. The loss of nuclear staining for MLH1 and MSH2 strongly correlates with MSI-H and suggests HNPCC in the appropriate clinical setting [PMID15749237]. Almost all PCR-proven cases of MSI-H had loss of 1 of these markers by immunohistochemistry, and 85% had loss of MLH1 [PMID15362369]. In the use of immunohistochemistry, MLH1 should be the first target of investigation, as its absence strongly suggests MSI-H and in an appropriate clinical setting essentially establishes the diagnosis of HNPCC syndrome and obviates the need for further testing, though testing for methylation of the *MLH1* promoter might be desired for reasons to be discussed.

Loss of the MMR protein MSH6 (also called hMSH6) by immunohistochemistry is found in only a minority of cases of HNPCC, but this enzyme should be searched for if HPNCC is suspected and MLH1 and MSH2 are shown to be present. The addition of testing for the MMR protein PMS2, resulting in a 4-test panel of MLH1, MSH2, MSH6, and PMS2, provides excellent exclusion of MSI if there is unequivocal nuclear staining for all 4 proteins. MLH1 and PMS2 loss or retention tend to occur together because these 2 proteins form a complex. Likewise, MSH2 and MSH6 are usually either lost or retained together because they are associated.

A correlation between loss of nuclear immunohistochemical staining for one of the above MMR proteins and MSI has also been shown in the endometrium and ovary [PMID15528786], suggesting that loss of these MMR proteins may indicate MSI in other tissues as well.

In addition to the greater convenience of immunohistochemistry, another advantage of testing for MMR proteins over MSI is that in immunohistochemistry, normal tissue is not needed, and one can identify the culprit gene from the absence of staining for its protein product. Yet another advantage of immunohistochemistry for MMR proteins is that MSI is often considered a genetic test (ie, a direct test for a genetic abnormality), special permission is likely to be required, whereas immunohistochemistry for MMR enzymes is considered an indirect test and can be performed without special consent.

In most cases, the results of the immunohistochemical staining, in conjunction with the clinical situation, will not require MSI corroboration. Indeed, while MSI is still considered the "gold standard" of testing, now that many of the specific MMR enzymes have been identified, one can argue that MSI is actually the surrogate test. But if HNPCC is strongly suspected and all 4 proteins are present, one could obtain additional testing either by MSI or by sequencing the genes in case there is a missense mutation that results in a nonfunctional protein that still reacts with the antibody used in immunohistochemistry [PMID18556767]. In addition, rare cases of HNPCC associated with MSI and with mutations in transforming growth factor receptor II have been reported [PMID10690536], suggesting the MMR pathway, while overwhelmingly predominant in HNPCC, may not necessarily be the only pathway. Thus, in exceptional cases, MSI testing is still needed.

Different MMR enzymes appear to be affected by different degrees of germline mutation and somatic promoter hypermethylation. For example, in cases of HNPCC that involve *MLH1*, the culprit is more often somatic hypermethylation of both copies of the gene without any germline mutation. Indeed, 15% of *all* colorectal carcinomas are caused by acquired, somatic hyperpmethylation of the promoters of both copies of *MLH1*, and most of these cases are not part of HNPCC [PMID20420947]. These patients tend to be older and without a family history. Hypermethylation of both copies of *MLH1* will cause a clinical picture that is identical to that caused by a combination of a germline mutation and a somatic mutation, but these cases are not part of HNPCC and do not have genetic implications because both mutations are somatic.

Consequently, if the MLH1 protein is absent by immunohistochemistry, it is beneficial to go an extra step and determine the methylation status of the gene encoding for the missing enzyme. If both copies are hypermethylated, that patient may have HNPCC clinically, but if so, it is sporadic rather than familial, without implications for his or her relatives [PMID20489114]. On the other hand, if the protein is absent and neither copy of the gene is hypermethylated, there is probably a germline mutation, with implications for relatives. Sequencing the gene and demonstrating a departure from the normal sequence would accomplish the same goal, but is much more labor intensive.

ISBN 978-089189-5886

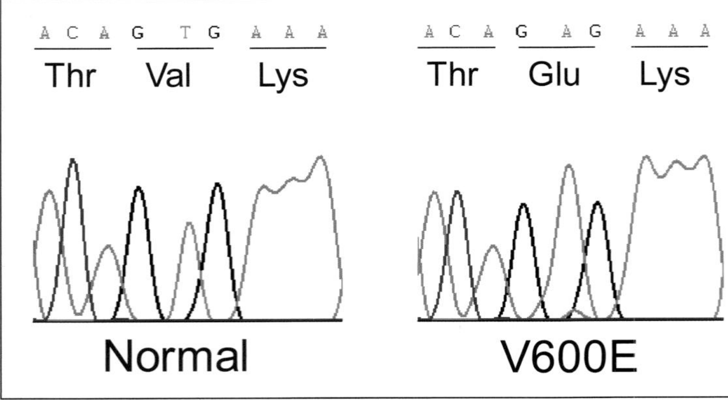

f46.2 A V600E (glutamate instead of valine at amino acid position 600) mutation in the *BRAF* gene in a sporadic colorectal carcinoma. The relevant codon is in the center and is a GTG on the left (coding for valine) but a mutated GAG (coding for glutamate) on the right.

The V600E mutation in the *BRAF* gene, which is also found in some cases of thyroid cancer, is found in about 1/2 of cases of sporadic colorectal carcinomas that have MSI and is strongly associated with promoter hypermethylation of the *MLH1* gene **f46.2**. In contrast, hereditary cases, in which there is a germline mutation in *MLH1*, do not have this mutation in *BRAF* [PMID20489114]. *BRAF* mutations can therefore be used to distinguish between sporadic MSI colorectal cancers and MSI colorectal cancers in Lynch syndrome, though assessment of *MLH1* promoter methylation is probably a more sensitive method.

On the other hand, with other MMR genes, at least 1 germline mutation is the rule, and the "2-hit" requirement for tumor suppressor genes (since both copies must be inactivated) is usually fulfilled by a combination of a germline mutation in 1 copy of the gene and somatic hypermethylation of the other gene's promoter [PMID20388775]. A convenient algorithm on the testing of possible MSI-associated colorectal carcinomas, beginning with immunohistochemistry and progressing to additional studies as needed, has been suggested [PMID21970482].

An interesting situation regarding *MSH2* came to light in 2009. A germline mutation in *TACSTD1*, which codes for epithelial cell adhesion molecule (Ep-Cam), resulting in deletion of the last exons of the gene, causes the hypermethylation (and silencing) of the promoter of *MSH2*, but only in tissues that express Ep-Cam (such as epithelia, including the epithelium of the colon) [PMID19098912]. This accounts for a minority of cases of Lynch syndrome.

Although a mutation in or silencing of a MMR gene is associated with an increased incidence of colon neoplasia, such neoplasms are often less clinically aggressive because the poor DNA repair will quickly cause the tumor to reach an unsustainable level of mutations. Paradoxically, colon tumors with MSI often are less aggressive because they "self-destruct" from their inability to repair their DNA. Although a significantly improved long-term survival benefit of MSI has not been shown, it appears likely [PMID15749237].

In addition to the possible implications for family members, the identification of MSI colon cancer cases is important because 5-fluorouracil, often used in colon carcinoma, is often less effective in MSI cases [PMID16106779]. Also, because of the lower aggressiveness of these tumors, chemotherapy may not be needed in situations where at the same clinical stage, it would be indicated in a carcinoma without MSI. For these reasons, it is important to be wary of a possible MSI colon cancer.

Julie et al found that the revised Bethesda guidelines may miss up to 25% of cases of HNPCC and recommend MSI testing of all colon carcinomas [PMID18759827]. It is not clear at this writing that the effort and expense of MSI testing of all colon carcinomas is cost-effective, but this study and others suggest that immunohistochemical testing for MMR proteins and/or testing for MSI should be employed more liberally. While the imperfect specificity of MSI for HNPCC may result in unnecessary screening of relatives, it provides for earlier screening of a high-risk population. If a patient has HNPCC with genetic implications (ie, not caused by methylation of both *MLH1* promoters), his or her asymptomatic relatives cannot be screened for MSI, as this requires both tumor and normal DNA. Asymptomatic relatives must be screened by direct sequencing of the MMR genes and/or earlier colonoscopic surveillance.

Familial Adenomatous Polyposis Is Another Major Hereditary Colon Cancer Syndrome

FAP (also called adenomatous polyposis coli or APC) is another example of a pathway to colon carcinoma involving loss of tumor suppressor activity. FAP is inherited in an autosomal dominant manner and demonstrates nearly complete penetrance (though about 1/4 of cases are de novo), and is characterized by nearly confluent adenomatous polyps throughout the colon. The enormous numbers of adenomatous polyps in these patients makes the eventual development of colon cancer virtually certain, and prophylactic colectomy is necessary.

β-catenin is a cytoplasmic protein that links transmembrane cell adhesion molecules, such as the cadherins, to the internal cytoskeleton. Normally, most β-catenin is complexed to E-cadherin. *APC* is a tumor suppressor gene on 5q whose protein product induces the degradation of the small amount of β-catenin that is not complexed to E-cadherin. Loss of function of *APC* leads to the accumulation of free β-catenin, which then migrates to the nucleus, complexes with transcription factors, and activates genes that induce proliferation, the result being innumerable colonic adenomatous polyps [PMID21483657].

FAP results from a germline loss of or mutations in 1 copy of *APC*, followed by a somatic mutation in the other copy. *APC* is a huge gene and mutations can be found anywhere within it, making a screening test difficult to develop. While there is appreciable overlap, mutations in the first 1/2 of the gene tend to result in a fully developed case, while those in the second 1/2 tend to cause an attenuated form (defined as 100 polyps or less). Because most mutations are truncating, the protein truncation test, which amplifies the DNA, then transcribes and translates the products, followed by the length determination of the resulting proteins by electrophoresis, can be helpful. The protein truncation test is occasionally performed on cDNA derived from mRNA by RT-PCR [PMID10425032]. This test is often done on the very large exon 15 of *APC*. As is the case with any large gene, a positive result requires only that the patient's children be tested for the particular region that is abnormal in the patient; testing of the entire gene need not be repeated.

Turcot syndrome is a combination of a colon cancer syndrome, either HNPCC or FAP, and a brain malignancy. If the colon cancer syndrome is HNPCC, the brain tumor is usually a glioblastoma. If it is FAP, it is usually a medulloblastoma. While sebaceous tumors are part of HNPCC, the presence of only sebaceous neoplasms and colon cancer suggests Muir-Torre syndrome. MYH -associated polyposis (MAP) is an autosomal recessive syndrome generally characterized by less than about a hundred adenomatous polyps. It arises from mutation is the *MYH* gene (on 1p34.3-p32.1), that codes for a base excision repair enzyme.

Hereditary Diffuse Gastric Cancer Syndrome Predisposes to Both Diffuse Gastric Cancer and Lobular Breast Cancer through Loss of E-Cadherin

Hereditary diffuse gastric cancer syndrome (HDGCS) is an autosomal dominant condition that is clinically suspected if a patient with diffuse gastric cancer has 1 or more first-degree relatives who also has this neoplasm, with at least 1 of the cases occurring before age 50, or if a patient has 2 or more first- or second-degree relatives with the disease, with any age of onset.

30-50% of patients with HDGCS have a germline defect that inactivates the *CDH1* gene on 16q22.1 that encodes for epithelial cadherin (E-cadherin), a transmembrane glycoprotein that is a cell-cell adhesion molecule. It is thought that loss of this gene product predisposes a cell to unrestrained proliferation by depriving it of contact inhibition [PMID16682529]. About 50 mutations in *CDH1* have been described. As is typical for mutations in tumor suppressor genes in hereditary cancer syndromes, most of these mutations are truncating (either by a premature stop codon, a nonsense substitution, or a frameshift mutation, which eventually causes a nonsense codon). Approximately 50% of patients with a mutation in *CDH1* will have diffuse gastric carcinoma, and many women patients with a mutation will also have lobular carcinoma of the breast, a neoplasm that also lacks E-cadherin. Cases of lobular carcinoma of the breast that are candidates for *BRCA1* and *BRCA2* testing and are negative for these mutations should be tested for *CDH1* [PMID17545690], and it is reasonable to test any patient who has both lobular carcinoma of the breast and diffuse gastric carcinoma.

BRCA1 and BRCA2 Are Involved in DNA Repair

5-10% of breast cancer cases occur as part of 1 of the hereditary breast cancer syndromes. Hereditary breast cancer syndrome is associated with *BRCA1* on 17q21 or *BRCA2* on 13q12.3. Whereas abnormalities in both *BRCA1* and *BRCA2* are associated with an increased incidence of carcinomas of the breast, ovary, and fallopian tube, mutations in *BRCA2* are also associated with increased incidences of adenocarcinomas of the prostate, pancreas, biliary tree, and stomach, as well as melanoma and head and neck squamous carcinomas [PMID14966099].

Since both *BRCA1* and *BRCA2* are tumor suppressor genes, both copies of one or the other must be lost for cancer to occur. In hereditary breast cancer syndrome, as in other cancer syndromes based on tumor suppressor gene mutations, there is a germline mutation in *BRCA1* or *BRCA2*, affecting all cells, but patients who inherit a germline mutation in *BRCA1/2* will not develop cancer unless they also inherit or develop a second somatic mutation in a specific tissue.

A germline defect in *BRCA1* or *BRCA2* is found in about 5% of breast cancer in the United States. Undesired proteins are marked for destruction when the enzyme ubiquitin ligase adds multiple ubiquitin molecules the unwanted protein molecules. The chain of ubiquitin molecules directs the protein to the proteasome for degradation. *BRCA1* is a large gene that encodes a ubiquitin ligase, so mutations in *BRCA1* impede the necessary destruction of senescent proteins. Specifically, the product of BRCA1 is a ubiquitin ligase that ubiquinates and destroys a phosphorylated histone during the repair of damaged DNA [PMID20936109]. *BRCA2* mutation also affects DNA repair, but by a different mechanism [PMID9660919].

In general, *BRCA* testing should be considered in patients who are under age 40, have bilateral breast carcinomas, other gynecologic malignancies, or a strong family history. Mutations in these genes may affect a number of regions, resulting in <100% sensitive testing. Breast carcinomas associated with *BRCA1/2* mutations often have a higher grade, and tend to be negative for estrogen and progesterone receptors and for *HER2* overexpression (ie, "triple negative") [PMID21050424], but it is the young age of the patient or a strong family history that indicates the need for genetic testing.

Over 1,600 mutations in *BRCA1* have been described and at least that many for *BRCA2*, making screening difficult. A number of screening methods are used, including the protein truncation test. At this writing, Myriad holds the patent for comprehensive *BRCA* testing.

Only about 25% of families with hereditary breast or ovarian carcinoma have mutations in *BRCA1* or *BRCA2* [PMID17885670] undoubtedly indicating as-yet undiscovered genes, so family members who have undergone *BRCA1/2* testing and been found to be negative should still undergo early conventional screening for breast and ovarian neoplasms.

Multiple Endocrine Neoplasia Type 2 is a Rare Form of Hereditary Cancer Syndrome That Is Associated with an Oncogene, Not a Tumor Suppressor Gene

Multiple endocrine neoplasia (MEN) type 1 is characterized by primary hyperparathyroidism, low-grade neuroendocrine neoplasms of the pancreas and gastrointestinal tract, pituitary adenomas, and occasionally other neoplasms [PMID21613050]. It is associated with loss of function of the tumor suppressor gene *MEN1*, which codes for the protein menin, whose function is not yet known.

MEN2 is subdivided into MEN2A, MEN2B, and familial medullary thyroid carcinoma (MTC) syndrome. MEN2A is diagnosed if the patient of a close relative has any 2 of the following 3 neoplasms: MTC, pheochromocytoma, or parathyroid adenoma/hyperplasia. While the latter 2 tumors are inconstant findings, MTC is virtually always present for the diagnosis of MEN2A. MEN2B is diagnosed if there is MTC in association with mucosal neuromas or ganglioneuromas of lips and mouth, pheochromocytoma, marfinoid habitus and a characteristic facies. Familial MTC syndrome (FMTC) is diagnosed if there are 4 or more cases of MTC in a family without the above associations (though testing is usually triggered by 2 such cases in a family).

All forms of MEN2 are strongly associated with mutations in the *RET* gene on 10q11.2 [PMID18402529]. Unlike most other genes implicated in hereditary cancer syndromes, *RET* is not a tumor suppressor gene, but rather is a proto-oncogene, the first such gene found to be responsible for a hereditary cancer syndrome [PMID15322516].

As is characteristic for cancers caused by oncogenes, there is a gain of function mutation in MEN2, often a missense mutation. *RET* codes for a receptor tyrosine kinase (ie, a transmembrane protein with a cytoplasmic tyrosine kinase) and actually has 2 intracellular tyrosine kinases. While there is imperfect correspondence, most cases of MEN2B have a mutation in the second tyrosine kinase domain of the *RET* gene (often Met918→Thr, a substitution of threonine for methionine at amino acid position 918), while *RET* mutations in MEN2A tend to be in a cysteine rich area in the extracellular portion. Mutations in familial MTC may be in the extracellular domain or in the first tyrosine kinase. Prophylactic thyroidectomy is recommended for patients in whom MEN 2 has been documented and there is an association of the specific mutation with the likely age of onset of MTC, so the precise mutation is considered in determining the age at which thyroidectomy is recommended.

Although sporadic cases of thyroid papillary carcinoma may also involve *RET*, the association of this gene with MTC (both familial and sporadic cases) and with MEN2 is much stronger.

Molecular Testing in Infectious Disease

Many organisms can now be studied by 1 or more molecular techniques and molecular pathology is revolutionizing the study of infectious disease, particularly now that commercial kits and self-contained nucleic acid amplification instruments are becoming available. In addition to a much more rapid identification than is possible with culture, advantages of nucleic acid identification include the ability to identify organisms that either cannot be cultured at all, or can only be cultured under fastidious conditions or in specialized laboratories. Antibiotic resistance and susceptibilities can often be obtained simultaneously, obviating the need for an additional delay.

The target of nucleic acid amplification in infectious diseases is often ribosomal RNA (rRNA) or the DNA that codes for rRNA. Eukaryotic ribosomes consist of 2 subunits called 40S and 60S (S is a unit derived from the speed at which a particle settles in ultracentrifugation; a larger S correlates with a greater mass). Because the centrifugation speeds of the 2 subunits are only roughly additive, the full eukaryote ribosome has a centrifugation speed of 80S, not 100S. Bacteria have ribosomes whose subunits are 30S and 50S, and the intact bacterial ribosome has a centrifugation speed of 70S. There are also differences in the size of the ribosomal RNA molecules that are found in bacterial and eukaryotic ribosomes. The smaller 30S subunit in bacteria has a ribosomal RNA molecule that is 16S, which may be present in >1 copy. The larger 50S subunit has ribosomal RNA molecules of 5S and 23S. On the bacterial DNA that codes for rRNA, the order of the genes is 16S, 23S, 5S, and there are noncoding internal transcribed spacers (ITSes) between the genes for each RNA, so the DNA sequence reads 16S, ITS1, 23S, ITS2, 5S.

For eukaryotes, the smaller 40S subunit has a ribosomal RNA molecule of 18S, and the larger 60S subunit contains 3 ribosomal RNA molecules with S values of 5, 5.8, and 28 (though the mitochondria of eukaryotes will have bacterial rRNAs). The 5S RNA is encoded by a separate region of DNA, but the other rRNA encoding regions are all adjacent on the DNA. In this long sequence, there is an external transcribed sequence (ETS) at both the 5' end and the 3' end of the rRNA, and there are 2 noncoding ITSes between the functional regions of rRNA, so that the full eukaryotic DNA sequence encoding for rRNA reads 5'ETS, 18S, ITS1, 5.8S, ITS2, 28S, 3'ETS. The DNA that encodes this sequence occurs as tandem repeats that are typically hundreds of copies long.

The DNA encoding rRNA is called rDNA. For example, the DNA encoding the 16S rRNA fragment in bacteria is called 16S rDNA and is often used in nucleic acid amplification in bacterial testing. Direct sequencing of 16S rDNA (1542 base pairs) is very promising not only in identification [PMID18402529], but also in strain typing. MicroSEQ, from Applied Biosystems, offers both a full sequencing of the 16S rDNA and a 527 base pair partial sequencing. Sequences that are obtained can be compared to databases, such as the Ribosomal Database Project, a subset of the large databases such as GenBank, EMBL, and DDBJ.

Clearly, this approach is more difficult for eukaryotic pathogens, though progress is being made in the gene encoding the 5.8S rRNA and the 18S subunit of RNA in fungi. A chromogenic-labeled probe constructed from locked nucleic acids, made from ribose nucleotides that have been modified by linking the 2'-oxygen and the 4'-carbon atoms of the ribose with a methylene unit, has been successful in identifying the 18S subunit of RNA in *Aspergillus* species in formalin-fixed, paraffin-embedded tissue [PMID19861892]. Progress has also been made in mycology in the comparison of the number of repeats in the genes encoding ITSes (ITS1 and ITS2) [PMID11173329] and in melting curve analysis of these spacers [PMID20007848]. In situ hybridization, using synthetic DNA probes directed at fungal rRNA, can be effective in formalin-fixed, paraffin-embedded tissue [PMID21228359].

Chlamydia

Chlamydia trachomatis can be identified by amplification of its nucleic acid by PCR (Roche COBAS), transcription-mediated amplification (Genprobe APTIMA), or an amplified strand displacement assay (ProbeTec by Becton-Dickinson). Any of these methods increases the sensitivity for *C trachomatis* detection and is now recommended over the previous gold standard of culture in McCoy cells, except in legal situations in some states where prevailing laws may still insist on culture.

There are 3 clinically important *Chlamydia* species. The most important of these is *Chlamydia trachomatis*, which causes urogenital infections and lymphogranuloma venereum, and may also cause conjunctivitis and pneumonia. The other *Chlamydia* species are *C pneumoniae* and *C psittaci*, both rare causes of pneumonia. *C pneumoniae* has been found in deposits of atherosclerosis, though no causative role has been shown.

Like other bacteria, *Chlamydia* have plasmids. In particular, almost all *C trachomatis* and most *C psittaci* have multiple copies of a cryptic plasmid—so called because its function is not known—though *C pneumoniae* appears to lack this plasmid. The cryptic plasmid is present throughout the life cycle of the organism.

Chlamydia exist in 2 forms The first is as small elementary bodies, which are not biologically active but which can exist as free units in the environment. Elementary bodies are not spores, but they share with spores the characteristics of biological inactivity and resistance to environmental stress. The second form is the reticulate body, which is the biologically active, intracellular form. Because only the reticulate body is pathogenic, *Chlamydia* are obligate intracellular parasites.

The endosome, or endocytic vesicle, is a plasma membrane-coated structure that conveys phagocytized external material into the cell, often to the lysosome for destruction. The endosome is the morphologic correlate of phagocytosis. *Chlamydia* infection begins when an elementary body attaches to the external surface of a eukaryotic host cell. The elementary bodies are internalized in an endosome, now called an inclusion or an inclusion body, but the organisms are able to circumvent the usual phagocytic pathway, which ends in destruction in a lysosome, and instead mediate their own endocytic entry in a process called internalization. It is probable that internalization is an evolutionary manipulation of phagocytosis, or vice versa.

The elementary bodies differentiate into reticulate bodies while still inside the inclusion. This differentiation is characterized by a larger amount of cytoplasm, many more ribosomes, and less tightly packed DNA. The unpacking of the DNA and the presence of ribosomes facilitate transcription. Reticulate bodies replicate by fission within the inclusion, completely filling and distending it until it occupies most of the cytoplasm. The reticulate bodies then reorganize into elementary bodies. The first step in this reorganization is a recondensation of the DNA into a more tightly packed form (this first step generates what is sometimes called an intermediate body), after which the parasitic cell loses much of its cytoplasm and almost all of its ribosomes, completing the transformation back to elementary bodies. Reticulate bodies may give rise to 1 or >1 elementary body.

The inclusion, stuffed with elementary bodies, fuses with the plasma membrane, disgorging its contents into the extracellular environment and destroying the cell. *Chlamydia* are not only intracellular pathogens, but in fact live the entire intracellular portion of their life cycle inside a single inclusion.

In addition to the gene encoding 23S rRNA, the cryptic plasmid within the elementary body of the organism is also a frequent target of molecular testing, largely because this plasmid is already present in multiple copies and is therefore easy to amplify. Testing is generally performed on urine, endocervical swabs, or urethral swabs. The sensitivity of urine testing is comparable to that of other sources [PMID15941699].

Neisseria gonorrhoea

The same specimens that are acceptable for *Chlamydia* testing (urine, endocervical swabs, or urethral swabs) are also acceptable in testing for *Neisseria gonorrhoea*. With both *Chlamydia* and *Neisseria gonorrhoea* testing, prompt transfer in appropriate media is required. GenProbe, using transcription-mediated amplification, is also used for this organism, targeting 23S rRNA. Rare cross-reactivity with other strains of *Neisseria* may occur. PCR is also a good test, targeting M-Ngo PII, and is a methylated form of a restriction endonuclease that is thought to be specific for *Neisseria gonorrhoea* (many restriction endonucleases are often modulated by methylation).

Mutations of the *PenB* gene (unlike human genes, bacterial genes are denoted in lowercase letters) in *Neisseria gonorrhoea* confer penicillin resistance and mutations in the gene *GyrA* confer resistance to fluoroquinolones (antibiotics that inhibit bacterial gyrase and topoisomerase, examples of which include levofloxacin, moxifloxacin, and gatifloxicin).

Enterococcus

Enterococcus is growing in importance because it is often hospital-acquired and resistant to vancomycin. *E faecalis* is the most common species. While the organism can be readily cultured, time-criticality makes nucleic acid testing much superior, especially in cases of possible vancomycin-resistant *Enterococcus* (VRE). The cell walls of Gram-positive bacteria consist of alternating units of N-acetylglucosamine (NAG) and N-acetylmurmanic acid (NAM). A peptide of 5 amino acids extends from each NAM molecule. The last 2 of these are D-alanine (D-alanyl-D-alanine). These 2 D-Ala residues crosslink with amino acids attached to other NAM molecules, stabilizing the wall. Vancomycin binds to these 2 D-Ala amino acids and prevents this crosslinking f46.3.

High-level resistance to vancomycin in *Enterococcus* species, such as is seen in *E faecium* and *E faecalis*, is associated with the presence of the genes *VanA*, *VanB*, and sometimes *VanD*. *VanA* and *VanB* produce enzymes that favor the synthesis of D-alanyl-D-lactate over D-alanyl-D-alanine. D-alanyl-D-lactate is still incorporated into the cell wall, but does not bind vancomycin to any significant extent [PMID16323116].

Lower levels of resistance occur when D-alanyl-D-alanine is replaced by D-alanyl-D-serine, rather than by the D-alanyl-D-lactate. Vancomycin does bind to D-alanyl-D-serine, though with only 1/6 the affinity that it has for D-alanyl-D-alanine [PMID15616270].

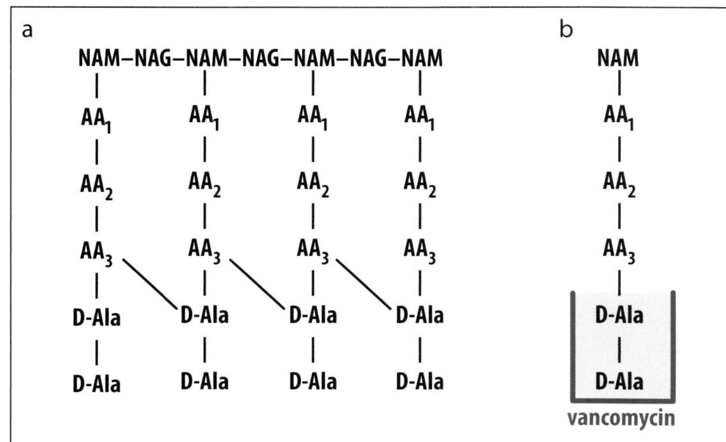

f46.3 **a** A simplified diagram of a Gram-positive bacteria cell wall. The cell walls of Gram-positive bacteria consist of alternating units of N-acetylglucosamine (NAG) and N-acetylmurmanic acid (NAM). 5 amino acids extend from each NAM molecule. The last 2 of these are D-alanine (D-Ala). D-Ala residues bind to amino acids extending from the adjacent NAM molecules, providing stabilization. **b** Vancomycin binds to the 2 terminal D-Ala amino acids, preventing them from binding to other amino acids and stabilizing the structure.

Staphylococcus aureus

The β-lactam ring of penicillin **f46.4a,b** inhibits cell wall synthesis, but many species of bacteria, including most strains of *S aureus*, have developed a β-lactamase that degrades penicillin [PMID21417998]. Later antibiotics, such as methicillin and oxacillin, are not susceptible to β-lactamase, but methicillin-resistant *S aureus* (MRSA; also called oxacillin-resistant *S aureus* [ORSA]) has developed a means of overcoming methicillin and oxacillin. MRSA is a common example of the huge problem of antibiotic resistance. Infections with MRSA begin with simple colonization and may remain indefinitely in that innocuous state. However, colonization may progress to a mild to moderate infection. If this progression occurs and is unchecked, the result is an invasive infection. At this writing, almost 100,000 new cases of invasive MRSA occur each year, resulting in nearly 20,000 deaths.

Jensen and Lyon offer an excellent review of antimicrobial resistance in *S aureus*, including methicillin and other antibiotics [PMID19492967]. MRSA can be hospital acquired (HA-MRSA) or community acquired (CA-MRSA). 85% of invasive cases are hospital acquired, but both HA-MRSA and CA-MRSA are caused by the *mecA* gene. *MecA* is a mobile genetic element that codes for a penicillin binding protein (PBP2a). The sole vector of *mecA* is a mobile genetic element called the staphylococcal chromosome cassette (SCC) [PMID10817707]. For this reason, the gene is sometimes called *SCCmecA*. SCC is inserted into the chromosome at a site called orfX (open reading frame of unknown function), and some tests for MRSA are based on finding the DNA for orfX. Rarely, there will be a SCC that is inserted into the chromosome but does not have the *mecA* element. These situations are called empty cassette or *mecA* dropout.

CA-MRSA is strongly associated with skin infections or lesions and is disproportionately seen in athletes and individuals who have been incarcerated. At this time, CA-MRSA is easier to treat because additional antibiotic resistance is usually limited to erythromycin, while HA-MRSA is also resistant to a variety of other antibiotics. For example, CA-MRSA is often susceptible to clindamycin, tetracyclines, and trimethoprim-sulfamethoxazole, and testing for CA-MRSA for clindamycin susceptibility by the disk diffusion test (D-test) is often performed in cases of CA-MRSA.

SCCmecA is subdivided into 7 types. *SCCmecA* types 1, 4, 5, 6, and 7 are associated with resistance only to β-lactam antibiotics, while types 2 and 3 are larger genetic elements and also contain genes that confer resistance to other antibiotics, such as tetracycline, gentamycin, and bactrim. Types 2 and 3—especially type 2—are associated with HA-MRSA, accounting for its greater range of antibiotic resistance, while the more innocuous types 4 and 5 are associated with CA-MRSA. However, CA-MRSA is becoming more prevalent, and we must assume that its increasing prevalence will eventually correlate with greater antibiotic resistance, diminishing the demarcation between HA-MRSA and CA-MRSA.

In addition to the above classification systems, based on HA-MRSA, CA-MRSA, and *SCCmecA*, the CDC has classified all MRSA isolates (ie, the entire organism, not just *mecA*) into 12 groups, based on pulsed field gel electrophoresis, a technique discussed in Chapter 45 [PMID19608582]. These are numbered USA100 to USA1200. In this system, the main HA-MRSA groups are USA100 and USA200, followed by USA500 and USA800. Among the CA-MRSA, USA300 and USA400 are the most common. USA300 is the strain of CA-MRSA that is particularly increasing in prevalence and about which more must be learned to prevent a serious epidemic of CA-MRSA. Methicillin-intermediate *S aureus* (MISA) is also recognized.

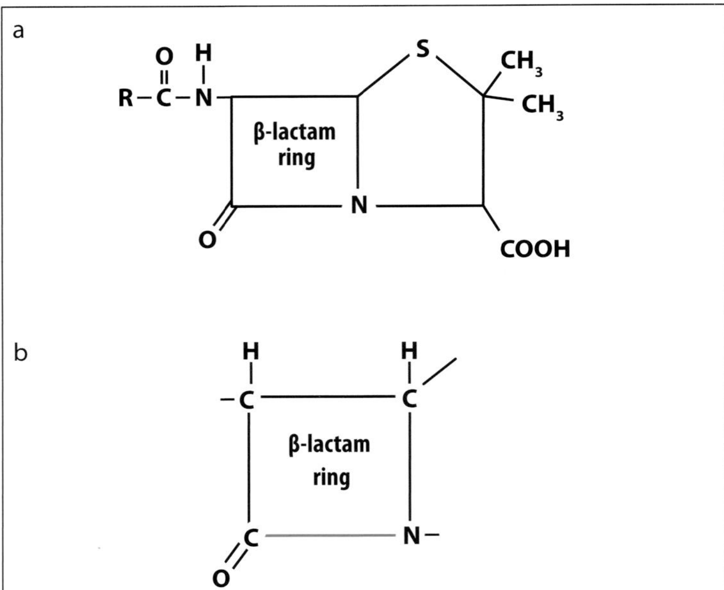

f46.4 a Structure of penicillin. Note the β-lactam ring, common to penicillins, cephalosporins, imipenem and clavulanate.
b Detail of the β-lactam ring structure. *Staphylococcus aureus* and other bacteria produce various β-lactamases, enzymes that break the β-lactam ring at the bond shown in red, inactivating some forms of these drugs.

Vancomycin is the safety net drug in all cases of MRSA, especially those of hospital origin. Of great concern is that rare cases of vancomycin-resistant *S aureus* (VRSA) have been described. These have the *VanA* gene, as is found in VRE. Fortunately, VRSA is rare, but vancomycin-intermediate *S aureus* (VISA) is clearly and ominously increasing. At this writing, VISA cannot be diagnosed by molecular testing because the mutations have not yet been determined.

In addition to obvious concerns about HA-MRSA, hospitals must address the issue of screening all incoming patients for CA-MRSA. Mupirocin is an antibiotic that is used topically in some cases of impetigo and intranasally in some cases of MRSA. Unfortunately, 5-10% of MRSA are also resistant to Mupirocin. Such resistance is caused by a gene called *ileS2* (originally called *MupA*), encoded on transferable plasmids.

Screening for MRSA is done by a variety of techniques, ranging from PCR to latex agglutination. PCR systems, such as GeneXpert by Cepheid and GenOhm by Becton-Dickinson, are commonly used in many laboratories.

In addition to antibiotic resistance, MRSA may also be associated with virulence factors. For example, Panton-Valentine leukocidin (PVL) is a leukocidin, coded by the genes *LukS* and *LukF*, that is associated with some strains of *S aureus*, especially CA-MRSA (PVL is rare in HA-MRSA). PVL is also implicated in many cases of extensive necrosis of the skin and subcutaneous tissue and in some cases of necrotizing pulmonary infections. PVL is a pore-forming exotoxin whose DNA is actually derived from integrated bacteriophage DNA that has infected the *S aureus* [PMID17146447].

S aureus causes toxic shock syndrome (TSS), though *Streptococcus pyogenes* causes a related condition called toxic shock-like syndrome. TSS is caused by TSS toxin 1 (TSST-1). Rare antigens, called superantigens, can bypass the usual pathway for an immune response and can simultaneously bind to the T-cell receptor and to an HLA class II molecule, directly stimulating the T cell without being broken down and presented by antigen presenting cells. Such binding causes an outpouring of cytokines. TSST-1 is such a superantigen, and like other superantigens, after binding to the T cell and the antigen-presenting cell, it initiates a cytokine storm.

Enterobacteriaceae, Extended Spectrum β-Lactamases, and Carbapenem-Resistant Enterobacteriaceae

Members of the family enterobacteriaceae commonly express β-lactamases, encoded by plasmids, that confer resistance to penicillins but not to cephalosporins. Examples of these enzymes include TEM-1, TEM-2, SHV-1, and CTX-M. TEM-1 is the most commonly encountered β-lactamase. SHV-1 is structurally similar to TEM-1 and shares 2/3 of its amino acids. Extended spectrum β-lactamases (ESBLs), also often encoded by plasmids, convey a broad range of antibiotic resistance to many enterobacteriaceae, including resistance to third generation cephalosporins [PMID20594363]. Most ESBLs are derived from mutations in the genes that encode for TEM-1, TEM-2, SHV-1, and CTX-M, creating slightly different enzymes [PMID20181902].

The carbapenems are a relatively new class of antibiotics that have a modified β-lactam ring **f46.5** and are effective against a wide range of both Gram-positive and Gram-negative bacteria. The carbapenems are usually resistant to ESBL but some enterobacteriaceae are becoming resistant to the carbapenems [PMID20615191]. Carbapenem-resistant enterobacteriaceae (CRE), of which carbapenem-resistant *Klebsiella pneumoniae* is the most common, produce the enzyme carbapenemase, which is usually encoded by the *KPC* gene on a plasmid [PMID20594363]. CRE are typically resistant to a wide variety of drugs [PMID20181902].

Resistance to carbapenem in Gram-negative enterobacteriaceae based on a different mechanism—the enzyme metallo-β-lactamase 1—has recently been reported. Because this enzyme was first acquired in New Delhi, it is sometimes called New Delhi metallo-β-lactamase 1 (NDM-1) [PMID20705517, PMID21129630].

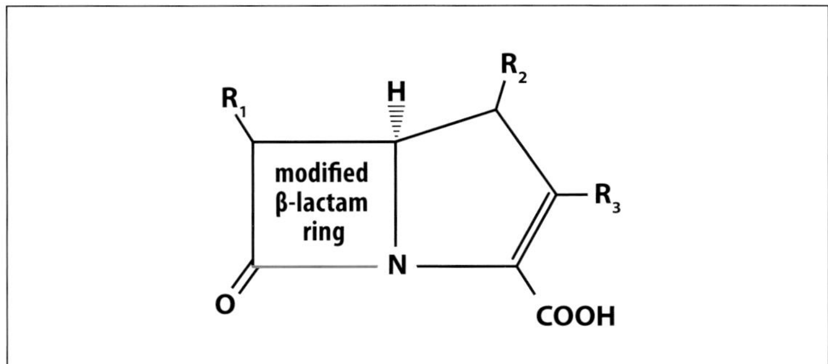

f46.5 Backbone structure of carbapenem antibiotics, with modified β-lactam ring. The red bond indicates the site of action of β-lactamases. Because the angles of the bonds are different in the modified β-lactam ring, many β-lactamases that can inactivate penicillins are not active against carbapenems.

Macrolide Resistance

3 chemically related classes of antibiotics have elaborate ring structures and inhibit prokaryotic protein synthesis by targeting the 23S rRNA—macrolides (eg, erythromycin), lincosamides (eg, clindamycin), and the streptogramins (especially streptogramin B) [PMID20645886]. These 3 groups together constitute the macrolide-lincosamide-streptogramin B (MLS) group.

Resistance to the macrolides is an increasing problem in *Streptococcus pneumoniae* and *Streptococcus pyogenes*, but most macrolide resistance is in *Staphylococcus* species. Almost all strains of *S aureus* that are resistant to erythromycin are also resistant to other MLS antibiotics.

MLS resistance often occurs after clindamycin use and occurs via 1 of 3 mechanisms. First, the product of the *erm* gene methylates the target 23 S rRNA, precluding antibiotic binding. Second, there is active efflux of the antibiotic out of the cell (especially for streptogramin B and antibiotics of the macrolide group). Third, streptogramin-B can be directly modified and inactivated by the product of the *SBH* gene, while the products of the *LinA* gene can inactivate the lincosamides [PMID10774259]. Of these mechanisms, the emergence of *erm* genes, particularly of *ermC*, appears to be the most important [PMID16261929].

Clostridium difficile

Clostridium difficile is an anaerobic, Gram-negative bacillus that is a major cause of hospital and nursing home-acquired diarrhea and abdominal pain, transmitted by the fecal-oral route. Increasingly, some cases appear to be acquired in the community [PMID21704273].

Clostridium difficile produces many toxins, the 2 most important of which are toxins A and B, encoded by 2 genes, *tcdA* and *tcdB*, that are both located at the pathogenicity locus (PaLoc) on the chromosome **f46.6**. Both of these toxins enter the cell through endocytosis via specific receptors and inhibit proteins of the Rho family of GTP-binding proteins, resulting in abnormalities of the actin microfilaments [PMID18289919, PMID20597005].

The first studies suggested that toxin A was the pathogenic protein. Subsequent studies on purified toxin proteins then suggested that either toxin can be pathogenic alone, but DNA studies under in vivo conditions similar to those in patients have suggested that toxin B is the real culprit and is required for pathogenicity [PMID19252482]. The PaLoc has a negative regulator, *tcdC* **f46.6**, whose product inhibits the expression of both toxins A and B.

C difficile hypervirulence is an emerging problem in which there is resistance to fluoroquinolones. This hypervirulent strain is called by various names, depending on the technique used to identify it, such as NAP1, B1, or 027, or as 027/BI/NAP1. Hypervirulent strains express much higher levels of both toxins A and B. A number of mutations of the negative

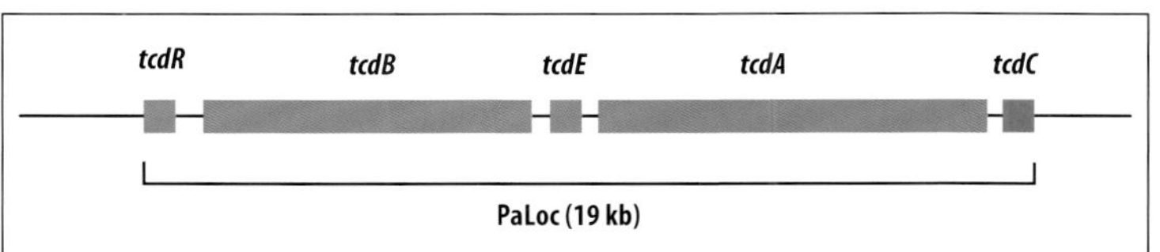

f46.6 Excerpt of the genome of *Clostridium difficile*.

regulator *tcdC* have been found, resulting in an ineffective or truncated protein. In particular, the hypervirulent strain has an 18 base pair deletion in the *tcdC* gene [PMID19303565]. Whereas in most cases of *C difficile* enterocolitis, most clinicians will stop a causative antibiotic and wait for several days, instituting metronidazole (flagyl) or vancomycin only if there is no improvement after this time, the finding of a hypervirulent strain will usually cause the immediate administration of one of these antibiotics.

In addition, some *C difficile* strains produce a third toxin, called binary toxin or CDT, at a different locus from PaLoc. This third toxin has not yet been shown to be pathogenic in humans, though it is found in about 10% of cases and there is some feeling that it may be involved in hypervirulence by augmenting the activity of toxins A and B [PMID20547099].

Prior to DNA testing, first line testing for *C difficile* was usually done by an immunoassay for the toxin A and toxin B. This was very specific, but only about 68% sensitive [PMID20117349], far less than DNA methods. Antigen testing (for glutamate dehydrogenase) is unable to distinguish between the pathogenic toxin-forming organisms and those that do not form toxins. For these reasons, DNA testing is emerging as the new gold standard, especially in cases of suspected hypervirulence.

A little-remembered public health point about *C difficile* is that since it is a spore-forming organism, it is not killed by the common alcohol-based hand sanitizers that we see in hospitals and public places.

Tuberculosis

Mycobacterium tuberculosis is an evolutionarily recent organism that consists of 3 primary genetic groups—GG1, GG2, and GG3—based on polymorphisms of codon 95 of the *gyr*A gene and codon 463 of the *kat*G gene [PMID9275218]. Rapid detection of mycobacteria can be done by transcription-mediated amplification or PCR, targeting the genes that code for rRNA.

Rifampicin inhibits the bacterial DNA-dependent RNA polymerase by binding to the β subunit of the enzyme. The mechanism of action of isoniazid is quite complex. It is a pro-drug that is bioactivated by the bacterial enzyme katG, which couples isoniazid to NADH. This complex then inhibits the gene *InhA*, whose product, inhA, is required for fatty acid synthesis. The end result is that mycolic acid, required for the bacterial cell wall, is not available [PMID8284673].

Multidrug-resistant TB (MDR-TB) are strains that are resistant to both of the first line drugs, isoniazid and rifampicin. Resistance to rifampicin is associated with a mutation in the β subunit of RNA polymerase (rpoB), while resistance to isoniazid is associated with a mutation in the genes for the enzymes katG or inhA [PMID20448341]. Mutations in katG prevent the bioactivation of isoniazid, while mutations in inhA make the bacterium resistant to inhibition by the complex of isoniazid and NADH. Extensive (or extreme) drug-resistant TB (XDR-TB) strains are defined by resistance to both rifampicin and isoniazid, and also to multiple second line drugs [PMID20448341].

At this writing, susceptibility testing is still largely phenotypic. This raises a larger question: Should antibiotic resistance be determined phenotypically or genotypically (ie, with molecular methods)? Phenotypic assays more closely approach the actual in vivo clinical situation, and it is not productive to use molecular methods to detect nonfunctional DNA. But phenotypic assays are not a perfect model for in vivo conditions, and genotypic assays can uncover subtle mutations that may have clinical relevance and that may be missed in an in vitro phenotypic assay. Molecular testing for RNA, whose presence is almost certainly clinically significant, or advances in proteomics will likely result in better susceptibility testing, but at this writing, there is a role for the phenotypic evaluation in occasional cases.

Strain Typing and Molecular Epidemiology

Many of the DNA techniques we have examined have been used in epidemiologic studies and have proven useful in identifying genetic similarities in pathogenic organisms from different patients, indicating a common source. This is called strain typing, species genotyping, genomic fingerprinting, or molecular epidemiology. There are many ways to perform strain typing, and different methods are better suited for different organisms (eg, food-borne bacteria vs *Mycobacterium* species). We will briefly consider 6 methods which were developed for *Mycobacteria* [PMID18599139, PMID11168781]. The first is direct DNA sequencing, which is laborious, though restricted sequencing of the 16S rDNA, if fully developed, would alleviate this drawback considerably. Indeed, complete sequencing of the 16S rDNA may emerge as the gold standard in prokaryotic phylogeny.

A second method is restriction fragment length polymorphism (RFLP) analysis, based largely on insertion sequence 6110 [PMID17154049]. Because IS6110 is found only in *M tuberculosis* and *M bovis*, strain typing by RFLP is limited to these 2 species. Almost all isolates of *M tuberculosis* have at least 1 copy of IS6110, and most have multiple copies. As discussed in Chapter 45, RFLP requires the labor intensive use of electrophoresis and Southern blotting, after which detection of bands is by a labeled probe. Because insertion sequences are scattered throughout the genome without tandem repetition, after restriction enzyme cutting, the fragments containing them will be of different lengths and will settle at different locations in a gel after electrophoresis. After blotting, a probe that hybridizes to IS6110 will disclose bands in different locations. For the same restriction enzyme and conditions, different strains will have different numbers of IS6110 numbers and migration patterns. Different isolates of *M tuberculosis* or *M bovis* that have the same number and migration pattern of IS6110 sequences likely arose from the same source. In addition to the labor-intensiveness of the RFLP process, IS6110 analysis is further delayed by the need to culture the organism.

A third method of strain typing of mycobacterium isolates is pulsed field gel electrophoresis (PFGE) [PMID10325348]. In PFGE, bacteria are embedded in a plug of agarose, after which they are subjected to a detergent (usually sodium dodecyl sulfate) to lyse the cells and a proteinase (usually proteinase K) to inhibit DNase enzymes. The DNA is then subjected to a restriction endonuclease that is chosen so that it will cut the DNA in only a few places, resulting in long strands of nucleic acid. The agarose plugs are then removed and placed into a PFGE apparatus. As discussed in Chapter 45, in PFGE, fragments of DNA are subjected to a constantly changing electric field. These changes in polarity cause constant reorientation of the large DNA fragments. Larger fragments take longer to reorient, resulting in a size-dependent migration that is not possible in ordinary electrophoresis because large fragments of DNA do not migrate in a purely size-dependent manner and may not even be able to enter the gel. After Southern blotting of the gel or staining with ethidium bromide, the position of the bands identifies each unique strain of mycobacterium. PFGE has proven to be of value in the identification of a source during an outbreak and in preventing outbreaks by identifying isolates of potentially pathogenic bacteria.

In addition being used in strain typing of *Mycobacterium* species, PFGE is the technique used by PulseNet, a network of public health laboratories that monitor food-borne infections [PMID16602975]. PulseNet laboratories perform PFGE on all isolates of *Salmonella typhimurium*, *E coli* O157:H7, *Listeria monocytogenes*, and *Shigella sonnei*, and sends results to the CDC, which then compares them, looking for similarities that might indicate a source with the potential to cause an outbreak. In New York state, for example, hospital microbiology laboratories must send any isolates of the above 4 organisms to the Department of Health, which then performs PFGE on them for local comparison and for reporting to the CDC.

A fourth method of strain typing of mycobacterium isolates is the spacer oligonucleotide typing (spoligotyping) technique. The direct repeat region is composed of multiple repeating sequences of 36 base pairs that are interspersed with nonrepeating sequences called spacers, which vary in length from 35 to 41 base pairs. 43 different sequences of spacers have been identified, and these are the targets of spoligotyping. In spoligotyping, the entire direct repeat region is amplified and labeled by PCR [PMID7934856]. The presence and identity of any of 43 different spacers is then determined by the binding of the labeled amplicons to synthetic oligonucleotides that are spotted onto membranes. The direct repeat region in *Mycobacterium tuberculosis* and *M bovis* is the only known locus that shows significant variation among strains. The more spacers that are shared between 2 sources of *M tuberculosis* or *M bovis*, the more likely they are to have originated from the same source. Because one need not wait for culture, the spoligotyping technique is much faster than RFLP analysis of IS6110. In addition, it can be used to study nonviable organisms (thus rendering it suitable for the study of paraffin-embedded tissue and organisms retrieved from Ziehl-Neelsen stained slides). Spoligotyping has generated the largest database of *M tuberculosis* strain typing, called SpolDB4 [PMID20739484]. However it may not as sensitive as IS6110 or PFGE because it examines a sequence that is found in only one place in the genome. Occasionally, strains of *M tuberculosis* have the same spoligotype patterns, but are shown to have different IS6110 profiles.

A fifth method of strain typing of mycobacterium isolates is PCR of repetitive DNA elements (rep-PCR). Prokaryotes also have repetitive DNA sequences, and in rep-PCR, some of these areas are amplified and the resulting fragments are electrophoresed or subjected to a sophisticated separation process based on microfluidics. The number of repeating units identifies the specific strain. A number of well described repetitive sequences have been used, including the enterobacterial repetitive intergenic consensus (ERIC) sequence of 124-127 base pairs [PMID14559175]. Rep-PCR has also been used in identification of species, but is better suited for strain typing than routine identification.

Most recently, attention has focused on a sixth method of strain typing that is based on mycobacterial interspersed repetitive units (MIRU), a locus of variable number of tandem repeats (VNTRs) that is specific to *M tuberculosis* [PMID10844663]. MIRU analysis is similar to that used for VNTR elsewhere. The MIRU sequences are amplified by PCR, after which the amplicons are subjected to gel or capillary electrophoresis. Strain typing is by the number of repeats, as indicated by the position of bands in a gel.

As is the case for so much of molecular pathology, methodology is moving toward real-time techniques that do not require culture, endonuclease digestion, blotting, or electrophoresis. Spoligotyping, for example, has been adapted to a microbead platform. As this trend continues, we can expect a movement towards microarray-based methods and towards the use of single nucleotide polymorphisms (SNPs), followed by a trend toward direct sequencing as it becomes cheaper and easier. Strain typing has also been adapted to individual patients to determine if their infection is a reactivation of a previous strain or a new infection, or to ascertain if a patient is infected by 2 different strains [PMID21420561].

Viruses

Viruses are the simplest organisms on earth, so simple in fact that many question if they are true life forms. A growing number believe that viruses are not living because they do not possess a true cellular structure and they do not have their own metabolism. These are very legitimate arguments, but the question of whether or not viruses are life forms is nearly unapproachable because there is no universally accepted definition of life. We must also remember that while viruses do not have a cellular structure, they do possess the 2 key constituents of cells—nucleic acid and proteins—in an orderly and useful arrangement. It is true that viruses do not have their own metabolism, but we must remember that some incontestable organisms, such as *Chlamydia*, are heavily dependent on host metabolism.

In any event, viruses have only nucleic acid and a few key proteins (some have a lipid envelope which is derived from the host in which they have reproduced but which has become intrinsic to the virus and its life cycle). The nucleic acid may be either DNA or RNA, and there are 2 types of each kind. Type I DNA viruses are double-stranded, while type II are single-stranded [PMID17501915]. Some RNA viruses have a positive sense strand and can be directly translated, while others have a negative sense strand that must copy itself before it can be translated. If the RNA has a positive sense, it exists as naked strands, but negatively sensed RNA exists in complex ribonucleoproteins that are required for the synthesis of a complementary copy of the RNA [PMID21358279]. The RNA in RNA viruses may also be double stranded [PMID18770617].

ISBN 978-089189-5886

A retrovirus is a special type of RNA virus. All retroviruses are RNA viruses, but not all RNA viruses are retroviruses. Retroviruses have 2 identical strands of RNA and they have envelopes. Retroviruses replicate via a reverse transcriptase enzyme that is coded for by viral nucleic acid. Reverse transcriptase synthesizes cDNA from viral RNA. This cDNA, called proviral DNA, is then incorporated into the host's genome by an integrase enzyme, also coded by viral nucleic acid. The integrated viral DNA replicates with the host genome via host DNA polymerase and uses host RNA polymerase for its transcription, after which other viral proteins reconstitute intact retroviral particles.

The Human Immunodeficiency Virus

The human immunodeficiency virus (HIV) is a retrovirus that has unleashed a plague in some parts of the world that is almost comparable to the Great Plague of the 14th century, and which is an immediate imperative of modern medicine. The HIV virus has a lipid coat, derived from host cells, in which are embedded glycoproteins, the 2 most important of which are gp120 and gp41, the latter of which is transmembrane. The core is inside the coat and contains 2 identical strands of RNA. The RNA codes for 9 genes, though the products of 2 of these genes, gag and pol, will subsequently be cleaved to yield multiple proteins.

The gag (group-specific antigen) gene encodes structural proteins while the pol gene codes for the enzymes of the virus, including reverse transcriptase, protease, and integrase. The env gene codes for the envelope proteins that are embedded in the viral envelope and are important to attachment to the host cell. There are also 2 regulatory proteins, Tat and Rev, that bind to the TAR and RRE sequences of viral RNA, respectively, and 4 accessory proteins, Vpu, Vpr, Vif, and Nef.

The life cycle of HIV is typical for a retrovirus. The order of the genes on the RNA is gag-pol-env. Gag and pol are usually transcribed and translated together by host enzymes, including host RNA polymerase, after which the protease from the pol gene frees itself from the combined protein and then cleaves at additional sites to free other enzymes such as reverse transcriptase and integrase. The protease also cleaves the gag transcript to form the smaller structural proteins that are used in assembly of the virus.

There are 3 major groups of HIV-1: M (main), O (outlier), and N (new). Group M is most common and important. It is divided into subtypes A-H. Subtype B is almost the only subtype found in North America and is also common in South America. The word "clade" is usually synonymous for subtype but is occasionally used synonymously with group and therefore is perhaps best avoided in clinical use.

Therapy is usually directed at either the reverse transcriptase, the protease, or both. Reverse transcriptase inhibitors can be either nucleoside analogues such as AZT or nonnucleoside analogues such as Nevirapine, Delavirdine, and Efavirenz. At this writing, the most common approach in developed nations is to direct therapy to both the reverse transcriptase and the protease. This is called highly active antiretroviral therapy (HAART) and has shown great promise.

The virus inhabits macrophages, dendritic cells, and CD4 T lymphocytes, but replication occurs only in CD4 T cells. Binding of HIV to the CD4 lymphocyte is mediated through the attachment of the gp 120 protein in the viral envelope to the CD4 receptor on the T cell. In addition, viral attachment requires 1 of 2 coreceptors, CCR5 or CXCR4, both of which are chemokine receptors [PMID15647694]. Indeed, a deletion in the DNA that codes for CCR5 leads to partial resistance to HIV. The requirement for coreceptors opens new therapeutic avenues, as blockade of either coreceptor could prevent viral entry. Progress is being made in blocking both the CCR5 coreceptor [PMID19339945] and the CXCR4 [PMID18624812] coreceptor.

While lytic replication in CD4 T cells, with consequent destruction of the cell, is a primary mechanism for the loss of cell mediated immunity that is the hallmark of the disease, HIV can apparently kill CD4 positive T lymphocytes via several other mechanisms. These have not been completely worked out, but it is known that they include apoptosis and the killing of CD4 cells by CD8 positive cytotoxic lymphocytes. There is also an interesting mechanism whereby an HIV-infected cell appears to be able to kill T4 lymphocytes that are not infected by HIV. In this scenario, the envelope proteins of the virus bind to the CXCR4 receptor of a bystander T4 lymphocyte and induce apoptosis [PMID16886061].

A vaccine for HIV has proven elusive because antibodies to HIV—which patients readily develop—are of minimal benefit, since the reservoirs of the virus are intracellular. Cellular immunity is desperately needed in AIDS because the virus is inside cells. Cytotoxic CD8 T cells are able to kill infected CD4 T cells that display HIV proteins, but the problem is that the viral proteins mutate, largely because the viral reverse transcriptase cannot proofread (viral polymerases generally lack proofreading ability). A secondary cause of mutation is that if >1 HIV virus infects a cell, they can exchange RNA. Cytotoxic CD8 T cells are only able to kill cells displaying the original HIV proteins. Cells of the immune system can only respond to the proteins they were originally "trained" to respond to. This leaves a relatively unopposed path for the cells that are infected by viruses whose proteins have mutated, and it is these viruses that are the primary clinical problem. The exquisite specificity of the immune system—normally our great ally—becomes our ironic enemy.

EIA screening for antibodies is still the first line of testing, with PCR confirmation of positive results. In newborns, one may employ a qualitative PCR assessment for the proviral DNA as an initial test. CD4 T-cell counts and viral load testing (quantitative RNA test) are the primary tools for following patients. qPCR, nucleic acid based sequence amplification, and branched nucleic acid technology are the 3 main methods for quantitating HIV viral load. Of these techniques, qPCR is emerging as the standard and can now be used for HIV, hepatitis B, hepatitis C, cytomegalovirus (CMV), EBV, and polyomavirus BK. Most qPCR quantitative testing for HIV is targeted at the gag gene, though Abbott targets the integrase. Because opportunistic infections can affect viral load, it is prudent to wait a month after such an infection has cleared before performing a viral load test.

Standards have been a problem in quantitation of viruses, and the relative lack of universally accepted standards has resulted in interlaboratory variation and difficulty in comparing results over time, even when the same technology is used. HIV and hepatitis C were the first viruses for which reliable external standards were developed. The initial standards were purified nucleic acid from the organism to be tested. This is still often the case, but it is likely that synthetic nucleotides may serve as readily available standard material for many viral quantitation tests in the near future [PMID20075208].

The development of drug resistance is a particular problem with HIV and suggests that a mutation has occurred. The most important mutations are those affecting the protease and reverse transcriptase, as these are the targets of most therapies. Resistance is often detected by sequencing the pol gene that codes for these enzymes [PMID20844809]. The potential difficulty of this approach is that if a previously uncharacterized mutation is detected, one will not know if it conveys drug resistance or not, though an educated guess can be made from the nature of the mutation and the clinical situation. Also, sequencing only 1 or 2 enzymes does not shed light on protein interactions, gene expression, or the overall in vivo behavior of the virus.

While many patients develop resistance after therapy, it is important to note that some patients are infected de novo with a resistant strain, without ever receiving therapy, and it is generally wise to genotype pol before commencing therapy to identify patients who may have a resistant strain. There is a database of known mutations for HIV, and sequencing some portion of the viral genome before treatment permits an educated guess about potentially effective therapies and also affords an opportunity to subtype the virus.

As is the case for tuberculosis, resistance can also be assayed phenotypically. Phenotypic testing for HIV drug resistance is performed by cultivating mononuclear cells from the patient (which contain the HIV) and a donor in the presence of increasing amounts of the retroviral drug to be tested. Drug susceptibility is measured by the levels of free p24 (1 of the core proteins in HIV) or diminished numbers of plaques in in vitro assays [PMID19940949]. The reverse transcriptase from the patient's virus can also be extracted and placed in an HIV whose reverse transcriptase has been removed, after which the virus is exposed to increasing doses of the drug to be tested.

As is the case for tuberculosis, both phenotypic and genotypic testing have advantages and disadvantages. Unlike sequencing, phenotypic assays permit an overall assessment of the virus's virulence, based on the entire molecular biology of the virus and its interactions with the host. However, they are labor-intensive and depend on an extrapolation of in vitro findings to an in vivo setting. There is no assurance that the more "complete" information obtained from in vitro phenotypic assays translates into clinically more useful information. Molecular methods offer the potential of more reliably predicting resistance by finding the responsible gene or genes without having to culture. Moreover, they provide the potential for identifying and targeting those portions of the genome that are differentially expressed during a pathogenic state.

In addition to the development of drug resistance, another problem with anti-HIV therapy is that it is never curative and the virus will almost always return if therapy is stopped. The reason for this is that the virus is able to "hide" in cells that antiretroviral drugs cannot reach. Memory T cells, which have both HIV proteins on the surface and HIV RNA integrated in their genomes, are the primary source of HIV in the blood of patients that have stable HIV infection, but infected antigen-presenting cells, such as macrophages and interdigitating dendritic cells, are also able to "fly under the radar" with regard to both an immune response and drug therapy.

The Hepatitis Viruses

Hepatitis C

Hepatitis C (HCV) is a positively single-stranded RNA virus with an envelope surrounding a core region. There is a 5' nontranslated region (NTR; also called UTR for untranslated region) at one end of the RNA and a 3' NTR at the other end. Between the NTRs, there are 10 major genes, 3 of which are structural and 7 of which are nonstructural. The structural genes are C (core) and E1 and E2 (envelope). The nonstructural genes are NS1, NS2, NS3, NS4a, NS4b, NS5a, and NS5b.

Approximately 10% of HCV patients have acquired the virus through unknown means. Only 20% of patients will be able to clear the virus without treatment, and of the 80% who cannot clear the virus spontaneously, about 1 in 4 will develop cirrhosis if not treated.

HCV screening is currently based on finding antibodies to core antigen by EIA. Serum IgM antibodies, normally indicative of active infection and absent in past infection, may still be present in chronic HCV infection, negating the usefulness of any attempt to identify acutely infected patients by separate IgM-IgG assays [PMID17013450]. Because of low specificity, positive EIA tests are confirmed by the identification and quantitation of viral nucleic acid.

There are 6 distinct genotypes of HCV, of which type 1 is most commonly encountered. Genotyping is generally based on sequencing the 5' NTR, but sometimes also on sequencing the core region or NS5b. After conversion of the RNA to cDNA, detection is by hybridization to commercially available reference probes. Quantitation of HCV is by conversion of a portion of the viral RNA (often a proprietary portion) to cDNA, followed by qPCR.

Historically, quantitation of HCV has often been performed by techniques other than PCR (such as branched chain methodology), the results of which are not comparable to quantitations obtained by PCR. As is the case for other viruses, reliable quantitation of HCV by qPCR has been delayed by the lack of universal standards, and even currently, as PCR methods move to the fore, there is suboptimal reproducibility among laboratories and difficulty in measuring small changes. Standards and reference material will be central to solving this problem, as has been reviewed [PMID20075208].

Treatment of HCV is with α interferon, which is usually pegylated (conjugated to polyethylene glycol) to increase its serum half-life. Ribavirin, a guanosine analogue, may also be used. In 2011, the FDA approved the protease inhibitors boceprevir (Victrelis) and telaprevir (Incivek), in combination with peginterferon and ribavirin, for genotype 1.

No drug resistance has yet been reported for hepatitis C, so there is currently no molecular testing for this. Patients with genotype 1 who have not been previously treated and who have either of 2 SNPs on chromosome 19q13, rs12979860 or rs8099917 (every confirmed polymorphism in the Single

Nucleotide Polymorphism Database receives an accession number that begins with "rs") respond better to treatment [PMID19684573, PMID20399780, PMID21704279]. These 2 SNPs are located just upstream of the gene that codes for IL28B, which is a newly discovered interferon called type III (or λ) interferon [PMID20624172].

Hepatitis B

Hepatitis B (HBV) is a DNA virus. It does not have an envelope and therefore is completely dependent on phagocytosis to gain entry into the cell. The surface antigen is the outermost portion of the virus. The core antigen encircles the DNA. The E antigen is just inside the surface antigen. The E antigen is a nonparticulate form of the core antigen and is of unknown function. It is also called the precore or basal core antigen.

The DNA of HBV is circular, with a portion that is single stranded and a portion that is double stranded. The DNA codes for its own polymerase. The most important genes in the life cycle of the virus are those that code for the surface and core antigens, and for the DNA polymerase. During the life cycle of the virus, some of the RNA is coded into DNA by a reverse transcriptase of viral origin, so this virus actually replicates partially as a retrovirus.

About 1/3 of patients with HBV have contracted it via an unknown mechanism. It is not transmitted through breast milk. Exposure is often asymptomatic, with only elevation of transaminases. In sharp contrast to hepatitis C, only about 10% of untreated exposed adult patients will enter into a chronic phase. Of these, about 2/3 will be mild cases (what was once called chronic persistent hepatitis; characterized only by persistent elevations of the transaminases ALT and/or AST). The other 1/3 will be a so-called chronic active hepatitis, with risk of cirrhosis and hepatocellular carcinoma. In young children and neonates, however, a much higher percentage of patients exposed to hepatitis B—about 90%—will develop a chronic form [PMID19575488].

In addition to the intact virus (the Dane particle), aggregates of surface antigen may also be found in blood and tissues. There are some 8 genotypes of the virus (A-H), determined by sequencing, but genotyping is less important in HBV than in HCV because it does not influence therapy. The major genotype in North America is A. The initial diagnosis of HBV is by serological detection of antibodies, with confirmation by PCR, usually targeting the genes that code for the core or surface antigens [PMID17942654].

A G1896A mutation in the E antigen, resulting in a stop codon, confers a favorable prognosis. Unfortunately, this mutation is rare in genotype A. 2 mutations in the E antigen (A1762T and G1764A; found together in tandem) appear to convey a higher incidence of chronic carrier status and hepatocellular carcinoma [PMID20846420]. Major drugs used in treating hepatitis B include lamivudine, telbuvidine, emtricitabine, and adefovir. Interferon is not used. Results are not as good as for the treatment of hepatitis C. Resistance occurs in about a third of patients, largely because of mutations arising from the reverse transcriptase's lack of proofreading ability. Because many of the reading frames in the viral genome overlap, a mutation may affect >1 gene. 2 tandem mutations (L180M and M204V) in the DNA polymerase appear to confer multidrug resistance [PMID20074155]. Vaccination to HBV is directed to the surface antigen. Mutations in this antigen, called vaccine escape mutations, may diminish the response to vaccination.

Hepatitis D (δ)

Hepatitis D is a defective RNA virus that cannot replicate without the surface antigen of hepatitis B. The 2 viruses together are clinically more aggressive than infection with hepatitis B alone. There are 8 genotypes of hepatitis D. The virus has been refractory, to treatment, and only PEGylated α interferon has been at all effective [PMID20460901]. At this writing, hepatitis D is rarely a target of molecular testing.

The Human Papillomavirus Family

Human papillomavirus (HPV) is a small double stranded DNA virus. At this writing, over 100 genotypes of HPV have been characterized, 15 of which (16, 18, 31, 33, 35, 39, 45, 51, 52, 56, 58, 59, 68, 73, and 82) are considered to be high risk. 3 additional types (26, 53, 66) are probably high risk [PMID12571259]. The products of the early genes E1 and E2 facilitate the integration of viral DNA into that of the host, as well as the replication and transcription of HPV DNA. The L1 and L2 genes code for viral capsid proteins. Because the virus cannot be easily cultured, identification and genotyping are done by a number of molecular means. Most molecular assays intended to subtype HPV are directed to L1 or one of the E genes [PMID22072858].

80% of women who are sexually active will have 1 subtype of high-risk HPV by age 50, and many will simultaneously have multiple subtypes. Infection is common in men, but is asymptomatic except for anal cancer, which is almost exclusively seen in gay men, so screening men for HPV (the so-called male Pap test) is unlikely to be rewarding from a public health standpoint. The Gardasil vaccine directly protects against types 6, 11, 16, and 18, and has cross-reactivity to several other types, including 31. The Cervarix vaccine is directed to types 16 and 18, but shows cross-reactivity to a number of other types [PMID19943762].

The study of human papillomavirus provides an opportunity to examine the cell cycle and the process of malignant transformation. The resting cell is said to be in G0. The cell cycle begins with a G1 phase, in which the cell is committed to DNA replication and cell division. The cycle continues with an S phase in which DNA is replicated, a G2 phase in which the DNA content of the cell is tetraploid instead of the normal diploid, a mitosis phase, in which 1/2 of the DNA is segregated to each pole of the cell, and with only rare exceptions, a final stage of cell division that restores diploid DNA content and G0 or G1 status to the daughter cells.

There are 4 principal stages at which the cell cycle is regulated—entry into the S phase (the G1-S checkpoint), in the S phase, entry into mitosis (the G2-M checkpoint), and in mitosis [PMID11063129]. Each of these stages is regulated by a specific protein or group of proteins. The most important checkpoints are G1-S and G2-M. To understand the control of the cell cycle and the pathogenesis of HPV, we must understand something about 5 groups of proteins.

The first of these groups are the cyclins, proteins that regulate entry into, progression through, and exit from the cell cycle. The major cyclin classes are A, B, C, D, and E, and there are isoforms of some of these classes (eg, there are 3 D cyclins,

D1, D2 and D3). The cyclin proteins work together in sequential deregulations to permit the cell cycle to unfold.

The cyclins activate kinase enzymes called cyclin-dependent kinases (CDKs), the second group of proteins important in cell cycle regulation. Kinases are enzymes that add a phosphate group to a protein. Binding of a cyclin to a cyclin-dependent kinase activates that kinase. The important CDKs are CDK-1, CDK-2, CDK-4, and CDK-6. There are associations between individual cyclins and cyclin dependent kinases [PMID15549091]. For example, all 3 forms of cyclin D interact with CDK4 and CDK6. The 2 forms of cyclin E, E1 and E2 (not to be confused with the E1 and E2 genes of HPV), both affiliate with CDK2, while cyclin A binds to CDK2 or to CDK1 and cyclin B binds only to CDK1.

Cyclin D is activated early in G1, before the S phase, and before other cyclins, except possibly cyclin C. The complex of cyclin D/CDK4/6 controls entry into the early stages of cell division [PMID16259056]. The cyclin B/CDK1 complex functions later and controls entry into G2-M [PMID11063129]. The roles of cyclins C, E and A, and the CDKs they bind to, are less well understood than those of cyclins D and B [PMID16236519]. Cyclin C has been more recently described and may interact with CDK3 even before cyclin D interacts with CDK 4/6.

Current thinking is that as the cell cycle begins, there is first activation of cyclin C/CDK3 in G1, followed by the activation of cyclin D/CDK4/6, then activation of cyclin E/CDK2 slightly later in G1. There is evidence that cyclin E facilitates entry into S phase, both by interacting with CDK2 and by independent actions [PMID17218276]. These early-acting cyclin/CDK complexes are sensitive to extracellular signals such as hormones, cytokines, and growth factors. Once the cell has progressed into the S phase, it is less sensitive to extracellular signals. Cyclin A/CDK2 is activated immediately upon entering the S phase. Cyclin A/CDK1 and cyclin B/CDK1 are activated during G2 and permit entry into and completion of mitosis [PMID19075565].

The third group of proteins is those that inhibit the CDKs. Binding of an inhibitor to a cyclin-dependent kinase will stop its kinase activity, even in the presence of an appropriate cyclin. 2 classes of proteins that inhibit CDKs have been elucidated. The first class of CDK inhibitors consists of members of the INK4 family, and includes p15, p16, p18, and p19. The second class is those of the members of CIP/KIP family, examples of which include p21, p27, and p57. The INK4 molecules specifically interact and inhibit the complex of cyclin D-CDK4/6, while the CIP/KIP family interacts with other complexes of cyclin-CDK [PMID16259056, PMID18298566].

The fourth group of proteins is tumor suppressor proteins whose normal function is to control DNA synthesis or cell division. Foremost among these are the retinoblastoma protein (Rb) and the p53 protein. Normally, unphosphorylated Rb binds to and inactivates a family of transcription factors called E2F. E2F is necessary for progression through the cell cycle, and because unphosphorylated Rb protein has inactivated it, the cell cycle cannot be traversed.

Phosphorylation of Rb turns off its suppressor activity of E2F, allowing the cell to proceed from G1 into the S phase. Rb is phosphorylated several times by cyclin-dependent kinases as the cell cycle progresses, suggesting that it requires multiple phosphorylations for the cell cycle to proceed normally [PMID1531876]. CDK4 or CDK6, bound to and activated by cyclin D1, and CDK1, bound to cyclin B, are the principal kinases that phosphorylate and inhibit Rb, releasing the inhibition of E2F and possibly of other proteins as well, and permitting the cell cycle to proceed [PMID19550046]. This is why p16 is an important tumor suppressor protein—by inhibiting CDK4 and 6, it largely prevents the phosphorylation of Rb. By keeping Rb in an unphosphorylated state, p16 keeps E2F in an inhibited state so the cell cycle cannot unfold.

The p53 protein, probably the most studied of all tumor suppressor proteins, is a transcription factor whose normal function has antiproliferative effects that function in a variety of ways to restrain inappropriate entry into the cell cycle and unwanted proliferation [PMID20066118]. P53 is a particularly important regulator of entry into the S phase in cells that have been damaged [PMID1323840], and either restricts entry into S phase of damaged cells until the damage can be repaired or initiates apoptosis if repair is not possible [PMID8939848].

P53 also functions, via different pathways, to either arrest the proliferation of or kill cells that have undergone malignant transformation [PMID20183804]. Oncogenesis apparently induces increased expression of p53 as a cellular defense mechanism, but almost 1/2 of cancers have some means of circumventing this increase [PMID19776747]. The *P53* gene is mutated or lost, or its protein product is inhibited, in about 1/2 of cancers [PMID20206267].

The details of how p53 suppresses proliferation in damaged or transformed cells remain unclear, but one mechanism for the antitumor effect of p53 is that it induces the p21 protein. The p21 protein inactivates complexes of cyclin/CDK, preventing them from phosphorylating tumor suppressor proteins such Rb. This keeps proteins such as Rb in their unphosphorylated (active) state, where they impede the cell cycle. The p21 protein, therefore, is a tumor suppressor protein that tends to keep cells in G1 [PMID16259056].

Now we can consider HPV, and as we do so, we encounter the fifth group of proteins, those made by the virus (or to speak more correctly, those made by the host cell in response to infection by the virus). While there are exceptions in both directions, in most cases of CIN, the virus remains episomal, but in most cases of invasive cancer, it is integrated into host DNA [PMID19055056, PMID18478264]. The major oncogenic proteins of HPV are E6 and E7, and increased expression of these proteins is seen in CIN and invasive carcinoma. There is much to be learned about the mechanism of oncogenesis of HPV, but it is known that integration of the virus into host DNA, which is accomplished by the E1 and E2 viral proteins, increases the likelihood of invasive carcinoma and results in constitutive expression of E6 and E7.

It is known that the E6 gene product of high-risk HPV types binds to the p53 tumor suppressor protein and facilitates its degradation via the ubiquitin pathway (in low-risk HPV subtypes, the E6 gene product does not have this effect on p53), while the E7 gene product of high-risk HPV types binds to Rb and inactivates or degrades it [PMID1321031]. The binding of E6 to the p53 protein and E7 to Rb effectively inactivates these tumor suppressor proteins and allows the cell to bypass critical cell-cycle checkpoints, resulting in a prolonged and inappropriate S-phase [PMID19721808, PMID17645777].

Interestingly, the HPV proteins E6 and E7 also induce the expression of the tumor suppressor protein p16 [PMID11790875], opposing their tumor-promoting actions on p53 and Rb. p16 is not normally expressed in cervical epithelium [PMID16462152], and because its presence inhibits the ability of the cyclin D1-CDK4/6 complex to phosphorylate Rb, one would expect that the presence of p16 would lead the cell away from dysplasia. For reasons that are not clear, however, p16 is not typically found in normal cervical epithelium but is found in cervical dysplasia and carcinoma. A number of theories have been advanced to explain this apparent paradox [PMID16259056], one of which is that increased levels of p16 are a compensatory mechanism of the cell under attack by HPV. While the details of this matter await clarification, it is important to remember that p16 is a normal protein with tumor suppressive function, but it is not typically found in normal cervical epithelium and its presence is a point for cervical dysplasia or carcinoma.

HPV cannot be diagnosed serologically, and cell culture is very impractical. Hence, the great importance of cytologic screening and the molecular techniques that identify the high-risk HPV genome. The hybrid capture method of detecting HPV is discussed in Chapter 30. A newer method to detect HPV is employed by the Cervista Invader technology, based on the enzyme cleavase, which detects hairpin structures caused by the junction of single-stranded and double-stranded DNA. In the Invader technology, probes are used to create a hairpin structure that is recognized and cleaved by cleavase. A probe, called an invader, is used that will hybridize at the 3' end, but not at the 5' end of the target HPV DNA sequence **f46.7ab**. The dangling 5' end is cleaved **f46.7c**, and then amplified, after which it incubates with a U-shaped synthetic oligonucleotide, constructed to be complementary to the 5' end, that carries a label at one end **f46.7d**. The 5' fragment binds to the synthetic oligonucleotide in such a way that the end portion carrying the probe is displaced **f46.7e**. A second cleavase reaction frees the probe and allows its fluorescence to be measured **f46.7f**. Like hybrid capture, the Invader method can be employed on the same vial as was used to generate the Pap smear. The 2 methods are comparable, with the Invader method perhaps having slightly better specificity [PMID18367578].

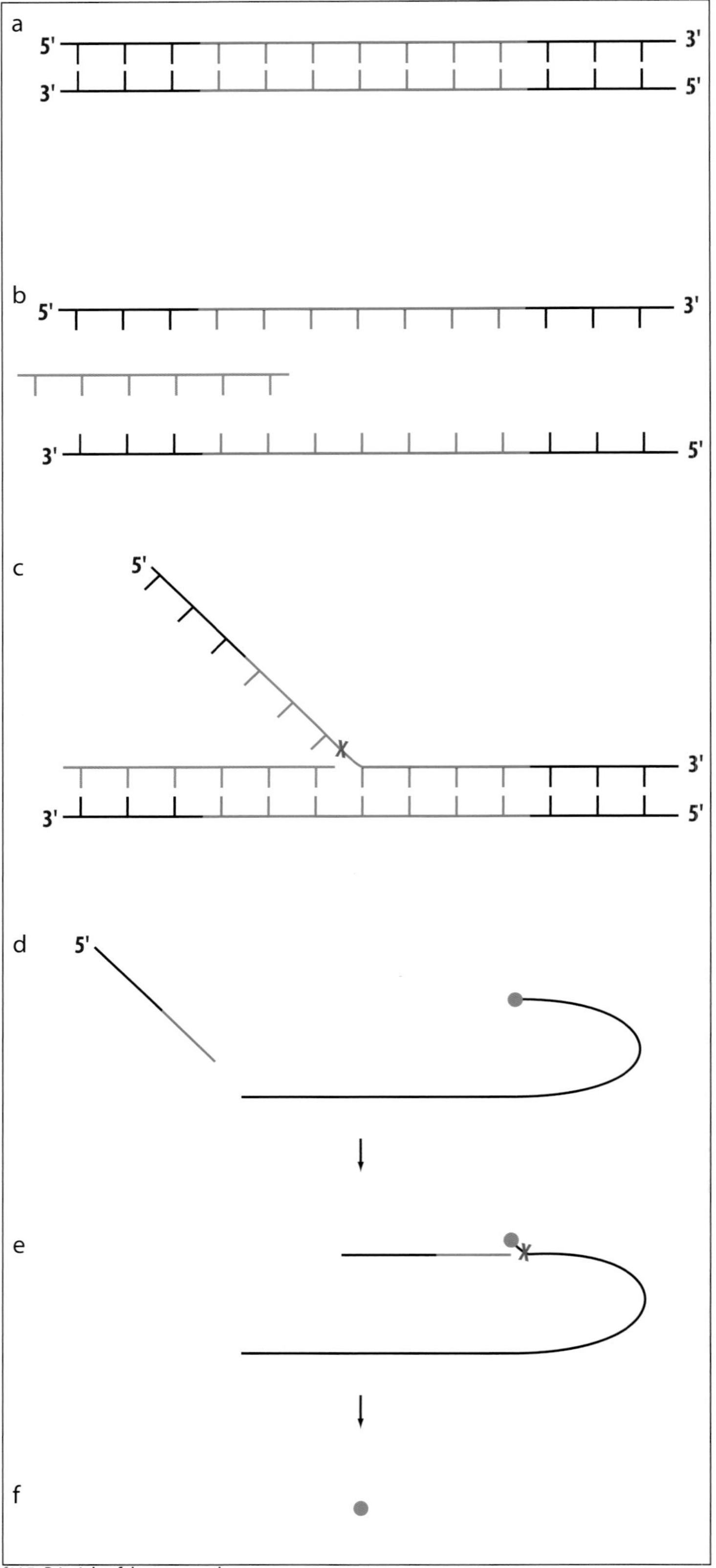

f46.7 Principle of the enzyme cleavase.
a Double-stranded HPV DNA.
b An invader probe, shown in green, hybridizes at the 3' end, but not at the 5' end of the target HPV DNA sequence.
c The dangling 5' end is cleaved, and then amplified.
d The cleaved 5' end incubates with a U-shaped synthetic oligonucleotide, constructed to be complementary to the 5' end, that carries a label at one end, shown as a green circle.
e The amplified 5' fragments bind to the synthetic oligonucleotide, displacing the fluorescent label.
f A second cleavase reaction detaches the label, allowing quantitation of its fluorescence.

The Human Herpesviruses Family

There are at least 8 described members of the human herpesvirus (HHV) family. Types 1 and 2 are called herpes simplex virus (HSV) 1 and 2. Other members of the HHV family include varicella-zoster (type 3), EBV (type 4), CMV (type 5), types 6 and 7, and human herpesvirus 8 (HHV-8). All members of the HHV family are nearly identical in basic structure, with a linear double-stranded DNA surrounded by an icosahedral capsid. A tegument (also called internal matrix) surrounds the capsid. The outermost portion of the virus is an envelope derived from previous hosts.

During infection, the viral DNA travels to the nucleus and circularizes, forming the viral episome. New viral particles may be produced (productive infection), or there may be latency. In either case, however, the viral genome remains episomal and does not integrate. Rare examples of integration have been reported, but the herpes family is unusual among pathogenic viruses in a nearly complete absence of integration [PMID20844040].

HSV-1 causes most cases of oral herpes, and tends to be self-limiting in this area. HSV-1 also causes about 1/4 of genital herpes cases, but those tend to be less severe and less likely to recur than genital HSV-2 cases. With occasional exceptions, most serious HSV infections are in neonatal patients, where symptoms are systemic and often include encephalitis.

Culture of HSV requires appreciable time and has poor sensitivity in cerebrospinal fluid [PMID11724856], so the diagnosis of HSV is by detection of viral DNA by PCR or demonstration of viral proteins by immunohistochemistry. Serology and the old Tzanck test are of limited value. Many laboratories diagnose HSV by PCR, usually targeting the DNA polymerase or glycoprotein B. Because these 2 genes have nearly identical sequences between HSV-1 and HSV-2, PCR does not separate HSV-1 and HSV-2. Melting curve analysis is one method of achieving this distinction [PMID15072751].

Acyclovir, valacyclovir, and famcyclovir are used for treatment of HSV. Acyclovir must be phosphorylated by host thymidine kinase to become active, and deficiencies or mutations of thymidine kinase can be tested for if drug resistance is suspected.

The EBV can cause a variety of diseases by either a primary infection or reactivation, as well as by either a lytic or latent life cycle in the host cell. Among the primary infections are infectious mononucleosis and hemophagocytic syndrome. A partial list of malignancies for which EBV is strongly and causally associated include Burkitt lymphoma, posttransplant lymphoproliferative disorder, and extranodal natural killer cell lymphoma of the nasal type [PMID15551754].

Important EBV antigens in the lytic phase include membrane antigen, viral capsid antigen, and early antigen [PMID9453844]. Membrane antigen consists of the glycoproteins gp 350, gp 250, and gp85, which are part of the viral envelope and are also found on the cell membranes of infected cells. Membrane antigen mediates attachment of the virus to the cell. Viral capsid antigen is a group of proteins, synthesized late in the lytic cycle, that comprises the structural proteins of the capsid. Early antigen is a group of proteins whose function is unknown.

Antigens that are expressed during the latent phase include Epstein-Barr nuclear antigen (EBNA) and latent membrane protein [PMID15551754]. EBNA is a complex of at least 6 proteins—EBNA-1, 2, 3A, 3B, 3C, and LP—of which EBNA-3C appears necessary to immortalize B cells [PMID19237563]. Latent membrane protein is a membrane-associated protein of unknown function. Lytic antigens will be expressed if there is a transition from a latent to a lytic mode of infection.

EBV can be diagnosed by the immunohistochemical identification of its proteins or by the in situ hybridization identification of RNA that is encoded by its DNA. qPCR is increasingly used for both diagnosis and viral load testing on patients with EBV-related tumors [PMID20375356].

CMV has the same general structure of other viruses of the herpes family, with DNA surrounded by a capsid, which in turn is surrounded by a tegument and an envelope [PMID9130048]. Glycoprotein B in the envelope is an important protein because it mediates entrance into cells and is a target of antibodies [PMID14607617]. Most people are infected by CMV in childhood and are asymptomatic, but like all members of the herpes family, CMV can reactivate. CMV infection can simulate mononucleosis.

Neonatal CMV can be difficult to diagnose because the mothers are asymptomatic. Time-honored TORCH titers in the mother (for antibodies to *Toxoplasma gondii*, rubella, CMV, and HSV) may help, but it is difficult to distinguish between past and current infection.

Serology is not very useful in diagnosis of CMV infection because of the inability to distinguish between present and past infection. Culture and immunofluorescence testing for the antigen are good tests, but are being replaced by molecular methods, generally PCR. Because of the latency inherent in all herpesvirus, the finding of low levels of CMV DNA does not mean active infection. Active infection can be established in the molecular laboratory by the finding of levels of DNA above a cutoff or the finding of the CMV tegument protein pp65. The pp65 test is an immunofluorescent test in which the protein is identified on the surface of neutrophils [PMID18627578]. At this time, quantitation of CMV has proven more difficult than for HCV and HIV, but progress is being made [PMID20075208].

Ganciclovir, a guanosine analogue that inhibits the viral DNA polymerase, is the drug of choice for CMV. Other drugs include foscarnet and cidofovir. Resistance to ganciclovir may occur from mutations in the viral polymerase gene or in the *UL97* gene, which codes for a viral phosphotransferase that must phosphorylate ganciclovir before it is active.

The Polyomavirus Family

Like all members of the polyomavirus family, the BK virus is icosahedral, unenveloped, and contains double-stranded DNA. Early proteins are nonstructural, while genes that are expressed later code for structural proteins. One of the early genes encodes for the large and small T antigens, which when present in high levels shut off early gene expression to pave the way for the expression of structural proteins.

Infection with BK virus is common and generally asymptomatic but can be a problem in immunocompromised patients, especially renal transplant patients (the name of the virus is derived from the initials of a renal transplant patient). BK virus is found in about 5% of renal transplants and can lead to BK nephropathy. In about 1/2 of affected patients, graft failure results. Many PCR tests target the large T antigen. While urine is the most likely material in which to find BK virus, it can be found in urine secondary to immunosuppression without indicating nephropathy. The best indication of BK virus-induced nephropathy in transplant patients is finding viral DNA in plasma, in conjunction with a compatible clinical situation [PMID19832926].

The JC virus is also a polyomavirus that is important in transplant patients. It is neurotrophic and causes progressive multifocal leukoencephalopathy (PML).

The Influenza Viruses

The influenza viruses are RNA viruses (a useful mnemonic is that except for adenovirus, most upper respiratory tract viruses are RNA). There are 3 major types of influenza virus, A, B, and C, of which type A is the major pathogen and is responsible for most epidemics. Influenza A consists of 8 strands of negatively polarized RNA (ie, a complementary copy must be synthesized) in a ribonucleoprotein complex. Because influenza is not a retrovirus, the complement is still RNA, not DNA. The complementary RNA is then processed to allow it to function as a messenger RNA in the host cell, permitting translation of viral proteins. The major proteins of the influenza virus are its RNA polymerase, hemagglutinin (HA) and neuramidase (NA). HA attaches the virus to the cell membrane, while NA permits its release after replication. Viruses are designated by the HA and NA numbers (eg, H1N1).

Wild fowl are the natural host. Small changes (usually point mutations) in the HA and NA molecules account for antigenic *drift*. Antigenic drift is usually caused by chance rather than by natural selection. Antigenic drifts are associated with epidemics and are the reason for yearly vaccinations for seasonal flu.

Much larger changes account for antigenic *shift* and are associated with pandemics. Only type A is affected in shifts, so only type A can give rise to a pandemic. A shift occurs every 20-30 years; these shifts were responsible for the pandemics of 1918 (H1N1), 1957 (H2N2), 1968 (H3N2), and another H1N1 pandemic in 2009.

Antigenic shift is a complete replacement of some genes by those from other subtypes of type A and usually requires a host that can incubate multiple subtypes of influenza A from different species. This host is usually swine, though some birds can also do this. Thus, pandemics are often colloquially called "bird flu" or "swine flu." Pandemics secondary to incubation in birds often begin in poultry markets, often in Hong Kong, where the selling of multiple species of live birds is an integral part of the economy. Transfer from ducks to chickens seems particularly important in these pandemics.

There are a number of nucleic acid amplification methods for detecting influenza [PMID22122441]. A common procedure is to use reverse transcriptase to generate cDNA from viral RNA, after which qPCR identifies a unique portion of this cDNA [PMID20455681].

The 2 major anti-influenza drugs are oseltamivir (tamiflu) and zanamivir (relenza), both neuramidase inhibitors. There are currently no tests for resistance to these drugs. Amantadine (symmetrel) is rarely used now because it must be given within 24 hours of infection and it targets a matrix protein that is not present in influenza B.

The *Enterovirus* Genus

The *Enterovirus* genus is a member of the picornavirus family, a group of small RNA viruses (hence, the name: pico RNA). Species within the *Enterovirus* genus include the polioviruses (3 serotypes), coxsackieviruses (23 serotypes of coxsackie A and 6 serotypes of coxsackie B), and echoviruses (28 serotypes).

Viruses are the most common identifiable cause of meningitis or encephalitis and enteroviruses are included in this group, along with herpes, zoster, and West Nile virus [PMID19889944]. Detection of the enteroviruses by nucleic acid amplification generally targets the 5' untranslated region that is common to the group and that is conserved [PMID19583870].

Molecular Testing for Other Pathogenic Organisms

A number of other bacteria can be identified with molecular techniques. Each of these bacteria has unique targets that are amenable to molecular identification. *Streptococcus pyogenes* (a group A strep) can be quickly recognized by a direct probe, often a chemiluminescent DNA probe that binds to rRNA (this is the Accuprobe technology from Gen-Probe), or by PCR amplification. *Streptococcus agalatiae* is the group B strep that is critical in neonatal infections. qPCR is as sensitive as culture for this organism [PMID21077984].

Anaplasma species (the new name for *Ehrlichia* species) are obligate intracellular Gram-negative bacteria that for all practical purposes cannot be cultured. Many targets are available for molecular identification, but the gene for 16S rRNA is perhaps the most common.

Tropheryma whippelii, the causative organism of Whipple disease, can be identified much more sensitively with molecular testing than with culture or the traditional and very poor PAS stain. There are a number of targets, including 16S rDNA (ie, the gene for 16S rRNA) [PMID20113556].

Bartonella is a Gram-negative bacillus that is very difficult to identify by conventional culture. It is the cause of bacillary angiomatosis and cat scratch disease, and is routinely missed in tissue sections, even with special stains. It is also an under-appreciated cause of bacterial endocarditis. 16S rDNA is a common target in PCR testing for *Bartonella* [PMID19685089].

Bordetella pertussis and *Bordetella parapertussis* have often been identified by direct fluorescent antibody more than by culture, but qPCR is more sensitive and specific than either of these. Major targets of *Bordetella* testing include the insertion sequence 481 [PMID18440175], though good results have also been obtained for *B pertussis* by targeting the sequences BP283 and BP485 [PMID18753352].

For years, testing for Lyme disease has been problematic. PCR testing for the spirochete *Borrelia burgdorferi*, the causative agent, has been directed at a number of targets, including rRNA and the proteins flagellin, outer surface protein A (Osp A), and heat shock protein GroEL. This has much improved the situation, but PCR testing still suffers from surprisingly low sensitivity (ranging from 40% in blood to about 70% in synovial fluid) [PMID16020686]. For this reason, there is still a role for antibody testing. Indeed, in the latter stages, the sensitivity of antibody testing approaches 100%. Antigen testing is not recommended.

Older, but still used methods for the detection of *Trichomonas vaginalis* include wet mount, direct immunofluorescence, and culture. Newer nucleic acid amplification methods include a transcription mediated nucleic acid amplification test from Genprobe, and PCR methods hold promise [PMID16809958].

Molecular testing for eukaryotic pathogens is far more difficult because their cell biology very closely matches that of the human host. At this writing, molecular testing is developing for the dimorphic fungi (*Blastomyces*, *Coccidioides*, and *Histoplasma*), as well as for *Aspergillus* and *Candida* [PMID15489939]. Testing is also developing for a number of parasites. PCR testing for *Plasmodium* species, often targeting the 18S rDNA, is far superior to blood smear examination and should replace it whenever possible [PMID18814727]. Likewise,

PCR testing for *Toxoplasma* is more sensitive than serology or immunofluorescent methods [PMID15715713].

Molecular Testing of Infectious Diseases—Closing Comments

6 comments complete our discussion of the vast and rapidly expanding area of molecular testing of infectious disease. First, molecular testing is replacing cytochemical special stains for organisms in formalin fixed, paraffin-embedded tissue. Infectious organisms in tissue sections will soon be sought by nucleic acid identification rather than by cytochemical stains such as acid fast, GMS, or PAS stains. Molecular methods are not only more sensitive, they also reduce interobserver variability and will be able to provide speciation.

Second, organisms, like tumors, produce distinctive and unique combinations of proteins [PMID18782034]. Techniques in proteomics, especially mass spectrometry (discussed in Chapter 47) will soon identify the unique protein signatures of infectious organisms.

Third, a promising area in the molecular study of infectious disease is the development of better vaccines. In DNA vaccines, a fragment of DNA encoding for a protein of interest from the organism is cloned in a plasmid, after which the plasmid is introduced into the target cells, causing those cells to produce the antigen intracellularly. With molecular techniques, multiple areas of an organism's genome that are responsible for pathogenicity can be inserted into the plasmid, often along with other sequences that may cause a more robust immune response. Unlike traditional vaccines, DNA vaccines do not require refrigeration and can therefore be used in the field or in developing countries.

Fourth, there are occasional discordant results between 2 molecular assays, or between a molecular method and a conventional method. After first eliminating clerical errors and specimen mix-ups, the specific target of the molecular methods should be determined. If an organism has a mutation in the gene that a particular molecular method targets, it might be invisible to tests directed at that gene.

Fifth, many infectious organisms express a membrane protein that functions as a multidrug pump, transporting antibiotics out of the cell (cancer cells often have a similar protein called Gpg, for P-glycoprotein, that pumps chemotherapeutic agents out of the cell). It is to be hoped that molecular studies will allow the characterization of both of these pumps and variations in their expression during pathogenesis, eventuating in the development of inhibitors.

Sixth, lost in the discussion of emerging drug resistance of bacteria and viruses is that it is proof positive not only of the fact of evolution, but also of the mechanism of natural selection, whereby those individuals that are best adapted to their environment have a reproductive advantage. Darwinian evolution through natural selection occurs all around us every day in the prokaryotic world.

Pharmacogenetics

Pharmacogenetics (PGX) is the assessment of DNA polymorphisms, often manifest as enzyme variations, which affect drug metabolism or a patient's response to medications. In conjunction with information about of the gene expression profile of a particular neoplasm or of a particular patient in a particular situation, PGX will hopefully permit the adjustment of drug dosages or even the construction of drugs that are tailor-made to individual patients. This is the exciting field of personalized medicine, still in its infancy but of enormous promise.

The biological effect of a drug on a patient depends on dosage, absorption, distribution, metabolism, half-life, and excretion (pharmocokinetics) as well as the actual intracellular actions of the drug (pharmacodynamics) **f46.8**. Some drugs require partial metabolism to be converted into an active form (bioactivation).

Most drugs are metabolized in the liver in a series of steps. In phase 1, the drug is made more polar and hydrophilic and undergoes reactions such as oxidation (removal of electrons), reduction (addition of electrons), or hydrolysis. The most common phase 1 reaction is oxidation. The purpose of phase 1 metabolism is to permit the conjugation that will occur in phase 2.

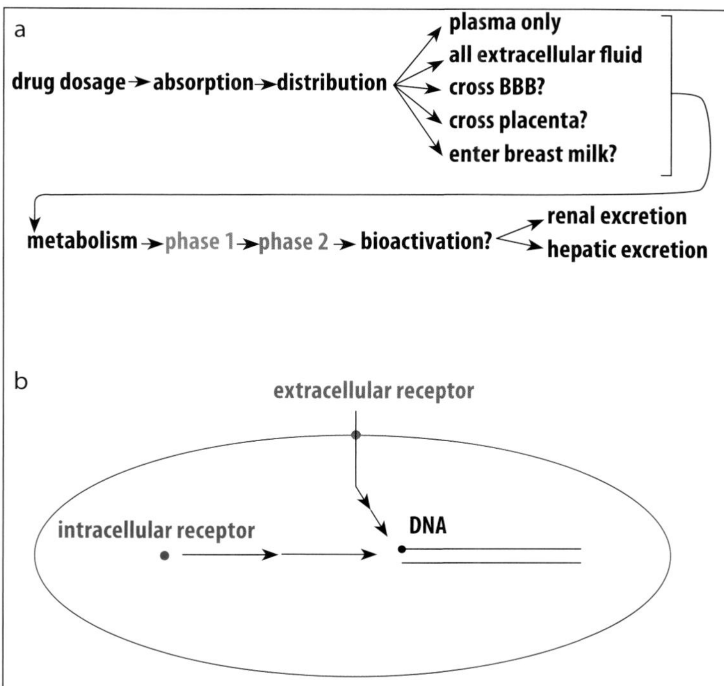

f46.8 The divisions of pharmacogenetics (PGX) and the life cycle of a drug
a Pharmacokinetics is the absorption, distribution, metabolism, and excretion of a drug. For a given drug dose, absorption varies with food intake and status of the GI tract. Major factors in distribution include whether the drug is restricted to the plasma or leaves the vascular space to distribute throughout the extracellular fluid. Does it cross the blood brain barrier (BBB) or the placenta, and does it enter the breast milk? Most drugs metabolize in a 2-step process. Bioactivation is a special kind of metabolism in which the metabolite is more active than the original compound. Excretion of most drugs is via the kidneys or the liver.
b Pharmacodynamics is the action of a drug inside a cell or on the cell surface. Most drugs bind to receptors, usually on the outside of the cell because the water-soluble drug is distributed in the extracellular fluid and cannot pass through the lipid-based cell membrane. A minority of drugs (eg, steroids) can pass through the cell membrane and bind directly to receptors in the cytoplasm or nucleus.
In either case, the actions of the drug involve a change in the shape, actions, or interactions of the receptor, initiating a series of reactions eventuating in a therapeutic effect, shown here as a modification of DNA transcription.

ISBN 978-089189-5886

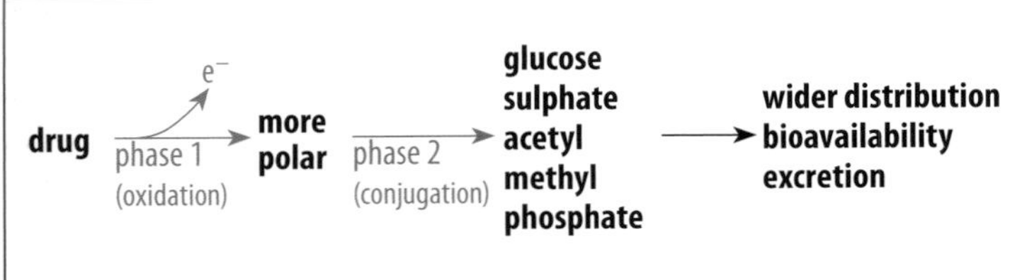

f46.9 Phase 1, depicted here as a loss of electrons (oxidation), makes the drug marginally more water soluble, but is primarily intended to allow phase 2 to occur. In Phase 2, the drug is conjugated to another compound that sharply increases its polarity and water solubility. The end result is wider distribution, great bioavailability, and easier excretion.

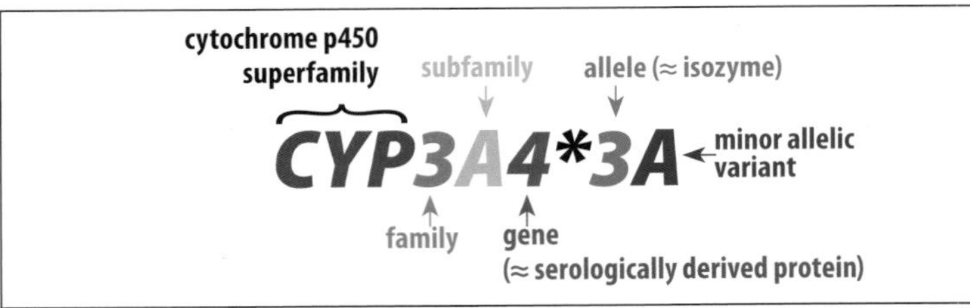

f46.10 *CYP* refers to the cytochrome p450 superfamily. The first number refers to the family, the next letter to the subfamily, and the second number to a specific gene. The number to the right of the asterisk denotes a specific allele at a given locus, and the final letter is a minor variant of the allele specified by its number.

In phase 2, there is conjugation of the drug to another compound (glucuronidation, sulphation, acetylation, methylation, etc), using enzymes, usually transferases, that are specific for those processes **f46.9**. After phase 2, the drug is water soluble and therefore much more easily distributed and excreted.

Most Enzymes of Phase 1 Metabolism Are Members of the Cytochrome P450 System

Cytochromes are a huge superfamily of iron-containing, membrane-bound enzymes with an enormous array of functions. Many are involved in electron transport. The P450 family of cytochromes, so called because its members absorb at 450 nanometers, is the largest and best characterized drug-metabolizing enzyme system. The cytochrome P450 system (abbreviated CYP450 or simply CYP in the context of PGX) is the major mechanism for phase 1 metabolism of many drugs, accounting for about 75% of all phase 1 reactions. The cytochrome P450 enzymes are found primarily in the liver and are usually associated with the endoplasmic reticulum.

CYP consists of 57 genes, 15 of which have been shown to be involved in drug metabolism. These genes are divided into families, subfamilies, and individual genes. For example, *CYP3A4* refers to family 3, subfamily A, gene 4. For each gene, there may be many allelic variants, denoted by an asterisk followed by a number. For example, *CYP3A4*3* (pronounced CYP 3A4 "star" 3), is the third-recognized allele of the *CYP3A4* gene **f46.10**. A given allele often corresponds to a known clinical variant of an enzyme. The collection of allelic variants of a gene is called a star family. *1 is usually the wild type. Higher numbered alleles refer to non-wild-type alleles and are numbered in their order of discovery. Occasionally, there will be a letter following the star allele referring to a slight variant that has the same clinical manifestation (eg, *CYP3A4*3A* is an asymptomatic variant of *CYP3A4*3*).

Although there are exceptions, the wild-type allele is usually more efficient at metabolizing a drug than other alleles. Patients with 2 copies of a wild-type allele are said to have extensive metabolism or to be extensive metabolizers (the term "rapid metabolizer" is also used). Those with 1 copy of wild-type gene and 1 allele that has suboptimal function are intermediate metabolizers. Those with 2 copies of a suboptimal allele are poor metabolizers, with minimal enzymatic activity. Occasionally, some patients will have increased metabolism, either from a hyperactive allele, from a duplication, or from a mutation in a promoter that increases the expression of wild-type alleles. These patients are said to have ultra-rapid metabolism.

Among the many drugs metabolized via the *CYPs* are selective serotonin reuptake inhibitors (SSRIs), tricyclic antidepressants (TCAs), some benzodiazepines, some antipsychotic medications, codeine (metabolized to morphine via *CYP2D6*), the breast cancer drug tamoxifen, and warfarin (coumadin). The website http://medicine.iupui.edu/clinpharm/ddis/ has a list of all drugs whose metabolism is known to be affected by *CYP* polymorphisms.

Slightly >50% of drugs are metabolized by members of the *CYP3* family and most of the remainder are metabolized by the *CYP2* family. The most important individual P450 enzymes in drug metabolism are *CYP3A4/CYP3A5*, responsible for about 50% of the drug metabolism of the *CYP* group, and *CYP2D6*, responsible for 20% of P450's drug metabolism, followed by *CYP2C9* and *CYP2C19* [PMID10319190].

Although *CYP3* metabolizes the highest percentage of drugs in the *CYP* system, it has not been as well described as *CYP2*, and most current *CYP* PGX focuses on *CYP2*. *CYP2D6*, *CYP2C9*, and *CYP2C19* are important in the metabolism of SSRIs, TCAs, other psychotherapeutic medications, and medications of other types. The FDA has approved a microarray-based assay for polymorphisms in *CYP2D6* and *CYP2C19*, called AmpliChip CYP450 (Roche). The AmpliChip identifies 27 different alleles of *CYP2D6* and 3 alleles of *CYP2C19* [PMID19169185].

Proton pump inhibitors (PPIs), used in the treatment of gastroesophageal reflux, are metabolized primarily via *CYP2C19* and *CYP3A4*. The wild-type allele of *CYP2C19* (*1) codes for an enzyme that metabolizes PPIs efficiently. Patients who are homozygous for this allele (ie, *CYP2C19*1/*1*) are rapid metabolizers. These patients are less likely to receive therapeutic benefit from standard doses and account for a high percentage of the 10-20% of patients who have a poor response to PPIs. Those with 1 *1 allele and a second allele that is *2 or *3 are intermediate metabolizers, and those without a *1, such as *CYP2C19*2/*2* or *CYP2C19*2/*3*, etc are slow metabolizers. Intermediate and slow metabolizers are more likely to respond clinically. They will have a higher gastric pH for a given dose and often need a smaller dose [PMID15988117].

CYP2C9 is involved in the metabolism of antiepileptic drugs, and it is the major phase I metabolizer of coumadin (warfarin). Coumadin is a mixture of the R and S forms of warfarin, but the S form has greater biologic activity. Complications of coumadin are a major contributor to emergency department visits and the reasons for the large variation in individual responsiveness to the drug are finally coming into view.

Variant forms of *CYP2C9* (*CYP2C9*2* and *CYP2C9*3*) are less efficient at metabolizing coumadin than *CYP2C9*1*, and patients with these alleles require lower doses. In *CYP2C9*2*, there is a cysteine at position 144 instead of the normal arginine in the enzyme (R144C). This isozyme is 10-12% as active as the wild-type isozyme. In *CYP2C9*3*, there is a leucine at position 359 instead of the normal isoleucine in the enzyme (I359L), resulting in an isozyme that is <5% as active as the wild-type. About 19% of Caucasians are heterozygous *CYP2C9*1/*2* and 3% are homozygous *CYP2C9*2/*2*. Patients in the former group are intermediate metabolizers of coumadin, while the latter are poor metabolizers. About 15% of patients are heterozygous *CYP2C9*1/*3*, and about 1% are homozygous *CYP2C9*3/*3*. Because of the very low activity of the *3 allele, even patients who are heterozygous for this allele are poor metabolizers, while those who are homozygous *3/*3 are very poor. The poorer the metabolism of coumadin, the more likely a given dose will cause hemorrhagic complications [PMID19955245]. Variant alleles not only affect dosage, but also time to steady state in the serum, this being longer in the *2 and *3 heterozygous states.

Another cause of unexpected response to coumadin has been elucidated from its mechanism of action. The vitamin K-dependent coagulation factors are II, VII, IX, and X, as well as factors C and S. All of these must undergo posttranslational carboxylation of glutamic acid residues to become biologically active. The enzyme γ-glutamyl carboxylase (γGCX) carboxylates the glutamic acid moieties in the vitamin K dependent proteins, in the process converting the reduced form of vitamin K, vitamin K hydroquinone, to its oxidized form, vitamin K epoxide. For this process to continue, there must be a conversion of vitamin K epoxide back to vitamin K hydroquinone. This is achieved by the vitamin K epoxide reductase complex (VKORC), especially subunit 1 of this complex (VKORC1). Coumadin inhibits VKORC1, preventing the regeneration of vitamin K hydroquinone and inhibiting further carboxylation of vitamin K-dependent proteins, thus preventing bioactivation of these coagulation factors.

In addition to abnormalities in the *CYP* system, variant forms of VKORC1 may result in either coumadin sensitivity or resistance, depending on how the variation affects coumadin binding and the subsequent inhibition of the enzyme. Variations in VKORCI affect coumadin dose more than variations in *CYP2C9*. For example, the *VKORC1*2* allele, common in Asians, leads to a form of the enzyme that binds coumadin more readily or is more inhibited by it, permitting the same therapeutic effect with a lower dose [PMID17635701]. *VKORC1*2* is also called the A/B haplotype or 1639G>A (ie, guanine to adenine transversion at nucleotide position 1639). The wild-type is not 2 copies of 1639G, but 1 each of 1639G and 1639A. Patients with 2 copies of 1639G have ultra-rapid metabolism and need larger doses of coumadin. While monitoring of the international normalized ratio (INR; derived from the prothrombin time) remains the mainstay of coumadin dosing, a number of algorithms have been published that predict coumadin dose based on PGX findings in *CYP2C9* and VKORC enzymes [PMID20228265]. These algorithms are slightly different, but all incorporate some combination of *CYP2C9* and *VKORC* testing, as well as the age, ethnicity, weight, body surface area, and gender of the patient [PMID19324988].

The individual variations in the response to coumadin, the serious potential complications, and the need to constantly monitor the INR has elicited a search for an alternative that has a more predictable response and does not require monitoring. In 2010, the FDA approved the first such drug: dabigatran (pradaxa), an oral thrombin antagonist. In 2011, the FDA approved rivaroxaban (xarelto), an orally administered Xa inhibitor, for prevention of deep vein thrombosis and seems certain to grant approval for atrial fibrillation in the near future.

CYP metabolizes the SSRIs. In addition, polymorphisms in the genes that code for the serotonin receptors HTR2A and HTR2C are important in the response to SSRIs. For example, polymorphisms in HTR2A often lead to increased drug levels and increased side effects, while polymorphisms in either locus can increase the risk of tardive dyskinesia, a side-effect of these drugs [PMID11134668].

Tamoxifen undergoes bioactivation to its active form, endoxifen, primarily by *CYP2D6*, and also by *CYP3A4/5*. More than 70 alleles of *CYP2D6* exist, many of which affect bioactivation [PMID19644023]. Most patients on tamoxifen undergo *CYP2D6* testing. Another concern with tamoxifen is that some SSRI drugs may reduce the activity of *CYP2D6* and lead to decreased bioactivation of tamoxifen [PMID20142325].

The P2Y12 receptor on platelets is activated by ADP and thromboxane and sets in motion many of the reactions necessary for platelet activation. Clopidogrel (plavix) inhibits the P2Y12 receptor, but it must first be bioactivated by a number of CYP enzymes, and its utility has been limited by a high percentage of patients with resistance. While the mechanism(s) of this resistance is not completely elucidated, it is established that variations in *CYP2C19*, especially *CYP2C19*2*, can result in suboptimal response to the drug [PMID21718233].

Pharmacogenetics of Drugs Not Metabolized by CYP

The antineoplastic agent Irinotecan (Campto) is bioactivated to its active form, SN-38, by carboxyesterase enzymes. SN-38 is a topoisomerase inhibitor that inhibits the uncoiling of DNA. SN-38 is then conjugated by UDP-glucuronosyltransferase and excreted [PMID19644023]. Polymorphisms in the gene that codes for UDP-glucuronosyltransferase, *UGT1A1*, can compromise excretion of SN-38 and lead to toxicity. The promoter for the *UGT1A1* gene has repeating units of TA , the usual number of such repeats being 6. Most of the known polymorphisms involve a variable number of TA repeats in the promoter region of *UGT1A1*. Patients who are homozygous for 7 or 8 repeats will have diminished expression of the gene, decreased levels of UDP-glucuronosyltransferase, and are prone to toxicity with irinotecan use because of diminished excretion. The asterisk terminology employed in the *CYP* system is also used in other system, and homozygous 7 TA repeats in *UGT1A1* are called the *28 allele [PMID20602618]. Other variants of *UGT1A1* lead to Gilbert and Crigler-Najjar syndromes, disorders of bilirubin conjugation. Gilbert syndrome is usually caused by the same 7 repeats of TA in the promoter that compromise metabolism of irinotecan [PMID17496722]. Crigler-Najjar syndrome is a more serious deletion of exons 2-5.

Another example of PGX involves the thiopurine family, which includes 6-thioguanine, 6-mercaptopurine, and azothioprine (imuran, which is bioactivated to 6-mercaptopurine). The enzyme thiopurine methyltransferase (TPMT) performs phase II metabolism by methylating and thereby inactivating members of the thiopurine family. Clearance is reduced in patients with deficient activity of TPMT, leading to toxicity. The activity of TPMT may also be increased, leading to an inadequate clinical response to any of these drugs because of increased methylation. The wild-type form of the enzyme is denoted as TPMT*1, while the major abnormalities causing slow methylation are TPMT*2, TPMT*3A and TPMT*3C. Clinical utility of this knowledge has been limited by imperfect correlation between genotypic and phenotypic assays of TPMT [PMID19663675].

5-fluorouracil (5FU) is metabolized primarily by dihydropyrimidine dehydrogenase (DPD) and deficiencies of this enzyme are associated with toxicity from 5FU [PMID15377401]. Polymorphisms in the corresponding gene, *DPYD*, have been shown, but it is not yet clear which of these are clinically relevant. In the meantime, assays of DPD or serum levels of 5FU have been suggested, but have not been shown to be clinically relevant [PMID17350823].

Cyclophosphamide (cytoxan) is used in both neoplastic and autoimmune disorders. It undergoes bioactivation, primarily by the enzyme aldehyde dehydrogenase. Because serum levels of this enzyme vary, cytoxan is variably metabolized by patients [PMID19786984].

Succinylcholine is metabolized by the enzyme butyrylcholinesterase (also called pseudocholinesterase or serum cholinesterase). 1 in 2,500 people are homozygous for a deficient enzyme and may therefore be inadvertently overdosed in anesthesia. Assay for butyrylcholinesterase is generally done enzymatically rather than genotypically. In a common assay, dibucaine is used as an inhibitor. Dibucaine inhibits the wild-type enzyme more than the mutated form. The percent inhibition of dibucaine is called the dibucaine number and for most patients, it is about 80. A lower dibucaine number, indicating reduced inhibition, suggests a mutation in the enzyme [PMID12689511]. A PCR for the mutated form of butyrylcholinesterase has also been described [PMID8014977].

Malignant hyperthermia (MHS) is an inherited disorder in which hyperthermia, hyperkalemia, and acidosis occur during or immediately after administration of certain anesthetic agents. In MHS, the calcium channels in the sarcoplasmic reticulum, the principal intracellular store of calcium in muscle cells, stay open too long, leading to excessive entry of calcium into the cytoplasm, resulting in extreme muscle contraction. The diagnosis is usually established by an in vitro test performed on a muscle biopsy, but several genes have been linked to the disorder. By far the most common culprit gene is *MHS1*, which codes for ryanodine receptor (RYR1), a major component of the calcium channel in the sarcoplasmic reticulum [PMID1967823]. Other genes implicated in malignant hyperthermia are *MHS3* and *MHS5*, also linked to the calcium channel.

Variations in HLA have been associated with hypersensitivity reactions to drugs. The most important of these hypersensitivity reactions is toxic epidermal necrolysis (Stevens-Johnson syndrome), often secondary to the drug carbamazepine (tegretol) and often associated with HLA-B*1502 (ie, the second allele in the 15th family of the HLA-B locus) [PMID20479057]. HLA-B*5701 is associated with a hypersensitivity reaction to the antiretroviral drug abacavir and HLA-B*5801 has been linked to a reaction to allopurinol.

N-acetyltransferase (NAT2) is an enzyme involved in acetylation during the phase II metabolism of many drugs, such as isoniazid, hydralazine, sulfonamide, and procainamide. Deficiencies of NAT2 cause slow acetylation and make the patient prone to toxicity, while gain of function mutations cause drug resistance [PMID20183529].

Glucose-6-phosphate dehydrogenase deficiency is the most common symptomatic enzyme deficiency in the world. It is inherited in an X-linked recessive manner and is clinically manifest primarily as anemia. Because of deficient production of NADPH in glycolysis, these patients are prone to anemic episodes if given an oxidative drug. The prototype offending drug is primaquine, an antimalarial [PMID19769422].

The Central Nervous System in Dementia

Mild cognitive impairment (MCI), though apparently an appropriate diagnosis for a huge percentage of the population, especially those in politics, is a specific neurologic diagnosis based on detailed criteria. There are different forms of MCI and not all will progress to Alzheimer disease (AD) [PMID21188312], but about 75% of patients with MCI will develop AD, at a rate of roughly 10% per year. A minority of patients with MCI will improve.

AD, the prototype for dementia disorders, is morphologically associated with 2 abnormal collections of proteins, 1 intracellular and 1 extracellular. Neurofibrillary tangles are intracellular and consist of paired helical filaments that are composed largely of tau (τ), a protein associated with microtubules (dephosphorylation of τ promotes microtubule assembly, while its phosphorylation leads to microtubule disassembly). Neurofibrillary tangles are not specific for AD, but in that disorder, one of the findings is excessive phosphorylation of τ. This causes depolymerization of microtubules, but more importantly, hyperphosphorylated τ forms filaments on its own, which become neurofibrillary tangles [PMID20101720]. Neurofibrillary tangles are a form of amyloid and stain with Congo red.

In contrast to neurofibrillary tangles, plaques are extracellular deposits, though neurites (axons and dendrites) containing neurofibrillary tangles are often wrapped around them. Plaques are also a form of amyloid. The extracellular amyloid in plaque is largely composed of β amyloid peptide (Aβ), which is made from a larger molecule called β amyloid precursor protein (βAPP or APP) by proteolytic cleavage [PMID20101720].

Approximately 90% of βAPP is cleaved by the enzyme α-secretase, producing harmless peptides, but cleavage by either β-secretase or γ-secretase is more problematic, and the consequences of their action depend on the precise nature of their cleavage. Cleavage by β-secretase or γ-secretase results in Aβ protein, a protein not found after cleavage by α-secretase [PMID21547213], but this does not necessarily ensure the accumulation of extracellular amyloid since there are several kinds of Aβ protein. Aβ40 is a peptide of 40 amino acids that is of unknown function but is innocuous and does not contribute to extracellular amyloid, while Aβ42 and Aβ43, consisting of 42 or 43 amino acids, respectively, lead to the production of extracellular amyloid and are implicated in the plaques of AD.

The factors that result in the production of Aβ40, as opposed to the production of Aβ42 and Aβ43, when cleavage is performed by cleavage by β-secretase or γ-secretase, are not fully understood. One possibility is the location within the cell in which cleavage occurs. The early endosome is an organelle that receives plasma-membrane bound vesicles and channels the contents to the lysosome, back to the plasma membrane, or to the Golgi apparatus [PMID19924646]. There is some evidence that if β-secretase or γ-secretase cleaves βAPP within the endosome, the harmless Aβ40 results. In contrast, if the cleavage by β-secretase or γ-secretase takes place in the endoplasmic reticulum or Golgi complex, the potentially problematic Aβ42 or Aβ43 results [PMID20232515]. However, it is not established that the location of cleavage is the sole determinant of the nature of the product. In any event, although a definitive causative relationship between Aβ42 and Aβ43, and AD has not been proven, both of these peptides aggregate into extracellular amyloid and appear to be toxic to neurons [PMID21725313].

While most cases of AD are multifactorial and largely idiopathic, approximately 10% of cases are familial, with an autosomal dominant mode of inheritance. In many cases of familial AD, there are mutations in βAPP near the site of α-secretase cleavage, which prevent this enzyme from creating the harmless products that it normally generates, opening the door to cleavage by β-secretase or γ-secretase. This does not necessarily cause familial AD since cleavage by either the β or the γ form of secretase may create the harmless protein Aβ40. In addition to any possible role in the location of cleavage by the β and γ secretases, the proteins presenilin 1 and presenilin 2 appear to shift production toward Aβ40. Normal presenilin 1 is a cofactor for γ-secretase and further cleaves its product, resulting in Aβ40. Mutated forms of presenilin 1 cleave several amino acids distal to the proper site, resulting in Aβ42 or Aβ43 [PMID21086758], and familial AD is also associated with mutations in presenilin 1. Presenilin 2 is apparently similar to presenilin 1 in its actions, and mutations in it account for a smaller percentage of familial AD. Thus, familial AD can result from mutations in βAPP that prevent the action of α-secretase, in conjunction with mutations in presenilin 1 or in presenilin 2 that favor the production of Aβ42 or Aβ43 instead of Aβ40 [PMID20955934].

Although the gold standard for the diagnosis of AD is still postmortem brain examination, there are 2 premortem tests that show promise. First, τ may be increased in the cerebrospinal fluid in a number of conditions, but an increased amount of hyperphosphorylated τ in CSF suggests AD [PMID19661632]. Second, people who are either homozygous or heterozygous for the e4 form of apoprotein E (ApoE4) have an increased risk of AD. The reason for this is not known, but ApoE4 homozygosity causes a 19-fold increase, while E4 heterozygosity causes about a 4 fold increase [PMID18948255]. Early work suggests that apoprotein E binds β amyloid and facilitates its clearance, and that the e4 allele is less able to do this. The e2 allele of apoprotein E might be protective.

In addition to these 2 tests, newer MRI imaging holds promise in the premortem diagnosis of AD. There is also preliminary evidence that positron emission tomography (PET) scanning can distinguish between AD, MCI, and subjects with no cognitive impairment [PMID17182990]. PET scanning with Pittsburgh compound B (PiB), an analog of thioflavin T (a fluorescent alternative to Congo red staining in the identification of amyloid in surgical and biopsy specimens), shows promise in detecting β amyloid in the brain and may assist in the premortem diagnosis of AD.

Neurofibrillary tangles and plaques are found in normal brains, and there are no universally agreed on criteria for the number of tangles and plaques needed to make the diagnosis of AD. Tables have been published on proposed "cutoffs" for normal numbers of tangles and plaques, but to my mind, the demonstration of any significant increase tangles or plaques in the right clinical context, with the exclusion of other causes of dementia, is more important than a specific number in the postmortem diagnosis of AD.

Other Causes of Dementia Share Clinical and Histologic Characteristics with AD

Deposits of the τ protein are also found in other neurodegenerative disorders, called tauopathies. Some regard tauopathies as inherently distinct from AD and require an absence of a significant number of plaques for the diagnosis of a tauopathy, but others regard AD as a tauopathy [PMID20942789]. Whether one includes AD as a tauopathy or not, potentially new therapeutic avenues are opening in these disorders by targeting the phosphorylation of τ proteins.

Lewy bodies are intracellular basophilic structures, often surrounded by a halo. They are composed of a number of proteins, primarily α-synuclein, and are seen in 2 groups of neurodegenerative diseases—Parkinson disease (PD) and dementia with Lewy bodies (the latter condition is occasionally called diffuse Lewy body disease or the Lewy body variant of AD) [PMID20963199].

PD is characterized by large neuronal losses in the substantia nigra. As is the case for AD, most cases of PD are sporadic, but a small minority have a genetic (autosomal recessive) basis. In these cases, there are mutations in the genes that encode for α-synuclein, or for other proteins, such as DJ-1 and parkin [PMID18267242]. DJ-1 is a protein of unknown function, but it is somehow neuroprotective, and its loss predisposes to early onset PD. Parkin, encoded by the *PARK2* gene, is a component of the E3 ubiquitin ligase complex, and mutations in the gene encoding for this protein undoubtedly lead to deficient ubiquitin-mediated processing of unwanted proteins.

There is both clinical and histopathologic overlap between AD, PD, and dementia with Lewy bodies. Patients with dementia with Lewy bodies have Alzheimer-like dementia, with or without Parkinson symptoms, but Lewy bodies are found in a number of locations in addition to the substantia nigra, including the neocortex [PMID8909416]. Immunohistochemical staining for α-synuclein often reveals a larger number of Lewy bodies than had been suspected. Although plaques and tangles are usually present, they are in insufficient numbers for the diagnosis of AD.

Vascular insufficiency may simulate the dementias caused by any of the above disorders. Some asymptomatic patients with evidence of carotid artery stenosis who do well on initial mental status testing may have cognitive impairment if given more intense testing [PMID20055242]. This suggests that so-called asymptomatic stenosis may not be truly asymptomatic and hints that some cases of apparent AD or MCI may have more of a vascular component than has been realized.

Prion Disease—Infectious Proteins?

Since their description by Prusiner [PMID6801762], prions have been one of the great enigmas of biological science. Since the days of the central dogma of molecular biology (DNA is transcribed into RNA, which is then translated into protein), it had been an unquestioned postulate that proteins alone could not be infectious.

All known prion diseases result from an abnormal 3-dimensional conformation of a membrane protein called PrP, a small glycoprotein of unknown function that is primarily secreted and then anchored to the external surface of the cell membrane via glycosyl phosphatidyl inositol (GPI) [PMID19196429]. The normal form is PrP(C). The prion form is an isoform designated as PrP(Sc). The structure of the human PrP(C) has been elucidated with nuclear magnetic resonance and shown to be largely helical [PMID10618385]. The structure of PrP(Sc) is less well understood, but it is established that there is appreciable unfolding of the helical structure and it is widely believed that PrP(Sc) is primarily in a β-pleated sheet conformation [PMID19860662].

There are 3 groups of prion diseases. The first is the 6 forms of inherited disease, all very rare (an example is fatal familial insomnia). The inherited forms arise from mutations of the *PRNP* gene, which codes for PrP(C). There is extensive amyloid formation in this group. The second group of prion diseases is naturally occurring, and includes Kuru, Creutzfeldt-Jakob disease (CJD), and Scrapie. A third class is food-borne CJD, which is a variant of naturally occurring CJD. The nonhereditary forms of prion diseases arise from the ingestion of PrP(Sc), which then causes a conformational change in PrP(C) by an unknown mechanism. There is little amyloid formation in the noninherited forms.

Applications of Microsatellite Analysis

Identity Testing

In addition to MSI that is associated with some hereditary cancer syndromes, a major application of microsatellite analysis is identity testing, which includes primarily paternity testing and judicial DNA profiling.

There are 2 critical postulates in paternity testing—there must be no question as to the identity of the mother, and no men who are genetically related to the alleged father could possibly have had intercourse with the mother during the time period under consideration.

The initial test is a blood typing to exclude men who could not possibly have furnished DNA to the child (eg, a man with group O blood could not have fathered a child of group A blood by a woman with group O blood). If exclusion is not achieved, a number of loci are studied at the DNA level in the mother, the child, and the alleged father. While these loci can theoretically be a variety of DNA sequences, including functional genes, microsatellites are typically used. In microsatellites, the term "allele" refers to varying numbers of repeating units at a given locus. For a given microsatellite, if 1 chromosome has 10 repeats of a basic unit and the other chromosome has 15 repeated units at the same locus, it is said that there are 2 alleles for that locus, and that the individual is heterozygous.

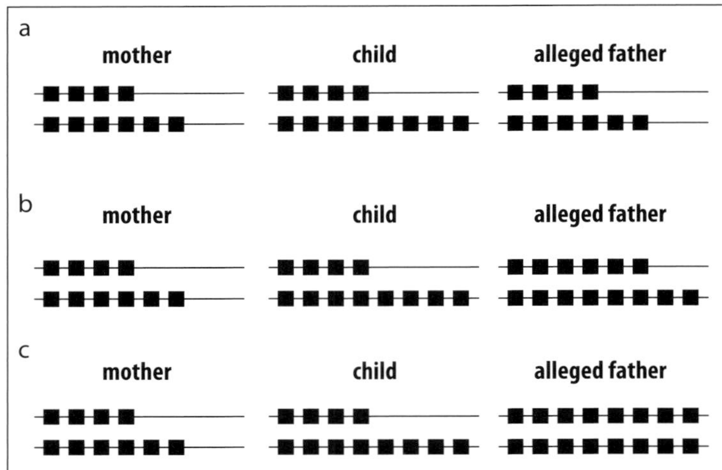

f46.11 Paternity testing. **a** Paternity is excluded because the child's father must have had at least 1 chromosome with 8 repeating units at this locus. A band found in the child but not in either adult excludes the alleged father.
b The alleged father is not excluded because he could have passed down a chromosome with 8 repeating units at this locus to complement a chromosome from the mother that contains 4 repeating units. The allele that is present in the child but not in the mother (ie, 8 repeating units) is now studied further. As the alleged father is heterozygous for that allele, the probability that he could have passed it to the child is 0.5. This value is compared to the probability that a random man of the same ethnicity could have passed the allele down, which is the frequency of that allele in the same population as the alleged father. The paternity index for this locus is 0.5 divided by the allele frequency in that population.
c The situation is similar to f46.11a in that paternity is not excluded. But the alleged father is homozygous, so the probability of passing it down is 1.0. The paternity index is 1.0 divided by the allele frequency in that population.

The number of repeating units at several well-characterized loci is determined for the 3 people involved, often by PCR and electrophoresis. Because each person has 2 chromosomes, they each have 2 alleles for each microsatellite (ie, they each have 2 possible lengths of the repeating subunit). The entire repeated segment on each chromosome of each person is amplified by PCR. The amplified segment from each chromosome will run as a single, distinct band in electrophoresis. Any bands possessed by the child but not by the mother must have come from the biological father. A band found in the child but not in either adult excludes the father, as it must have come from another man. For example, for a single microsatellite and a single pair of chromosomes, if the mother has bands indicating 4 repeating subunits in 1 chromosome and 6 in the other, the child has bands indicating 4 repeating subunits in 1 chromosome and 8 in the other, and the alleged father has bands indicating 6 repeating units in 1 chromosome and 8 in the other, paternity is possible if the mother passed down a chromosome containing 4 repeats and the man passed down a chromosome containing 8 repeats **f46.11a**. On the other hand, if the man's 2 chromosomes have 4 and 6 repeating units, he is excluded because those 2 adults could not have produced a child with 8 repeating units in 1 chromosome **f46.11b**.

For each microsatellite, a paternity index (PI) is calculated. In calculating a PI, it is critical to take into account the ethnicity of the alleged father, as ethnicity influences gene frequencies, including the number of repeats of microsatellite subunits. The PI compares the likelihood that the man under investigation, upon mating with the mother, could have fathered a child with this genotype with the likelihood that a random man *of the same race and ethnicity as the alleged father* could have done so. To calculate the PI for each microsatellite, one starts by identifying an allele possessed by the child that is not present in the mother (ie, a microsatellite with a different number of repeating units in the child from the number found in either chromosome in the mother). This allele must have come from the child's biological father. If the alleged father has not been excluded, the probability that he passed that allele to the child is 0.5 if he is heterozygous for it or 1.0 if he is homozygous. The probability that a random man of the same race and ethnicity as the alleged father could pass on that allele is simply the frequency of that allele in that population and is published for all genetic loci that are used in testing. If we find that the alleged father is heterozygous for an allele that the child possesses and the mother does not, and if we know that the frequency of that allele in that particular racial and ethnic population is 0.1 (ie, 10% of people have that gene), then the PI for that particular locus is 0.5 divided by 0.1, or 5.0.

If we find another locus for which the child has an allele the mother does not and we find that the alleged father is homozygous for that allele f46.11c, with a gene frequency in that population of 0.2, the PI for that gene is 1.0 divided by 0.2, again 5.0. If the alleged father is heterozygous at a third such locus, with a gene frequency in his population of 0.05, the PI for that third locus is 0.5 divided by 0.05, or 10.

Most paternity tests examine between 3 and 16 markers. The combined paternity index (CPI) is the product of the individual PIs. In this example, the CPI is 5 times 5 times 10, or 250. This is a statistical odds ratio. A CPI of 250 means that the alleged father is 250 times more likely to have fathered the child than a random man from his racial and ethnic group.

The probability of paternity (PP) is based on the CPI and the prior probability, which is a measure of social factors that might impact paternity, such as opportunity of contact, what is known about the personal feelings about the mother and the alleged father, etc. Since the factors involved in prior probability are unknown to the laboratory, it assumed that the alleged father had the same probability of having intercourse with the mother as a random man. Laboratories do not get involved in issues that are not genetically based and assume a prior probability of 50%, such that only genetic factors are calculated. If a court determines that the prior probability is not 50%, the probability of paternity will need to be calculated by a more complex formula using Bayesian statistics. The PP, calculated on a purely genetic basis, is the CPI divided by 1 plus the CPI:

$$PP = CPI/(1+CPI)$$

In this example, the PP is 250 divided by 251, which is 0.996, indicating a probability of paternity of 99.6. A PP of 1.0 can never be achieved.

The Principles of DNA Profiling Are Very Similar to Those of Paternity Testing

Alec Jeffreys inaugurated judicial DNA profiling (formerly called DNA fingerprinting) in 1984 by an RFLP analysis of minisatellites. Today, PCR analysis of microsatellites has replaced RFLP analysis of minisatellites in judicial DNA profiling and offers the huge advantage of being feasible on much smaller DNA samples because of the amplification step. In addition to blood, semen, saliva, sweat, and microsamples of tissue (eg, fingernail scrapings) may be used, and any of these can be recovered from an object at the scene or from personal items of the suspect.

The basic principle is very similar to that employed in paternity testing. As is the case in paternity testing, experience has demonstrated a few short tandem repeat loci whose repeat pattern is sufficiently polymorphic and easily studied to be useful. Most criminal DNA profiling is based on a set of 13 loci of short tandem repeats called the Combined DNA Index System (CODIS), inaugurated in 1998. European law enforcement services use a set of 10 markers, 8 of which are among the 13 used in the United States and 2 of which are not routinely used in the US. These loci are commonly used in both criminal and paternity work because they have been well characterized and testing for them can be performed with commercially available kits.

As is the case for paternity testing, it is critical to compare the person of interest to others of his or her ethnic/racial group, but these loci have been typed in a variety of populations commonly encountered in the United States, so that baseline frequencies have been established for almost any ethnic group a suspect may belong to.

The procedure is essentially the same as that employed for paternity testing and has been reviewed numerous times. Of the many good reviews on this subject, a good start is the summary by Butler [PMID16566758]. The website http://www.dna.gov discusses the forensic use of DNA and also has links to online instructional modules in forensic training.

Following PCR amplification of these loci, the size of the locus (a function of the number of repeating units) is obtained from electrophoresis (generally capillary rather than gel) by comparison to known standards. In many cases, microsatellites that differ by only a single repeat unit can be effectively separated. The number of repeating units at these loci in the suspect can be compared to the number found in the DNA at the crime scene or from the victim. In a manner very similar to that used in paternity testing, the probability that the DNA came from the individual of interest, relative to others of his or her ethnic/racial group, is calculated for each microsatellite locus. The product of all such calculations is a combined probability.

One must be careful in drawing conclusions from faint bands that are very close to a primary band because of the possibility of stutter bands, which are artifactual bands, usually indicating 1 repeating unit less than a primary band, caused by misalignment during PCR amplification. Fortunately, the commonly used alleles in forensic studies have been sufficiently characterized that stutter bands are rarely a problem in most situations. In addition to stutter bands, which differ from the primary band from which they are derived by a whole number of repeat units (usually just 1),

ISBN 978-089189-5886

one occasionally encounters bands that have sizes that are not whole number multiples of the basic unit (eg, 10.2 repeating units). Many of these situations are due to small insertions or deletions in the regions of DNA that flank the repeating subunit and which are included in the amplification.

While initial PCR DNA profiling relied on gel electrophoresis, the process has now been substantially automated using capillary electrophoresis and fluorescent probes to the repeated segment, followed by quantitation of signal with software [PMID15532568]. As is the case in all DNA work, databases available on the Internet are invaluable in any work with microsatellites. One of the best is the National Institute of Standards and Technology (NIST) Short Tandem Repeat Internet Database (the STRBase), the URL for which is http://www.cstl.nist.gov/biotech/strbase/.

As for any laboratory analyses, periodic comparison to known standards is essential for quality assurance. The NIST has issued Standard Reference Material (SRM) for forensic DNA work [PMID11451239, PMID19377837]. At least once per year, a laboratory performing this type of work must check its results against 1 of these standards. The primary standard for most laboratories is NIST SRM 2391b, which contains a certified number of repeating units for all 13 loci in CODIS. NIST has also developed standard material for work in mitochondrial DNA. The National Forensic Science Technology Center (NFSTC) and the American Society of Crime Lab Directors/Laboratory Accreditation Board (ASCLD/LAB) have issued quality assurance documents (http://www.nfstc.org/programs/quality-documents/) that must be adhered to by any laboratory wishing to be heard in an American court. Both the NFSTC and the ASCLD/LAB offer accreditation of laboratories performing forensic DNA work. The Scientific Working Group on DNA Analysis Methods (SWGDAM) proposes revisions to guidelines, which can be seen on their website (http://www.nfstc.org/pdi/Subject10/pdi_s10_m03_01_d.htm). In addition, traditional Levey-Jennings charts and Westgard rules, as used in testing in the traditional clinical laboratory, can be used in PCR-based microsatellite analysis [PMID18258922].

As is the case for many areas of DNA technology, we can expect a movement towards SNPs (discussed subsequently) [PMID18474034], followed in all probability by a movement toward direct DNA sequencing.

A final word in judicial DNA profiling is that a common mistake is to consider only the odds of a match. A probability of a match by chance of 1 in a 1,000,000 sounds incriminating, but if there are 10,000,000 people in the relevant metropolitan area, 10 of them will match, and the actual probability of innocence, based only on DNA evidence, is 9 in 10, not 1 in 1,000,000. A DNA match by itself is not incriminating unless the probability of a match by chance is 1 in many millions.

There Are Many Other Applications of Microsatellites

In addition to paternity testing and judicial DNA profiling, microsatellite analysis has numerous other applications. One of these, also an example of identity testing, is in surgical pathology to clarify situations in which there has been a potential specimen mix-up or mislabeling. DNA can be extracted from the sample in question and compared to that of the patient or patients from whom it is thought to have been obtained. A good match provides sufficient certainty of specimen identification that the findings in the specimen can be used to treat the patient [PMID8685211, PMID21173135].

There are also applications of microsatellite analysis that do not pertain to identity testing. Microsatellite analysis can be used to provide information on which of the 2 chromosomes a given parent has passed down to the child. Microsatellites can be used to determine if a tumor is a new primary or a metastasis from a previous tumor. Although metastatic foci often have a somewhat different appearance from a primary tumor, they will generally have the same number of repeats in their microsatellites as the primary tumor, while new primaries tend to have a different number of repeating units [PMID19094981].

Yet another use of microsatellite analysis is in bone marrow transplants to determine if the bone marrow cells are those of the donor (desired), remain those of the recipient (undesired), or are a combination of the 2 **f46.12** [PMID19582766].

Single Nucleotide Polymorphisms

A current frontier in molecular pathology is SNPs, sites where the DNA sequence of individuals differs by only 1 nucleotide. SNPs are often called point mutations, but these terms are not necessarily synonymous. A polymorphism (of an allele or of a nucleotide) is a variant of normal that is found in 1% or more of the population. Only if an SNP is found in <1% would it be abnormal (ie, a mutation) and therefore synonymous with a point mutation. Because most SNPs that have so far been detected are not found in such low numbers, an SNP is usually not a mutation.

About every 1,000 base pairs, there is a polymorphism wherein a given individual has a base pair that is different from the general population. More than 5,000,000 SNPs have been identified. Many millions of people will share any given SNP, but the combination of millions of SNPs is an important part of what makes us unique. It is thought that each SNP occurred a very few times—possibly only once—in human evolution. Because of reproduction through hundreds of generations since the formation of any given SNP, many SNPs now have a frequency of 10-50%. The frequency of any given SNP can vary between populations or may be present in only certain ethnic groups, depending on when in our evolutionary history it arose.

Along with copy number variation and repetitive DNA (both discussed in Chapter 45), SNPs are a major cause of DNA variation between any 2 individuals. People share 99.9% of the genome, and the 0.1% that is different is largely in the form of SNPs. SNPs constitute the majority of human DNA polymorphisms and are the most common and predictable variations in the human genome. Because of the unclear function of other sources of polymorphisms, such as satellite DNA, and the fact that polymorphisms in satellite DNA are often clinically silent, SNPs are probably the most clinically significant form of polymorphism.

SNPs may result in a premature stop codon, truncating the protein product, or they may result in a missense codon that codes for a different amino acid. Missense codons are

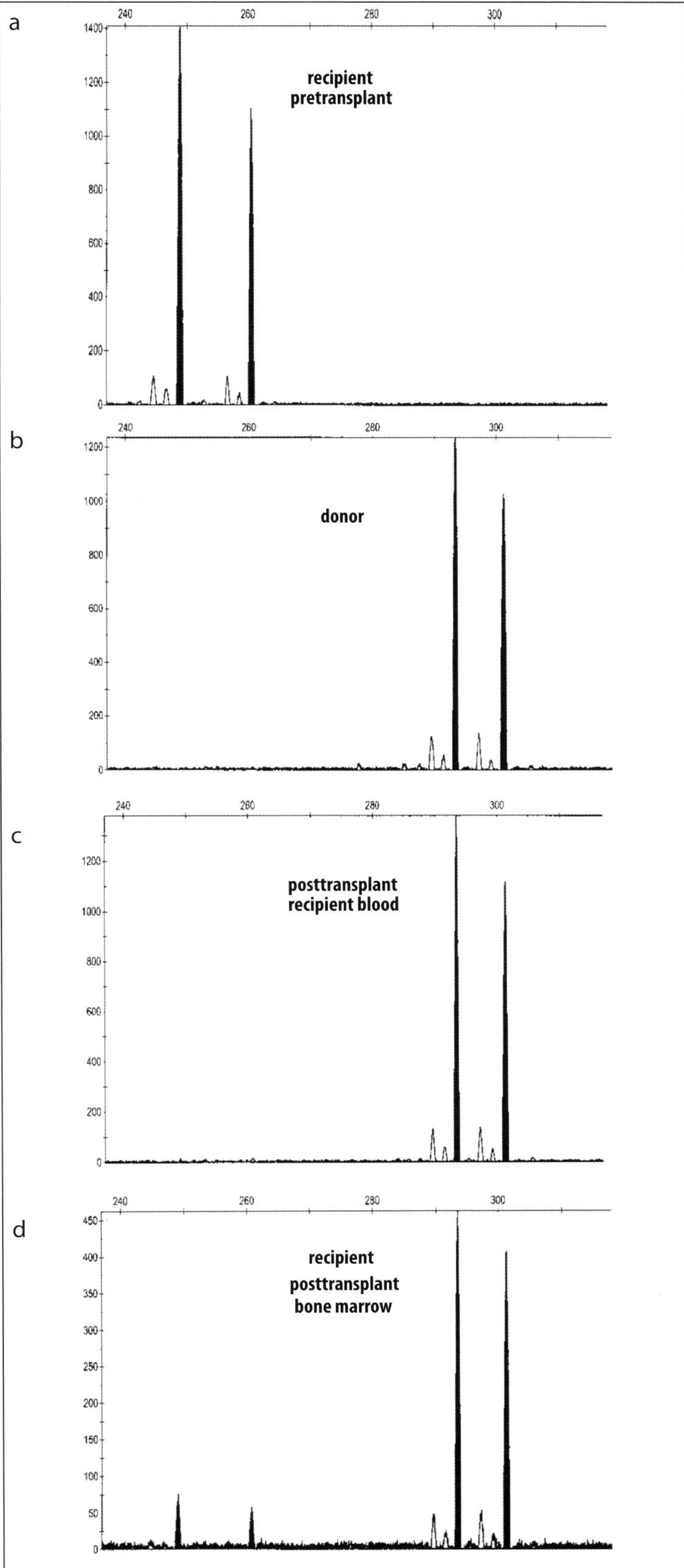

f46.12 Use of microsatellites in a bone marrow transplant patient. **a** and **b** represent the number of repeating units of a microsatellite in the recipient and donor, respectively.
c After transplant in the blood, only the donor's microsatellites are seen, indicating full engraftment in the blood.
d In the marrow, donor microsatellites predominate, but there are a few from the recipient. This is called chimerism.

said to be synonymous if the new codon codes for the same amino acid. Synonymous SNPs can occur because of the redundancy of the genetic code and often occur at the third base position since this is often not necessary to specify a specific amino acid (wobble hypothesis). Nonsynonymous missense SNPs code for a different ammo acid, resulting in a different gene product. Nonsynonymous SNPs often involve the first or second of the 3 codon positions, since these are more important in determining the amino acid than the third position.

Nonsynonymous SNPs, in turn, can be conservative (substitution by a related amino acid such that the overall final gene product is substantially similar, with minimal or no clinical consequences) or nonconservative (substitution by a fundamentally different amino acid, resulting in a significantly different gene product). Any SNP that changes the charge in an amino acid, such as the D816V mutation (a substitution of the neutral and nonpolar amino acid valine for the negatively charged aspartic acid) in mastocytomas, is almost certain to be nonconservative because it will affect the 3-dimensional conformation of the protein. A "built-in" safety mechanism for nonsynonymous missense mutation is that they often result in an unstable RNA that is degraded without translation. SNPs may also influence promoter activity, splicing, the stability of mRNA, or the trafficking of mRNA or proteins to their proper intracellular location [PMID19768584].

SNPs can be studied by allele-specific PCR, melt curve analysis, and microarrays. They are emerging as the technique of choice in many DNA studies because they are more frequent than microsatellites and therefore more likely to be associated with the gene that is of interest. Also, many SNPs are in the gene of interest rather than simply close to it, so unlike most microsatellite analysis, SNP studies are rarely surrogate testing. Moreover, unlike microsatellite analysis, SNP analysis does not require electrophoresis and is technically simpler and faster, making it more suitable as a screening technique, especially now that microarray methods are available. At this writing, for example, Affymetrix has a microarray platform that is able to interrogate over 900,000 of the approximately 5,000,000 known SNPs.

The Single Nucleotide Polymorphism Database, dbSNP, is maintained by the National Center for Biotechnology Information (NCBI). In addition to cataloguing SNPs, dbSNP also catalogues other polymorphisms, including microsatellites, short deletions, and insertions. The dbSNP supplements GenBank, 1 of the 3 major databases of DNA sequence information. Every submitted SNP polymorphism receives a submitter accession number that begins with "ss," for "submitted SNP." After the polymorphism is confirmed, the accession number is prefaced by "rs," for "reference SNP" (so there will be many "ss" accessions for each "rs" accession number). An example is rs12979860, which confers a better response to treatment in patients with genotype 1 hepatitis C. By early 2010, dbSNP had compiled over 60,000,000 SNPs and other polymorphisms from dozens of species, including humans.

The Tendency for SNPs to Remain Together during Evolution Is the Basis of the HapMap

A haplotype (short for haploid genotype) is a set of alleles on a segment of a chromosome that tend to be inherited together. Haplotypes can be tracked through generations and have been invaluable in the genetic analysis of diseases. SNPs tend to be inherited as a group or block, and in the context of SNPs, a haplotype (also called a haplotype block or a linkage disequilibrium block) refers to a particular group of SNPs from a single chromosome that are generally inherited together [PMID15660514]. Each SNP haplotype is thought to be indicative of descent from 1 or a very small number of individual ancestral chromosomes.

Because of genetic recombination in germ cells, one would expect that SNP haplotypes would not be stable and would become smaller as fewer and fewer SNPs are able to stay together over generations. But haplotypes are longer than expected, indicating some protection from recombination, because recombination preferentially occurs in specific areas on the chromosome. The SNPs in a haplotype block tend to be inherited together even in the face of recombination because haplotype blocks are relatively spared from recombination.

Even at this early stage in DNA sequencing, where only a small number of people have had their DNA completely sequenced, it is already clear that certain SNP haplotypes are associated with certain diseases or with responses to certain drugs, reminiscent of the association of certain diseases with HLA haplotypes. Because identifying SNPs is much cheaper and easier than completely sequencing each patient's genome, it seems likely that SNP testing will replace much laboratory testing that is currently performed by other means. The first such area may be blood banking, as SNP testing can replace traditional hemagglutination studies in blood group polymorphisms [PMID20431033].

Many SNPs tend to occur in recognizable associations. For example, if there is a substitution of an A for a G in 1 location, it is likely that there will be a substitution of a G for an A about 1,000 base pairs later, followed by a substitution of a C for a T 1,000 or so base pairs after that, etc. Therefore, the identification of a few SNPs in a haplotype—called tag SNPs or tagging SNPs—will usually permit an educated guess about the composition of the entire haplotype. Tag SNPs greatly simplify genetic analysis because only a small portion (perhaps 5%) of the SNPs in a haplotype must be actually determined. The rest can be safely postulated from known associations, allowing the rapid determination of most of an individual's entire genome.

The International HapMap Project is working to develop a haplotype map of the human genome, called the HapMap [PMID20194478]. The HapMap is a database of known SNP associations in 4 ethnic groups—European, Han Chinese, West African, and Japanese. Tag SNPs are not a perfect representation of haplotypes, and one of the goals of the HapMap is to determine how effectively a given tag SNP reflects an entire haplotype and to develop the most effective set of tag SNPs. Likewise, there is slight variation among these 4 ethnic groups in the number of nucleotides between SNPs, and a challenge of the HapMap is to learn more about these variations and to determine if the same tag SNPs can be used for all population subgroups. The homepage of the HapMap project is http://www.Hapmap.org.

The HapMap project has confirmed the essential identity of DNA from different populations, and in particular, it has shown that there are blocks of highly conserved DNA that are invariant among the 4 populations studied [PMID17943122]. There is very strong linkage disequilibrium (ie, association) of these blocks. Incidentally, in addition to its enormous importance in medicine, HapMap has shown that there is slightly greater variability and slightly smaller conserved blocks in the West African population, suggesting that this population is slightly older than the other 3. This supports the Out of Africa model of human evolution, which holds that modern *Homo sapiens* arose only in Africa and not from *Homo erectus* or Neanderthal populations that were scattered around the world.

Another reason for SNP analysis is that because of incomplete annotation of the genome (ie, incomplete understanding of intron-exon boundaries, the start and stop locations of genes, the probable products, regulatory features), not all genes are located and fully understood, even though the entire DNA sequence is known. Consequently, it is well worthwhile to understand SNPs, the leading cause of human polymorphism. The 1,000 Genomes Project is currently sequencing the DNA of 1,000 individuals from diverse populations so that new SNPs can be identified and rare SNPs can be better characterized.

SNPs can be detected by allele-specific PCR using sequence-specific primers, microarrays, mass spectrometry, or direct sequencing. Another method for detecting SNPs is by immobilized mismatch binding protein. In one version of this technique, a protein that recognizes the imperfect structure of mismatched DNA is immobilized on a substrate (usually the MMR enzyme MutS from *E coli* is used). The DNA under investigation is then incubated with a labeled probe that is complementary to the wild-type sequence. If there is a perfect match, MutS does not bind the sequence and the duplex of test DNA and labeled probe is not bound to the substrate. If there is an imperfect match (ie, an SNP), the MutS binds the labeled duplex and holds it to the substrate.

Molecular Pathology of Inherited Disorders

We begin our consideration of molecular testing of inherited diseases with 2 comments. First, as mentioned at the opening of this chapter, testing for hereditary disease often requires a special consent beyond a general consent for testing and treatment. Second, as mentioned at the close of Chapter 45, a general principle in genetic testing is that it is wise to determine the specific mutation in any patient before testing family members. Because the risk, if any, to a family member is based on the passage of a specific mutation, family members need only be tested for the specific mutation that is found in the patient. If the family member does not have that mutation, he or she is no more likely to be a carrier than a random person.

Cystic Fibrosis

The incidence of cystic fibrosis (CF) varies among ethnic groups, but is overall about 1 per 3,500 births [PMID21708286]. CF is caused by a defect in the *CFTR* (CF transmembrane conductance regulator) gene, which codes for a transmembrane chloride ion channel and is a member of the ATP-binding cassette superfamily of transmembrane proteins that transport a variety of compounds through the cell membrane [PMID12644668]. The CFTR protein has 5 domains. 2 of these span the cell membrane and form the actual chloride channel, 2 are nucleotide binding domains in the cytoplasm (NBD1 and NBD2) that bind and cleave ATP, and the fifth is a regulatory domain [PMID20653506].

CFTR, on the long arm of chromosome 7, is 250,000 base pairs in length and has 27 exons. As is often the case, these exons are not sequentially numbered because the order of their discovery does not correspond to their arrangement on the chromosome. For example, there are only 24 numbered exons, but there is a 14A and a 14B exon.

CF has only 1 mode of inheritance—autosomal recessive—but there may be multiple types of mutations within the gene. This necessitates multiple tests and results in a testing sensitivity of <100%. For example, a 3 nucleotide deletion that removes a phenylalanine at position 508 (ΔF508) in NBD1 is responsible for 70% of CF in Caucasian patients, but there are >1,500 other known alterations of *CFTR*, about 1,200 of which are pathogenic. Most of these involve only 1 or a few nucleotides. These mutations can be manifest anywhere in the very long and complicated CFTR protein. Some of the mutations preclude synthesis of the protein, while others impede its maturation, prevent the protein from reaching its proper apical location within the cell, or diminish proper function of the protein once it reaches its appropriate intracellular destination [PMID21708286]. The common ΔF508 has multiple effects [PMID20653506].

The term "compound heterozygote" refers to different mutations of the same gene on different chromosomes. Compound heterozygosity is relatively common in CF. The degree of clinical disease in a compound heterozygote depends on the location of the 2 mutations and the effect on protein structure and function. If they are both serious, a severe phenotype will occur because neither chromosome can produce a working copy of the protein product, but if 1 abnormality is mild, then 1 of the 2 chromosomes can produce a partially functioning protein and a lesser clinical presentation is to be expected.

The impact of dysfunctional *CFTR* varies from organ to organ. In the sweat glands, the impaired chloride pump fails to resorb chloride as sweat passes down the duct to its opening. Since sodium follows passively, salt is not resorbed as perspiration moves along the duct, accounting of the familiar finding that these patients have increased salt in their perspiration.

In the pancreas, there is a similar mechanism, but there is impaired chloride transport into the duct rather than out of it, as is the case for sweat glands. Diminished chloride transport leads to a reduction in the passive transfer of sodium and water into the duct. The result is viscous secretions and diminished passage of pancreatic enzymes, causing dilatation and fibrosis of ducts, accounting for the name of the disease. Exocrine pancreatic insufficiency occurs in 85% of patients, causing malabsorption. 15% of adults with CF will develop diabetes from destruction of β cells in the islets.

In other organs, especially in the lung, not all symptoms can be explained by a simple loss of chloride transport, but there is mucus accumulation in bronchi, causing bronchiectasis and a predisposition to infections. Lung transplantation may be necessary in severe cases. Other symptoms involve increased viscosity in the gastrointestinal or biliary tracts, leading to meconium ileus or jaundice.

The vas deferens has the highest requirement of the CFTR protein and almost all male patients have partial or complete agenesis of the vas deferens, making this the most likely phenotype in male patients, regardless of the mutation. The pancreas has the second highest CFTR protein requirement, and the lung third. For example, homozygous ΔF508 is more serious than homozygous R117H, and patients in the former group always have pancreatic disease, while patients in the latter group are usually pancreatic sufficient. A ΔF508-R117H compound heterozygote will have intermediate manifestations.

Pulmonary symptoms are not as amenable to prediction in this manner. Lung symptoms depend on polymorphisms in intron 8 of *CFTR*. There is a locus in intron 8 that has 5, 7, or 9 thymines in a row. Normal splicing occurs with either 7 or 9 repeats, but 5 thymines leads to abnormal splicing and is considered a mild mutation [PMID16126774]. This polymorphism is not a cause of CF, but modifies its pulmonary expression. A patient who is homozygous for the relatively mild R117H and who has either 7 or 9 repeats of thymine may have reasonable lung function. If such a patient is female, she may be relatively asymptomatic, and if male, he may have only congenital bilateral absence of vas deferens (CBAVD).

From a carrier viewpoint, if a patient is positive for R117H mutation, but has 5 thymines in Cis (ie, on the same chromosome as the R117H), then that chromosome is compromised and the patient is a full carrier. On the other hand, if R117H and the 5 thymines are in trans (ie, on different chromosomes), neither chromosome is seriously affected, and even if the patient's partner is a carrier and transmits his or her abnormal chromosome, only a mild manifestation of CF is to be expected. For reasons such as these, older people with an attenuated form of the disorder will occasionally present with pulmonary symptoms or recurrent, previously unexplained sinus infections.

Carrier frequency for CF varies among ethnic groups but is highest in Ashkenazi Jews and Caucasians, being about 1 in 29 in both groups. Carrier screening for CF is frequently offered to pregnant women during routine prenatal visits. There is controversy as to which of the enormous number of mutations should be tested for, and regulations vary from state to state, but there is a general consensus that any mutation that occurs with a rate of 0.1% or more should be included in the analysis, unless its innocuous nature has been shown. 23 mutations fulfill these criteria. A negative carrier screening test for these 23 mutations drops the risk in an Ashkenazi Jew to 1:930 but only to 1:140 in a patient of southern European descent.

There are a number of methods used in CF carrier screening [PMID20638569], including amplification refractory mutation detection systems, oligonucleotide ligation assays (OLAs), and a method based on the Invader technology [PMID14711349]. The

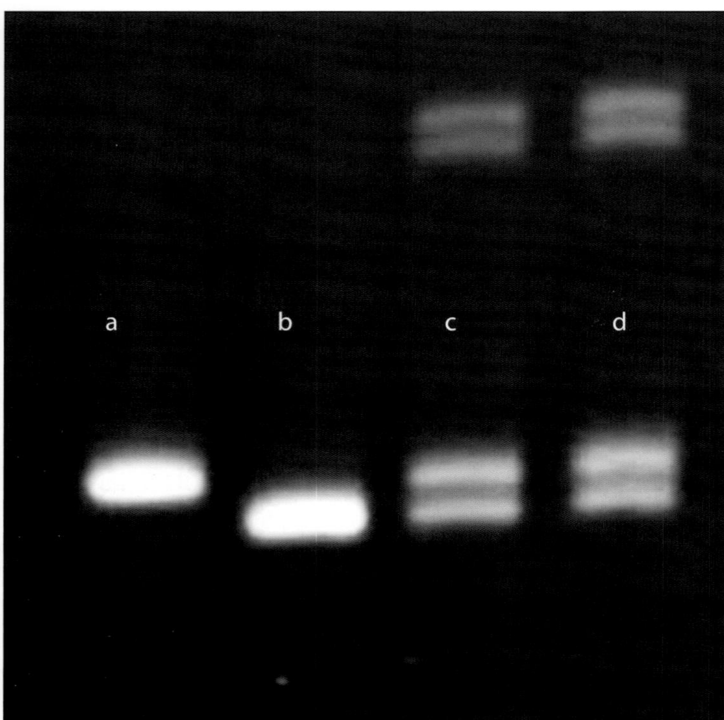

f46.13 Cystic fibrosis testing for ΔF508 by PCR. PCR is carried out across the region of DNA that contains the codon that codes for amino acid 508.
a Homozygous normal patient. There is a single band of 98 base pairs (bp).
b Homozygous patient for ΔF508. There is a single band of 95 bp, which runs slightly ahead of the normal band.
c, d Patients who are heterozygous for ΔF508. Both the 98 and 95 bp bands are seen. The 2 fainter bands at the top of the gel are heteroduplex bands, formed by the hybridization of 1 strand of an abnormal DNA and 1 strand of normal DNA. This is amplicon-amplicon binding, rather than amplicon-primer binding. Because these heteroduplex bands have an abnormal 3-dimensional conformation, they run more slowly in a gel.

common ΔF508 mutation may be specifically investigated as a first step, often via PCR using primers that flank the DNA that includes codon 508. A deletion generates a slightly shorter amplicon that runs just ahead of the normal amplicon **f46.13**. But because there are so many mutations, testing often uses a multiplex assay. One method is OLA, a form of ligation-dependent PCR, of which there are several variants [PMID12636046]. In a common use of OLA, a collection of commercial probes is employed in pairs of hemiprobes, 1 pair for each potentially abnormal area. An abnormality in the patient sample that precisely matches a pair of DNA hemiprobes will permit the hemiprobes to bind to immediately adjacent areas. The hemiprobes will then be close enough for DNA ligase to form a single probe, which can then undergo PCR amplification. After all such pairs of hemiprobes are allowed to hybridize to the patient sample, and all opportunities of DNA ligase to ligate any matches have occurred, PCR is performed and the amplicons, if any, are subjected to capillary electrophoresis. PCR products, corresponding to abnormal alleles, are detected as they pass by a laser. If there are no abnormalities in the gene, there will be no hybridizations of hemiprobes, no ligations, no amplifications, and no amplicons will be detected by electrophoresis. If there are 1 or more mutations, they are identified by the electrophoretic mobility of the products (ie, amplicons derived from ΔF508 pass the laser in a capillary electrophoresis system at a different time from those secondary to R117H).

A variant of OLA sequences the amplicons rather than separating them by electrophoresis. Another variant of OLA testing in CF uses a fluorescently labeled common hemiprobe that will hybridize to normal DNA and to DNA from any known abnormality. It will hybridize to the patient's DNA under any circumstances and is used with a series of sequence-specific hemiprobes, one of which will hybridize to each sequence of abnormal DNA that is to be tested for. The common hemiprobe does not have a mobility modifier, but the sequence-specific hemiprobes each have mobility modifiers (stuffer sequences) that are of different lengths. If there are no mutations, none of the sequence-specific hemiprobes will bind, there is no ligation, and there are no amplicons. If there is a mutation, the corresponding hemiprobe, with its unique length, will bind, after which there will be ligation and amplification. After capillary electrophoresis, the position of the amplicons permits the identification of the mutation. Heterozygotes can be detected by the finding of 2 bands.

Allele-specific PCR amplification (also called amplification refractory mutation system [ARMS]) is also used in CF carrier testing [PMID19645745]. After allele-specific amplification, the amplicons, if any, are run on a gel. Any abnormal band indicates an abnormality at the DNA level, and its location provides the identity. In a typical allele-specific amplification test, sequences known to contain mutations of both long and short length are added. These should always amplify, proving that amplification can occur over any range of sizes. There is also a control with a normal phenylalanine in position 508. This testing does not distinguish between homozygosity and heterozygosity.

Yet another technique for CF carrier testing is allele-specific oligohybridization (ASO), based on older dot-blot procedures [PMID12636046]. In one form of ASO, labeled synthetic oligonucleotide probes, each capable of hybridizing to 1 mutation, are immobilized on a membrane in known locations. The patient DNA sample is amplified by PCR, denatured, and then applied to the membrane. A washing step removes any normal DNA because it has not hybridized to any of the oligonucleotides. If the patient sample contains an abnormality, it will hybridize to the relevant probe and adhere to the membrane. The location divulges the specific mutation.

If 2 known carriers are already pregnant, prenatal testing is possible. A potential problem with any prenatal testing is that fetal cells from amniocentesis or chorionic villus sampling may be contaminated by maternal cells, but such contamination can usually be identified by concurrent testing of maternal DNA obtained from blood or buccal cells, and comparison to the putative fetal source [PMID21227389].

Newborn CF screening usually does not begin with DNA testing, as described above for carrier testing. Rather, in a typical 2-tiered screening program, newborn screening begins with serum levels of immunoreactive trypsinogen (IRT). If elevated levels of this enzyme are found, the infant then undergoes traditional DNA screening, as in carrier screening [PMID20521170].

CF transmembrane conductance regulator-related disorders stem from an abnormality of proteins that interact with CFTR or are also involved in the functioning of the chloride channel. These patients have a less aggressive course than most CF patients [PMID22020151].

Spinal Muscular Atrophy

Spinal muscular atrophy (SMA) is the second most common lethal autosomal recessive disorder after CF [PMID21227388]. The overall carrier frequency is 1 in 50, and the incidence is about 1 in 6,000. 4 forms are recognized ranging in severity from the lethal type I (Werdnig-Hoffman) to the adult onset type IV. Histologic changes of SMA are those of denervation, ie, atrophic rounded fibers, with scattered normal or hypertrophic fibers, with increased perimysial connective tissue.

The most frequent mutation in SMA is a deletion in the survival of motor neuron gene (*SMN*) on 5q. There are actually 2 versions of the *SMN* gene, *SMN1* and *SMN2*, differing by only 5 base pairs. *SMN1* is telomeric to *SMN2* and is transcribed at much higher levels. It is the more important gene and deletions in it are responsible for most cases of SMA [PMID20057317]. *SMN1* has 9 exons. Most deletions are in exon 7. Screening is based on the detection of deletions in *SMN1*, but care must be taken because either *SMN1* or *SMN2* may be present in extra copies and some testing may not distinguish between these 2 genes [PMID21362338]. Consider a patient who has 1 normal chromosome and 1 in which there is both a deletion in *SMN1* and an extra copy of *SMN2*, and who is studied by a test that does not distinguish between the 2 genes. Since there is a working copy of *SMN1*, the patient will be asymptomatic. If testing does not distinguish between *SMN1* and *SMN2*, the 2 copies of *SMN2* on the abnormal chromosome will be indistinguishable from the normal situation of 1 copy of *SMN1* and 1 copy of *SMN2*, and the patient will appear normal on screening. She will appear to have 1 copy of *SMN1* and 1 copy of *SMN2* on each chromosome. But since *SMN2* is transcribed at a low level, the function of the chromosome with the deletion in *SMN1* and 2 copies of *SMN2* will be compromised, and the patient is actually an undetected carrier. Rarely, there may be 2 copies of *SMN1* on 1 chromosome and none on the other. These patients will also be asymptomatic but will also be missed carriers unless screening tests each chromosome individually because 2 copies of *SMN1* will be detected. Many feel that newborn SMA screening should be mandatory [PMID20808230], but the patent held by Athena Diagnostics complicates widespread testing [PMID21227388].

Inherited Hypercoagulability

Protein C is a vitamin K-dependent protein and is activated by the complex of thrombin-thrombomodulin, after which it degrades the activated forms of factors V and VIII, exerting an antithrombotic effect on the coagulation cascade [PMID20423310]. The free form of protein S is vitamin K-dependent and has anticoagulant activities of its own, but also enhances the activity of activated protein C. Deficient *response* to activated protein C is the leading cause of a genetic predisposition to hypercoagulability, but the problem is rarely due to protein C itself or to protein S. Much more commonly, the problem is a defective factor V, called factor V Leiden, that is resistant to activated protein C.

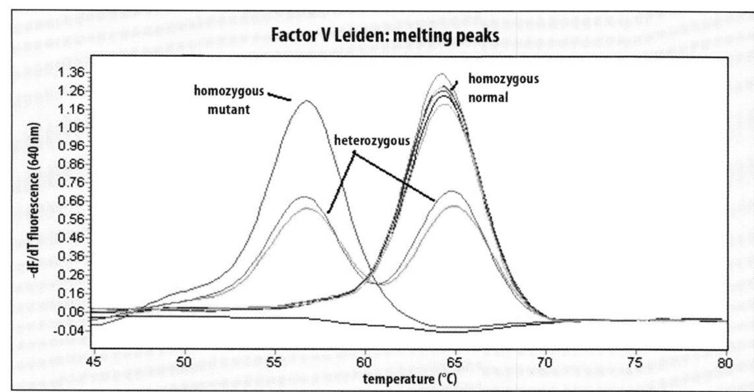

f46.14 Following melting curve analysis, the patient's DNA is amplified and exposed to a fluorescent probe that is homologous to the normal sequence. Because the probe binds the normal sequence more strongly, and because fluorescence decreases upon dissociation of the 2 strands, fluorescence decreases at a lower temperature in the abnormal allele. A homozygous normal patient is seen at right (at high temperature); a homozygous abnormal at left, and a heterozygous patient in the middle.

Factor V Leiden is the most common cause of inherited hypercoagulability. It is caused by a single point mutation of guanine to adenine at the nucleotide position 1691 (1691G>A) in the gene, resulting in the substitution of glutamine for arginine at amino acid position 506 in the protein. Of those with an abnormal activated protein C assay, about 94% are heterozygous for factor V Leiden, so testing for factor V genotype should precede protein C testing in most patients. 3-5% of people are heterozygous for factor V Leiden, and these patients may well be symptomatic, with a 5- to 10-fold increase in the incidence of venous thrombosis. 20% of individuals with an initial diagnosis of venous thrombus and 60% of those with recurrent thrombi are heterozygotes for the factor V Leiden mutation. Women who are heterozygous for factor V Leiden have a 20-30 fold increase in venous thrombi if they are on oral contraceptives [PMID11309638].

A less common cause of functional factor V deficiency is 4070A>G, a replacement of adenine by guanine at nucleotide position 4070 in the gene. This form of factor V is distinct from factor V Leiden, though also incapable of an optimal response to protein C.

The leading method of detecting factor V Leiden is allele-specific PCR, in which primers are chosen so that only the allele of interest (the abnormal one) can support amplification. There are other methodologies, such as OLA, a cleavase method, and melting curve analysis **f46.14**.

The second most common cause of hereditary coagulopathy is a mutation of the prothrombin gene, usually caused by 20210G>A (a substitution of a guanine by an adenine at base pair 20210 in the gene) [PMID18574041]. Abnormalities of the prothrombin gene are usually detected by PCR followed by RFLP, allele-specific PCR, or by melting curve analysis [PMID20162544].

Achondroplasia, Hypochondroplasia, and Craniosynostosis Syndromes

These disorders are discussed together because they all result from a defect in the fibroblast growth factor receptor (*FGFR*) gene. There are 4 *FGFR* genes in humans: *FGFR1*, *FGFR2*, *FGFR3*, and *FGFR4*, all of which encode a transmembrane receptor/tyrosine kinase. These 4 genes are paralogous (similar genes at different locations, likely derived from duplication and subsequent slight divergence).

FGFR3 is the culprit in achondroplasia [PMID20601886]. Achondroplasia is inherited in an autosomal dominant manner, though remarkably, 80% of cases are spontaneous new mutations. The homozygous condition in this disorder is lethal. 99% of mutations are 1138G>A (ie, guanine to adenine transversion at nucleotide position 1138). This results in a glycine to arginine substitution at amino acid position 380 in the FGFR3 protein. FGFR3 restrains the proliferation of chondrocytes, so that endochondral bone formation proceeds in an orderly manner. In the mutated form of the gene, there is gain of function that causes excessive inhibition of chondrocyte proliferation. Without sufficient chondrocytes, endochondral bone formation is retarded, accounting for the characteristic stature of these patients and the fact that the smaller bones, which are not dependent on endochondral ossification, are unaffected.

Hypochondroplasia is a milder form of achondroplasia. While most cases of hypochondroplasia are associated with *FGFR3*, a minority are not. Of those cases in which the *FGRF3* is the problem, about 70% have a 1620C>A mutation, resulting in asparagine to lysine change at amino acid position 540 in the protein [PMID9055906].

Craniosynostosis results from premature closure of the sutures in the skull. The incidence of craniosynostosis is almost 1 in 2,000 live births. Beyond the cosmetic effects, the abnormally shaped skull in may impede brain development or predispose to cerebral hypertension. Surgery can be highly effective in some cases.

Some cases of craniosynostosis are sporadic, but about 150 syndromes involving craniosynostosis have been described, depending on which suture or sutures are affected. Only about 15-20% of the syndromic forms are related to mutations in 1 of the 4 *FGFR* genes. The most common craniosynostosis syndromes are Pfeiffer, Apert, and Crouzon syndromes, all of which are linked to mutations in one of the *FGFR* genes, but the specific gene that is mutated varies from syndrome to syndrome [PMID21042516]. For example, about 2/3 of Apert syndrome are due to mutations in the *FGFR2* gene, with most cases caused by either 934C>G in the gene, resulting in a substitution of tryptophan for serine at amino acid position 252 in the protein, or 937C>G, causing an arginine for proline substitution at amino acid position 253 in the protein. Pfeiffer syndrome can be associated with mutations in *FGFR2* and *FGFR1*. Syndromic forms often involve abnormalities in other areas, such as the limbs, and are generally autosomal dominant. Genetic testing is available for some of the craniosynostosis syndromes, both to identify carriers and in prenatal use.

Muscular Dystrophy

Duchenne muscular dystrophy (DMD) is the most common X-linked recessive lethal condition, affecting about 1 in every 3,500 newborns. The pattern of development of weakness is leg before arm and proximal before distal. In muscle biopsies of early DMD, there is variable diameter of muscle fibers. In later stages, there is degeneration and dropout of fibers, with replacement by fat and fibrous tissue. Nuclei are found in the interior instead of their normal peripheral location. If additional evidence is needed for the diagnosis, an immunohistochemical stain for dystrophin is available and, in normal muscle, demonstrates a strong cell membrane staining pattern, while staining is absent in DMD and reduced in either Becker muscular dystrophy (BMD) or in asymptomatic carriers [PMID1358314].

BMD is much milder and much rarer, affecting only about 1 in 100,000 live births. Symptoms do not appear until about age 5, and by definition, these patients are ambulatory until age 16. Some have no symptoms until the fourth decade. Nevertheless, life expectancy is reduced.

Both DMD and BMD stem from abnormalities in the dystrophin gene, the largest gene known in humans, which codes for the dystrophin protein. DMD patients lack a functional dystrophin protein altogether, while BMD patients either have a diminished amount or an altered form. The dystrophin gene has 79 exons and a transcript that is 14 kilobases.

Dystrophin is expressed in all forms of muscle, including the heart. Almost all DMD patients will also have cardiac abnormalities, such as fibrosis of the posteriobasal wall of the left ventricle and intra-atrial conduction. 90% of patients have abnormal ECGs. Although many will be clinically asymptomatic from a cardiac standpoint throughout most of their lives, with improved treatment of respiratory failure, heart failure secondary to loss of cardiac muscle cells is now a leading cause of death [PMID21258567]. Female carriers are asymptomatic except that some will have cardiac manifestations, and about 1/2 will have elevated serum creatine kinase.

Even as large as it is, the dystrophin protein is part of a huge complex called the dystrophin complex, in which dystrophin links extracellular proteins to the cytoskeletal matrix. The nature of this complex, which has been elucidated largely by Campbell and colleagues [PMID2188135, PMID1913804, PMID8349731], has been the subject of numerous reviews [PMID8541869, PMID9146999]. Dystrophin is a cytoskeletal protein whose amino terminus associates with actin and whose carboxy terminus associates with proteins in the sarcolemma (cell membrane), especially with the cytoplasmic portion of a transmembrane protein called β dystroglycan (dystrophin-associated glycoprotein). The extracellular portion of β dystroglycan binds the external protein α dystroglycan, which in turn binds laminin in the extracellular matrix. The intramembranous portion of β dystroglycan interacts with the sarcoglycans, a series of transmembrane proteins. The function of the sarcoglycans is not known, but mutations in them are implicated in the limb girdle muscular dystrophies, a group of disorders that is distinct from DMD and BMD, and that is not linked to dystrophin [PMID21496623]. The cytoplasmic portion of β dystroglycan interacts with dystrophin, completing a complex association between the extracellular matrix and actin.

Dystrophin is also expressed in the brain, and 20% of DMD patients have cognitive impairment, usually primarily manifest in verbal abilities. The precise function of dystrophin in the brain is not understood, and the structure of the dystrophin complex is somewhat different in brain [PMID20625423].

Screening for the carrier state of DMD is difficult for a number of reasons. First, the disease can be caused by several types of mutations in the dystrophin gene. It is usually secondary to large deletions, often in exons 44-53. The size of the deletion does not correlate with severity of symptoms in DMD. A smaller number of cases involve duplications, and a still smaller subset is caused by point mutations (usually premature stop codons). A well-known point mutation cause of DMD occurs in exon 76 of the dystrophin gene and may affect the actin binding site. Second, about 1/3 of cases result from new mutations. Third, in about 4% of cases, the mutation cannot be detected by DNA analysis, even sequencing, but can only be found by study of the mRNA [PMID19959795]. Fourth, there are many polymorphisms in the dystrophin gene, most of which are innocuous, so a detected variant may not have clinical significance. There is no other gene that is as large, with as many different mutations of different types, often requiring multiple modalities to effectively study. Perhaps the only "easy" aspect of screening for DMD carrier status is that there are no significant differences among ethnic groups in the mutations.

Testing for mutations in the dystrophin gene is usually done by PCR across a portion of the dystrophin gene, followed by electrophoresis. A normal and an abnormal control are run. Missing bands relative to the normal control imply deletions. Other methods may be needed for other types of mutations, and rarely, Southern blotting may be necessary [PMID16049303].

Neurofibromatosis

There are 2 types of neurofibromatosis (NF): NF1 and NF2. NF1 (von Recklinghausen disease) is more common and is associated with multiple neurofibromas and an increased incidence of malignant nerve sheath tumors relative to the general population (though only about 10% or less of NF1 patients will get a malignant nerve sheath tumor). There are also numerous nonneoplastic manifestations, including café-au-lait spots on the skin and Lisch nodules in the iris. NF1 is associated with loss of function of the *NF1* gene, an extremely large gene on 17q11.2 that codes for the protein neurofibromin. Neurofibromin is a tumor suppressor protein that exerts control over the regulatory protein ras [PMID19348714]. It is not known how a defect in this tumor suppressor protein leads to the many nonneoplastic manifestations of the disorder. NF1 is inherited in an autosomal dominant manner, though *NF1* has a very high spontaneous mutation rate, and about 50% of cases of neurofibromatosis are sporadic because of these spontaneous mutations [PMID19348714]. Most mutations are truncating point mutations, but about 10% are microdeletions [PMID19767589]. Because of the great size of the *NF1* gene and the absence of "hotspots" that are more prone to mutation, testing is a daunting task that is usually accomplished by the use of multiple methods on each sample [PMID19348714].

NF2 is rare and results from mutations in the *NF2* tumor suppressor gene. Its clinical manifestations are usually restricted to neurofibromas of the eighth cranial nerve (often, but incorrectly called acoustic neuromas, since they are not neuromas) and tumors of the central nervous system [PMID19476995]. *NF2* codes for the protein merlin (also called schwannomin), a cytoskeletal protein that is made in Schwann cells and that is important in a number of functions, one of which is maintenance of contact inhibition [PMID20491622].

Osteogenesis Imperfecta

There are over 20 types of collagen, but type I collagen is the matrix upon which bone is mineralized. Type I collagen is made from a triple helix of 3 type I procollagen chains, each consisting of 2 $\alpha1$ subunits, encoded by the gene *COL1A1*, and 1 $\alpha2$ chain, encoded by the gene *COL1A2*.

Osteogenesis imperfecta is a group of related disorders characterized by brittle bones and skeletal abnormalities. 4 types were initially recognized by Sillence et al [PMID458828], based on the mode of inheritance, and clinical and radiographic findings. As more has been learned about the responsible genes, the classification has expanded to 7 types and some recognize 8 types. Types I-V are inherited in an autosomal dominant manner. Other types are generally inherited in an autosomal recessive manner, but there is some uncertainty about type VI [PMID20301472].

All forms of osteogenesis imperfecta are related to defects in the collagenous matrix of bone, not to the actual mineralization. Types I-IV are associated with mutations in *COL1A1* or *COL1A2*, while other genes are involved in types V-VII. Type I osteogenesis imperfecta, a milder form, results from a diminished *amount* of procollagen production, usually because of a premature stop codon in 1 of the 2 copies of *COL1A1* [PMID15110498]. The usual result is bone with 1/2 of the normal amount of type I procollagen. Because a large number of mutations have been described in *COL1A1* and *COL1A2* (in many cases a mutation appears unique to one family), direct sequencing, either of genomic DNA or of cDNA, is the technique of choice. On the other hand, types II, III, and IV are more severe forms that result from *defective* type I procollagen. Osteogenesis imperfecta is an exception to the general rule that it is better to have a defective protein than no protein. In this group of disorders, it is better to have a diminished amount of the collagen matrix than to have a defect in the matrix. This exception is often seen in structural proteins that are polymerized, because polymerization amplifies any defective function, whereas deficient amounts are less subject to such amplification during polymerization.

Hearing Loss

Vibrations are transmitted mechanically to the inner ear, after which the displacement of the membranes in the inner ear causes motion of the sensory hair cells. This motion opens the ion channels, causing an influx of potassium ions from the endolymph into the cell, depolarizing it. This depolarization opens calcium channels, resulting in an influx of calcium into the hair cell. Calcium triggers the release of a neurotransmitter, causing an action potential in the adjacent neuron and beginning the auditory neuronal pathway. The potassium must then leave the cell so it can be repolarized. While the precise details of potassium efflux and recycling are not clear, it is believed that during repolarization, the potassium leaves the hair cell and enters supporting cells. The potassium ions then leave these supporting cells through gap junctions that are formed by connexin proteins and diffuse into the stria vascularis (vascular tissue in the wall of the cochlea), to make their way back to the endolymph, so the process can repeat [PMID19942739, PMID19741536].

1 in 1,000 newborns is deaf. 60% of these cases are genetic, while the remainder is caused by infection or environmental factors. Of the genetic cases, all forms of inheritance have been described, and there are both syndromic and nonsyndromic forms. Genetic testing can be valuable in the early identification of other clinical problems that might be found in syndromic cases. Pendred syndrome is one of the most common syndromic forms and is characterized by a mutation in the *PDS* gene on chromosome 7 that encodes the protein pendrin, an ion transporter thought to be needed to recondition endolymphatic fluid so that there can be further depolarization of hair cells [PMID19608655]. Patients with Pendred syndrome also have goiter since the pendrin protein is present in the apical portion of thyrocytes and is thought to facilitate the transport of iodide into the follicle [PMID16444159].

Many genetic cases of hearing impairment are caused by defects in the connexin proteins that compose gap junctions because the ability of potassium to leave the hair cell after depolarizing it is impeded, so there can be no further depolarization. Connexin proteins are transmembrane proteins arranged concentrically in groups of 6 to form structures called connexons that have miniscule pores in the center. Opposed connexons in 2 adjacent cells form a gap junction, allowing nearly instant passage of ions between the 2 cells. At this writing, 21 connexin proteins have been identified in humans, but differing combinations of connexins allow for many types of connexons. Connexins are given numbers that correspond to their molecular weights (eg, connexin 26 has a molecular weight of 26,000 Daltons).

GJB2, the gene on 13q that codes for the connexin 26 protein, is the primary culprit among the connexin disorders in genetic deafness. Over 100 abnormalities in *GJB2* have been described, many of which lead to autosomal recessive nonsyndromic sensineural hereditary hearing loss. The most common of these is nonsyndromic hearing loss and deafness (DFNB1), which results from 35delG, a deletion of a single guanine base that results in a frameshift [PMID11603757]. Mutations in *GJB6*, which codes for connexin 30, may also cause hearing impairment.

Genetic Screening in Ashkenazi Jews

To understand appropriate genetic screening in Ashkenazi Jews, we must first understand founder mutations. The Hardy-Weinberg law states that gene frequencies are stable, but the law is based on a number of assumptions, one of which is that the size of the population is reasonably large and that mating is random. Random chance is more important in small populations and can lead to genetic changes, called genetic drift, that may be greater than changes caused by natural selection. As an analogy, if we flip a coin 100 times, we are likely to get something close to 50 heads and 50 tails, but if we flip it only 10 times, we could easily get 6 heads and 4 tails or even 7 heads and 3 tails.

Small gene pools are the equivalent of flipping a coin only 5 or 10 times. Any time a small group of individuals from a particular population becomes isolated, mutations caused by chance are more likely to be perpetuated rather than being diluted out as they would be in a larger population. These are called founder mutations. Founder mutations are accentuated by what geneticists call population bottlenecks, which occur when a large population is significantly reduced in size because of migration or death, forcing a small number of people ("founders") to reconstitute the population. Bottlenecks can either enhance or reduce the frequency of rare alleles, depending on the frequency of those alleles in the founders relative to the frequency in the population prior to the traumatic event. Because of the numerous forced relocations, population bottlenecks, and isolated communities of the Jewish people, especially Ashkenazi Jews, they have a greater preponderance of founder mutations.

In addition to CF, about 17 other diseases occur in increased incidence in Ashkenazi Jews [PMID15516842]. These include Tay Sachs disease, Neimann-Pick, Bloom syndrome, Canavan disease, Fanconi anemia type C, familial dysautonomia, mucolipidosis type IV, glycogen storage disease type 1A (von Gierke), and Gaucher disease. The American College of Medical Genetics recommends screening patients of Ashkenazi Jewish descent for all of these diseases except von Gierke, and by any estimation, an essential panel for this population, in addition to CF, includes Tay Sachs, Canavan, and familial dysautonomia [PMID20494256].

Tay Sachs disease is one of the lysosomal storage disorders [PMID15686451] and results from the accumulations of GM2 ganglioside (a complex lipid) secondary to deficient activity of the enzyme β-hexosaminidase A caused by a mutation in the *Hex A* gene on chromosome 15 [PMID17015493]. The severe infantile forms are caused by an insertion of TATC at position 1278 in exon 11 or an abnormality at a splice site in intron 12. In addition to the severe forms, there is a milder adult-onset form of Tay Sachs that is caused by partial deficiency of hexosaminidase A activity resulting from G269S (substitution of serine for glycine at amino acid position 269).

The carrier frequency of Tay Sachs disease among Ashkenazi Jews is 1 in 28, similar to that of CF [PMID15686451]. DNA testing centers on exon 11, intron 12, and, in the adult form, exon 5. Maximum sensitivity and specificity of screening occur when DNA testing is combined with serum assay of the enzyme [PMID17015493].

The carrier frequency of Canavan disease in Ashkenazi Jews is 1 in 40. Like Tay Sachs, Canavan disease is a neurodegenerative lysosomal storage disease. Symptoms are caused by the accumulation of N-acetyl aspartic acid in the brain. The defect is in deficient activity of the enzyme aspartoacylase, which is encoded by a gene on chromosome 17 [PMID16802706]. Almost all mutations result in either E285A (a substitution of alanine for glutamate at amino acid position 285) or Y231X (a substitution of any of a number of amino acids or an unknown amino acid for tyrosine at position 231) in the protein [PMID17391648]. A305E (a substitution of glutamate for alanine at position 305) is the most common mutation in patients who are not of Ashkenazi Jewish descent [PMID17391648] and is often tested for if either partner is not of that genetic lineage.

Familial dysautonomia is not a lysosomal storage disease, but a defect in the autonomic nervous system caused by diminished levels of a protein called IκB kinase complex-associated protein (IKAP), the function of which is not clear, but it may modify transcription. IKAP is made by a gene called inhibitor of κ light polypeptide gene enhancer in

B cells kinase complex-associated protein (*IKBKAP*) on chromosome 9. In familial dysautonomia, there is a mutation in an intronic region of *IKBKAP*. This mutation is IVS20+6T>C (also written as c.2204+6T>C). This is a substitution of cytosine for thymine at position 6 of intron 20, which is also the sixth base after the 2,204th coding nucleotide in the complementary DNA. This mutation causes exon 20 to be deleted from the IKAP protein [PMID11179021, PMID20301359] The carrier frequency of familial dysautonomia in Ashkenazi Jews is about 1 in 30.

Trinucleotide Repeat Disorders

The trinucleotide repeat disorders are the major group within a broader category of disorders in which the basic subunit of a microsatellite, consisting of only a few nucleotides, has the potential to be present in a greater number of repeats with passing generations. Rare examples involve 4, 5, or 12 repeating nucleotides in noncoding segments of DNA. The terms "unstable expanding repeats," "repeat expansion diseases," or "dynamic mutations" are used to describe these disorders [Strachan ISBN978-0815341499].

Trinucleotide repeats are a type of microsatellite. The trinucleotide repeat disorders encompass approximately 12 rare, autosomal dominant, and primarily neurological diseases. These are characterized by microsatellites whose basic unit is composed of 3 nucleotides, but which have a greater number of that basic unit than usual. The repeats are usually located within a gene, and most of them code for a glutamine residue. The greater the number of repeated units, the more severe is the expression of the disease.

Examples of trinucleotide repeat disorders include Huntington disease, fragile X, myotonic dystrophy type 1, spinocerebellar ataxias, spinobulbar muscular atrophy, dentatorubral pallidoluysian atrophy, and Friedreich ataxia. These are all inherited in an autosomal dominant manner, except for spinobulbar muscular atrophy, which is X-linked recessive.

Huntington disease is caused by repeated sequences of CAG, which code for glutamine, in the Huntington gene (*HTT*) on 4p16 [PMID21496570]. More than 36 repeats of CAG in *HTT* will result in Huntington disease. *HTT* spans over 200,000 base pairs and has 67 exons. The normal function of the Huntingtin protein is unknown, but in the disease, the expanded tract of glutamine amino acids causes it to be misshapen, leading to its accumulation within neurons. However, it has not been established whether this accumulation is the primary pathogenic event, leads to another event that is more directly etiologic, or may even be a protective mechanism [PMID21209075].

In fragile X syndrome, there is an amplification of a CGG triplet near the *FMR1* gene on Xq27.3. *FMR1* codes for the FMR1 protein (sometimes called FMRP), which binds to mRNA molecules and facilitates their intracellular localization and translation [PMID16006558]. The triplet CGG does not code for an amino acid, but amplification of the number of CGG repeats (which is normally <45) results in hypermethylation of the promoter region of *FMR1* and decreased transcription [PMID19804849]. Diminished levels of FMR1 protein result in hereditary mental retardation in males, and less commonly, in females.

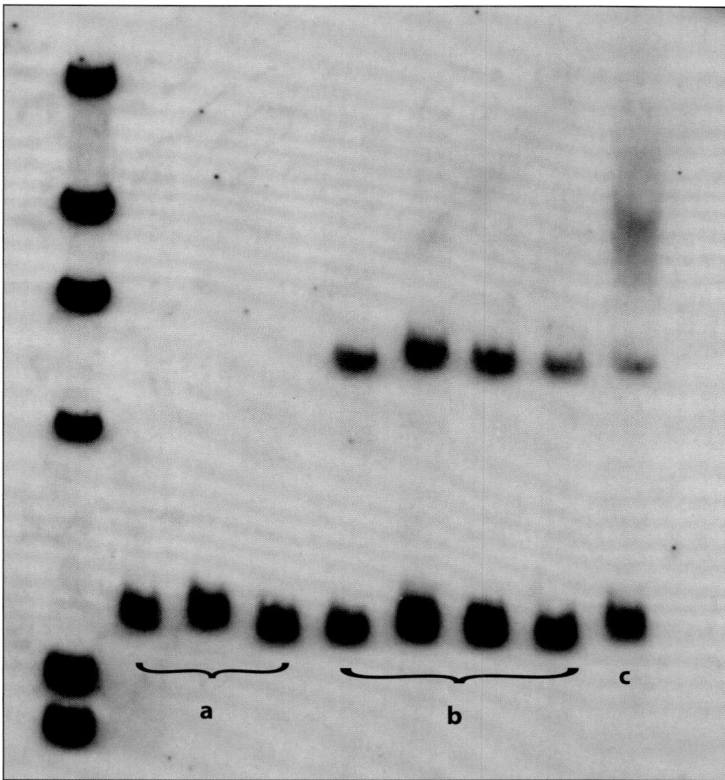

f46.15 Testing for fragile X by testing for methylation of the *FMR1* gene. High levels of methylated DNA indicate a high number of repeats of the CGG triplet. Patient DNA is amplified and subjected to 2 restriction enzymes, one of which will not cleave methylated DNA. The well at far left is a standard.
a is 3 wells from normal males. Because there is no methylated DNA, there is only 1 band, at ~2.8 kB.
b is 4 wells from normal females. Because 1 of the X chromosomes is inactivated by methylation, 1 of the 2 restriction enzymes does not cleave the DNA, resulting in 2 bands: the ~2.8 kB seen in males and a ~5.2 kB band higher on the gel.
c is a sample from a woman who has a high number of repeats of CGG. In addition to the 2 bands expected in females, there is a blurry region in the gel above the ~5.2 kB band resulting from large fragments of DNA because the large number of CGG repeats has resulted in methylation, and 1 of the 2 enzymes could not cleave the methylated DNA.

Testing for fragile X can either be by PCR, testing for the actual size of the repeated segment, or by searching for methylation of *FMR1* by using a methylation-dependent restriction enzyme **f46.15**. The latter method may correlate more closely with the patient's symptoms since methylation directly controls the production of the protein.

Trinucleotide Repeat Disorders Have Anticipation and Grey Zones

It is characteristic of the trinucleotide repeat disorders that the repeated region may undergo expansion after fertilization, either in somatic cells or in germ cells. This results in a clinical phenomenon called anticipation, wherein the age of onset becomes less and the disease becomes more severe in successive generations because the number of repeating units of the 3 base subunit has increased. In some cases, anticipation means that an asymptomatic individual, with a tolerable number of repeats, will have a symptomatic child with a larger number of repeats. Anticipation is a type of variable expression, which is often seen in autosomal dominant conditions.

A grey zone in the trinucleotide repeat disorders is a range of repeating units that is prone to expansion, but not to enough expansion to cause full expression in the next generation. For example, in fragile X, most consider up to 44 repeats of the relevant trinucleotide CGG to be normal and stable, with little likelihood that the number of repeating units will increase in the next generation. 45-54 repeating units is a grey zone that will likely lead to a greater number of repeats in the next generation, but usually not to a degree sufficient to cause full expression in that generation. Prior to 2009, when a case was reported in which 56 repeats expanded sufficiently from mother to son to cause full expression of the disease [PMID19525339], it had been thought that at least 59 repeats were necessary for an expansion to a full clinical manifestation in the next generation. 100 or more repeats is sure to lead to a greater number of repeats in the next generation and is likely to cause full expression in any male children, and 200 repeats will surely do so.

Core Points for Molecular Pathology III: Applications and Diagnoses

- Genetic testing: ethical, legal, and social implications (ELSI) for patient and family members.
  - Regulations from many organizations.
- Oncogenes: normal genes with a gain of function mutation that causes unrestrained cellular proliferation.
  - Account for most somatic mutations that cause cancer.
  - Act in a dominant manner—only 1 copy suffices to cause the cancer.
  - Examples: *MYC*, *HER2*, *ABL*, *C-KIT*, *RET*, *BCL-1* (cyclin D1), *BCL-2*, and the *RAS* family.
- Tumor suppressor genes: normally restrain proliferation.
  - Mutations usually act in a recessive manner because both copies must be lost or nonfunctional.
  - Examples: *p53*, retinoblastoma gene (*RB*), *p16*, *APC* (adenomatous polyposis coli), *CDH1* (E-cadherin gene), *VHL* (von Hippel Lindau), *NF1*, *MSH2*, *MLH1*, *MSH6* (DNA mismatch repair proteins), *BCL-2*, *BRCA1*, and *BRCA2*.
  - But most hereditary cancer syndromes are caused by mutations in tumor suppressor genes, not oncogenes.
    - Demonstrate autosomal dominant inheritance because a germline mutation of one tumor suppressor gene is strongly associated with a second mutation in a somatic line of the other tumor suppressor gene.
- DNA testing offers much faster and more sensitive method of identifying infectious agents.
  - Also for detecting drug-resistant strains, such as MRSA and VRE.
  - And monitoring response to therapy.
  - There are many targets of nucleic acid amplification—most often ribosomal RNA or DNA codes for rRNA (rDNA).
  - DNA techniques have also permitted strain typing for public health and epidemiology.
- 4 major stages in which the cell cycle is regulated: entry into the S phase (the G1-S checkpoint), in the S phase, entry into mitosis (the G2-M checkpoint), and in mitosis.
- Phase I of drug metabolism: oxidation, reduction, or hydrolysis.
  - Often mediated by enzymes of the cytochrome P450 system (CYP), and a number of additional enzyme systems have also been described.
- Phase II conjugates the drug to another compound, for greater water solubility.
- Pharmacogenetics (PGX): assessment of DNA polymorphisms that affect drug metabolism by coding for variant forms of the enzymes needed to metabolize the drug.
  - Allows for adjustment of drug doses to facilitate therapeutic effect and minimize side effects.
  - A foundation of personalized medicine.
- Microsatellites are used in identity testing, such as in paternity testing and judicial applications.
  - Paternity index (PI) is calculated for each of a number of well-understood microsatellites.
    - For each microsatellite, the PI is the likelihood that the alleged father, upon mating with the mother, could have fathered a child who has the observed number of repeating units in the microsatellite relative to the likelihood that a random man of the same race and ethnicity could have done so.
    - Combined paternity index (CPI) is the product of the individual PIs and is used to calculate the probability of paternity.
- Single nucleotide polymorphisms (SNPs): may result in a premature stop codon or an incorrect amino acid.
  - Major cause of DNA variation.
  - Until direct DNA sequencing becomes practical for all applications, SNP testing can be a substitute.
- Cystic fibrosis: prototype of a genetic disease for which effective screening is available.
  - Some genetic diseases can be screened during pregnancy via amniocentesis or chorionic villus sampling.
  - Testing for fetal nucleic acid in maternal plasma is a frontier.
- Ashkenazi Jewish patients: testing particularly important because the forced relocations, population bottlenecks, and genetic isolation of that group has resulted in founder mutations.
- Trinucleotide repeat disorders: an increased number of a 3 base pair subunit in microsatellites.
  - Screening is a form of microsatellite analysis.
  - Subject to anticipation, whereby the number of repeating units may increase in succeeding generations,
    - and if there is expression, it is often more severe and occurs at an earlier age.

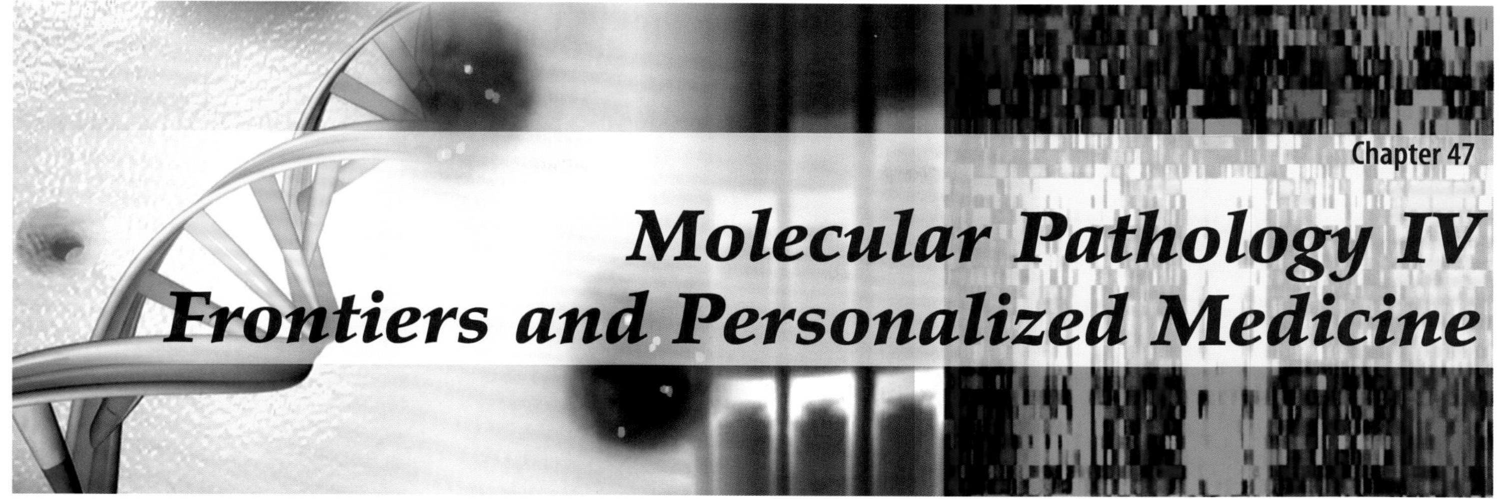

The future has come upon us with a suddenness that is breathtaking and exciting, but also bewildering and disconcerting. Here, we discuss how continued developments in molecular biology will change how medicine of the near future will be practiced.

Epigenetic Regulation of the Genome

"Epigenetic regulation" refers to long-term regulation of DNA expression that does not depend directly on the DNA sequence. The key word is "directly," for the processes of epigenetics involve enzymes, which are ultimately specified by the DNA sequence. Indeed, there can be no regulation of DNA and no biological activity that is not ultimately in some way dependent on the sequence of base pairs in DNA.

Given that the Human Genome Project found that there are only approximately 30,000 genes (about the same number as in rodents) instead of the expected 100,000, much of our complexity must reside in how those genes are regulated, and epigenetic mechanisms undoubtedly account for much of the gene regulation that impacts phenotype.

Unlike regulation that is directly controlled by DNA sequence, epigenetic regulation can be modified by environmental factors and may be amenable to therapy. The primary forms of epigenetic regulation of DNA expression include modification of histones, DNA methylation (which prevents transcription, especially if it occurs at promoters), and RNA interference, which includes microRNAs. RNA interference was discussed in Chapter 44, so we will now consider histone modification and DNA methylation.

Histone modification often takes the form of acetylation or methylation. In histones, acetylation is the better characterized of these processes and is known to facilitate transcription and increase gene expression by uncoiling DNA and, indeed, is often essential for transcription [PMID21234331]. In most cases, acetylation of histones works with chromatin remodeling complexes to allow greater access of transcription factors and enzymes to the double helix.

Histone modification is often studied by chromatin immunoprecipitation. In immunoprecipitation, an antibody specific to the protein of interest is added to a solution or a lysate of cells. Subsequent capture of the antibody (for example, by passing it by a substrate to which is bound an antibody to that antibody) will also capture the protein. In chromatin immunoprecipitation, proteins known to bind to DNA (such as histones, transcription factors, etc) are cross-linked to the DNA, usually by formaldehyde (such cross-linking is necessary because DNA-associated proteins bind with low affinity). The cells are then lysed, and the lysate is sonicated to break the DNA into small fragments. The antibody to the protein of interest is then added, and an antibody capture step is performed, allowing the protein and the DNA to which it has bound to be separated f47.1. Although useful in many studies of protein-DNA interaction, chromatin immunoprecipitation has been particularly useful in studying histones, their interaction with DNA, and their modification of transcription.

Unlike acetylation, methylation usually works on DNA (especially promoters), not on histones, and usually diminishes transcription. Eukaryotic DNA is not normally methylated, but some parts of the genome, such as repetitive regions, pseudogenes, and transposable elements are heavily methylated. Methylation usually occurs at CpG islands (CpG indicates that there are consecutive cytosine and guanine bases on one strand, as opposed to a C-G pair involving both strands). The base cytosine, over the course of evolution, has tended to become methylated, then deaminated, resulting in thymine. Vertebrate DNA therefore has much less of the dinucleotide CpG than bacteria since many such areas have become TpG. The CpG that remains is often clustered into CpG islands, which are associated with promoters.

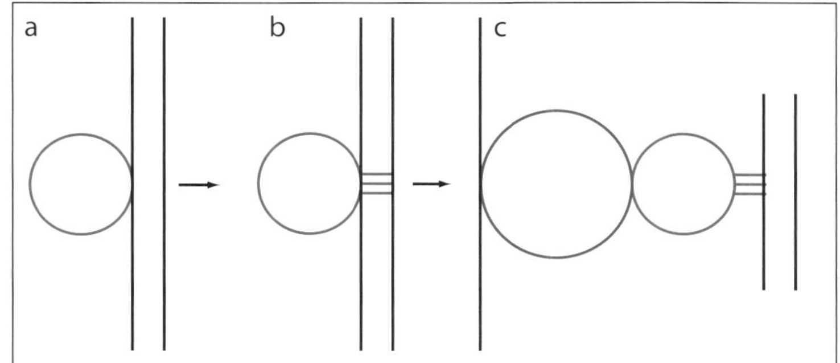

f47.1 Chromatin immunoprecipitation. In **a**, a protein, such as a histone or a transcription factor, denoted as a red circle, is loosely bound to DNA. In **b**, the binding has been made stronger by the addition of an agent such as formalin. In **c**, after breaking up of the cell and fragmentation of the DNA, the lysate is passed through a column to which is bound an antibody, depicted as a blue circle, to the protein of interest. The antibody captures the protein and the DNA to which it has bound, allowing them to be isolated and studied.

ISBN 978-089189-5886

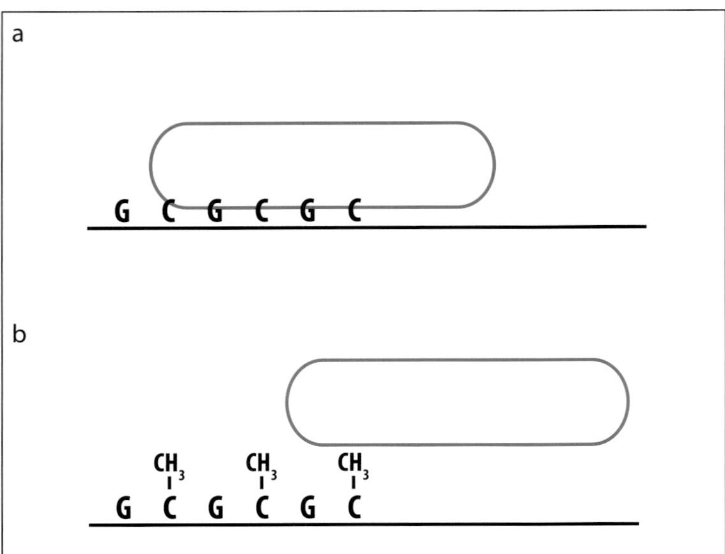

f47.2 **a** GpC island in a promoter. The transcription factor, depicted as a red capsule, can bind normally. **b** Methylation of the cytosine bases in a GpC island. The transcription factor cannot bind, and transcription does not occur.

Methyl groups may bind to the cytosines in CpG islands of promoters, preventing the binding of transcription factors and preventing transcription f47.2.

Detection of methylation requires that methylated and unmethylated DNA be discriminated, and that the methylated form then be amplified. Methylation can be detected by the synchronized use of 2 restriction enzymes, HpaII and MspI. Both of these cleave CCGG, but the former cuts only an unmethylated sequence, whereas the latter cuts both methylated and unmethylated sequences, resulting in 2 different products if there has been methylation.

Another means of detecting methylated sequences is to use sodium bisulfite, which converts cytosine to uracil, but only if the cytosine is not methylated. This results in a change in sequence that permits specific polymerase chain reaction (PCR) primers to distinguish the methylated from unmethylated DNA based on the presence or absence of uracil. In the Methylight detection system [PMID10734209], sodium bisulfite is used, after which the DNA is amplified and detected by fluorescence-based qPCR. One can also sequence after bisulfite treatment [PMID19541921].

DNA methylation can also be studied by methylated DNA immunoprecipitation, which is similar in principle to chromatin immunoprecipitation except that the capture antibody is directed against 5'-methylcytidine instead of a protein and cross-linking is not performed. Newer methods, including microarrays and multiplex ligation-dependent probe amplification (MLPA), are also available to study DNA methylation.

Methylation is an integral part of differentiation. Stem cells experience methylation, with subsequent silencing of much of its genome, as they differentiate. The function of DNA methylation in the differentiated cell is not well understood, and the number of methylated genes is small. But methylated genes are disproportionately concerned with the regulation of cell growth and DNA methylation is implicated in some malignancies. Most cancer cells have sharply diminished overall methylation, making them metabolically more active, but the DNA of the promoters of tumor suppressor genes may be hypermethylated in cancers, reducing the expression of these genes. A small number of genes have been identified whose hypermethylation is associated with neoplasia [PMID17167179]. The role of hypermethylation of the tumor suppressor gene *MLH1* in HNPCC was discussed in Chapter 46. Hypermethylation of a number of tumor suppressor genes, including *BRCA1* and *P16*, has been shown in sporadic breast cancer [PMID17264521].

Likewise, *hypomethylation* of an oncogene's promoter could account for its overexpression. Clarification of the role of methylation in malignancy is critical since methylation does not involve the actual DNA sequence and is therefore amenable to therapy.

Fragile X is a trinucleotide repeat disorder, with an excessive number of repeats of CGG. These excessive repeats methylate and transcriptionally silence the *FMR* gene, whose product, FMR1 protein (or FMRP) is important in learning and development, making fragile X both a trinucleotide repeat disorder and an example of inappropriate methylation.

Another consequence of methylation is imprinted genes. Imprinting involves a small number of genes that are differentially methylated in parental germ cells, such that the allele from one parent is methylated and inactive, while the allele from the other parent is unmethylated and active. In imprinting, the cell somehow recognizes which parent a gene came from and then specifically silences 1 copy of that gene. Imprinting is a form of monoallelic expression that is dependent on parental origin. Imprinting may be differentially expressed in different tissues and is therefore a source of phenotypic heterogeneity.

Imprinting is completely reset in gametes. In meiosis, methylation is removed and reestablished. By an unknown mechanism, the person's gender determines whether a particular gene in a gamete is imprinted or not. Once this decision is made, imprinting becomes a permanent feature of the gene. This can even be tracked across generations, where a gene is alternately turned on and off as a man has a daughter who has a son, etc.

Among vertebrates, only animals with placentas exhibit imprinting. Currently, about 100 imprinted genes are known [PMID20822494]. Neither the purpose nor the mechanism of imprinting is well understood, but inappropriate imprinting is an occasional cause of several rare syndromes, such as Prader-Willi syndrome and Angelman syndrome. Failure to inherit a working *paternal* copy of a gene or set of genes on chromosome 15 causes Prader-Willi syndrome, while failure to inherit a functional *maternal* copy at the same gene locus causes the much more serious Angelman syndrome.

75% of cases of Prader-Willi result from del15q11.2-q13 of paternal DNA, and approximately 25% of these cases are caused by the very rare phenomenon of uniparental disomy (UPD), in which all or part of both chromosomes 15 come only from the mother. The most common cause of this UPD is nondisjunction. While microdeletions and UPD are the most common causes of Prader-Willi syndrome, less common causes include gene mutations and abnormal methylation (ie, abnormalities in imprinting) [PMID20803659]. Abnormalities of the small nuclear ribonucleoprotein polypeptide N gene (*SNRPN*) are implicated in many cases of Prader-Willi. In normal patients, 1 copy of *SNRPN* should be methylated, but in some cases of Prader-Willi, both copies are methylated [PMID20803659].

As is the case for Prader-Willi, most cases of Angelman syndrome stem from del15q11.2-q13, but it is a deletion in the *maternal* allele. The specific gene involved in Angelman syndrome is *UBE3A*, which codes for ubiquitin protein ligase 3A, the enzyme that attaches ubiquitin to the protein targeted for destruction, so that it will be channeled to the proteasome to be degraded [PMID20803659]. In addition to deletions, about 5% of cases of Angelman syndrome are caused by UPD, such as may result from nondisjunction (paternal UPD rather than the maternal UPD that is a rare cause of Prader-Willi). About 10% of cases of Angelman syndrome result from a mutation in the maternal copy of *UBE3A* and another 5% are imprinting errors (inappropriate methylation of the maternal allele of *UBE3A*).

Cases of Prader-Willi and Angelman syndromes that are caused by microdeletions can be detected by FISH, but because FISH cannot determine on which chromosome the microdeletion has occurred, only clinical correlation can distinguish between the 2 syndromes if a microdeletion is found. FISH cannot identify cases of Prader-Willi syndrome or Angelman syndrome that are caused by UPD, mutation, or imprinting.

Another condition that can result from imprinting is Beckwith-Wiedemann syndrome. A number of abnormalities have been found in 11p15 in Beckwith-Wiedemann syndrome. About half of cases are secondary to a methylation defect in insulin-like growth factor 2, and 20% of cases result from paternal UPD of 11p15 [PMID20803657].

Another possible example of imprinting, or actually, a possible *release* from imprinting, is Rett syndrome, an inherited form of mental retardation that is X-linked dominant and, therefore, found almost exclusively in females. In Rett syndrome, mutations in the *MECP2* gene on Xq28 cause a defect in the protein product, MeCP2. Little is known of MeCP2, but it is known that it binds methylated DNA at CpG sites and recruits histone deacetylases [PMID19058783]. Because DNA methylation and histone deacetylation both diminish transcription, Rett syndrome may be caused by inappropriate activation of genes that should be silent.

Imprinting is one cause of monoallelic expression. Additional causes of monoallelic expression include microdeletions in one chromosome, UPD secondary to nondisjunction, loss of function mutations affecting only 1 allele, and the inactivation of one X chromosome in females (called lyonization after its discover, Mary Lyon). Lyonization is caused by DNA methylation, and unlike imprinting, is initially random, but once the exclusion of one parental X chromosome is made in early development, the pattern is maintained in all daughter cells.

The Human Epigenome Project is a public and private consortium that is attempting to identify the methylation positions in the genome, and their variation and consequences [PMID15347255]. Early data suggest that methylation variable positions (MVPs) may function in a manner analogous to single nucleotide polymorphisms (SNPs) [PMID19004867]. In addition, some SNPs may themselves show allele-specific methylation.

Transcription: Key to Complexity

Functional genomics and transcriptomics are already suggesting that transcription, not translation, may be the key to complexity. The sequencing of the human genome was a triumph, but as is always the case, a triumph is a beginning. Sequencing is only the beginning of the task of understanding the nature of DNA and its products. Full annotation, composed of structural and functional annotation as discussed in Chapter 45, is the new frontier. Functional annotation is essentially synonymous with functional genomics and is the study of the function and interaction of all RNA and protein molecules, including the collections of mRNAs (the transcriptome), noncoding RNAs, and all proteins (the proteome). Functional genomics encompasses transcriptomics and proteomics and will explain the enormous amount of DNA that does not code for proteins or ribosomal RNA. Full annotation and functional genomics will allow us to truly understand the 3 billion base pairs that determine who we are.

ENCODE (Encyclopedia of DNA Elements) is an international consortium intended to identify all functional parts of the genome. ENCODE began in 2004 with an attempt to take a small fraction of the genome (about 1%) and characterize every RNA molecule that is transcribed from it, whether it is translated or not [PMID19920125]. The project was expanded to address the entire genome in 2007 and has also expanded to study every function pertaining to transcription, including transcription factors, histones, and chromatin properties during transcription. Some of the best results have come from studies of *Drosophila* [PMID21177974].

ENCODE will be more challenging than the Human Genome Project for many reasons, one of which is that noncoding RNA does not have distinct stop and start codons. The results of the pilot project have already changed the way DNA expression is understood [PMID17567987]. It has been learned, for example, that while only a small portion of DNA is eventually translated into protein, most of it is transcribed into RNA. Nongenic transcription refers to RNA that is never translated. Introns, constituting a third of the genome, are transcribed but not translated. Transfer RNA, ribosomal RNA, and microRNA are additional types of noncoding RNA. But even allowing for these forms of RNA, there are still thousands of genes (defining a gene as a discrete area of DNA that is transcribed) that are not translated. These are called RNA genes or noncoding RNA. RNA genes appear to be involved in regulation of gene expression [PMID16183745, PMID19859665].

Early results from ENCODE have also shown that often, both strands of DNA are transcribed, whereas it had been thought that only 1 strand was transcribed. It has long been known that promoter and enhancers are physically separate from the actual transcribed DNA, but ENCODE has shown that some of the exons themselves may be separate from the bulk of the DNA that is transcribed. Early ENCODE data has also confirmed that some exons are transferred between genes (exon shuffling). ENCODE has shown that DNA transcription works more like an alphabet—with combinations from noncontiguous locations and the use of components in multiple genes—than a simple linear assembly line.

Only about 2% of the genome actually encodes for specific proteins. It has been proposed that phenotypic variation in species comes as much or more from differences in RNA as

ISBN 978-089189-5886

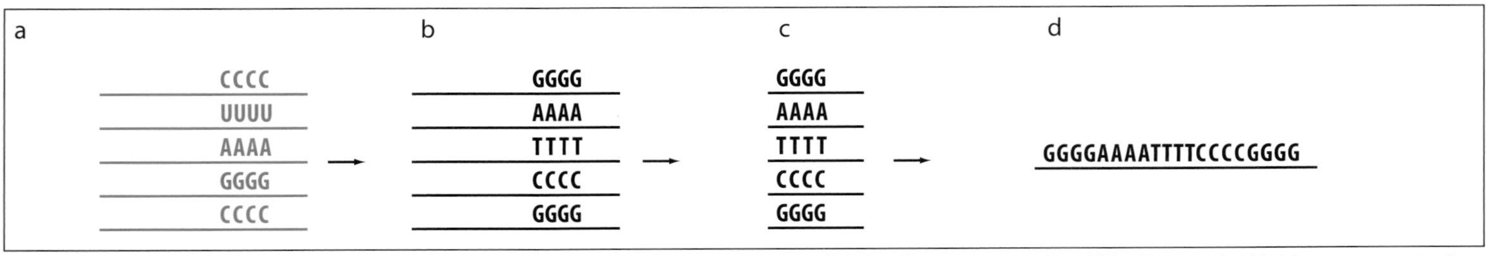

a		b		c		d
CCCC		GGGG		GGGG		
UUUU		AAAA		AAAA		
AAAA	→	TTTT	→	TTTT	→	GGGGAAAATTTTCCCCGGGG
GGGG		CCCC		CCCC		
CCCC		GGGG		GGGG		

f47.3 A simplified example of serial analysis of gene expression (SAGE). In **a**, there are 5 mRNA molecules, for each of which a 4-base sequence is indicated. We will assume that this 4-base sequence uniquely identifies each mRNA molecule. In **b**, these mRNA molecules have been converted to cDNA by reverse transcriptase. In **c**, a restriction enzyme has isolated the 4-base sequences of the cDNA molecules. In **d**, these sequences are concatenated into 1 DNA molecule, which has been sequenced. Because the sequence GGGG occurs twice, at each end of the DNA molecule, there must have been 2 copies of the mRNA molecule containing the sequence CCCC, indicating that this mRNA has been transcribed at twice the amount of the other mRNA molecules.

from differences in DNA sequence or in proteins [PMID11713189]. In fact, though the number of genes that code for proteins varies much less with complexity than would be expected, the amount of noncoding RNA—much of which is apparently regulatory—*does* seem to correspond with complexity [PMID16651366]. ENCODE results so far support the concept that the origin of our complexity is likely to be at the transcriptional level rather than at the translational level.

These developments have shifted the functional unit of DNA away from a unit that is significant because it is ultimately *translated* and toward a unit that is important because it is *transcribed*. Even this can only be an incomplete solution because only about 1/6 of the genome is transcribed into mRNA. We may eventually find that a "gene" is a unit of DNA with a specific function that may be regulation, genetic variation, transcription without translation, or, in a minority of cases, transcription with translation.

Another immediate issue in functional genomics is that in some way that we do not understand, many portions of DNA must be capable of participating in the production of multiple proteins. This seems particularly true since there are only about 30,000 human genes, instead of the 100,000 that had been thought.

Study of Gene Expression Begins Functional Genomics

Gene expression (ie, which portions of DNA are transcribed and to what extent) can be studied by or comparative genomic hybridization or microarrays, as discussed in Chapter 45. Another useful technique for studying gene expression is serial analysis of gene expression (SAGE), wherein many RNA transcripts can be analyzed simultaneously [PMID7570003]. In SAGE, multiple RNA molecules are converted to complementary double-stranded DNA. A portion of each cDNA, called a tag, is then obtained by restriction endonuclease digestion. Although a tag is only 9-15 base pairs long, it usually uniquely identifies the mRNA transcript from which it was derived (rarely, different genes may have enough homology to share a tag). The tags are then joined together, often through linker DNA, to generate a cDNA concatemer. This concatemer is sequenced, and software is used to count the number of separate tags. The more times a particular portion of DNA has been transcribed, the more copies of its mRNA will exist, the more copies of cDNA will be made, and the more tags of that cDNA will be in the final concatemer **f47.3**. The number of times that each tag is present indicates the level of expression of that gene.

Yet another method of studying gene expression employs a massively parallel format, similar to that used in DNA sequencing. In gene expression analysis, massively parallel format is called massively parallel signature sequencing (MPSS). MPSS can be used to quantify the number of mRNA molecules that are transcribed from each gene [PMID10835600, PMID15251069]. In large measure, MPSS follows the same principles as in its use in DNA sequencing. mRNA is converted to double-stranded cDNA, which is then cleaved by an endonuclease and cloned in a plasmid vector in such a way that each cDNA molecule is attached to a 32-base pair tag. The use of a 32-base pair tag permits almost 17 million distinct tags. This generates a library of cDNA inserts, each of which has a unique 32-base pair tag. These fragments are then PCR-amplified and exposed to myriad microbeads, each of which contains 1 and only 1 of the nearly 17 million tags, but it contains that one tag in great numbers. The result is that each microbead will capture only 1 of the millions of cDNA molecules, but it will capture many copies of it.

In the subsequent sequencing phase, a type IIs endonuclease digests the cDNA sequences on the beads in such a way as to produce an overhang of 4 base pairs. The bead is then exposed to a set of labeled adaptor molecules of known sequence, one of which will hybridize to any 4 base pair overhanging sequence. The adaptor that hybridizes is identified by its fluorescence and indicates the sequence of the overhang. The adaptor is then removed with an endonuclease, with the generation of another 4 base overhang, and the process is repeated with another set of labeled adaptors, one of which will hybridize to any 4 base overhang. Because the sequence of the adaptors is known and because that sequence indicates the sequence of the 4 base overhang, sequential iterations of the process provide information on the sequence of the cDNA on the bead. Although only a small number of bases can be determined from each bead, the additive information permits the sequencing of long sequences, and MPSS can study nearly all of the mRNA in the cell. An advantage of MPSS is that the information is collected and analyzed digitally.

As is the case for genomics, there are a number of databases concerned with transcriptomics. In addition to the Stanford Microarray Database, these include ArrayExpress repository at the European Bioinformatics Institute (EBI), Gene Expression Omnibus at the National Center for Biotechnology Information (NCBI), and SymAtlas of the Novartis Research Foundation. In addition, the Jackson Laboratory in Maine operates the Gene Expression Database, which is dedicated to data obtained from mice.

Proteomics

Although only a small minority of DNA is transcribed and translated, there are still many thousands of proteins in each cell. Understanding the definitive structure, function, and interaction of all of these proteins—proteomics—is much more complex and will be much more difficult than the human genome project. There are many good reviews on proteomics, one of which is that by Wong et al [PMID19385940].

The first challenge of proteomics is understanding the precise 3-dimensional (3D) structure of proteins. Knowing a protein's amino acid sequence (the primary structure) is the first step in understanding its 3D structure, and an additional advantage of the sequencing of the genome is that it affords an excellent estimate of the amino acid sequence of many proteins. However, a protein's 3D conformation can be only partially elucidated from the amino acid sequence because we have a poor understanding of how a known amino acid sequence will fold in 3 dimensions in vivo. We also have an incomplete understanding of the many posttranslational modifications (ie, glycosylation, methylation, phosphorylation, etc) that proteins must undergo to be functional, and how these modifications affect 3D structure and interactions.

The second challenge is the determination of the function of a protein and how it carries out that function. The amino acid sequence of a protein is a good start in understanding its probable function, but it is important to find a protein of known function with a closely related structure or to be able to place the protein in a known family. Sometimes, a clue to the function of a protein can be obtained by studying its interaction with other proteins. The third great challenge of proteomics is to elucidate how multiple proteins affiliate and interact.

As is the case with studies involving DNA, many techniques are used in proteomics, often in combination. Immunohistochemistry and fluorescent tagging of proteins can determine the presence or absence of a protein, and its location within the cell, and furnish an estimate of the amount of the protein, but they provide no insight into the structure, function, and interactions of the protein, and they can only be used for proteins that have previously been characterized and to which a monoclonal antibody or a fluorescent tag are available.

A commonly used technique is 2-dimensional (2D) electrophoresis, in which proteins are separated on the basis of both size and charge f47.4. Depending on the protein's amino acid sequence and 3D structure, there will be one pH at which it is overall neutral. In the first electrophoretic procedure, termed "isoelectric focusing," the proteins will migrate in a pH gradient until they come to rest at the one pH at which they have no net charge (the isoelectric point). The proteins, which form a horizontal row based on their *charges*, are then treated with sodium dodecyl sulfate (SDS), a negatively charged compound that denatures the proteins and conveys a negative charge to the them (SDS is also called sodium lauryl sulfate and is the active ingredient in bath soap). The denatured proteins are then subjected to another electric current at right angles to the first, so that they run vertically. Because of the negative charge conveyed by the SDS, the proteins migrate towards the positive electrode in accordance with their *size*, not their charge (SDS is not needed in nucleic acid electrophoresis because the phosphate groups make nucleic acids intrinsically negatively charged). Whereas many proteins will have the same size, only very rarely will 2 proteins have both the same isoelectric point and the same size f47.4. In 2D electrophoresis, proteins that eventually settle in very close proximity are likely to be related and may represent posttranslational modification of a single protein.

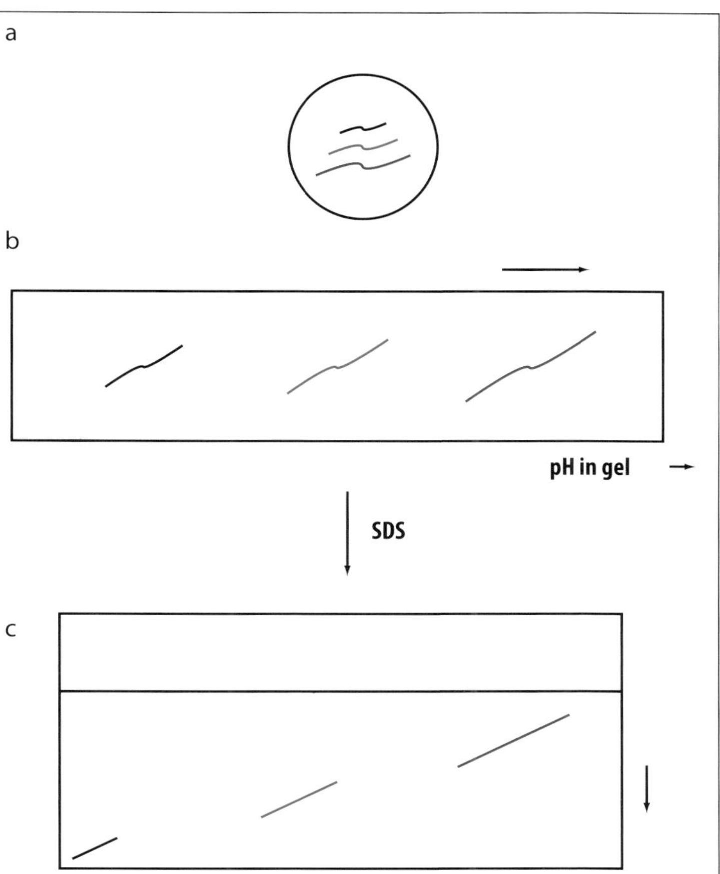

f47.4 2-dimensional electrophoresis. In **a**, there are a collection of 3 proteins that differ from each other in both charge and size. In **b**, these proteins, in their native state, are subjected to an electric field that causes them to migrate to the right in a gel of increasing pH. The arrow indicated the direction of migration. The proteins come to rest at a point where they have no net charge at a particular pH. In **c**, the gel has been layered on top of another gel containing SDS, which separates the proteins into their subunits. They migrate downward in an electric field and are now separated by their size, with the smaller fragments moving further into the gel. The proteins are maximally separated.

Unlike immunohistochemistry, 2D electrophoresis can identify previously unknown proteins. 2D electrophoresis is often combined with mass spectrometry (MS). For example, a protein may be run on a 2D gel, after which the band is cut out and the protein is digested with trypsin, then ionized and analyzed by MS.

2D difference in gel electrophoresis (2D DIGE) is a variant on 2D gel electrophoresis in which 2 protein samples (typically a control sample and the sample to be tested, such as serum from a normal patient and from one with a particular tumor) are labeled with fluorochromes of differently colors. The investigator can lightly label the proteins with a fluorochrome that binds to only some of the lysine residues or heavily label them with a fluorochrome that binds to all of the cysteine residues. The former approach causes minimal interference with the electrophoretic migration of the proteins, but the latter method is more sensitive. After 2D electrophoresis, the gel is scanned at the wavelengths of the 2 fluorochromes. Statistical analysis can furnish information about differences in the quantity of any protein (a spot on the gel) between the 2 samples. One may find, for example, that a given protein is expressed much more in a tumor sample than in a control. Because monoclonal antibodies are not used in the identification of proteins by 2D DIGE, it is well suited for the discovery of previously unknown proteins that are expressed by a neoplasm or an experimental state. Any unusual proteins found in 2D DIGE (eg, those that are expressed in the tumor sample but not in the normal sample) can be cut out of the gel and studied by MS. A particularly exciting development has been the ability to combine 2D DIGE with laser microdissection of patient samples in paraffin blocks [PMID17406554].

Chromatography (of which there are several kinds) and x-ray crystallography are among the many other techniques in proteomics. Magnetic resonance imaging, commonly used in radiology, can also be used to study the structure of individual macromolecules [PMID21214860]. These techniques are often used in combination and can be used both to study proteins and to purify them so that they can be studied by other methods. Another method of removing unwanted proteins is immunodepletion, wherein antibodies bind to unwanted proteins, facilitating their removal.

Mass Spectrometry (MS)

MS is often used as a final technique after proteins have been studied by other methods. There are 2 reasons for employing MS as a final technique. First, the proteins are vaporized and ionized in MS and are unsuitable for further studies afterward. Second, MS requires a highly purified sample, necessitating other techniques as preliminary measures. While many techniques are used to purify samples for MS, gas and liquid chromatography are often employed.

MS determines properties of proteins by measuring the charge-to-mass ratio, and therefore the proteins to be analyzed—however they are obtained and whatever previous studies may have been performed on them—must be ionized. These ions are positively charged and migrate in an electric field to a negative grid. As they migrate to the grid, the ions are exposed to a magnetic field. Moving charged particles follow a curved path in a magnetic field, and the degree of curvature depends on their charge and mass. Protein molecules of different charges and masses follow curved pathways of different radii to the detector. The radius of curvature permits a determination of the charge-to-mass ratio of the protein molecule. Because different molecules contact the detector at different locations, it is also possible to physically separate and count the molecules **f47.5**.

There are 3 major parts to a mass spectrometer. The first part ionizes the sample. The second part uses electric and magnetic fields to sort the ions, and the third part is a detector. In tandem MS, the output from one MS becomes the input to another.

There are a number of techniques to achieve the necessary ionization for MS, including electrospray ionization (ESI), matrix-assisted laser desorption ionization (MALDI), surface-enhanced laser desorption/ionization (SELDI), collision-induced dissociation (CID), and electron transfer dissociation (ETD) [PMID20029632, PMID19082706, PMID19086863, PMID21698312].

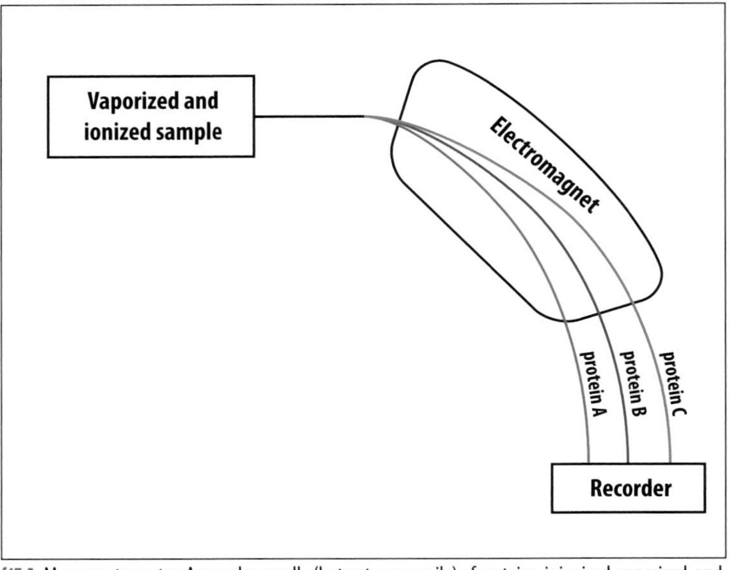

f47.5 Mass spectrometry. A sample, usually (but not necessarily) of proteins, is ionized, vaporized, and accelerated in an electric field and then subjected to a magnetic field. This causes the molecules to assume a curved path, the radius of which depends on the molecule's charge-to-mass ratio.

In ESI, a solution of proteins is passed through a metal-coated capillary tube and subjected to a high voltage. This voltage causes the formation of positively charged droplets emerging in a fine spray that can be studied by MS.

In MALDI, a light-absorbing compound is added to the protein solution, after which the solution is spotted onto a metal plate. After evaporation, the protein molecules are embedded in a crystalline matrix composed of the light-absorbing compound. The application of a laser then gently generates ions (the light absorbing compound protects the protein from complete destruction by the laser and ensures gentle ionization).

MALDI has also been adapted for use with tissue samples, called imaging MS (MALDI IMS) [PMID17901873]. Most applications of MALDI IMS involve frozen sections, as formalin causes precipitation and cross-linking that make the attainment of an ionized sample difficult. However, enzymatic digestion has been successfully used to counteract these effects of formalin and permit formalin-fixed, paraffin-embedded sections to be used [PMID18712763, PMID17291023].

SELDI is a variation of MALDI in which the protein solution is allowed to dry onto a selective surface. Some proteins will adhere, while others will not and are removed by washing. After washing, a matrix is applied. This matrix then crystallizes with the adherent proteins and the sample is exposed to a laser which ionizes the protein.

In CID, a neutral gas is collided with the protein to cleave the peptide bond and produce ions. In ETD, electrons are transferred from anions to the proteins. These electrons break the peptide bond in a different way from that used in CID. While both CID and ETD have advantages and disadvantages, ETD preserves posttranslational modifications of proteins [PMID21542796].

In MS, there are several technologies to analyze the ions once they have been generated. 2 of the most common are time of flight (TOF) and quadrupole. In TOF MS, the ions are accelerated in an electromagnetic field, then allowed to drift to a detector. Drift time (TOF) is a function of mass. Ions generated by MALDI and SELDI are often analyzed by the TOF method (MALDI-TOF and SELDI-TOF). In quadrupole MS, the ions pass between 4 parallel metals rods. At any instant, one diagonally opposed pair is positively charged, and the other is negatively charged. These charges are rapidly alternated, so that only ions of a particular mass-to-charge ratio will pass through the rods to reach the detector. Ions with other mass-to-charge ratios will collide with the rods and will not be detected [PMID21917684].

In the detection phase of MS, the detector can be broadly set in a comprehensive analysis if the identities of the analytes are not known, but more targeted parameters are used if a specific analyte is sought.

Like 2D electrophoresis, MS can identify proteins that were not previously known. MS began as a qualitative method, but quantitative applications are now promising [PMID19957301]. In proteomic studies of neoplasms, it will hopefully be possible not only to ascertain if a tumor produces a particular protein, perhaps identifying proteins that are unique to particular tumors, but also to determine abnormal amounts or ratios of proteins that may indicate a specific type of neoplasm.

MS is 1 of several techniques that offer the opportunity to obtain potential biomarkers directly from tissue samples [PMID19385940], but candidate biomarker proteins must be confirmed by additional methods such as immunohistochemistry in tumor tissue and ultimately by correlation studies of patients and controls.

In addition to potential applications in proteomics and tumor biomarkers, MALDI-TOF has been proposed as a means of identifying microorganisms, since each organism has a unique proteomic profile [PMID11835304].

Medical applications of MS are not limited to proteins. Both MALDI-TOF [PMID17082249] and SELDI-TOF [PMID20186013] have been used in SNP analysis of PCR-amplified DNA fragments, and MALDI-TOF has been developed for screening in cystic fibrosis [PMID20616359]. A multiplex MS assay to simultaneously screen for multiple mutations shows promise in identifying the many cancer cases that have multiple mutations [PMID21726664].

As is the case for genomics and transcriptomics, comparison to an ever-increasing collection of bioinformatic databases of known protein structure and function is important for interpretation of data in proteomics [PMID21370076]. These databases are devoted to slightly different aspects of proteomics and differ in their precise content, their structure, and how they are accessed. For example, there are several databases that are dedicated to helping investigators with data obtained from MS. Pfam and Interpro are primarily devoted to the tabulation of data concerning protein domains and families (a domain is a part of a protein that can function and evolve independently from the rest of the protein; domains are typically involved in the binding of key components, such as metals, ions, coenzymes, etc). The Pfam database has been useful in demonstrating the antiquity and evolution of the immunoglobulin superfamily [PMID19614588]. The Structural Classification of Proteins (SCOP) database also deals with protein domains. The Families of Structurally Similar Proteins (FSSP) database is devoted to proteins that are related and contain similar regions. The Worldwide Protein Data Bank (wwPDB, available at http://www.wwpdb.org/) is the world's largest store of information regarding protein structure and is primarily concerned with the 3D structure of proteins. It consists of a number of interacting databases, foremost among which are the Protein Databank (RCSB PDB, available at http://www.rcsb.org) and the BMRB from the United States, the PDBe from Europe, and the PDBj from Japan. The Proteome Browser from the University of California at Santa Cruz is linked to that institution's Genome Browser database, allowing investigators to examine information from DNA and protein simultaneously.

Some protein databases have merged. Uniprot is a large database devoted to protein sequence and function, obtained by the merging of several other databases. As such mergers continue, we can expect more consolidation, as has been the case for the major genomics databases. An idea of the many types of protein databases can be obtained by visiting http://www.ebi.ac.uk/Databases/protein.html or http://biology.unm.edu/biology/maggieww/Public_Html/ANALYSIS.HTM.

Any interested individual can participate in proteomics through 2 distributive computing projects that allow a personal computer to assist in calculating protein structure when it is in screensaver mode. Middleware software is then used to assemble the data from the myriad personal computers into a form that is usable to the researchers. The Folding@Home project (http://folding.stanford.edu/) concentrates on protein folding and interactions. The structure and function of proteins is one of the projects of World Community Grid (http://www.worldcommunitygrid.org/). There are a number of others of equal interest and importance.

Proteomics

Proteomics offers the opportunity to identify collections of proteins that are associated with a neoplasm rather than a single protein. Protein markers in the serum have long been used to monitor certain types of cancers (eg, PSA for prostate carcinoma or CA125 for some types of ovarian carcinoma) and were the initial foray into the molecular classification of tumors. The best serum protein markers for any disease are those proteins that are normally secreted, as these have the best chance of being detected in the blood. Some of the best known serum tumor markers, such as CEA and CA125, are actually membrane-bound proteins that are not normally secreted. The effectiveness of serum assays depends on both the uniqueness of the protein to a particular tissue and on the tumor's propensity to secrete significantly more of the protein than normal tissue. For example, CEA is elevated in a variety of neoplastic and nonneoplastic conditions. On the other hand, PSA is nearly specific to prostatic tissue but is secreted by the normal prostate almost as much as by prostatic carcinoma. While proteins such as PSA are excellent in following patients who have already been diagnosed and treated, it has been almost impossible to find a serum marker that is effective in diagnosis.

Because malignant tumors often express and secrete characteristic groups of proteins, a close study of serum proteins by the techniques of proteomics may reveal unique collections of proteins or altered relative concentrations of proteins, which would be a far better screening test than the single proteins that are currently associated with some tumors [PMID12465452]. For example, a new area being investigated in patients at risk for ovarian carcinoma is the mass spectrometric analysis of the entire gamut of serum proteins, and its comparison to patients with known ovarian carcinoma and to normal controls [PMID18595727].

Progress is also being made in the diagnosis and staging of cancer by the detection in the serum of the mRNA that codes for proteins of interest. For example, a promising avenue of early detection and staging of colon cancer is serum levels of mRNA coding for the protein S100A4 (also called metastasin), a member of the S100 family that facilitates the development and metastasis of colon carcinoma by multiple pathways, including binding to cytoskeletal proteins, decreasing cell adhesion, and suppression of tumor suppressor proteins [PMID21354054].

One occasionally encounters the term "peptidomics," which is the branch of proteomics concerned with low-molecular-weight proteins. Likewise, the term "metabolomics" (or metabolic profiling) refers to the study of the smaller molecules that derive from intermediary metabolism. Examples include glucose, fatty acids, cholesterol, and other molecules that participate in biochemical pathways. While many of these molecules are critical in the diagnosis of specific diseases (such as elevated glucose in diabetes), these molecules represent final common pathways for many processes, and it is unlikely that metabolomics will play an expanded role in molecular medicine. Indeed, molecular medicine is shifting the diagnostic effort away from small molecules and toward macromolecules such as DNA, RNA, and proteins.

Molecular Phenotyping of Cancers

Following from the famous "central dogma" of molecular biology (proteins arise from transcription of DNA into RNA, followed by translation of RNA into proteins), molecular characterization of tumors can be performed at the DNA, RNA, or protein level. We now know that the expression of DNA can be modified by epigenetic factors, and this furnishes yet another means of characterizing tumors at the molecular level. The characterization of a tumor by any of these means is a form of molecular phenotyping.

While characterization of a tumor's DNA, called oncogenomics or oncogenomic profiling, can theoretically be done by complete sequencing of the tumor's DNA, in practice there are limitations. First, because fully sequencing DNA is labor intensive and expensive, the responsible gene must be known and localized, and even when it is, restricted sequencing of that area of the genome is still laborious and expensive. Second, while many neoplasms arise from 1 or a small number of well defined mutations, many others are associated with a very large number of mutations. For example, over 1,600 mutations in over 1,100 genes are associated with carcinomas of the breast and bowel [PMID16959974]. Many of these mutations are in multiple locations, defeating the strategy of targeted sequencing. Moreover, many mutations found in a cancer are undoubtedly incidental. The Cancer Genome Atlas (http://cancergenome.nih.gov), discussed in Chapter 46, is a database that will eventually tabulate the etiologic genetic changes in human malignancies.

Molecular phenotyping of neoplasms has not only demonstrated that many tumors that are similar in their H&E appearance are different at the molecular level, it has also shown that even within an individual tumor, there are different clones. In particular, there is now evidence that a small clone of cells within a given tumor is particularly able to undergo transformation into a malignant population and attain immortality. This clone is also more able to invade and metastasize, and more resistant to therapy. At this time, this group of tumor cells, apparently the instigators of tumorigenesis, is called cancer stem cells [PMID22070916]. Breast cancer stem cells seem to have the immunophenotype of CD44+, and CD24– or weak, and also express aldehyde dehydrogenase type 1 [PMID21957977, PMID21680574]. Evidence for cancer stem cells has been uncovered in other cancers, especially those of the head and neck [PMID22070916].

Molecular phenotyping is a potential method of identifying tumors of unknown primary [PMID16594740] but, at this writing, has not yet been added to the time-honored trio that must be used to determine a primary site—clinical/radiographic correlation, H&E appearance, and immunohistochemical characteristics.

Molecular phenotyping may also assist in determining which drugs a neoplasm will respond to. Both specific and nonspecific resistance mechanisms exist. Multidrug resistance (MDR) is a nonspecific resistance mechanism in which membrane proteins pump a variety of chemotherapeutic drugs out of the cell. These pumps are called P-glycoproteins (Pgp), and are overexpressed in cancers that have MDR. Pgp has the remarkable capacity to export hundreds of molecules that are apparently unrelated to each other [PMID19442049]. Some tumors inherently have MDR from the beginning, while other tumors acquire this capacity. There has been progress in inhibiting Pgp [PMID11172691]. Currently, third-generation inhibitors are being investigated and show promising potency and specificity for Pgp.

Breast Cancer Is the Best Developed Example of Molecular Phenotyping

The treatment of breast cancer illustrates how advances in molecular biology are finding clinical application. The first partially effective, commonly used combination of chemotherapeutic agents for breast cancer was cyclophosphamide, methotrexate, and 5-fluorouracil (CMF). Studies then demonstrated an added advantage for the addition of anthracycline agents, which work by intercalating between base pairs in DNA and RNA (adriamycin is an example). The taxanes were added. The use of these drugs was largely empirical. Herceptin, employed in cases that overexpress *HER2*, was the first breast cancer drug to come into clinical use from basic science.

Oncogenomics is occasionally used in the study of breast cancers. Variations in mRNA expression in breast cancers have prognostic significance [PMID15591335]. Characterization of tumors at the mRNA level is called oncotranscriptomics or oncotranscriptomic profiling. This relies heavily on RT-PCR,

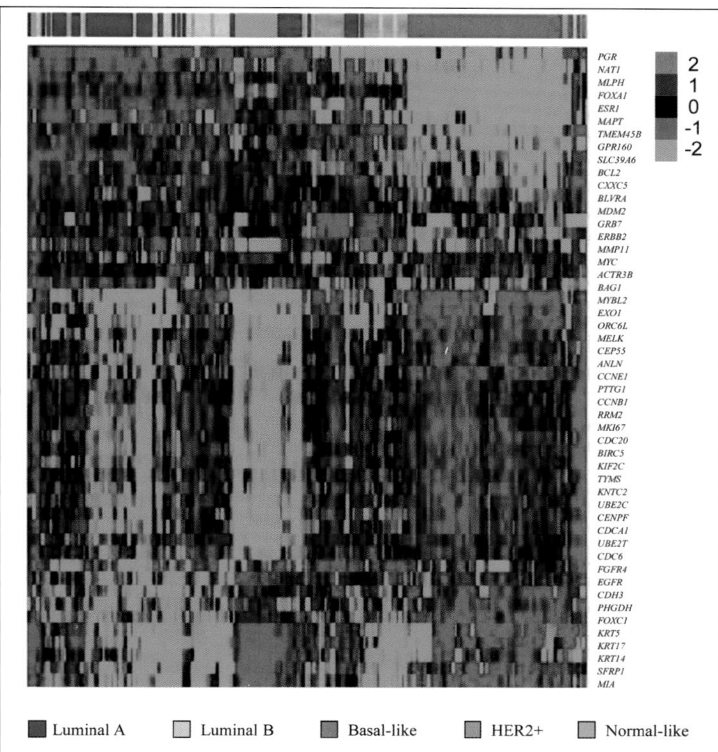

f47.6 A reverse transcriptase PCR study of 202 breast cancers, from formalin-fixed, paraffin-embedded specimens. 50 genes (indicated on the right) were studied using quantitative RT-PCR. Red signals indicate high levels of gene expression while green signals indicate low levels of expression. The data are presented in an unsupervised format, where samples with similar results are adjacent to each other. Different types of breast cancer, as identified by morphology and immunohistochemistry, have different patterns of gene expression (luminal-C cancers were not studied).

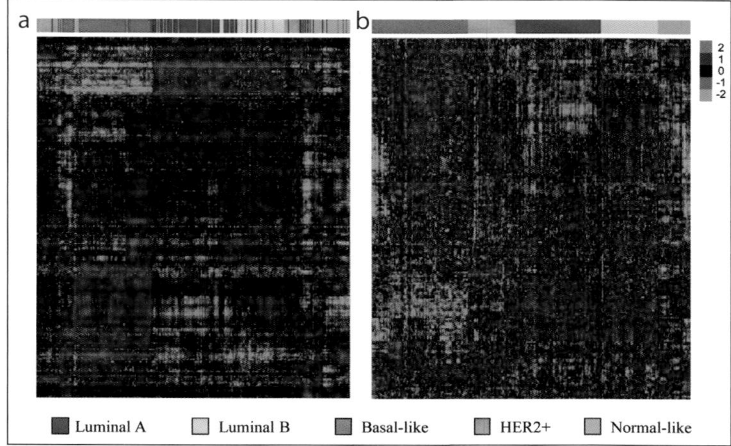

f47.7 A microarray study of the expression of 326 genes in 294 breast cancers.
a Individual samples from the cancers are on the X axis. The cancers are classified by type on the basis of morphology and immunohistochemistry, and each type is assigned a color as indicated at the bottom of the figure. The color bar at the top of the figure indicates the type of cancer at a given location on the X axis. The genes are on the Y axis. Red signals indicate high levels of gene expression while green signals indicate low levels of expression. The cancers that have the most similar gene expression pattern are adjacent (unsupervised data presentation).
b The same data as in the unsupervised figure, but the data have been arranged to show all the cancers of the same morphologic and molecular type together (this is supervised clustering; note that there is no intermingling of colors in the color bar at the top of the figure).
Both unsupervised and supervised clustering show that there are significant differences in gene expression among these 5 types of breast cancer (luminal-C cancers were not studied).

microarray analysis, or SAGE. There are a number of proprietary molecular profiles, designed to predict local recurrence or distant metastases and based on an examination of mRNA by reverse transcription PCR. For example, the Oncotype DX assay is proprietary to Genomic Health, Inc, and is a reverse transcriptase PCR-based set of tests that assays the levels of mRNA for a variety of potentially important proteins. While Oncotype DX can be helpful, it is limited to node-negative, hormone receptor positive breast cancer [PMID20665886] and is not performed in metastatic foci, which is the tumor tissue for which one would most like to have molecular and prognostic information. It has not been shown to provide superior prognostic information relative to ER, PR, Ki-67, and Her2 status [PMID21990413], but has been shown to decrease the use of chemotherapy by identifying a low-risk group [PMID22585699]. MammaPrint, marketed by Agendia BV, has also received Food and Drug Administration approval for prognostication but, again, only in node-negative cases. It compares the amount of mRNA in tumor cells with the amount in normal cells for 70 genes. Gene expression by microarrays has also shown promise in prognostication [PMID11823860].

However, as is the case with most types of tumors, most of what we know about the molecular biology of breast cancers is at the protein level (oncoproteomics), and has been primarily learned through immunohistochemistry, the foray into proteomics. Breast cancers can be divided into 4 main classes by immunohistochemistry. These are luminal-like (meaning that they express cytokeratins 8 and 18, which are often found in normal epithelial cells near the lumen, not in basal or myoepithelial cells), basal-like (expressing cytokeratins 5 and 6, and perhaps also cytokeratins 14 or 17, which are usually found in normal basal epithelium), normal-like (expressing keratins that are similar to those of normal breast epithelium, with no preference for either luminal-like or basal-like keratins), and *HER2*-amplified [PMID10963602, PMID16643655].

Subsequent work then indicated 3 subtypes of luminal cancers—luminal-A, luminal-B, and luminal-C—each of which preferentially expresses a set of proteins but which all tend to be positive for estrogen receptor or progesterone receptor (indeed, many of the proteins expressed by luminal breast carcinomas are involved in lipid metabolism and steroid hormone signaling, as might be expected in estrogen-responsive tissue). For example, a luminal-A carcinoma is positive for ER or PR and negative for Her2 (the protein by immunohistochemistry) and *HER2* (amplification of the DNA), while a luminal-B tumor is positive for ER or PR and positive for Her2 or *HER2* [PMID11553815]. Invasive ductal carcinomas can thus be divided into 6 subtypes—luminal-A, luminal-B, luminal-C, basal-like (usually triple negative), *HER2*-amplified, and normal-like. Gene expression studies by both reverse transcriptase PCR (RT-PCR) **f47.6** and microarrays **f47.7a,b** have affirmed the subtypes, and the number will grow as more is learned at the nucleic acid level.

Because cytokeratin 5 is expressed more frequently than cytokeratin 6, this antibody alone is more sensitive and specific than a 5/6 cocktail in the identification of basal-like breast carcinomas [PMID18854264]. Basal-type carcinomas tend to be of higher histologic grade, sometimes with metaplastic areas, and occur disproportionately in younger and African-American women. Although basal tumors and those with *HER2* overexpression may initially respond better to chemotherapy, luminal-A cancers ultimately have a better long-term survival than either of these groups [PMID19082617].

The terms "triple negative" (ER–, PR–, no overexpression of *HER2*) and "basal-like" are often used synonymously. In most cases, this is appropriate, but in actuality, triple-negative carcinomas of the breast are a heterogeneous group, of which basal-like carcinomas are a subset [PMID18398844, PMID19089739].

About 16% of triple-negative tumors are not basal-like in their epithelial expression [PMID19855377], and there are basal-like carcinomas that are not triple negative [PMID21076464]. In patients with triple-negative cancers and negative lymph nodes, basal phenotype was an important negative prognostic factor, and the relatively few triple-negative, node-negative carcinomas that did not have basal epithelium were less aggressive [PMID17146782].

Even apart from expression of basal epithelium, there are differences in clinical behavior among triple-negative carcinomas. Distant metastases in triple-negative tumors are associated with central fibrosis and a small number of lymphocytes within the tumor, while the absence of fibrosis and an abundant lymphocytic infiltrate were associated with fewer metastases [PMID17910759]. In addition, there are differences among triple-negative carcinomas in expression of epidermal growth factor receptor and c-kit [PMID17885672], further confirming the heterogeneous nature of these neoplasms.

Triple-negative carcinomas tend to be of high nuclear grade and to have minimal gland formation, with a solid growth pattern. They are associated with defective DNA repair, making them theoretically vulnerable to chemotherapeutic agents that damage DNA and to inhibitors of DNA repair enzymes, such as those of the poly ADP-ribose polymerase (PARP) family. The PARP inhibitor iniparib has been shown to be of benefit in metastatic triple negative breast cancers. Interestingly, iniparib also may benefit breast cancers arising from the BRCA1/2 pathway [PMID21208101].

While in most cases, molecular characterization has not yet added significantly to information already available from H&E and immunohistochemical evaluation, it is clear that we are rapidly approaching a time when the final diagnosis will be made in a new way. The expectation is that what now appear to be specific forms of cancer (such as invasive ductal adenocarcinoma of the breast) will be shown to be a heterogeneous group of neoplasms, as has already been shown for diffuse large B-cell lymphoma. Eventually, the molecular profile of each tumor, in conjunction with a better understanding of the individual patient's metabolism of therapeutic agents (pharmacogenetics), will make possible a specific therapeutic regimen that is tailor-made for that tumor, an example of personalized medicine.

Molecular Pathology: Closing Comments

"Orphan" diseases are those that receive little attention because they are rare, and it is hoped that advances in molecular pathology will allow more attention to be given to these diseases. Because molecular methods can be rapidly applied to any specimen, regardless of the rarity of its abnormality, it is to be hoped that all diseases will soon be characterized at the DNA level, making possible diagnostic and therapeutic applications of molecular pathology in the orphan diseases. Likewise, increasing automation will hopefully lead to decreasing costs and greater availability of molecular methods in developing countries.

The Association of Molecular Pathology (AMP) can be contacted at 301-634-7939, or at molecularpathology.org. The American College of Medical Genetics can be contacted at 301-718-9603, acmg@acmg.net, or their website at http://www.acmg.net. The *Journal of Molecular Diagnostics*, free with AMP membership, is a leading journal in this field.

In the near future, the final diagnosis will come from molecular methods, not from a microscope. Molecular medicine will make possible personalized medicine, treatments that are based on the gene expression of a particular neoplasm or of a particular patient to an infectious agent, and the pharmacogenetics of that patient. We are privileged to live in this era of transition.

Core Points for Molecular Pathology IV: Frontiers and Personalized Medicine

- Epigenetics: regulation of DNA expression that does not directly depend on the DNA sequence.
  - Can be modified by environmental factors.
  - Major forms include modification of histones and DNA methylation.
  - Histone modification: often by acetylation.
    - Allows greater access of transcription factors and enzymes, facilitating transcription.
  - DNA methylation: often on promoters.
    - Inhibits transcription.
    - Sequential turning on and off of DNA methylation is an important part of differentiation.
    - Cancers may be associated with hypermethylation of the promoters of tumor suppressor genes, rendering those genes less active.
    - Methylation may also cause imprinting, wherein genes are expressed or silenced depending on whether they are derived from the individual's mother or father.
- Annotation of the genome: understanding information beyond the sequence, such as start and stop points and the regulation of transcription.
- Functional genomics: study of RNA molecules, and the function and interaction of proteins.
- Only a very small minority of DNA is transcribed and translated.
  - Many portions of DNA are apparently capable of contributing to the production of more than one protein.
  - Findings will require a new definition of a gene, probably based on a portion of DNA that has a specific function.
- Proteomics: study of the structure, function, and interaction of all proteins.
  - Challenges: understanding 3D structure of proteins, their function, how structure is related to function, and protein interactions.
  - Techniques: 2D gel electrophoresis, chromatography, and x-ray crystallography, magnetic resonance imaging, mass spectrometry (MS).
  - 2D gel electrophoresis: proteins separated first on their charge, then on their size.
  - MS: often used as a final procedure after other techniques.
    - Requires that the proteins be positively ionized so that they will migrate to a negative electrode.
    - During migration, ions are exposed to a magnetic field and will follow a curved path.
    - Degree of curvature depends on the charge-to-mass ratio.
- As for genomics and transcriptomics, bioinformatics databases are critical in proteomics.
- Many cancers are actually heterogeneous groups of disorders.
  - Examples: diffuse large B-cell lymphomas and breast cancers.
  - Breast cancers: luminal-like, basal-like, HER2-amplified, and normal-like.
    - Basal-like cancers: not strictly synonymous with "triple negative" cancers, but most triple negative breast cancers are of basal-like immunophenotype and are aggressive.
- Analysis of groups of proteins secreted by malignant tumors, rather than a single protein, and detection of tumor nucleic acids will augment molecular phenotyping.
  - Will lead to better identification of tumors of unknown primary.
  - Also more specific therapy.

ISBN 978-089189-5886

Index

*Images are in **bold;** figures are in *italics*.

A

α chain disease
Abetalipoproteinemia, 242
Abl, 46, 511
Abortions, hydropic, 309, **312**
Abscesses, 84
  crypt, **251**
  Munro, 413, **420**
  Pautrier, **418**
  tubo-ovarian (TOA), 357
Acantholysis, 414
Acantholytic acanthoma, 406
Acanthomas, 406, **417**
Acanthotic epidermis, 408
Accelerated maturation, 304
Accessory tragus, 159
Accuprobe, 484
Acetylation, 464
aCGH, 504-505
Achondroplasia syndrome, 543-544
Achromatic lenses, 2
Acinar cell tumors, 175, **177**, **273**
Acinic cell tumors, 175, **177**, **273**
Acinus, 274
Acne lesions, 84
Acoustic neuromas, 160, **162**
Acquired immunity, 76
Acquired immunodeficiency syndrome (AIDS), lymph nodes in patient with, **123**
Acrocentric chromosomes, 446, 501
Acromegaly, 423
Acrospiroma, 406
ACTH, 423
Actin, 14
Actinic keratosis of conjunctiva, 160
Activation-induced deaminase (AID), 100
Actonel, 31
Acute basophilic leukemia, 142
Acute cellular rejection, 369, **374**
Acute erythroid leukemia, 142
Acute inflammation, 76-81
Acute leukemia, 135
Acute lymphocyte (lymphoblastic) leukemia, 146-147
Acute lymphoid (lymphoblastic) leukemia, 141, 445, 513
Acute megakaryoblastic leukemia, 142
Acute myelogenous leukemia, 138, 140-142, **154**, **155**
  of ambiguous lineage, 141
  cytogenetic abnormalities and, 141
  with multilineage dysplasia, 141, **154**
  subgroups of, 141-142
Acute myelomonocytic leukemia, 141, **155**
Acute promyelocytic leukemia (APL), **153**
Acyclovir, 529
Adaptive immunity, 76, 88-105
Adenine, 453
Adenocarcinoma, *see specific type or organ*
Adenoid basal carcinoma, 325, **331**
Adenoid cystic adenocarcinoma, 325
Adenoid cystic carcinoma, 48-49, 174-175, **177**, 317
Adenomas
  double, 67
  follicular, 65
  medullary, 66
  metanephric, 377
  nephrogenic, 377-378
  nipple, 39
  tubular, 39
Adenomatoid malformation, 191
Adenomatoid odontogenic tumor, 167, **170**
Adenomatous hyperplasia, 291, 336, 388
Adenomatous polyposis coli, 261, 516-517
Adenomatous polyps, 234, **238**, **255**, **264**
  dysplasia in, 259
Adenomyomas, 346
  of gallbladder, 274, **285**
Adenomyosis, 337, 346, **348**
Adenopathy, 109
Adenosine, 453
Adenosine monophosphate (AMP), 453
Adenosis, **52**, 387-388
  apocrine, 38-39
  florid form of, 38
  localized form of, 38
  microglandular, 39, **52**
  of breast, 38-39
  of prostate, **393**
  vaginal adenosis, 317, 320
Adenosquamous carcinoma of endometrium, **344**
Adnexal neoplasms, 406
Adrenal cortex, 68
Adrenal cortical tumors, 68
Adrenal glands, 68-69
Adrenal paragangliomas, 61
Adrenocortical adenomas, **74**
Adrenogenital syndrome, 399
Adult respiratory distress syndrome (ARDS), 198
Adult T-cell leukemia/lymphoma (ATCL), 408
Adventitial dermis, 405
Affinity, 88
Affinity maturation, 100
African Americans, prostate carcinoma in, 384
Agarose, 469
AIP, 198-199
Alagille syndrome, 275
Alcoholic fatty liver disease, 281-282, **289**, **290**
ALK/EML translocation, **204**
ALK, 512
Allantois, 301
Allele-specific oligohybridization (ASO), 542
Allele-specific oligonucleotide hybridization (ASO), 504
Allele-specific polymerase chain reaction, 477-478, 543

ISBN 978-089189-5886

Allele-specific polymerase chain reaction amplification, cystic fibrosis carrier testing, 542
Allelic heterogeneity, 439
Allergic bronchopulmonary aspergillosis, 179, 199
Allergic fungal sinusitis, 179
Allotypes, 101
Allred score, 7
α-1-antitrypsin (α1AT) deficiency, nonneoplastic liver and, 277
α DNA, 501
Alternative promoters, 460
Alveolar rhabdomyosarcoma, **23**
Alzheimer disease, 534
Amebiasis, 248, **256**
Ameloblastic fibroma, 167, **171**
Ameloblastomas, 166-167, **170**, 423
Ameloblasts, 165
Amenorrhea, 423
Amino acids, 465
Amniocentesis, 306
Amnion, 301, 302
Amnion-chorion fusion, **307**
Amplicon-amplicon hybridization, 477
Amplicon-primer hybridization, 477
Amplicons, 477, 478
Amplification, 469, 476, 485, 499
  bias in, 477
  COLD-PCR, 478
  DNA, 482, *483*, 484
  isothermal nucleic acid, 484-485, *485*
  polymerase chain reaction, *476*, 476-482
  signal, 485
Amplification refractory mutation system (ARMS), 477
  cystic fibrosis carrier testing, 542
Amyloid, 407
Amyloid deposition, 368
Amyloidosis, 368, 407
β Amyloid precursor protein (βAPP), 534-535
Anal canal, 262
Anal canal intraepithelial neoplasia (ACIN), 262
Anal canal squamous carcinomas, 262
Anal intraepithelial neoplasia, **268**
Analyte specific reagent (ASR) disclaimer, 509
Anaphase, 459
Anaphase lag, 445
Anaplasia in Wilms tumor, 372
Anaplasma species, 530
Anaplastic carcinoma, **73**, 192
Anaplastic lymphoma kinase (ALK), 195
Anaplastic lymphomas, 120, **132**, 408, 511
Anaplastic meningiomas, 424
Anaplastic seminoma, 397
Anaplastic thyroid carcinoma, 66
Anastrozole (Arimidex), 45
Anatomic pathology
  analytic phase of, 429
  postanalytic phase of, 429
  preanalytic stage of, 429
  quality assurance in, 429-434
    mistakes of documentation, 432-433
    mistakes of identification, 429-430
    mistakes of interpretation, 430-432
    mistakes of omission, 430
    surgical pathology critical values, 433-434
  testing in, 429
Androgen-deprivation therapy, 389
Anemia
  megaloblastic, **155**
  refractory, 139
  sickle cell, 465
  sideroblastic, 139
Aneuploidy, 445
Aneurysmal bone cyst (ABC), 32, **35**
Angelman syndrome, 446, 551
Angiocentric lymphoma, 182
Angiodysplasia, 249
Angiofibroma, 180, **183**
Angiofollicular hyperplasia, 109
Angiogenesis, 87
Angioimmunoblastic lymphadenopathy, **132**
  with dysproteinemia, 121
Angiolipoma, 13
Angiolymphoid hyperplasia with eosinophilia, 15
Angiomatoid fibrous histiocytoma, 19
Angiomatosis, bacillary, 15
Angiomyofibroblastoma, 11, 316, **318**
Angiomyolipomas, 369-370, **374**
Angiomyxoma, 11, 316
  aggressive, **318**
Angiosarcoma, 16, 51, 192
  epithelioid, **24**
  high-grade, **24**, **59**
  of liver, **300**
Annotation of the genome, 500, 551
Annular pancreas, 269
Ano-rectal carcinomas, 260
Antibodies to *Saccharomyces cerevisiae* (ASCA), 244
Antibody dependent cell-mediated cytotoxicity (ADCC), 106
Antibody molecule, structure of, *88*
α-1-Antichymotrypsin, 384
Anticipation in trinucleotide repeat disorders, 547
Antigenic shift, 530
Antigen-presenting cells (APCs), 89
Antigens
  reaction with monoclonal antibodies, 5
  T cell-independent, 104
Antimicrosomal antibodies, 63
Antimitochondrial antibodies, 275
Antineutrophilic cytoplasmic antibody (ANCA), 181-182, 220-221
Antinuclear antibodies, 275
Antisense ribonucleic acid, 461
Antisense therapy, 462, 478
Antismooth muscle antibodies, 275
Antitransglutaminase IgA antibodies, 242
α-1-antitrypsin deficiency, **286**
APC, 261, 512
APC tumor suppressor pathway, 12
Apert syndrome, 544
Aphthous ulcers, 243, **252**
Apochromatic lenses, 2
Apocrine adenosis, 38-39
Apocrine carcinoma of breast, **56**
Apocrine lesions, 48
Apoptosis, 462, 511
Appendectomy, **256**
Appendiceal mucinous neoplasms, 261
Appendicitis, 248-249
  granulomatous, 248-249
Appendix, 248-249, 261, 353
Arachidonic acid, 80
Arachidonic acid metabolites, 76
Archaea, differences between bacteria and, 453
ArmFISH, 497

Array comparative genomic hybridization (aCGH), 505, *505*

ArrayExpress repository at the European Bioinformatics Institute (EBI), 552

Arrays, *see* Microarrays

Arteriovenous malformation, 15

Arteritis, 220

Arthritis, 30

Artifactual ectocervical hyperplasia, **329**

Asbestosis, 199

Ashkenazi Jews, genetic screening in, 546-547

Ask-Upmark kidney, 368

Association studies (analysis), 447-450

Astrocytoma, 424, **427**, **428**

Atelectasis, 199

ATP2A2, 414

ATP7B, 276

Atrophic endometrium, **340**

Atrophy, 322

Atypical adenomatous hyperplasia (AAH), 193, 387

Atypical decubital fibroplasia, 11

Atypical fibroxanthoma (AFX), 406, 407, **418**

Atypical glandular cells, 325

Atypidal hyperplasia
- of breast, 40
- of prostate, 388

Atypical lobular hyperplasia (ALH), 49

Atypical small acinar proliferation (ASAP), 388, **394**

Auer rods, **154**

Autoimmune disorder, lymph nodes in, 108

Autoimmune enteropathy, 242

Autoimmune hepatitis, 280-281, **288**

Autoimmune liver disease, 275, 279

Autoimmune oophoritis, 350

Autoimmune pancreatitis, 269-270

Autoimmune sialadenitis, 269

Autoimmune subepidermal bullous disorders, 414

Automated deoxyribonucleic acid extraction, 469

Autosomal dominant polycystic disease
- of liver, 296
- of kidney (ADPKD), 367, **374**

Autosomal recessive disorders, 291, 541-543, *542*

Autosomal recessive and dominant inheritance, 437- 439

Autosomal recessive polycystic kidney disease (ARPKD), **296**, 367

Avidin, 5

Avidin-biotin complex (ABC) method, 5

Avidity, 88

Axillary dissection, potential difficulty with, 45

5-Azacytidine, 513

Azothioprine (Imuran), 369

Azurophilic granules, **154**

B

B-1 cells, 104

B-2 cells, 104

Bacillary angiomatosis, 15

Backwash ileitis, 243

Bacteria, differences between archaea and, 453

Bacterial artificial chromosomes (BACs), 474

Bacterial vaginosis, 315

Bacteriophage, 473

Bacteroides, 315

Baker cysts, 30

Barrett esophagus, 224, **229**, **230**, 244
- dysplasia in, 226

Bartholin duct cyst, **318**

Bartholin glands, 315

Bartonella, 530

Basal cell adenocarcinoma of salivary glands, 174, **177**

Basal cell carcinoma, 386, 406

Basal cell hyperplasia, 387, **393**

Basal endometrium, **341**

Basal lamina, 86

Basaloid neoplasms of skin, 406

Basaloid squamous carcinoma
- of larynx, 187, **189**, 192
- of lung, 192
- of vulva, 317

Basaloid tumors of skin, 227, 403

Base flipping, 458

Basement membrane, 86, **163**

Basic Local Alignment Search Tool (BLAST), 500

Basophils, 78, 138

Bayesian analysis in Mendelian inheritance, 439-442

B-cell antigen receptor, synthesis of, 91-93, *92*

B-cell coreceptor complex, 103

B-cell lymphoma, 215, 399
- diffuse large cell, 116-117, **130**, **240**
- T-cell-rich, **130**
- treatment with monoclonal antibody to CD20, 118

B-cell neoplasms, WHO classification of, 112-121

B-cell receptor complex, 102-103

B cells, 78
- activation of, 99-104, *100*, *101*, *102*, *103*
- maturation of, *93*

BCL-1, 511

BCL-2, 113, 511, 512

BCR/ABL translocation, 512

Becker muscular dystrophy (BMD), 544

Beckwith-Wiedemann syndrome, 551

Benign processes that mimic invasive carcinoma, 38-39

Benign sarcoma-like proliferations, 10-12

Benzodiazepines, 532

β-hemolytic streptococci, 86

β-lactam ring of penicillin, 520

Bethesda guidelines
- for Pap smears, 66-67
- revised, for testing for microsatellite instability, 515

Bile, 274

Bile canaliculi, 274

Bile duct hamartoma, 291, **296**

Bile ductules, 274-275

Biliary hamartomas, 291

Bilineal acute leukemia, 141

Bioactivation of drugs, 531

Biofilm, 241

Bioinformatics, 500

Biopsies, *see specific organ or tissue*

Biotin, 488, 499, *499*

Bird flu, 530

Birefringent material, 3

Bisphosphonates, 31

Bizarre parosteal osteochondromatous proliferation of bone (BPOP), 33

BK virus, 529

Bladder, **382**
- benign neoplasms and neoplasm-like conditions of, 377-378
- biopsy of, **382**
- core points for, 381
- inflammatory conditions of, 377
- invasive urothelial (transitional cell) carcinoma, 379
- inverted papilloma of, **382**
- nephrogenic adenoma of, **382**
- normal, 328
- papillary urothelial lesions, 378-379
- urothelial carcinoma, 379-380
- urothelial dysplasia and carcinoma in situ, 378

Blast crisis in chronic myelogenous leukemia, 143
BLAST-Like Alignment Tool (BLAT), 500
Blastocyst, 301
Bleeding, dysfunctional uterine, 335, **341**
Blocking DNA, 488-489, 494, 502
Blood, unusual conditions found in, 149-150
Blood vessels, 219-221
Bloom-Richardson system, 48, 385
Bloom syndrome, 546
Blotting in molecular pathology, 470
- northern, 470
- Southern, 470, 472, 502
- western, 470

Blue nevus, 411-412
Blunt duct adenosis, 49
B lymphocytes, 78, 88, 96
- maturation of, 93, *93*

Bone marrow, 138-150, **151-158**
- biopsies of, **152**
- core points for, 150
- hypocellular, **151**
- myelodysplastic syndromes, 138-140
- nonneoplastic processes in, 138
- normal, 138, **151**
- in reactive hyperplasia, **151**
- recovering, **153**
- unusual conditions found in, 149-150

Bone marrow fibrosis, 144
Bone marrow transplants, application of microsatellite analysis in, 538
Bones and joints, 30-33
- core points for, 33
- masses and neoplasms of, 31-33
- metabolic bone and joint disease, 31
- traumatic and degenerative conditions, 30
  - arthritis, 30
  - osteonecrosis, 31

Borderline ovarian neoplasm, **360**
Bordetella parapertussis, 530
Bordetella pertussis, 247, 530
Bowel, unusual conditions in, 249
Bowenoid papulosis, 316
Bowman membrane, 160
Brachytherapy, 389
Bradykinin, 80
BRAF, 511, 516, *516*
Brainerd diarrhea, 245
Branched chain nucleic acid technology, 485
Branched nucleic acid detection, 485
BRCA1/2-associated hereditary breast and ovarian cancer syndrome, 514
BRCA1/2 mutations, 365, 512
BRCA1/2 DNA repair, 517
BRCA1/2 testing, 513
Breakage-prone regions, 436
Break apart fluorescent **in situ** hybridization (FISH), 8, **8**, 490, *490*, 492
Breast, 38-51, **52-59**
- assessment of invasive ductal adenocarcinoma, 43-47, *46*
- benign processes mimicking invasive carcinoma, 38-39
- biopsy of, 42-43
- core points for, 51

Breast Imaging Reporting and Data System (BIRADS), 42
Brenner tumors, 354, **361**
Brightfield ISH, 487
Bronchiolar adenocarcinoma, 193
Bronchiolar carcinoma, 192-193, **203**
Bronchiolitis, 199
Bronchiolitis obliterans with organizing pneumonia (BOOP), 193, 198, 199, 200, **208**
Bronchocentric granulomatosis, 197
Bronchogenic cyst, 191
Bronchopulmonary dysplasia, 197-198
Brown bowel syndrome, 249
Brunner gland hyperplasia, **251**, 257
Brunner glands, 241, **251**
Brunn nests, 377, 380, **382**, **383**
Bullous keratopathy, 160, **163**
Bullous pemphigoid, 414, **421**
Bullous/vesicular disorders of skin, 414-415
Burkitt leukemia, 147
Burkitt lymphoma, 117-118, **131**, 510-511
Bursa, 30

C

C282Y, 275
CA125, 351, 353, 354
CAAT box, 460
Cadherins, 49, 84
Cajal cells, 235
Calcifying fibrous pseudotumor, 213
Calcineurin, 369
Calcium hydroxyapatite, 31
Calcium pyrophosphate, 31, **35**
Call-Exner bodies, 354
Calretinin, 354, 365
Calymmatobacterium granulomatis, 315
Canalicular adenoma, 174, **177**
Canavan disease, 546
Cancer Genome Atlas (TCGA), 513, 556
Cancer Sequence Genome Atlas, 500
Candida, 165, 315
Capillary electrophoresis, 479, 484, 498
Carbapenem, 521
Carbapenem-resistant Enterobacteriaceae (CRE), 521
Carbohydrates, complex, 464
Carboxylation, 464
Carcinoid tumor, 60, 215
Carcinoma, *see specific tissue or organ*
Carcinoma ex pleomorphic adenoma, **176**
Carcinoma showing thymus-like elements (CASTLE), 66, **73**
Caroli disease, 291, **296**
Carpel tunnel syndrome, 30
Cartilaginous tumors, 17-18
Caseating granuloma, 86, **124**
Castleman disease, **124**, 173, 213, **216**, 269
- hyaline vascular variant of, 109, **124**
- multicentric, 109
- plasma cell variant of, 109, 117
- types of, 109

Cast nephropathy, 368
Cataract, 160
Catarrhal exudate, 77
Catecholamines, 60
β-Catenin, 12, 516
Cat scratch disease, **124**
C-banding, 445
C cell hyperplasia, 66

CD8 T cells, 98
CD10 stains, 317, 338, 350, **359**
CD21, 103, 113, 355
CD31, 14, 364
CD34, 14, 235
CD56, 60
CD68, 397, 424
CD117, 235-236, 369
CD146 (Mel-CAM), 310
CDH1, 512
CEA, 326, 351, 353, 354
Cecal kick, 243
Celiac disease, 241-242, **251**
Cell adhesion molecules, 84-86, *85*, 167
Cell cycle, 457, *457*, 458
Cell division, 457
Cell-mediated immunity, 76, 105
Cellular blue nevi, 411, **420**
Cellular bronchiolitis, 199
Cellulitis, 86
Cementoblastoma, **171**
Cementoma, 167
Cemento-ossifying fibroma, 166
Centers for Disease Control (CDC), 509
Centers for Medicare and Medicaid Services (CMS), 509
Central giant cell granuloma, **169**
Central necrosis, **29**
Central nervous system, 423-426, **427-428**
  core points for, 426
  dementia and, 423, 534-536
  inflammatory and degenerative conditions of muscles, 425
  neoplasms of, 424-425
  nonneoplastic disorders of, 423
  WHO classification of tumors in, 424-425
Central tolerance, 105
Centroblastic large cell lymphomas, 116
Centroblasts, 102, *102*
Centrocytes, 102
Centrosome, 459
Ceroidosis, 249
Ceruloplasmin, 276-277
Ceruminous gland adenocarcinoma, 159
Cervical atrophy, **329**
Cervical intraepithelial neoplasia (CIN), 321-323, **328-332**
Cervista Invader technology, 528
Cervix, 321-327, **328-332**, 364
  cervical intraepithelial neoplasia, 321-323
  core points for, 326
  endocervical lesions and, 325-326
  invasive squamous cell carcinoma of, 324-325
  pap smear, 323-324
Chain disease, 149, 257-258
Chain termination method, 497
Chalazion, 160, **163**
Chancre, 315, **318**
Chaperones, 464
Charcot joint, 30
Chargaff, Erwin, 452
Chemiluminescence, 471
Chemokine receptors, 84
Chemokines, 82-83
Cholecystitis, 274
χ^2 test, 449
Chiasma, 436
ChIP-chip, 506
Chlamydia pneumoniae, 518-519
Chlamydia psittaci, 518-519
Chlamydia trachomatis, 315, 518-519
  detection of, 485
Cholangiocarcinoma, primary, 293
Cholecystitis, 274
  follicular, **285**
Cholesteotoma, 159-160
Chondroblastoma, 32, **35**
Chondrodermatitis, **162**
Chondrodermatitis nodularis helicis, 159
Chondromalacia, 159
Chondromatosis, synovial, **35**
Chondromyxoid fibroma, 32, **35**
Chondrosarcomas, 17, 32-36, **25**, **35**, **36**
Chorangioma, 304, **308**
Chorangiosis, 304, **308**
Chorioamnionitis, 303-304, **307**
Choriocarcinoma, 311, **313**, 356, 396-398, **402**
  gestational, 309, 311, **313**
Chorion, 301, 302, 305
Chorionic villus sampling, 305, 306
Chromatic aberration, 2
Chromatids, 435
  nonsister, 436
  sister, 435
Chromatin immunoprecipitation (ChIP), 505, 549, *549*
Chromatography, 554
Chromogenic (color) detection, 471
Chromogranin, 60
Chromophobe carcinoma of kidney, 369, 371-372, **376**
Chromosomal aberrations, 444
Chromosomal nondisjunction, 447
Chromosome, marker, 446
Chromosome banding
  cytogenetics and, 444-447
  nomenclature for, 445
Chromosome combing, 493
Chromosome enumerator probes (CEP), 492, *492*
Chromosome libraries, 493
Chromosome packing, degree of, 456
Chromosomes and Morphology Collaborative Study Group (CHAMP), 10
Chromosome walking, 474
Chronic Epstein-Barr virus (EBV) infection, 118
Chronic granulomatous disease (CGD), 77
Chronic idiopathic myelofibrosis (CIMF), 142, **156**
Chronic ischemia, 246, 304
Churg-Strauss syndrome, 197, 199, 219, 221
Ciliated metaplasia, **342**
Ciprofloxacin, 457
Circumferential trophoblastic hyperplasia, **312**
Cirrhosis, 279-280, 282
Cis-acting, 460
Cisterns, 309
CK7, 353
CK20, 351, 353, 378
C-KIT, 511
CKX2, 351
Clarke leveling, 409-410
Classical choriocarcinomas, 398
Classical Hodgkin disease, 110-111, **125**, 135
Class/isotype switching, 101
Clear cell adenocarcinoma, 317, **344**
Clear cell carcinoma, 338, **344**, 353-354, **361**
Clear cell hidradenoma, 406

ISBN 978-089189-5886

Clear cell sarcoma, 20, **29**, 372, **376**
Clear cell variant of hepatocellular carcinoma (HCC), **297**
Cleavase, 470
Cleavase fragment length polymorphism (CFLP), 470
Clinging carcinoma, 40, **53**
Clinical genetics, 435-451
  chromosome banding and cytogenetics in, 444-447
  evolution of X and Y chromosomes, 450
  linkage and association in, 447-450
  Mendelian inheritance in, 437-443
  non-Mendelian inheritance secondary to multifactorial inheritance in, 443-444
Clinical Laboratory Improvement Act (CLIA) (1988), 509
Clinical Laboratory Improvement Advisory Committee (CLIAC), 509
Clinical Network Scoring System, 281
Clonality, 112
  assessment of, 104, *104*
Clone, 447
Cloning expression, 475
  genomic, 472-473
Clostridium difficile, 247, 248, 521-522
Cluster designation (CD), 5
Coagulative necrosis, 346, **349**
Codeine, 532
Codon, 462
Cohesive end sites (COS), 474
Cohort (prospective) studies, 449
COLD-PCR, 478
ColE1, 472
Colectomy specimen, 260
Colitis
  acute infectious, **255**
  acute ischemic, **254**
  chronic ischemic, **254**
  collagenous, 245-246, **254**
  diversion, 245, **253**
  dysplasia in ulcerative, 244-245
  focal active, 243
  indeterminate, 244
  infectious, 247-248
  ischemic, 246
  lymphocytic, 245-246, **254**
  microscopic, 245
  ulcerative, **252**, **253**
Collagen, 86
Collagenous colitis, 245-246, **254**
Collagenous fibroma, 11
Collagenous sprue, 242
Collecting duct carcinoma, 372, **376**
College of American Pathologists (CAP)
  publication of quality improvement manual by, 432
  on testing for estrogen and progesterone receptors, 45
  use of research use only kits, 509-510
Collision-induced dissociation (CID), 554
Colonic adenocarcinoma, **266**
Colonic medullary carcinoma, **267**
Colonic polyps and adenocarcinoma, 258-259
Colonography, 259
Colonoscopy, 243
  screening, 225
Colorectal cancer, 259-262
  molecular pathology of, 262
Colorimetric ISH (CISH), 487
Columnar cell lesions of breast, 49
Columnar cells, 363
Columnar cell variant of papillary thyroid carcinoma, **71**
Combinatorial labeling, 495, *495*
Combined DNA Index System (CODIS), 537
Combined paternity index (CPI), 537
Community acquired *Staphylococcus aureus* (CA-MRSA), 520
Comparative C_T method, 481
Comparative genomic hybridization (CGH), 491, 493-495, *494*, 504-505, *505*
Complement, 80
Complementarity determining regions (CDRs), 92, *92*, 101
Complementary DNA (cDNA) library, 473
Complementation, 475
Complex carbohydrates, 464
Complex hyperplasia, **342**
Complex inheritance, 443, 444
Complex odontoma, **171**
Complex sclerosing lesion, 39
Compound heterozygote, 541
Compound nevi, 409
Compound odontoma, **171**
Conception, products of, 305
Concomitant endometriosis, 353
Conditional probability, 440, 441
Condyloma, 316, 405
  immature, 322
  of vulva, **319**
Condyloma latum, 315, **318**
Condylomatous carcinoma, 403
Congenital bronchiectasis, 191
Congenital hepatic fibrosis, **296**
Congenital lobar emphysema, 191
Conjugative plasmids, 467-468
Conjugative transposons, 467, 468
Conjunctiva, 160-161
Connexin proteins, 546
Conn syndrome, 68, 367
Consanguinity, 438
Constitutive heterochromatin, 456
Conventional G-banding, 444-445, 505
Conventional karyotyping, 505
Copy number polymorphisms, 505
Copy number variants (CNVs), 484, 510
Cornea, lesions of, 160
Corpora albicans, 351
Corpora lutea, 351
Corpus cavernosum urethral, 403
Corpus luteum, 350
Corpus spongiosum, 403
Corrugated parakeratosis, 166
Cosmid, 474
Cot-1, 488, 494, 502
Coumadin, 532, 533
Councilman bodies, 277, **286**
Cowper glands, 386
COX-1, 80-81
COX-2, 80-81
CpG islands, 549-550, *550*
CpG sequence, 78
Craniopharyngioma, 423
  with fibrous stroma, **427**
Craniosynostosis syndrome, 543-544
C-reactive protein (CRP), 83
Creutzfeldt-Jakob disease (CJD), 536
Crick, Francis, 452-453
Cri-du-Chat, 446
Crigler-Najjar syndrome, 533
Crohn disease, 242-244, **252**
Crossing over, 436
Crossover threshold, C_T, 481
Crouzon syndrome, 544

Crush artifact, **205**
Cryoglobulinemic vasculitis, 219
Cryoprobe-assisted lumpectomies, 44
Cryotherapy, 389
Crypt abscesses, **251**
Cryptocidins, 76
Cryptogenic organizing pneumonia, 198
Cryptorchidism, 396
Cryptorchid testis, 395, **401**
Crypts, 241
Crystals of Reinke, 350
Cushing syndrome, 68, 367, 423
Cutaneous B-cell lymphoid proliferations, 409
Cutaneous lymphoproliferative disorders, 407-412
Cutaneous melanoma, 410
Cutaneous neoplasms and masses, 405-407
Cutaneous neuroendocrine tumors, 60
Cycle threshold, 481
Cyclin D, 527
Cyclin D1, 326
Cyclins, 114
  overexpression of, 511
Cyclooxygenase (COX), 80-81
Cyclophosphamide (cytoxan), 534
Cyclophosphamide and mycophenolate (CellCept), 369
Cyclosporine, 369
CYLD, 406
Cylindroma, **417**
CYP, pharmacogenetics of drugs not metabolized by, 533-534
CYP2C9, 532
*CYP3A4**3, 532
Cystadenofibroma of ovary, **360**
Cystadenoma of pancreas, **272**
Cystic fibrosis, 249, 439, 441, 442, 541-543, *542*
Cystic fibrosis transmembrane conductance regulator gene, 541
Cystic fibrosis transmembrane conductance regulator-related disorders, 542-543
Cystic formation hyaline fibrosis, 16
Cystic nephroma, 370, **374**
Cystic renal cell carcinoma, 370, **375**
Cystic thymoma, 213, 214, **217**
Cystic tumors of pancreas, 270
Cystitis, 377-378
  cystica, 377
  glandularis, 377
Cytidine, 453
Cytidine monophosphate (CMP), 453
Cytidine triphosphate (CTP), 453
Cytochemical stains, 2
Cytochrome C, 105
Cytochrome p450 system, enzymes of phase 1 metabolism as member of, 532-533
Cytogenetic microarray analysis (CMA), 505
Cytogenetics, 489, 491, 493, 505
Cytogenic abnormalities, soft tissue neoplasms associated with, 10-20
Cytokeratin, 398
Cytokeratin 5, 557
Cytokeratin 5/6, 227, 365, 387, 388
Cytokeratin 7, 196, 351, 387
Cytokeratin 18, 310
Cytokeratin 20, 354, 406
Cytokine receptors, 81
Cytokines, 76, 81-84, *82*
  DNA coding for, 84
Cytokinesis, 457
Cytokine storm, 83
Cytopenia, 109
  with multilineage dysplasia, refractory, **152**
Cytoplasmic tyrosine kinases, 46
Cytosine, 453, 549
Cytotrophoblasts, 302, 309

D

D2-40, 44
DAB complex, 460
DAG (diacylglyceral), 98
D-alanine, 519
DAPI, 489
Darier disease, 414, **421**
Dark-field microscopy, 3
Darwinian evolution, 531
Database of Chromosomal Imbalance and Phenotype in Humans (DECIPHER), 505
Database of Genomic Variants (DGV), 505
Decubital fibroplasia, **21**
Deep-penetrating nevus, 412
Deep perivascular inflammation, 414
Deep sequencing, 499
Defensins, 76
Degenerative joint disease, 30
Degenerative schwannoma, **25**
Delavirdine, 524
Deletions, 444
Dementia
  causes of, 535-536
  central nervous system in, 423, 534-536
Dendritic cells, plasmacytoid, 96
Denosunab, 31
De novo chromosomal aberrations, 443
De novo mutation, 437
Dense core vesicles, 60
Dental laminae, 165
Dentatorubral pallidoluysian atrophy, 547
Dentigerous cysts, **169**
Deoxyribose, 453
De Quervain disease, 63
Derivative chromosome, 446
Dermatitis, **421**
  acute, 413-414, **420**
  chronic, 413-414, **420**
  photoallergic, 413
  photocontact, 413
  seborrheic, 413
  stasis, **421**
  subacute, 413, **420**
Dermatitis herpetiformis, 242, **421**
Dermatofibroma, 18, **418**
  bizarre, 406-407
  cellular, 406, **418**
Dermatofibrosarcoma protuberans, 18, 406-407, **415**, **418**
Dermatomyositis, 415, 425
Dermatopathic lymphadenitis, 108, **123**
Dermis, 405
Dermoid cysts, 160, 356
Descemet membrane, 160, **163**
Desmin, 14, 338
Desmoid, 12
Desmoplastic fibroma, 11
Desmoplastic hepatocellular carcinoma, **297**
Desmoplastic medulloblastoma, 424
Desmoplastic melanomas, 410, **419**
Desmoplastic mesothelioma, 209
Desmoplastic small round cell tumor, **29**, 365, **366**
Desmoplastic Spitz nevus, 411

ISBN 978-089189-5886

Desquamative interstitial pneumonitis, 199, **208**
Detection methods in immunohistochemistry, 5-6
Detergents, 469
Developmental vascular lesions, 15
Diabetic glomerular disease, 368
Diabetic mastopathy, 50, **58**
Diabetic nephropathy, 368
Diaminobenzidine (DAB), 5-6
Diandric triploidy, 310
Diapedesis, 77
Diethylstilbestrol (DES), 317
Diffuse alveolar damage (DAD), 198
Diffuse astrocytoma, 424
Diffuse gastric cancer, 517
Diffuse hyperplasia, 108
Diffuse interstitial pneumonitis, 198
Diffuse large cell B-cell lymphomas, 116-117, **130**, **240**
DiGeorge syndrome, 446, 491
Digital photoimaging system, 471
Digoxigenin, 488
Dihydropyrimidine dehydrogenase (DPD), 534
Diploid cell, 435
Direct deoxyribonucleic acid (DNA) sequencing, 522
Direct detection, 471
Direct labeling, 488, 492
Direct sequencing, 450
Dirofilaria immitus organism, **296**
Discoid lupus, **422**
Disease odds ratio, 449
Disordered proliferative endometrium, **341**
Dispermy, 309-310, 445
Dispersed neuroendocrine system (DNS), 60
Displaced epithelium, invasive adenocarcinoma versus, 247
Displacement loop
  mutations in, 443
  replication, 442
Disseminated peritoneal leiomyomatosis, **366**
Disuse colitis, 245
Diversion colitis, 245, **253**
Diverticulitis, 246
Diverticulosis, 246
Dizygotic (fraternal) twins, 305, 444
DNA (deoxyribonucleic acid), 469
  abnormalities in, 465
  blocking, 488-489, 494, 502
  central dogma of, 453
  complementary, 473
  detection of, 471-472
  differences between ribonucleic acid and, 453
  discovery of, 452
  double-stranded, 470
  enzymes that repair damaged or mismatched, 458
  fingerprinting, 537
  genetic information carried by, 452
  hypervariable minisatellite, 502
  intactness of, 469
  interspersed repetitive, 501
  methylation of, 456
  packing, 456, *456*
  polymerase, 457, 458
  polymorphism, 447
  posttranslocation, 490
  profiling, 502, 537-538
  proviral, 482
  repetitive, 500-503
  replication, 457
  satellite, 501
  sequencing, 496-498
  single-stranded, 470
  structure of, 452, 453-457
  variations in, 472
  vertebrate, 549
DNA amplification, 482, *483*, 484
DNA-associated proteins, 549
DNA Database of Japan, 500
DNA fingerprinting, 502
DNA polymerase, 457-458
DNA polymerase Taq, 477
DNA (deoxyribonucleic acid) repair
  BRCA1/2 in, 517
  mismatch repair enzymes, 458
DNA replication, 435, *435*, 442, 457-459, 502
DNA reprogramming, 476
DNA sequencing, 497, *497*, 498, 513, 538
  newer methods, 513, 522, 552
  Sanger method of, 498
  synthesis as basis of, *498*, 498-499
DNA testing, 509
DNA transcription and translation, 459-466
DNA vaccines, 106-107, 531
Documentation, mistakes of, 432
DOG1, 235
Domain, 453
Dominant trait, 437
Donovan bodies, 315
Double adenomas, 67
Double fusion strategy in FISH, 8, 490, *490*
Double minutes, 445
Double negative thymocytes, 94
Double-stranded RNA, 78
Double-strand sequence specific conformation polymorphism assays (DSSCP), 470
Down syndrome, 305, 444
Drug-induced hepatitis, 282
Dual-approach immunohistochemistry, 388
Dual-fusion fluorescent in situ hybridization (FISH), 8, **8**, **128**
Duchenne muscular dystrophy, 544
Ductal carcinoma in situ (DCIS)
  diagnosis of high-grade, 39
  intracystic papillary, 41
  lobular extension of, **56**
  micropapillary low-grade, 39
Duct obstruction and atresia, 275
Duodenal mucosa, normal, **251**
Duplication, 444, 466, 484, 501, 503
Duplication cyst, 249
Dyad, 435
Dye-terminator methods of sequencing, 498-499
Dynamic mutations, 547
Dyneins, 459
Dysautonomia, familial, 546-547
Dysgerminoma, 351, 354
Dyskeratotic cells, 322
Dysplasia, 321, **330**
  ectocervical, 321-323
  endocervical, 323
  gastric, 234
  hepatocyte, 292, **297**
  high-grade, 226, 234, 244, **253**
  low-grade, 226, 234, 244-245, **253**
  in adenomatous polyps, 259
  in Barrett esophagus, 232, 234
  in ulcerative colitis, 244-245
  urothelial, 378

Dysplasia-associated lesion or mass (DALM), 244-245, **253**
Dysplastic nevi, 409, 410-411, **419**
Dystrophin, 544-545

E

Ear(s), **162**, **163**
  core points for, 161
  external, 159-160
  inner, 160
  middle, 159-160
Ear canal, 159
Eburnation, 30
E-cadherin, 49, 50
  loss of, 517
Eccrine spiradenoma, **417**
Echinococcal (hydatid) cyst of liver, **296**
Echinoderm microtubule-associated protein-like 4 (*EML4*), 195
EcoRI, 472
Ectocervical epithelium, **328**
Ectoderm, 301
Ectopic decidua, 350
Ectopic glial tissue, **162**
Ectopic parathyroid tissue, 215
Eczema, 413
Efavirenz, 524
EGFR, 511
Elastin, 86
Electron microscopy, 3
Electron transfer dissociation (ETD), 554
Electrophoresis
  capillary, 479, 484
  microchip-based, 479
  types of, 470-471
Electrospray ionization (ESI), 554
Embryo, 301
Embryogenesis, 301, 438
Embryonal carcinoma, 396, 398, **402**
Embryonal rhabdomyosarcoma, **23**, 316
Embryonic stem cells, 301, 475
Embryonic teratomas, 356
Empty plasmids, 472
Encephalitis, 530
Encountered mature cystic teratoma, **362**
Encyclopedia of DNA Elements (ENCODE), 551
Endocervical dysplasia, 325, **331**
Endocervical intraepithelial neoplasia, 323
Endocervical lesions, 325-326
Endocervicosis, 364
Endocrine tumor, 271
Endoderm, 301
Endolymphatic sac papillary tumor, 159
Endometrial adenocarcinoma, **343**, **344**
  endometrium and, 336-338
  unusual types of, 337-338
Endometrial intraepithelial neoplasia (EIN), 336
Endometrial metaplasia, 335
Endometrial polyps, 336, **341**
Endometrial stromal histogenesis, 338
Endometrial stromal sarcoma, 338, **345**
Endometrioid adenocarcinoma of ovary, 353
Endometrioid carcinoma, 353, **361**
Endometriosis, 317, 350, 364, **366**
  concomitant, 353
Endometritis, 334-335, **341**
Endometrium, 333-339, **340-345**
  core points for, 339
  effect of exogenous hormones on, 334
  endometritis and, 334-335
  hyperplasia of, 335-336
  in dysfunctional uterine bleeding, 335
  metaplasia and, 335
  normal histology and dating, 333-334
Endonucleases, restriction, *471*, 471-472
Endoplasmic reticulum (ER), 464
Endosalpingiosis, 317, 364, **366**
Endothelium, 160
End-stage renal disease, 368
Enhancer-binding proteins, 460
Enhancers, 460
Entamoeba histolytica, 248
Enteric duplication cyst, 249
Enterobacteriaceae, 521
Enterococcus, 519
Enterocytozoon bieneusi, 248
Enteropathy-associated T-cell lymphoma (EATCL), 258, **263**
Enterovirus genus, 530
Enucleation, 160-161
Enzyme immunoassay tests, 275
Eosin, 2
Eosinophilia-myalgia syndrome, 11
Eosinophilic cystitis, 377
Eosinophilic esophagitis (EE), 224, **230**
Eosinophilic fasciitis, 11
Eosinophilic gastrointestinal disorders (EGIDs), 227
Eosinophilic granuloma, 199
Eosinophilic inflammation, 224
Eosinophilic metaplasia, **342**
Eosinophilic pneumonia, 199
Eosinophils, 77, 78, 138, 224, 227
Ependymoma, 425
  with pseudorosettes, **428**
Epidermal growth factor receptor (EGFR), 46, 82, 194, 261
Epidermal hyperplasia, 405
Epidermal nevus, 405
Epidermis, 405
Epigenetic regulation of genome, 549-551
Episomes, 472
Epithelial hyperplasia, **172**, 316
  of larynx, 186
  of vulva, **319**
Epithelial malignant mesothelioma, **211**
Epithelial membrane antigen (EMA), 354, 363, 397
Epithelial mesothelioma, 209, **211**
Epithelial-myoepithelial carcinoma, 175, **177**
Epithelial neoplasms, 213-214, 351, 406
Epithelial predominant thymoma, **216**
Epithelial tumors, 351
Epithelioid angiosarcoma, **24**
Epithelioid hemangioendothelioma, 16, 197, **207**, 294, **300**
Epithelioid hemangioma, 15
Epithelioid leiomyoma, **349**
Epithelioid leiomyosarcoma, 310, **349**
Epithelioid macrophages, 86
Epithelioid sarcoma, 20, **29**
Epithelioid smooth muscle tumors, 347
Epithelioid trophoblastic tumor (ETT), 309, 310, **313**
Epstein-Barr virus (EBV), 103, 510
  in cervical lymph node infection, **123**
  chronic infection from, 118
  in hemophagocytic syndromes, 149
  in infectious mononucleosis, 108
Epulis, 166
Epulis fissuratum, 166
ERB-B family of genes, 261
Erythema induratum, 416

Erythema nodosum, 415, **422**
Erythropoietin, 84
Escherichia coli, 247
Escherichia coli O157:h7, 248
Esophageal biopsies, 227, **231**
Esophageal webs, 224
Esophagus, 224-228, **229-231**
  Barrett, 224-227
  carcinomas of, 227
  core points for, 228
  gastroesophageal reflux disease and, 224-227
Essential thrombocythemia, 142
Essential thrombocytosis, 145
Esthesioneuroblastoma, 180
Estrogen receptor, β form of, 45
Estrogen receptor positive carcinomas, hormonal therapy for, 45
Ethical issues in molecular pathology, 509-510
Ethidium bromide, 469, 470
  staining with, 478
Euchromatin, 456
Eukaryotes, 458, 459, 462
  distinction between prokaryotes and, 453
Eukaryotic evolution, 443
Eukaryotic ribonucleic acid, modifications of, 461-462
Eukaryotic transcription, 461
European Bioinformatics Institute (EBI), 507
European Molecular Biology Laboratory (EMBL), 500
Evolution, eukaryotic, 443
Ewing sarcoma, 20, **29**, 365, 511
EWS/FLI-1 translocation, 512
EWS, 512
Excision repair enzymes, 458
Exemestane (Aromasin), 45
Exenteration, 161
Exogenous hormones, effect of, on endometrium, 334
Exon shuffling, 461
5' Exonuclease assay, 480
Exonucleases, 471
Expression cloning, 475
Expression vectors, 506
Expressivity, 437
Extended chromatin fibers (fiber-FISH), 493
External ear adenoma, 159
External hordeolum, 160
Extraadrenal paraganglia, 61
Extraadrenal pheochromocytoma, 61
Extracellular matrix, 76
Extramedullary myeloid tumors, 121, **133**
Extranodal natural killer cell lymphoma, 180, **184**
Extraskeletal myxoid chondrosarcoma, **25**
Exudate, 77
Eye(s), 160-161, **163-164**
Eyelids, lesions of, 160

F

Factor P, 80
Factor V Leiden, 543
Facultative heterochromatin, 456
Fallopian tubes, **362**, 364
  inflammation of, 357
  neoplasms of, 357
  nonneoplastic conditions of, 357
Famcyclovir, 529
Familial adenomatous polyposis, 259, 261, 514, 516-517
Familial aggregation, 444
Familial dysautonomia, 546-547
Familial enteropathy, 242
Families of Structurally Similar Proteins (FSSP) database, 555
Fas-associated death domain (FADD), 105
Fasciitis, 10-11
FASTA, 500
Fatal familial insomnia, 536
Fat necrosis, 51, **59**
Female adnexal tumor of probable Wolffian origin (FATWO), 357, **362**
Ferruginous bodies, 199
FGF9, 395
FGFR3, 378, 511
  in achondroplasia, 544
Fibrillation, 30
Fibrin degradation products (FDP), 80
Fibrinogen, 80
Fibrinoid necrosis, **185**, 368
Fibrinous exudation, 77
Fibrinous pleuritis, **212**
Fibrin split products, 80
Fibromuscular hyperplasia, 246
Fibroadenolipoma, **58**
Fibroadenomas, 191
  juvenile, 50
Fibroadenomatoid hyperplasia, 50
Fibroblast growth factor, 82
Fibrocystin/polyductin (FPC), 367
Fibroepithelial lesion, **58**
  with cellular stroma, 50
Fibroid polyps, **238**
Fibrolamellar variant of hepatocellular carcinoma, **297**
Fibrolipoma, 13
Fibroma, 11
Fibromatosis, 12, **21**, 370
  aggressive, 12
  nuclear uniformity of, **21**
  retroperitoneal, 269
Fibromyxoid sarcoma, 19, **26**
Fibromyxoid stroma, **171**
Fibronectins, 87
Fibro-osseous lesion of the jaw, **170**
Fibro-osseous pseudotumor, 11
Fibrosarcomas, 12, **22**, 370
Fibrosing colonopathy, 249
Fibrosing epulis, 166, **170**
Fibrosing interstitial pneumonitis, 198
Fibrosing pancreatis, chronic, **272**
Fibrosis, 377, 410
  idiopathic, 138
  lobular, **289**, **290**
Fibrotic orbital pseudotumor, 269
Fibrous dysplasia, 33, **36**, 166
Fibrous histiocytoma
  of skin, 406-407
  of soft tissue, 18-19
FIGO system of classification of endometrial adenocarcinomas, 336-337
Finasteride, 391
Fine needle aspiration of thyroid, 66-67
Fissural cysts, 166, **169**
Fissuring ulcers, 243
Fixation of tissues, 1
Flagellin, 78
Flaring (sandwich effect), 496
Flat epithelial atypia, 40
Flexner-Wintersteiner rosettes, 161, **164**
Floret cells, 13

Fluorescein, 487
Fluorescein isothiocyanate (FITC), 470-471, 487, 492
Fluorescence, 470
Fluorescence intensity profile, 496
Fluorescence microscopy, 8
Fluorescence resonance energy transfer (FRET) probes, 480
Fluorescent in situ hybridization (FISH), 7-8, *8*, 10, 445, 477, 482, 486-489, 493
  break apart, 8, *8*
  characterized abnormalities and, 489-493, *490*, *492*
  combining with immunohistochemistry, 493
  dual-fusion, 8, *8*
  limitations of, 487-497
  multicolor (M-FISH), 495, *495*
  multiple probe, 493
  reverse, 491
Fluorite objectives, 2
5-Fluorouracil (5FU), 534
FMRP, 547
Focal acantholytic dyskeratosis (FAD), 414
Focal active colitis, 243
Focal cemento-osseous dysplasia, 166
Focal nodular hyperplasia, 291, **296**
Focal nuclear atypia, 347
Follicle-associated epithelial cells, 241
Follicle-within-follicle formation, 63
Follicular adenomas, 65, **71**
Follicular atrophy, 63
Follicular carcinoma of thyroid, minimally invasive, **72**
Follicular center cell lymphomas, 116
Follicular cholecystitis, **285**
Follicular dendritic cells, immunohistochemical stains for, 109
Follicular gastritis, **237**
Follicular hyperplasia, 108, **123**, 213
Follicular involution, **123**
Follicular lymphoid hyperplasia, **216**
Follicular lymphoma, 108, 112-114, **127**, **128**
Follicular neoplasms, 65
Follicular variant of papillary carcinoma, 64
Food and Drug Administration, (FDA), 509
Food-borne Creutzfeldt-Jakob disease, 536
Forbes-Albright syndrome, 423
Formalin, 1, 5
Formamide, 489
Fosamax, 31
Fosmid, 474
Founder mutations, 546
Foveola, **237**
Fox-Fordyce, 315
F-plasmid, 474
Fragile X syndrome, 484, 547, 548
  testing for, 547, *547*
  as trinucleotide repeat disorder, 550
Frameshift mutation, 461
Free radical, 77
French-American-British (FAB) classification of myelodysplastic syndromes, 139
Frenulum, 403
FRET probes, 480
Friedreich ataxia, 547
Fuch dystrophy, 160, **163**
Functional annotation, 500, 551
Functional genomics and transcriptomics, 551-552
Function mutation, tumor suppressor gene and, 512-513
Fundic gland polyp, **238**
Fungiform papillomas, 179, **183**
Funisitis, 304

G

Galactorrhea, 423
Gallbladder, 274
  adenocarcinoma of, 274, **285**
  adenomyoma of, 274, **285**
  core points for, 284
  Rokitansky-Aschoff sinus of, **285**
Ganciclovir, 529
Gangliocytic paragangliomas, 61, **62**
Ganglion cyst, 30
Ganglioneuroblastoma, 69, **75**
Ganglioneuroma, **75**, **218**
  of colon, **265**
Gap junctions, 84
Gardnerella, 315
Gardnerella vaginalis, 315
Gardner syndrome, 259
Gartner duct, 315, 317
  cysts of, 315, **318**
Gastric acid, 241
Gastric adenocarcinoma, 234-235
Gastric antral vascular ectasia (GAVE), 233
Gastric dysplasia, 234
Gastric lymphoid proliferations, 234
Gastric marginal zone lymphoma, **239**
Gastric stromal tumors, 235-236
Gastric xanthoma, 233, **238**
Gastritis, 232-233
  acute, 232, **237**
  chronic, **237**
    Whitehead system for, 232
  chronic atrophic, 232, **237**, **420**
  chronic superficial, 232
  follicular, **237**
  Helicobacter, 233
  lymphocytic, 232
Gastroesophageal reflux disease, 186, 224
Gastrointestinal autonomic nerve tumor (GANT), 235
Gastrointestinal stromal tumors (GISTs), 257, **263**
Gastrointestinal tract, 241
Gastrulation, 301
Gaucher disease, 134, **136**, 138, 546
  bone marrow in, **151**
G-banding, 444, 445, 488, 491
  conventional, 444-445, 505
GC box, 460
GCDFP-15, 47, **298**
Gel electrophoresis, 469
GenBank, 500
Gene(s)
  defined, 466-468
  naming, 466
  targeting, 475
  tracing, 447-450
  transcriptional silencing of, 460-461
Gene amplification, 445
Gene chips, 503
Gene conversion, 101
Gene expression, 460-461, 480
  analysis of, 18
  profiling, 506
  study of, 552
Gene Expression Database, 552
Gene expression library, 473

ISBN 978-089189-5886

Gene Expression Omnibus at the National Center for Biotechnology Information (NCBI), 552
Gene knockin, 475
Gene knockout, 475
Gene mapping, 447
Gene modification, in molecular pathology techniques, 475-476
Gene probes, 7
Generalized colitis cystica profunda, 247
Gene rearrangement, 101
GeneTests, 510, 511
Gene therapy, 475, 476
Genetic code, 463-464
Genetic counseling, 439
Genetic distances, 436
Genetic drift, 546
Genetic engineering, 107
Genetic family history, 436-437
Genetic Information Nondiscrimination Act (2008), 510
Genetic linkage, 447
Genetics. *See also* Clinical genetics
  Mendelian, 442
  molecular biology link to, 435
Genetic testing, 509, 510
  in Ashkenazi Jews, 546-547
Genetic variability, 436
Gene transfer with retroviruses, 475-476
GeneXpert, 520
GenOhm, 520
Genomes
  annotation of, 500
  prokaryotic, 472-473
Genome-wide association studies (GWAS), 450
Genomic cloning, 472-473
Genomic islands, 467, 468
Genomic library, 472
Genotypes, 437
Geographic tongue, 165
Germ cell neoplasms, 396-399
Germ cell tumors, 215, 351, 356
  of ovary, 356
  of testes, 396
Germinal centers
  centroblastic area of normal, **127**
  lymphocyte maturation in, 123
  progressive transformation of, 109, **124**
Germline mutation, 514, 515
Gestational choriocarcinoma, 309, 311, **313**
Gestational trophoblastic disease, 309-311, **312-314**
Giant cell arteritis, 219
Giant cell epulis, 166
Giant cell granulomas, **170**
  reparative, 166
Giant cell tumors, 32
  of bone, **35**
Giant cell undifferentiated pleomorphic sarcoma (UPS), **26**
Giant condyloma, 404, **404**
Giardia, 242
Giemsa method of chromosome banding, 444, 445
Gigantism, 423
Gilbert syndrome, 533
Gingivitis, 165
  acute necrotizing, 165
GJB2, 546
Glandular cells
  atypical, 325
  in vagina, 317
Glandular dysplasia, 226-227, *See also* Dysplasia
Gleason grading system, 385-386, 389, **392**, **393**
α-Gliadin, 241
Glial cells, **362**
Glial fibrillary acidic protein (GFAP), 424
Glial tissue, 160
Glioblastoma multiforme, 424, **428**
Glioblastomas, 424
Glioma, 424
Gliomatosis cerebri, 424
Gliosis, reactive, **427**
Global glomerulosclerosis, 368
Glomeruli, 368
Glomerulonephritis, 221, 369
Glomerulopathy, acute renal transplant, 368-369
Glomerulosclerosis, 368
Glossitis, benign migratory, 165
Glottis, 186
Glucose-6-phosphate dehydrogenase deficiency, 534
Glucose transport protein-1, 363
Gluten-sensitive enteropathy, 241-242
Glycogen storage disease, 546
Glycoprotein B, 529
Glycoproteins, 464
Glycosaminoglycans (GAGs), 87, *87*, 464
Glycosylation, 464
Glycosylphosphatidylinositol (GPI), 81
Glypican 3, 292, 398
Goblet cell carcinoid, 261
Goblet cells, 224, **229**, **230**
  significance of, in biopsies, 225
Golgi apparatus, 464
Gomori methenamine silver (GMS), 2
Gonadoblastoma, 357, 399
Gonococci, 77
Goodpasture syndrome, 219
Gout, 31
Gouty tophus, **34**
Gp91 glycoprotein complex, 77
Gp100 (or Pmel17), 409
Gpg, 531
G-protein-coupled receptors, 79, 82
G-proteins, 82
Graft vs host disease, 249, **256**, 283
  transplantation pathology of liver and, 283
Granular cell tumors, 19, **27**
Granulocyte colony-stimulating factor (G-CSF), 84
Granulocyte monocyte colony-simulating factor (GM-CSF), 84
Granulocytes, 138
Granulocytes neutrophils basophils, 77
Granuloma, 86
  overt, 415
  types of, 108
Granuloma annulare, 415, **422**
Granuloma inguinale, 315
Granulomatous inflammation, 86
Granulosa cell tumor, 354, 399
Granulosa-stromal cell tumor, 357
Graves disease, 63, **70**
Gross cystic disease fluid protein 15 (GCDFP-15), 194
Gross examination, 1
Group II introns, 468
Grover disease, 414
Guanine, 453
Guanosine, 453
Guanosine monophosphate (GMP), 453
Guide strand, 462
Gynandroblastoma, 357

H

Haemophilus ducreyi, **126**, 315
Hairy cell leukemia, 135, **137**, **158**
HAM-56, 424
Hamartoma, 50
  lung, **202**
  splenic, **136**
Hamman-Rich syndrome, 198
Haploid cell, 435
Haplotype, 89, 436, 448
Hardy-Weinberg law, 438, 546
Hashimoto thyroiditis, 63, **70**
Hassall corpuscles, 213, 214, **216**
HBME-1, cell membrane staining for, 64
H-caldesmon, 338
Healed arteritis, 220
Health and Human Services, U.S. Department of, Secretary's Advisory Committee on Genetic Testing (SACGT) of, 509
Health Insurance Portability and Accountability Act (1966) (HIPPA), 433
Hearing loss, 545-546
Heat shock proteins (HSPs), 464
Heffner tumor, 159-160, **162**
Helicases, 457
Helicobacter infections, 233, 234
Helicos Bioscience, 499
HeliScope, 499
α Helix, 464
Hemangioblastoma, 425, **428**
Hemangioendothelioma, 15-16
  epithelioid, 16, 294
  infantile, 16
  juvenile, 15, 16
  retiform, 15-16
Hemangioma, **58**, 134
  cellular, 15
  epithelioid, 15
  juvenile, 15
  lobular, 15
  lobular capillary, 15
  Masson, 15
  spindle cell, 15
Hemangiopericytoma, 16, **24**, 179, **183**, **212**, 424
Hematein, 1
Hematogones, 147
Hematologic neoplasms, 32
Hematopoietic colony stimulating factors (CSFs), 82
Hematoxylin, 1, 2
Hematoxylin and eosin (H & E), 1-2
Hemochromatosis, 276
Hemoglobin S, 449, 465
HEMOJUVELIN, 276
Hemolytic uremic syndrome, 368
Hemophagocytic syndromes, 149-150, **158**
Hemorrhagic colitis syndrome, 247-248
Hemorrhagic cystitis, 377
Hemorrhagic cysts, **359**
Hemorrhagic endovasculitis, 304, **308**
Hemorrhagic endovasculopathy, 304
Hemosiderin macrophages, 246, 317
Hemostasis, secondary, 80
Henoch-Schönlein purpura, 219
Hepatic activity index (HAI), 278
Hepatic adenomas, 291-292, **297**
Hepatic cysts, 291, 367
Hepatic iron concentration, 276
Hepatic iron index, 276
Hepatic masses, 291-292
Hepatitis
  acute, **186**, 277, **286**, **289**
  autoimmune, 280-281, **288**
  chronic, 277, **286**, **287**
  drug-induced, 282
  neonatal, 283, **290**
  unusual forms of, 283
  viral, 277-279
Hepatitis A, 277
Hepatitis B, 277, 278, 279
Hepatitis B virus, 526
Hepatitis C, 277-278, 279, 482
Hepatitis C virus, 525-526
Hepatitis D, 277, 526
Hepatocellular carcinoma, **204**, 291, 292, 294, **297**, **298**
  clear cell variant of, **297**
  fibrolamellar variant of, **297**
Hepatocyte dysplasia, 292
HEPCIDIN, 276
HER2, 445, 511, 512, 513
  testing for, 492, *492*, 513
Her2 protein, 82
  action of, 46
Herceptin, 512
Hereditary cancer syndromes, 513-518
Hereditary coagulopathy, 543
Hereditary diffuse gastric cancer syndrome, 517
Hereditary hemochromatosis, 275-276, **285**
Hereditary nonpolyposis colon cancer syndrome, 259, 261, 503, 513, 514-518
Herpes, 138, 165, 315
Herpes gestationalis, 414
Herpes simplex virus (HSV) 1, 528
Herpes simplex virus (HSV) 2, 528
Herpetic inclusions, **151**
Herpetic infection in vulva, **318**
Heterochromatin, 456
Heteroduplex assays, 470
Heteroduplexes, 478
Heteroplasmy, 443
Heterotopic gastric mucosa, 257, **263**
Heterotopic pancreas, 257, 269
Heterotopic pancreatic tissue in duodenum, **263**
Heterozygosity, 437
Heterozygote, compound, 541
HFE, 275-276
Hibernoma, 13
Hidradenitis suppurativa, 315, **318**
Hidradenoma papilliferum, 316, **318**
Highly active antiretroviral therapy (HAART), 524
High molecular weight keratin (CK903), 40-41, 227
High-resolution typing, 91
Hilus cell hyperplasia, 350
Hirschsprung disease, 249, 511
Histamine, 76, 79
Histiocytes, 78, 108
Histiocytes X, 199
Histiocytic necrotizing lymphadenitis, 108
Histiocytomas, 18-19, *see specific tissue or organ*
Histiocytosis, sinus, 108, **123**
Histiocytosis X, 19
Histone modifications, 549
Histopathology, hematoxylin use in, 1
2-hit hypothesis, 512, 513, 516
HLA-B*5701, 534
HLA-DQ2, 241-242
HLA-G, 305

ISBN 978-089189-5886

HMB-45, 409, 410

Hodgkin disease, **125**, **137**, 138, 214, 215
- classical, 110-111, **125**, 135
- lymphocyte-depleted, 110, **125**
- lymphocyte-rich classical, 110
- mixed cellularity, **125**
- nodular lymphocyte predominant, 111
- nodular sclerosing, 110
- WHO classification of, 109-110

Homer Wright rosettes and pseudorosettes, 68, 161

Homogeneously staining regions (HSRs), 445

Homologous recombination, 475

Homozygosity, 437

Honeycomb lung, 198

Hordeolum, 160

Horizontal transfer, 466

Hospital acquired *Staphylococcus aureus* (HA-MRSA), 520

HpaII, 550

HPV cytopathic effect, **328**

H-score, 7

Human chorionic gonadotropin, 302, 305, 309, 311

Human epidermal growth factor receptor type 2 (Her2 or Her2/neu), 46

Human Epigenome Project, 551

Human genome, sequencing of, 472, 551

Human Genome Project, 474, 498, 510, 549, 551

Human herpesvirus 8 (HHV 8), 15, 109, 511

Human immunodeficiency virus (HIV), 482, 524-525

Human lymphocyte antigen (HLA), *89*, 89-93
- testing by DNA methods, 91
- variations in, 534

Human papillomavirus (HPV), 321, 323, 526-528
- cytopathic effect, 322

Human placental lactogen (HPL), 302, 310

Humoral immunity, mechanisms of, 105-106

Humoral rejection, 368

Humoral response, 106

Hunner cystitis, 377

Huntington disease, 484, 547

Hyaline membrane formation, **208**

Hyalinizing necrosis, 346, **348**

Hybridization
- gene probes, *7*
- in situ, 7-8, 471, 486-487, *495*

Hybridization protection assay, 484

Hydatidiform mole, **312**
- complete, 309
- partial, 309-310

Hydralazine, 534

Hydrocele, 396

Hydrogen peroxide, 77

Hydropic abortions, 309, **312**

Hydroxyapatite, 31

Hymenal cysts, 315

Hyperacute rejection, 368

Hypercalcemia, 81

Hypercellular bone marrow in reactive hyperplasia, **151**

Hypercellularity, 11

Hypercellular septae, 13

Hyperchromasia, 226, 379

Hyperdiploid, 491

Hypereosinophilic syndrome, 142

Hypergammaglobulinemia, 109

Hypergranulosis, 405

Hyperkeratosis, 186

Hyperparathyroidism, 166

Hyperplasia, 39, 67, 309, **343**
- angiolymphoid, 15
- atypical, 40, 388
- benign epidermal, 405
- benign lymphoid, 108
- cellular, 64
- complex, **342**
- diffuse, 108
- endometrium and, 335-336
- follicular, 108, **123**
- interfollicular, 108
- intraductal, 40
- microglandular, 326
- paracortical, 108
- simple, **342**

Hyperplastic polyps, 233-234, **238**, 258, **264**, **265**

Hyperreactio luteinalis, 350-351, **359**

Hypersensitivity pneumonitis, 200, **208**

Hypersensitivity reactions, 106

Hyperthecosis, 355

Hypertrophic hypersecretory gastropathy, 233

Hyperuricemia, 31

Hypervariable minisatellite DNA, 501-502

Hypocellular bone marrow, **151**

Hypochlorite, 77

Hypochondroplasia syndrome, 543-544

Hypodiploid, 491

Hypodiploidy, 147

Hypomethylation, of oncogenes promoter, 550

Hypoxia, 303

I

Identification, mistakes of, 429-430

Identity testing, 502, 536-537
- microsatellites in, 538

Idiopathic cystic chondromalacia, 159

Idiopathic eosinophilic esophagitis (EE), 224

Idiopathic fibrosis, 138

Idiopathic midline destructive disease, 182

Idiopathic pulmonary fibrosis (IPF), 198

Idiopathic scrotal calcinosis, 403, **404**

IgA, 100

IgD, 100

IgE, 100

IgG, 100

IgG4-associated lymphadenopathy, 109

IgG4-related autoimmune disorders, 269

IgG4-related sclerosing sialadenitis, 173

IgG4 syndrome, 11

IgM, 100, 101

I$_K$B kinase complex-associated protein (IKAP), 546-547

IL-2, 88

IL-7, 93

Ileitis, backwash, 243

Illumina Solexa Genome Analyzer, 499

Immune function, normal, 76

Immune response
- components of, 76
- to parasites, 106
- to viruses, 106

Immunity
- acquired, 76
- adaptive, 76, 88-105
- cell-mediated, 76
- gastrointestinal system as integral part of, 241
- innate, 76-86
- specific, 76

Immunoblastic lymphadenopathy (IBL), 121
Immunocompromised patients, lymphoproliferative disorders in, 118
ImmunoCyt assay, 380
Immunoglobulin gene rearrangement, 91-93, *92*
Immunoglobulin synthesis, 436
Immunohistochemistry, 1, 4-7
 detection methods in, 5-6
 fluorescent in situ hybridization (FISH) in combining with, 493
 in lymphomas, 109
Immunological synapse, 97
Immunologic memory, 76
Immunoproliferative small-intestinal disease, 257-258
Imprinted genes, 550
Imprinting, 309, 550-551
Inclusion body myositis, 425
Incomplete penetrance, 437
Independent assortment, 436
Independent segregation, 436
Indeterminate colitis, 244
Indian filing in breast cancer, 50
Indolent myeloma, 148
Infectious colitis, 247-248
Infectious diseases, 242
 molecular testing in, 518-530, 531
Infectious mononucleosis, 118
 Epstein-Barr virus as cause of, 108
Infertility, testes and, 396
Infiltrating carcinoma
 cribriform, 48-49
 lobular, **56**
Inflammation
 acute, 76-81
 chronic, 86
 molecular mediators of, *79*, 79-81, *80*
Inflammatory bowel disease, 242-245, **252**
 quiescent, **252**
Inflammatory cloacogenic polyp, 246
Inflammatory myofibroblastic tumor, 11-12, **21**, 179
Inflammatory pseudopolyp in ulcerative colitis, **253**
Inflammatory response, participants in acute, 76
Influenza viruses, 529-530
Informed consent, 510
Inheritance
 autosomal dominant, 437
 autosomal recessive, 438
 Mendelian, 437-443
 mitochondrial, 442-443
 X-linked, 437, 438
 Y-linked, 439
Inherited disorders, molecular pathology of, 540-547
Inherited hypercoagulability, 543, *543*
Inhibin, 310, 355
Initiation codon, 463
Initiation factors, 463
Innate immunity, 76-86
In situ hybridization, *7*, 7-8, 471, 486-487, **495**
Insular carcinoma of thyroid, 66, **73**
Insulin-like growth factor, 82
Integrins, 84
Intensity-modulated radiation therapy (IMRT), 389
Intercellular adhesion molecules (ICAMs), 84
Interferons (IFNs), 82, 96-97
Interleukins, 82
Intermediate filaments, 84
International Cancer Genome Consortium (ICGC), 513
International HapMap Project, 540
International Mouse Knockout Consortium, 475, 476
International Prognostic Scoring System (IPSS), 140
International System for Human Cytogenetic Nomenclature (ISCN), 445, 491
Interphase cytogenetics, 491
Interpretation, mistakes of, 430-432
Interspersed nuclear elements (LINEs), 501
Interspersed repetitive DNA, 501
Interstitial cystitis, 377, **382**
Interstitial fibrosis of kidney, 199, 368, 369
Interstitial lung disease, 198-199
Intestinal carcinomas, with neuroendocrine differentiation, 260-261
Intestinal lymphoid proliferations, 257-258
Intestinal metaplasia, 225, **229**
Intestinal neoplasms, 257-262, **263-268**
 colonic polyps and adenocarcinoma, 258-259
 colorectal cancer screening, 259-260
 core points for, 262
 dysplasia in adenomatous polyps, 259
 lymphoid proliferations, 257-258
 molecular pathology in colorectal cancer, 261-262
 stromal, 257
 unusual, 261
Intimal hyperplasia, **222**
Intracytoplasmic sperm injection (ICSI), 396
Intraductal carcinoma of breast, 39-40, 42, **53**
Intraepithelial neoplasia, 186-187, 321, 322, 325, 336
Intrahepatic biliary atresia, 275, **285**
Intralobular proliferations of breast, 49
Intramucosal carcinoma of colon, 259, **265**
Intratubular germ cell neoplasia, **401**
Intravascular lymphoma, 117, **130**
Intravenous leiomyomatosis, 347, **349**
Intronic mutation, 465-466
Introns, 468
 classes of, 461
 mutations in, 465-466
 splicing of, 461-462
Intussusception, 246
Invasive omental implant, **360**
Inversions, 444
 fluorescent in situ hybridization (FISH) in detecting, 490-491
Inverted papilloma, 377
 of bladder, **382**
 of sinus, **183**
Inverted repeat, 468
Involucrum, 31
Iris diaphragm, 2
Iron overload syndromes in liver, 275-276, **285**
Irritable bowel syndrome, 244
Ischemic colitis, 246, **254**
Ischemic fasciitis, 11
Ishak modification of Knodell system, 278, 281
Islet cell tumor, 271
Isochromosome, 446
Isoniazid, 534
Isospora, 248
Isothermal nucleic acid amplication techniques, 484-485, *485*
Isotopic labeling, 471

ISBN 978-089189-5886

J

JC virus, 529
Joint probability, 440
Joints. *See* Bones and joints
Juvenile fibroadenomas, 50, **57**
Juvenile granulosa cell tumor, 354, **361**
Juvenile hemangioendothelioma, 15, 16
Juvenile hemangioma, 15
Juvenile hemochromatosis, 276
Juvenile myelomonocytic leukemia, 146
Juvenile papillomatosis
  of breast, 50, **57**
  of larynx, 186, **189**
Juvenile polyps, 258, **264**

K

Kallikrein, 80
Kamino bodies, 411
Kaposi sarcoma, 15, **23**, **24**, 117, 192, 511
Karyogram, 444
Karyorrhectic debris, 108
Karyotyping, 444, 505
  spectral (SKY), 495, *495*
Kawasaki disease, 219
Keratin, 76, 347, 364, 405
Keratin CK903, 187
Keratinization, 405
Keratoconus, 160, **163**
Keratosis follicularis, 414
Keratosis obturans, 159
Ki-67, 321, 322, 323, 326, **330**, 424
Kidney, 367-373, **374-376**
  benign renal neoplasms and, 369-370
  chronic pyelonephritis and, 367-368
  clear cell sarcoma of, 372, **376**
  congenital disorders in, 367
  core points for, 373
  malignant renal neoplasms and, 370-372
  nonneoplastic conditions, 368
  in transplantation, 368-369
  vascular changes in, 367, **374**
Kikuchi disease, 108, **123**
Kimmelstiel-Wilson nodule, 368, **374**
Kimura disease, 15
Kinesins, 459
Kinetochore microtubules, 459
Klatskin tumor, 293
Klebsiella oxytoca, 248
Kleiner and Brunt system in steatotic liver disease, 282
Klenow fragment, 488
Klinefelter syndrome, 396, 399, **401**
Knockout gene, 476
Knodell system, 278, 281
Köhler illumination, 2
Koilocytic atypia, 322
K-RAS, 261, 511
Kuru, 536

L

Labeling of probes, 488
  direct, 488
  isotopic, 471
  probe, 488
Laboratory-developed test (LDT), 510
Lac (lactose) operon, 460
Lacrimal caruncle, 160
Lactobacillus, 315
Lacunar cells in nodular sclerosing Hodgkin disease, **125**
Langerhans cell histiocytosis, 19, 20, **28**, 135, 199, **208**
Langerhans cells, 108, 180
Lapatinib (Tykerb), 46, 512
Large cell carcinoma
  lung, 60
  undifferentiated, 196
Large cell variant of anaplastic lymphoma, **132**
Large plaque parapsoriasis, 408
Laryngeal carcinoma
  sarcomatoid, 187
  squamous, **189**
Laryngeal nodules, 186
Larynx, 186-187, **188-190**
  core points for, 187
  epithelial hyperplasia of, 186
  intraepithelial neoplasia of, 186-187
  laryngeal neoplasia of, 186-187
  nonneoplastic processes in, 186
  papillomatosis, 186, **188**
Laser-assisted microdissection, 493
Laser capture microdissection, 493
Lateral periodontal cyst, 165
Lauren classification of gastric carcinoma, 234
Leber Congenital Amaurosis, 476
Lectins, 79
Legal issues in molecular pathology, 509-510
Leiomyoma, 14, **265**, 370
  benign, **348**
  metastasizing, 191
Leiomyosarcoma, 346, **349**
Lenses, 2-3
Lentigo maligna, 411, **419**
Lethal midline granuloma, 181
Leukemia
  acute, 135
  acute vs megaloblastic anemia, 155
  acute basophilic, 142
  acute erythroid, 142
  acute lymphoid (lymphoblastic), 141, 146-147
  acute megakaryoblastic, 142
  acute myelogenous, 140-142
  acute myelomonocytic, 141, **155**
  bilineal acute, 141
  chronic eosinophilic, 142, 144
  chronic lymphoid (chronic lymphocytic [CLL]), 147-149, 157
  chronic myelogenous (CML), 135, **137**, 142, 146, **155-156**
  chronic myelomonocytic (CMML), **157**
  chronic myeloproliferative neoplasms, 142-146
  chronic neutrophilic, 142, 144
  hairy cell, 135, **158**
  precursor B-cell, 146
  pure erythroid, **155**
  T-cell prolymphocytic, 149
Leukocytes, 76, 77, 84
  migration of, 77
  types and functions of, *78*, 78-79
Leukocytoclastic vasculitis, 219, 220, **223**
Leukodystrophy, 423
Leukoencephalopathy, 423
Leukoplakia, 167
Leukotriene B4, 81
Leu-M1, 354
Levey-Jennings charts, 538
Lewy bodies, 535
Lewy body disease, 535
Leydig cell hyperplasia, 396, **401**
Leydig cells, 395
Leydig cell tumor, 355, 399, **402**

L & H lymphocytic and histiocytic cells, 111

Libraries
- chromosome, 493
- complementary DNA, 473
- gene expression, 473
- genomic, 472
- plasmid, 473

Lichenoid inflammation, 414

Lichenoid keratosis, **421**

Lichenoid mucositis, 165

Lichen planus, 165, **421**

Lichen sclerosis et atrophicus (LS&A), 320, 403

Lichen sclerosus, 316

Lichen simplex chronicus, 413, **420**

Li-Fraumeni syndrome, 513

Ligase chain reaction (LCR), 482

Ligation-dependent PCR (LD-PCR), 482-483

Light, polarized, 3

Light chain disease, **158**, 368

Light microscopy, 1

Linkage, 452
- analysis of, 447, 450

Linkage and association in clinical genetics, 447-450

Linkage disequilibrium, 448

Linkage equilibrium, 448

Lipid cell tumors, 355

Lipid rafts, 97

Lipoadenoma of parathyroid, 67

Lipoblastoma, 13, **22**

Lipoma, 12-14
- atypical, 13, **22**
- pleomorphic, 13, **22**
- sclerosing, 13
- spindle cell, 12-13
- types of, 13

Lipopolysaccharide, 78, 104

Liposarcoma
- dedifferentiated, 14, **22**
- high-grade, **22**
- myxoid, 13-14, 17-18, **23**
- pleomorphic, 14, 18, **22**
- round cell, 13
- well-differentiated, **23**

Lipoxygenase, 81

Littoral cell angioma, **136**

Liver
- core points for, 284, 295
- echinococcal (hydatid) cyst of, **296**
- graft vs host disease and, 283
- hepatocellular carcinoma on core biopsy, 292
- hepatocyte dysplasia, 292
- masses and neoplasms, 291-295, 296-300
- malignant biopsy, primary or metastatic, 293-294
- nonepithelial primary liver masses, 294
- undifferentiated (embryonal) sarcoma of, 294

Liver masses and neoplasms, 291-295, **296-300**
- benign hepatic masses, 291-292
- clearly malignant biopsy of liver mass, 293-294
- hepatocellular carcinoma on core biopsy, 292
- hepatocyte dysplasia and, 292
- nonepithelial primary liver neoplasms and, 294

Lobular breast cancer, hereditary diffuse gastric cancer syndrome (DHGCS) and, 517

Lobular capillary hemangioma, 15

Lobular carcinoma, **57**
- in situ, 49, **56**

Lobular extension of ductal carcinoma in situ (DCIS), **56**

Lobular hemangioma, 15

Lobular hyperplasia, 49, **56**

Lobular panniculitis, 415

Lobular steatosis, **289**

Lobule, 274

Localized colitis cystica profunda, 246

Localized fibrous tumor, 363

Locked nucleic acids (LNAs), 478

Locus heterogeneity, 439, 465

LOD scores, 448

LOH/microsatellite analysis, 502-503

Long-acting thyroid stimulator, 63

Longitudinal ulcers in Crohn disease, 243

Long-range PCR, 477

Long terminal repeats (LTRs), 502

Loose bodies in joints, 31

Loss of heterozygosity, 502-503

Low malignant potential ovarian neoplasms, 351, **360**

Low-resolution HLA typing, 90-91

LPS-binding protein, 78

Luminal-type cancers, 557

Lumpectomies, cryoprobe-assisted, 44

Lung, 191-201, **202-208**
- benign masses in, 191-192
- core points for, 200
- hamartoma of, **202**
- interstitial disease, 198
- malignant neoplasms in, 192
- metastatic carcinoma to, 193-194
- mutations in non-small carcinomas of, 194-195
- neoplasms in, 197
- neuroendocrine carcinomas of, 195-196
- nonneoplastic masses in, 191
- non-small cell carcinoma, 192-195
- unusual inflammatory conditions, 197-198

Luteinized solitary follicle cyst of pregnancy and puerperium, 350, **359**

Lyme disease, testing for, 530

Lymphadenitis, dermatopathic, 108

Lymphadenopathy
- angioimmunoblastic, **132**
  - with dysproteinemia, 121
- benign, 108-109, 213
- IgG4-associated, 109

Lymphangioleiomyoma, 347

Lymphangioleiomyomatosis, 191, 369

Lymphangiomas, 213

Lymphangiomyoma, 191, **202**

Lymphatic spaces, tumor invasion into, 44

Lymph node pathology, 108-122, **123-133**, *see also* Lymphomas
  - angioimmunoblastic lymphadenopathy with dysproteinemia, 121
  - core points for, 122
  - extramedullary myeloid tumors, 121
  - immunoblastic lymphadenopathy (IBL), 121

Lymph nodes
- in autoimmune disorders, 108
- metastatic neoplasms in, 109-112
- normal function of, 88-105
- vascular transformation of sinuses, **123**
- very rare neoplasms of, 121

Lymphocyte activation, 97

Lymphocytes, 10, 78, **157**, 227
- activated, 102

Lymphocytic colitis, 245-246, **254**

Lymphocytic esophagitis, 227

Lymphocytic gastritis, 232

Lymphocytic thyroiditis, 63

ISBN 978-089189-5886

Lymphoepithelial cysts, 173

Lymphoepithelioma-like variant of urothelial carcinoma, 379

Lymphogranuloma venereum, 315

Lymphoid follicles, **127**, 241

Lymphoid hyperplasia, 108, **263**

Lymphoid interstitial pneumonia, 198, 199-200, **208**

Lymphoid nodules, **151**

Lymphoma/immunocytoma, 148
 lymphoplasmacytic, 116-118

Lymphomas, 138, 242, 257, 399
 anaplastic, 120, **132**, 408, 511
 angiocentric, 182
 B-cell, 118, **130**, 215, 399
 Burkitt, 117-118, **131**, 510-511
 centroblastic large cell, 116
 common non-Hodgkin, 135
 of conjunctiva and orbit, 161
 cutaneous T-cell, 408
 diffuse large cell B-cell, 116-117, **130**
 enteropathy-associated T-cell, 258, **263**
 extranodeal natural killer cell, 180, **184**
 follicular, 108, 112-114, **127**, **128**
 follicular center cell, 116
 gastric marginal zone, **239**
 hepatosplenic γ-δ T-cell, 120
 immunohistochemistry in, 109
 intravascular, 117, **130**
 lymphoblastic, 20
 lymphoplasmacytic/immunocytoma, **130**
 mantle cell, 114-115, **128**, **129**
 marginal zone, 115, 116, **129**, 161
 microvillous, 117
 natural killer cell, **132**
 NK-cell, 120
 plasmablastic, 117, **130**
 precursor T-lymphoblastic, 119-120
 primary effusion, 117
 primary mediastinal large B-cell, 117, **130**
 small cell variant of anaplastic, **132**
 small lymphocytic, 115-116, **130**, **157**
 splenic, 135
 T-cell, **131**
 T-lymphoblastic, **131**
 treatment with monoclonal antibody to CD20, 118-119
 WHO classification
  of B-cell neoplasms, 112-121
  of T-cell neoplasms, 119

Lymphomatoid granulomatosis, 197, **207**

Lymphomatoid papulosis, 408, **418**

Lymphoproliferative disorders in immunocompromised patients, 118

Lymphotoxin, 83

Lynch syndrome, 259, 337, 503, 514, 516

Lyonization, 438, 551

Lysogeny, 473-474

M

μ chain disease, 149

Macrodeletion syndromes, 446

Macroglobulinemia, Waldenström, 116

Macrolide resistance, 521

Macromolecules, helical structure of, 452

Macrophages, 10, 78, 79, 96, **375**, 424
 epithelioid, 86
 hemosiderin, 246

Magnification, 2

Major hereditary colon cancer syndrome, 516-517

Major histocompatibility complex, 89

Malakoplakia, 368, 370, 396, 397

Malignant cells, characteristics of, 4

Malignant fibrous histiocytoma, 12
 benign and low-grade, 18

Malignant hyperthermia, 534

Malignant mesothelioma, **212**

Mallory bodies, 281, **286**

Malpighian corpuscle, 134, **136**

MALTomas, 66, 115, 257

Mammaglobin, 47, 194, **298**

MammaPrint, 557

Mannose-binding lectin, 79

Mantle cell lymphoma, 114-115, **128**, **129**, 258

Mantle zone lymphoma of colon, **263**

Marfan syndrome, 86

Marginal zone lymphoma, 115, 116, **129**, 161, 409

Marker chromosome, 446

Marker DNA fragments, 469-470

Marsh system in celiac disease, 242

Massively parallel sequencing, 552

Massive ovarian edema, 351

Masson hemangioma, 15

Mass spectrometry, 531, 554-556

Mast cell leukemia, 145

Mast cells, 377

Mastocytosis, **133**, **135**, 137
 with fibrosis, **133**
 systemic, 135, **137**

Mastopathy, diabetic, 50, **58**

Maternal floor infarct, **308**

Maternally derived deoxyribonucleic acid, 436

Matrix-assisted laser desorption ionization (MALDI), 554

Mature (peripheral) T-cell and NK-cell neoplasm, 120-121

M-banding, 496-497, *497*

McCune-Albright syndrome, 166

Meckel diverticulum, 249, **256**

Meconium macrophage, 303

Meconium passage, 303

Meconium staining, 303

Medial calcific sclerosis, 220

Medial fibroplasia, 367

Medial umbilical ligament, 301

Mediastinal bronchogenic cysts, 213

Mediastinum, 191, 213-215, **216-218**
 core points for, 215
 epithelial neoplasms of anterior, 213-214
 middle and posterior lesions, 215
 nonepithelial neoplasms of anterior, 214-215
 nonneoplastic anterior lesions, 213

Mediterranean lymphoma, 257-258

Medullary adenomas, 66

Medullary carcinoma
 of breast, 48, **55**
 of colon, 261, **267**
 of kidney, 372, **376**
 of thyroid (and MTC syndrome), 60, 66, **72**, **73**

Medulloblastoma, 424, **427**

Megakaryocytes, 138

Megaloblastic anemia, **155**

Megaloblastic leukemia, **155**

Meibomian glands, 160

Meiosis, *435*, 435-436

Melan-A, 354, 410

Melan-A/MART-1, 369

Melan-A positivity, 399

Melanocytes, 409

Melanocytic proliferations, 409-412

Melanocytoma, 161

Melanoma, 409, **418**

desmoplastic, 410, **419**
minimal deviation, 410
polypoid or exophytic, 410
reexcising, 410
in situ, 411
spindle cell, 410
uveal, 161, **163**
Mel-CAM, 305
Melting, 8, 476
Melting curve analysis, 486, *486*, *487*
Membrane attack complex, 80
Mendelian genetics, 442
Mendelian inheritance, 476
Bayesian analysis in, 439-442
in clinical genetics, 437-443
in humans, 437
Mendelian traits, 437
Menetrier disease, 233
Meningiomas, 160, 424, **427**
Meningitis, 530
Meningococci, 77
Meniscectomy, 30
Meniscus, 30
Menstrual endometrium, **341**
Merkel cell carcinoma, 60, 406, **417**
Merkel cell polyomavirus tumor antigen, 406
Mesenchymal chondrosarcoma, 32-33, **35**, **36**
Mesenchymal hamartomas, 291, **296**
Mesenteric fibromatosis, 257, **263**
Mesenteric thrombi, 246
Mesoblastic nephroma, 370, **374**
Mesoderm, 301
Mesonephric adenoma, 377
Mesonephric cysts, 315
Mesonephric metaplasia, 377
Mesonephric remnants, 317
Mesothelial cells, **212**
Mesothelial hyperplasia, 363-364
Mesothelial-lined cysts, 213
Mesothelial proliferation, **366**
Mesothelioma, 194, 257, 363-364, 399
Mesothelium, 363
Messenger ribonucleic acid (mRNA), 461, 463, 506
cloning and, 473
translation into protein, 462
Metabolomics, 556
Metamyelocytes, 78
Metanephric adenoma, 370, **375**, 377
Metaphase, 459
Metaplasia, 322
transitional cell, 322
Metaplastic carcinoma, 48, **55**, **56**
Metastasin, 556
Metastasizing benign mixed tumor, 174
Metastatic adenocarcinoma, **151**, **212**, 353
Metastatic tumors, 138, 257
Methicillin, 520
Methicillin-resistant *Staphylococcus aureus* (MRSA), 481, 520
Methionine, 463
α-Methylacyl-coenzyme A racemase (αMACR), 370, 384, 387
Methylation, 464, 549-550
Methylation variable positions (MVPs), 551
Methylene glycol, 1
Meyenburg complex, 291
M-FISH (multicolor FISH), 495, *495*
MGMT, 512
Michaelis-Gutman bodies, 368
Microarray Experiment (MIAME), 507
Microarray Gene Expression Database Group (MEGD), 507
Microarrays, 446, 462, 499, 503-507, *504*, 550
comparative genomic hybridization, 505
normalization of data, 507
Microcalcifications, 174
Microchip-based electrophoresis, 479
Microdeletion analysis, 489-490
Microdeletion syndromes, 446
Microfollicular variant of adult granulosa cell tumor with Call-Exner bodies, **361**
Microglandular adenosis, 39, **52**
Microglandular hyperplasia, 326, **331**
Microinvasion, 41, 324, 352, 379
Micrometastasis, 44
Micropapillae, benign, 39
Micropapillary adenocarcinoma of breast, invasive, 48
Micropapillary carcinoma of breast, 39
Micropapillary low-grade ductal carcinoma in situ (DIC) of breast, 39
MicroRNAs, 270, 462
Microsatellite analysis, applications of, *536*, 536-538
Microsatellite instability (MSI), 337, 503, 514
testing for, 513, 515
Microsatellites, 501-503, 538, *539*
Microscopic colitis, 245
Microscopic polyangiitis, 219, 221
Microscopy
dark-field, 3
electron, 3
fluorescence, 8
phase contrast, 3
specimen examination in, 4
tissue appearance in, 3-4
Microvillous inclusion disease (MID), 242
Microvillous lymphoma, 117
Middle and posterior mediastinal lesions, 215
Middle ear, 159-160
Midfacial necrotizing lesions, 181
Midsecretory endometrium, **340**
Migratory glossitis, 165
Mikulicz disease, 173
Mild cognitive impairment, 534
Miller-Dieker syndrome, 446
Minimal deviation adenocarcinoma, 325
Minimal deviation melanoma, 410
Minimal residual disease (MRD), 142
Minisatellites, types of, 501-502
Minute tubules, **171**
Mismatch repair enzymes, 458
Misplaced epithelium, invasive adenocarcinoma vs, 247
Missense codons, 538-539
Mitochondrial deoxyribonucleic acid, *443*
Mitochondrial inheritance, 442-443
Mitogen-activated protein (MAP) kinases, 98, 511
Mitomap database, 443
Mitosis, 409, 457, 458-459, *459*
counting of, 44
Mitotic spindle, 459
Mixed cellularity Hodgkin disease, **125**
Mixed epithelial-stromal renal tumor (MEST), 370
Mixed lineage leukemia (MLL), 147
Mixed neuroendocrine carcinoma, 261, **267**

ISBN 978-089189-5886

MLH1, 515
Mobile genetic elements, *466*, 466-468, *467*
Modifications, posttranslational, 464
Molar pregnancy, **312**
Molecular beacon, 478
Molecular biology, 1
  central dogma of, 459
  link to genetics, 435
Molecular mediators of inflammation, *79*, 79-81, *80*
Molecular pathology, 452-548
  amplification in, 476
    DNA amplification, 482, *483*, 484
    isothermal nucleic acid, 484-485, *485*
    melting curve analysis, 486, *486*, *487*
    polymerase chain reaction, *476*, 476-482
    signal, 485
    in situ hybridization, 486-487
  blotting in, 470
  cloning in, 472
    vectors, 472-475, *473*
  in colorectal cancer, 261-262
  dementia in, 534-536
  DNA replication and, 457-459
  DNA structure in, 453-457
  DNA transcription and translocaton in, 459-466
  epigenetic regulation of genome and, 549-551
  fluorescent in situ hybridization in, 487-497
    preparation, 487-489
  functional genomics and transcriptomics, 551-552
  genes in, 466-468, 475-476
  hereditary cancer syndromes, 513-518
  historical background of, 452-453
  infectious disease testing in, 518-530
    Chlamydia trachomatis, 518-519
    Clostridium difficile, 521-522
    Enterobacteriaceae, 521
    Enterococcus, 519
    Enterovirus genus, 530
    Hepatitis B virus (HBV), 526
    Hepatitis C virus (HCV), 525-526
    Hepatitis D, 526
    human immunodeficiency virus (HIV), 524-525
    human papillomavirus, 526-528
    influenza viruses, 529-530
    Macrolide resistance, 521
    Neisseria gonorrhoeae, 519
    polyomavirus family, 529
    Staphylococcus aureus, 520-521
    strain typing and epidemiology, 522-523
    tuberculosis, 522
    viruses, 523-524
    viruses of herpes family, 528-529
  inherited disorders in, 540-547
    achondroplasia syndrome, 543-544
    craniosynostosis syndrome, 543-544
    cystic fibrosis, 541-543, *542*
    genetic screening in Ashkenazi Jews, 546-547
    hearing loss, 545-546
    hypercoagulability, 543, *543*
    hypochondroplasia syndrome, 543-544
    muscular dystrophy, 544-545
    neurofibromatosis, 545
    osteogenesis imperfecta, 545
    spinal muscular atrophy, 543
  mass spectrometry in studying proteins, 554-556
  microsatellite analysis in, *536*, 536-538
  multiple-probe fluorescent in situ hybridization (FISH), 493
    bioinformatics and public DNA databases, 499-500
    comparative genomic hybridization, 493-495, *494*
    deoxyribonucleic acid (DNA) sequencing, 497, *497*, 498
    multicolor, special karyotyping, 495-497
  nucleases in, *471*, 471-472
  nucleic acid studies in, 469-470
  oncogenes and tumor suppressor genes in, 510-513
  pathogenic organism testing in, 530-531
  pharmacogenetics in, *531*, 531-534, *532*
  phenotyping in, 556-557
  proteomics and, 553-554
  regulatory, ethical, and legal issues in, 509-510
  single nucleotide polymorphisms in, 538-540
  trinucleotide repeat disorders in, 547-548
  types of electrophoresis in, 470-471
Molecular phenotyping, 556-557
Molecular testing, 7-9
  in chronic myelogenous leukemia, 143
  for eukaryotic pathogens, 530-531
  in infectious diseases, 518-530, 531
    Chlamydia trachomatis, 518-519
    Clostridium difficile, 521-522
    Enterobacteriaceae, 521
    Enterococcus, 519
    Enterovirus genus, 530
    Hepatitis B virus (HBV), 526
    Hepatitis C virus (HCV), 525-526
    Hepatitis D, 526
    human immunodeficiency virus (HIV), 524-525
    human papillomavirus, 526-528
    influenza viruses, 529-530
    Macrolide resistance, 521
    Neisseria gonorrhoeae, 519
    polyomavirus family, 529
    Staphylococcus aureus, 520-521
    strain typing and epidemiology, 522-523
    tuberculosis, 522
    viruses, 523-524
    viruses of herpes family, 528-529
  for other pathogenic organisms, 530-531
  principles of, 469
  reference material in, 510
Molluscum contagiosum, 405
Monckeberg medial stenosis, 220
Monoallelic expression, imprinting as cause of, 551
Monoclonal antibodies, 369
Monoclonal antibodies renal cell carcinoma, 371
Monoclonal gammopathy of undetermined significance (MGUS), 148
Monocytes, 78
Monocytoid appearance, **129**
Mononucleosis, 108
Monophasic synovial sarcoma, **27**
Monophosphate, 453
Monosomy, 444
  fluorescent in situ hybridization (FISH) in detection, 489
Monozygotic (identical) twins, 305, 444
Morphea, 415, **422**
Morphea profundus, 11
Morton neuroma, 30
Morula, 301
Mosaicism, 446, 447, 475
MSH2, 512
MSH6, 512
MspI, 550

MUC2, 353
MUC6, 387
Mucinous adenocarcinoma of appendix, **267**
Mucinous adenoma of ovary, **360**
Mucinous carcinoma, 48, **55**, **360**
Mucinous cystadenomas, 351
Mucinous low malignant potential neoplasms of ovary, 352-353, **361**
Mucinous neoplasms, 351
  cystic, 270, **272**
  epithelial, 351
Mucocutaneous lymph node syndrome, 219
Mucoepidermoid carcinoma, 175, **178**
Mucolipidosis type IV, 546
Mucor mycosis, **183**
Mucosal prolapse, 246-247, 259, **265**
Mucosal prolapse simulating ulcerative proctitis, **254**
Muir-Torre syndrome, 517
Mullerian ducts, 364
Mullerian duct syndrome, 395
Mullerian-inhibiting substance, 395
Multicolor banding, 496-497
Multicolor fluorescent in situ hybridization (M-FISH), 495-497, *495*
Multidrug resistance (MDR), 556
Multifactorial inheritance, 443, 444, 447
Multifocality, 399
Multilocular cysts of thymus, 363, **216**, **217**
Multinodular hyperplasia of thyroid, **70**
Multiple endocrine neoplasias syndromes, 271, 517-518
Multiple fluorochromes, 481
Multiple lymphoepithelial cysts, **176**
Multiple myeloma, 148-149, **158**
Multiple-probe fluorescent in situ hybridization, 493-495, **497**
  multicolor (M-FISH) and spectral karyotyping (SKY), 495-497, *495*
Multiple sclerosis, 423, **427**
Multiplex ligation-dependent probe amplification (MLPA), 482, 484, 550
Munro abscesses, 413, **420**
Muscle(s)
  biopsies of, 425, **428**
  inflammatory and degenerative conditions of, 425
  tumors of, 14
Muscular dystrophy, 544-545
Mutations, 437
  in the D-loop, 443
  dynamic, 547
  founder, 546
  frameshift, 461
  germline, 514, 515
  in colorectal cancer, 261
  in introns, 465-466
  in non-small cell cancer, 194
  point, 510, 511, 538
  somatic, 510, 511, 513
  spontaneous, 438
Mutation-selection hypothesis, 449
Myasthenia gravis, 213
MYC, 445, 511
Mycobacterium avium intracellulare (MAI), 248
Mycobacterium tuberculosis, 522
Mycosis fungoides, 408-409
Myeloblasts, 140, **152**
Myelocytes, 78
Myelodysplastic/myeloproliferative neoplasms, 146
Myelodysplastic syndromes, 138-140
Myelofibrosis, **153**
Myeloma, 149
  plasmacytic type of, **158**
Myeloma cast, **374**
Myeloma cast nephropathy, 368
Myeloma kidney, 368
Myeloperoxidase, 77
Myelophthisis, 138
Myocardial infarct, early diagnosis of, 462
Myoepithelial cells, 38
Myoepithelioma, 174, **177**
Myofibroblastoma, 50-51, **58**
  palisaded, **133**
Myofibroblasts, 14
Myometrial infiltration, 347
Myometrium, 346-347, **348-349**
  adenomyosis and, 346
  core points for, 347
  uterine smooth muscle neoplasms, 346-347
Myositis ossificans, 11
Myospherulosis, 179, **183**
Myotonic dystrophy type 1, 547
Myxofibrosarcoma, 12, 18
Myxoid chondrosarcoma, 17, **25**, **349**
Myxoid leiomyoma, 11, **349**
Myxoid leiomyosarcomas, 347
Myxoid liposarcomas, 13-14, 17-18, **23**, 316
Myxoid neurofibroma, 11
Myxoid stroma, **24**, 347
Myxoid tumors, 316
  nerve sheath, 17
  smooth muscle, 316, **349**
Myxoid undifferentiated pleomorphic sarcoma/malignant fibrous histiocytoma, 316
Myxoma, 316

N

N-acetyltransferase (NAT2), 534
Nanometastases, 44, 196
Napsin A, 193, 196
Nasal polyps, 179, **183**
Nasopharyngeal carcinoma, 110
Nasopharynx. *See also* Nose, sinuses, oropharynx, and nasopharynx
  malignant neoplasms of, 180-181
National Center for Biotechnology Information, maintenance of Single Nucleotide Polymorphism Database by, 539-540
National Forensic Science Technology Center (NFSTC), 538
National Institute of Standards and Technology (NIST), Standard Reference Material (SRM) for, 538
National Institutes of Health (NIH), 507
  guidelines on definition, scope, purpose, and regulation of genetic testing, 509
National Marrow Donor Program, 91
Natural killer cell lymphomas, 119-120, **132**, 180, 182
Natural killer cell lymphoproliferative disorders, 120
Natural selection, 531
N-cadherin, 49
Necrobiosis lipoidica diabeticorum, 415
Necrosis, 6, 39, 187, **205**, **313**, 346, 385
Necrotizing fasciitis, causes of, 11
Necrotizing granuloma, **124**
Necrotizing sialometaplasia, 167, **172**
Neimann-Pick disease, 546
Neisseria gonorrhoeae, 519
  detection of, 485

ISBN 978-089189-5886

Neonatal hepatitis, 283, **290**
Nephrogenic adenoma, 377-378, **382**, 387
Nephrogenic rests, 370, **375**
Nerve growth factor, 82
Nerve sheath tumors, 16-17, 215
Neural cell adhesion molecule (NCAM), 84
Neural crest, 61
Neuroblastic tumors, 68
Neuroblastomas, 68
  differentiating, 68-69, **75**
  with Homer Wright pseudorosettes, **75**
  poorly differentiated, 68
  undifferentiated, 74
Neuroectodermal tumor, **29**
Neuroendocrine carcinoma, 60, **62**, 187, 191, 196, **202**, **205**, **267**
  of lung, 195
Neuroendocrine cells, 60, 224
Neuroendocrine differentiation, 260-261
Neuroendocrine neoplasms, 60, 191
Neuroendocrine system, 60-61, **62**
Neuroendocrine tumors, 257
  neural group of, 60
Neurofibrillary tangles, 534
Neurofibroma, 16, **25**, 215, 316
Neurofibromatosis, 514, 545
Neuromas, 30
  acoustic, 160, **162**
  Morton, 30
Neuron-specific enolase (NSE), 196
Neurosecretory vesicles, 60
Neutral buffered formalin, 1
Neutrophils, 78, 138
Nevi
  cellular blue, **420**
  compound, 409
  deep-penetrating, 412
  dysplastic, 409, 410-411, **419**
  Spitz, 412, **420**
Nevus sebaceous, **417**
New Delhi metallo-β-lactamase 1 (NDM-1), 521
NF1, 512
NFkB, 31
N-formyl-methionyl, 79
Nick translation, 488
Niemann-Pick disease, 134, **136**
Night sweats, 109
Nipple adenoma, 39, **53**
Nitric oxide, 76, 81
NOD2, 244
Nodular fasciitis, 10-11, **21**
Nodular glomerulosclerosis, 368
Nodular hyperplasia of thyroid, 63-64, **70**
  regenerative, 291, **296**
Nodular lymphocyte predominant Hodgkin disease, 109, 111, **126**, **127**
Nodular sclerosing Hodgkin disease, 110, **124**, **218**
  syncytial form of, **125**
Nodular tenosynovitis, 32
Nodular vasculitis, 416
Nomarski optics, 3
Nonautoimmune bullous disorders, 414
Noncaseating nonnecrotizing granuloma, **151**
Noncoding ribonucleic acid (RNA), 551
Nondisjunction, 445
Non-Hodgkin lymphomas (NHLs), 110-112, **125**, 135
Nonkeratinizing carcinoma
  nasopharyngeal, 181
  oropharyngeal squamous cell, 181
  undifferentiated, **184**, **185**
Non-Mendelian inheritance secondary to multifactorial inheritance, 443-444
Nonprocessed pseudogenes, 467
Nonseminomatous mixed germ cell tumor, **402**
Nonsister chromatids, 436
Non-small cell lung carcinomas, 192, **203**
Nonspecific interstitial pneumonia (NSIP), 198
Nonsynonymous single nucleotide polymorphisms, 539
Nora lesion, 33
Normalization in microassays, 507
Northern blotting, 470
Nose, sinuses, oropharynx, and nasopharynx, 179-182, **183-185**
  benign neoplasms and neoplasm-like conditions, 179-180
  core points for, 182
  inflammatory and infectious reactions, 179
  malignant neoplasms of nasopharynx, 181
  malignant neoplasms of oropharynx, 181
  malignant sinonasal neoplasms, 180
  Wegener and its differential diagnosis, 181-182
Nottingham index in breast cancer, 41, 44, 50
NPM1, 512
  mutations in, 141
Nuclear activator of activated T cells (NFAT), 98
Nuclear ISH, 491
Nuclear staining with hematoxylin, 2
Nuclear transplantation (cloning), 472
Nuclear truncation artifact, 492-493
Nucleases in molecular pathology techniques, *471*, 471-472
Nucleic acid, isolation of, 469
Nucleic acid, 109
  amplification, 469
  extraction and measurement of, 469-470, 477
  isolation of, 469
  purification of, 469
  sequence-based, 484, *485*
  testing of, 109
Nucleic acid extraction and measurement, 469-470, 477
Nucleic acid purification, 469
Nucleoside, 453, *454*
Nucleoside triphosphates, 454
Nucleosomes, 456
Nucleotide, 453
Numerical aperture, 2-3

O

Oblimersen (Genasense), 462
Obliterative vasculopathy, 304
Occult blood, stool testing for, 260
OCT3/4, 397, 398
Odontoblasts, 165, 167
Odontogenic cysts, 165-166
Odontogenic fibroma, 167
Odontogenic keratocyst, 165-166, **169**
Odontogenic myxoma, 167, **171**
Odontogenic neoplasms in oral cavity, 166-167
Odontomas, 167
Oil immersion lenses, 3
Okazaki fragments, 457
Olfactory neuroblastoma, 180, **183**, **184**
Oligodendrogliomas, 424-425, **428**
Oligonucleotide ligation assay, 482
  in screening for cystic fibrosis, 541-542
Oligonucleotides, 462, 478

Oncocytomas, 173, 369, 370-371, **375**
Oncogenes, 511-512
as cause of transformation, 511
transformation of proto-oncogene into, 512
tumor suppressor genes and, 510-513
Oncogenomic profiling, 556
Oncogenomics, 556
Oncotranscriptomics, 556
profiling in, 556
Oncotype DX, 557
1-gene-1 enzyme hypothesis, 452, 453
1,000 Genomes Project, 540
Online Mendelian Inheritance in Man (OMIM), 437
Oocyte, 350
Oophoritis, autoimmune, 350
Open reading frame, 463
Operon, 460
Opportunistic infections, 369
Opsonin, 80
Oral cavity, 165-168, **169-172**
benign odontogenic neoplasms in, 166-167
core points for, 168
inflammatory lesions in, 165
nonneoplastic mass lesions of, 166
odontogenic cysts in, 165-166
proliferations of squamous epithelium in, 167-168
Oral hairy leukoplakia, 168
Oral intraepithelial neoplasia (OIN), 167
Orchitis, 396
Organoid nevus, 405
Oriental cholangiohepatitis, 283
Oropharyngeal carcinoma, 181
Oropharynx. *See also* Nose, sinuses, oropharynx, and nasopharynx
malignant neoplasms of, 181
Orphan diseases, 557
Oseltamivir (Tamiflu), 530
Osseous dysplasia, 166
Ossifying fibroma, 166
Osteitis deformans, 31
Osteoarthritis, 30, **34**
Osteoblastic reactive atypia, 33
Osteochondritis dessicans, 31
Osteogenesis imperfecta, 545
Osteomyelitis, 31, **34**
Osteonecrosis, 31, **34**
Osteonectin, 87
Osteoporosis, 31
Osteosarcoma, **37**, 166
diagnosis of, 33
parosteal, 33, **36**
telangiectatic variant of, 33
treatment of, 33
Otitis media, chronic, 159
Otosclerosis, 159, **162**
Ovarian cysts, **359**
Ovarian endometriosis, **359**
Ovarian fibromas, 355, **362**
Ovarian fibromatosis, 355
Ovarian teratomas, 356
Ovary, 350-358, **359-362**
core points for, 358
endometrioid adenocarcinoma of, 353
epithelial neoplasms and, 351, 353-354
germ cell tumors of, 356
mucinous low malignant potential neoplasms and, 352-353
nonneoplastic stromal processes and, 350-351
normal function and histology, 350
primary adenocarcinoma versus metastatic adenocarcinoma, 353
serous and mucinous epithelial neoplasms and, 351
serous low malignant potential and, 351-352
sex cord-stromal neoplasms and, 354-356
small cell carcinoma, 357, **362**
teratomas, 356
unusual neoplasms and, 356-357
Overlap syndrome in autoimmune liver disease, 281, **288**
Ovulation, 350
Ovum, 350
Oxacillin, 520
Oxacillin-resistant *Staphylococcus aureus* (ORSA), 520
Oxygen-dependent pathways, 77
Oxytocin receptor, 338

P

P, 174
P2Y12 receptor, 533
P16, 323, **330**, 512
P27, 512
P53, 261, 326, 354, 378, 512, 513, 527
P57kip2, 309
P63, 187, 193, 196, 227, **330**
P504S, 384, 387
Pacental ischemia, acute, 304
PACE system, 484
PACs, 474
Paget disease, 31, **34**, 409
of bone, 159
of nipple, 47
Pagetoid invasion of epidermis, 409
Pagetoid reticulosis, 408
Painful bladder syndrome, 377
Palatal papillomatosis, 167, **172**
Palisaded myofibroblastoma, **133**
Pancreas, 269-271, **272-273**
acinar (or acinic) cell tumors of, **273**
core points for, 271
developmental anomalies of, 269
heterotopic, 269
neoplasms and, 270-271
nonneoplastic conditions of, 269-270
solid-pseudopapillary tumor of, **273**
Pancreas divisum, 269
Pancreatic acinar cell tumors, 270-271
Pancreatic adenocarcinoma, 270
ductal, 270
Pancreatic intraepithelial neoplasia, 270
Pancreatic islet cell tumor, 60
Pancreatic neoplasia, pancreas and, 270-271
Pancreatic neuroendocrine tumors, 271, **273**
Pancreatic pseudocysts, 269
Pancreatitis
acute, 269
autoimmune, 269-270
chronic, 269
chronic fibrosing, **272**
Paneth cells, 224
Panmyelosis, acute, 139, 142
Panniculitis conditions, 415-416
Pannus, **34**
Panton-Valentine leukocidin, 520
Papillary carcinoma, 64-65
follicular variant, 64
intraductal, 41, 42, **54**
renal cell, 371
squarmous, 186, **189**, **404**
urothelial, **383**

ISBN 978-089189-5886

Papillary dermis, 405
Papillary mesothelial hyperplasia, 363
Papillary microtumor, 65
Papillary syncytial metaplasia, **342**
Papillary urothelial lesions, 378-379
Papillary urothelial neoplasm of low malignant potential, 378
Papillomas, 41, 316
Papillomatosis, 405
  juvenile, 50, **57**
Pap smears, 322, 323-324
  Bethesda system for, 66-67
Paracentric inversion, 446
Paracortical hyperplasia, 108, **123**
Paracortical necrosis, 108
Paraffin, 1
Paraganglia, 60-61, **62**
  extraadrenal, 61
Paragangliomas, 159, **162**, 215, 380
  adrenal, 61
  core points for, 61
  gangliocytic, 61, **62**
  zellballen pattern, 61, **62**
Parakeratosis, **169**, 186
Paraphimosis, 403
Parasites, immune response to, 106
Parathyroid adenomas, 67, **74**
Parathyroid gland, 67-68
  core points for, 69
  normal, **74**
Parathyroid hyperplasia, **74**
Parathyroid tumors, 215
Paratubal cysts, 357
Paraurethral cysts, 315
Parkinson disease, 535
Parosteal osteosarcoma, 33, **36**
Paroxysmal nocturnal hemoglobinuria, 150
PARP inhibitor, 557
Partial endonuclease digestion, 474
Partial hydatidiform mole, 309-310, **312**
Paternity testing, 537-538
Pathogenic candidiasis, 165
Pathogenicity islands, 467
Pathwork Tissue of Origin Test (Pathwork Diagnostics), 506
Paucicellular myxoid stroma of vulvar aggressive angiomyxoma, **318**
Pauling, Linus, 452
Pautrier abscess, **418**
PAX2, 387
PAX8, 65
PAX8/PPARγ translocations, 65
PCA3 urine assay, 384
PCR/electrophoresis analysis, 503
PE-10, 196
PEComas, 191
Pedigrees, 436-437, 447
Pelvic inflammatory disease, 357
Pemphigoid, 165
Pemphigoid gestationis, 414
Pemphigus, 165, **421**
PenB, mutations of, 519
Pendred syndrome, 546
Penetrance, 437
Penis
  core points for, 404
  neoplasms of, 403-404
  papillary squamous cell carcinoma of, **404**
Pentoses, 453
Peptide bond, 463
Peptide nucleic acids, 477-478
  properties of, 478
Peptide nucleic acids oligonucleotides, 478
Peptides, 76
Peptidomics, 556
Periapical cemental dysplasia, 166, 167
Periapical cementoma, 167
Periapical cysts, 165, **169**
Periarteritis nodosa, 220, **223**
Pericentric inversion, 446
Perineural invasion, 386
  in adenoid cystic carcinoma, **177**
Perineurioma, 17
Perinuclear halos, 322, **328**
Periodic acid-Schiff (PAS), 2
Periostitis, reactive, **36**
Peripheral cutaneous T-cell lymphoma lymphoma, 408
Peripheral giant cell granuloma, 166, **170**
Peritoneal implants, 352
Peritoneal inclusion cysts, 363, **366**
Peritoneum, 363-365, **366**
  core points for, 365
  inclusion cysts, 363
  mesothelioma and mesothelial hyperplasia, 363-364
  normal serosa, 363
  pseudomyxoma peritonei, 364
  reactive fibrosis, 363
  secondary Mullerian system, 364-365
  unusual peritoneal neoplasms, 365
Perivascular epithelioid cell tumor, 347, 369
Persistent trophoblastic disease, 311
Peutz-Jeghers polyps, 258, **264**
Pfaffl method in qPCR, 481
Pfeiffer syndrome, 544
Pfu, 477
P-glycoprotein, 531
Phagocytic cells, 78, 87
Phagocytic system, 276
Phagocytosis, 77
Pharmacogenetics, 465
  in molecular pathology, *531*, 531-534, *532*
Pharmocokinetics, 531
Phase 1 metabolism, enzymes of, 532-533
  as member of cytochrome p450 system, 532-533
Phase contrast microscopy, 3
Pheochromocytoma, 60-61, 69, **75**
  composite, 69
  extraadrenal, 61
  with zellballen pattern, **75**
Philadelphia chromosome, 143, 146
Phimosis, 403
Phosphatidylinositol triphosphate (PIP3), 98
Photoallergic dermatitis, 413
Photocontact dermatitis, 413
Photodynamic therapy, 227
Photofrin, 227
Photomicrographs, **185**
Phthisis bulbi, 161, **164**
Phyllodes tumor, 50, **57-58**
Pick adenoma, 395
PIG-A, 150
Pigmented spindle cell nevus, 411
Pigmented villonodular synovitis, 32, **35**
Pill esophagitis, **231**
Pineoblastomas, 424
Pingueculum, 160
Pituitary adenoma, 180
Pituitary gland, 423
  normal, **427**
Pityriasis rosea, 413
PKD1, 291, 367
PKD2, 291, 367
PKHD1, 291

Placenta, 301-305, **306-308**
core points for, 306
development of, *301*, 301-302
gross examination of, 302-303
ischemia, 246, 304
microscopic examination of, 303-305
products of conception and, 305
testing in pregnancy, 305-306
twin, **308**
Placenta accreta, 309
Placenta increta, 309
Placental abruption, acute, 304
Placental alkaline phosphatase (PLAP), 354, 397
Placental infarct, acute, **307**
Placental site nodules, 305, 310
Placental site trophoblastic tumor (PSTT), 309, 310, **313**
Planapochromatic lenses, 2
Plaque, 474
Plasmablastic lymphoma, 117, **130**
Plasmacytoid dendritic cells, 96
Plasma proteins, 76
Plasmid libraries, 473
Plasmids, 472
conjugative, 467-468
empty, 472
Platelet aggregation, 80
Platelet-derived growth factor, 82
Platelet derived growth factor receptor (PDGFR), 46
Platelet-derived growth factor receptor α (PDGFRA), 235
Platelet-endothelial cell adhesion molecule (PECAM), 84
β Pleated sheet, 464
Pleomorphic adenoma, 173-174, **176**
Pleomorphic fibroma, 11
Pleomorphic lipoma, 13, **22**
Pleomorphic liposarcoma, 14, 18, **22**
Pleomorphic rhabdomyosarcoma, **23**
Pleomorphism, 379
Pleura, 209-210, **211-212**, 363
core points for, 210
malignant mesotheliomas and their mimics, 209-210
mesothelial cells versus metastatic carcinoma, 209
solitary fibrous tumors, 210
Pleural plaque, 210, **212**
Pleuropulmonary blastoma, 197, **207**
Plexiform spindle cell nevus, 411
Ploidy analysis, 310
Pneumatosis cystoides intestinalis, 247, **255**
Pneumococcal antigens, 4-5
Pneumococci, 77
Pneumocystis carinii, 197, **207**
Pneumocyte proliferation, atypical, 193, 203
Pneumocytomas, 192
Point mutations, 510, 511, 538
Polarized light, 3
Polonies, 499
Polyacrylamide, 469
Polyangiitis overlap syndrome, 221
Polycystic kidney disease, 291
Polycystic ovary disease, 351, **359**
Polycystin-1, 291
Polycythemia vera, 142, **156**, 465
Polygenic inheritance, 444
Polymerase chain reaction (PCR), 8-9, 104, *476*, 476-482
advent of, 469
allele-specific, 477-478, 543
amplification, 478
clamping, 477-478
COLD, 478
ligation-dependent, 482-483
long-range, 477
multiple, 479
quantitative (qPCR), 480-482, *481*
reverse, 44, 462, 470, 479-480, 506, 512
reverse transcriptase (RT-PCR), 479-480
sequence-specific, 477
testing, 510
2-step nested, 479
weakness of, 477
Polymorphism, 89, 465
Polymorphous low-grade adenocarcinoma (PLGA), 175, **178**
Polymyositis, 425
Polyomavirus family, 529
Polypeptide, coding for, 466
Polyploidy, 445
Polypoid melanoma, 410
Polyps
adenomatous, **238**, 258, 264
colonic, 258
dysplasia in, **259**
fundic gland, **238**
hyperplastic, **238**, **264**
inflammatory fibroid, 238
juvenile, 258, **264**
Peutz-Jeghers 258, **264**
Popliteal fossa, cysts of, 30
Populations, 447
Population stratification, 449
Poromas, 406
Portal hypertension, 291
Port-wine stain, 15
Posterior probability, 440
Postirradiation vascular, **59**
Postoperative spindle cell nodule, 385
Posttranscriptional silencing, 460, 462
Posttranslational modifications, 464
Posttransplant lymphoproliferative disorder, 118, **131**, 369
Potter system of renal cystic disease, 367
Pouchitis, **253**
diversion colitis and, 245
Poulson phenomenon, 278
PPARγ, 65
Prader-Willi syndrome, 446, 550-551
Preauricular skin tag, 159
Pre-B cell, 93
Precursor B-cell leukemia, 146
Precursor T-lymphoblastic lymphoma, 119-120
Predictive autoantibodies, 384
Pregnancy, testing in, 305-306
Pregnancy luteoma, 350, **359**
Preinitiation, 460
Preleukemia conditions, 138
Premature ovarian failure, 350
Primary adenocarcinoma versus metastatic adenocarcinoma of ovary, 353
Primary biliary cirrhosis, 279-280, **288**
nonneoplastic liver and, 279-280
Primary effusion lymphoma, 117
Primary hyperparathyroidism, **169**
Primary mediastinal large B-cell lymphoma, 117, **130**, **218**
Primary ovarian adenocarcinoma, metastatic adenocarcinoma versus, 353

Primary peritoneal carcinoma, 364-365
Primary protein structure, 464
Primary recurrent pyogenic cholangitis, 283
Primary ribonucleic acid, 461
Primary sclerosing cholangitis, 279, **287**
Primary sex cords, 395
Primitive neuroectodermal tumor, 511
Prion disease, 536
Prior probability, 439
Probability of paternity, 537
Probe, 503
Probe labeling, 488
ProbeTec assay, 485
Procainamide, 534
Processed pseudogenes, 467
Proctitis, chronic radiation, 249, **256**
ProExC, 323
Prognostic Scoring System (WPSS), 140
Prokaryotes, 458, 463
  distinction between eukaryotes and, 453
Prokaryotic genomes, 472-473
Prolactin, secretion of, 423
Prolactinomas, secretion of, 423
Proliferations of squamous epithelium in oral cavity, 167-168
Proliferative endometrium, **340**
Proliferative fasciitis, 11
Proliferative verrucous leukoplakia (PVL), 167
Promoter hypermethylation, 513
Promoters, 459, 460
  alternative, 460
Properdin, 80
Prophase, 459
Propidium iodide, 489
Prostaglandin G2 (PGG2), 80-81
Prostaglandins, 81
Prostate
  adenosis of, **393**
  basal cell carcinoma of, 386
  cancer of, 384, 449
  sclerosing adenosis of, **394**
  transitional metaplasia of, **392**
Prostatectomy, 386
  radical, 389-390
Prostate gland, 384-391, **392-399**
  benign, **392**
  biopsy of, 384-386, **393**
    after treatment for carcinoma, 389
  cancer screening for, 384
  carcinoma in
    in metastatic sites, 391
    prevention of, 391
  core points for, 391
  immunohistochemistry of prostatic tissue, 387-388
  mimics of prostatic adenocarcinoma, 387
  normal histology, **392**
  prostatic intraductal neoplasia, 388
  radical prostatectomy and, 389-390
  transurethral resection, 390
  urethral polyp, 385
Prostate specific antigen (PSA) test, 384
Prostate specific antigen (PSA) test index, 384
Prostatic adenocarcinoma, 386, **392**, **393**, **394**
  ductal, 386, **393**
  mimics of, 387
Prostatic intraductal neoplasia (PIN), 385, 388, **394**
Prostatic tissue, normal, **392**
Protamines, 456
Proteasome, 465
Protein C, 543
Protein crosslinking, 5
Protein Databank (RCSB PDB), 555
Protein kinase C (PKC), 98
Proteins
  DNA-associated, 549
  mass spectrometry in studying, 554-556
  properties of, 464, *464*
  3-dimensional structure of, 553
  transport to correct intracellular location, 464-466, *465*
Protein synthesis, 459
Protein transcription factors, 460
Protein truncation test, 516-517
Proteolytic cascade, 79, 80
Proteome, 465
Proteome Browser, 555
Proteomics, 465, 531
  molecular pathology and, 553-554
  opportunities offered by, 555-556
Proton pump inhibitors, 532
Proto-oncogene, 511
  transformation of, into oncogene, 512
Proviral deoxyribonucleic acid, 482, 524
Psammoma bodies, **71**, **360**, 363
Psammoma carcinoma, 351
Pseudoautosomal regions, 450
Pseudodecidualized stroma, **341**
Pseudodiploid, 491
Pseudofollicles, 115
Pseudogenes, 91, 466, 467
  nonprocessed, 467
  processed, 467
Pseudo-Giemsa banding, 494
Pseudogoblet cells, 224, 225, **229**
Pseudogout, 31
Pseudomembranous inflammation, 84
Pseudomyxoma peritonei, 352-353, **361**, 364
Pseudotumor, fibro-osseous, 11
Psoriasis, 413
PTEN, 337, 378, 512
Pterygium, 160, **163**
Public DNA databases, bioinformatics and, 499-500
Pulmonary adenocarcinoma, 192
Pulmonary blastoma, 197, **207**
Pulmonary hamartoma, 191, **202**
Pulmonary hyalinizing granuloma, 191, **202**
Pulmonary meningothelial-like nodules (PMLNs), 191
Pulmonary sequestration, 191
Pulmonary small cell carcinoma, 406
Pulsed field gel electrophoresis, 470
  in strain typing, 522-523
PulseNet, 523
Punnett squares, 436, 442
Purulent exudate, 77
PVNS/diffuse tenosynovial giant cell tumor, 32
Pyelonephritis, chronic, 367-368, **374**
Pyogenic bacteria, 77
Pyogenic granuloma, 15, 166, **170**
Pyrogram, 498, *498*
Pyrosequencing, 498, 499

Q

Q-banding, 444
Quantitative polymerase chain reaction (qPCR), 480-482, *481*
Quaternary structure, 464

R

Radiation in treating prostate carcinoma, 389
Radiation proctitis, 249, **256**
Radical prostatectomy prostate gland and, 389-390
Raloxifene (Evista), 45
RANKL, 31
Rapamycins, 369
Rapid amplification of cDNA ends (RACE), 479
RAS, 378, 511
RasGDP, 98
Ras proteins, 511
Rb, phosphorylation of, 527
RB, 378, 513
R-banding, 445
Reactivation syndromes, 118
Reactive periostitis, 32, **36**
Reactive pneumocytes, 193
Reactive pneumocytes hyperplasia, 193
Reactive thrombocytosis, 145
Reactive vascular lesions, 15
REAL classification system of lymphomas, 111-112
Receptor tyrosine kinases, 46
Reciprocal translocation, 446
Reclast, 31
Recombinant immunoblot assay (RIBA), 279
Recombination, 436, 447, 450
Recombination activating genes 1 and 2, 94
Recombination signal sequence (RSS), 92, 94
Rectal adenocarcinoma, **266**
5α-Reductase inhibitors, side effects of, 391
Reed-Sternberg cells, 110-111, 135, **137**, **152**, 214, **218**
  classic, **125**
Reflux nephropathy, 368
Refractory anemia, 139
Refractory cytopenia with multilineage dysplasia, 139, **152**
Region-specific partial chromosome paints (RPCP), 496
Regulatory issues in molecular pathology, 509-510
Regulatory T-cells (T-regs), 99
Relapsing polychondritis, 159
Relative probability, 440
Relative risk ratio, 448, 449
Renal allograft rejection, 374
Renal artery dysplasia, 367
Renal artery stenosis, 367
Renin-secreting juxtaglomerular cell tumor, 367
Repetitions, types of, 468
Repetitive DNA, 488, 494, 501-502
Replacement vector, 473
Replication slippage, 467, 468
Replicative segregation, 443
Residual risk, 440
Resistant ovary syndrome, 350
Respiratory bronchiolitis, 199
Respiratory burst, 77
Respiratory epithelial adenomatoid hamartoma, 179, 180, **183**
Restriction endonucleases, 471, *471*, 471-472
Restriction fragment length polymorphism (RFLP), 91, 472
  analysis of, in strain typing, 522
RET, 511
Rete pegs, 405
Reticuloendothelial system, 276
Retiform hemangioendothelioma, 15-16
Retinitis pigmentosa, 439
Retinoblastoma, 161
  with Flexner-Wintersteiner rosettes, **164**
Retroelements, 466
Retrogene, 467
Retroperitoneal fibromatosis, 269
Retroperitoneal fibrosis, 269, 363
Retrotransposition, 466, 467
Retrotransposons, 466
Retroviruses, 524
  gene transfer with, 475-476
Rett syndrome, 438, 551
Reverse chromosome painting, 493
Reverse-DAPI, 496
Reverse fluorescent in situ hybridization (FISH), 491, 495
Reverse transcriptase, 467, 473
Reverse transcriptase-polymerase chain reaction (RT-PCR), 44, 462, 470, 479-480, 506, 512
Reversible dye-terminator techniques, 499
Rhabdoid tumor, 372, **376**
Rhabdomyosarcoma, 14, 316
  alveolar, **23**
  embryonal, **23**
  pleomorphic, **23**
Rheumatoid arthritis, 30
Rheumatoid nodules, 415
Rheumatoid vasculitis, 219
Rhinoscleroma, 179
Rhinosporidiosis, 179
Rhodamine, 487
Ribonucleic acid (RNA)
  antisense, 461
  primary, 461
  structure of, 459
  trafficking, 462
Ribonucleic acid (RNA) genes, 551
Ribonucleic acid (RNA) interference, 462, 549
Ribonucleic acid (RNA) polymerase, 453, 460
Ribonucleic acid (RNA) splicing, 461
Riboprobes, 323
Riboproteins, 462
Ribose, 453
Ribosomal Database Project, 518
Ribosomal ribonucleic acid (RNA), 453
Ribosomes, 453
Ribozymes, 461, 462
Richter syndrome, **157**
Riedel thyroiditis, 63, 269
Rifampicin, 522
Ring chromosome, 446
Risedronate, 31
RNA-induced silencing complex (RISC), 462
RNA interference (RNAi), 475
Robertsonian translocation, 446
Roche/454 FLX Pyrosequencer, 499
Roche LightCycler, 486
Rokitansky-Aschoff sinus of gall bladder, 274, **285**
Rosai-Dorfman disease, 19, **28**, 180
rosebud, 587
Rosettes
  in ependymoma, 425
  in retinoblastoma, 425

ISBN 978-089189-5886

S

S-100, 410
Salivary duct carcinoma, 175, **178**
Salivary gland, 173-175, **176-178**
  benign neoplasms in, 173-174
  core points for, 175
  malignant neoplasms in, 174-175
  nonneoplastic processes in, 173
Salpingitis, **362**
Salpingitis isthmica nodosa, 357, **362**
Sandwich effect, 496
Sanger method of DNA sequencing, 498
Sarcoidosis, 86, 138, **151**, 200
Sarcoma, systems of grading, 10
Sarcomatoid carcinoma, 197
  renal cell, 369
Sarcomatous mesotheliomas, 209, *211*, 364
Satellite DNA, 501
Scarff-Bloom-Richardson system, 44
SCCmecA, 520
Schatzki rings, 224
Scheuer system, 278, 280, 281
Schiller-Duval bodies, **401**
Schneiderian papillomas, 179
Schwannoma, 16, **24**, **162**, 215, **218**
  cellular, 16-17, **25**
  degenerative, 16-17, **25**
Scientific Working Group on DNA Analysis Methods, 538
Scleroderma, 415
Sclerosing adenosis, 388
  of breast, **52**
  of prostate, 388, **394**
Sclerosing atypical lipoma, 13
Sclerosing cholangitis, 269, 363
Sclerosing hemangioma of lung, 191, 192, **202**
Sclerosing mediastinitis, 213, **216**, 269, 363
Sclerosing mesenteritis, 257, **263**, 363
Sclerosing peritonitis, 363
Sclerosing sialadenitis, 173
Sclerosing stromal tumor, 355
Scrapie, 536
Scrotum, 403, 404
Sebaceous lymphadenoma of parotid, **176**
Seborrheic dermatitis, 413
Seborrheic keratosis, 316, 405, **417**
Secondary Mullerian system, 364-365
Secondary sex cords, 395
Secondary vasculitis, **222**
Secretogranins, 60
Secretory carcinoma
  of breast, 49, **56**
  of endometrium, 338, **340**
Selectins, 84
Selective serotonin reuptake inhibitors (SSRIs), 532
Self-splicing, 468
Self-sustained sequence replication, 484, *485*
Sella turcica, 423
Seminal vesicle tissue, 387, **393**
Seminoma, **218**, 396, 397
  anaplastic, 397
  spermatocytic, 397
Sentinel lymph nodes, examination of, 44-45
Septic shock, 83
Septin 9, 260
Sequence comparison, 500
Sequence-specific oligonucleotide probe (SSOP), 478
Sequence-specific polymerase chain reaction, 477
Sequence-specific primers (SSP), 477
Sequencing of DNA, 472
  by synthesis, 498
Sequential hybridization, 474
Sequestrum, 31
Serial analysis of gene expression (SAGE), 552
Serous carcinoma of ovary, 351, **362**
Serous epithelial neoplasms of ovary, 351
Serous low malignant potential, 351-352
Serous tubal intraepithelial carcinoma (STIC), 357
Serrated adenoma, **264**
Sertoli cell-only syndrome, 396
Sertoli cells, 396
Sertoli cell tumors, 355, 395, 397, 399, **402**
  stromal, 357
Sertoli differentiation, 357
Sertoli-Leydig cell tumor, 355, **361**
Serum testing in pregnancy, 305
Severe combined immunodeficiency (SCID), 88, 476
Sex chromosomes, 456
Sex cord-stromal neoplasms, 351, 354-356, 399
Sex reversal, 395
Sézary syndrome, 408
Shigella dysenteriae, 247
Short interfering RNA, 462
Short interspersed nuclear elements (SINEs), 501
Short tandem repeats (STR), 502
Shotgun sequencing, 474
Sialadenitis, autoimmune, 269
Sialadenoma papilliferum, 167
Sicca syndrome, 173
Sickle cell anemia, 465
Sideroblastic anemia, 139
Signal amplification techniques, 485
Signal transduction, 81
Signet ring adenocarcinoma, **240**, **267**
Silencers, 461
Silver staining, 471
Simple sequence repeat polymorphisms (SSRP), 502
Single fusion strategy in FISH, 490, 492
Single nucleotide polymorphism, 447-448, 449, 478, 539, 551
Single Nucleotide Polymorphism Database, 525-526, 539-540
Single-strand conformation polymorphism (SSCP), 470
Single-stranded DNA, 470
Sinonasal adenocarcinoma, 179, 180
Sinonasal hemangiopericytomas, 179
Sinonasal undifferentiated carcinoma, 180
Sinuses. *See* Nose, sinuses, oropharynx, and nasopharynx
Sinus histiocytosis, 108, **123**
  with massive lymphadenopathy, 180
Sinusitis, 179
Sister chromatids, 435
Sjögren syndrome, 173, **176**
Skene duct cysts, 315
Skin, 405-416, **417-422**
  acute and chronic dermatitis, 413-414
  autoimmune disorders of, 415
  bullous/vesicular disorders, 414-415
  core points for, 416
  cutaneous lymphoproliferative disorders, 407-412
  epithelial neoplasms of, 406
  infectious and granulomatous conditions of, 415
  inflammatory lesions (dermatoses), 412-413
  normal structure of, 405, **417**

Skin tags, 316
  preauricular, 159
SKY (spectral karyotyping), 495, *495*
Slides, interchange among laboratories, 1
SMAD4, 261
Small cell carcinoma, 60, **205**, **206**, **207**
  of lung, 195
Small cell lymphomas, 112-116
Small lymphocytic lymphoma, 115-116, **130**, **157**
Small nuclear ribonucleoproteins, 461
Small vessel vasculitis, 219, 220
Smooth muscle actin (SMA), 14
SN-38, 533
Sodium dodecyl sulfate (SDS), 553
Soft tissue, 10-20, **21-29**
Soft tissue neoplasms, with cytogenetic abnormalities, 10-20
Solid-pseudopapillary tumor of pancreas, 270, **273**
Solitary fibrous tumor, 210, **212**, 363-364
Solitary infantile hemangioendotheliomas, 294
Solitary rectal ulcer syndrome, 246
Somatic hypermutation, 100, 101, *101*, 104
Somatic mosaicism, 447
Somatic mutation, 510, 511, 513
Somatic promoter hypermethylation, 515
Southern blotting, 470, 472, 502
SOX9, 395
SP1, 460
Spacer oligonucleotide typing (spoligotyping) technique, in stain typing, 523
Spectral karyotyping (SKY), 495-497
Spectrophotometry, purity determination by, 469
Spermatocele, 396
Spermatocytic seminoma, 397, **401**
Spermatogenesis, 396
Spermatogonia, 395
Spherical aberration, 2
Spinal muscular atrophy, 543
Spindle cell hemangioma, 15
Spindle cell lipoma, **22**, 316
Spindle cell melanoma, 410
Spindle cell thymoma, **216**
Spindle cell variant of Spitz nevus, **420**
Spinobulbar muscular atrophy, 547
Spinocerebellar ataxias, 547
Spitz nevi, 411, 412, **420**
Spleen, 134-135, **136-137**
  benign lesions of, 134-135
  core points for, 135
  malignant lesions of, 135
  vascular pattern of, 134
Splenic cysts, 134
Splenic hamartoma, **136**
Splenic lymphomas, 135
Splenic marginal zone lymphoma (SMZL), 135, **137**
Splice donor, 461
Spliceosomes, 461
Spontaneous mutations, 438
Squamous carcinoma, 167, 181, **268**
  basaloid type of, 186, 187, **203**, 317, 325
  keratinizing, 316
Squamous intraepithelial lesions, 324
Squamous metaplasia simulating CIN, **329**
Squamous odontogenic tumor, 167
SRY, 395, 439
Stacking, 488
Stanford Microarray Database, 507, 552
Staphylococci, 77
Staphylococcus aureus, 520-521
Start codon, 463
Starting probability, 439
Stasis dermatitis, 415, **421**
Statistical testing, 449
Steatohepatitis, 282
Stellate reticulum, 167
Stem line, 447
Steroid cell tumor, 355, **362**
Stevens-Johnson syndrome, 534
Stomach, 232-236, **237-240**
  core points for, 236
  gastric adenocarcinoma and, 234-235
  gastric dysplasia and, 234
  gastric lymphoid proliferations and, 234
  gastric stromal tumors and, 236
  gastritis, 232-233
  nonneoplastic and polypoid conditions of, 233-234
  normal histology of, 232
Stool testing for occult blood, 260
Stop codon, 463
Strain typing and molecular epidemiology, 522-523
Strand displacement amplification (SDA), 485, *485*
Stratification of population, 438, 449
Strawberry nevus, 15
Streaming in benign breast masses, 39
Streptococcus agalatiae, 530
Streptococcus pyogenes, 530
Stromal hyperplasia of ovary, 351
Stromal hyperthecosis, 351, **359**
Stromal luteinization, **359**
Stromal luteoma, 355
Structural annotation, 500
Structural Classification of Proteins (SCOP) database, 555
Strumal carcinoid, **362**
Struma ovarii, 356
Stutter bands, 503
Subacute dermatitis, 413, **420**
Subcellular localization of staining, 109
Subchondral bone cysts, 30
Subcutaneous panniculitis-like T-cell lymphoma, 408
Subepidermal bullae, 414
Subglottis, ulceration of, **188**
Substage condenser, 2
Succinylcholine, 534
Sugar tumor, 191, **202**
Sulfonamide, 534
Superficial and deep perivascular inflammation, 413, 414
Superficial perivascular inflammation with plasma cells, 414
Suppressor of cytokine signaling (SOCS) proteins, 84
Suppurative exudate, 77
Supraglottis, 186
Surface-enhanced laser desorption/ionization (SELDI), 554
Surgical specimens, steps in examining, 1-4
Swine flu, 530
Swiss cheese disease, 50
SYBR green, 470, 480, 486
Sydney system of gastritis, 232
Syk, 46
Symplastic leiomyoma, 346
Synaptic vesicles, 60
Synaptophysin, 60, 354
Syncytial form of nodular sclerosing Hodgkin disease (NSHD), **125**
Syncytioma, 310

ISBN 978-089189-5886

Syncytiotrophoblastic giant cells, 302
Syncytiotrophoblasts, 302, **307**, 309, 397
Synovial chondromatosis, 31, **35**
Synovial sarcomas, 19, **28**
Synthetic oligonucleotide arrays, 503
Syphilis, 315
Systemic inflammatory response syndrome (SIRS), 83

T

Tacrolimus, 369
Takayasu arteritis, 219, 220
Tamoxifen, 45, 532, 533
Tamoxifen-associated endometrial adenocarcinomas, 45
Tandem direct repeat, 468
Tandem duplications, 501
TaqMan assay, 480
Targeted arrays, 505
TATA box, 460
TATA box binding protein (TBP), 460
Tauopathies, 535
Tay-Sachs disease, 546
T:B lymphocyte ratio, 138
T-cell activation, 95-96, 100, 369
T-cell-independent antigens, 104
T-cell lymphoma, **131**, 197
  cutaneous, 408
  enteropathy-associated, 258, **263**
T-cell prolymphocytic leukemia (T-PLL), 120, 149
T-cell receptor gene rearrangement, *94*, 94-99
T-cell receptors, 94
T-cell-rich B-cell lymphomas (TCRBCL), **130**, 197
  vs Hodgkin disease, 111, 117
Telomerase, 323
Temporal arteritis, 219, 220, **222**
Teratocarcinoma, 398
Terminal deoxynucleotidyl transferase (TdT), 92
Terminal duct/lobular unit (TDLU), 45
Terminal villus, **307**
Testes, 395-400, **401-402**
  core points for, 400
  cryptorchid, 395, **401**
  disorders of development and location, 395-396
  infertility and, 396
  neoplasms of, 396-400, **402**
  nonneoplastic conditions, 396
  normal development and structure, 395
  testicular neoplasms and, 396-399
Testicular choriocarcinomas, 398
Testicular neoplasia, 396-399
Testicular seminoma, **401**
Testicular teratomas, 356
Testosterone, 391, 395
Texas red, 487
TH-3 cells, 99
Thecoma, **362**
Therapy-related myeloid neoplasms, 141
THEROS CancerTYPe ID (bioTheranostics), 506
ThinPrep system, 324
Thiopurine methyltransferase (TPMT), 534
Thrombomodulin, 365
Thrombotic microangiopathy conditions, 368
Thrombotic thrombocytopenic purpura (TTP), 368
Thromboxane, 81
Thymic carcinoma, 214, **217**
Thymic cysts, 213, **216**
Thymic hyperplasia, 213
Thymic neoplasms, 214
Thymolipoma, 215, **218**
Thymomas, 214
Thyroid carcinoma, unusual forms of, 66
Thyroid gland, 63
  core points for, 69
  fine needle aspiration of, 66-67
  frozen sections of, 67
  inflammatory and autoimmune conditions of, 63
  mass lesions of, 63-67
  nonepithelial neoplasms of, 66
Thyroiditis, 63
Thyroid transcription factor (TTF-1), 47, 192
T lymphoblastic lymphoma, **131**
Tolerance, immunologic, 105
Toll-like receptors (TLRs), 78
Tooth formation, 165
Topoisomerases, 457
Toxic shock syndrome (TSS), 521
TRAb, 63
Trachea, 186-187, **188-190**
  intraepithelial neoplasia, 186-187
  laryngeal neoplasia, 186-187
  nonneoplastic processes, 186
Traits, Mendelian, 437
Tram-tracking, 368-369
Trans-acting, 460
Transcribed strands, 459
Transcription, 459-461
Transcriptional activator proteins, 460
Transcriptional silencing of gene, 460-461
Transcription-initiation complex, 460
Transcription-mediated amplification, 484, *485*
Transcriptomics, 465
Transduction, 468, 476
Transfection, 473, 476
Transfer ribonucleic acid (tRNA), 453, 468
Transformation, 468, 472, 476
  oncogenes as cause of, 511
Transforming growth factor-β (TGF-β), 4, 82
Transgenic animal, 475
Transglutaminase, 241
Transient acantholytic dermatosis, 414
Transitional cell carcinoma, 379
Transitional cell metaplasia, 322
Transitional meningioma, **427**
Transitional metaplasia of prostate, 385, **392**
Translation, 462-464, *463*
Transmembrane proteins, 81
Transplantation
  kidney in, 368-369
  liver in, 294
  testing for solid organs, 91
Transposons, 466
Transrectal prostate biopsy, 385
Transrectal ultrasound, 384
Transudate, 77
Trastuzumab (Herceptin), 46
Trichoepithelioma, 406, **417**
Trichofolliculoma, 406
Trichomonas, 315
Trichomonas vaginalis, detection of, 530
Tricyclic antidepressants (TCAs), 532
Trinucleotide repeat disorders, 547-548
Tripartite tree of life, 453
Triple-negative carcinomas, 557

Triploidy, 310, 445

Trisomies, 444, 510
  fluorescent in situ hybridization in detection of, 489

Trisomy 21, 444

Tropheryma whippelii, 530

Trophoblastic hyperplasia, **312**

Trophoblasts, 301-302, 305, 309
  abnormalities of intermediate, 310

True natural killer cell lymphomas, 182

True vocal cords, 186

Tryptophan repressor operon, 460

Tubal intraepithelial carcinoma (TIC), 357

Tuberculosis, 522

Tuberous sclerosis retroperitoneum, 191

Tubo-ovarian abscess (TOA), 357

Tubular adenoma of breast, 39, **52**

Tubular carcinoma of breast, 48, **55**

Tubules, 368

Tubulitis, 369

Tumor cell necrosis, 346, 347

Tumorlets, 191, 192, **202**

Tumor necrosis factor (TNF), 82, 83

Tumor suppressor genes, 512-513

Tumor suppressor proteins, 527

Tunica albuginia, 395, 396

Tunica vaginalis, 395

Turcot syndrome, 517

Turner syndrome, 444

Twins, 437

Twin-twin transfusion syndrome (TTTS), 305

2-dimensional electrophoresis, 553-554

2-step nested PCR, 479

Tympanosclerosis, 159

Typhlitis, 248

Tyrosine-based activation motif (ITAM), 102

Tyrosine kinases, types of, 46

U

UBE3A, 551

Ubiquitin, 96, **343**

Ubiquitin-specific protease-6 (*USP6*), 32

UDP-glucuronosyltransferase, 533

UGT1A1, 533

Ulcerative colitis, 242-245, **252**, **253**
  dysplasia in, 244

Ulcerative proctitis, 243

Ulcers, 84
  aphthous, 243, **252**
  fissuring, 243
  longitudinal, 243

Umbilical cord, 301

Umbilical cord vasculitis, 304

Undifferentiated retinoblastoma without Flexner-Wintersteiner rosettes, **164**

Unicameral bone cyst, 32

Unilocular thymic cyst, 213, **216**

Uniparental disomy (UPD), 550

Upper gastrointestinal screening, 225

Urachal carcinoma, 379

Uracil, 453, 462-463

Urethral caruncle, 378, **382**

Uric acid crystals, deposition of, **34**

Urine cytology, 380

Uroplakin III, 379

Urothelial carcinoma, 369, 370, 372, *see also* Bladder

Urothelial dysplasia and carcinoma in situ, 378

Urothelial papilloma, 378

UroVysion, 380

Urticaria pigmentosum, 407

Usual interstitial pneumonia, 198, **208**

Uterine bleeding, dysfunctional, 335, **341**

Uterine papillary serous carcinoma, 337-338, **344**

Uterine smooth muscle neoplasms, 346-347
  hyalinizing necrosis, **348**

Uveal melanomas, 161, **163**

V

V600E mutation in *BRAF*, 64, 67, 516

Vaccines, 106-107
  DNA, 106-107, 531

Vagina, 315-317, **318-320**
  adenosis, 317, 320
  core points for, 317
  Gartner duct cyst in, **318**
  glandular cells in, 317
  inflammatory/infectious processes of, 315
  vaginal intraepithelial neoplasia (VAIN), 316, 319

Vaginal adenosis, 317, **320**

Vaginal intraepithelial neoplasia, 316, **319**

Valacyclovir, 529

Vancomycin-resistant *Enterococcus* (VRE), 519

Vancomycin-resistant *Staphylococcus aureus* (VRSA), 520

Van Nuys system in breast carcinoma, 41

Variable expressivity, 437

Variable number of tandem repeats (VNTRs), 501, 502

Vascular cell adhesion molecule (VCAM), 84

Vascular ectasia of colon, 249

Vascular endothelial growth factor, 82

Vascular lesions, 15

Vascular neoplasms, 15, 407

Vasculitis, 219, **219-223**, 246
  leukocytoclastic, **223**
  temporal arteritis, 219-220, **222**

Vasectomy, 396

Vasitis nodosum, 357

Vectors, 472-475, *473*
  expression in microarrays, 506
  in cloning, 473

Verocay body, **25**

Verruca vulgaris, 405, **417**

Verrucous carcinoma
  of anal canal, 262, **268**
  of oral canal, 168, **172**
  of penis, 403-404
  of vulva, 317

Verrucous epidermal hyperplasia, 405

Verrucous epithelial hyperplasia, 168

Verrucous hyperplasia, 168

Vertebrate deoxyribonucleic acid (DNA), 549

Vibrio cholerae, 247

Villitis, chronic, 304-305

Villoglandular adenocarcinoma of endometrium, **344**

Villoglandular carcinoma, 337-338

Villous dysmaturity, 304

Villous edema, 309, **312**

Vimentin, 260, 355, 365

Viral hepatitis, 277-279

Viral load quantitation, 279, 482

Viral load testing, 481-482

ISBN 978-089189-5886

Viruses, 523-530
Enterovirus genus, 530
hepatitis, 525
herpes, 528-529
HIV, 524
immune response to, 106
influenza, 529
papillomavirus, 529
polyomavirus, 529
Vitamin E deficiency, 249
Vitamin K epoxide reductase complex (VKORC), 533
Vocal cords, 186, **188**
Volvulus, 246
Von Hippel-Lindau syndrome, 160
Von Recklinghausen disease, 545
Vulva, 315-317, **318-320**
benign neoplasms of, 316
carcinoma of, 317
core points for, 317
herpetic infection in, **318**
inflammatory/infectious processes of, 315
Vulvar intraepithelial neoplasia (VIN), 315, 316, **319**
Vulvar vestibulitis syndrome, 315

W

Waldenström macroglobulinemia, 116, 148, 149, **158**
Warfarin, 532
Warthin tumor, 173
Warty dyskeratoma, 406
Weber-Christian panniculitis, 416
Wegener granulomas, 181, 219, 220
Wegener granulomatosis, **185**, 197
Western blotting, 470
Westgard rules, 538
Whipples disease, 248
Whitehead system for chronic gastritis, 232
WHO/EORTC system for primary cutaneous lymphomas, 112, 407-408, 409
Whole chromosome painting, 493, 495
Whole genome amplification (WGA), 507
Whole genome arrays, 505
Wilms tumor, 372, **376**
Wilson disease, 276-277, **286**
Winkler disease, 159
WNT4, 395
Wobble hypothesis, 463
Woese, Carl, 453
Wolffian (mesonephric) duct, 395
World Health Organization (WHO) classification, 111-112
of acute myelogenous leukemia (AML), 140
of B-cell neoplasms, 112-121
angioimmunoblastic lymphadenopathy with dysproteinemia, 121
extramedullary myeloid tumors, 121
follicular lymphomas, 112-114
immunoblastic lymphadenopathy (IBL), 121
lymphoplasmacytic lymphoma/immunocytoma, 116-118
mantle cell lymphoma, 114-115
marginal zone lymphoma, 115
precursor T-lymphoblastic lymphoma, 119-120
small lymphocytic lymphoma, 115-116
treatment with monoclonal antibody to CD20, 118-119
of tumors of nervous system, 424
Worldwide Protein Data Bank (wwPDB), 555
Wound healing, sequence of events in, 87-88
W-Z system of sex determination, 450

X

χ^2 test, 449
Xanthelasma, 233, 248
Xanthogranulomatous pyelonephritis, 368, 370, **375**
Xanthoma, 248
gastric, **238**
X chromosomes, 435, 439, 444
evolution of, 450
Xeroderma pigmentosum, 458
X-linked recessive and dominant conditions, 118, 437, 438-440
X-ray crystallography, advances in, 452-453
X-Y system of sex determination, 450

Y

YAC vector, 474
Y chromosomes, 435, 439
evolution of, 450
Y-linked inheritance, 439
Yolk sac, 301
tumor of, 397, **401**

Z

Zanamivir (relenza), 530
ZAP-70, 46, 103
Zidovudine (AZT), 524
Zoledronic acid, 31
Zollinger-Ellison syndrome, 233
Zona fasciculata, 68
Zona glomerulosa, 68
Zona reticularis, 68
Zuckerkandl, organ of, 61